Ninth Edition

Nutrition & Diet Therapy

Linda Kelly DeBruyne

Kathryn Pinna

Ellie Whitney

CENGAGE
Learning

Australia • Brazil • Japan • Korea • Mexico • Singapore • Spain • United Kingdom • United States

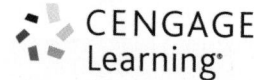
CENGAGE
Learning·

Nutrition & Diet Therapy, **Ninth Edition**
Linda Kelly DeBruyne, Kathryn Pinna,
Ellie Whitney

Product Director: Mary Finch

Senior Product Team Manager: Yolanda Cossio

Senior Product Manager: Peggy Williams

Content Developer: Elesha Hyde

Product Assistant: Chelsea Joy

Senior Media Developer: Miriam Myers

Marketing Manager: Tom Ziolkowski

Senior Content Project Manager: Carol Samet

Art Director: John Walker

Manufacturing Planner: Karen Hunt

Production and Composition Service:
MPS Limited

Photo Researcher: Lumina Datamatics

Text Researcher: Lumina Datamatics

Copy Editor: MPS Limited

Text Designer: Tani Hasegawa

Cover Designer: John Walker

Cover Image: Maximilian Stock Ltd./Getty

For product information and technology assistance, contact us at
Cengage Learning Customer & Sales Support, 1-800-354-9706.

For permission to use material from this text or product,
submit all requests online at **www.cengage.com/permissions**.
Further permissions questions can be e-mailed to
permissionrequest@cengage.com.

Library of Congress Control Number: 2014940083

ISBN-13: 978-1-305-11040-3

ISBN-10: 1-305-11040-4

Cengage Learning
20 Channel Center Street
Boston, MA 02210
USA

Cengage Learning is a leading provider of customized learning solutions with office locations around the globe, including Singapore, the United Kingdom, Australia, Mexico, Brazil, and Japan. Locate your local office at **www.cengage .com/global**.

Cengage Learning products are represented in Canada by Nelson Education, Ltd.

To learn more about Cengage Learning Solutions, visit **www.cengage.com**.

Purchase any of our products at your local college store or at our preferred online store **www.cengagebrain.com**.

Printed in the United States of America
Print Number: 01   Print Year: 2015

Contents in Brief

Contents

17 Foods and Food Consistency for Upper GI Disorders 469

18 Fiber-Modified Diets for Lower Gastrointestinal Tract Disorders 494

19 Carbohydrate- and Fat-Modified Diets for Malabsorption Disorders 512

20 Nutrition Therapy for Liver and Gallbladder Diseases 531

21 Carbohydrate-Controlled Diets for Diabetes Mellitus 552

How To Features Appear on the Following Pages

Case Study Features Appear on the Following Pages

Preface

Numerous discoveries in nutrition science over the past few years have continued to benefit the field of health care. In revising this ninth edition of *Nutrition and Diet Therapy*, we have been pleased at the number of new findings we have been able to incorporate into these pages. As always, major goals of this textbook are to present both core nutrition information and guidelines about the prevention of, and care during, illness. Another mission is to help nutrition students evaluate information and products available from the media, colleagues, and the marketplace.

As in the previous edition of this book, Chapters 1 through 10 introduce basic concepts in nutrition and explain how sound nutrition supports health. Chapters 11 to 13 apply nutrition principles to individuals during different stages of life, from pregnancy and birth through old age. The second half of the book addresses the concerns of individuals who are at risk of illness or have medical conditions that require medical nutrition therapy. A hallmark of the text is the "Nutrition in Practice" section located at the end of every chapter: these sections provide coverage of current research topics, advanced subjects, or specialty areas.

Changes for This Edition

Each chapter of this book is based on current nutrition knowledge and the latest clinical practice guidelines, and features new learning objectives for each major section. Some major content changes in this edition include the following:

Chapter 1 Introduced the new MyPlate figure and discussion, added definitions of solid fats, added sugars, and nutrient profiling, added a brief discussion of nutrient profiling, included a new discussion of portion sizes, added a discussion and new figure of the proposed updated Nutrition Facts panel on food labels, added new figures of Facts Up Front and label claims, and added the definition of registered dietitian nutritionist in the Nutrition in Practice.

Chapter 2 Added a new figure showing glycogen and starch molecules and their branching, reorganized and enhanced the discussion of blood glucose regulation, reorganized the section "Health Effects of Sugars and Alternative Sweeteners," added a discussion of sugar and heart disease, placed new emphasis on the term *nonnutritive sweeteners* rather than *artificial sweeteners* as per the Academy of Nutrition and Dietetics, added a new How To box: "How to Reduce Added Sugar Intake," updated and reorganized the table of nonnutritive sweeteners, and added a little more information about glycemic load in the Nutrition in Practice.

Chapter 3 Added brief discussion and definition of conjugated linoleic acid, increased the emphasis on and explanation of solid fats, added a table of solid fats on food labels, and added a new figure about replacing saturated fat with unsaturated fat in the Nutrition in Practice.

Chapter 4 Enhanced the discussion of proteins as antibodies, reorganized the section on protein deficiency, introduced and defined the WHO term *severe acute malnutrition* and defined chronic malnutrition, added a table comparing severe acute malnutrition and chronic malnutrition, and enhanced the glossary of terms to describe vegetarian diets.

Chapter 5 Added the Food Safety Modernization Act to the discussion in the Nutrition in Practice and reorganized and shortened the foodborne illness table to include the pathogens that cause most foodborne illnesses.

Chapter 6 Deleted a margin note about the "3500-kcal rule" and downplayed its exactness in the text with references, included information from the American Heart Association/American College of Cardiology Guidelines for the Management of Overweight and Obesity in Adults, and added information about and a definition of RED-S (relative energy deficiency in sport) from the International Olympic Committee to replace the female athlete triad.

Chapter 7 Introduced and defined screen time, food deserts, satiation, and satiety, added a new section on "Neighborhood Obstacles to Physical Activity and Healthy Foods," streamlined the obesity drug discussion and simplified and updated FDA-approved obesity drugs information, separated and enhanced tables of weight-loss and weight-gain strategies, addressed new thinking and research about the "3500-kcalorie rule," enhanced and updated the table "Popular Diets Compared," added a new table called "Tips for Identifying Fad Diets and Weight-Loss Scams," and added a brief discussion of protein and kcalorie restriction.

Chapter 8 Added a new table comparing fat-soluble and water-soluble vitamins, updated figures of good sources of vitamins (A, folate, and C) using current USDA nutrient data, added definitions of vitamin D_2 and D_3, added a brief note about tocotrienols in the vitamin E discussion, and added a new table in the Nutrition in Practice providing tips for consuming phytochemicals.

Chapter 9 Added a new table, "Top Contributors of Sodium in the Diet," added a section on potassium and hypertension, added more food sources of calcium, added information on magnesium and disease, added information on iron excess and oxidative stress, and added information on and a definition of hepcidin, the iron-regulating hormone.

Chapter 10 Reorganized and rewrote parts of the beginning of the chapter, added new tables comparing intensities of physical activity and symptoms of heat stroke and hypothermia, updated the hydration table, rewrote and reorganized the Nutrition in Practice, and added a discussion of beta-alanine to the Nutrition in Practice.

Chapter 11 Added a new table on the benefits of breastfeeding and personalized the table of strategies for successful breastfeeding.

Chapter 12 Added new tables listing protective factors in breast milk and providing tips for picky eaters, enhanced the table of food skills for preschoolers, added a figure to highlight MyPlate resources for children, included new National School Lunch/Breakfast requirements, added a table of new USDA standards for foods and beverages sold in schools, added a new table of physical activities for children and adolescents, and modified and simplified the feature "How to Protect against Lead Toxicity."

Chapter 13 Added a new table comparing signs of Alzheimer's and typical age-related changes, defined health care communities as per the Academy of Nutrition and Dietetics, added a brief discussion of the obesity/food insecurity paradox in the Nutrition in Practice, and enhanced the feature about thrifty meal planning, "How to Stretch Food Dollars and Reduce Waste."

Chapter 14 Reorganized the table on information included in a nutrition screening, included a discussion of the multiple-pass method for conducting a 24-hour dietary recall interview, added a paragraph about C-reactive protein in the section on biochemical analyses, revised the SOAP note figure, and updated names for diets in the "Modified Diets" section to more closely match current dietetics terminology.

Chapter 15 Modified the paragraph on isoniazid and vitamin B_6 in the "Diet-Drug Interactions" section, modified several paragraphs about the effectiveness and safety of herbal supplements, and modified and expanded the table listing examples of herb-drug interactions.

Chapter 16 Introduced oral supplements in the beginning of the chapter, reorganized the middle two sections of the chapter so that the discussion of tube feeding candidates and tube feeding routes precedes the section on enteral formulas, added new photos of a current feeding tube and transnasal tube placement in an adult, simplified the presentation of tube feeding initiation and advancement, introduced the term *cyclic feedings* in the section on formula delivery methods, revised the section on fluids and electrolytes in parenteral solutions, clarified the difference between continuous and cyclic parenteral nutrition, shortened the section on discontinuing parenteral nutrition, and expanded the section on hyperglycemia in parenteral nutrition. In the Nutrition in Practice on inborn errors, revised the introductory paragraph about PKU, added a photo showing phenylalanine-free formula, and updated the medical foods and treatments used in phenylketonuria.

Chapter 17 Modified the table of suggestions for managing dry mouth, expanded the discussion about food thickeners, updated the box that describes ways to improve acceptance of mechanically altered foods, updated the diet-drug interactions box, and modified the discussions on dumping syndrome and bariatric surgery. In the Nutrition in Practice about oral health, modified several sections and added a table listing suggestions for preventing oral diseases.

Chapter 18 Revised some paragraphs in the sections on inflammatory bowel diseases, irritable bowel syndrome, and diverticular disease of the colon; and updated the diet-drug interactions box.

Chapter 19 Replaced the Schilling test with the xylose absorption test in the section on evaluating malabsorption; revised some material in the sections on acute and chronic pancreatitis, cystic fibrosis, celiac disease, and short bowel syndrome; and updated the diet-drug interactions box.

Chapter 20 Revised the introduction to fatty liver and the descriptions of the different types of hepatitis viruses, modified several sections on cirrhosis complications and the table on stages of hepatic encephalopathy, revised the sections on the medical treatment and nutrition therapy for cirrhosis, introduced the *transjugular intrahepatic portosystemic shunt* and eliminated the *peritoneovenous shunt* in the discussion about ascites treatment, modified the section about risk factors for gallstone disease, and updated the diet-drug interactions box.

Chapter 21 Updated statistics throughout the chapter; expanded paragraphs on prediabetes, long-term glycemic control, and diabetic pregnancy; added a note about the types of insulin used in the Diabetes Control and Complications Trial; updated sections on nutrition therapy according to newly released nutrition guidelines from the American Diabetes Association; reorganized the discussion about body weight concerns by moving the topic of weight gain in type 1 diabetes to the insulin therapy section and the topic on weight loss for type 2 diabetes to the nutrition therapy section; expanded the table on antidiabetic drugs; updated the diet-drug interactions box; and updated several sections in the Nutrition in Practice on metabolic syndrome.

Chapter 22 Reorganized the chapter introduction; revised several paragraphs on the causes of atherosclerosis; expanded and modified the discussions of CHD risk assessment and lifestyle management, including recent (2013) guidelines from the American Heart Association and American College of Cardiology; added a new discussion about cholesterol and egg intakes; modified the introduction to hypertension and some sections on the risk factors and treatment of hypertension, including recent guidelines by the Eighth Joint National Committee (JNC 8) released in 2013; and updated the diet-drug interactions box.

Chapter 23 Modified sections related to the nephrotic syndrome, updated the section on nutrition therapy for acute kidney injury, updated the section on the evaluation of chronic kidney disease to reflect new clinical practice guidelines, clarified and updated some sections related to the nutrition therapy for chronic kidney disease to reflect current recommendations, modified the section on prevention of calcium oxalate stones, updated the table on food sources of oxalates, and updated the diet-drug interactions box.

Chapter 24 Modified the discussion about the systemic effects of inflammation, updated the discussion about the clinical effects of altering omega-6 and omega-3 fatty acid intakes based on recent analyses, revised the section about estimating energy needs during acute stress, added the concept of hypocaloric feedings for obese critical care patients, changed the table on using disease-specific stress factors for estimating energy needs to a "How to" box, and updated the diet-drug interactions box with current drug treatments for COPD.

Chapter 25 Rearranged the sections related to the consequences of cancer, introduced the term *oral mucositis*, modified the section on hematopoietic stem cell transplantation and introduced the term *graft-versus-host disease*, revised the paragraph about protein and energy intakes for cancer patients, modified the introductory paragraphs in the HIV/AIDS section, rearranged and revised some sections related to the consequences of HIV infection, revised some sections related to the nutrition therapy for HIV infection, and updated the diet-drug interactions box.

Features of this Text

Throughout the book, the readable text and pedagogic features should help to facilitate students' understanding and retention of the material. For example, **definitions of key terms** appear in the margins. **"How to" skill boxes** help readers work through calculations or give practical suggestions for applying nutrition information. **Learning objectives** (new for this edition) and **"In Summary"** statements at the beginning and end of each major chapter section help students assimilate the material and assess reading comprehension.

Study tools include the **"Self Check"** at the end of each chapter, which helps readers test their understanding of the chapter material. **"Your Diet"** exercises ask students to apply nutrition information from each chapter to their own diets. **Case studies** in the later chapters challenge readers to apply chapter information to clinical situations.

"Clinical Applications" provide practice with mathematical calculations and help students understand the impact of nutrition-related issues on health care professionals and their clients.

"Nutrition Assessment Checklists" summarize assessment parameters relevant to different stages of the life cycle or groups of disorders. **"Diet-Drug Interaction"** boxes point out interactions relevant to the medications described in each chapter. The **appendixes** include a wealth of information on the contents of foods and enteral formulas, U.S. nutrient intake recommendations and the exchange system, Canadian guidelines and food guides, physical activity and energy requirements, additional information about nutrition assessment, and aids to calculations.

We hope that as you discover the many fascinating aspects of nutrition, you will enthusiastically apply the concepts in both your professional and your personal life. To access additional course materials including Course Mate, please visit **www.cengagebrain.com.** At the CengageBrain.com home page, search for the ISBN of your title (from the back cover of your book) using the search box at the top of the page. This will take you to the product page where these resources can be found.

Ancillaries

- **CourseMate** helps you make the grade. It includes an interactive eBook with highlighting, note taking, and search capabilities; interactive learning tools including quizzes, flash cards, and videos; and more! Go to cengagebrain.com to access these resources.

- A test bank is available through **Cengage Learning Testing Powered by Cognero,** a flexible online system that allows instructors to author, edit, and manage test bank content from multiple Cengage Learning solutions; create multiple test versions in an instant; and deliver tests from an LMS, a classroom, or wherever the instructor wants.

- The password-protected **Instructor Companion Site** offers everything an instructor needs for the course in one place! This collection of book-specific lecture and class tools is available online via www.cengage.com/login. Access and download Power-Point presentations, images, an instructor's manual, videos, and more.

Acknowledgments

Among the most difficult words to write are those that express the depth of our gratitude to the many dedicated people whose efforts have made this book possible. A special note of appreciation to Sharon Rolfes for her numerous contributions to the chapters and Nutrition in Practice sections as well as to the Dietary Reference Intakes on the inside front cover and the appendices. Many thanks to Fran Webb for sharing her knowledge, ideas, and resources about the latest nutrition developments. Thanks also to David L. Stone for his assistance with multiple sections in the clinical chapters. Elesha Hyde's critical eye, numerous suggestions, and unceasing support were especially helpful in revising both the normal nutrition and the clinical chapters. We also wish to acknowledge the efforts of the folks at Axxya for their assistance in creating the food composition appendix. We are indebted to our editorial team, Peggy Williams and Elesha Hyde, and our production team, especially Carol Samet, for seeing this project through from start to finish. We would also like to acknowledge Tom Ziolkowski for his marketing efforts. To the many others involved in designing, indexing, typesetting, dummying, and marketing, we offer our thanks. We are especially grateful to our associates, family, and friends for their continued encouragement and support and to our reviewers who consistently offer excellent suggestions for improving the text.

Reviewers

Dr. Suman Ahuja
Lincoln University

Heather T. Casale, MS, RD, CNSC
Merritt College

Dr. Julie K. Collins
Eastern Oklahoma State College

Kelly K. Eichmann, PhD, RD
University of Phoenix

Deborah A. Hutcheon, MS, RD, LD
Bob Jones University

About the Authors

Linda Kelly DeBruyne, M.S., R.D., received her B.S. in 1980 and her M.S. in 1982 in nutrition and food science at Florida State University. She is a founding member of Nutrition and Health Associates, an information resource center in Tallahassee, Florida, where her specialty areas are life cycle nutrition and fitness. Her other publications include the textbooks *Nutrition for Health and Health Care,* and *Health: Making Life Choices* and a multimedia CD-ROM called *Nutrition Interactive.* She is a registered dietitian and maintains a professional membership in the Academy of Nutrition and Dietetics.

Kathryn Pinna, Ph.D., R.D., received her M.S. and Ph.D. degrees in nutrition from the University of California at Berkeley. She has taught nutrition, food science, and human biology courses in the San Francisco Bay Area for over 25 years and has also worked as an outpatient dietitian, Internet consultant, and freelance writer. Her other publications include the textbooks *Understanding Normal and Clinical Nutrition* and *Nutrition for Health and Health Care.* She is a registered dietitian and a member of the American Society for Nutrition and the Academy of Nutrition and Dietetics.

Ellie Whitney, Ph.D., grew up in New York City and received her B.A. and Ph.D. degrees in English and biology at Radcliffe/Harvard University and Washington Universities, respectively. She has taught at both Florida State University and Florida A&M University, has written newspaper columns on environmental matters for the *Tallahassee Democrat*, and has authored almost a dozen college textbooks on nutrition, health, and related topics, many of which have been revised multiple times over the years. In addition to teaching and writing, she has spent the past three-plus decades exploring outdoor Florida and studying its ecology. Her latest book is *Priceless Florida: The Natural Ecosystems* (Pineapple Press, 2004).

Dedication

To my husband Tom, Can t wait to see where the
next part of our journey takes us.
—Linda Kelly DeBruyne

To David Stone, who shares my passion for nutrition, science,
old-time fiddle music, and swallowtail butterflies.
—Kathryn Pinna

To the memory of my parents, Edith Tyler Noss and Henry H. B. Noss,
who supported me with love, discipline, and pride.
—Ellie Whitney

1

Overview of Nutrition and Health

Jack Hollingsworth/ Photodisc/ Getty Images

1.1 Food Choices

LO 1.1 Describe how various factors influence personal food choices.

1.2 The Nutrients

LO 1.2 Name the six major classes of nutrients and identify which are organic and which yield energy.

1.3 Nutrient Recommendations

LO 1.3 Define the four categories of the DRI, the Estimated Energy Requirement (EER), and the Acceptable Macronutrient Distribution Ranges (AMDR), and explain their purposes.

1.4 National Nutrition Surveys

LO 1.4 Describe the kinds of information researchers collect from nutrition surveys and explain how the information is used.

1.5 Dietary Guidelines and Food Guides

LO 1.5 Explain how each of the dietary ideals can be used to plan a healthy diet, and how the *Dietary Guidelines* and USDA Food Patterns help make diet planning easier.

1.6 Food Labels

LO 1.6 Compare the information on food labels to make selections that meet specific dietary and health goals.

1.7 Nutrition in Practice: Finding the Truth about Nutrition

LO 1.7 Recognize misinformation and describe how to identify reliable nutrition information.

$\mathbf{E}$very day, several times a day, you make choices that will either improve your **health** or harm it. Each choice may influence your health only a little, but when these choices are repeated over years and decades, their effects become significant.

The choices people make each day affect not only their physical health but also their **wellness**—all the characteristics that make a person strong, confident, and able to function well with family, friends, and others. People who consistently make poor lifestyle choices on a daily basis increase their risks of developing diseases. Figure 1-1 shows how a person's health can fall anywhere along a continuum, from maximum wellness on the one end to total failure to function (death) on the other.

As health care professionals, when you take responsibility for your own health by making daily choices and practicing behaviors that enhance your well-being, you prepare yourself physically, mentally, and emotionally to meet the demands of your profession. As health care professionals, however, you have a responsibility to your clients as well as to yourselves.* You have unique opportunities to make your clients aware of the benefits of positive health choices and behaviors, to show them how to change their behaviors and make daily choices to enhance their own health, and to serve as role models for those behaviors.

This text focuses on how nutrition choices affect health and disease. The early chapters introduce the basics of nutrition to promote good

health: a range of states with physical, mental, emotional, spiritual, and social components. At a minimum, health means freedom from physical disease, mental disturbances, emotional distress, spiritual discontent, social maladjustment, and other negative states. At a maximum, health means *wellness*.

wellness: maximum well-being; the top range of health states; the goal of the person who strives toward realizing his or her full potential physically, mentally, emotionally, spiritually, and socially.

*Health care professionals generally use either *client* or *patient* when referring to an individual under their care. The first 13 chapters of this text emphasize the nutrition concerns of people in good health; therefore, the term *client* is used in these chapters.

We as health care professionals must be role models.

make others aware of benefits of positive health choices.

responsibility for health = being prepared physically, mentally & emotionally.

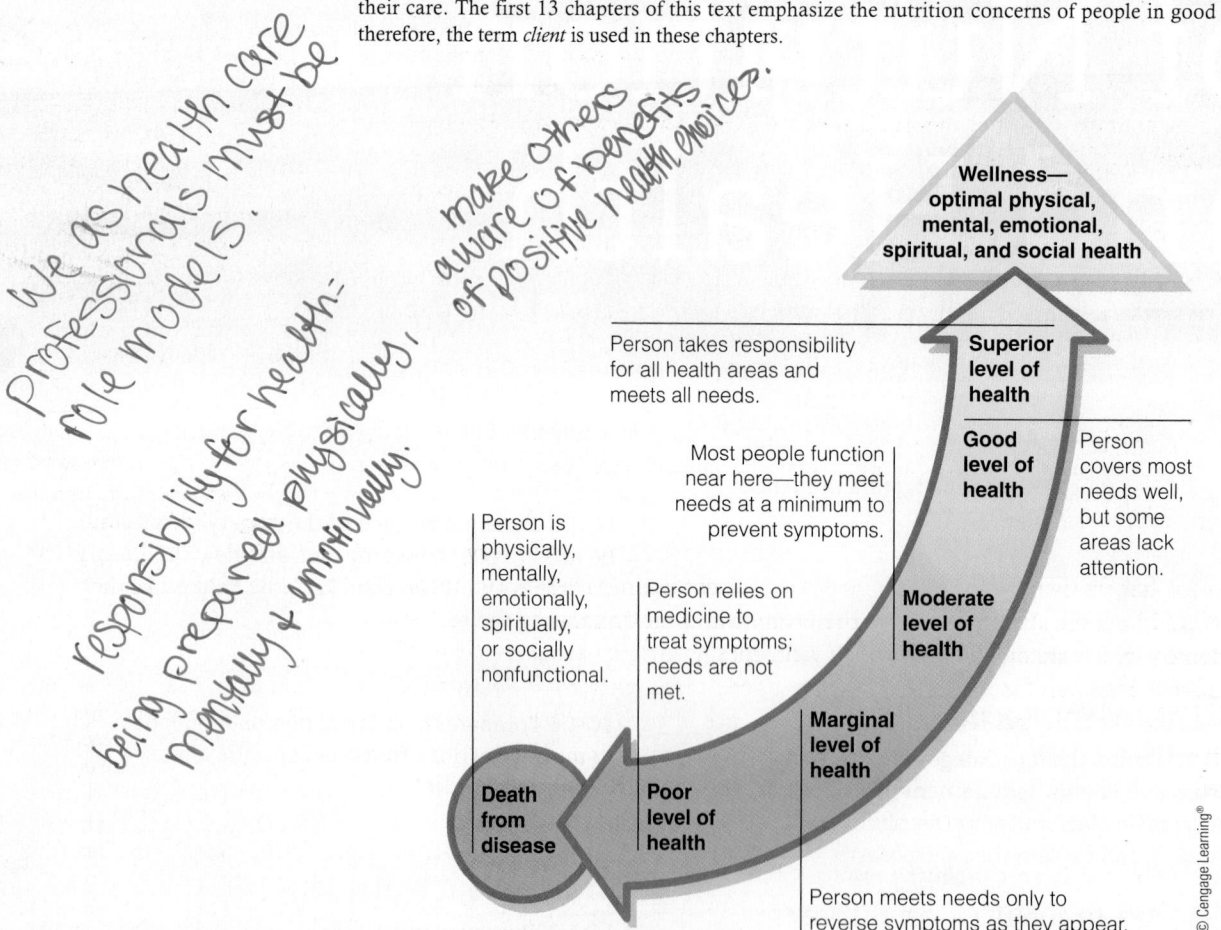

FIGURE 1-1 The Health Line
No matter how well you maintain your health today, you may still be able to improve tomorrow. Likewise, a person who is well today can slip by failing to maintain health-promoting habits.

2

health and reduce disease risks. The later chapters emphasize medical nutrition therapy and its role in supporting health and treating diseases and symptoms.

1.1 Food Choices

LO 1.1 Describe how various factors influence personal food choices.

Sound **nutrition** throughout life does not ensure good health and long life, but it can certainly help to tip the balance in their favor. Nevertheless, most people choose foods for reasons other than their nourishing value. Even people who claim to choose foods primarily for the sake of health or nutrition will admit that other factors also influence their food choices. Because food choices become an integral part of their lifestyles, people sometimes find it difficult to change their eating habits. Health care professionals who help clients make diet changes must understand the dynamics of food choices, because people will alter their eating habits only if their preferences are honored. Developing **cultural competence** is an important aspect of honoring individual preferences, especially for health care professionals who help clients to achieve a nutritious diet.[1]

Preference Why do people like certain foods? One reason, of course, is their preference for certain tastes. Some tastes are widely liked, such as the sweetness of sugar and the savoriness of salt.[2] Research suggests that genetics influence people's taste preferences, a finding that may eventually have implications for clinical nutrition.[3] For example, sensitivity to bitter taste is an inheritable trait. People born with great sensitivity to bitter tastes tend to avoid foods with bitter flavors such as broccoli, cabbage, brussels sprouts, spinach, and grapefruit juice. These foods, as well as many other fruits and vegetables, contain **bioactive food components—phytochemicals** and nutrients—that may reduce the risk of cancer. Thus, the role that genetics may play in food selection is gaining importance in cancer research.[4] Nutrition in Practice 8 addresses phytochemicals and their role in disease prevention.

Habit Sometimes habit dictates people's food choices. People eat a sandwich for lunch or drink orange juice at breakfast simply because they have always done so.

Associations People also like foods with happy associations—foods eaten in the midst of warm family gatherings on traditional holidays or given to them as children by someone who loved them. By the same token, people can attach intense and unalterable dislikes to foods that they ate when they were sick or that were forced on them when they weren't hungry.

Ethnic Heritage and Regional Cuisines Every country, and every region of a country, has its own typical foods and ways of combining them into meals. The **foodways** of North America reflect the many different cultural and ethnic backgrounds of its inhabitants. Many foods with foreign origins are familiar items on North American menus: tacos, egg rolls, lasagna, sushi, and gyros, to name a few. Still others, such as spaghetti and croissants, are almost staples in the "American diet." North American regional cuisines like Cajun and TexMex blend the traditions of several cultures. Table 1-1 (p. 4) presents selected **ethnic diets** and food choices.

Values Food choices may reflect people's environmental ethics, religious beliefs, and political views. By choosing to eat some foods or to avoid others, people make statements that reflect their values. For example, people may select only foods that come in containers that can be reused or recycled. A concerned consumer may boycott fruit or vegetables picked by migrant workers who have been exploited. People may

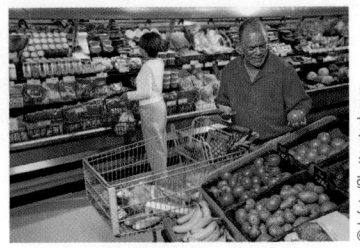
© lofoto/Shutterstock.com

Nutrition is only one of the many factors that influence people's food choices.

[handwritten notes:]
why we choose food
① preference   ⑪ medical conditions
② habit
③ associations   ⑫ health + nutrition
④ ethnic heritage
⑤ values
⑥ social interaction
⑦ emotional state
⑧ availability/conveinence
⑨ age
⑩ body weight/image

nutrition: the science of foods and the nutrients and other substances they contain, and of their ingestion, digestion, absorption, transport, metabolism, interaction, storage, and excretion. A broader definition includes the study of the environment and of human behavior as it relates to these processes.

cultural competence: an awareness and acceptance of one's own and others' cultures, combined with the skills needed to interact effectively with people of diverse cultures.

bioactive food components: compounds in foods (either nutrients or phytochemicals) that alter physiological processes in the body.

phytochemicals (FIGH-toe-CHEM-ih-cals)**:** compounds in plants that confer color, taste, and other characteristics. Some phytochemicals are bioactive food components in functional foods. Nutrition in Practice 8 provides details.

foodways: the eating habits and culinary practices of a people, region, or historical period.

ethnic diets: foodways and cuisines typical of national origins, races, cultural heritages, or geographic locations.

TABLE 1-1 Selected Ethnic Cuisines and Food Choices

	Grains	Vegetables	Fruits	Protein Foods	Milk
Asian	Millet, rice, rice or wheat noodles	Amaranth, baby corn, bamboo shoots, bok choy, cabbages, mung bean sprouts, scallions, seaweed, snow peas, straw mushrooms, water chestnuts, wild yam	Kumquats, loquats, lychee, mandarin oranges, melons, pears, persimmon, plums	Pork, poultry, fish and other seafood, squid, soybeans, tofu, duck eggs, cashews, peanuts	Soy milk
Mediterranean	Bulgur, couscous, focaccia, Italian bread, pastas, pita pocket bread, polenta, rice	Cucumbers, eggplant, grape leaves, onions, peppers, tomatoes	Dates, figs, grapes, lemons, melons, olives, raisins	Beef, gyros, lamb, pork, sausage, chicken, fish and other seafood, fava beans, lentils, almonds, walnuts	Feta, goat, mozzarella, parmesan, provolone, and ricotta cheeses; yogurt
Mexican	Taco shells, tortillas (corn or flour), rice	Cactus, cassava, chayote, chilies, corn, jicama, onions, tomatoes, tomato salsa, yams	Avocado, bananas, guava, lemons, limes, mango, oranges, papaya, plantain	Beef, chorizo, chicken, fish, refried beans, eggs	Cheese, flan (caramel custard)

buy vegetables from local farmers to save the fuel and environmental costs of foods shipped from far away. Labels on some foods carry statements or symbols—known as ecolabels—that imply that the foods have been produced in ways that are considered environmentally favorable.

Religion also influences many people's food choices. Jewish law sets forth an extensive set of dietary rules. Many Christians forgo meat on Fridays during Lent, the period prior to Easter. In Islamic dietary laws, permitted or lawful foods are called *halal*. Other faiths prohibit some dietary practices and promote others. Diet planners can foster sound nutrition practices only if they respect and honor each person's values.

Social Interaction Social interaction is another powerful influence on people's food choices. Meals are social events, and the sharing of food is part of hospitality. It is often considered rude to refuse food or drink being shared by a group or offered by a host. Food brings people together for many different reasons: to celebrate a holiday or special event, to renew an old friendship, to make new friends, to conduct business, and many more. Sometimes food is used to influence or impress someone. For example, a business executive invites a prospective new client out to dinner in hopes of edging out the competition. In each case, for whatever the purpose, food plays an integral part of the social interaction.

Emotional State Emotions guide food choices and eating behaviors.[5] Some people cannot eat when they are emotionally upset. Others may eat in response to a variety of emotional stimuli—for example, to relieve boredom or depression or to calm anxiety. A depressed person may choose to eat rather than to call a friend. A person who has returned home from an exciting evening out may unwind

Ethnic meals and family gatherings nourish the spirit as well as the body.

with a late-night snack. Eating in response to emotions can easily lead to overeating and obesity but may be appropriate at times. For example, sharing food at times of bereavement serves both the giver's need to provide comfort and the receiver's need to be cared for and to interact with others as well as to take nourishment.

Availability, Convenience, and Economy The influence of these factors on people's food selections is clear. You cannot eat foods if they are not available, if you cannot get to the grocery store, if you do not have the time or skill to prepare them, or if you cannot afford them. Consumers who value convenience frequently eat out, bring home ready-to-eat meals, cook meals ahead at storefront meal preparation sites, or have food delivered. Whether decisions based on convenience meet a person's nutrition needs depends on the choices made. Eating a banana or a candy bar may be equally convenient, but the fruit provides more vitamins and minerals and less sugar and fat.

Rising food costs have shifted some consumers' priorities and changed their shopping habits.[6] They are less likely to buy higher-priced convenience foods and more likely to prepare home-cooked meals. Those who frequently prepare their own meals eat fast food less often and are more likely to meet dietary guidelines for fat, calcium, fruits, vegetables, and whole grains. It is not surprising that, when eating out, consumers choose low-cost fast-food outlets over more expensive fine-dining restaurants. Foods eaten away from home, especially fast-food meals, tend to be high in kcalories, sodium, total fat, saturated fat, and *trans* fat—which can contribute to a variety of health problems.[7]

Some people have jobs that keep them away from home for days at a time, require them to conduct business in restaurants or at conventions, or involve hectic schedules that allow little or no time for meals at home. For these people, the kinds of restaurants available to them and the cost of eating out so often may limit food choices.

Age Age influences people's food choices. Infants, for example, depend on others to choose foods for them. Older children also rely on others but become more active in selecting foods that taste sweet and are familiar to them and rejecting those whose taste or texture they dislike. In contrast, the links between taste preferences and food choices in adults are less direct than in children. Adults often choose foods based on health concerns such as body weight. Indeed, adults may avoid sweet or familiar foods because of such concerns.

Body Weight and Image Sometimes people select certain foods and supplements that they believe will improve their physical appearance and avoid those they believe might be detrimental. Such decisions can be beneficial when based on sound nutrition and fitness knowledge but may undermine good health when based on fads or carried to extremes. Eating disorders are the topic of Nutrition in Practice 6.

Medical Conditions Sometimes medical conditions and their treatments (including medications) limit the foods a person can select. For example, a person with heart disease might need to adopt a diet low in certain types of fats. The chemotherapy needed to treat cancer can interfere with a person's appetite or limit food choices by causing vomiting. Allergy to certain foods can also limit choices. The second half of this text discusses how diet can be modified to accommodate different medical conditions.

Health and Nutrition Finally, of course, many consumers make food choices they believe will improve their health.[8] Food manufacturers and restaurant chefs have responded to scientific findings linking health with nutrition by offering an abundant selection of health-promoting foods and beverages. Foods that provide health benefits beyond their nutrient contributions are called **functional foods.**[9] Whole foods—as natural and familiar as oatmeal or tomatoes—are the simplest functional foods. In other cases, foods have been modified through fortification, enrichment, or

functional foods: whole, fortified, enriched, or enhanced foods that have a potentially beneficial effect on health when consumed as part of a varied diet on a regular basis at effective levels.

enhancement. Examples of these functional foods include orange juice fortified with calcium to build strong bones, bread enriched with folate to promote normal fetal development, and margarine enhanced with a plant sterol to lower blood cholesterol. Nutrition in Practice 8 offers more discussion of functional foods.

Consumers typically welcome new foods into their diets, provided that these foods are reasonably priced, clearly labeled, easy to find in the grocery store, and convenient to prepare. These foods must also taste good—as good as the traditional choices. Of course, a person need not eat any "special" foods to enjoy a healthy diet; many "regular" foods provide numerous health benefits as well. In fact, foods such as whole grains; vegetables and legumes; fruits; meats, seafood, poultry, eggs, nuts, and seeds; and low-fat milk products are among the healthiest choices a person can make.

IN SUMMARY

▌ A person selects foods for many different reasons.

▌ Food choices influence health—both positively and negatively. Individual food selections neither make nor break a diet's healthfulness, but the balance of foods selected over time can make an important difference to health.

▌ In the interest of health, people are wise to think "nutrition" when making their food choices.

1.2 The Nutrients

LO 1.2 Name the six major classes of nutrients and identify which are organic and which yield energy.

You are a collection of molecules that move. All these moving parts are arranged in patterns of extraordinary complexity and order—cells, tissues, and organs. Although the arrangement remains constant, the parts are continually changing, using **nutrients** and energy derived from nutrients.

Almost any food you eat is composed of dozens or even hundreds of different kinds of materials. Spinach, for example, is composed mostly of water (95 percent), and most of its solid materials are the compounds carbohydrates, fats (properly called lipids), and proteins. If you could remove these materials, you would find a tiny quantity of minerals, vitamins, and other compounds.

Six Classes of Nutrients

Water, carbohydrates, fats, proteins, vitamins, and minerals are the six classes of nutrients commonly found in spinach and other foods. Some of the other materials in foods, such as the pigments and other phytochemicals, are not nutrients but may still be important to health. The body can make some nutrients for itself, at least in limited quantities, but it cannot make them all, and it makes some in insufficient quantities to meet its needs. Therefore, the body must obtain many nutrients from foods. The nutrients that foods must supply are called **essential nutrients.**

Carbohydrates, Fats, and Proteins Four of the six classes of nutrients (carbohydrates, fats, proteins, and vitamins) contain carbon, which is found in all living things. They are therefore **organic** (meaning, literally, "alive").[†] During metabolism, three of

[†]Note that this definition of *organic* excludes coal, diamonds, and a few carbon-containing compounds that contain only a single carbon and no hydrogen, such as carbon dioxide (CO_2).

nutrients: substances obtained from food and used in the body to provide energy and structural materials and to serve as regulating agents to promote growth, maintenance, and repair. Nutrients may also reduce the risks of some diseases.

essential nutrients: nutrients a person must obtain from food because the body cannot make them for itself in sufficient quantities to meet physiological needs.

organic: in chemistry, substances or molecules containing carbon-carbon bonds or carbon-hydrogen bonds. The four organic nutrients are carbohydrate, fat, protein, and vitamins.

these four (carbohydrates, fats, and proteins) provide energy the body can use.[‡] These **energy-yielding nutrients** continually replenish the energy you spend daily.

Vitamins, Minerals, and Water Vitamins are organic but do not provide energy to the body. They facilitate the release of energy from the three energy-yielding nutrients. In contrast, minerals and water are **inorganic** nutrients. Minerals yield no energy in the human body, but, like vitamins, they help to regulate the release of energy, among their many other roles. As for water, it is the medium in which all of the body's processes take place.

kCalories: A Measure of Energy

The amount of energy that carbohydrates, fats, and proteins release can be measured in **calories**—tiny units of energy so small that a single apple provides tens of thousands of them. To ease calculations, energy is expressed in 1000-calorie metric units known as **kilocalories** (shortened to **kcalories,** but commonly called "calories"). When you read in popular books or magazines that an apple provides "100 calories," understand that it means 100 kcalories. This book uses the term *kcalorie* and its abbreviation *kcal* throughout, as do other scientific books and journals.[§] kCalories are not constituents of foods; they are a measure of the energy foods provide. The energy a food provides depends on how much carbohydrate, fat, and protein the food contains.

Carbohydrate yields 4 kcalories of energy from each gram, and so does protein. Fat yields 9 kcalories per gram. Thus, fat has a greater **energy density** than either carbohydrate or protein. Chapter 7 revisits energy density with regard to weight management. If you know how many grams of each nutrient a food contains, you can derive the number of kcalories potentially available from the food. Simply multiply the carbohydrate grams times 4, the protein grams times 4, and the fat grams times 9, and add the results together (Box 1-1 on p. 8 describes how to calculate the energy a food provides).

Energy Nutrients in Foods Most foods contain mixtures of all three energy-yielding nutrients, although foods are sometimes classified by their predominant nutrient. To speak of meat as "a protein" or of bread as "a carbohydrate," however, is inaccurate. Each is rich in a particular nutrient, but a protein-rich food such as beef contains a lot of fat along with the protein, and a carbohydrate-rich food such as cornbread also contains fat (corn oil) and protein. Only a few foods are exceptions to this rule, the common ones being sugar (which is pure carbohydrate) and oil (which is pure fat).

Energy Storage in the Body The body first uses the energy-yielding nutrients to build new compounds and fuel metabolic and physical activities. Excesses are then rearranged into storage compounds, primarily body fat, and put away for later use. Thus, if you take in more energy than you expend, whether from carbohydrate, fat, or protein, the result is an increase in energy stores and weight gain. Similarly, if you take in less energy than you expend, the result is a decrease in energy stores and weight loss.

Alcohol, Not a Nutrient One other substance contributes energy: alcohol. The body derives energy from alcohol at the rate of 7 kcalories per gram. Alcohol is not a nutrient, however, because it cannot support the body's growth, maintenance, or repair. Nutrition in Practice 20 discusses alcohol's effects on nutrition.

[‡]*Metabolism* is the set of processes by which nutrients are rearranged into body structures or broken down to yield energy.

[§]Food energy can also be measured in kilojoules (kJ). The kilojoule is the international unit of energy. One kcalorie equals 4.2 kJ.

---

energy-yielding nutrients: the nutrients that break down to yield energy the body can use. The three energy-yielding nutrients are carbohydrate, protein, and fat.

inorganic: not containing carbon or pertaining to living organisms. The two classes of nutrients that are inorganic are minerals and water.

calories: a measure of *heat* energy. Food energy is measured in **kilocalories** (1000 calories equal 1 kilocalorie), abbreviated **kcalories** or kcal. One kcalorie is the amount of heat necessary to raise the temperature of 1 kilogram (kg) of water 1°C. The scientific use of the term *kcalorie* is the same as the popular use of the term *calorie*.

energy density: a measure of the energy a food provides relative to the amount of food (kcalories per gram).

To calculate the energy available from a food, multiply the number of grams of carbohydrate, protein, and fat by 4, 4, and 9, respectively. Then add the results together. For example, one slice of bread with 1 tablespoon of peanut butter on it contains 16 grams of carbohydrate, 7 grams of protein, and 9 grams of fat:

16 g carbohydrate × 4 kcal/g = 64 kcal
7 g protein × 4 kcal/g = 28 kcal
9 g fat × 9 kcal/g = 81 kcal
Total = 173 kcal

From this information, you can calculate the percentage of kcalories each of the energy nutrients contributes to the total.

To determine the percentage of kcalories from fat, for example, divide the 81 fat kcalories by the total 173 kcalories:

81 fat kcal ÷ 173 total kcal = 0.468 (rounded to 0.47)

Then multiply by 100 to get the percentage:

0.47 × 100 = 47%

Dietary recommendations that urge people to limit fat intake to 20 to 35 percent of kcalories refer to the day's total energy intake, not to individual foods. Still, if the proportion of fat in each food choice throughout a day exceeds 35 percent of kcalories, then the day's total surely will, too. Knowing that this snack provides 47 percent of its kcalories from fat alerts a person to the need to make lower-fat selections at other times that day.

IN SUMMARY

▌ Foods provide nutrients—substances that support the growth, maintenance, and repair of the body's tissues.

▌ The six classes of nutrients are water, carbohydrates, fats, proteins, vitamins, and minerals.

▌ Vitamins, minerals, and water do not yield energy; instead they facilitate a variety of activities in the body.

▌ Foods rich in the energy-yielding nutrients (carbohydrates, fats, and proteins) provide the major materials for building the body's tissues and yield energy the body can use or store.

▌ Energy is measured in kcalories.

1.3 Nutrient Recommendations

LO 1.3 Define the four categories of the DRI, the Estimated Energy Requirement (EER), and the Acceptable Macronutrient Distribution Ranges (AMDR), and explain their purposes.

Nutrient recommendations are used as standards to evaluate healthy people's energy and nutrient intakes. Nutrition experts use the recommendations to assess nutrient intakes and to guide people on amounts to consume. Individuals can use them to decide how much of a nutrient they need to consume.

Dietary Reference Intakes

Defining the amounts of energy, nutrients, and other dietary components that best support health is a huge task. Nutrition experts have produced a set of standards that define the amounts of energy, nutrients, other dietary components, and physical activity that best support health. These recommendations are called **Dietary Reference Intakes (DRI)** and reflect the collaborative efforts of scientists in both the United States and Canada.*[10] The inside front covers of this book present the DRI values.

Dietary Reference Intakes (DRI): a set of values for the dietary nutrient intakes of healthy people in the United States and Canada. These values are used for planning and assessing diets.

*The DRI reports are produced by the Food and Nutrition Board, Institute of Medicine of the National Academies, with active involvement of scientists from Canada.

(A set of nutrient recommendations developed by the World Health Organization for international use is presented in Appendix B.)

Setting Nutrient Recommendations: RDA and AI One advantage of the DRI is that they apply to the diets of individuals. The DRI committee offers two sets of values to be used as nutrient intake goals by individuals: a set called the **Recommended Dietary Allowances (RDA)** and a set called **Adequate Intakes (AI).**

Based on solid experimental evidence and other reliable observations, the RDA are the foundation of the DRI. The AI values are based on less extensive scientific findings and rely more heavily on scientific judgment. The committee establishes an AI value whenever scientific evidence is insufficient to generate an RDA. To see which nutrients have an AI and which have an RDA, turn to the inside front cover.

In the last several decades, abundant new research has linked nutrients in the diet with the promotion of health and the prevention of chronic diseases. An advantage of the DRI is that, where appropriate, they take into account disease prevention as well as an adequate nutrient intake. For example, the RDA for calcium is based on intakes thought to reduce the likelihood of osteoporosis-related fractures later in life.

To ensure that the vitamin and mineral recommendations meet the needs of as many people as possible, the recommendations are set near the top end of the range of the population's estimated average requirements (see Figure 1-2). Small amounts above the daily **requirement** do no harm, whereas amounts below the requirement may lead to health problems. When people's intakes are consistently **deficient,** their nutrient stores decline, and over time this decline leads to deficiency symptoms and poor health.

Facilitating Nutrition Research and Policy: EAR In addition to the RDA and AI, the DRI committee has established another set of values: **Estimated Average Requirements (EAR).** These values establish average requirements for given life stage and gender groups that researchers and nutrition policymakers use in their work. Nutrition scientists may use the EAR as standards in research. Public health officials may use them to assess nutrient intakes of populations and make recommendations. The EAR values form the scientific basis on which the RDA are set.

Establishing Safety Guidelines: UL The DRI committee also establishes upper limits of intake for nutrients posing a hazard when consumed in excess. These values, the **Tolerable Upper Intake Levels (UL),** are indispensable to consumers who take supplements. Consumers need to know how much of a nutrient is too much. The UL are also of value to public health officials who set allowances for nutrients that are added to foods and water. The UL values are listed on the inside front cover.

Using Nutrient Recommendations Each of the four DRI categories serves a unique purpose. For example, the EAR are most appropriately used to develop and evaluate nutrition programs for *groups* such as schoolchildren or military personnel. The RDA (or AI, if an RDA is not available) can be used to set goals for *individuals*. The UL help to keep nutrient intakes below the amounts that increase the risk of toxicity. With these understandings, professionals can use the DRI for a variety of purposes.

In addition to understanding the unique purposes of the DRI, it is important to keep their uses in perspective. Consider the following:

- The values are recommendations for safe intakes, not minimum requirements; except for energy, they include a generous margin of safety. Figure 1-3 (p. 10) presents an accurate view of how a person's nutrient needs fall within a range, with marginal and danger zones both below and above the range.

- The values reflect daily intakes to be achieved on average, over time. They assume that intakes will vary from day to day, and they are set high enough to

FIGURE 1-2 Nutrient Intake Recommendations

The nutrient intake recommendations are set high enough to cover nearly everyone's requirements (the boxes represent people).

[a]Estimated Average Requirement

RDA is most accurate

Recommended Dietary Allowances (RDA): a set of values reflecting the average daily amounts of nutrients considered adequate to meet the known nutrient needs of practically all healthy people in a particular life stage and gender group; a goal for dietary intake by individuals.

Adequate Intakes (AI): a set of values that are used as guides for nutrient intakes when scientific evidence is insufficient to determine an RDA.

requirement: the lowest continuing intake of a nutrient that will maintain a specified criterion of adequacy.

deficient: in regard to nutrient intake, describes the amount below which almost all healthy people can be expected, over time, to experience deficiency symptoms.

Estimated Average Requirements (EAR): the average daily nutrient intake levels estimated to meet the requirements of half of the healthy individuals in a given age and gender group; used in nutrition research and policymaking and as the basis on which RDA values are set.

Tolerable Upper Intake Levels (UL): a set of values reflecting the highest average daily nutrient intake levels that are likely to pose no risk of toxicity to almost all healthy individuals in a particular life stage and gender group. As intake increases above the UL, the potential risk of adverse health effects increases.

Naive view   Accurate view

FIGURE 1-3 Naive versus Accurate View of Nutrient Intakes

The RDA or AI for a given nutrient represents a point that lies within a range of appropriate and reasonable intakes between toxicity and deficiency. Both of these recommendations are high enough to provide reserves in times of short-term dietary inadequacies, but not so high as to approach toxicity. Nutrient intakes above or below this range may be equally harmful.

ensure that body nutrient stores will meet nutrient needs during periods of inadequate intakes lasting a day or two for some nutrients and up to a month or two for others.

- The values are chosen in reference to specific indicators of nutrient adequacy, such as blood nutrient concentrations, normal growth, and reduction of certain chronic diseases or other disorders when appropriate, rather than prevention of deficiency symptoms alone.

- The recommendations are designed to meet the needs of most healthy people. Medical problems alter nutrient needs, as later chapters describe.

- The recommendations are specific for people of both genders as well as various ages and stages of life: infants, children, adolescents, men, women, pregnant women, and lactating women.

Setting Energy Recommendations In contrast to the vitamin and mineral recommendations, the recommendation for energy, called the **Estimated Energy Requirement (EER),** is not generous because excess energy cannot be excreted and is eventually stored as body fat. Rather, the key to the energy recommendation is balance. For a person who has a body weight, body composition, and physical activity level consistent with good health, energy intake from food should match energy expenditure, so the person achieves energy balance. Enough energy is needed to sustain a healthy, active life, but too much energy leads to obesity. The EER is therefore set at a level of energy intake predicted to maintain energy balance in a healthy adult of a defined age, gender, weight, height, and physical activity level.* Another difference between the requirements for other nutrients and those for energy is that each person has an obvious indicator of whether energy intake is inadequate, adequate, or excessive: body weight. Because *any* amount of energy in excess of need leads to weight gain, the DRI committee did not set a Tolerable Upper Intake Level.

Acceptable Macronutrient Distribution Ranges (AMDR)

As noted earlier, the DRI committee considers prevention of chronic disease as well as nutrient adequacy when establishing recommendations. To that end, the committee established healthy ranges of intakes for the energy-yielding nutrients—carbohydrate, fat, and protein—known as **Acceptable Macronutrient Distribution Ranges (AMDR).** Each of these three energy-yielding nutrients contributes to a person's total energy (kcalorie) intake, and those contributions vary in relation to each other. The DRI committee has determined that a diet that provides the energy-yielding nutrients in the following proportions provides adequate energy and nutrients and reduces the risk of chronic disease:

- 45 to 65 percent of kcalories from carbohydrate

- 20 to 35 percent of kcalories from fat

- 10 to 35 percent of kcalories from protein

Estimated Energy Requirement (EER): the dietary energy intake level that is predicted to maintain energy balance in a healthy adult of a defined age, gender, weight, and physical activity level consistent with good health.

Acceptable Macronutrient Distribution Ranges (AMDR): ranges of intakes for the energy-yielding nutrients that provide adequate energy and nutrients and reduce the risk of chronic disease.

IN SUMMARY

- The Dietary Reference Intakes (DRI) are a set of nutrient intake values that can be used to plan and evaluate dietary intakes for healthy people.

- The Estimated Average Requirement (EAR) defines the amount of a nutrient that supports a specific function in the body for half of the population.

*The EER for children, pregnant women, and lactating women includes energy needs associated with the deposition of tissue or the secretion of milk at rates consistent with good health.

- The Recommended Dietary Allowance (RDA) is based on the EAR and establishes a goal for dietary intake that will meet the needs of almost all healthy people.

- An Adequate Intake (AI) serves a similar purpose as the RDA when an RDA cannot be determined.

- The Tolerable Upper Intake Level (UL) establishes the highest average daily nutrient intake level that appears safe for almost all healthy people.

- The Estimated Energy Requirement (EER) defines the energy intake level needed to maintain energy balance in a healthy adult of a defined age, gender, weight, height, and physical activity level.

- The Acceptable Macronutrient Distribution Ranges (AMDR) define the proportions contributed by carbohydrate, fat, and protein to a healthy diet.

1.4 National Nutrition Surveys

LO 1.4 Describe the kinds of information researchers collect from nutrition surveys and explain how the information is used.

How do nutrition experts know whether people are meeting nutrient recommendations? The Dietary Reference Intakes and other major reports that examine the relationships between diet and health depend on information collected from nutrition surveys. Researchers use nutrition surveys to learn which foods people are eating and which supplements they are taking, to assess people's nutritional health, and to determine people's knowledge, attitudes, and behaviors about nutrition and how these relate to health. The resulting wealth of information can be used for a variety of purposes. For example, Congress uses this information to establish public policy on nutrition education, assess food assistance programs, and regulate the food supply. The food industry uses the information to guide decisions in public relations and product development. Scientists use the information to establish research priorities. One of the first nutrition surveys, taken before World War II, suggested that up to a third of the U.S. population might be eating poorly. Programs to correct **malnutrition** have been evolving ever since.

[handwritten margin note: relationships between diet & health, & what people are eating]

Coordinating Nutrition Survey Data

The National Nutrition Monitoring program coordinates the many nutrition-related activities of various federal agencies. All major reports that examine the contribution of diet and nutrition status to the health of the people of the United States depend on information collected and coordinated by this national program. A national food and nutrient intake survey, called *What We Eat in America,* collects data on the kinds and amounts of foods people eat. Researchers then calculate the energy and nutrients in the foods and compare the amounts consumed with standards such as the DRI. *What We Eat in America* is conducted as part of a larger research effort, the National Health and Nutrition Examination Surveys (NHANES), which examine the people themselves using nutrition assessment methods. The data provide valuable information on several nutrition-related conditions such as growth retardation, heart disease, and nutrient deficiencies. These data also provide the basis for developing and monitoring national health goals.

National Health Goals

Healthy People is a program that identifies the nation's health priorities and guides policies that promote health and prevent disease. At the start of each decade, the program sets goals for improving the nation's health during the following 10 years.

malnutrition: any condition caused by deficient or excess energy or nutrient intake or by an imbalance of nutrients.

Healthy People: a national public health initiative under the jurisdiction of the U.S. Department of Health and Human Services (DHHS) that identifies the most significant preventable threats to health and focuses efforts toward eliminating them.

TABLE 1-2 Leading Causes of Death in the United States

The diseases in bold italics are nutrition related.

1. ***Heart disease***
2. ***Cancers***
3. Chronic lung diseases
4. ***Strokes***
5. Accidents
6. Alzheimer's disease
7. ***Diabetes mellitus***
8. Pneumonia and influenza
9. Kidney disease
10. Suicide

Source: D.L. Hoyert and J. Xu, Deaths: Preliminary data for 2011, *National Vital Statistics* 61 (2012): 1–52.

overnutrition: overconsumption of food energy or nutrients sufficient to cause disease or increased susceptibility to disease; a form of malnutrition.

undernutrition: underconsumption of food energy or nutrients severe enough to cause disease or increased susceptibility to disease; a form of malnutrition.

chronic diseases: diseases characterized by slow progression, long duration, and degeneration of body organs due in part to such personal lifestyle elements as poor food choices, smoking, alcohol use, and lack of physical activity.

eating pattern: customary intake of foods and beverages over time.

adequacy: the characteristic of a diet that provides all the essential nutrients, fiber, and energy necessary to maintain health and body weight.

balance: the dietary characteristic of providing foods in proportion to one another and in proportion to the body's needs.

kcalorie (energy) control: management of food energy intake.

nutrient density: a measure of the nutrients a food provides relative to the energy it provides. The more nutrients and the fewer kcalories, the higher the nutrient density.

Nutrition is one of 38 topic areas of Healthy People 2020, each with numerous objectives (www.healthypeople.gov).

IN SUMMARY

▮ Nutrition surveys measure people's food consumption and evaluate the nutrition status of populations.

▮ Information gathered from nutrition surveys serves as the basis for many major diet and nutrition reports, including Healthy People.

1.5 Dietary Guidelines and Food Guides

LO 1.5 Explain how each of the dietary ideals can be used to plan a healthy diet, and how the *Dietary Guidelines* and USDA Food Patterns help make diet planning easier.

Today, government authorities are as concerned about **overnutrition** as they once were about **undernutrition.** Research confirms that dietary excesses, especially of energy, sodium, certain fats, and alcohol, contribute to many **chronic diseases,** including heart disease, cancer, stroke, diabetes, and liver disease.[11] Only two common lifestyle habits have more influence on health than a person's choice of diet: smoking and other tobacco use, and excessive drinking of alcohol. Table 1-2 lists the leading causes of death in the United States; notice that three of the top four are nutrition related (and related to tobacco use). Note, however, that although diet is a powerful influence on these diseases, they cannot be prevented by a healthy diet alone; genetics, physical activity, age, gender, and other factors also play a role. Within the range set by genetic inheritance, however, disease development is strongly influenced by the foods a person chooses to eat.

Sound nutrition does not depend on the selection of any one food. Instead, it depends on the overall **eating pattern**—the combination of many different foods and beverages at numerous meals over days, months, and years.[12] So how can health care professionals help people select foods to create an eating pattern that supplies all the needed nutrients in amounts consistent with good health? The principle is simple enough: encourage clients to eat a variety of foods that supply all the nutrients the body needs. In practice, how do people do this? It helps to keep in mind that a nutritious diet achieves six basic ideals.

Dietary Ideals ADEQUACY + BALANCE

A nutritious diet has the six characteristics listed in Box 1-2. The first, **adequacy,** was already addressed in the earlier discussion on the DRI. An adequate diet has enough energy and enough of every nutrient (as well as fiber) to meet the needs of healthy people. Second is **balance:** the food choices do not overemphasize one nutrient or food type at the expense of another. Balance in the diet helps to ensure adequacy.

The essential minerals calcium and iron illustrate the importance of dietary balance. Meat is rich in iron but poor in calcium. Conversely, milk is rich in calcium but poor in iron. Use some meat for iron; use some milk for calcium; and save some space for other foods, too, because a diet consisting of milk and meat alone would not be adequate. For other nutrients, people need to consume other protein foods, whole grains, vegetables, and fruit.

The third characteristic is **kcalorie (energy) control:** the foods provide the amount of energy needed to maintain a healthy body weight—not more, not less. The key to kcalorie control is to select foods that deliver the most nutrients for the least food energy. This fourth characteristic is known as **nutrient density.** Nutrient density promotes adequacy and kcalorie control. Consider foods containing calcium, for example. You can get about 300 milligrams of calcium from either 1½ ounces of cheddar cheese or 1 cup of fat-free milk, but the cheese delivers about twice as much food energy (kcalories) as the milk. The fat-free milk, then, is twice as calcium dense as the cheddar cheese; it offers the same amount of calcium for half the kcalories. Both foods are excellent choices for adequacy's sake alone, but to achieve adequacy while controlling kcalories, the fat-free milk is the better choice. (Alternatively, a person could select a low-fat cheddar cheese providing kcalories comparable to fat-free milk.)

Just as a financially responsible person pays for rent, food, clothes, and tuition on a limited budget, healthy people obtain iron, calcium, and all the other essential nutrients on a limited energy (kcalorie) allowance. Success depends on getting many nutrients for each kcalorie "dollar." For example, a can of cola and handful of grapes may both provide about the same number of kcalories, but grapes deliver many more nutrients. A person who makes nutrient-dense choices, such as fruit instead of cola, can meet daily nutrient needs on a lower energy budget. Such choices support good health.

Foods that are notably low in nutrient density—such as potato chips, candy, and colas—are called **empty-kcalorie foods.** The kcalories these foods provide are called "empty" because they deliver a lot of energy (from added sugars, solid fats, or both) but little or no protein, vitamins, or minerals.

The concept of nutrient density is relatively simple when examining the contributions of one nutrient to a food or diet. With respect to calcium, milk ranks high and meats rank low. With respect to iron, meats rank high and milk ranks low. But which food is more nutritious? Answering that question is a more complex task because we need to consider several nutrients—those that may harm health and those that may be beneficial.[13] Ranking foods based on their overall nutrient composition is known as **nutrient profiling.** Researchers have yet to agree on an ideal way to rate foods based on the nutrient profile, but when they do, nutrient profiling will be quite useful in helping consumers identify nutritious foods and plan healthy diets.[14]

The fifth characteristic of a nutritious diet is **moderation.** Moderation contributes to adequacy, balance, and kcalorie control. Foods rich in fat and sugar often provide enjoyment and energy but relatively few nutrients. In addition, they promote weight gain when eaten in excess. A person who practices moderation eats such foods only on occasion and regularly selects foods low in **solid fats** and **added sugars,** a practice that automatically improves nutrient density. Returning to the example of cheddar cheese and fat-free milk, the milk not only offers more calcium for less energy, but also it contains far less fat than the cheese.

Finally, the sixth characteristic of a nutritious diet is **variety:** the foods chosen differ from one day to the next. A diet may have all the virtues just described and still lack variety if a person eats the same foods day after day. People should select foods from each of the food groups daily and vary their choices within each food group from day to day, for a couple of reasons. First, different foods within the same group contain different arrays of nutrients. Among the fruits, for example, strawberries are especially rich in vitamin C while apricots are rich in vitamin A. Variety improves nutrient adequacy. Second, no food is guaranteed entirely free of substances that, in excess, could be harmful. The strawberries might contain trace amounts of one contaminant, the apricots another. By alternating fruit choices, a person will ingest very little of either contaminant.

Dietary Guidelines for Americans

What should a person eat to stay healthy? The answers can be found in the *Dietary Guidelines for Americans*. These guidelines translate the *nutrient* recommendations of the DRI into *food* recommendations.[15] The *Dietary Guidelines for Americans 2010* provide evidence-based advice to help people attain and maintain a healthy weight, reduce the risk of chronic diseases, and promote overall health through diet and physical activity.[16] Table 1-3 (p. 14) presents the key recommendations of the *Dietary Guidelines for Americans 2010*, clustered into four major topic areas. The first area focuses on

13

BOX 1-2

A nutritious diet has the following six characteristics:

- Adequacy
- Balance
- kCalorie (energy) control
- Nutrient density
- Moderation
- Variety

empty-kcalorie foods: a popular term used to denote foods that contribute energy but lack protein, vitamins, and minerals.

nutrient profiling: ranking foods based on their nutrient composition.

moderation: the provision of enough, but not too much, of a substance.

solid fats: fats that are not usually liquid at room temperature; commonly found in most foods derived from animals and vegetable oils that have been hydrogenated. Solid fats typically contain more saturated and *trans* fats than most oils (Chapter 4 provides more details).

added sugars: sugars, syrups, and other kcaloric sweeteners that are added to foods during processing or preparation or at the table. Added sugars do not include the naturally occurring sugars found in fruits and milk products.

variety (dietary): consumption of a wide selection of foods within and among the major food groups (the opposite of monotony).

TABLE 1-3 Key Recommendations of the *Dietary Guidelines for Americans 2010*

Balancing kCalories to Manage Weight

- Prevent and/or reduce overweight and obesity through improved eating and physical activity behaviors.
- Control total kcalorie intake to manage body weight. For people who are overweight or obese, this will mean consuming fewer kcalories from foods and beverages.
- Increase physical activity and reduce time spent in sedentary behaviors.
- Maintain appropriate kcalorie balance during each stage of life—childhood, adolescence, adulthood, pregnancy and breastfeeding, and older age.

Foods and Food Components to Reduce

- Reduce daily sodium intake to less than 2300 milligrams, and further reduce intake to 1500 milligrams among persons who are 51 and older and those of any age who are African American or have hypertension, diabetes, or chronic kidney disease. The 1500 milligrams recommendation applies to about half of the U.S. population, including children and the majority of adults.
- Consume less than 10 percent of kcalories from saturated fatty acids by replacing them with monounsaturated and polyunsaturated fatty acids.
- Consume less than 300 milligrams per day of dietary cholesterol.
- Keep *trans* fatty acid consumption as low as possible by limiting foods that contain synthetic sources of *trans* fats, such as partially hydrogenated oils, and by limiting other solid fats.
- Reduce the intake of kcalories from solid fats and added sugars.
- Limit the consumption of foods that contain refined grains, especially refined grain foods that contain solid fats, added sugars, and sodium.
- If alcohol is consumed it should be consumed in moderation—up to one drink per day for women and two drinks per day for men—and only by adults of legal drinking age.

Foods and Nutrients to Increase

- Increase vegetable and fruit intake.
- Eat a variety of vegetables, especially dark-green and red and orange vegetables and beans and peas.
- Consume at least half of all grains as whole grains. Increase whole-grain intake by replacing refined grains with whole grains.
- Increase intake of fat-free or low-fat milk and milk products, such as milk, yogurt, cheese, or fortified soy beverages.
- Choose a variety of protein foods, which include seafood, lean meat and poultry, eggs, beans and peas, soy products, and unsalted nuts and seeds.
- Increase the amount and variety of seafood consumed by choosing seafood in place of some meat and poultry.
- Replace protein foods that are higher in solid fats with choices that are lower in solid fats and kcalories and/or are sources of oils.
- Use oils to replace solid fats where possible.
- Choose foods that provide more potassium, dietary fiber, calcium, and vitamin D, which are nutrients of concern in American diets. These foods include vegetables, fruits, whole grains, and milk and milk products.

Building Healthy Eating Patterns

- Select an eating pattern that meets nutrient needs over time at an appropriate kcalorie level.
- Account for all foods and beverages consumed and assess how they fit within a total healthy eating pattern.
- Follow food safety recommendations when preparing and eating foods to reduce the risk of foodborne illnesses.

Note: These guidelines are intended for adults and healthy children aged 2 and older.
Source: Dietary Guidelines for Americans 2010, available at www.dietaryguidelines.gov.

balancing kcalories to manage a healthy body weight by improving eating habits and engaging in regular physical activity. The second area advises people to reduce their intakes of such foods and food components as sodium, solid fats (and the saturated fats, *trans* fats, and cholesterol they contain), added sugars, refined grain products, and alcoholic beverages (for those who partake). The third area encourages consumers to select a variety of fruits and vegetables, whole grains, low-fat milk products, and protein foods (including seafood). The fourth area helps consumers build healthy eating patterns that meet energy and nutrient needs while reducing the risk of foodborne illnesses. Together, the *Dietary Guidelines for Americans 2010* point the way toward longer, healthier, and more active lives.

IN SUMMARY

▍ A well-planned diet delivers adequate nutrients, a balanced array of nutrients, and an appropriate amount of energy.

▍ A well-planned diet is based on nutrient-dense foods, moderate in substances that can be detrimental to health, and varied in its selections.

▍ The *Dietary Guidelines* apply these principles, offering practical advice on how to eat for good health.

Matthew Farruggio

A portion of grains is 1 ounce, yet most bagels today weigh 4 ounces or more—meaning that a single bagel can easily supply four or more portions of grains, not one, as many people assume.

The USDA Food Patterns

To help people achieve the goals set forth by the *Dietary Guidelines for Americans* (see Table 1-3), the USDA provides a **food group plan**—the **USDA Food Patterns**—that builds a diet from categories of foods that are similar in vitamin and mineral content. Thus, each group provides a set of nutrients that differs somewhat from the nutrients supplied by the other groups. Selecting foods from each of the groups eases the task of creating an adequate and balanced diet. The DASH Eating Plan, presented in Chapter 22, is another dietary pattern that meets the goals of the *Dietary Guidelines for Americans*.

Figure 1-4 (on pp. 16–17) presents the USDA Food Patterns. The USDA Food Patterns assign foods to five major food groups—fruits, vegetables, grains, protein foods, and milk and milk products—and recommend daily amounts of foods from each group to meet nutrient needs. The judicious use of oils is also described in the USDA Food Patterns. In addition to presenting the food groups, Figure 1-4 indicates the most notable nutrients of each group, the cup or ounce equivalents, and the foods within each group.

Recommended Amounts All food groups offer valuable nutrients, and people should make selections from each group daily. Table 1-4 specifies the amounts of food needed from each group daily to create a healthful diet for several energy (kcalorie) levels. A person needing 2000 kcalories a day, for example, would select 2 cups of fruit; 2½ cups of vegetables; 6 ounces of grain foods; 5½ ounces of protein foods; and 3 cups of milk or milk products.[††] Additionally, a small amount of unsaturated oil, such as vegetable oil or the oils of nuts, olives, or fatty fish, is required to supply needed nutrients. Estimated daily kcalorie needs for sedentary and active men and women are

all food groups offer valuable nutrients, & people should make selections from each group daily.

food group plan: a diet-planning tool that sorts foods into groups based on nutrient content and then specifies that people should eat certain amounts of food from each group.

USDA Food Patterns: the USDA's food group plan for ensuring dietary adequacy that assigns foods to five major food groups.

[††]Milk and milk products also can be referred to as dairy products.

TABLE 1-4 USDA Food Patterns: Recommended Daily Amounts from Each Food Group

Food Group	1600 kcal	1800 kcal	2000 kcal	2200 kcal	2400 kcal	2600 kcal	2800 kcal	3000 kcal
Fruits	1½ c	1½ c	2 c	2 c	2 c	2 c	2½ c	2½ c
Vegetables	2 c	2½ c	2½ c	3 c	3 c	3½ c	3½ c	4 c
Grains	5 oz	6 oz	6 oz	7 oz	8 oz	9 oz	10 oz	10 oz
Protein foods	5 oz	5 oz	5½ oz	6 oz	6½ oz	6½ oz	7 oz	7 oz
Milk	3 c	3 c	3 c	3 c	3 c	3 c	3 c	3 c
Oils	5 tsp	5 tsp	6 tsp	6 tsp	7 tsp	8 tsp	8 tsp	10 tsp
Discretionary kcalorie allowance	121 kcal	161 kcal	258 kcal	266 kcal	330 kcal	362 kcal	395 kcal	459 kcal

© 2016 Cengage Learning®

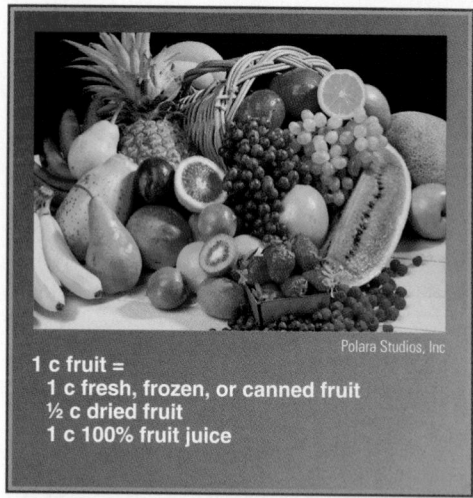

1 c fruit =
1 c fresh, frozen, or canned fruit
½ c dried fruit
1 c 100% fruit juice

Polara Studios, Inc

Fruits contribute folate, vitamin A, vitamin C, potassium, and fiber.

Consume a variety of fruits, and choose whole or cut-up fruits more often than fruit juice.

Apples, apricots, avocados, bananas, blueberries, cantaloupe, cherries, grapefruit, grapes, guava, honeydew, kiwi, mango, nectarines, oranges, papaya, peaches, pears, pineapples, plums, raspberries, strawberries, tangerines, watermelon; dried fruit (dates, figs, prunes, raisins); 100% fruit juices

Limit these fruits that contain solid fats and/or added sugars:
Canned or frozen fruit in syrup; juices, punches, ades, and fruit drinks with added sugars; fried plantains

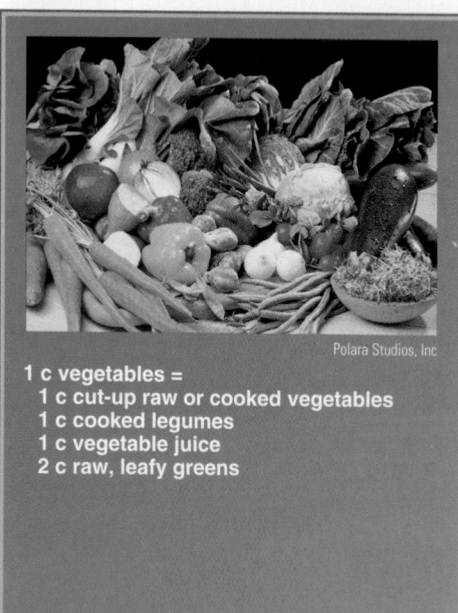

1 c vegetables =
1 c cut-up raw or cooked vegetables
1 c cooked legumes
1 c vegetable juice
2 c raw, leafy greens

Polara Studios, Inc

Vegetables contribute folate, vitamin A, vitamin C, vitamin K, vitamin E, magnesium, potassium, and fiber.

Consume a variety of vegetables each day, and choose from all five subgroups several times a week.

Dark-green vegetables: Broccoli and leafy greens such as arugula, beet greens, bok choy, collard greens, kale, mustard greens, romaine lettuce, spinach, turnip greens, watercress

Red and orange vegetables: Carrots, carrot juice, pumpkin, red bell peppers, sweet potatoes, tomatoes, tomato juice, vegetable juice, winter squash (acorn, butternut)

Legumes: Black beans, black-eyed peas, garbanzo beans (chickpeas), kidney beans, lentils, navy beans, pinto beans, soybeans and soy products such as tofu, split peas, white beans

Starchy vegetables: Cassava, corn, green peas, hominy, lima beans, potatoes

Other vegetables: Artichokes, asparagus, bamboo shoots, bean sprouts, beets, brussels sprouts, cabbages, cactus, cauliflower, celery, cucumbers, eggplant, green beans, green bell peppers, iceberg lettuce, mushrooms, okra, onions, seaweed, snow peas, zucchini

Limit these vegetables that contain solid fats and/or added sugars:
Baked beans, candied sweet potatoes, coleslaw, french fries, potato salad, refried beans, scalloped potatoes, tempura vegetables

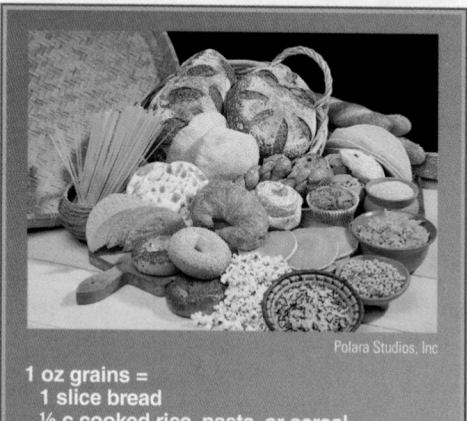

1 oz grains =
1 slice bread
½ c cooked rice, pasta, or cereal
1 oz dry pasta or rice
1 c ready-to-eat cereal
3 c popped popcorn

Polara Studios, Inc

Grains contribute folate, niacin, riboflavin, thiamin, iron, magnesium, selenium, and fiber.

Make most (at least half) of the grain selections whole grains.

Whole grains: amaranth, barley, brown rice, buckwheat, bulgur, cornmeal, millet, oats, quinoa, rye, wheat, wild rice and whole-grain products such as breads, cereals, crackers, and pastas; popcorn

Enriched refined products: bagels, breads, cereals, pastas (couscous, macaroni, spaghetti), pretzels, white rice, rolls, tortillas

Limit these grains that contain solid fats and/or added sugars:
Biscuits, cakes, cookies, cornbread, crackers, croissants, doughnuts, fried rice, granola, muffins, pastries, pies, presweetened cereals, taco shells

© 2016 Cengage Learning®

FIGURE 1-4 USDA Food Patterns: Food Groups and Subgroups

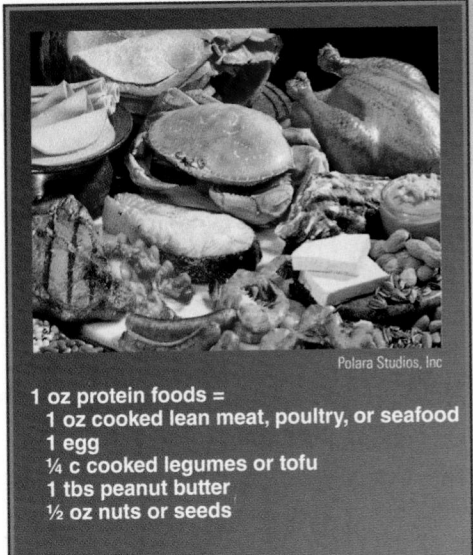

1 oz protein foods =
1 oz cooked lean meat, poultry, or seafood
1 egg
¼ c cooked legumes or tofu
1 tbs peanut butter
½ oz nuts or seeds

Polara Studios, Inc

Protein foods contribute protein, essential fatty acids, niacin, thiamin, vitamin B6, vitamin B12, iron, magnesium, potassium, and zinc.

Choose a variety of protein foods from the three subgroups, including seafood in place of meat or poultry twice a week.

Seafood: Fish (catfish, cod, flounder, haddock, halibut, herring, mackerel, pollock, salmon, sardines, sea bass, snapper, trout, tuna), shellfish (clams, crab, lobster, mussels, oysters, scallops, shrimp)

Meats, poultry, eggs: Lean or low-fat meats (fat-trimmed beef, game, ham, lamb, pork, veal), poultry (no skin), eggs

Nuts, seeds, soy products: Unsalted nuts (almonds, cashews, filberts, pecans, pistachios, walnuts), seeds (flaxseeds, pumpkin seeds, sesame seeds, sunflower seeds), legumes, soy products (textured vegetable protein, tofu, tempeh), peanut butter, peanuts

Limit these protein foods that contain solid fats and/or added sugars:
Bacon; baked beans; fried meat, seafood, poultry, eggs, or tofu; refried beans; ground beef; hot dogs; luncheon meats; marbled steaks; poultry with skin; sausages; spare ribs

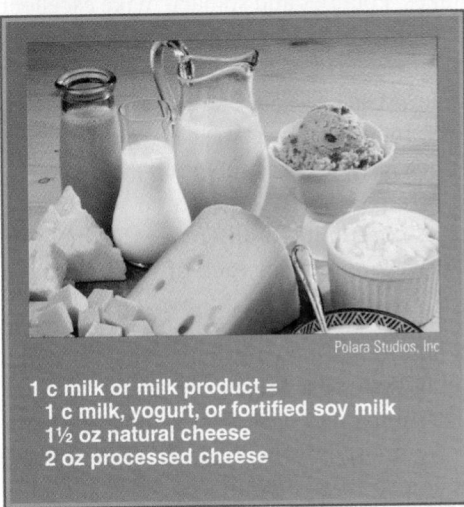

Polara Studios, Inc

1 c milk or milk product =
1 c milk, yogurt, or fortified soy milk
1½ oz natural cheese
2 oz processed cheese

Milk and milk products contribute protein, riboflavin, vitamin B12, calcium, potassium, and, when fortified, vitamin A and vitamin D.

Make fat-free or low-fat choices. Choose other calcium-rich foods if you don't consume milk.

Fat-free or 1% low-fat milk and fat-free or 1% low-fat milk products such as buttermilk, cheeses, cottage cheese, yogurt; fat-free fortified soy milk

Limit these milk products that contain solid fats and/or added sugars:
2% reduced-fat milk and whole milk; 2% reduced-fat and whole-milk products such as cheeses, cottage cheese, and yogurt; flavored milk with added sugars such as chocolate milk, custard, frozen yogurt, ice cream, milk shakes, pudding, sherbet; fortified soy milk

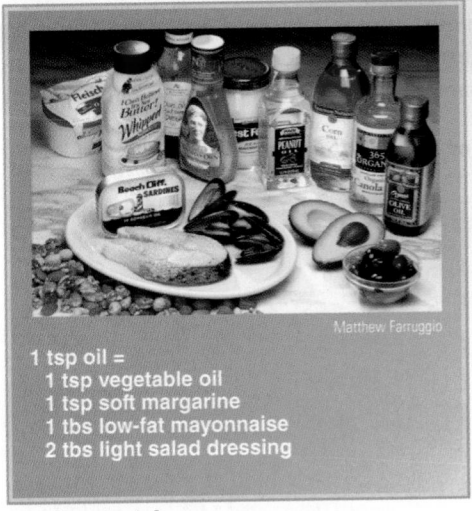

Matthew Farruggio

1 tsp oil =
1 tsp vegetable oil
1 tsp soft margarine
1 tbs low-fat mayonnaise
2 tbs light salad dressing

Oils are not a food group, but are featured here because they contribute vitamin E and essential fatty acids.

Use oils instead of solid fats, when possible.

Liquid vegetable oils such as canola, corn, flaxseed, nut, olive, peanut, safflower, sesame, soybean, sunflower oils; mayonnaise, oil-based salad dressing, soft *trans*-free margarine; unsaturated oils that occur naturally in foods such as avocados, fatty fish, nuts, olives, seeds (flaxseeds, sesame seeds), shellfish

Limit these solid fats:
Butter, animal fats, stick margarine, shortening

© 2016 Cengage Learning®

FIGURE 1-4 (continued)

TABLE 1-5 Estimated Daily kCalorie Needs for Adults

	Sedentary[a]	Active[b]
Women		
19–30 yr	2000	2400
31–50 yr	1800	2200
51+ yr	1600	2100
Men		
19–30 yr	2500	3000
31–50 yr	2300	2900
51+ yr	2100	2600

© Cengage Learning®

[a]*Sedentary* describes a lifestyle that includes only the activities typical of day-to-day life. [b]*Active* describes a lifestyle that includes physical activity equivalent to walking more than 3 miles per day at a rate of 3 to 4 miles per hour, in addition to the activities typical of day-to-day life. kCalorie values for active people reflect the midpoint of the range appropriate for age and gender, but within each group older adults may need fewer kcalories and younger adults may need more. In addition to gender, age, and activity level, energy needs vary with height and weight (see Chapter 6).

[Handwritten notes in left margin:]
veg groups
① dark green - B vitamin folate
② red + orange - vitamin A
③ legumes - iron + protein
④ starchy - carbohydrate energy
⑤ other veg - fill in gaps + add more nutrients

legumes (lay-GYOOMS, LEG-yooms)**:** plants of the bean and pea family with seeds that are rich in protein compared with other plant-derived foods.

shown in Table 1-5. Chapter 6 explains how to determine energy needs.

All vegetables provide an array of vitamins, fiber, and the mineral potassium, but some vegetables are especially good sources of certain nutrients and beneficial phytochemicals. For this reason, the vegetable group is sorted into five subgroups. The dark green vegetables deliver the B vitamin folate; the red and orange vegetables provide vitamin A; legumes supply iron and protein; the starchy vegetables contribute carbohydrate energy; and the other vegetables fill in the gaps and add more of these same nutrients.

[Handwritten note in right margin:] *5 groups veggies*

In a 2000-kcalorie diet, then, the recommended 2½ cups of daily vegetables should be varied among the subgroups over a week's time. In other words, eating 2½ cups of potatoes or even nutrient-rich spinach every day for seven days does *not* meet the recommended vegetable intakes. Potatoes and spinach make excellent choices when consumed in balance with vegetables from the other subgroups. One way to help ensure selections for all of the subgroups is to eat vegetables of various colors—for example, green broccoli, orange sweet potatoes, black beans, yellow corn, and white cauliflower. Intakes of vegetables are appropriately averaged over a week's time—it isn't necessary to include every subgroup every day.

For similar reasons, the protein foods group is sorted into three subgroups. Perhaps most notably, each of these subgroups contributes a different assortment of fats. Table 1-6 presents the recommended *weekly* amounts for each of the subgroups for vegetables and protein foods.

Notable Nutrients As Figure 1-4 notes, each food group contributes key nutrients. This feature provides flexibility in diet planning because a person can select any food from a food group (or its subgroup) and receive similar nutrients. For example, a person can choose milk, cheese, or yogurt and receive the same key nutrients. Importantly, foods provide not only these key nutrients, but also small amounts of other nutrients and phytochemicals as well.

Legumes contribute the same key nutrients—notably protein, iron, and zinc—as meats, poultry, and seafood. They are also excellent sources of fiber, folate, and potassium, which are commonly found in vegetables. To encourage frequent consumption

TABLE 1-6 USDA Food Patterns: Recommended Weekly Amounts from the Vegetable and Protein Foods Subgroups

Vegetable Subgroups	1600 kcal	1800 kcal	2000 kcal	2200 kcal	2400 kcal	2600 kcal	2800 kcal	3000 kcal
Dark green	1½ c	1½ c	1½ c	2 c	2 c	2½ c	2½ c	2½ c
Red and orange	4 c	5½ c	5½ c	6 c	6 c	7 c	7 c	7½ c
Legumes	1 c	1½ c	1½ c	2 c	2 c	2½ c	2½ c	3 c
Starchy	4 c	5 c	5 c	6 c	6 c	7 c	7 c	8 c
Other	3½ c	4 c	4 c	5 c	5 c	5½ c	5½ c	7 c
Protein Foods Subgroups								
Seafood	8 oz	8 oz	8 oz	9 oz	10 oz	10 oz	11 oz	11 oz
Meats, poultry, eggs	24 oz	24 oz	26 oz	29 oz	31 oz	31 oz	34 oz	34 oz
Nuts, seeds, soy products	4 oz	4 oz	4 oz	4 oz	5 oz	5 oz	5 oz	5 oz

© Cengage Learning®

Note: Table 1-4 specifies the recommended amounts of total vegetables and protein foods per *day*. This table shows those amounts dispersed among five vegetable and three protein foods subgroups per *week*.

of these nutrient-rich foods, legumes are included as a sub-group of both the vegetable group and the protein foods group. Thus, legumes can be counted in either the vegetable group or the protein foods group.[17] In general, people who regularly eat meat, poultry, and seafood count legumes as a vegetable, and vegetarians and others who seldom eat meat, poultry, or sea-food count legumes in the protein foods group.

The USDA Food Patterns encourage greater consumption from certain food groups to provide the nutrients most often lacking in the diets of Americans—dietary fiber, vitamin D, calcium, and potassium. In general, most people need to eat:

- *More* vegetables, fruits, whole grains, seafood, and fat-free or low-fat milk and milk products.

- *Less* sodium, saturated fat, *trans* fat, and cholesterol, and *fewer* refined grains and foods and beverages with solid fats and added sugars.

FIGURE 1-5 Discretionary kCalories in a 2000-kCalorie Diet

Nutrient-Dense Choices A healthy eating pattern emphasizes nutrient-dense options within each food group. By consistently selecting nutrient-dense foods, a person can obtain all the nutrients needed and still keep kcalories under control. In contrast, eating foods that are low in nutrient density makes it difficult to get enough nutrients without exceeding energy needs and gaining weight. For this reason, consumers should select low-fat foods from each group and foods without added fats or sugars—for example, fat-free milk instead of whole milk, baked chicken without the skin instead of hot dogs, green beans instead of french fries, orange juice instead of fruit punch, and whole-wheat bread instead of biscuits. Notice that Figure 1-4 indicates which foods *within each group* contain solid fats and/or added sugars and therefore should be limited. Oil is a notable exception: even though oil is pure fat and therefore rich in kcalories, a small amount of oil from sources such as nuts, fish, or vegetable oils is necessary every day to provide nutrients lacking from other foods. Consequently, these high-fat foods are listed among the nutrient-dense foods (see Nutrition in Practice 3 to learn why).

(handwritten note: low-fat foods can help prevent weight gain.)

Discretionary kCalories People who consistently choose nutrient-dense foods may be able to meet their nutrient needs without consuming their full allowance of kcalories. The difference between the kcalories needed to supply nutrients and those needed to maintain weight might be considered **discretionary kcalories** (see Figure 1-5). Table 1-4 includes discretionary kcalories for each kcalorie level.

Discretionary kcalories allow a person to choose whether to:

(handwritten note: —where we need to focus...)

- Eat additional nutrient-dense foods, such as an extra serving of skinless chicken or a second ear of corn.

- Select a few foods with fats or added sugars, such as reduced-fat milk or sweetened cereal.

- Add a little fat or sugar to foods, such as butter or jelly on toast.

- Consume some alcohol. (Nutrition in Practice 20 explains why this may not be a good choice for some individuals.)

Alternatively, a person wanting to lose weight might choose to:

- *Not* use discretionary kcalories.

Cup and Ounce Equivalents Recommended daily amounts for fruits, vegetables, and milk are measured in cups, and those for grains and protein foods in ounces. Figure 1-4 provides the equivalent measures for foods that are not readily measured in cups and ounces. For example, 1 ounce of grains is considered equivalent to 1 slice of bread or ½ cup of cooked rice.

> **discretionary kcalories:** the kcalories remaining in a person's energy allowance after consuming enough nutrient-dense foods to meet all nutrient needs for a day.

BOX 1-3

- ¼ c dried fruit or nuts = a golf ball
- 1 c fruit or vegetables = a baseball
- 3 oz meat = a deck of cards
- 2 tbs peanut butter = a ping-pong ball

Consumers using the USDA Food Patterns can learn how to estimate the cups or ounces in their personal **portion sizes** by determining the answers to questions such as these: What portion of a cup is a small handful of raisins? Is a "helping" of mashed potatoes more or less than a half cup? How many ounces of cereal do you typically pour into the bowl? How many ounces is the steak at your favorite restaurant? How may cups of milk does your glass hold? For quick and easy estimates, visualize each portion as being about the size of one of the common objects listed in Box 1-3.

Mixtures of Foods Some foods—such as casseroles, soups, and sandwiches—fall into two or more food groups. With a little practice, users can learn to divide these foods into food groups. From the USDA Food Patterns' point of view, a taco represents four different food groups: the taco shell from the grains group; the onions, lettuce, and tomatoes from the vegetable group; the ground beef from the protein foods group; and the cheese from the milk group.

Vegetarian Food Guide Vegetarian diets are plant-based eating patterns that rely mainly on grains, vegetables, legumes, fruits, seeds, and nuts. Some vegetarian diets include eggs, milk products, or both. People who do not eat meats or milk products can still use the USDA Food Patterns to create an adequate diet.[18] The subgroups for protein foods have been reorganized to eliminate meats, poultry, and seafood (see Table NP 4-1 on p. 104). The other food groups and the recommended daily amounts for each food group remain the same. Nutrition in Practice 4 defines vegetarian terms and provides details on planning healthy vegetarian diets.

Ethnic Food Choices People can use the USDA Food Patterns and still enjoy a diverse array of culinary styles by sorting ethnic foods into their appropriate food groups. For example, a person eating Mexican foods would find tortillas in the grains group, jicama in the vegetable group, and guava in the fruit group. Table 1-1 (p. 4) features ethnic food choices.

MyPlate

The USDA created an educational tool called MyPlate to illustrate the five food groups and remind consumers to make healthy food choices. The MyPlate icon, shown in Figure 1-6, divides a plate into four sections, each representing a food group—fruits, vegetables, grains, and protein foods. The sections vary in size, indicating the relative proportion each food group contributes to a healthy diet. A circle next to the plate represents the milk group (dairy).

The MyPlate icon does not stand alone as an educational tool. A wealth of information can be found at the MyPlate website (chooseMyPlate.gov). The USDA's MyPlate online suite of information makes applying the USDA Food Patterns easier. Consumers can create a personal profile to estimate kcalorie needs and determine the kinds and amounts of foods they need to eat each day based on their height, weight, age, gender, and activity level. Information is also available for children, pregnant and lactating women, and vegetarians. In addition to creating a personal plan, consumers can find daily tips to help them improve their diet and increase physical activity. A key message of the website is to enjoy food, but eat less by avoiding oversized portions.

FIGURE 1-6 MyPlate
Note that vegetables and fruits occupy half the plate and that the grains portion is slightly larger than the portion of protein foods.

Source: USDA, www.choosemyplate.gov.

IN SUMMARY

- Food group plans such as the USDA Food Patterns help consumers select the types and amounts of foods to provide adequacy, balance, and variety in the diet.

- Each food group contributes key nutrients, a feature that provides flexibility in diet planning.

- MyPlate is an educational tool used to illustrate the five food groups.

portion size: the quantity of food served or eaten at one meal or snack; *not* a standard amount.

1.6 Food Labels

LO 1.6 Compare the information on food labels to make selections that meet specific dietary and health goals.

Today, consumers know more about the links between diet and disease than they did in the past, and they are demanding still more information on disease prevention. Many people rely on food labels to help them select foods with less saturated fat, *trans* fat, cholesterol, and sodium and more vitamins, minerals, and dietary fiber.[19] Food labels appear on virtually all packaged foods, and posters or brochures provide similar nutrition information for fresh fruits, vegetables, and seafoods. Packages of meat cuts, ground meats, and poultry also must display nutrition information.[20] A few foods need not carry nutrition labels: those contributing few nutrients, such as plain coffee, tea, and spices; foods produced by small businesses; and foods prepared and sold in the same establishment. Producers of some of these items, however, voluntarily use food labels.

The Ingredient List

All packaged foods must list *all* ingredients on the label in descending order of predominance by weight. Knowing that the first ingredient predominates by weight, consumers can glean much information. Compare these products, for example:

- A beverage powder that contains "sugar, citric acid, natural flavors . . ." versus a juice that contains "water, tomato concentrate, concentrated juices of carrots, celery . . . ."

- A cereal that contains "puffed milled corn, sugar, corn syrup, molasses, salt . . ." versus one that contains "100 percent rolled oats. . . ."

In each comparison, consumers can tell that the second product is the more nutrient dense.

Nutrition Facts Panel

The Food and Drug Administration (FDA) requires food labels to include key nutrition facts. The "Nutrition Facts" panel provides such information as serving sizes, Daily Values, and nutrient quantities. Because knowledge about nutrition science has advanced greatly during the two decades or more since food labels were first introduced, the FDA has recently proposed updates to the Nutrition Facts panel to make it easier for consumers to make informed decisions about the foods they eat.[21] The updated panel will also include a refreshed design that displays kcalories and serving size information more prominently to emphasize parts of the label that are most important in addressing public health concerns such as obesity, diabetes, and heart disease. Manufacturers may take up to 2 years to change their labels, so Figure 1-7 (p. 22) illustrates and compares both the original "Nutrition Facts" panel and the proposed panel.

Serving Sizes Food labels must identify the serving size (food quantity) for which nutrition information is presented. The FDA has established specific serving sizes for various foods and requires that all labels for a given product use the same serving size. By law, serving sizes must be based on the amounts of food or beverage people actually consume, not what they "should" consume. In general, people are eating and drinking more today than 20 years ago when the label was first designed, so the FDA proposes updating the reference values for serving sizes that manufacturers use, to better reflect what people really eat and drink. For example, the serving size for all ice creams may be changed from ½ cup to 1 cup. The use of specific serving sizes for various foods facilitates comparison shopping. Consumers can see at a glance which brand has more or fewer kcalories or grams of fat, for example. However, these serving sizes

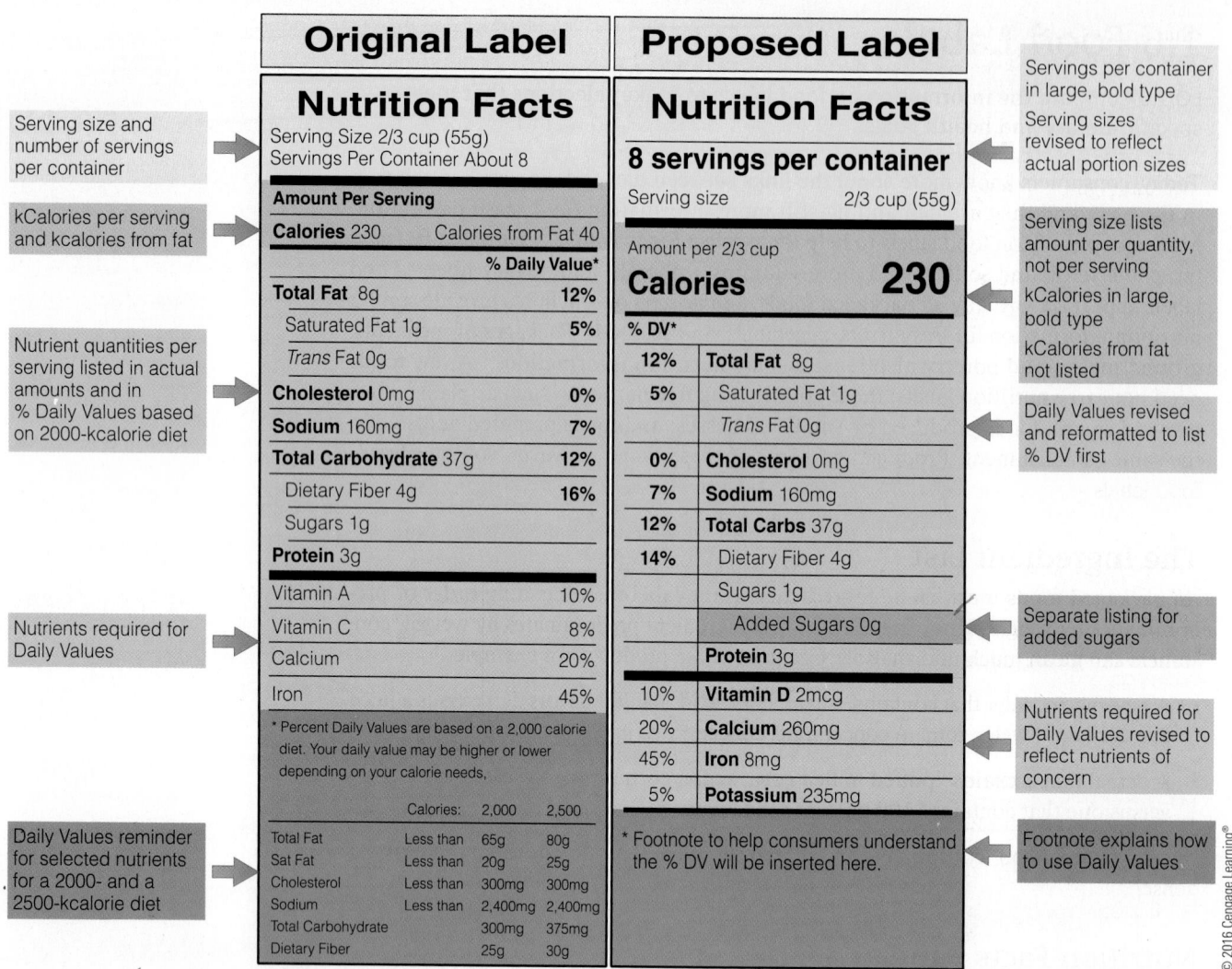

FIGURE 1-7 Original and Proposed Nutrition Facts Panel

The figure labels (left to right):

Left side (Original Label):
- Serving size and number of servings per container
- kCalories per serving and kcalories from fat
- Nutrient quantities per serving listed in actual amounts and in % Daily Values based on 2000-kcalorie diet
- Nutrients required for Daily Values
- Daily Values reminder for selected nutrients for a 2000- and a 2500-kcalorie diet

Original Label:

Nutrition Facts
Serving Size 2/3 cup (55g)
Servings Per Container About 8

Amount Per Serving

Calories 230   Calories from Fat 40

	% Daily Value*
Total Fat 8g	12%
Saturated Fat 1g	5%
Trans Fat 0g	
Cholesterol 0mg	0%
Sodium 160mg	7%
Total Carbohydrate 37g	12%
Dietary Fiber 4g	16%
Sugars 1g	
Protein 3g	
Vitamin A	10%
Vitamin C	8%
Calcium	20%
Iron	45%

* Percent Daily Values are based on a 2,000 calorie diet. Your daily value may be higher or lower depending on your calorie needs.

		Calories:	2,000	2,500
Total Fat	Less than		65g	80g
Sat Fat	Less than		20g	25g
Cholesterol	Less than		300mg	300mg
Sodium	Less than		2,400mg	2,400mg
Total Carbohydrate			300mg	375mg
Dietary Fiber			25g	30g

Proposed Label:

Nutrition Facts
8 servings per container

Serving size   2/3 cup (55g)

Amount per 2/3 cup

Calories   **230**

% DV*

12%	**Total Fat** 8g	
5%	Saturated Fat 1g	
	Trans Fat 0g	
0%	**Cholesterol** 0mg	
7%	**Sodium** 160mg	
12%	**Total Carbs** 37g	
14%	Dietary Fiber 4g	
	Sugars 1g	
	Added Sugars 0g	
	Protein 3g	
10%	**Vitamin D** 2mcg	
20%	**Calcium** 260mg	
45%	**Iron** 8mg	
5%	**Potassium** 235mg	

* Footnote to help consumers understand the % DV will be inserted here.

Right side (Proposed Label):
- Servings per container in large, bold type
- Serving sizes revised to reflect actual portion sizes
- Serving size lists amount per quantity, not per serving
- kCalories in large, bold type
- kCalories from fat not listed
- Daily Values revised and reformatted to list % DV first
- Separate listing for added sugars
- Nutrients required for Daily Values revised to reflect nutrients of concern
- Footnote explains how to use Daily Values

© 2016 Cengage Learning®

TABLE 1-7 Household and Metric Measures

- 1 teaspoon (tsp) = 5 milliliters (mL)
- 1 tablespoon (tbs) = 15 mL
- 1 cup (c) = 240 mL
- 1 fluid ounce fl (fl oz) = 30 mL
- 1 ounce (oz) = 28 grams (g)

© Cengage Learning®

Note: The Aids to Calculation section at the back of the book provides additional weights and measures.

Daily Values: reference values developed by the FDA specifically for use on food labels.

do not provide a standard for desirable consumption. Standard serving sizes are expressed in both common household measures, such as cups, and metric measures, such as milliliters, to accommodate users of both types of measures (see Table 1-7).

In addition to updating serving sizes for certain products, the FDA may require some food and beverages previously labeled as more than one serving to be labeled as a single serving because people typically eat or drink them in one sitting. Examples are a 20-ounce soda or a 15-ounce can of soup. Certain larger packages may have a two-column label because some people may consume them in one sitting while others may consume them in two or three sittings. For example, a 24-ounce can of soda or a 19-ounce can of soup might be one serving for one person but not for another.

When examining the nutrition information on a food label, consumers need to compare the serving size on the label with how much they actually eat and adjust their calculations accordingly. For example, if the serving size is four cookies and you only eat two, then you need to cut the nutrient and kcalorie values in half; similarly, if you eat eight cookies, then you need to double the values. The number of servings per container is listed just above the serving size on the updated label.

The Daily Values To help consumers evaluate the information found on labels, the FDA created a set of nutrient standards called the **Daily Values** specifically for use on food labels. The Daily Values do two things: they set adequacy standards for nutrients that are desirable in the diet such as protein, vitamins, minerals, and fiber, and they set moderation standards for other nutrients that must be limited, such as fat, saturated fat, cholesterol, and sodium.

The "% Daily Value" column on a label provides a ballpark estimate of how individual foods contribute to the total diet. It compares key nutrients in a serving of food with the daily goals of a person consuming 2000 kcalories. Although the Daily Values are based on a 2000-kcalorie diet, people's actual energy intakes vary widely; some people need fewer kcalories, and some people need many more. This makes the Daily Values most useful for comparing one food with another and less useful as nutrient intake targets for individuals. By examining a food's general nutrient profile, however, a person can determine whether the food contributes "a little" or "a lot" of a nutrient, whether it contributes "more" or "less" than another food, and how well it fits into the consumer's overall diet.

The proposed label will include updated Daily Values for calcium, potassium, sodium, dietary fiber, and vitamin D. The Daily Value footnote will better explain the standards to consumers.

Nutrient Quantities In addition to the serving size and the servings per container, the FDA requires that the Nutrition Facts panel on a label present nutrient information in two ways—in quantities (such as grams) and as percentages of the Daily Values. The proposed Nutrition Facts panel must provide the nutrient amount, percent Daily Value, or both for the following:

- Total food energy (kcalories)
- Total fat (grams and percent Daily Value)—note that the proposed revision does not include kcalories from fat
- Saturated fat (grams and percent Daily Value)
- *Trans* fat (grams)
- Cholesterol (milligrams and percent Daily Value)
- Sodium (milligrams and percent Daily Value)
- Total carbs, including starch, sugar, and fiber (grams and percent Daily Value)
- Dietary fiber (grams and percent Daily Value)
- Sugars, which includes both those naturally present in and those added to the foods (grams)
- Added sugars (grams)—note that the original label does not include a line for added sugars
- Protein (grams)
- The following vitamins and minerals (percent Daily Value): vitamin D, potassium, iron, and calcium

[handwritten margin note: Nutritional Facts panels must contain]

Food energy from fat will no longer be required to appear on the label because research shows that the type of fat is more important than the amount. Note that vitamin D and potassium will be required because these are nutrients of concern for consumers, whereas vitamins A and C, once mandatory, will no longer be required but can be included on a voluntary basis.

The FDA developed the Daily Values for use on food labels because comparing nutrient amounts against a standard helps make them meaningful to consumers. A person might wonder, for example, whether 1 milligram of iron or calcium is a little or a lot. As Table 1-8 (p. 24) shows, the Daily Value for iron is 18 milligrams, so 1 milligram of iron is enough to take notice of: it is more than 5 percent. But because the current Daily Value for calcium on food labels is 1000 milligrams (and the proposed is 1300), 1 milligram of calcium is a negligible amount.

TABLE 1-8 Daily Values for Food Labels

Food labels must present the "% Daily Value" for these nutrients.

Food Component	Original Daily Value	Proposed Daily Value
Fat (total)	65 g	65 g
Saturated fat	20 g	20 g
Cholesterol	300 mg	300 mg
Carbohydrate (total)	300 g	300 g
Fiber	25 g	28 g
Vitamin D	Not required	20 μg
Sodium	2400 mg	2300 mg
Potassium	Not required	4700 mg
Calcium	1000 mg	1300 mg
Iron	18 mg	18 mg

© Cengage Learning®

Note: Daily Values were established for adults and children over 4 years old. The values for energy-yielding nutrients are based on 2000 kcalories a day. The original label includes vitamins A and C, but the proposed label does not.

Front-of-Package Labels Some consumers find the many numbers on Nutrition Facts panels overwhelming. They want an easier and quicker way to interpret information and select products. Food manufacturers responded by creating front-of-package labels that incorporate text, color, and icons to present key nutrient facts.[22] Without any regulations or oversight, however, different companies used a variety of different symbols to describe how healthful their products were. To calm the chaos and maintain the voluntary status of front-of-package labels, major food industry associations created a standardized presentation of nutrient information called Facts Up Front (see Figure 1-8). Whether consumers find this approach to be the most helpful remains to be seen.[23] The FDA is currently evaluating the program and reviewing recommendations from the Institute of Medicine to determine the best way to present front-of-package information.[24]

Claims on Labels

In addition to the Nutrition Facts panel, consumers may find various claims on labels. These claims include nutrient claims, health claims, and structure-function claims.

Nutrient Claims Have you noticed phrases such as "good source of fiber" on a box of cereal or "rich in calcium" on a package of cheese? These and other **nutrient claims** may be used on labels only if the claims meet FDA definitions, which include the conditions under which each term can be used. For example, in addition to having less than 2 milligrams of cholesterol, a "cholesterol-free" product may not contain more than 2 grams of saturated fat and *trans* fat combined per serving. Table 1-9 defines nutrient terms on food labels, including criteria for foods described as "low," "reduced," and "free."

[handwritten note in left margin:] A cholesterol-free product may not contain more than 2 grams sat. fat & trans fat COMBINED per serving

FIGURE 1-8 Facts Up Front

This example of front-of-package labeling (created by the Grocery Manufacturers Association and the Food Marketing Institute) presents key nutrient facts.

nutrient claims: statements that characterize the quantity of a nutrient in a food.

TABLE 1-9 **Terms Used on Food Labels**

GENERAL TERMS

free: "nutritionally trivial" and unlikely to have a physiological consequence; synonyms include *without*, *no*, and *zero*. A food that does not contain a nutrient naturally may make such a claim but only as it applies to all similar foods (for example, "applesauce, a fat-free food").

good source of: the product provides between 10 and 19 percent of the Daily Value for a given nutrient per serving.

healthy: a food that is low in fat, saturated fat, cholesterol, and sodium, and that contains at least 10 percent of the Daily Values for vitamin D, iron, calcium, potassium, protein, or fiber.

high: 20 percent or more of the Daily Value for a given nutrient per serving; synonyms include *rich in* or *excellent source of*.

less: at least 25 percent less of a given nutrient or kcalories than the comparison food (see individual nutrients); synonyms include *fewer* and *reduced*.

light or lite: one-third fewer kcalories than the comparison food; 50 percent or less of the fat or sodium than the comparison food; any use of the term other than as defined must specify what it is referring to (for example, "light in color" or "light in texture").

low: an amount that would allow frequent consumption of a food without exceeding the Daily Value for the nutrient. A food that is naturally low in a nutrient may make such a claim but only as it applies to all similar foods (for example, "fresh cauliflower, a low-sodium food"); synonyms include *little*, *few*, and *low source of*.

more: at least 10 percent more of the Daily Value for a given nutrient than the comparison food; synonyms include *added* and *extra*.

organic (on food labels): at least 95 percent of the product's ingredients have been grown and processed according to USDA regulations defining the use of fertilizers, herbicides, insecticides, fungicides, preservatives, and other chemical ingredients.

ENERGY

kcalorie-free: fewer than 5 kcalories per serving.

low kcalorie: 40 kcalories or less per serving.

reduced kcalorie: at least 25 percent fewer kcalories per serving than the comparison food.

FAT AND CHOLESTEROL[a]

percent fat free: may be used only if the product meets the definition of *low fat* or *fat free* and must reflect the amount of fat in 100 grams (for example, a food that contains 2.5 grams of fat per 50 grams can claim to be "95 percent fat free").

fat free: less than 0.5 gram of fat per serving (and no added fat or oil); synonyms include *zero-fat*, *no-fat*, and *nonfat*.

low fat: 3 grams or less fat per serving.

less fat: at least 25 percent less fat than the comparison food.

saturated fat free: less than 0.5 gram of saturated fat and 0.5 gram of *trans* fat per serving.

low saturated fat: 1 gram or less saturated fat and less than 0.5 gram of *trans* fat per serving.

less saturated fat: at least 25 percent less saturated fat and *trans* fat combined than the comparison food.

***trans* fat free:** less than 0.5 gram of *trans* fat and less than 0.5 gram of saturated fat per serving.

cholesterol free: less than 2 milligrams cholesterol per serving and 2 grams or less saturated fat and *trans* fat combined per serving.

low cholesterol: 20 milligrams or less cholesterol per serving and 2 grams or less saturated fat and *trans* fat combined per serving.

less cholesterol: at least 25 percent less cholesterol than the comparison food (reflecting a reduction of at least 20 milligrams per serving), and 2 grams or less saturated fat and *trans* fat combined per serving.

extra lean: less than 5 grams of fat, 2 grams of saturated fat and *trans* fat combined, and 95 milligrams of cholesterol per serving and per 100 grams of meat, poultry, and seafood.

lean: less than 10 grams of fat, 4.5 grams of saturated fat and *trans* fat combined, and 95 milligrams of cholesterol per serving and per 100 grams of meat, poultry, and seafood. For mixed dishes such as burritos and sandwiches, less than 8 grams of fat, 3.5 grams of saturated fat, and 80 milligrams of cholesterol per reference amount customarily consumed.

CARBOHYDRATES: FIBER AND SUGAR

high fiber: 5 grams or more fiber per serving. A high-fiber claim made on a food that contains more than 3 grams fat per serving and per 100 grams of food must also declare total fat.

sugar-free: less than 0.5 gram of sugar per serving.

SODIUM

sodium free and **salt free:** less than 5 milligrams of sodium per serving.

low sodium: 140 milligrams or less per serving.

very low sodium: 35 milligrams or less per serving.

[a]Foods containing more than 13 grams total fat per serving or per 50 grams of food must indicate those contents immediately after a cholesterol claim. As you can see, all cholesterol claims are prohibited when the food contains more than 2 grams saturated fat and *trans* fat combined per serving.

© Cengage Learning®

OVERVIEW OF NUTRITION AND HEALTH

TABLE 1-10 Reliable Health Claims on Food Labels

- Calcium and reduced risk of osteoporosis
- Sodium and reduced risk of hypertension
- Dietary saturated fat and cholesterol and reduced risk of coronary heart disease
- Dietary fat and reduced risk of cancer
- Fiber-containing grain products, fruits, and vegetables and reduced risk of cancer
- Fruits, vegetables, and grain products that contain fiber, particularly soluble fiber, and reduced risk of coronary heart disease
- Fruits and vegetables and reduced risk of cancer
- Folate and reduced risk of neural tube defects
- Sugar alcohols and reduced risk of tooth decay
- Soluble fiber from whole oats and from psyllium seed husk and reduced risk of heart disease
- Soy protein and reduced risk of heart disease
- Whole grains and reduced risk of heart disease and certain cancers
- Plant sterol and plant stanol esters and reduced risk of heart disease
- Potassium and reduced risk of hypertension and stroke

© Cengage Learning®

Some descriptions *imply* that a food contains, or does not contain, a nutrient. Implied claims are prohibited unless they meet specified criteria. For example, a claim that a product "contains no oil" implies that the food contains no fat. If the product is truly fat free, then it may make the no-oil claim, but if it contains another source of fat, such as butter, it may not.

Health Claims **Health claims** describe the relationship of a food or food component to a disease or health-related condition. In some cases, the FDA authorizes health claims based on an extensive review of the scientific literature. For example, the health claim that "diets low in sodium may reduce the risk of high blood pressure," is based on enough scientific evidence to establish a clear link between diet and health. Such reliable health claims still appear on food labels, and they have a high degree of scientific validity (see Table 1-10).

In cases where there is emerging—but not established—evidence for a relationship between a food or food component and disease, the FDA allows the use of *qualified* health claims that must use specific language indicating that the evidence supporting the claim is limited. A qualified health claim might state that "Very limited and preliminary research suggests that eating one-half to one cup of tomatoes and/or tomato sauce a week may reduce the risk of prostate cancer. The FDA concludes that there is little scientific evidence supporting the claim." Unfortunately, many consumers are not knowledgeable enough to distinguish between scientifically reliable claims and those that are best ignored.

Structure-Function Claims **Structure-function claims** describe the effect that a substance has on the structure or function of the body but do not make reference to a disease—for example, "calcium builds strong bones." Unlike health claims, which require food manufacturers to collect scientific evidence and petition the FDA, structure-function claims can be made without any FDA approval. Product labels can claim to "slow aging," "improve memory," and "support immunity and digestive health" without any proof. The only criterion for a structure-function claim is that it must not mention a disease or symptom. Unfortunately, structure-function claims can be deceptively similar to health claims. Consider these statements:

- "May reduce the risk of heart disease." — *must have FDA approval*
- "Promotes a healthy heart." — *no approval needed*

[handwritten margin notes: Implied claims are prohibited unless they meet specified criteria. i.e. - "contains no oil" implies NO FAT! if it contains butter it cannot make this claim]

health claims: statements that characterize the relationship between a nutrient or other substance in food and a disease or health-related condition.

structure-function claims: statements that describe how a product may affect a structure or function of the body; for example, "calcium builds strong bones." Structure-function claims do not require FDA authorization.

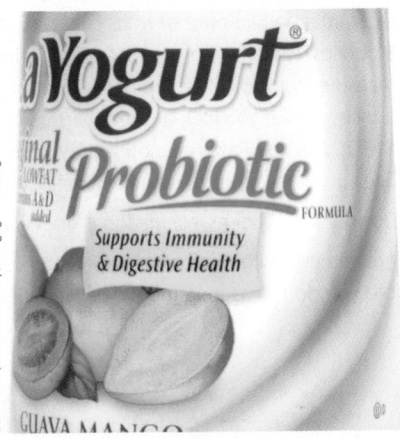

Nutrient claims characterize the level of a nutrient in the food—for example, "fat free" or "less sodium."

Health claims characterize the relationship of a food or food component to a disease or health-related condition—for example, "soluble fiber from oatmeal daily in a diet low in saturated fat and cholesterol may reduce the risk of heart disease" or "a diet low in total fat may reduce the risk of some cancers."

Structure-function claims describe the effect that a substance has on the structure or function of the body and do not make reference to a disease—for example, "supports immunity and digestive health" or "calcium builds strong bones."

FIGURE 1-9 Label Claims

Although most consumers do not distinguish between these two types of claims, the first is a health claim that requires FDA approval, whereas the second is an unproven, but legal, structure-function claim. Figure 1-9 compares the three types of label claims.

IN SUMMARY

health claims require FDA approval - this is where product "lowers rise of heart disease"

structure function claim- "promotes healthy heart" - no FDA approval needed.

▌ Food labels list the ingredients, the serving size, the number of kcalories provided, and the key nutrient quantities in a food—information consumers need to select foods that will help them meet their nutrition and health goals.

▌ Daily Values are a set of nutrient standards created by the FDA for use on food labels.

▌ Reliable health claims are backed by the highest standards of scientific evidence.

Your Diet

The secret to making healthy food choices is learning to incorporate the *Dietary Guidelines* (Table 1-3 on p. 14) and the USDA Food Patterns (Figure 1-4 on pp. 16–17) into your decision-making process. Before completing this assignment, you may want to review the section called "Mixtures of Foods" on p. 20 to see where foods such as casseroles or soups fall in the food group plan.

▌ Keep a record of the foods and beverages you eat for 24 hours. Record both the types and amounts of foods eaten.

▌ Enter your food record information into an online diet analysis tool such as Cengage Learning's *Diet and Wellness Plus* or the USDA's SuperTracker (www.supertracker.usda.gov). If you have not used the application before, you will need to first enter

some personal information (such as height, weight, age, gender, and activity level) to create a profile.

▌ What is your estimated daily kcalorie need based on your profile information in the diet analysis tool? How does this compare to your estimated needs based on Table 1-5 on p. 18? (Chapter 6 offers a more individualized approach to estimating your kcalorie needs).

▌ Compare the foods you ate with the USDA Food Patterns recommendations for your energy needs (see Table 1-4 on p. 15) by viewing the appropriate reports in the diet analysis tool. (Keep a copy of all the reports from the tool for later reference.) For example, if you need 2400 kcalories a day, the recommended amount of fruits is 2 cups, while that of grains is 8 ounces. Figure 1-4 on pp. 16–17 provides equivalent measures for foods that are not readily measured in cups or ounces. When you look at the report comparing your intake to the USDA Food Patterns, notice how your food choices have been converted into these equivalents.

▪ Do your food choices include foods from each of the food groups?

▪ Are some food groups over- or underrepresented? If so, what can you do to ensure a more balanced diet?

▪ Do you eat a variety of foods within each group? If not, suggest ways to enhance the variety in your diet.

▪ Did you choose at least some whole-grain foods from the grain group, and fat-free or low-fat foods from the milk and milk products group and the protein foods group? List the foods you selected that are whole grain (grain group), fat free, and low fat (milk and protein foods groups).

Clinical Applications

1. Make a list of the foods and beverages you've consumed in the past two days. Look at each item on your list and consider why you chose the particular food or beverage you did. Did you eat cereal for breakfast because that's what you always eat (habit), or because it was the easiest, quickest food to prepare (convenience)? Did you put fat-free milk on the cereal because you want to control your energy intake (nutrition)? In going down your list, you may be surprised to discover exactly why you chose certain foods.

2. As a health care professional, you can uncover clues about a client's food choices by paying close attention. You may be surprised to discover why a client chooses certain foods, but you can then use this knowledge to serve the best interests of the client. For example, an elderly, undernourished widower may eat the same sandwich for lunch every day. In talking with the client, you discover that this is what he and his wife fixed together each day. Consider ways you might be able to help the client learn to eat other foods and vary his choices.

3. Using the list of foods and beverages from exercise #1, compare your day's intake with the USDA Food Patterns. Did you vary your choices within each food group? Did your intake match the daily recommended amounts from each group? If not, list some changes you could have made to meet the recommendations.

Self Check

1. When people eat the foods typical of their families or geographic area, their choices are influenced by:
   a. occupation.
   b. nutrition.
   c. emotional state.
   d. ethnic heritage or regional cuisine.

2. The energy-yielding nutrients are:
   a. fats, minerals, and water.
   b. minerals, proteins, and vitamins.
   c. carbohydrates, fats, and vitamins.
   d. carbohydrates, fats, and proteins.

3. The inorganic nutrients are:
   a. proteins and fats.
   b. vitamins and minerals.
   c. minerals and water.
   d. vitamins and proteins.

4. Alcohol is not a nutrient because:
   a. the body derives no energy from it.
   b. it is organic.
   c. it is converted to body fat.
   d. it does not contribute to the body's growth or repair.

5. The nutrient standards in use today include all of the following except:
   a. Recommended Dietary Allowances (RDA).
   b. Adequate Intakes (AI).
   c. Daily Minimum Requirements (DMR).
   d. Tolerable Upper Intake Levels (UL).

6. Which of the following is consistent with the *Dietary Guidelines for Americans*?
   a. Limit intakes of fruits, vegetables, and whole grains.
   b. Increase physical activity and reduce time spent in sedentary activities.
   c. Choose a diet with plenty of whole-milk products.
   d. Eat an abundance of foods to ensure nutrient adequacy.

7. In a food group plan such as the USDA Food Patterns, foods within a given food group are similar in their contents of:
   a. energy.
   b. proteins and fibers.
   c. vitamins and minerals.
   d. carbohydrates and fats.

8. A slice of apple pie supplies 350 kcalories with 3 grams of fiber; an apple provides 80 kcalories and the same 3 grams of fiber. This is an example of:
   a. kcalorie control.
   b. nutrient density.
   c. variety.
   d. essential nutrients.

9. According to the USDA Food Patterns, which of the following fruits/vegetables should be limited?
   a. Carrots
   b. Avocados
   c. Baked beans
   d. Potatoes

10. Food labels list ingredients in:
    a. alphabetical order.
    b. ascending order of predominance by weight.
    c. descending order of predominance by weight.
    d. manufacturer's order of preference.

Answers to these questions appear in Appendix H.

Notes

1. M. Truong, Y. Paradies, and N. Priest, Interventions to improve cultural competency in healthcare: A systematic review of reviews, *BMC Health Services Research* 14 (2014): 99; C. J. Heiss and coauthors, Preparing dietetics practitioners to effectively serve the Hispanic population, *Journal of the Academy of Nutrition and Dietetics* 113 (2013): S24–S28; K. Stein, Navigating cultural competency: In preparation for an expected standard in 2010, *Journal of the American Dietetic Association* 110 (2010): S13–S20.

2. A. Drewnowski and coauthors, Sweetness and food preference, *Journal of Nutrition* 142 (2012): 1142S–1148S; J. E. Hayes, B. S. Sullivan, and V. B. Duffy, Explaining variability in sodium intake through oral sensory phenotype, salt sensation and liking, *Physiology and Behavior* 100 (2010): 369–380.

3. E. R. Grimm and N. I. Steinle, Genetics of eating behavior: Established and emerging concepts, *Nutrition Reviews* 69 (2011): 52–60; J. E. Hayes and R. S. Keast, Two decades of supertasting: Where do we stand? *Physiology and Behavior* 104 (2011): 1072–1074.

4. Position of the Academy of Nutrition and Dietetics: Nutritional genomics, *Journal of the Academy of Nutrition and Dietetics* 114 (2014): 299–313.

5. C. Jacquier and coauthors, Improving the effectiveness of nutritional information policies: Assessment of unconscious pleasure mechanisms involved in food-choice decisions, *Nutrition Reviews* 70 (2012): 118–131.

6. Food Marketing Institute, US grocery shopper trends 2012: Executive summary, www.fmi.org /research, 2012.

7. A. Jaworowska and coauthors, Nutritional challenges and health implications of takeaway and fast food, *Nutrition Reviews* 71 (2013): 310–318.

8. International Food Information Council Foundation, *2013 Food & Health Survey*, www.foodinsight.org.

9. Position of the Academy of Nutrition and Dietetics: Functional foods, *Journal of the Academy of Nutrition and Dietetics* 113 (2013): 1096–1103.

10. S. A. Atkinson, Defining the process of Dietary Reference Intakes: Framework for the United States and Canada, *American Journal of Clinical Nutrition* 94 (2011): 655S–657S.

11. A. S. Go and coauthors, Heart disease and stroke statistics—2014 update: A report from the American Heart Association, *Circulation* 129 (2014): e28–e292; M. A.H. Hendriksen and coauthors, Potential effect of salt reduction in processed foods on health, *American Journal of Clinical Nutrition* 99 (2014): 446–453; R. H. Eckel and coauthors, 2013 AHA/ACC Guidelines on lifestyle management to reduce cardiovascular risk: A report of the American College of Cardiology/American Heart Association Task Force on Practice Guidelines, http://circ .ahajournals.org/content/early/2013/11/11/01 .cir.0000437740.48606.dl.citation; Position of the Academy of Nutrition and Dietetics: The role of nutrition in health promotion and chronic disease prevention, *Journal of the Academy of Nutrition and Dietetics* 113 (2013): 972–979; A. B. Evert and coauthors, Position statement: Nutrition therapy recommendations for the management of adults with diabetes, *Diabetes Care* 36 (2013): 3821–3842; L. H. Kushi and coauthors, American Cancer Society guidelines on nutrition and physical activity for cancer prevention, *CA: Cancer Journal for Clinicians* 62 (2012): 30–67; L. J. Appel and coauthors, The importance of population-wide sodium reduction as means to prevent cardiovascular disease and stroke: A call to action from the American Heart Association, *Circulation* 123 (2011): 1138–1143.

12. Position of the Academy of Nutrition and Dietetics, Total diet approach to healthy eating, *Journal of the Academy of Nutrition and Dietetics* 113 (2013): 307–317.

13. A. Drewnowski and V. L. Fulgoni, Nutrient density: Principles and evaluation tools, *American Journal of Clinical Nutrition* 99 (2014): 1223S–1228S; A. Drewnowski and coauthors, Achieve better health with nutrient-rich foods, *Nutrition Today* 47 (2012): 23–29.

14. Drewnowski and Fulgoni, Nutrient density: Principles and evaluation tools, 2014; Drewnowski and coauthors, Achieve better health with nutrient-rich foods, 2012; C. Kapica, The science behind current nutrition profiling systems to promote consumer intake of nutrient-dense foods, *American Journal of Clinical Nutrition* 91 (2010): entire supplement.

15. D. Mozaffarian and D. S. Ludwig, Dietary guidelines in the 21st century: A time for food, *Journal of the American Medical Association* 304 (2010): 681–682.

16. U.S. Department of Agriculture and U.S. Department of Health and Human Services, *Dietary Guidelines for Americans, 2010,* www .dietaryguidelines.gov.

17. U.S. Department of Agriculture, Vegetables: Peas and beans are unique foods, www.choosemyplate .gov/food-groups/vegetables-beans-peas.html, accessed March 24, 2014.

18. Position of the American Dietetic Association: Vegetarian diets, *Journal of the American Dietetic Association* 109 (2009): 1266–1282.

19. J. Ollberding, R. L. Wolf, and I. Contento, Food label use and its relation to dietary intake among US adults, *Journal of the American Dietetic Association* 111 (2011): S47–S51; D. Schorr and coauthors, Nutrition facts you can't miss: The evolution of front-of-pack labeling, *Nutrition Today* 45 (2010): 22–32.

20. R. M. Bliss, Nutrient data in time for the new year, *Agricultural Research* January 2012, pp. 20–21.

21. U. S. Food and Drug Administration, Proposed changes to the Nutrition Facts label, www.fda.gov/Food/GuidanceRegulation /GuidanceDocumentsRegulatoryInformation /LabelingNutrition/ucm385663.htm, updated March 7, 2014.

22. J. C. Hersey and coauthors, Effects of front-of-package and shelf nutrition labeling systems on consumers, *Nutrition Reviews* 71 (2013): 1–14.

23. K. D. Brownell and J. P. Koplan, Front-of-package nutrition labeling—An abuse of trust by the food industry? *New England Journal of Medicine* 364 (2011): 2373–2375.

24. E. A. Wartella and coauthors, *Front-of-Package Nutrition Rating Systems and Symbols: Promoting Healthier Choices* (Washington, D.C.: National Academies Press, 2011), available at www.iom .edu/Reports/2011/Front-of-Package-Nutrition -Rating-Systems-and-Symbols-Promoting -Healthier-Choices.aspx.

LO 1.7 Recognize misinformation and describe how to identify reliable nutrition information.

Nutrition and health receive so much attention on television, on the radio, in the popular press, and on the Internet that it is easy to be overwhelmed with inconsistent, unclear information.[1] More than two-thirds of U.S. consumers are interested in the relationship between nutrition and health, but the majority of them agree that such information is often confusing and conflicting.[2] Determining whether nutrition information is accurate can be a challenging task. It is also an important task because nutrition affects a person both professionally and personally.

A person watches a nutrition report on television and then reads a conflicting report in the newspaper. Why do nutrition news reports and claims for nutrition products seem to contradict each other so often?

The problem of conflicting messages arises for several reasons:

▪ Popular media, often faced with tight deadlines and limited time or space to report new information, rush to present the latest "breakthrough" in a headline or a 60-second spot. They can hardly help omitting important facts about the study or studies that the "breakthrough" is based on.

▪ Despite tremendous advances in the past few decades, scientists still have much to learn about the human body and nutrition. Scientists themselves often disagree on their first tentative interpretations of new research findings, yet these are the very findings that the public hears most about.

▪ The popular media often broadcast preliminary findings in hopes of grabbing attention and boosting readership or television ratings.

▪ Commercial promoters turn preliminary findings into advertisements for products or supplements long before the findings have been validated—or disproved. The scientific process requires many experiments or trials to confirm a new finding. Seldom do promoters wait as long as they should to make their claims.

▪ Promoters are aware that consumers like to try new products or treatments even though they probably will not withstand the tests of time and scientific scrutiny.

So how can a person tell what claims to believe?

Valid nutrition information derives from scientific research, which has the following characteristics:

▪ Scientists test their ideas by conducting properly designed scientific experiments. They report their methods and procedures in detail so that other scientists can verify the findings through replication.

▪ Scientists recognize the inadequacy of personal testimonials.

▪ Scientists who use animals in their research do not apply their findings directly to human beings.

▪ Scientists may use specific segments of the population in their research. When they do, they are careful not to generalize the findings to all people.

▪ Scientists report their findings in respected scientific journals. Their work must survive a screening review by their peers before it is accepted for publication.

With each report from scientists, the field of nutrition changes a little—each finding contributes another piece to the whole body of knowledge. Table NP1-1 features 9 red flags of junk science to help consumers distinguish valid from misleading nutrition information.

Because nutrition misinformation harms the health and economic status of consumers, the **Academy of Nutrition and Dietetics** (formerly the Academy of Nutrition and Dietetics) works with health care professionals and educators to present sound nutrition information to the public and to actively confront nutrition misinformation.[3] Table NP1-2 offers a list of credible sources of nutrition information.

TABLE NP1-1 Warning Signs of Nutrition Quackery

1. **Quick and easy fixes.** Even proven treatments take time to be effective.

2. **Personal testimonials.** Hearsay is the weakest form of scientific validity.

3. **One product does it all.** No one product can treat every disease and condition.

4. **Natural.** Natural is not necessarily safer or better. Any product strong enough to be effective is strong enough to cause side effects.

5. **Time-tested or latest innovation.** Such findings would be widely publicized and accepted by health professionals.

6. **Satisfaction guaranteed.** Marketers of fraudulent products may make generous promises, but consumers won't be able to collect on them.

7. **Paranoid accusations.** These claims suggest that health professionals and legitimate drug manufacturers are conspiring with each other to promote drug companies' products for financial gain.

8. **Meaningless medical jargon.** Phony terms hide the lack of scientific proof.

9. **Too good to be true.** If it sounds too good to be true, it probably isn't true.

TABLE NP1-2 Credible Sources of Nutrition Information

Government agencies, volunteer associations, consumer groups, and professional organizations provide consumers with reliable health and nutrition information. Credible sources of nutrition information include:

- Nutrition and food science departments at a university or community college

- Local agencies such as the health department or County Cooperative Extension Service

- Government resources such as:

  - Centers for Disease Control and Prevention (CDC) — www.cdc.gov

  - Department of Agriculture (USDA) — www.usda.gov

  - Department of Health and Human Services (DHHS) — www.hhs.gov

  - *Dietary Guidelines for Americans* — www.dietaryguidelines.gov

  - Food and Drug Administration (FDA) — www.fda.gov

  - Health Canada — http://www.hc-sc.gc.ca/fn-an/index-eng.php

  - Healthy People — www.healthypeople.gov

  - Let's Move! — www.letsmove.gov

  - MyPlate — www.choosemyplate.gov

  - National Institutes of Health — www.nih.gov

  - *Physical Activity Guidelines for Americans* — www.health.gov/paguidelines

- Volunteer health agencies such as:

  - American Cancer Society — www.cancer.org

  - American Diabetes Association — www.diabetes.org

  - American Heart Association — www.americanheart.org

- Reputable consumer groups such as:

  - American Council on Science and Health — www.acsh.org

  - Federal Citizen Information Center — www.usa.gov

  - International Food Information Council — www.foodinsight.org

- Professional health organizations such as:

  - Academy of Nutrition and Dietetics — www.eatright.org

  - American Medical Association — www.ama-assn.org

  - Dietitians of Canada — www.dietitians.ca

- Journals such as:

  - *American Journal of Clinical Nutrition* — www.ajcn.org

  - *Journal of the Academy of Nutrition and Dietetics* — www.andjrnl.org/

  - *New England Journal of Medicine* — www.nejm.org

  - *Nutrition Reviews* — www.ilsi.org

TABLE NP1-3 Evaluating the Reliability of Websites

To determine whether an Internet site offers reliable nutrition information, answer the following questions:

- Who is responsible for the site? Clues can be found in the three-letter "tag" that follows the dot in the site's name. For example, "gov" and "edu" indicate government and university sites, respectively, which are usually reliable sources of information.

- Do the names and credentials of information providers appear? Is an editorial board identified? Many legitimate sources provide e-mail addresses or other ways to obtain more information about the site and the information providers behind it.

- Are links with other reliable information sites provided? Reputable organizations almost always provide links with other similar sites because they want you to know of other experts in their area of knowledge. Caution is needed when you evaluate a site by its links, however. Anyone, even a quack, can link a web page to a reputable site without the organization's permission. Doing so may give the quack's site the appearance of legitimacy, just the effect for which the quack is hoping.

- Is the site updated regularly? Nutrition information changes rapidly, and sites should be updated often.

- Is the site selling a product or service? Commercial sites may provide accurate information, but they also may not. Their profit motive increases the risk of bias.

- Does the site charge a fee to gain access to it? Many academic and government sites offer the best information, usually for free. Some legitimate sites do charge fees, but before paying up, check the free sites. Chances are good you will find what you are looking for without paying.

- Some credible websites include

  - National Council Against Health Fraud: www.ncahf.org

  - Stephen Barrett's Quackwatch: www.quackwatch.com

What about nutrition and health information found on the Internet? How does a person know whether the websites are reliable?

With hundreds of millions of websites on the Internet, searching for nutrition and health information can be daunting. The Internet offers no guarantee of the accuracy of the information found there, and much of it is pure fiction. Websites must be evaluated for their accuracy, just like every other source. Table NP1-3 provides clues to identifying reliable nutrition information sites and lists some credible sites.

One of the most trustworthy sites used by scientists and others is the National Library of Medicine's PubMed (www.ncbi.nlm.nih.gov/pubmed), which provides free access to more than 10 million abstracts (short descriptions) of research papers published in scientific journals around the world. Many abstracts provide links to websites where full articles are available.

Promoters of fraudulent "health" products use the Internet as a primary means to sell their wares. Agencies such as the Food and Drug Administration (FDA) take action against fraudulent marketing of supplements and health products on the Internet.[4] The latest actions target unscrupulous companies that use the Internet to promote products to the most vulnerable consumers—those with diseases such as cancer or AIDS. Of greatest concern are those products that not only make false promises but also are potentially dangerous. For example, herbal products touted as safe treatments for serious illnesses such as cancer may interact with and impair the effectiveness of medications. The FDA advises consumers to be suspicious of:

■ Claims that a product is "natural" or "nontoxic." "Natural" or "nontoxic" does not always mean safe.

■ Claims that a product is a "scientific breakthrough," "miraculous cure," "secret ingredient," or "ancient remedy."

■ Claims that a product cures a wide range of illnesses.

■ Claims that use impressive-sounding medical terms.

■ Claims of a "money-back" guarantee.

■ Consumers with questions or suspicions about fraud can contact the FDA on the Internet at www.FDA.gov or by telephone at (888) INFO-FDA.

Everyone seems to be giving advice on nutrition. How can a person tell whom to listen to?

Registered dietitian nutritionists (RDNs), also called **registered dietitians (RDs),** and nutrition professionals with advanced degrees (M.S., Ph.D.) are experts (see Box NP1-1). These professionals are probably in the best position to answer a person's nutrition questions. On the other hand, a "**nutritionist**" may be an expert or a quack, depending on which state the person practices in. Some states require people who use this title to meet strict

standards. In other states, a "nutritionist" may be any individual who claims a career connection with the nutrition field. There is no accepted national definition for the term *nutritionist*.

Other purveyors of nutrition information may also lack credentials. A health-food store owner may be in the nutrition business simply because it is a lucrative market. The owner may have a background in business or sales and no education in nutrition at all. Such a person is not qualified to provide nutrition information to customers. For accurate nutrition information, seek out a trained professional with a college education in nutrition—an expert in the field of **dietetics.**

What about nurses and other health care professionals?

All members of the health care team share responsibility for helping each client to achieve optimal health, but the registered dietitian nutritionist is usually the primary nutrition expert. Each of the other team members has a related specialty. Some physicians are specialists in clinical nutrition and thus are also experts in the field. Other physicians, nurses, and **dietetic technicians** often assist dietitians in providing nutrition information and may help to administer direct nutrition care. Nurses play central roles in client care management and client relationships. Visiting nurses and home health care nurses may become intimately involved in clients' nutrition care at home, teaching them both theory and cooking techniques. Physical therapists can provide individualized exercise programs related to nutrition—for example, to help control obesity. Social workers may provide practical and emotional support.

What roles might these other health care professionals play in nutrition care?

Some of the responsibilities of the health care professional might be:

■ Helping people understand why nutrition is important to them.

■ Answering questions about food and diet.

■ Explaining to clients how modified diets work.

■ Collecting information about clients that may influence their nutritional health.

■ Identifying clients at risk for poor nutrition status (see Chapter 14) and recommending or taking appropriate action.

■ Recognizing when clients need extra help with nutrition problems (in such cases, the problems should be referred to a dietitian or physician).

Health care professionals may routinely perform these nutrition-related tasks:

■ Obtaining diet histories.

■ Taking weight and height measurements.

■ Feeding clients who cannot feed themselves.

■ Recording what clients eat or drink.

■ Observing clients' responses and reactions to foods.

BOX NP1-1 GLOSSARY OF NUTRITION EXPERTS

Academy of Nutrition and Dietetics: the professional organization of dietitians in the United States; formerly the Academy of Nutrition and Dietetics. The Canadian equivalent is Dietitians of Canada, which operates similarly.

dietetic technicians: persons who have completed a minimum of an associate's degree from an accredited college or university and an approved dietetic technician program. A dietetic technician, registered (DTR) has also passed a national examination and maintains registration through continuing professional education.

dietetics: the application of nutrition principles to achieve and maintain optimal human health.

nutritionists: all registered dietitians are nutritionists, but not all nutritionists are registered dietitians. Some state licensing boards set specific qualifications for holding the title. For states that regulate this title, the definition varies from state to state. To obtain some "nutritionist" credentials requires little more than a payment.

registered dietitian nutritionists (RDNs): food and nutrition experts who have earned a minimum of a bachelor's degree from an accredited university or college after completing a program of coursework approved by the Academy of Nutrition and Dietetics (or Dietitians of Canada); also called *registered dietitians (RDs)*. The dietitians must serve in an approved, supervised internship or coordinated program to practice the necessary skills, pass the registration examination, and maintain competency through continuing education. Many states require licensing for practicing dietitians. Licensed dietitians (LDs) have met all state requirements to offer nutrition advice.

registered dietitian (RD): an alternative term for an RDN.

- Helping clients mark menus.

- Monitoring weight changes.

- Monitoring food and drug interactions.

- Encouraging clients to eat.

- Assisting clients at home in planning their diets and managing their kitchen chores.

- Alerting the physician or dietitian when nutrition problems are identified.

- Charting actions taken and communicating on these matters with other professionals as needed.

Thus, although the dietitian assumes the primary role as the nutrition expert on a health care team, other health care professionals play important roles in administering nutrition care.

Notes

1. D. Quagliani and M. Hermann, Practice paper of the Academy of Nutrition and Dietetics: Communicating accurate food and nutrition information, *Journal of the Academy of Nutrition and Dietetics* 112 (2012): 759.

2. D. Schor and coauthors, Nutrition facts you can't miss: The evolution of front-of-pack labeling, *Nutrition Today* 45 (2010): 22–32.

3. Quagliani and Hermann, 2012.

4. Food and Drug Administration, 6 tip-offs to rip-offs: Don't fall for health fraud scams, www.fda.gov /FoorConsumers/ConsumerUpdates/ucm341344.htm, updated November 18, 2013.

2

Carbohydrates

2.1 The Chemist's View of Carbohydrates

LO 2.1 Identify the monosaccharides, disaccharides, and polysaccharides common in nutrition and list their major food sources.

2.2 Regulation of Blood Glucose

LO 2.2 Explain how hormones control blood glucose concentrations.

2.3 Health Effects of Sugars and Alternative Sweeteners

LO 2.3 Describe how added sugars can contribute to health problems and how alternative sweeteners may help to limit kcalories and sugar intake.

2.4 Health Effects of Starch and Dietary Fibers

LO 2.4 Identify the health benefits of, and recommendations for, starches and fibers.

2.5 Nutrition in Practice: The Glycemic Index in Nutrition Practice

LO 2.5 Describe the glycemic index and explain why its use in disease prevention is controversial.

Most people would like to feel good all the time. Part of the secret of feeling good is replenishing the body's energy supply with food. Carbohydrate is the preferred energy source for many of the body's functions. As long as carbohydrate is available, the human brain depends exclusively on it as an energy source. Athletes eat a "high-carb" diet to store as much muscle fuel as possible, and dietary recommendations urge people to eat carbohydrate-rich foods for better health. Some people, however, mistakenly think of carbohydrate-rich foods as "fattening" and avoid them when trying to lose weight. This strategy may be helpful if the carbohydrates are the concentrated sugars of soft drinks, candies, and cookies, but it is counterproductive if the carbohydrates are from whole grains, vegetables, legumes, and fruit. These plant foods provide carbohydrate and fiber with little or no fat. Milk is the only animal-derived food that contains significant amounts of carbohydrate. Thus, people who wish to lose fat, maintain lean tissue, and stay healthy can best do so by being physically active, paying close attention to portion sizes, and designing an eating pattern based on foods that supply fiber-rich carbohydrate in balance with other energy nutrients.[1]

This chapter on carbohydrates is the first of three on the energy-yielding nutrients. Fats are the topic of Chapter 3 and protein is featured in Chapter 4. Nutrition in Practice 20 addresses one other contributor of energy to the human diet, alcohol. Alcohol, of course, has well-known undesirable side effects when used in excess.

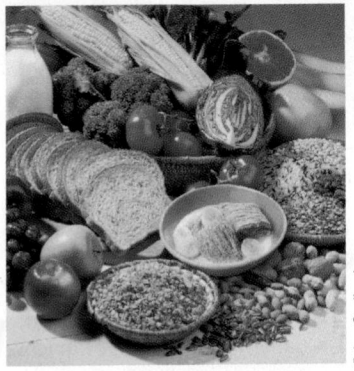

Grains, vegetables, legumes, fruits, and milk offer ample carbohydrate.

carbohydrate-rich foods are not always fattening…

monosaccharides: simple sugars. disaccharides: double sugars. polysaccharides: chains of monosaccharides

2.1 The Chemist's View of Carbohydrates

LO 2.1 Identify the monosaccharides, disaccharides, and polysaccharides common in nutrition and list their major food sources.

The dietary **carbohydrates** include the sugars, starch, and fiber. Chemists describe the sugars as:

- **Monosaccharides** (single sugars).
- **Disaccharides** (double sugars).

Starch and fiber are:*

- **Polysaccharides**—compounds composed of chains of monosaccharide units.

All of these carbohydrates are composed of the single sugar **glucose** and other compounds that are much like glucose in composition and structure. Figure 2-1 (p. 36) shows the chemical structure of glucose.

Monosaccharides

Three monosaccharides are important in nutrition: glucose, fructose, and galactose. All three monosaccharides have the same number and kinds of atoms but in different arrangements.

Glucose Most cells depend on glucose for their fuel to some extent, and the cells of the brain and the rest of the nervous system depend almost exclusively on glucose for their energy. The body can obtain this glucose from carbohydrates. To function

---

*Monosaccharides and disaccharides (sugars) are sometimes called *simple carbohydrates*, and the polysaccharides (starch and fiber) are sometimes called *complex carbohydrates*.

carbohydrates: energy nutrients composed of monosaccharides.

carbo = carbon

hydrate = water

monosaccharides (mon-oh-SACK-uh-rides): single sugar units.

mono = one

saccharide = sugar

disaccharides (dye-SACK-uh-rides): pairs of sugar units bonded together.

di = two

polysaccharides: long chains of monosaccharide units arranged as starch, glycogen, or fiber.

poly = many

glucose: a monosaccharide; the sugar common to all disaccharides and polysaccharides; also called *blood sugar* in the body or *dextrose* in foods.

fructose: a monosaccharide; sometimes known as *fruit sugar*.

fruct = fruit

galactose: a monosaccharide; part of the disaccharide lactose.

FIGURE 2-1 Chemical Structure of Glucose
On paper, the structure of glucose has to be drawn flat, but in nature the five carbons and oxygen are roughly in a plane, with the H, OH, and CH₂OH extending out above and below it.

optimally, the body must maintain blood glucose within limits that allow the cells to nourish themselves. A later section describes blood glucose regulation.

Fructose Fructose is the sweetest of the sugars. Fructose occurs naturally in fruits, in honey, and as part of table sugar. However, most fructose is consumed in sweet beverages such as soft drinks, in ready-to-eat cereals, and in other products sweetened with **high-fructose corn syrup** or other **added sugars**. Glucose and fructose are the most common monosaccharides in nature.

Galactose The third single sugar, galactose, occurs mostly as part of lactose, a disaccharide also known as milk sugar. During digestion, galactose is freed as a single sugar.

Disaccharides

In disaccharides, pairs of single sugars are linked together. Three disaccharides are important in nutrition: maltose, sucrose, and lactose. All three contain glucose as one of their single sugars. As Table 2-1 shows, the other monosaccharide is either another glucose (in maltose), fructose (in sucrose), or galactose (in lactose). The shapes of the sugars in Table 2-1 reflect their chemical structures as drawn on paper.

Sucrose Sucrose (table, or white, sugar) is the most familiar of the three disaccharides and is what people mean when they speak of "sugar." This sugar is usually obtained by refining the juice from sugar beets or sugarcane to provide the brown, white, and powdered sugars available in the supermarket, but it occurs naturally in many fruits and vegetables. When a person eats a food containing sucrose, enzymes in the digestive tract split the sucrose into its glucose and fructose components.

Lactose Lactose is the principal carbohydrate of milk. Most human infants are born with the digestive enzymes necessary to split lactose into its two monosaccharide parts, glucose and galactose, so as to absorb it. Breast milk thus provides a simple, easily digested carbohydrate that meets an infant's energy needs; many formulas do, too, because they are made from milk. Many people lose the ability to digest lactose after infancy. This condition, known as lactose intolerance, is discussed in Chapter 19.

Maltose The third disaccharide, **maltose**, is a plant sugar that consists of two glucose units. Maltose is produced whenever starch breaks down—as happens in plants when they break down their stored starch for energy and start to sprout and in human beings during carbohydrate digestion.

Polysaccharides

Unlike the sugars, which contain the three monosaccharides—glucose, fructose, and galactose—in different combinations, the polysaccharides are composed almost

high-fructose corn syrup: a widely used commercial kcaloric sweetener made by adding enzymes to cornstarch to convert a portion of its glucose molecules into sweet-tasting fructose.

added sugars: sugars, syrups, and other kcaloric sweeteners that are added to foods during processing or preparation or at the table. Added sugars do not include the naturally occurring sugars found in fruits and milk products. Also called *carbohydrate sweeteners,* they include glucose, fructose, high-fructose corn syrup, concentrated fruit juice, and other sweet carbohydrates. Also defined in Chapter 1.

sucrose: a disaccharide composed of glucose and fructose; commonly known as *table sugar, beet sugar,* or *cane sugar.*

  sucro = sugar

lactose: a disaccharide composed of glucose and galactose; commonly known as *milk sugar.*

  lact = milk

maltose: a disaccharide composed of two glucose units; sometimes known as *malt sugar.*

TABLE 2-1 The Major Sugars

Monosaccharides		Disaccharides	
Glucose	⬢	Sucrose (glucose + fructose)	⬢⬠
Fructose	⬠	Lactose (glucose + galactose)	⬠⬢
Galactose	⬢	Maltose (glucose + glucose)	⬢⬢
(found primarily as part of lactose)			

Glycogen

A glycogen molecule contains hundreds of glucose units in highly branched chains.

Starch (branched)

Starch (unbranched)

A starch molecule contains hundreds of glucose molecules in either occasionally branched chains or unbranched chains.

FIGURE 2-2 Glycogen and Starch Compared

entirely of glucose (and, in some cases, other monosaccharides). Three types of polysaccharides are important in nutrition: glycogen, starch, and fibers.

Glycogen is a storage form of energy for human beings and animals; starch plays that role in plants; and fibers provide structure in stems, trunks, roots, leaves, and skins of plants. Both glycogen and starch are built entirely of glucose units; fibers are composed of a variety of monosaccharides and other carbohydrate derivatives.

Glycogen Glycogen molecules are made of chains of glucose that are more highly branched than those of starch molecules (see the left side of Figure 2-2). Glycogen is found in meats only to a limited extent and not at all in plants.* For this reason, glycogen is not a significant food source of carbohydrate, but it does play an important role in the body. The human body stores much of its glucose as glycogen in the liver and muscles.

Starch Starch is a long, straight or branched chain of hundreds or thousands of glucose units linked together (see the middle and right side of Figure 2-2). These giant molecules are packed side by side in grains such as rice or wheat, in root crops and tubers such as yams and potatoes, and in legumes such as peas and beans. When a person eats the plant, the body splits the starch into glucose units and uses the glucose for energy.†

All starchy foods come from plants. Grains are the richest food source of starch. In most human societies, people depend on a staple grain for much of their food energy: rice in Asia; wheat in Canada, the United States, and Europe; corn in much of Central and South America; and millet, rye, barley, and oats elsewhere. A second important source of starch is the legume (bean and pea) family. Legumes include peanuts and "dry" beans such as butter beans, kidney beans, "baked" beans, black-eyed peas (cowpeas), chickpeas (garbanzo beans), and soybeans. Root vegetables (tubers) such as potatoes and yams are a third major source of starch, and in many non-Western societies, they are the primary starch sources. Grains, legumes, and tubers not only are rich in starch but may also contain abundant dietary fiber, protein, and other nutrients.

*Glycogen in animal muscles rapidly breaks down after slaughter.
†The short chains of glucose units that result from the breakdown of starch are known as *dextrins*. The word sometimes appears on food labels because dextrins can be used as thickening agents in foods.

glycogen (GLY-co-gen): a polysaccharide composed of glucose, made and stored by liver and muscle tissues of human beings and animals as a storage form of glucose. Glycogen is not a significant food source of carbohydrate and is not counted as one of the polysaccharides in foods.

starch: a plant polysaccharide composed of glucose and digestible by human beings.

Starch · Cellulose

© 2016 Cengage Learning®

FIGURE 2-3 **The Bonds of Starch and Cellulose Molecules Compared (Small Segments)**

Human enzymes can digest starch, but they cannot digest cellulose because the bonds that link the glucose units together in cellulose are different.

Fibers **Dietary fibers** are the structural parts of plants and thus are found in all plant-derived foods—vegetables, fruits, **whole grains**, and legumes. Most dietary fibers are polysaccharides—chains of sugars—just as starch is, but in fibers the sugar units are held together by bonds that human digestive enzymes cannot break. Consequently, most dietary fibers pass through the body, providing little or no energy for its use. Figure 2-3 illustrates the difference in the bonds that link glucose molecules together in starch and those found in the plant fiber cellulose. In addition to cellulose, fibers include the polysaccharides hemicellulose, pectins, gums, and mucilages, as well as the nonpolysaccharide lignins.

Cellulose is the main constituent of plant cell walls, so it is found in all vegetables, fruits, and legumes. Hemicellulose is the main constituent of cereal fibers. Pectins are abundant in vegetables and fruits, especially citrus fruits and apples. The food industry uses pectins to thicken jelly and keep salad dressing from separating. Gums and mucilages have similar structures and are used as additives or stabilizers by the food industry. Lignins are the tough, woody parts of plants; few foods people eat contain much lignin.

A few starches are classified as fibers. Known as **resistant starches**, these starches escape digestion and absorption in the small intestine. Starch may resist digestion for several reasons, including the individual's efficiency in digesting starches and the food's physical properties. Resistant starch is common in whole or partially milled grains, legumes, raw potatoes, and unripe bananas. Cooked potatoes, pasta, and rice that have been chilled also contain resistant starch. Similar to some fibers, resistant starch may support a healthy colon.[2]

Although cellulose and other dietary fibers are not broken down by human enzymes, some fibers can be digested by bacteria in the human digestive tract. Bacterial **fermentation** of fibers can generate some absorbable products that can yield energy when metabolized. Food fibers, therefore, can contribute some energy (1.5 to 2.5 kcalories per gram), depending on the extent to which they break down in the body.

Fibers are divided into two general groups by their chemical and physical properties.* In the first group are fibers that dissolve in water (**soluble fibers**). These form gels (are **viscous**) and are more readily digested by bacteria in the human large intestine (are easily fermented). Commonly found in barley, legumes, fruits, oats, and vegetables, these fibers are often associated with lower risks of chronic diseases (as discussed in a later section). In foods, soluble fibers add a pleasing consistency; for example, pectin puts the gel in jelly, and gums are added to salad dressings and other foods to thicken them.

Other fibers do not dissolve in water (**insoluble fibers**), do not form gels (are not viscous), and are less readily fermented. Insoluble fibers, such as cellulose and many hemicelluloses, are found in the outer layers of whole grains (bran), the strings of celery, the hulls of seeds, and the skins of corn kernels. These fibers retain their structure and rough texture even after hours of cooking. In the body, they aid the digestive system by easing elimination.[3]

*The DRI committee has proposed these fiber definitions: the term *dietary fibers* refers to naturally occurring fibers in intact foods, and *functional fibers* refers to added fibers that have health benefits; *total fiber* refers to the sum of fibers from both sources.

dietary fibers: a general term denoting in plant foods the polysaccharides cellulose, hemicellulose, pectins, gums, and mucilages, as well as the nonpolysaccharide lignins, which are not digested by human digestive enzymes, although some are digested by GI tract bacteria.

whole grains: grains or foods made from them that contain all the essential parts and naturally occurring nutrients of the entire grain seed (except the inedible husk).

resistant starches: starches that escape digestion and absorption in the small intestine of healthy people.

fermentation: the anaerobic (without oxygen) breakdown of carbohydrates by microorganisms that releases small organic compounds along with carbon dioxide and energy.

soluble fibers: indigestible food components that readily dissolve in water and often impart gummy or gel-like characteristics to foods. An example is pectin from fruit, which is used to thicken jellies.

viscous: having a gel-like consistency.

insoluble fibers: the tough, fibrous structures of fruits, vegetables, and grains; indigestible food components that do not dissolve in water.

IN SUMMARY

- Carbohydrate is the body's preferred energy source. Six sugars are important in nutrition: the three monosaccharides (glucose, fructose, and galactose) and the three disaccharides (sucrose, lactose, and maltose).

- The three disaccharides are pairs of monosaccharides; each contains glucose paired with one of the three monosaccharides. The polysaccharides (chains of monosaccharides) are glycogen, starches, and fibers.

- Both glycogen and starch are storage forms of glucose—glycogen in the body and starch in plants—and both yield energy for human use.

- The dietary fibers also contain glucose (and other monosaccharides), but their bonds cannot be broken by human digestive enzymes, so they yield little, if any, energy.

Starch- and fiber-rich foods are the foods to emphasize.

2.2 Regulation of Blood Glucose

LO 2.2 Explain how hormones control blood glucose concentrations.

If blood glucose falls below normal, a person may become dizzy and weak; if it rises substantially above normal, the person may become fatigued. **Diabetes**, a disorder characterized by elevated blood glucose, is the topic of Chapter 21. Left untreated, fluctuations to the extremes—either high or low—can be fatal. Blood glucose **homeostasis** is regulated primarily by two hormones: **insulin**, which moves glucose from the blood into the cells, and **glucagon**, which brings glucose out of storage when blood glucose falls (as occurs between meals).

Insulin After a meal, as blood glucose rises, the pancreas is the first organ to respond. It releases the hormone insulin, which signals body tissues to take up surplus glucose. Muscle tissue responds to insulin by taking up excess blood glucose and using it to make glycogen. The liver takes up excess blood glucose, too, but it needs no help from insulin to do so. Instead, the liver cells respond to insulin by speeding up their glycogen production. Adipose (fat) tissue also responds to insulin by both taking up blood glucose and slowing its release of the fat stored within its cells.[4] Simply put, insulin regulates blood glucose by:

- Facilitating blood glucose uptake by the muscles and adipose tissue.

- Stimulating glycogen synthesis in the liver.

The muscles hoard two-thirds of the body's total glycogen to ensure that glucose, a critical fuel for physical activity, is available for muscular work. The brain stores a tiny fraction of the total, thought to provide an emergency glucose reserve sufficient to fuel the brain for an hour or two in severe glucose deprivation. The liver stores the remainder and is generous with its glycogen, making it available as blood glucose for the brain or other tissues when the supply runs low. Without carbohydrate from food to replenish it, the liver glycogen stores can be depleted in less than a day. Balanced meals and snacks, eaten on a regular schedule, help the body to maintain its blood glucose. Meals with starch and soluble fiber combined with some protein and a little fat slow digestion so that glucose enters the blood gradually at an ongoing, steady rate.

The Release of Glucose from Glycogen The glycogen molecule is highly branched with hundreds of ends bristling from each molecule's surface (review this structure in Figure 2-2 on p. 37). When blood glucose starts to fall too low, the hormone glucagon is released into the bloodstream and triggers the breakdown of liver glycogen to single glucose molecules. Enzymes in liver cells respond to glucagon by attacking a multitude of glycogen ends simultaneously to release a surge of glucose into the blood for use by all the body's cells. Thus, the highly branched structure of glycogen uniquely suits the purpose of releasing glucose on demand.

---

diabetes (DYE-uh-BEE-teez): metabolic disorders characterized by elevated blood glucose resulting from insufficient insulin, ineffective insulin, or both; the complete medical term is *diabetes mellitus* (MELL-ih-tus or mell-EYE-tus).

homeostasis (HOME-ee-oh-STAY-sis): the maintenance of constant internal conditions (such as chemistry, temperature, and blood pressure) by the body's control system.

homeo = the same

stasis = staying.

insulin: a hormone secreted by the pancreas in response to (among other things) high blood glucose. It promotes cellular glucose uptake for use or storage.

glucagon (GLOO-ka-gon): a hormone that is secreted by special cells in the pancreas in response to low blood glucose concentration and that elicits release of glucose from storage.

[Handwritten margin notes:]

glucagon – a hormone secreted by special cells in the pancreas.

homeostasis – maintenance of constant internal conditions by the body's control system

HOMEO = the same

STASIS = stay equal balance

glucagon brings glucose into the blood stream when glucose is low

glycogen – stored glucose

■ Blood glucose concentrations are regulated primarily by two hormones: insulin, which moves glucose from the blood into the cells, and glucagon, which brings glucose out of storage when blood glucose falls.

2.3 Health Effects of Sugars and Alternative Sweeteners

LO 2.3 Describe how added sugars can contribute to health problems and how alternative sweeteners may help to limit kcalories and sugar intake.

Fiber-rich carbohydrate foods such as vegetables, whole grains, legumes, and fruits should predominate in people's diets; the **naturally occurring sugars** in these foods and in milk are acceptable because they are accompanied by many nutrients. In contrast, concentrated sweets such as candy, cola beverages and other soft drinks, cookies, pies, cakes, and other foods with added sugars add kcalories, but few, if any, other nutrients or fiber. The *Dietary Guidelines for Americans* offer clear advice on added sugars: reduce intake.[5] People who want to limit their use of sugar may choose from two sets of alternative sweeteners: sugar alcohols and nonnutritive sweeteners.

Sugars

Recent decades have seen a dramatic upward trend in consumption of added sugars. Sugary foods and beverages taste delicious, cost little money, and are constantly available, making overconsumption extremely likely. Though people are adding less sugar in the kitchen, food manufacturers are adding plenty to foods during processing. Soft drinks and other sugar-sweetened beverages are a major source of added sugars in the diets of U.S. consumers.[6] An estimated 75 percent of the packaged foods in the United States contain sweeteners, mostly added sugars.[7] On average, U.S. adults consume almost 15 percent of their daily energy intake from added sugars.[8] Most people can afford only a little added sugar in their diets if they are to meet nutrient needs within kcalorie limits.

The U.S. population is not alone in increasing sugar consumption. The trend is a worldwide phenomenon. In response, the World Health Organization has also taken a stand on sugar intake: consume less than 10 percent of total kcalories from added sugars. The World Health Organization further suggests that consuming less than 5 percent will provide additional health benefits.*

The increase in sugar consumption has raised many questions about sugar's effects on health. In moderate amounts, sugars add pleasure to meals without harming health.[9] In excess, however, sugars can be detrimental, and the average American diet currently delivers excessive amounts. Mounting evidence links high intakes of added sugars with obesity and other chronic diseases.[10] Sugars can also contribute to nutrient deficiencies by supplying energy (kcalories) without providing nutrients and to tooth decay, or **dental caries**.

Sugar and Obesity Over the past several decades, as obesity rates increased sharply, consumption of added sugars reached an all-time high—largely because high-fructose corn syrup use, especially in beverages, surged.[11] High-fructose corn syrup is composed of fructose and glucose in a ratio of about 50:50. Compared with sucrose, high-fructose corn syrup is less expensive, easier to use, and more stable. In addition to being used

Sugary soft drinks are the leading source of added sugars in the United States; cakes, cookies, pies, and other baked goods come next; and sweetened fruit drinks and punches follow closely behind.

naturally occurring sugars: sugars that are not added to a food but are present as its original constituents, such as the sugars of fruit or milk.

dental caries: the gradual decay and disintegration of a tooth.

*The World Health Organization uses the term *free sugars* to mean all monosaccharides and disaccharides added to foods by the manufacturer, cook, or consumer, plus the naturally occurring sugars in honey, syrups, and fruit juices.

in beverages, high-fructose corn syrup sweetens candies, baked goods, and hundreds of other foods. The use of high-fructose corn syrup sweetener parallels unprecedented increases in the incidence of obesity, but does this mean that the increasing sugar intakes are responsible for the increase in body fat and its associated health problems?[12] Excess sugar in the diet may be associated with more fat on the body.[13] When they are eaten in excess of need, energy from added sugars contributes to body fat stores, raising the risk of weight gain.[14] When total energy intake is controlled, however, *moderate* amounts of sugar do not *cause* obesity. Thus, to the extent that sugar contributes to an excessive energy intake, it can play a role in the development of obesity.

Because swallowing liquids requires little effort, the liquid form of sugar in soft drinks makes it especially easy to overconsume kcalories. Sugar-sweetened beverages are energy-dense, providing more than 150 kcalories per 12-ounce can, and many people drink several cans a day. The sugar kcalories of sweet beverages also cost less than many other energy sources, and they are widely available. The convenience, economy, availability, and flavors of sugary foods and beverages encourage overconsumption.

Limiting selections of foods and beverages high in added sugars can be an effective weight-loss strategy, especially for people whose excess kcalories come primarily from added sugars. Replacing a can of cola with a glass of water every day, for example, can help a person lose a pound (or at least not gain a pound) in one month.[15] That may not sound like much, but it adds up to more than 10 pounds a year, for very little effort.

Sugar and Heart Disease Added sugars also influence the balance between the body's fat-making and fat-clearing mechanisms, a balance that plays critical roles in the development of heart disease.[16] Fructose stimulates the body's fat-making pathways and impairs its fat-clearing pathways in ways that could lead to an unhealthy build-up of blood lipids (triglycerides, discussed in Chapter 4).[17]

To determine whether added sugars raise blood lipids, researchers studied more than 6000 healthy adults. They observed that people with higher intakes of added sugars had blood lipid values indicating an increased risk of heart disease.[18] In another study, young adults who consumed more sugar-sweetened beverages had greater abdominal fatness, more harmful blood lipids, and higher blood pressure than those who drank fewer.[19] It may not take an unrealistic amount of added sugars to cause this effect. As little as the equivalent of one or two fructose- or sucrose-sweetened soft drinks a day consumed for only a few weeks significantly changes blood lipids in ways that may pose risks to the heart and arteries.[20]

Sugar and Nutrient Deficiencies Empty-kcalorie foods that contain lots of added sugars such as cakes, candies, and sodas provide the body with glucose and energy, but few, if any, other nutrients. By comparison, foods such as whole grains, vegetables, legumes, and fruits that contain some natural sugars and lots of starches and fibers also provide protein, vitamins, and minerals.

A person spending 200 kcalories of a day's energy allowance on a 16-ounce soda gets little of value for those kcalories. In contrast, a person using 200 kcalories on three slices of whole-wheat bread gets 9 grams of protein, 6 grams of fiber, plus several of the B vitamins with those kcalories. For the person who wants something sweet, a reasonable compromise might be two slices of bread with a teaspoon of jam on each. The amount of sugar a person can afford to eat depends on how many discretionary kcalories are available beyond those needed to deliver indispensable vitamins and minerals.

By following the USDA Food Patterns and making careful food selections, a typical adult can obtain all the needed nutrients within an allowance of about 1500 kcalories. Some people have more generous energy allowances. For example, an active teenage boy may need as many as 3000 kcalories a day. If he eats mostly nutritious foods, then he may have discretionary kcalories available for cola beverages and other "extras." In contrast, an inactive older woman who is limited to fewer than 1500 kcalories a day can afford to eat only the most nutrient-dense foods—with few, or no, discretionary kcalories available.

Added sugars contribute to nutrient deficiencies by displacing nutrients. For nutrition's sake, the appropriate attitude to take is not that sugar is "bad" and must be avoided, but that nutritious foods must come first. If nutritious foods crowd sugar out of the diet, that is fine—but not the other way around. As always, balance, variety, and moderation guide healthy food choices.

Sugar and Dental Caries Does sugar contribute to dental caries? The evidence says yes. Any carbohydrate-containing food, including bread, bananas, or milk, as well as sugar, can support bacterial growth in the mouth. These bacteria produce the acid that eats away tooth enamel. Of major importance is the length of time the food stays in the mouth. This, in turn, depends on the composition of the food, how sticky the food is, how often a person eats the food, and especially whether the teeth are brushed afterward. Total sugar intake still plays a major role in caries incidence; populations whose diets provide no more than 10 percent of kcalories from sugar have a low prevalence of dental caries. The Academy of Nutrition and Dietetics and the *Dietary Guidelines for Americans* recommend a combined approach to prevent dental caries—practicing good oral hygiene, drinking fluoridated water, and reducing the amount of time sugars and starches are in the mouth.[21] Nutrition in Practice 17 discusses nutrition and oral health.

Recommended Sugar Intakes Moderate sugar intakes are not harmful and make eating more enjoyable, but the average U.S. intake is well above moderate. Thus, the *Dietary Guidelines for Americans* urge people to "reduce the intake of kcalories from added sugars." These added sugar kcalories (and those from solid fats and alcohol) are considered discretionary kcalories—and most people need to limit their intake. The USDA Food Patterns suggest about 8 teaspoons of sugar, about the amount in one 12-ounce soft drink, in a nutrient-dense 2000-kcalorie eating pattern. The USDA Food Patterns recommendations for sugar represent about 5 to 10 percent of the day's total energy intake. As noted earlier, the World Health Organization agrees that people should restrict their consumption of added sugars to less than 10 percent of total energy and that reducing added sugar intake to less than 5 percent of total energy would have additional health benefits. Box 2-1 provides strategies for reducing the intake of added sugars.

The DRI committee did not set a Tolerable Upper Intake Level for added sugars, but, as mentioned, excessive intakes can interfere with sound nutrition and good health. Few people can eat lots of sugary treats and still meet all of their nutrient needs without exceeding their kcalorie allowance. Instead, the DRI committee suggests that added sugars should account for no more than 25 percent of the day's total energy intake.[22] One out of eight in the U.S. population exceeds this rather high maximum intake.[23] For a person consuming 2000 kcalories a day, 25 percent

How To BOX 2-1 REDUCE INTAKES OF ADDED SUGARS

- Use less table sugar when preparing meals and at the table.
- Use your sugar kcalories to sweeten nutrient-dense foods (such as oatmeal) instead of consuming empty-kcalorie foods and beverages (such as candy and soda).
- Replace empty kcalorie-rich regular sodas, sports drinks, energy drinks, and fruit drinks with water, fat-free milk, 100% fruit juice, or unsweetened tea or coffee.
- Use sweet spices such as cinnamon, nutmeg, allspice, or clove.

- Select fruit for dessert. Eat less cake, cookies, ice cream, other desserts, and candy. If you do eat these foods, have a small portion.
- Warm up sweet foods before serving (heat enhances sweet tastes).
- Read the Nutrition Facts on labels to choose foods with less sugar and less added sugar.

represents 500 kcalories from added sugars—the equivalent of 40 ounces of cola, ½ cup of honey, 125 jelly beans, 23 marshmallows, or 30 teaspoons of sugar. Perhaps an athlete in training whose energy needs are high can afford the added sugars from sports drinks without compromising nutrient intake, but most people would do better following recommendations to limit added sugar consumption to less than 10 percent of the day's total energy intake.

Recognizing Sugars People often fail to recognize sugar in all its forms and so do not realize how much they consume. To help your clients estimate their sugar intakes, tell them to treat all of the following concentrated sweets as equivalent to 1 teaspoon of white sugar (4 grams of carbohydrate):

- 1 teaspoon brown sugar, candy, jam, jelly, any corn sweetener, syrup, honey, molasses, or maple sugar or syrup

- 1 tablespoon ketchup

- 1½ ounces carbonated soft drink

These portions of sugar all provide about the same number of kcalories. Some are closer to 10 kcalories (for example, 14 kcalories for molasses), whereas some are more than 20 kcalories (22 kcalories for honey), so an average figure of 16 kcalories is an acceptable approximation. Box 2-2 presents the multitude of names that denote sugar on food labels.

People often ask: What is the difference between honey and white sugar? Is honey, by virtue of being natural, more nutritious? Honey, like white sugar, contains glucose and fructose. The difference is that, in white sugar, the glucose and fructose are bonded together in pairs, whereas in honey some of them are paired and some are free single sugars. When you eat either white sugar or honey, though, your body breaks all of the sugars apart into single sugars. It ultimately makes no difference, then, whether you eat single sugars linked together, as in white sugar, or the same sugars unlinked, as in honey; they will end up as single sugars in your body.

BOX 2-2 GLOSSARY OF ADDED SUGARS

brown sugar: refined white sugar with molasses added; 95 percent pure sucrose.

concentrated fruit juice sweetener: a concentrated sugar syrup made from dehydrated, deflavored fruit juice, commonly grape juice; used to sweeten products that can then claim to be "all fruit."

confectioner's sugar: finely powdered sucrose; 99.9 percent pure.

corn sweeteners: corn syrup and sugar solutions derived from corn.

corn syrup: a syrup, mostly glucose, partly maltose, produced by the action of enzymes on cornstarch. It may be dried and used as *corn syrup solids.*

dextrose, anhydrous dextrose: forms of glucose.

evaporated cane juice: raw sugar from which impurities have been removed.

granulated sugar: white sugar.

high-fructose corn syrup (HFCS): a widely used commercial kcaloric sweetener made by adding enzymes to cornstarch to convert a portion of its glucose molecules into sweet-tasting fructose.

honey: a concentrated solution primarily composed of glucose and fructose; produced by enzymatic digestion of the sucrose in nectar by bees.

invert sugar: a mixture of glucose and fructose formed by the splitting of sucrose in an industrial process. Sold only in liquid form and sweeter than sucrose, invert sugar forms during certain cooking procedures and works to prevent crystallization of sucrose in soft candies and sweets.

malt syrup: a sweetener made from sprouted barley.

maple syrup: a concentrated solution of sucrose derived from the sap of the sugar maple tree, mostly sucrose. This sugar was once common but is now usually replaced by sucrose and artificial maple flavoring.

molasses: a thick, brown syrup left over from the refining of sucrose from sugarcane. The major nutrient in molasses is iron, a contaminant from the machinery used in processing it.

raw sugar: the first crop of crystals harvested during sugar processing. Raw sugar cannot be sold in the United States because it contains too much filth (dirt, insect fragments, and the like). Sugar sold as "raw sugar" is actually evaporated cane juice.

turbinado (ter-bih-NOD-oh) sugar: raw sugar from which the filth has been washed; legal to sell in the United States.

white sugar: granulated sucrose or "table sugar," produced by dissolving, concentrating, and recrystallizing raw sugar; 99.9 percent pure.

TABLE 2-2 Sample Nutrients in Sugars and Other Foods

The indicated portion of any of these foods provides approximately 100 kcalories. Notice that—for a similar number of kcalories and grams of carbohydrate—milk, legumes, fruits, grains, and vegetables offer more of the other nutrients than do the sugars.

	Size of 100 kCal Portion	Carbohydrate (g)	Protein (g)	Calcium (mg)	Iron (mg)	Vitamin A (µg)	Vitamin C (mg)
Foods							
Milk, 1% low-fat	1 c	12	8	300	0.1	144	2
Kidney beans	½ c	20	7	30	1.6	0	2
Apricots	6	24	2	30	1.1	554	22
Bread, whole wheat	1½ slices	20	4	30	1.9	0	0
Broccoli, cooked	2 c	20	12	188	2.2	696	148
Sugars							
Sugar, white	2 tbs	24	0	trace	trace	0	0
Molasses, blackstrap	2½ tbs	28	0	343	12.6	0	0.1
Cola beverage	1 c	26	0	6	trace	0	0
Honey	1½ tbs	26	trace	2	0.2	0	trace

Honey does contain a few vitamins and minerals, but not many. Honey is denser than crystalline sugar, too, so it provides more energy per spoonful. Table 2-2 shows that honey and white sugar are similar nutritionally—and both fall short of milk, legumes, fruits, grains, and vegetables. Honey may offer some health benefits, however: It seems to relieve nighttime coughing in children and reduce the severity of mouth ulcers in cancer patients undergoing chemotherapy or radiation.

Some sugar sources are more nutritious than others, though. Consider a fruit such as an orange. The orange provides the same sugars and about the same energy as a tablespoon of sugar or honey, but the packaging makes a big difference in nutrient density. The sugars of the orange are diluted in a large volume of fluid that contains valuable vitamins and minerals, and the flesh and skin of the orange are supported by fibers that also offer health benefits. A tablespoon of honey offers no such bonuses. Of course, a cola beverage, containing many teaspoons of sugar, offers no advantages either.

IN SUMMARY

- In moderation, sugars pose no major health threat except for an increased risk of dental caries.

- Excessive sugar intakes may displace needed nutrients and fiber and may contribute to obesity.

- A person deciding to limit daily sugar intake should recognize that it is the added sugars in concentrated sweets, which are high in kcalories and relatively lacking in other nutrients, that should be restricted. Sugars that occur naturally in fruits, vegetables, and milk are acceptable.

You receive about the same amount and kinds of sugars from an orange as from a tablespoon of honey, but the packaging makes a big nutrition difference.

CHAPTER TWO

Alternative Sweeteners: Sugar Alcohols

The **sugar alcohols** are carbohydrates, but they trigger a lower glycemic response and yield slightly less energy (2 to 3 kcalories per gram) than sucrose (4 kcalories per gram) because they are not absorbed completely.[24] The sugar alcohols are sometimes called **nutritive sweeteners** because they do yield some energy. One exception, erythritol, cannot be metabolized by human enzymes and so is kcalorie free.

The sugar alcohols occur naturally in fruits and vegetables; they are also used by manufacturers to provide sweetness and bulk to cookies, sugarless gum, hard candies, and jams and jellies. Unlike sucrose, sugar alcohols are fermented in the large intestine by intestinal bacteria. Consequently, side effects such as gas, abdominal discomfort, and diarrhea make the sugar alcohols less attractive than the nonnutritive sweeteners.

The advantage of using sugar alcohols is that they do not contribute to dental caries. Bacteria in the mouth metabolize sugar alcohols much more slowly than sucrose, thereby inhibiting the production of acids that promote caries formation. They are therefore valuable in chewing gums, breath mints, and other products that people keep in their mouths awhile. The Food and Drug Administration (FDA) allows food labels to carry a health claim (see p. 26 in Chapter 1) about the relationship between sugar alcohols and the nonpromotion of dental caries as long as certain FDA criteria, including those for sugar-free status, are met. Figure 2-4 presents labeling information for products using sugar alternatives.

Alternative Sweeteners: Nonnutritive Sweeteners

The **nonnutritive sweeteners** sweeten with minimal or no carbohydrate or energy. The human taste buds perceive many of them as extremely sweet, so just tiny amounts are

sugar alcohols: sugarlike compounds in the chemical family *alcohol* derived from fruits or manufactured from carbohydrates; sugar alcohols are absorbed more slowly than other sugars, are metabolized differently, and do not elevate the risk of dental caries. Examples are maltitol, mannitol, sorbitol, isomalt, lactitol, and xylitol.

nutritive sweeteners: sweeteners that yield energy, including both the sugars and the sugar alcohols.

nonnutritive sweeteners: synthetic or natural food additives that offer sweet flavor but with negligible or no kcalories per serving; also called *artificial sweeteners, intense sweeteners, noncaloric sweeteners,* and *very-low-calorie sweeteners.*

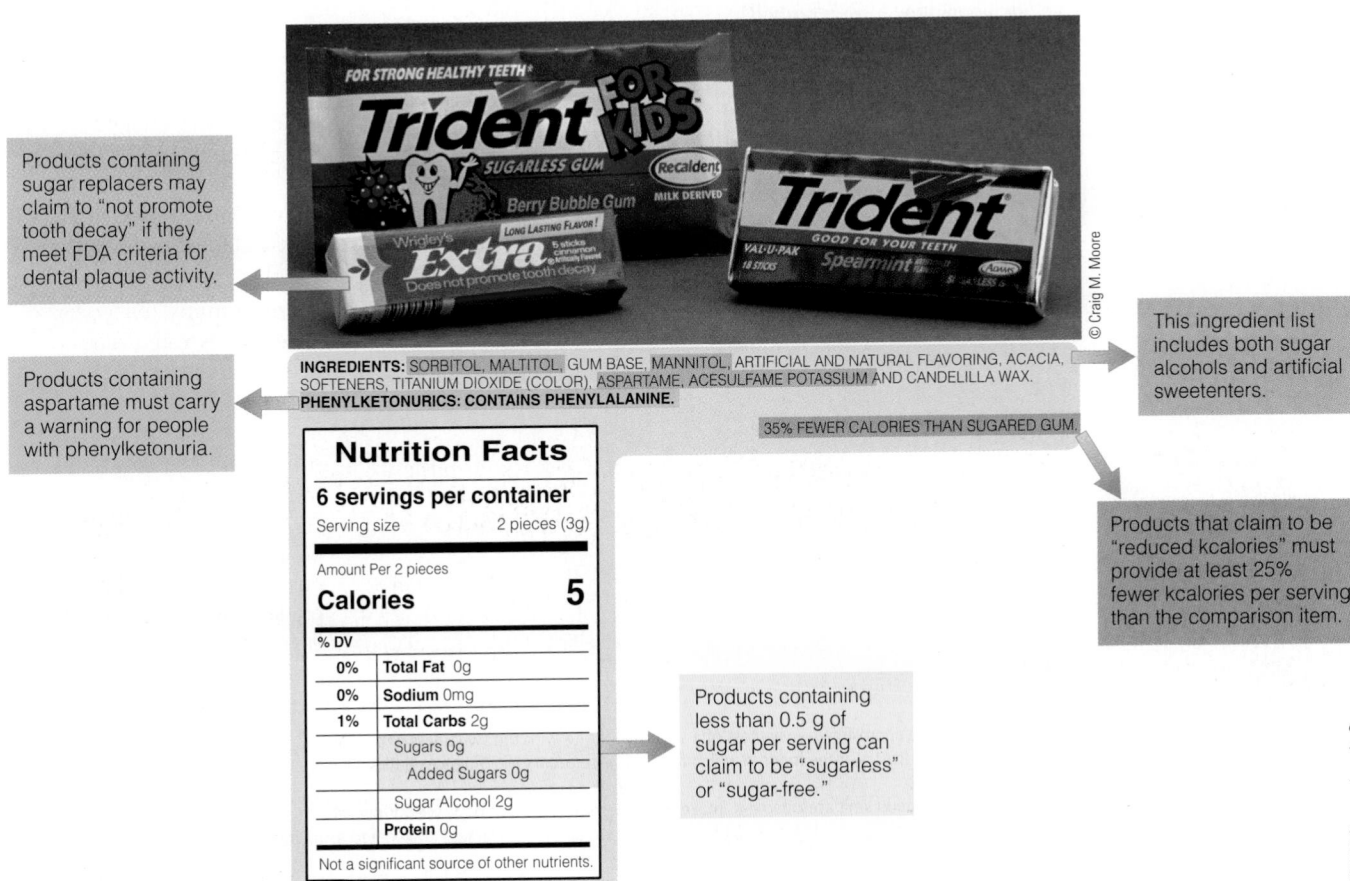

Products containing sugar replacers may claim to "not promote tooth decay" if they meet FDA criteria for dental plaque activity.

Products containing aspartame must carry a warning for people with phenylketonuria.

INGREDIENTS: SORBITOL, MALTITOL, GUM BASE, MANNITOL, ARTIFICIAL AND NATURAL FLAVORING, ACACIA, SOFTENERS, TITANIUM DIOXIDE (COLOR), ASPARTAME, ACESULFAME POTASSIUM AND CANDELILLA WAX.
PHENYLKETONURICS: CONTAINS PHENYLALANINE.

This ingredient list includes both sugar alcohols and artificial sweetenters.

35% FEWER CALORIES THAN SUGARED GUM.

Nutrition Facts

6 servings per container

Serving size	2 pieces (3g)

Amount Per 2 pieces	
Calories	**5**

% DV		
0%	**Total Fat** 0g	
0%	**Sodium** 0mg	
1%	**Total Carbs** 2g	
	Sugars 0g	
	Added Sugars 0g	
	Sugar Alcohol 2g	
	Protein 0g	

Not a significant source of other nutrients.

Products containing less than 0.5 g of sugar per serving can claim to be "sugarless" or "sugar-free."

Products that claim to be "reduced kcalories" must provide at least 25% fewer kcalories per serving than the comparison item.

© Craig M. Moore

© 2016 Cengage Learning®

FIGURE 2-4 Sugar Alternatives on Food Labels

added to foods to achieve the desired sweet taste.[25] The FDA endorses nonnutritive sweeteners as safe for use over a lifetime within **Acceptable Daily Intake (ADI)** levels. Like the sugar alcohols, nonnutritive sweeteners make foods taste sweet without promoting tooth decay. Table 2-3 offers details about nonnutritive sweeteners, including ADI levels.

TABLE 2-3 U.S.-Approved Nonnutritive Sweeteners

Sweetener	Chemical Composition	Digestion/ Absorption	Sweetness Relative to Sucrose[a]	Energy (kcal/g)	Acceptable Daily Intake (ADI) and Estimated Equivalent[b]	Approved Uses
Acesulfame potassium or acesulfame-K (Sunette, Sweet One)	Potassium salt	Not digested or absorbed	200	0	15 mg/kg body weight[c] (30 cans diet soda)	General use, except in meat and poultry. Tabletop sweeteners. Heat stable.
Aspartame (NutraSweet, Equal, others)	Amino acids (phenylalanine and aspartic acid) and a methyl group	Digested and absorbed	180	4[d]	50 mg/kg body weight[e] (18 cans diet soda)	General use in all foods and beverages; warning to population with PKU. Degrades when heated.
Luo han guo	Curcurbine, glycosides from monk fruit extract	Digested and absorbed	150–300	1	No ADI determined	GRAS[f]; general use as a food ingredient and tabletop sweetener.
Neotame	Aspartame with an additional side group attached	Not digested or absorbed	7000	0	18 mg/day	General use, except in meat and poultry.
Saccharin (SugarTwin, Sweet'N Low, others)	Benzoic sulfimide	Rapidly absorbed and excreted	300	0	5 mg/kg body weight (10 packets of sweetener)	Tabletop sweeteners, wide range of foods, beverages, cosmetics, and pharmaceutical products.
Stevia (Sweetleaf, Truvia, PureVia)	Glyosides found in the leaves of the *Stevia rebaudiana* herb	Digested and absorbed	200–300	0	4 mg/kg body weight	GRAS[f]; tabletop sweeteners, a variety of foods and beverages.
Sucralose (Splenda)	Sucrose with Cl atoms instead of OH groups	Not digested or absorbed	600	0	5 mg/kg body weight (6 cans diet soda)	Baked goods, carbonated beverages, chewing gum, coffee and tea, dairy products, frozen desserts, fruit spreads, salad dressing, syrups, tabletop sweeteners.
Tagatose[g] (Nutralose, Nutrilatose, Tagatesse)	Monosaccharide similar in structure to fructose; naturally occurring or derived from lactose	Not well absorbed	0.9	1.5	7.5 g/day	GRAS[f]; bakery products, beverages, cereals, chewing gum, confections, dairy products, dietary supplements, energy bars, tabletop sweeteners.

© Cengage Learning®

[a]Relative sweetness is determined by comparing the approximate sweetness of a sugar substitute with the sweetness of pure sucrose, which has been defined as 1.0. Chemical structure, temperature, acidity, and other flavors of the foods in which the substance occurs all influence relative sweetness.
[b]Based on a person weighing 70 kg (154 lb).
[c]Recommendations from the World Health Organization limit acesulfame-K intake to 9 mg per kilogram of body weight per day.
[d]Aspartame provides 4 kcal/g, as does protein, but because so little is used, its energy contribution is negligible. In powdered form, it is sometimes mixed with lactose, however, so a 1-g packet may provide 4 kcal.
[e]Recommendations from the World Health Organization and in Europe and Canada limit aspartame intake to 40 mg per kilogram of body weight per day.
[f]Generally recognized as safe.
[g]Tagatose is a poorly digested sugar, and technically not a nonnutritive sweetener.

Nonnutritive Sweeteners and Weight Management Whether the use of nonnutritive sweeteners promotes weight loss or improves health by reducing total kcalorie intakes is not known with certainty.[26] Some research even suggests that their use may *promote* weight gain through unknown mechanisms; these are topics of current research.

When people reduce their energy intakes by replacing sugar in their diets with nonnutritive sweeteners and then compensate for the reduced energy at later meals, energy intake may stay the same or increase. Using nonnutritive sweeteners will not automatically lower energy intake; to successfully control energy intake, a person needs to make informed diet and activity decisions throughout the day.

Safety of Nonnutritive Sweeteners Through the years, questions have emerged about the safety of nonnutritive sweeteners, but these issues have since been resolved. For example, early research indicating that large quantities of saccharin caused bladder tumors in laboratory animals was later shown to be inapplicable to humans. Common sense dictates that consuming large amounts of saccharin is probably not safe, but consuming moderate amounts poses no known hazard.

Aspartame, a sweetener made from two amino acids (phenylalanine and aspartic acid) is one of the most thoroughly studied food additives ever approved, and no scientific evidence supports the Internet stories that accuse it of causing disease.[27] However, aspartame's phenylalanine base poses a threat to those with the inherited disease phenylketonuria (PKU). People with PKU cannot dispose of phenylalanine efficiently (see Nutrition in Practice 16). Food labels warn people with PKU of the presence of phenylalanine in aspartame-sweetened foods (see Figure 2-4). In addition, foods and drinks containing nonnutritive sweeteners have no place in the diets of even healthy infants or toddlers.

IN SUMMARY

▌ Two types of alternative sweeteners are sugar alcohols and nonnutritive sweeteners.

▌ Sugar alcohols are carbohydrates, but they yield slightly less energy than sucrose.

▌ Sugar alcohols do not contribute to dental caries.

▌ The FDA endorses the use of nonnutritive sweeteners within ADI levels as safe over a lifetime.

▌ The nonnutritive sweeteners sweeten with minimal or no carbohydrate and energy.

▌ Like the sugar alcohols, nonnutritive sweeteners do not promote tooth decay.

2.4 Health Effects of Starch and Dietary Fibers

LO 2.4 Identify the health benefits of, and recommendations for, starches and fibers.

Despite dietary recommendations that people should eat generous servings of starch- and fiber-rich carbohydrate foods for their health, many people still believe that carbohydrate is the "fattening" component of foods. Gram for gram, carbohydrates contribute fewer kcalories to the body than do dietary fats, so a moderate diet based on starch- and fiber-rich carbohydrate foods is likely to be lower in kcalories than a diet based on high-fat foods.

For health's sake, most people should increase their intakes of carbohydrate-rich foods such as whole grains, vegetables, legumes, and fruits—foods noted for their starch, fiber, and naturally occurring sugars.[28] In addition, most people should also limit their intakes of foods high in added sugars and the types of fats associated with heart disease (see Chapter 3). A diet that emphasizes whole grains, vegetables, legumes, and fruits is almost invariably moderate in food energy, low in fats that can harm health, and high in dietary fiber, vitamins, and minerals. All these factors working together can help reduce the risks of obesity, cancer, cardiovascular disease, diabetes, dental caries, gastrointestinal disorders, and malnutrition.

Carbohydrates: Disease Prevention and Recommendations

Fiber-rich carbohydrate foods benefit health in many ways. Foods such as whole grains, legumes, vegetables, and fruits supply valuable vitamins, minerals, and phytochemicals, along with abundant dietary fiber and little or no fat. The following paragraphs describe some of the health benefits of diets that emphasize a variety of these foods each day.

Heart Disease Diets rich in whole grains, legumes, and vegetables, especially those rich in whole grains, may protect against heart disease and stroke by lowering blood pressure, improving blood lipids, and reducing inflammation.[29] Such diets are generally low in saturated fat, *trans* fat, and cholesterol and high in dietary fibers, vegetable proteins, and phytochemicals—all factors associated with a lower risk of heart disease. (The role of saturated fat, *trans* fat, and cholesterol in heart disease is discussed in Chapter 3. The benefits of phytochemicals in disease prevention are presented in Nutrition in Practice 8). Foods rich in soluble fibers (such as oat bran, barley, and legumes) lower blood cholesterol by binding cholesterol compounds and carrying them out of the body with the feces.[30] High-fiber foods may also lower blood cholesterol indirectly by displacing fatty, cholesterol-raising foods from the diet. Even when dietary fat intake is low, research shows that high intakes of soluble fiber exert separate and significant blood cholesterol–lowering effects.

Diabetes High-fiber foods—and especially whole grains—play a key role in reducing the risk of **type 2 diabetes** (see Chapter 21).[31] The soluble fibers of foods such as oats and legumes can help regulate blood glucose following a carbohydrate-rich meal. Soluble fibers trap nutrients and delay their transit through the digestive tract, slowing glucose absorption and preventing the glucose surge and rebound often associated with diabetes onset.

The term **glycemic response** refers to how quickly glucose is absorbed after a person eats, how high blood glucose rises, and how quickly it returns to normal. Slow absorption, a modest rise in blood glucose, and a smooth return to normal are desirable (a low glycemic response). Fast absorption, a surge in blood glucose, and an overreaction that plunges glucose below normal are less desirable (a high glycemic response). Different foods have different effects on blood glucose. The **glycemic index**, a method of classifying foods according to their potential to raise blood glucose, is the topic of Nutrition in Practice 2.

GI Health Soluble and insoluble fibers, along with ample fluid intake, may enhance the health of the large intestine. The healthier the intestinal walls, the better they can block absorption of unwanted constituents. Soluble fibers help to maintain normal colonic bacteria necessary for intestinal health.[32] Insoluble fibers that both enlarge and soften stools such as cellulose (in cereal brans, fruits, and vegetables) ease elimination for the rectal muscles and thereby alleviate or prevent constipation and hemorrhoids.

Some fibers (again, such as cereal bran) help keep the contents of the intestinal tract moving easily. This action helps prevent compaction of the intestinal contents, which could obstruct the appendix and permit bacteria to invade and infect it. In addition, fibers stimulate the muscles of the gastrointestinal (GI) tract so that they retain their strength and resist bulging out in places, as occurs in diverticulosis.[33] Recommendations typically suggest increasing fiber to protect against diverticular disease, although research findings are inconsistent.[34]

type 2 diabetes: the type of diabetes that accounts for 90 to 95 percent of diabetes cases and usually results from insulin resistance coupled with insufficient insulin secretion.

glycemic response: the extent to which a food raises the blood glucose concentration and elicits an insulin response.

glycemic index: a method of classifying foods according to their potential for raising blood glucose.

Cancer Many studies show that, as people increase their dietary fiber intakes, their risk for colon cancer declines.[35] A recent meta-analysis using data from several studies exposed a strong, linear inverse association between dietary fiber and colon cancer.[36] People who ate the most fiber (24 grams per day) reduced their risk of colon and rectal cancer by almost 30 percent compared with those who ate the least (10 grams per day). Mid-range intakes (18 grams per day) reduced the risk by 20 percent. It is important to note that fiber from food but not from supplements demonstrates this association, possibly because fiber supplements lack the nutrients and phytochemicals of whole foods that may also help to protect against cancers.

All plant foods—vegetables, fruits, and whole-grain products—have attributes that may reduce the risks of colon and rectal cancers. Their fiber dilutes, binds, and rapidly removes potential cancer-causing agents from the colon. In addition, the colon's bacteria ferment soluble fibers, forming small fatlike molecules that lower the **pH**. These small fatlike molecules activate cancer-killing enzymes and inhibit inflammation in the colon.[37]

Other processes may also be at work. As research progresses, cancer experts recommend that fiber in the diet come from 2½ to 4½ cups of vegetables and fruit daily, along with generous portions of whole grains and legumes.

Weight Management Fiber-rich foods tend to be low in fat and added sugars and therefore prevent weight gain and promote weight loss by delivering less energy per bite.[38] In addition, fibers absorb water from the digestive juices; as they swell, they create feelings of fullness, delay hunger, and reduce food intake. Soluble fibers may be especially useful for appetite control. By whatever mechanism, as populations eat more refined low-fiber foods and concentrated sweets, body fat stores creep up.[39] In contrast, people who eat three or more ounces of whole grain foods each day tend to have lower body and abdominal fatness over time.[40]

Commercial weight-loss products often contain bulk-inducing fibers such as methylcellulose, but pure fiber compounds are not advised. High-fiber foods not only add bulk to the diet but are economical, are nutritious, and supply health-promoting phytochemicals—benefits that no purified fiber preparation can match. Figure 2-5 (p. 50) summarizes fibers and their health benefits.

Harmful Effects of Excessive Fiber Intake Despite fiber's benefits to health, when too much fiber is consumed, some minerals may bind to it and be excreted with it, without becoming available for the body to use. When mineral intake is adequate, however, a reasonable intake of high-fiber foods does not seem to compromise mineral balance.

People with marginal intakes who eat mostly high-fiber foods may not be able to take in enough food to meet energy or nutrient needs. The malnourished, the elderly, and young children adhering to all-plant (vegan) diets are especially vulnerable to this problem. Fibers also carry water out of the body and can cause dehydration. Advise clients to add an extra glass or two of water to go along with the fiber added to their diets. Athletes may want to avoid bulky, fiber-rich foods just prior to competition.

Recommended Intakes of Starches and Fibers The DRI committee advises that carbohydrates should contribute about half (45 to 65 percent) of the energy requirement. A person consuming 2000 kcalories a day should therefore obtain 900 to 1300 kcalories' worth of carbohydrate, or between 225 and 325 grams. This amount is more than adequate to meet the RDA for carbohydrate, which is set at 130 grams per day based on the average minimum amount of glucose used by the brain.[41]

When it established the Daily Values that appear on food labels, the FDA used a guideline of 60 percent of kcalories in setting the Daily Value for carbohydrate at 300 grams per day. For most people, this means increasing total carbohydrate intake. To this end, the *Dietary Guidelines for Americans* encourage people to choose fiber-rich whole grains, vegetables, fruits, and legumes daily.

Recommendations for fiber encourage the same foods just mentioned: whole grains, vegetables, fruits, and legumes, which also provide vitamins, minerals, and

pH : the concentration of hydrogen ions. The lower the pH, the stronger the acid. Thus, pH 2 is a strong acid; pH 6 is a weak acid; pH 7 is neutral; and a pH above 7 is alkaline.

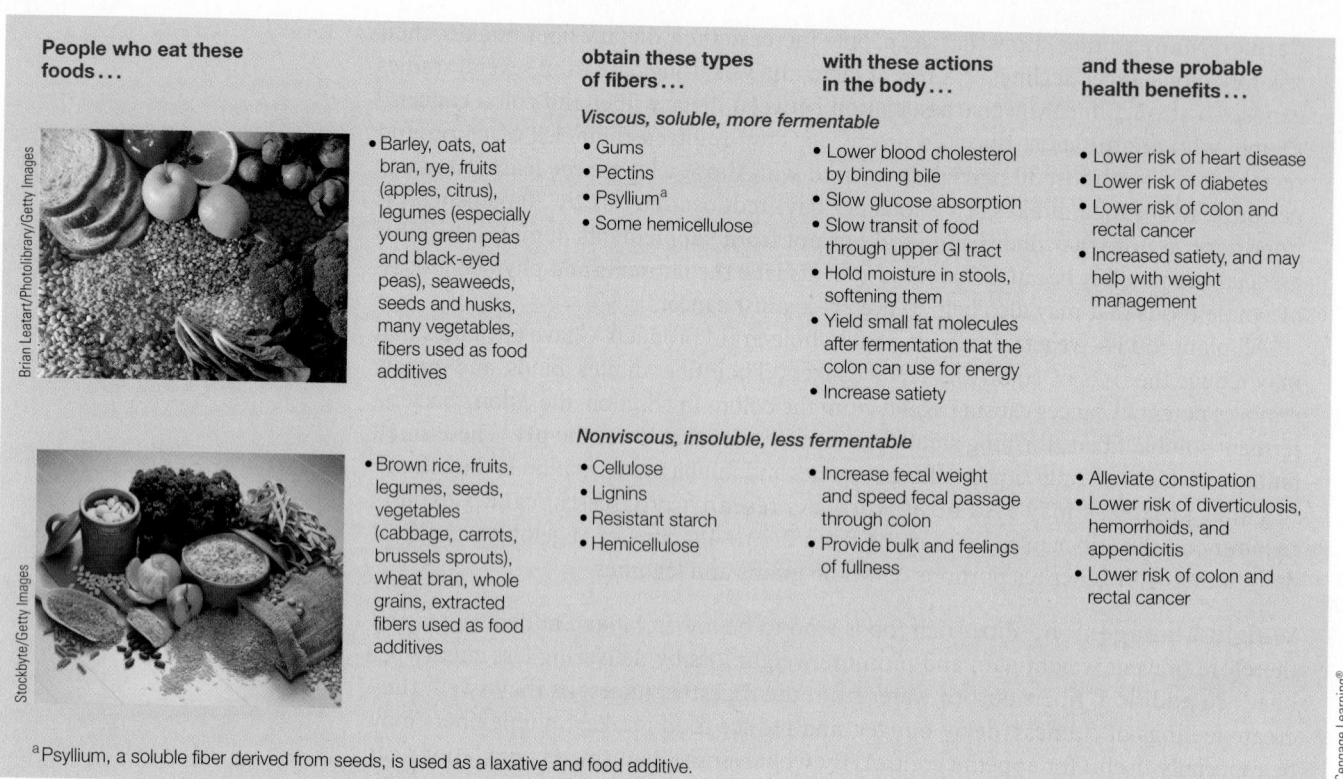

People who eat these foods...	obtain these types of fibers...	with these actions in the body...	and these probable health benefits...
• Barley, oats, oat bran, rye, fruits (apples, citrus), legumes (especially young green peas and black-eyed peas), seaweeds, seeds and husks, many vegetables, fibers used as food additives	**Viscous, soluble, more fermentable** • Gums • Pectins • Psyllium[a] • Some hemicellulose	• Lower blood cholesterol by binding bile • Slow glucose absorption • Slow transit of food through upper GI tract • Hold moisture in stools, softening them • Yield small fat molecules after fermentation that the colon can use for energy • Increase satiety	• Lower risk of heart disease • Lower risk of diabetes • Lower risk of colon and rectal cancer • Increased satiety, and may help with weight management
• Brown rice, fruits, legumes, seeds, vegetables (cabbage, carrots, brussels sprouts), wheat bran, whole grains, extracted fibers used as food additives	**Nonviscous, insoluble, less fermentable** • Cellulose • Lignins • Resistant starch • Hemicellulose	• Increase fecal weight and speed fecal passage through colon • Provide bulk and feelings of fullness	• Alleviate constipation • Lower risk of diverticulosis, hemorrhoids, and appendicitis • Lower risk of colon and rectal cancer

[a] Psyllium, a soluble fiber derived from seeds, is used as a laxative and food additive.

FIGURE 2-5 Characteristics, Sources, and Health Effects of Fibers

phytochemicals. The FDA set the Daily Value for fiber at 28 grams for a 2000-kcalorie intake. This is based on the DRI recommendation of 14 grams per 1000-kcalorie intake—roughly 25 to 35 grams of dietary fiber daily. These recommendations are almost two times higher than the usual intake in the United States.[42]

As health care professionals, you can advise your clients that an effective way to add dietary fiber while lowering fat is to substitute plant sources of proteins (legumes) for some of the animal sources of protein (meats and cheeses) in the diet. Another way to add fiber is to encourage clients to consume the recommended amounts of fruits and vegetables each day. People choosing high-fiber foods are wise to seek out a variety of fiber sources and to drink extra fluids to help the fiber do its job. Many foods provide fiber in varying amounts, as Figure 2-6 shows.

As mentioned earlier, too much fiber is no better than too little. The World Health Organization recommends an upper limit of 40 grams of dietary fiber a day.

IN SUMMARY

▌ A diet rich in starches and dietary fibers helps prevent heart disease, diabetes, GI disorders, and possibly some types of cancer. It also supports efforts to manage body weight.

▌ For these reasons, recommendations urge people to eat plenty of whole grains, vegetables, legumes, and fruits—enough to provide 45 to 65 percent of the daily energy from carbohydrate and 14 grams of fiber per 1000 kcalories.

Carbohydrates: Food Sources

A day's meals based on the USDA Food Patterns not only meet carbohydrate recommendations but also provide abundant fiber, too. Grains, vegetables, fruits, and legumes deliver dietary fiber and are noted for their valuable energy-yielding starches and dilute sugars.

50

Grains

Whole-grain products provide 1 to 2 g of fiber or more per serving:

- 1 slice whole wheat or rye bread (1 g)
- 1 slice pumpernickel bread (2 g)
- ½ c ready-to-eat 100% bran cereal (10 g)
- ½ c cooked barley, bulgur, grits, oatmeal (2 to 3 g)

Vegetables

Most vegetables contain 2 to 3 g of fiber per serving:

- 1 c raw bean sprouts
- ½ c cooked broccoli, brussels sprouts, cabbage, carrots, cauliflower, collards, corn, eggplant, green beans, green peas, kale, mushrooms, okra, parsnips, potatoes, pumpkin, spinach, sweet potatoes, swiss chard, winter squash
- ½ c chopped raw carrots, peppers

Fruits

Fresh, frozen, and dried fruits have about 2 g of fiber per serving:

- 1 medium apple, banana, kiwi, nectarine, orange, pear
- ½ c applesauce, blackberries, blueberries, raspberries, strawberries
- Fruit juices contain very little fiber

Legumes and Nuts

Many legumes provide about 8 g of fiber per serving:

- ½ c cooked baked beans, black beans, black-eyed peas, kidney beans, navy beans, pinto beans

Some legumes provide about 5 g of fiber per serving:

- ½ c cooked garbanzo beans, great northern beans, lentils, lima beans, split peas

Most nuts and seeds provide 1 to 3 g of fiber per serving:

- 1 oz almonds, cashews, hazelnuts, peanuts, pecans, pumpkin seeds, sunflower seeds

FIGURE 2-6 **Fiber in Selected Foods**

Each class of foods makes its own typical carbohydrate contribution. The USDA Food Patterns in Chapter 1 can help you and your clients choose carbohydrate-rich foods.

Grains Most foods in this group—a slice of whole-wheat bread, half an English muffin or bagel, a 6-inch tortilla, or ½ cup of rice, pasta, or cooked cereal—provide about 15 grams of carbohydrate per ounce equivalent, mostly as starch.* Be aware that some foods in this group, especially snack crackers and baked goods such as biscuits, croissants, and muffins, contain added sugars, solid fats, and sodium. When selecting from the grain group, limit refined grains and be sure at least half of the foods chosen are whole-grain products. People who eat more whole grains tend to have healthier diets.[43]

Vegetables Some vegetables are major contributors of starch in the diet. Just a small white or sweet potato or ½ cup of cooked dry beans, corn, peas, plantain, or winter squash provides 15 grams of carbohydrate, as much as in a slice of bread, though as a mixture of sugars and starch. One-half cup of carrots, okra, onions, tomatoes, cooked greens, or most other nonstarchy vegetables or a cup of salad greens provides about 5 grams as a mixture of starch and sugars. Each of these foods also contributes a little protein, some fiber, and no fat.

Fruits A half-cup equivalent of fruit contains an average of about 15 grams of carbohydrate, mostly as sugars, including the fruit sugar fructose. The amount of fruit equivalent to a half-cup varies depending on the form of the fruit: ½ cup of juice; a small banana, apple, or orange; ½ cup of most canned or fresh fruit; or ¼ cup of dried fruit. Fruits vary greatly in their water and fiber contents; therefore, their sugar concentrations vary also. No more than one-half of the day's fruit should come from juice. With the exception of avocado, which is high in fat, the fruits contain insignificant amounts of fat and protein.

Milk and Milk Products One cup of milk or yogurt or the equivalent (1 cup of buttermilk, ⅓ cup of dry milk powder, or ½ cup of evaporated milk) provides a generous 12 grams of carbohydrate. Among cheeses, cottage cheese provides about 6 grams of carbohydrate per cup, whereas most other types contain little, if any, carbohydrate. These foods also contribute high-quality protein as well as several important vitamins and minerals. Calcium-fortified soy beverages are options for providing calcium and about the same amount of carbohydrate as milk. All milk products vary in fat content, an important consideration in choosing among them; Chapter 3 provides the details.

Cream and butter, although dairy products, are not equivalent to milk because they contain little or no carbohydrate and insignificant amounts of the other nutrients important in milk. They are appropriately classified as solid fats.

Protein Foods With two exceptions, foods of this group provide almost no carbohydrate to the diet. The exceptions are nuts, which provide a little starch and fiber along with their abundant fat, and dry beans, which are excellent sources of both starch and fiber. Just ½ cup of beans provides 15 grams of carbohydrate, an amount equal to the richest carbohydrate sources. Among sources of fiber, beans and other legumes are outstanding, providing as much as 8 grams in ½ cup. The carbohydrate content of a diet can be determined by using a nutrient composition table such as that found in Appendix A, the food list system described in Chapter 21, or a computer diet analysis program.

Carbohydrates: Food Labels and Health Claims

Food labels list the amount, in grams, of total carbohydrate—including starch, fibers, and sugars—per serving. Grams of fiber and total sugars are listed separately. (With this information, consumers can calculate starch grams by subtracting the grams of fibers and sugars from the total carbohydrate.) As Chapter 1 described, once the updated Nutrition Facts panel is displayed on labels, added sugars will also be listed

*Gram values in this section are adapted from *Choose Your Foods: Food Lists for Diabetes*.

separately. Total carbohydrate and dietary fiber are also expressed as "% Daily Values" for a person consuming 2000 kcalories; there is no Daily Value for sugars.

The FDA authorizes four health claims on food labels concerning fiber-rich carbohydrate foods. One is for "fiber-containing grain products, fruits, and vegetables and reduced risk of cancer." Another is for "fruits, vegetables, and grain products that contain fiber, and reduced risk of coronary heart disease." A third is for "soluble fiber from whole oats and from psyllium seed husk and reduced risk of coronary heart disease," and a fourth is for "whole grains and reduced risk of heart disease and certain cancers." Chapter 1 describes the criteria foods must meet to bear these health claims.

IN SUMMARY

▌ Grains, vegetables, fruits, and legumes contribute dietary fiber and energy-yielding starches and dilute sugars to people's diets. One cup of milk or yogurt or the equivalent contributes a generous 12 grams of carbohydrate as well as protein and other important nutrients.

▌ Food labels list grams of total carbohydrate and also provide separate listings of grams of fiber and sugar.

Your Diet

Carbohydrates

Most of the energy people receive from foods comes from carbohydrates. Healthy choices provide carbohydrates rich in fiber, starches, vitamins, minerals, and naturally occurring sugars. A diet that is consistently low in dietary fiber and high in added sugar can lead to health problems. The table below displays related foods in categories that roughly indicate their fiber and sugar contents. Look back to the food record you completed for the Your Diet activity at the end of Chapter 1. Draw a table like the one below, listing

five of your carbohydrate choices in the appropriate column(s). If your food is not listed in the first column (High in Fiber/Low in Added Sugar), suggest an alternative selection to place in this column. As an example, if you consumed a Rice Krispies Treat® (low in fiber, high in added sugar), you could list the food in the third column and write "brown rice" in the first column. For any food with no obvious alternatives, such as candy or sweetened soda, circle the food and list an alternative choice below the table (for example, you can replace regular soda with diet soda or low-fat milk).

High in Fiber/Low in Added Sugar	Intermediate Fiber and/or Sugar	Low in Fiber/High in Added Sugar
Apple with peel	Applesauce, sweetened	Fruit drink, 10% apple juice
Oatmeal	Granola	Granola breakfast bar
Whole-wheat bread	Bagel, plain	Danish pastry
Corn on the cob	Creamed corn	Corn flakes, added sugar
Baked sweet potato	Candied sweet potato casserole	Sweet potato pie

Clinical Applications

1. Considering the health benefits of carbohydrate-rich foods, especially those that provide starch and fiber, what suggestions would you offer to a client who reports the following:

   ▌ Eats only three ounces of refined, sugary breads or cereals each day.

   ▌ Eats one cup of vegetables (usually french fries) each day.

   ▌ Drinks fruit juice once a day but never eats fruit.

   ▌ Eats cheese at least twice a day but does not drink milk.

   ▌ Eats large portions of meat at least twice a day.

   ▌ Eats hard candy two or three times a day.

Self Check

1. Which of the following foods is *not* a good source of carbohydrates?
   a. Plain yogurt
   b. Steak
   c. Brown rice
   d. Green peas

2. Polysaccharides include:
   a. galactose, starch, and glycogen.
   b. starch, glycogen, and fiber.
   c. lactose, maltose, and glycogen.
   d. sucrose, fructose, and glucose.

3. The chief energy source of the body is:
   a. sucrose.
   b. starch.
   c. glucose.
   d. fructose.

4. The primary form of stored glucose in animals is:
   a. glycogen.
   b. cellulose.
   c. starch.
   d. lactose.

5. The polysaccharide that helps form the cell walls of plants is:
   a. cellulose.
   b. starch.
   c. glycogen.
   d. lactose.

6. Which of the following terms on a food label may denote sugar?
   a. Corn syrup
   b. Aspartame
   c. Xylitol
   d. Cellulose

7. The two types of alternative sweeteners are:
   a. saccharin and cyclamate.
   b. sugar alcohols and nonnutritive sweeteners.
   c. sorbitol and xylitol.
   d. sucrose and fructose.

8. A diet high in carbohydrate-rich foods such as whole grains, vegetables, fruits, and legumes is:
   a. most likely low in fat.
   b. most likely low in fiber.
   c. most likely poor in vitamins and minerals.
   d. most likely disease promoting.

9. A fiber-rich diet may help to prevent or control:
   a. diabetes.
   b. heart disease.
   c. constipation.
   d. all of the above.

10. The DRI fiber recommendation is:
    a. 10 grams per 1000 kcalories.
    b. 15 to 25 grams per day.
    c. 14 grams per 1000 kcalories.
    d. 40 to 55 grams per day.

Answers to these questions can be found in Appendix H.

Notes

1. U.S. Department of Agriculture and U.S. Department of Health and Human Services, *Dietary Guidelines for Americans 2010*, www.dietaryguidelines.gov.

2. D. F. Birt and coauthors, Resistant starch: Promise for improving human health, *Advances in Nutrition* 4 (2013): 587–601.

3. A. Dilzer, J. M. Jones, and M. E. Latulippe, The family of dietary fibers: Dietary variety for maximum health benefit, *Nutrition Today* 48 (2013): 108–118; K. Raninen and coauthors, Dietary fiber type reflects physiological functionality: Comparison of grain fiber, insulin, and polydextrose, *Nutrition Reviews* 69 (2011): 9–21; Position of the American Dietetic Association: Health implications of dietary fiber, *Journal of the American Dietetic Association* 108 (2008): 1716–1731.

4. F. Magkos, S. Wang, and B. Mittendorfer, Metabolic actions of insulin in men and women, *Nutrition* 28 (2010): 686–691.

5. U.S. Department of Agriculture and U.S. Department of Health and Human Services, *Dietary Guidelines for Americans 2010*, www.dietaryguidelines.gov.

6. American Heart Association, Sugar 101, www.aha.org/HEARTORG/GettingHealthy/NutritionCenter/HealthyEating/Sugar-101_ucm_30624.Article.jsp, updated February 24, 2014.

7. S. W. Ng, N. M. Slining, and B. M. Popkin, Use of caloric and noncaloric sweeteners in US consumer packaged foods, 2005–2009, *Journal of the Academy of Nutrition and Dietetics* 112 (2012): 1828–1834.

8. Position of the Academy of Nutrition and Dietetics: Use of nutritive and nonnutritive sweeteners, *Journal of the Academy of Nutrition and Dietetics* 112 (2012): 739–758.

9. S. W. Rizkalla, Health implications of fructose consumption: A review of recent data, *Nutrition and Metabolism* 7 (2010): 82–98.

10. G. L. Ambrosini and coauthors, Prospective associations between sugar-sweetened beverage intakes and cardiometabolic risk factors in adolescents, *American Journal of Clinical Nutrition* 98 (2013): 327–334; V. S. Malik and coauthors, Sugar-sweetened beverages and weight gain in children and adults: A systematic review and meta-analysis, *American Journal of Clinical Nutrition* 98 (2013): 1084–1102; K. L. Stanhope, Role of fructose-containing sugars in the epidemics of obesity and metabolic syndrome, *Annual Review of Medicine* 63 (2012): 19.1–19.15; J. L. Sievenpiper and coauthors, Effect of fructose on body weight in controlled feeding trials: A systematic review and meta-analysis, *Annals of Internal Medicine* 156 (2012): 291–304; L. de Koning and coauthors, sugar-sweetened and artificially sweetened beverage consumption and risk of type 2 diabetes in men, *American Journal of Clinical Nutrition* 93 (2011): 1321–1327; R. D. Mattes and coauthors, Nutritively sweetened beverage consumption and body weight: A systematic review and meta-analysis of randomized experiments, *Obesity Reviews* 12 (2011): 346–365; K. J. Duffey and coauthors, Drinking caloric beverages increases the risk of adverse cardiometabolic outcomes in the Coronary Artery Risk Development in Young Adults (CARDIA) Study, *American Journal of Clinical Nutrition* 92 (2010): 954–959; V. S. Malik and coauthors, Sugar-sweetened beverages and risk of metabolic syndrome and type 2 diabetes; A meta-analysis, *Diabetes Care* 33 (2010): 2477–2483; F. B. Hu and V. S. Malik, Sugar-sweetened beverages and risk of obesity and

type 2 diabetes: Epidemiologic evidence, *Physiology and Behavior* 100 (2010): 47–54.

11. O. I. Bermudez and X. Gao, Greater consumption of sweetened beverages and added sugars is associated with obesity among US young adults, *Annals of Nutrition and Metabolism* 57 (2010): 211–218.

12. Malik and coauthors, 2013; K. L. Stanhope, 2012; Sievenpiper and coauthors, 2012; Mattes and coauthors, 2011.

13. Bermudez and Gao, 2010; Hu and Malik, 2010; V. S. Malik and coauthors, Sugar-sweetened beverages, obesity, type 2 diabetes mellitus, and cardiovascular disease risk, *Circulation* 121 (2010): 1356–1364.

14. L. Trappy and coauthors, Fructose and metabolic diseases: New findings, new questions, *Nutrition* 26 (2010): 1044–1049.

15. D. F. Tate and coauthors, Replacing caloric beverages with water or diet beverages for weight loss in adults: Main results of the Choose Healthy Options Consciously Everyday (CHOICE) randomized clinical trial, *American Journal of Clinical Nutrition* 95 (2012); 555–563.

16. M. Maersk and coauthors, Sucrose-sweetened beverages increase fat storage in the liver, muscle, and visceral fat depot: A 6-mo randomized interventions study, *American Journal of Clinical Nutrition* 95 (2012): 283–289; K. Sevastianova and coauthors, Effect of short-term carbohydrate overfeeding and long-term weight loss on liver fat in overweight humans, *American Journal of Clinical Nutrition* 96 (2012): 727–734; L. de Koning and coauthors, Sweetened beverages consumption, incident coronary heart disease and biomarkers of risk in men, *Circulation* 125 (2012): 1735–1741.

17. Stanhope, 2012; M. J. Dekker and coauthors, Fructose: A highly lipogenic nutrient implicated in insulin resistance, hepatic steatosis, and the metabolic syndrome, *American Journal of Physiology, Endocrinology and Metabolism* 299 (2010): E685–E694.

18. J. A. Welsh and coauthors, Caloric sweetener consumption and dyslipidemia among US adults, *Journal of the American Medical Association* 303 (2010): 1490–1497.

19. K. J. Duffy and coauthors, 2010.

20. I. Aeberli and coauthors, Low to moderate sugar-sweetened beverage consumption impairs glucose and lipid metabolism and promotes inflammation in healthy young men: a randomized controlled trial, *American Journal of Clinical Nutrition* 94 (2011): 479–485; K. L. Stanhope, Consumption of fructose and high fructose corn syrup increase postprandial triglycerides, LDL-cholesterol, and apolipoprotein-B in young men and women, *Journal of Clinical Endocrinology and Metabolism* 96 (2011): E1596–E1605.

21. Position of the Academy of Nutrition and Dietetics: Oral health and nutrition, *Journal of the Academy of Nutrition and Dietetics* 113 (2013): 693–701.

22. Standing Committee on the Scientific Evaluation of Dietary Reference Intakes, Food and Nutrition Board, Institute of Medicine, *Dietary Reference Intakes for Energy, Carbohydrate, Fiber, Fat, Fatty Acids, Cholesterol, Protein, and Amino Acids* (Washington D.C.: National Academies Press, 2005), p. 770.

23. B. P. Marriott and coauthors, Intake of added sugars and selected nutrients in the United States, National Health and Nutrition Examination Survey (NHANES) 2003–2006, *Critical Reviews in Food Science and Nutrition* 50 (2010): 228–258.

24. Position of the Academy of Nutrition and Dietetics: Use of nutritive and nonnutritive sweeteners, *Journal of the Academy of Nutrition and Dietetics* 112 (2012): 739–758.

25. Position of the Academy of Nutrition and Dietetics: Use of nutritive and nonnutritive sweeteners, 2012.

26. C. Gardner and coauthors, Nonnutritive sweeteners: Current use and health perspectives, *Diabetes Care* 35 (2012): 1798–1808.

27. Position of the Academy of Nutrition and Dietetics: Use of nutritive and nonnutritive sweeteners, 2012.

28. S. Chuang and coauthors, Fiber intake and total and cause-specific mortality in the European Prospective Investigation into Cancer and Nutrition cohort, *American Journal of Clinical Nutrition* 96 (2012): 164–174.

29. R. H. Eckel and coauthors, 2013 AHA/ACC guidelines on lifestyle management to reduce cardiovascular risk: A report of the American College of Cardiology/American Heart Association Task Force on Practice Guidelines, *Circulation*, http://circ.ahajournals.org/content/early/2013/11/11/01.cir.0000437740.48606.dl.citation; R. J. J. van de Laar and coauthors, Lower lifetime dietary fiber intake is associated with carotid artery stiffness: The Amsterdam Growth and Health Longitudinal Study, *American Journal of Clinical Nutrition* 96 (2012): 14–23; K. Raninen and coauthors, 2011; A. Fardet, New hypotheses for the health-protective mechanisms of whole-grain cereals: What is beyond fibre? *Nutrition Research Reviews* 23 (2010): 65–134; T. M. S. Wolever and coauthors, Physicochemical properties of oat ß glucan influence its ability to reduce serum LDL cholesterol in humans: A randomized clinical trial, *American Journal of Clinical Nutrition* 92 (2010): 723–732.

30. V. Kumar and coauthors, Dietary roles of non-starch polysaccharides in human nutrition: A review, *Critical Reviews in Food Science and Nutrition* 52 (2012): 899–935; R. A. Othman, M. H. Moghadasian, and P. J. Jones, Cholesterol-lowering effects of oat ß-glucan, *Nutrition Reviews* 69 (2011): 299–309; Raninen and coauthors, 2011.

31. T. Wirström and coauthors, Consumption of whole grain reduces risk of deteriorating glucose tolerance, including progression to prediabetes, *American Journal of Clinical Nutrition* 97 (2013): 179–187; Raninen and coauthors, 2011; J. A. Nettleton and coauthors, Interactions of dietary whole-grain intake with fasting glucose- and insulin-related genetic loci in individuals of European descent: A Meta-analysis of 14 cohort studies, *Diabetes Care* 33 (2010): 2684–2691.

32. A. M. Brownawell and coauthors, Prebiotics and the health benefits of fiber: Current regulatory status, future research, and goals, *Journal of Nutrition* 142 (2012): 962–974; J. E. Ravikoff and J. R. Korzenik, The role of fiber in diverticular disease, *Journal of Clinical Gastroenterology* 45 (2011): S7–S11.

33. S. Tarleton and J. K. Dibaise, Low-residue diet in diverticular disease: Putting an end to a myth, *Nutrition in Clinical Practice* 26 (2011): 137–142.

34. A. F. Peery and coauthors, Constipation and a low-fiber diet are not associated with diverticulosis, *Clinical Gastroenterology and Hepatology* 11 (2013): 1622–1627; C. Ünlü and coauthors, A systematic review of high-fibre dietary therapy in diverticular disease, *International Journal of Colorectal Disease* 27 (2012): 419–427; L. L. Strate, Lifestyle factors and the course of diverticular disease, *Digestive Diseases* 30 (2012): 35–45; A. F. Peery and coauthors, A high-fiber diet does not protect against asymptomatic diverticulosis, *Gastroenterology* 142 (2012): 266–272; F. L. Crowe and coauthors, Diet and risk of diverticular disease in Oxford cohort of European Prospective Investigation into Cancer and Nutrition (EPIC): Prospective study of British vegetarians and non-vegetarians, *British Medical Journal* 343 (2011): d4131; Ravikoff and J. R. Korzenik, 2011.

35. D. Aune and coauthors, Dietary fibre, whole grains, and risk of colorectal cancer: Systematic review and dose-response meta-analysis of prospective studies, *British Medical Journal* 343 (2011), doi: 10.1136/bmj.d6617; C. C. Dahm and coauthors, Dietary fiber and colorectal cancer risk: A nested case-control study using food diaries, *Journal of the National Cancer Institute* 102 (2010): 614–626.

36. Dahm and coauthors, 2010.

37. H. M. Chen and coauthors, Decreased dietary fiber intake and structural alteration of gut microbiota in patients with advanced colorectal adenoma, *American Journal of Clinical Nutrition* 97 (2013): 1044–1052; M. H. Pan and coauthors, Molecular mechanisms for chemoprevention of colorectal cancer by natural dietary compounds, *Molecular Nutrition and Food Research* 55 (2011): 32–45.

38. T. F. Turner and coauthors, Dietary adherence and satisfaction with a bean-based high-fiber weight loss diet: A pilot study, *ISRN Obesity*, October 29, 2013, doi: 10.1155/2013/915415.

39. H. Du and coauthors, Dietary fiber and subsequent changes in body weight and waist circumference in European men and women, *American Journal of Clinical Nutrition* 91 (2010): 329–336.

40. M. Kristensen and coauthors, Whole grain compared with refined wheat decreases the percentage of body fat following a 12-week, energy-restricted dietary intervention in postmenopausal women, *Journal of Nutrition* 142 (2012): 710–716; S. S. Jonnalagadda and coauthors, Putting the whole grain puzzle together: Health benefits associated with whole grains—Summary of American Society for Nutrition 2010 Satellite symposium, *Journal of Nutrition* 141 (2011): 1011S–1022S; K. A. Harris and P. M. Kris-Etherton, Effects of whole grains on coronary heart disease risk, *Current Atherosclerosis reports* 12 (2010): 368–376.

41. Standing Committee on the Scientific Evolution of Dietary Reference Intakes, 2005, p. 265.

42. D. E. King, A. G. Mainous, and C. A. Lambourne, Trends in dietary fiber intake in the United States, 1999-2008, *Journal of the Academy of Nutrition and Dietetics* 112 (2012): 642-648.

43. C. E. O'Neil and coauthors, Consumption of whole grains is associated with improved diet quality and nutrient intake in children and adolescents: The National Health and Nutrition Examination Survey 1999–2004, *Public Health Nutrition* 14 (2011): 347–355; C. E. O'Neil and coauthors, Whole-grain consumption is associated with diet quality and nutrient intake in adults: The National Health and Nutrition Examination Survey, 1999–2004, *Journal of the American Dietetic Association* 110 (2010): 1461–1468.

LO 2.5 Describe the glycemic index and explain why its use in disease prevention is controversial.

Carbohydrate-rich foods vary in the degree to which they elevate both blood glucose and insulin concentrations. Chapter 2 introduced the *glycemic index* (GI), a ranking of carbohydrate foods based on their glycemic effect after ingestion. The glycemic index may be of interest to people with diabetes who must regulate their blood glucose to protect their health. In diabetes treatment, however, the total amount of carbohydrate is more important than the type of carbohydrate consumed.[1] Thus, dietetics experts have debated the usefulness of the glycemic index for diabetes treatment. Despite some controversy, however, the American Diabetes Association encourages low-glycemic foods that are rich in fiber and other nutrients.[2] Furthermore, because some recent research shows that a low-glycemic index diet can improve blood glucose control in type 2 diabetes, the use of low-glycemic diets for this purpose may be gaining credibility.[3]

Researchers are also trying to determine whether low-GI diets may be helpful for improving risk factors for a number of other chronic diseases.[4] This Nutrition in Practice will describe the factors that contribute to a food's glycemic effect and the results of research studies that have examined the potential benefits of selecting mainly low-GI foods.

How is the glycemic index measured?

The glycemic index is essentially a measure of how quickly the carbohydrate in a food is digested and absorbed. Although testing methods vary to some degree, the most common protocol is to feed the test food—which contains a measured quantity of digestible carbohydrate—to research subjects and then measure blood glucose levels for two or three hours after the feeding. The increase in blood glucose over the two- or three-hour period is then compared to the blood glucose rise after an identical amount of digestible carbohydrate is ingested from a reference food such as pure glucose or white bread. Figure NP2-1 illustrates the difference in the blood glucose response to a low-GI food and a high-GI food. The blood glucose curve displays the surge in blood glucose above normal fasting levels after the food is consumed and the subsequent fall over several hours. Table NP2-1 lists the GIs of various carbohydrate-containing foods, arranged from highest to lowest within each food group listed.

The *amount* of carbohydrate consumed also influences the glycemic response. A food's total glycemic effect—expressed as the *glycemic load* (GL)—is the product of its GI and the amount of available carbohydrate from the portion consumed, divided by 100. For example, if the GI of sweet potato is 60, a 100-gram serving containing about 20 grams of carbohydrates would have a GL of 12. The GL is used to standardize GI values to the carbohydrate content and portion size of a food or a meal.[5]

What factors influence a food's glycemic effect?

Table NP2-1 shows that starchy foods such as bread and potatoes tend to have high GI values, whereas many fruits and legumes have low GI values. The main factors that influence the GI value of a food include the following:

■ *Starch structure.* Starch is present in foods as either a straight chain or branched chain of glucose molecules. Whereas digestion of the branched form tends to release glucose quickly, the straight chain is resistant to digestion. Thus, foods that contain mainly the branched form of starch tend to raise blood glucose levels more quickly and have a high GI value. Due to the subtle differences in starch among foods, different species of the same foods can have substantially different GI values; for example, current GI values for rice range from low (38 for parboiled white rice) to high (85 for Japanese sushi-style white rice).[6]

■ *Fiber content.* Certain types of dietary fibers (primarily soluble fibers) increase the viscosity of chyme, slowing the passage of food in the stomach and upper intestine and making it more difficult for enzymes to digest the food. Therefore, foods such as beans, fruits, and vegetables, which contain soluble fibers, tend to have lower GI values.

© 2016 Cengage Learning®

FIGURE NP2-1 Blood Glucose Response to High-GI and Low-GI Foods
Foods that are digested slowly have a low glycemic index. These foods cause a gradual and more moderate response in blood glucose than do foods with a high glycemic index.

TABLE NP2-1 Glycemic Index (GI) of Selected Foods[a]

Value	GI
High	≥70
Medium	56–69
Low	≤55

Food Item	Glycemic Index
Grains	
Cornflakes	81
Instant oatmeal, cooked	79
White bread, enriched	75
Whole-wheat bread	74
White rice	73
Bagel, white	69
Brown rice	68
Couscous	65
Popcorn	65
Bran flakes	63
Oatmeal, cooked	55
Spaghetti, white, boiled	49
Spaghetti, whole-meal, boiled	48
Corn tortilla	46
Oat bran bread; 50% oat bran	44
Barley	28
Milk products	
Ice cream	51
Yogurt, fruit	41
Whole milk	39
Nonfat milk	37
Soy milk	34
Legumes	
Lentils	32
Garbanzo beans	28

Food Item	Glycemic Index
Kidney beans	24
Soy beans	16
Vegetables	
Russet potato, baked	111
Potato, instant mash	87
Potato, boiled	78
Pumpkin, boiled	64
Potato, french fries	63
Sweet potato, boiled	63
Taro	53
Sweet corn	52
Green peas, boiled	51
Carrots, boiled	39
Fruits	
Watermelon	76
Pineapple	59
Bananas	51
Mangoes	51
Orange juice	50
Oranges	43
Apple juice	41
Apples	36
Snack Foods/Beverages	
Fruit punch	67
Soft drink/soda	59
Chocolate	56
Potato chips	40
Sugars	
Sucrose	65
Honey	61
Fructose	15

[a]Reference food: glucose = 100

Source: F. S. Atkinson, K. Foster-Powell, and J. C. Brand-Miller, International tables of glycemic index and glycemic load values: 2008. *Diabetes Care* (2008): 2281–2283.

▌ *Presence of fat and protein*. The fat in foods tends to slow stomach emptying, thus reducing the rate of digestion and absorption; hence, the presence of fat usually reduces a food's GI value. The protein in foods can also influence the GI because protein promotes insulin secretion, increasing the rate at which glucose is taken up from the blood.

▌ *Food processing*. The manner in which a food is processed and cooked influences the interactions among starch, protein, and fiber and thus affects the final GI value. For example, both pasta and bread are prepared from wheat flour, but pasta (cooked *al dente*) has a lower GI because the starch granules in pasta are surrounded by a sturdy protein barrier that hampers starch digestion. Cooking the pasta for longer periods can break down its structure and raise the GI value. As another example, the GI values for oatmeal vary according to the size and thickness of the oats used to prepare it: oatmeal prepared from steel-cut oats has a lower GI value than oatmeal prepared from quick oats. This is because the steel-cut oats are solid particles of grain, whereas "quick oats" are small, thin flakes.

▌ *Mixture of foods in a meal*. Because foods are rarely consumed in isolation, the GI value of an individual food may be less important than the combination of foods consumed at a meal. For example, in a cheese sandwich, the high GI of the bread is lowered by the addition of fat and protein in the cheese.

▌ *Individual glucose tolerance*. Cellular responses to insulin vary; thus, individual variability affects the glycemic response to foods. Persons with diabetes or prediabetes exhibit higher blood glucose levels after ingesting carbohydrate foods than do healthy individuals.[7]

What evidence suggests that a low-GI diet may influence chronic disease risk?

Some research shows that low-GI diets may reduce the risks of developing diabetes, heart disease, and obesity and help individuals

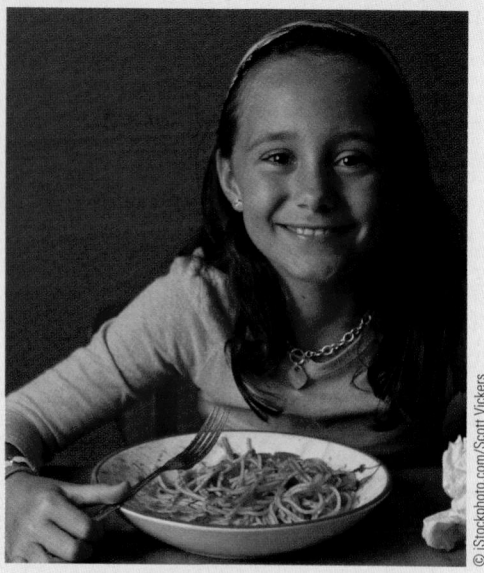

Pasta cooked *al dente* has a lower glycemic index than many other starchy foods.
Source: F. S. Atkinson, K. Foster-Powell, and J. C. Brand-Miller, International tables of glycemic index and glycemic load values: 2008. Diabetes Care (2008): 2281–2283.

lose weight.[8] Other studies, however, do not support such findings.[9] Studies are often difficult to interpret because low-GI foods often provide abundant soluble fiber, and soluble fiber slows glucose absorption, sustains feelings of fullness, and improves blood lipids. Therefore, it could be that soluble fiber, and not the low-GI diet, is responsible for any reported effects.[10] Because of mixed findings so far, health practitioners do not routinely recommend that patients consume low-GI diets to prevent or treat disease. An abundance of ongoing research to reveal specific relationships between low-GI diets and chronic disease risk, however, may change such thinking. Examples of research include the following:

▪ *Diabetes prevention.* Some researchers have proposed that a high glycemic load can increase the body's demand for insulin and eventually reduce pancreatic function, resulting in inadequate insulin secretion. Indeed, results of several studies suggest that low-GI diets might prevent or delay the onset of type 2 diabetes in those at risk.[11]

▪ *Heart disease risk.* Although some research suggests that low-GI diets may improve blood lipid levels, other research shows no consistent effects of low-GI diets on heart disease risk.[12]

▪ *Appetite and weight loss.* Some research shows that low-GI foods can slow the after-meal rise in blood glucose, supporting the hypothesis that such foods may promote satiety and suppress hunger.[13] Other research, however, shows no effect of low-GI foods on satiety.[14] Research results are also inconsistent regarding whether low-GI diets assist in weight loss.[15]

Given the mixed results of research studies on chronic disease prevention, are there any benefits associated with consuming low-GI foods?

Yes, if the low-GI foods are nutrient-dense, high-fiber foods. Not all low-GI foods meet these criteria: note that cakes, cookies, and candy bars may have a low GI due to their high fat content. Thus, a food's GI should be considered along with other nutrient criteria when assessing the health benefits.

The GI can be a helpful tool for choosing the most healthful food from a food group. For example, low-GI breakfast cereals tend to be high in fiber and low in added sugars, whereas high-GI cereals tend to be those that contain refined flours and significant amounts of added sugars. In other words, low-GI foods are often wholesome foods that have been minimally processed.

In general, should people avoid consuming high-GI foods?

Some people assume that starchy foods such as breads and potatoes should be avoided due to their high GI values. As mentioned earlier, these foods are rarely consumed in isolation, and their GI values are reduced in a mixed meal. For example, breads often have a GI greater than 70, but adding cheese or peanut butter reduces the GI to 55 or 59, respectively. Also worth considering is that GI values often vary considerably. For example, published values for white potatoes range from 24 to 101, and many samples have values in the mid-50s.[16] For these reasons and others, more studies are needed to confirm whether the GI is practical or beneficial for healthy people.

Given the complexity of the GI, what are the current recommendations?

The potential benefits associated with consuming low-GI diets are still under investigation. As discussed earlier, people with type 2 diabetes may benefit from limiting high-GI foods—those that produce too great a rise, or too sudden a fall, in blood glucose. Additional research is needed to justify the use of diets based on the GI for preventing or treating diseases such as heart disease, obesity, or other medical problems.

At present, many nutrition scientists advocate consuming a plant-based diet that contains minimally processed grains, legumes, vegetables, and fruits. Such a diet would include abundant fiber and limited amounts of solid fats and added sugars. Undoubtedly, meals consisting of these foods would tend to have low or medium GI values.

Notes

1. A. B. Evert and coauthors, American Diabetes Association, Position statement: Nutrition therapy recommendations for the management of adults with diabetes, *Diabetes Care* 35 (2013): 3821–3842.

2. American Diabetes Association, Standards of medical care in diabetes—2014, *Diabetes Care* 37 (2014): S14–S80; Evert and coauthors, American Diabetes Association, 2013.

3. Evert and coauthors, American Diabetes Association, 2013; O. Ajala, P. English, and J. Pinkney, Systematic review and meta-analysis of different dietary approaches to the management of type 2 diabetes, *American Journal of Clinical Nutrition* 97 (2013): 505–516; D. J. Jenkins and coauthors, Effect of legumes as part of a low glycemic index diet on glycemic control and cardiovascular risk factors in type 2 diabetes mellitus: A randomized controlled trial, *Archives of*

Internal Medicine 172 (2012): 1653–1660; A. Pande, G. Krishnamoorthy, and N. D. Moulick, Hypoglycaemic and hypolipidaemic effects of low GI and medium GL Indian diets in type 2 diabetics for a period of 4 weeks: A prospective study, *International Journal of Food Sciences and Nutrition* 63 (2012): 649–658; J. Brand-Miller and A. E. Buyken, The glycemic index issue, *Current Opinion in Lipidology* 23 (2012): 62–67; T. P. J. Solomon and coauthors, A low-glycemic index diet combined with exercise reduces insulin resistance, postprandial hyperinsulinemia, and glucose-dependent insulinotropic polypeptide responses in obese, prediabetic humans, *American Journal of Clinical Nutrition* 92 (2010): 1359–1368.

4. J. M. Jones, Glycemic index: The state of the science, part 3 Role in cardiovascular disease and blood lipids, *Nutrition Today* 48 (2013): 61–67; J. M. Jones, Glycemic index: The state of the science, part 4—Roles in inflammation, insulin resistance, and metabolic syndrome, *Nutrition Today* 48 (2013): 101–107; Brand-Miller and Buyken, 2012; I. Krog-Mikkelsen and coauthors, A low glycemic index diet does not affect postprandial energy metabolism but decreases postprandial insulinemia and increases fullness ratings in healthy women, *Journal of Nutrition* 141 (2011): 1679 1684.

5. J. M. Jones, Glycemic index: The state of the science, part 1—The measure and its variability, *Nutrition Today* 47 (2012): 207–213.

6. F. S. Atkinson, K. Foster-Powell, and J. C. Brand-Miller, International tables of glycemic index and glycemic load values: 2008, *Diabetes Care* 31 (2008): 2281–2283.

7. American Diabetes Association, Diagnosis and classification of diabetes mellitus, *Diabetes Care* 37 (2014): S81–S90.

8. L. M. Goff and coauthors, Low glycaemic index diets and blood lipids: A systematic review and meta-analysis of randomized controlled trials, *Nutrition, Metabolism, and Cardiovascular Diseases* 23 (2013): 1 10; G. Livesey and coauthors, Is there a dose-response relation of dietary glycemic load to risk of type 2 diabetes? Meta-analysis of prospective cohort studies, *American Journal of Clinical Nutrition* 97 (2013): 584–596; Brand-Miller and Buyken, 2012; M. L. Neuhouser and coauthors, A low-glycemic load diet reduces serum C-reactive protein and modestly increases adiponectin in overweight and obese adults, *Journal of Nutrition* 142 (2012): 369–374; O. Gögebakan and coauthors, Effects of weight loss and long-term weight maintenance with diets varying in protein and glycemic index on cardiovascular risk factors: The diet, obesity, and genes (DiOGenes) study: A randomized, controlled trial, *Circulation* 124 (2011): 2829–2838; G. M. Turner-McGrievy and coauthors, Decreases in dietary glycemic index are related to weight loss among individuals following therapeutic diets for type 2 diabetes,

Journal of Nutrition 141 (2011): 1469–1474; I. Sluijs and coauthors, Carbohydrate quantity and quality and risk of type 2 diabetes in the Europena Prospective Investigation into Cancer and Nutrition—Netherlands (EPIC-NL) study, *American Journal of Clinical Nutrition* 92 (2010): 905–911; Solomon and coauthors, 2010.

9. A. Mirrahimi and coauthors, The role of glycemic index and glycemic load in cardiovascular disease and its risk factors: A review of the recent literature, *Current Atherosclerosis Reports* 16 (2014): 381; A. S. Kristo, N. R. Matthan, and A. H. Lichtenstein, Effect of diets differing in glycemic index and glycemic load on cardiovascular risk factors: Review of randomized controlled-feeding trials, *Nutrients* 5 (2013): 1071–1080; I. Sluijs and coauthors, Dietary glycemic index, glycemic load, and digestible carbohydrate intake are not associated risk of type 2 diabetes in eight European countries, *Journal of Nutrition* 143 (2013): 93–99.

10. Jones, Glycemic index: The state of the science, part 3—Role in cardiovascular disease, 2013.

11. Livesey and coauthors, 2013; Brand-Miller and Buyken, 2012.

12. Kristo, Matthan, and Lichtenstein, 2013; Goff and coauthors, 2013; M. L. Wheeler and coauthors, Macronutrients, food groups, and eating patterns in the management of diabetes: A systematic review of the literature, 2010, *Diabetes Care* 35 (2012): 434–445; E. Denova-Gutierrez and coauthors, Dietary glycemic index, dietary glycemic load, blood lipids, and coronary heart disease, *Journal of Nutrition and Metabolism*, 2010, doi:10.1155/2010/170680; C. E. Finley and coauthors, Glycemic index, glycemic load, and prevalence of the metabolic syndrome in the Cooper Center Longitudinal Study, *Journal of the American Dietetic Association* 110 (2010): 1820–1829.

13. K. T. Chang and coauthors, Low glycemic load experimental diet more satiating than high glycemic load diet, *Nutrition and Cancer* 64 (2012): 666–673; Krog-Mikkelsen and coauthors, 2011.

14. A. Geliebter and coauthors, Satiety following intake of potatoes and other carbohydrate test meals, *Annals of Nutrition and Metabolism* 62 (2013): 37–43; A. G. Liu and coauthors, Reducing the glycemic index or carbohydrate content of mixed meals reduces postprandial glycemia and insulinemia over the entire day but does not affect satiety, *Diabetes Care* 35 (2012): 1633–1637.

15. J. M. Jones, Glycemic index: The state of the science, part 2—Roles in weight, weight loss, and satiety, 2013; Turner-McGrievy and coauthors, 2011.

16. Atkinson, Foster-Powell, and Brand-Miller, 2008.

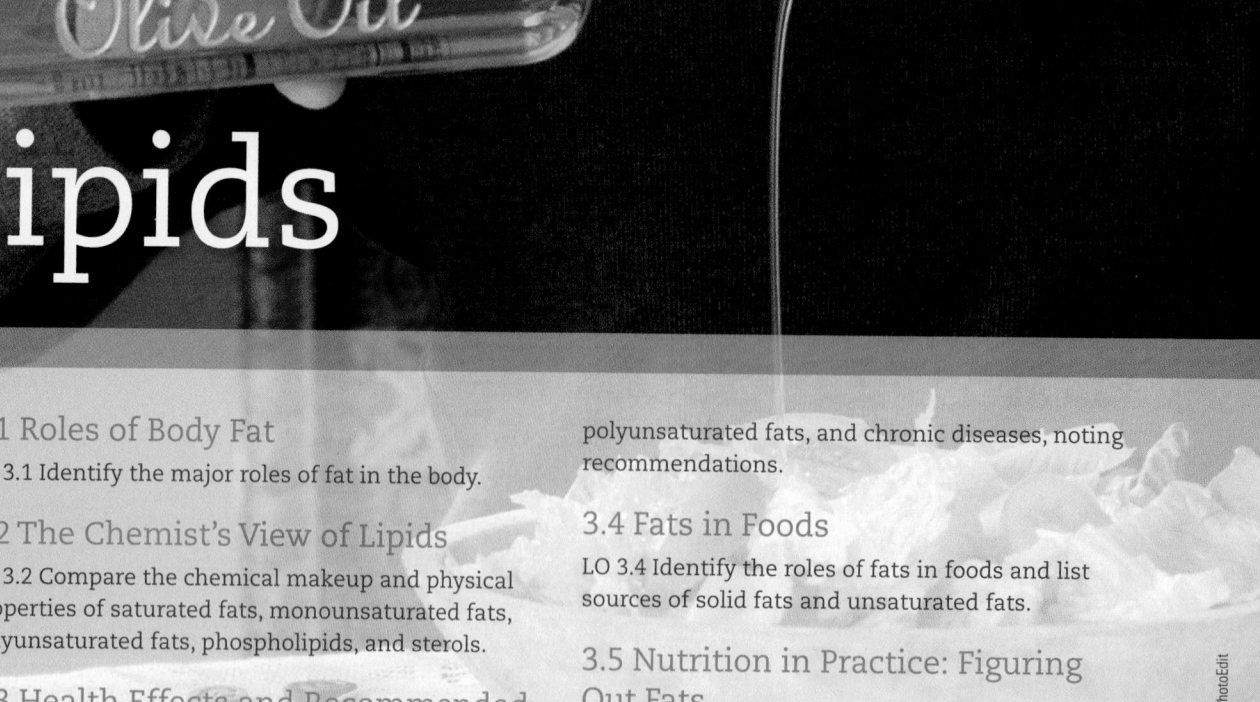

3

Lipids

3.1 Roles of Body Fat

LO 3.1 Identify the major roles of fat in the body.

3.2 The Chemist's View of Lipids

LO 3.2 Compare the chemical makeup and physical properties of saturated fats, monounsaturated fats, polyunsaturated fats, phospholipids, and sterols.

3.3 Health Effects and Recommended Intakes of Fats

LO 3.3 Explain the relationships among saturated fats, *trans* fat, cholesterol, monounsaturated and polyunsaturated fats, and chronic diseases, noting recommendations.

3.4 Fats in Foods

LO 3.4 Identify the roles of fats in foods and list sources of solid fats and unsaturated fats.

3.5 Nutrition in Practice: Figuring Out Fats

LO 3.5 Identify which fats support health and which may impair it.

Most people know that too much fat in the diet, especially certain kinds of fat, imposes health risks, but they may be surprised to learn that too little does, too. People in the United States, however, are more likely to eat too much fat than too little.

Fat is a member of the class of compounds called **lipids**. The lipids in foods and in the human body include triglycerides (**fats** and **oils**), phospholipids, and sterols.

3.1 Roles of Body Fat

LO 3.1 Identify the major roles of fat in the body.

Lipids perform many tasks in the body, but most importantly they provide energy. A constant flow of energy is so vital to life that, in a pinch, any other function is sacrificed to maintain it. Chapter 2 described one safeguard against such an emergency—the stores of glycogen in the liver that provide glucose to the blood whenever the supply runs short. The body's stores of glycogen are limited, however. In contrast, the body's capacity to store fat for energy is virtually unlimited due to the fat-storing cells of the **adipose tissue.** The fat cells of the adipose tissue readily take up and store fat, growing in size as they do so. Fat cells are more than just storage depots, however; fat cells secrete hormones that help to regulate the appetite and influence other body functions.[1] Figure 3-1 shows a fat cell.

The fat stored in fat cells supplies 60 percent of the body's ongoing energy needs during rest. The fat embedded in muscle tissue shares with muscle glycogen the task of providing energy when the muscles are active. During some types of physical activity or prolonged periods of food deprivation, fat stores may make an even greater energy contribution. The brain and nerves, however, need their energy as glucose, and, as explained in Chapter 6, fat is an inefficient source of glucose. After a long period of glucose deprivation (during fasting or starvation), brain and nerve cells develop

lipids: a family of compounds that includes triglycerides (fats and oils), phospholipids, and sterols. Lipids are characterized by their insolubility in water.

fats: lipids that are solid at room temperature (70°F or 21°C).

oils: lipids that are liquid at room temperature (70°F or 21°C).

adipose tissue: the body's fat, which consists of masses of fat-storing cells called adipose cells.

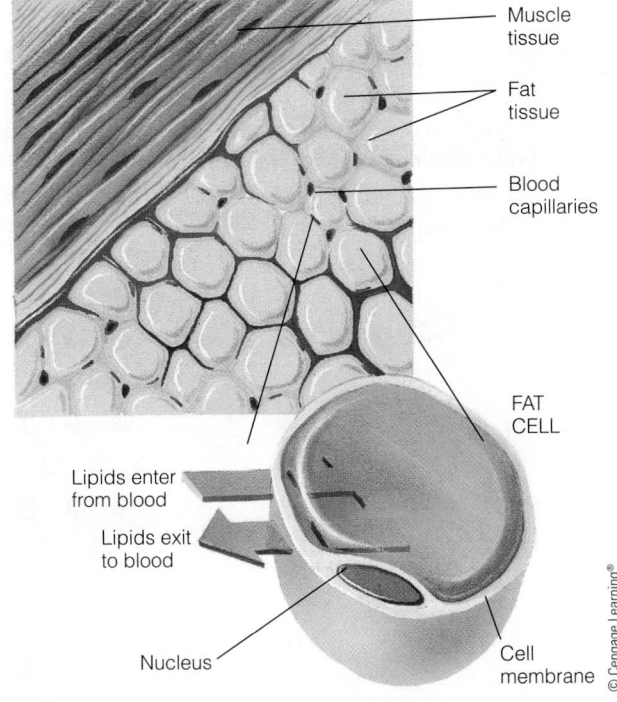

Muscle tissue

Fat tissue

Blood capillaries

FAT CELL

Lipids enter from blood

Lipids exit to blood

Nucleus

Cell membrane

© Cengage Learning®

FIGURE 3-1 A Fat Cell
Within the fat, or adipose, cell, lipid is stored in a droplet. This droplet can greatly enlarge, and the fat cell membrane will expand to accommodate its swollen contents.

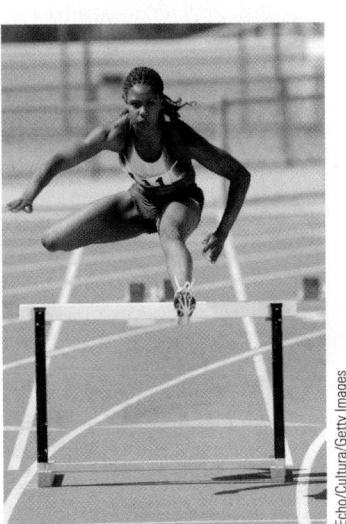

Echo/Cultura/Getty Images

Body fat supplies much of the fuel that muscles need to do their work.

[handwritten margin notes:] lipids- a family of compound that includes triglycerides (fats + oils), phospholipids, and sterols; characterized by their insolubility in water.

fats- lipids solid at room temperature

oils- lipids liquid at room temperature.

TABLE 3-1 The Functions of Fats in the Body

- *Energy stores.* Fats are the body's chief form of stored energy.

- *Muscle fuel.* Fats provide much of the energy to fuel muscular work.

- *Padding.* Fat pads inside the body cavity protect the internal organs from shock.

- *Insulation.* Fats insulate against temperature extremes by forming a fat layer under the skin.

- *Cell membranes.* Fats form the major material of cell membranes.

- *Raw materials.* Fats are converted to other compounds, such as hormones, bile, and vitamin D, as needed.

---

ketones (KEY-tones): acidic, water-soluble compounds produced by the liver during the breakdown of fat when carbohydrate is not available; technically known as *ketone bodies.*

triglycerides (try-GLISS-er-rides): one of the main classes of lipids; the chief form of fat in foods and the major storage form of fat in the body; composed of glycerol with three fatty acids attached.

  tri = three

  glyceride = a compound of glycerol

fatty acids: organic compounds composed of a chain of carbon atoms with hydrogen atoms attached and an acid group at one end.

glycerol (GLISS-er-ol): an organic compound, three carbons long, that can form the backbone of triglycerides and phospholipids.

---

the ability to derive about half of their energy from a special form of fat known as **ketones,** but they still require glucose as well. This means that people wanting to lose weight need to eat a certain minimum amount of carbohydrate to meet their energy needs, even when they are limiting their food intakes.

In addition to supplying energy, fat serves other roles in the body. Natural oils in the skin provide a radiant complexion; in the scalp, they help nourish the hair and make it glossy. The layer of fat beneath the skin insulates the body from extremes of temperature. A pad of hard fat beneath each kidney protects it from being jarred and damaged, even during a motorcycle ride on a bumpy road. The soft fat in a woman's breasts protects her mammary glands from heat and cold and cushions them against shock. The phospholipids and the sterol cholesterol are cell membrane constituents that help maintain the structure and health of all cells. Table 3-1 summarizes the major functions of fats in the body.

IN SUMMARY

> Lipids in the body not only serve as energy reserves but also protect the body from temperature extremes, cushion the vital organs, and provide the major material of cell membranes.

3.2 The Chemist's View of Lipids

LO 3.2 Compare the chemical makeup and physical properties of saturated fats, monounsaturated fats, polyunsaturated fats, phospholipids, and sterols.

The diverse and vital functions that lipids perform in the body reveal why eating too little fat can be harmful. As mentioned earlier, though, too much fat in the diet seems to be the greater problem for most people. To understand both the beneficial and harmful effects that fats exert on the body, a closer look at the structure and function of members of the lipid family is in order.

Triglycerides

When people talk about fat—for example, "I'm too fat" or "That meat is fatty"—they are usually referring to triglycerides. Among lipids, **triglycerides** predominate—both in the diet and in the body. The name *triglyceride* almost explains itself: three (*tri*) **fatty acids** attached to a **glycerol** "backbone." Figure 3-2 shows how three fatty acids combine with glycerol to make a triglyceride.

Glycerol

3 fatty acids of differing lengths

Triglyceride formed from 1 glycerol + 3 fatty acids

© Cengage Learning®

FIGURE 3-2 Triglyceride Formation
Glycerol, a small, water-soluble compound, plus three fatty acids, equals a triglyceride.

[handwritten note: glycerol can form the backbone of triglycerides & phospholipids.]

62

Fatty Acids

When energy from any energy-yielding nutrient is to be stored as fat, the nutrient is first broken into small fragments. Then the fragments are linked together into chains known as fatty acids. The fatty acids, three at a time, are then packaged with glycerol to make triglycerides.

Chain Length and Saturation Fatty acids may differ from one another in two ways—in chain length and in degree of saturation. The chain length refers to the number of carbons in a fatty acid. Saturation also refers to its chemical structure—specifically, to the number of hydrogen atoms the carbons in the fatty acid are holding. If every available carbon is filled to capacity with hydrogen atoms, the chain is called a **saturated fatty acid.** A saturated fatty acid is fully loaded with hydrogen atoms and has only single bonds between the carbons. The first zigzag structure in Figure 3-3 represents a saturated fatty acid.

Unsaturated Fatty Acids In some fatty acids, including most of those in plants and fish, hydrogen atoms are missing from the fatty acid chains. The places where the hydrogen atoms are missing are called points of unsaturation, and a chain containing such points is called an **unsaturated fatty acid.** An unsaturated fatty acid has at least one double bond between its carbons. If there is one point of unsaturation, the chain is a **monounsaturated fatty acid.** The second structure in Figure 3-3 is an example. If there are two or more points of unsaturation, then the fatty acid is a **polyunsaturated fatty acid** (see the third structure in Figure 3-3).

Hard and Soft Fat A triglyceride can contain any combination of fatty acids—long chain or short chain and saturated, monounsaturated, or polyunsaturated. The degree of saturation of the fatty acids in a fat influences the health of the body (discussed in a later section) and the characteristics of foods. Fats that contain the shorter chain or the more unsaturated fatty acids are softer at room temperature and melt more readily. A comparison of three fats—lard (which comes from pork), chicken fat, and

saturated fatty acid: a fatty acid carrying the maximum possible number of hydrogen atoms (having no points of unsaturation).

unsaturated fatty acid: a fatty acid with one or more points of unsaturation where hydrogen atoms are missing (includes monounsaturated and polyunsaturated fatty acids).

monounsaturated fatty acid (MUFA): a fatty acid that has one point of unsaturation; for example, the oleic acid found in olive oil.

polyunsaturated fatty acids (PUFA): fatty acids with two or more points of unsaturation. For example, linoleic acid has two such points, and linolenic acid has three. Thus, polyunsaturated *fat* is composed of triglycerides containing a high percentage of PUFA.

Saturated **Monounsaturated** **Polyunsaturated**

Point of unsaturation

Points of unsaturation

© Cengage Learning®

FIGURE 3-3 Three Types of Fatty Acids
The more carbon atoms in a fatty acid, the longer it is. The more hydrogen atoms attached to those carbons, the more saturated the fatty acid is.

safflower oil—illustrates these differences: lard is the most saturated and the hardest; chicken fat is less saturated and somewhat soft; and safflower oil, which is the most unsaturated, is a liquid at room temperature.

Stability Saturation also influences stability. Fats can become **rancid** when exposed to oxygen. Polyunsaturated fatty acids spoil most readily because their double bonds are unstable. The **oxidation** of unsaturated fats produces a variety of compounds that smell and taste rancid; saturated fats are more resistant to oxidation and thus less likely to become rancid. Other types of spoilage can occur due to microbial growth, however.

Manufacturers can protect fat-containing products against rancidity in three ways—none of them perfect. First, products may be sealed airtight and refrigerated—an expensive and inconvenient storage system. Second, manufacturers may add **antioxidants** to compete for the oxygen and thus protect the oil (examples are the additives **BHA** and **BHT** and vitamins C and E).* Third, manufacturers may saturate some or all of the points of unsaturation by adding hydrogen atoms—a process known as hydrogenation.

Hydrogenation **Hydrogenation** offers two advantages: it protects against oxidation (thereby prolonging shelf life) and also alters the texture of foods by increasing the solidity of fats. When partially hydrogenated, vegetable oils become spreadable margarine. Hydrogenated fats make piecrusts flaky and puddings creamy. A disadvantage is that hydrogenation makes polyunsaturated fats more saturated. Consequently, any health advantages of using polyunsaturated fats instead of saturated fats are lost with hydrogenation.

Trans-Fatty Acids Another disadvantage of hydrogenation is that some of the molecules that remain unsaturated after processing change shape from *cis* to *trans*. In nature, most unsaturated fatty acids are *cis*-fatty acids—meaning that the hydrogen atoms next to the double bonds are on the same side of the carbon chain. Only a few fatty acids in nature (notably a small percentage of those found in milk and meat products) are ***trans*-fatty acids**—meaning that the hydrogen atoms next to the double bonds are on opposite sides of the carbon chain (see Figure 3-4). These arrangements result in different configurations for the fatty acids, and this difference affects function: in the body, *trans*-fatty acids behave more like saturated fats, increasing blood cholesterol and the risk of heart disease (as a later section describes).[2]

Researchers are trying to determine whether the health effects of naturally occurring *trans* fats differ from those of commercially created *trans* fats.[3] In any case, the important distinction is that intake of naturally occurring *trans*-fatty acids is typically low. At current levels of consumption, naturally occurring *trans* fats are unlikely to have adverse effects on blood lipids. The naturally occurring *trans*-fatty acid **conjugated linoleic acid** may even have health benefits.[4]

rancid: the term used to describe fats when they have deteriorated, usually by oxidation. Rancid fats often have an "off" odor.

oxidation (OKS-ee-day-shun): the process of a substance combining with oxygen.

antioxidants: as a food additive, preservatives that delay or prevent rancidity of foods and other damage to food caused by oxygen.

BHA, BHT: preservatives commonly used to slow the development of "off" flavors, odors, and color changes caused by oxidation.

hydrogenation (high-dro-gen-AY-shun): a chemical process by which hydrogen atoms are added to monounsaturated or polyunsaturated fats to reduce the number of double bonds, making the fats more saturated (solid) and more resistant to oxidation (protecting against rancidity). Hydrogenation produces *trans*-fatty acids.

***trans*-fatty acids:** fatty acids in which the hydrogen atoms next to the double bond are on opposite sides of the carbon chain.

conjugated linoleic acid: a collective term for several fatty acids that have the same chemical formulas as linoleic acid but with different configurations.

Cis-fatty acid   *Trans*-fatty acid

© 2016 Cengage Learning®

FIGURE 3-4 *Cis*- and *Trans*-Fatty Acids Compared

*BHA is butylated hydroxyanisole; BHT is butylated hydroxytolvene.

CHAPTER THREE

Essential Fatty Acids Using carbohydrate, fat, or protein, the human body can synthesize all the fatty acids it needs except for two—**linoleic acid** and **linolenic acid.** Both linoleic acid and linolenic acid are polyunsaturated fatty acids. Because they cannot be made from other substances in the body, they must be obtained from food and are therefore called **essential fatty acids.** Linoleic acid and linolenic acid are found in small amounts in plant oils, and the body readily stores them, making deficiencies unlikely. From both of these essential fatty acids, the body makes important substances that help regulate a wide range of body functions: blood pressure, clot formation, blood lipid concentration, the immune response, the inflammatory response to injury, and many others.[5] These two essential nutrients also serve as structural components of cell membranes.

Linoleic Acid: An Omega-6 Fatty Acid Linoleic acid is an **omega-6 fatty acid,** found in the seeds of plants and in the oils produced from the seeds. Any diet that contains vegetable oils, seeds, nuts, and whole-grain foods provides enough linoleic acid to meet the body's needs. Researchers have long known and appreciated the importance of the omega-6 fatty acid family.

Linolenic Acid and Other Omega-3 Fatty Acids Linolenic acid belongs to a family of polyunsaturated fatty acids known as **omega-3 fatty acids,** a family that also includes **EPA** and **DHA.** EPA and DHA are found primarily in fish oils. As mentioned, the human body cannot make linolenic acid, but given dietary linolenic acid, it can make EPA and DHA, although the process is slow.

The importance of omega-3 fatty acids has been recognized since the 1980s, and research continues to unveil impressive roles for EPA and DHA in metabolism and disease prevention. The brain has a high content of DHA, and both EPA and DHA are needed for normal brain development.[6] DHA is also especially active in the rods and cones of the retina of the eye.[7] Today, researchers know that these omega-3 fatty acids are essential for normal growth and development and that they may play an important role in the prevention and treatment of heart disease.[8]

Phospholipids

Up to now, this discussion has focused on one class of lipids, the triglycerides (fats and oils), and their component parts, the fatty acids (see Table 3-2). Two other classes of lipids, the **phospholipids** and sterols, make up only 5 percent of the lipids in the diet, but they are nevertheless worthy of attention. Among the phospholipids, the lecithins are of particular interest.

Structure of Phospholipids Like the triglycerides, the **lecithins** and other phospholipids have a backbone of glycerol; they differ from the triglycerides in having only two fatty acids attached to the glycerol. In place of the third fatty acid, they have a phosphate group (a phosphorus-containing acid) and a molecule of **choline** or a similar compound. The fatty acids make the phospholipids soluble in fat; the phosphate group enables them to dissolve in water. Such versatility benefits the food industry, which uses phospholipids as **emulsifiers** to mix fats with water in such products as mayonnaise and candy bars.

Phospholipids in Foods In addition to the phospholipids used by the food industry as emulsifiers, phospholipids are also found naturally in foods. The richest food sources of lecithin are eggs, liver, soybeans, wheat germ, and peanuts.

Roles of Phospholipids Lecithins and other phospholipids are important constituents of cell membranes. They also act as emulsifiers in the body, helping to keep other fats in solution in the watery blood and body fluids. In addition, some phospholipids generate signals inside the cells in response to hormones, such as insulin, to help alter body conditions.

TABLE 3-2 The Lipid Family

Triglycerides (fats and oils)
▪ Glycerol (1 per triglyceride)
▪ Fatty acids (3 per triglyceride)
Saturated
Monounsaturated
Polyunsaturated
Omega-6
Omega-3
Phospholipids (such as the lecithins)
Sterols (such as cholesterol)

© Cengage Learning®

linoleic acid, linolenic acid: polyunsaturated fatty acids that are essential for human beings.

essential fatty acids: fatty acids that the body requires but cannot make and so must be obtained through the diet.

omega-6 fatty acid: a polyunsaturated fatty acid with its endmost double bond six carbons back from the end of its carbon chain. Linoleic acid is an example. Chemists use the term *omega*, the last letter of the Greek alphabet, to refer to the position of the last double bond in a fatty acid.

omega-3 fatty acids: polyunsaturated fatty acids in which the endmost double bond is three carbons back from the end of the carbon chain. Linolenic acid is an example.

EPA, DHA: omega-3 fatty acids made from linolenic acid. The full name for EPA is *eicosapentaenoic* (EYE-cosa-PENTA-ee-NO-ick) *acid.* The full name for DHA is *docosahexaenoic* (DOE-cosa-HEXA-ee-NO-ick) *acid.*

phospholipids: one of the three main classes of lipids; compounds that are similar to triglycerides but have *choline* (or another compound) and a phosphorus-containing acid in place of one of the fatty acids.

lecithins: one type of phospholipid.

choline: a nutrient that can be made in the body from an amino acid.

emulsifiers: substances that mix with both fat and water and that disperse the fat in the water, forming an emulsion.

65

Sterols

Sterols are large, complex molecules consisting of interconnected rings of carbon. Cholesterol is the most familiar sterol, but others, such as vitamin D and the sex hormones (for example, testosterone), are important, too.

Sterols in Foods Foods derived from both plants and animals contain sterols, but only those from animals—meats, eggs, fish, poultry, and dairy products—contain significant amounts of cholesterol. Organ meats, such as liver and kidneys, and eggs are richest in cholesterol; cheeses and meats have less. Shellfish contain many sterols but much less cholesterol than was previously thought.

Sterols other than cholesterol are naturally found in plants. Being structurally similar to cholesterol, plant sterols interfere with cholesterol absorption. Food manufacturers have fortified foods such as margarine with plant sterols, creating a functional food that helps to reduce blood cholesterol.

Cholesterol Synthesis Like the lecithins, cholesterol can be made by the body, so it is not an essential nutrient. Right now, as you read, your liver is manufacturing cholesterol from fragments of carbohydrate, protein, and fat. Most of the body's cholesterol ends up in the membranes of cells, where it performs vital structural and metabolic functions.

Cholesterol's Two Routes in the Body After it is made, cholesterol leaves the liver by two routes:

1. It may be incorporated into bile, stored in the gallbladder, and delivered to the intestine.
2. It may travel, via the bloodstream, to all the body's cells.

The bile that is made from cholesterol in the liver is released into the intestine to aid in the digestion and absorption of fat. After bile does its job, most of it is absorbed and reused by the body; the rest is excreted in the feces.

Cholesterol Excreted While bile is in the intestine, some of it may be trapped by soluble fibers or by some medications, which carry it out of the body in feces. The excretion of bile reduces the total amount of cholesterol remaining in the body.

Cholesterol Transport As described in Chapter 5, some cholesterol, packaged with other lipids and protein, leaves the liver via the arteries and is transported to the body tissues by the blood. These packages of lipids and proteins are called **lipoproteins.** As the lipoproteins travel through the body, tissues can extract lipids from them. Cholesterol can be harmful to the body when it forms deposits in the artery walls. These deposits contribute to **atherosclerosis,** a disease that can cause heart attacks and strokes.

IN SUMMARY

▌ Table 3-2 summarizes the members of the lipid family.

▌ The predominant lipids both in foods and in the body are triglycerides, which have glycerol backbones with three fatty acids attached.

▌ Fatty acids vary in the length of their carbon chains and their degree of saturation. Those that are fully loaded with hydrogen atoms are saturated; those that are missing hydrogen atoms and therefore have double bonds are unsaturated (monounsaturated or polyunsaturated).

▌ Most triglycerides contain more than one type of fatty acid.

▌ Fatty acid saturation affects the physical characteristics and storage properties of fats.

sterols: one of the main classes of lipids; includes cholesterol, vitamin D, and the sex hormones (such as testosterone).

lipoproteins: clusters of lipids associated with proteins that serve as transport vehicles for lipids in the lymph and blood.

atherosclerosis (ath-er-oh-scler-OH-sis): a type of artery disease characterized by accumulations of lipid-containing material on the inner walls of the arteries (see Chapter 22).

- Hydrogenation, which makes polyunsaturated fats more saturated, gives rise to *trans*-fatty acids, altered fatty acids that may have health effects similar to those of saturated fatty acids.

- Linoleic acid and linolenic acid are essential nutrients. In addition to serving as structural parts of cell membranes, they make powerful substances that help regulate blood pressure, blood clot formation, and the immune response.

- Phospholipids, including the lecithins, have a unique chemical structure that allows them to be soluble in both water and fat.

- In the body, phospholipids are major constituents of cell membranes; the food industry uses phospholipids as emulsifiers.

- Sterols include cholesterol, bile, vitamin D, and the sex hormones.

- Only animal-derived foods contain significant amounts of cholesterol.

3.3 Health Effects and Recommended Intakes of Fats

LO 3.3 Explain the relationships among saturated fats, *trans* fat, cholesterol, monounsaturated and polyunsaturated fats, and chronic diseases, noting dietary intake recommendations.

Of all the dietary factors related to chronic diseases prevalent in developed countries, high intakes of certain fats are by far the most significant. The person who chooses a diet too high in saturated fats or *trans* fats invites the risk of **cardiovascular disease (CVD),** and heart disease is the number-one killer of adults in the United States and Canada. As for cancer, evidence is less compelling than for heart disease, but it does suggest that a diet high in certain kinds of fat is associated with a greater-than-average risk of developing some types of cancer.[9] Conversely, some research suggests that omega-3 fatty acids from fish may protect against some cancers.[10] Nutrition and cancer is a topic of Chapter 25.

Obesity carries serious risks to health. A diet high in energy-rich fatty foods makes it easy for people to exceed their energy needs and encourages unneeded weight gain.[11] An increasing waistline, in turn, often increases blood triglycerides, which can indicate an increased risk of heart disease and other chronic diseases.[12] The health risks of obesity are described in Chapter 6, and Chapter 7 focuses on weight management. The links between diet and disease are the focus of much research. Some points about fats and heart health are presented here because they underlie dietary recommendations concerning fats. Nutrition and heart disease is the topic of Chapter 22.

Fats and Heart Health

As noted earlier, cholesterol travels in the blood within lipoproteins. Two of the lipoproteins, LDL and HDL, play major roles with regard to heart health and are the focus of most recommendations made for reducing the risk of heart disease. A high blood LDL cholesterol concentration is a predictor of the likelihood of suffering a fatal heart attack or stroke, and the higher the LDL, the earlier the episode is expected to occur. A *low* blood concentration of HDL cholesterol also signifies a higher disease risk.[13]

Most people realize that elevated blood cholesterol is an important risk factor for heart disease. Most people may not realize, though, that cholesterol in *food* is not the main influential factor in raising *blood* cholesterol.

cardiovascular disease (CVD): a general term for all diseases of the heart and blood vessels (see Chapter 22).

Saturated Fats and Blood Cholesterol The main dietary factors associated with elevated blood LDL cholesterol are high saturated fat and high *trans* fat intakes.*[14] High LDL cholesterol levels increase the risk of heart disease because high LDL concentrations promote the uptake of cholesterol in the blood vessel walls. Nutrition in Practice 3 examines various types of fats and their roles in supporting or harming heart health.

Solid fats, introduced in Chapter 1, are foods or ingredients in foods (such as shortening in cakes or pies) that provide abundant saturated fat, *trans* fat, and/or cholesterol and many kcalories. The current American diet delivers excessive amounts of solid fats—representing an average of almost one-fifth of the day's total kcalories.[15] The easiest way to lower saturated fat, then, is to limit solid fats in the diet. Grain-based desserts, pizza, cheese, and processed and fatty meats are major providers of solid fats. Solid fats from animal sources contribute a great deal of the saturated fat in most people's diets. Some vegetable fats (coconut oil, palm kernel oil, and palm oil) and hydrogenated fats such as shortening or stick margarine provide smaller amounts of saturated fats.

It is important to note that replacing dietary saturated fats with added sugars and refined starches is often counterproductive.[16] The best diet for health not only replaces saturated fats with polyunsaturated and monounsaturated oils (as discussed in a later section), but also is adequate, balanced, kcalorie controlled, and based on mostly nutrient-dense whole foods.

Trans-Fatty Acids and Blood Cholesterol Consuming commercially derived *trans* fat poses a risk to the health of the heart and arteries by raising LDL and lowering HDL cholesterol, and by producing inflammation.[17] Commercially derived *trans* fats are found in the partially hydrogenated oils used in some margarines, snack foods, and prepared desserts. The risk to heart health from *trans* fats is similar to or slightly greater than that from saturated fat, so the *Dietary Guidelines for Americans* suggest that people keep *trans* fat intake as low as possible.[18] Limiting the intake of *trans* fats can improve blood cholesterol and lower the risk of heart disease. To that end, many restaurants and food manufacturers have taken steps to eliminate or greatly reduce *trans* fats in foods.[19]

For example, margarine makers have reformulated their products to contain much less *trans* fat. Soft or liquid varieties are made from unhydrogenated oils, which are mostly unsaturated and so are less likely to elevate blood cholesterol than the saturated fats of butter. Some margarines contain olive oil, omega-3 fatty acids, or plant sterols (mentioned earlier), making these products preferable to butter and other margarines for the heart.† The words *hydrogenated vegetable oil* or *shortening* in an ingredients list indicate *trans*-fatty acids in the product.

In the past, most commercially fried foods, from doughnuts to chicken, delivered a sizeable amount of *trans* fats to consumers. Today, newly formulated commercial oils and fats perform the same tasks as the previously used hydrogenated fats but with fewer *trans*-fatty acids. Some manufacturers, however, merely substitute saturated fats—which pose well-established risks to heart health—for *trans* fats. When reformulating their products, food companies must consider not only the fat composition, but also the taste, texture, cost, and availability of materials. No health benefits can be expected when saturated fats replace *trans* fats in the diet.

Dietary Cholesterol and Blood Cholesterol Although its effect is not as strong as that of saturated fat or *trans* fat, dietary cholesterol may contribute to elevated blood cholesterol in some people. Less clear is its role in heart disease.[20] The *Dietary Guidelines* recommend limiting dietary cholesterol to less than 300 milligrams per day for healthy people (less than 200 milligrams for some people with or at high risk of heart disease). On average, women take in about 240 milligrams a day and men take in

solid fats: fats that are not usually liquid at room temperature; commonly found in most foods derived from animals and vegetable oils that have been hydrogenated. Solid fats typically contain more saturated and *trans* fats than most oils. Also defined in Chapter 1.

---

*It should be noted that not all saturated fatty acids have the same cholesterol-raising effect. Stearic acid, an 18-carbon fatty acid, does not seem to raise blood cholesterol.

†Two brand names of margarines with plant sterols currently on the market are *Benecol* and *Promise activ.*

about 350 milligrams.[21] Foods providing the greatest share of cholesterol to the U.S. diet are eggs and egg dishes, chicken and chicken dishes, beef and beef dishes, and all types of beef burgers.

In healthy people, evidence suggests no association between consuming one egg per day and increased risk of heart disease.[22] For individuals with or at high risk of heart disease, however, consuming one egg per day may worsen or accelerate the progression of heart disease. The cholesterol content of one egg is about 210 milligrams.

Monounsaturated Fatty Acids and Blood Cholesterol Replacing saturated and *trans* fats with monounsaturated fat such as olive oil may be an effective dietary strategy to prevent heart disease. The lower rates of heart disease among people in the Mediterranean region of the world are often attributed to their liberal use of olive oil, a rich source of monounsaturated fatty acids.[23] Olive oil also delivers valuable phytochemicals that help to protect against heart disease.[24] Nutrition in Practice 3 examines the role of olive oil and other fats in supporting or harming heart health.

Polyunsaturated Fatty Acids, Blood Cholesterol, and Heart Disease Risk Polyunsaturated fatty acids (PUFA) of the omega-3 families are potent protectors against heart disease. The omega-3 fatty acids EPA and DHA, which are found mainly in fatty fish, exert their beneficial effects by influencing the function of both the heart and blood vessels. Specifically, EPA and DHA protect heart health by:[25]

Food Collection/Stockfood America

- Lowering blood triglycerides.

- Preventing blood clots.

- Protecting against irregular heartbeats.

- Lowering blood pressure.

- Defending against inflammation.

The primary member of the omega-3 family, linolenic acid, may benefit heart health as well, but evidence for this effect is much less certain than for EPA and DHA. Table 3-3 names sources of omega-6 and omega-3 fatty acids.

Grilling or broiling fish, instead of frying them, preserves their beneficial omega-3 fatty acids while adding little or no saturated fat.

TABLE 3-3 **Food Sources of Omega-3 and Omega-6 Fatty Acids**

Omega-3	
Linolenic acid	Oils (canola, flaxseed, soybean, walnut, wheat germ, liquid or soft margarine made from canola or soybean oil) Nuts and seeds (flaxseeds, walnuts, soybeans) Vegetables (soybeans)
EPA and DHA	Human milk Fish and seafood: *>500 mg per 3.5-oz serving:* European seabass (bronzini), herring (Atlantic and Pacific), mackerel, oyster (Pacific wild), salmon (wild and farmed), sardines, toothfish (includes Chilian seabass), trout (wild and farmed) *150–500 mg per 3.5-oz serving:* black bass, catfish (wild and farmed), clam, cod (Atlantic), crab (Alaskan king), croakers, flounder, haddock, hake, halibut, oyster (eastern and farmed), perch, scallop, shrimp (mixed varieties), sole, swordfish, tilapia (farmed) *<150 mg per 3.5-oz serving:* cod (Pacific), grouper, lobster, mahi-mahi, monkfish, red snapper, skate, triggerfish, tuna, wahoo
Omega-6	
Linoleic acid	Seeds, nuts, vegetable oils (corn, cottonseed, safflower, sesame, soybean, sunflower), poultry fat

© 2016 Cengage Learning®

The *Dietary Guidelines* recommend choosing 8 to 12 ounces of a variety of seafood each week, or about one of every five ounces of protein foods, to provide an average of 250 milligrams of EPA and DHA per day along with the beneficial array of other nutrients that seafood provides.[26] Greater heart health benefits can be expected when fish is grilled, baked, or broiled, partly because the varieties prepared this way often contain more EPA and DHA than species used for fried fish in fast-food restaurants and frozen products.[27] Additionally, benefits are attained by avoiding commercial frying fats, which may be laden with *trans* fat and saturated fat. Further benefits arise when fish replaces high-fat meats or other foods rich in saturated fats in several meals each week.

Some species of fish and shellfish, however, may contain significant levels of mercury or other environmental contaminants. Most healthy people can safely consume most species of ocean fish several times a week, but for some, the risks are greater. Women who may become pregnant, pregnant and lactating women, and children are more sensitive to contaminants than others, but even they can benefit from consuming safer fish varieties within recommended limits (see Chapter 11 for details).

For everyone, consuming a variety of different types of fish to minimize exposure to any single toxin that may accumulate in a favored species is a good idea. The fish most heavily contaminated with mercury are: king mackerel, shark, swordfish, and tilefish (also called golden bass or golden snapper). Those lower in mercury are: catfish, pollock, salmon, sardines, and canned light tuna. Canned albacore ("white") tuna generally contains more mercury than light tuna. Consumers should check local advisories to determine the safety of freshwater fish caught by family and friends.

Omega-3 Supplements Fish, not fish oil supplements, is the preferred source of omega-3 fatty acids. High intakes of omega-3 polyunsaturated fatty acids may increase bleeding time, interfere with wound healing, raise LDL cholesterol, and suppress immune function. Evidence is mixed for people with heart disease—several studies show hopeful results, while others reveal no benefits from supplements.[28] Because supplements pose risks, such as excessive bleeding, those taking daily fish oil supplements need medical supervision.[29] The benefits and risks from EPA and DHA illustrate an important concept in nutrition: too much of a nutrient is often as harmful as too little.

Recommendations

Some fat in the diet is essential for good health. The *Dietary Guidelines for Americans* recommend that a portion of each day's total fat come from raw oils. Oils are naturally present in foods such as nuts, avocados, and seafood. In addition, many commonly used oils such as olive, peanut, safflower, soybean, and sunflower oils are extracted from plants. When choosing oils, alternate among the various types to obtain the benefits different oils offer. Peanut and safflower oils are especially rich in vitamin E. Olive oil contributes naturally occurring antioxidant phytochemicals with potential heart benefits (see Nutrition in Practice 3), and canola oil is rich in monounsaturated and essential fatty acids. An adequate intake of the needed fat-soluble nutrients can be ensured by a small daily intake of oil: 27 grams (6 tsp) for a 2,000-kcalorie diet, for example (see Table 1-4 for recommendations for other kcalorie levels).

Defining the exact amount of fat, saturated fat, or cholesterol that benefits health or begins to harm health, however, is not possible. For this reason, no RDA or UL has been set. Instead, the DRI and *Dietary Guidelines* suggest a diet that is low in saturated fat, *trans* fat, and cholesterol and provides 20 to 35 percent of the daily energy intake from fat. These recommendations recognize that diets with up to 35 percent of kcalories from fat can be compatible with good health if energy intake is reasonable and saturated and *trans* fat intakes are low. When total fat intake exceeds 35 percent of kcalories, saturated fat intakes increase to unhealthy levels. For a 2,000-kcalorie diet, 20 to 35 percent represents 400 to 700 kcalories from fat (roughly 45 to 75 grams). Fat and oil intakes below 20 percent of kcalories increase the risk of inadequate essential fatty acid intakes. The FDA established Daily Values for food labels using 30 percent of energy intake as the guideline for fat.

Part of the allowance for total fat provides for the essential fatty acids—linoleic acid and linolenic acid—and Adequate Intakes (AI) have been established for these two fatty acids (see the inside front cover). The DRI suggest that linoleic acid provide 5 to 10 percent of the daily energy intake, and linolenic acid 0.6 to 1.2 percent.

Recommendations urge people to eat diets that are low in saturated fat, *trans* fat, and cholesterol. Specifically, consume less than 10 percent of kcalories from saturated fat, keep *trans* fat intakes as low as possible, and consume less than 300 milligrams of cholesterol each day.[30] To help consumers meet these goals, the FDA established Daily Values for food labels using 10 percent of energy intake for saturated fat; the Daily Value for cholesterol is 300 milligrams, regardless of energy intake. There is no Daily Value for *trans* fat.

IN SUMMARY

■ High intakes of saturated or *trans* fats contribute to heart disease, obesity, and other health problems.

■ High blood cholesterol, specifically, poses a risk of heart disease, and high intakes of saturated fat and *trans* fat contribute the most to high blood cholesterol. Cholesterol in foods presents less of a risk.

■ Polyunsaturated fatty acids of the omega-6 and omega-3 families protect against heart disease.

■ When monounsaturated fat such as olive oil replaces saturated and *trans* fats in the diet, the risk of heart disease may be lessened.

■ Though some fat in the diet is necessary, health authorities recommend a diet moderate in total fat and low in saturated fat, *trans* fat, and cholesterol.

3.4 Fats in Foods

LO 3.4 Identify the roles of fats in food and list sources of solid fats and unsaturated fats.

Fats are important in foods as well as in the body. Many of the compounds that give foods their flavors and aromas are found in fats and oils. The delicious aromas associated with bacon, ham, and other meats, as well as with onions being sautéed, come from fats. Fats also influence the texture of many foods, enhancing smoothness, creaminess, moistness, or crispness. In addition, four vitamins—A, D, E, and K—are soluble in fat. When the fat is removed from a food, many fat-soluble compounds, including these vitamins, are also removed. Table 3-4 summarizes the roles of fats in foods.

Fats are also an important part of most people's ethnic or national cuisines. Each culture has its own favorite food sources of fats and oils. In Canada, canola oil (also known as rapeseed oil) is widely used. In the Mediterranean area, Greeks, Italians, and Spaniards rely heavily on olive oil. Both canola oil and olive oil are rich sources of monounsaturated fatty acids. Asians use the polyunsaturated oil of soybeans. Jewish people traditionally employ chicken fat. Everywhere in North America, butter and margarine are widely used.

TABLE 3-4 The Functions of Fats in Foods

■ *Nutrient.* Food fats provide essential fatty acids and other raw materials.

■ *Energy.* Food fats provide a concentrated energy source.

■ *Transport.* Fats carry fat-soluble vitamins A, D, E, and K along with some phytochemicals and assist in their absorption.

■ *Sensory appeal.* Fats contribute to the taste and smell of foods.

■ *Appetite.* Fats stimulate the appetite.

■ *Satiety.* Fats contribute to feelings of fullness.

■ *Texture.* Fats make fried foods crisp and other foods tender.

© 2016 Cengage Learning®

Finding the Fats in Foods

The remainder of this chapter and the Nutrition in Practice show you how to choose fats wisely, with the goals of providing optimal health and pleasure in eating. To achieve such goals, you need to know which foods offer unsaturated oils that provide the essential fatty acids and which foods are loaded with solid fats—the saturated and *trans* fats. Also important for many people is learning to control portion sizes, particularly portions of fatty foods that can pack hundreds of kcalories into just a few bites.

Keep in mind that, whether solid or liquid, essential or nonessential, all fats bring the same abundant kcalories to the diet, and excesses contribute to body fat stores. According to the *Dietary Guidelines for Americans,* no benefits can be expected when oil is added to an already fat-rich eating pattern. The following amounts of these fats contain about 5 grams of pure fat, providing 45 kcalories and negligible protein and carbohydrate:

- 1 teaspoon of oil or shortening
- 1½ teaspoons of mayonnaise, butter, or margarine
- 1 tablespoon of regular salad dressing, cream cheese, or heavy cream
- 1½ tablespoons of sour cream

The solid fat of some foods, such as the rim of fat on a steak, is visible (and therefore identifiable and removable). Other solid fats, such as those in candy, cheeses, coconut, hamburger, homogenized milk, and lunch meats, are invisible (and therefore easily missed or ignored). Equally hidden are the solid fats blended into biscuits, cakes, cookies, chip dips, ice cream, mixed dishes, pastries, sauces, and creamy soups, and integral to fried foods. Invisible fats supply the majority of solid fats in the U.S. diet.[31]

Milk and Milk Products Milk products go by different names that reflect their varying fat contents (see Table 3-5). A cup of homogenized whole milk contains the protein and carbohydrate of fat-free milk, but in addition it contains about 80 extra kcalories from butterfat, a solid fat. A cup of reduced-fat (2 percent fat) milk falls between whole milk and fat-free, with 45 kcalories from fat.

Note that cream and butter do not appear in the milk and milk products group. Milk and yogurt are rich in calcium and protein, but cream and butter are not. Cream and butter are solid fats, as are whipped cream, sour cream, and cream cheese. Other cheeses, grouped with milk products, vary in their fat contents and are major contributors of saturated fat in people's diets.

Protein Foods Meats conceal a good deal of the fat—and much of the solid fat—that people consume. To help "see" the fat in meats, it is useful to think of them in three categories according to their fat contents: lean, medium-fat, and high-fat meats (as the Food Lists in Appendix C group them). Meats in all three categories contain about equal amounts of protein, but their fat, saturated fat, and kcalorie amounts vary significantly. Table 1-9 on p. 25 in Chapter 1 provided definitions for common terms used to describe the fat contents of meats.

The USDA Food Patterns suggest that most adults limit their intake of protein foods to about 5 to 7 ounces per day. For comparison, the smallest fast-food hamburger weighs about 3 ounces. A steak served in a restaurant often runs 8, 12, or 16 ounces, more than a whole day's meat allowance. You may have to weigh a serving or two of meat to see how much you are eating.

People think of meat as a protein food, but calculation of its nutrient content reveals a surprising fact. A big (4-ounce) fast-food hamburger sandwich contains 24 grams of protein and 18 grams of fat, 7 of them saturated fat. Because protein offers 4 kcalories per gram and fat offers 9, the sandwich provides 96 kcalories from

TABLE 3-5 Fat Options among Milk and Milk Products

Fat-free and low-fat options	Fat-free (skim) or 1% (low-fat) milk or yogurt (plain)
Reduced-fat options	2% milk or yogurt (plain)
High-fat options	Whole milk, yogurt Most cheeses

© 2016 Cengage Learning®

protein but 162 kcalories from fat. Hot dogs, fried chicken sandwiches, and fried fish sandwiches also provide hundreds of fat kcalories, mostly from invisible solid fat. Because so much meat fat is hidden from view, meat eaters can easily and unknowingly consume a great many grams of solid fat from this source.

When choosing beef or pork, look for lean cuts named *loin* or *round* from which the fat can be trimmed, and eat small portions. Chicken and turkey flesh are naturally lean, but commercial processing and frying add solid fats, especially in "patties," "nuggets," "fingers," and "wings." Chicken wings are mostly skin, and a chicken stores most of its fat just under its skin. The tastiest wing snacks have also been fried in cooking fat (often a hydrogenated, saturated type with *trans*-fatty acids); smothered with a buttery, spicy sauce; and then dipped in blue cheese dressing, making wings an extraordinarily high-fat snack. People who snack on wings may want to plan on eating low-fat foods at several other meals to balance them out.

Vegetables, Fruits, and Grains Choosing vegetables, fruits, whole grains, and legumes helps lower the saturated fat, cholesterol, and total fat content of the diet. Most vegetables and fruits naturally contain little or no fat; avocados and olives are exceptions, but most of their fat is unsaturated, which is not harmful to heart health. Most grains contain only small amounts of fat. Some refined grain *products* such as fried taco shells, croissants, and biscuits are high in saturated fat, so consumers need to read food labels. Similarly, many people add butter, margarine, or cheese sauce to grains and vegetables, which raises their saturated and *trans* fat contents. Because fruits are often eaten without added fat, a diet that includes several servings of fruit daily can help a person meet the dietary recommendations for fat.

A diet rich in vegetables, fruits, whole grains, and legumes offers abundant vitamin C, folate, vitamin A, vitamin E, and dietary fiber—all important in supporting health. Consequently, such a diet protects against disease both by reducing saturated fat, cholesterol, and total fat and by increasing nutrients. It also provides valuable phytochemicals that help defend against heart disease.

Cutting Solid Fats and Choosing Unsaturated Fats

Meeting today's lipid guidelines can be challenging. Reducing intakes of saturated and *trans* fatty acids, for example, involves identifying food sources of these fatty acids—that is, foods that contain solid fats. Then, replacing them appropriately involves identifying unsaturated oils. To help simplify these tasks, the *Dietary Guidelines* suggest:

1. Selecting the most nutrient-dense foods from all food groups. Solid fats and high-kcalorie choices can be found in every food group.
2. Consuming fewer and smaller portions of foods and beverages that contain solid fats.
3. Replacing solid fats with liquid oils whenever possible.
4. Checking Nutrition Facts labels and selecting foods with little saturated fat and no *trans* fat.

Such advice is easily dispensed but not easily followed. The first step in doing so is learning which foods contain heavy doses of solid fats. Table 3-6 lists some terms that indicate solid fats in a food label ingredients list.

Box 3-1 (p. 74) offers strategies for making heart-healthy choices, food group by food group. The best diet for heart health is also rich in fruits, vegetables, nuts, and whole grains that offer many health advantages by supplying abundant nutrients, fiber, and phytochemicals.

TABLE 3-6 Solid Fat Ingredients Listed on Food Labels

- Beef fat (tallow)
- Butter
- Chicken fat
- Coconut oil
- Cream
- Hydrogenated oil
- Milk fat
- Palm kernel oil; palm oil
- Partially hydrogenated oil
- Pork fat (lard)
- Shortening
- Stick margarine

Source: U.S. Department of Agriculture and U.S. Department of Health and Human Services, *Dietary Guidelines for Americans 2010,* available at www .dietaryguidelines.gov.

In General

▌ Select the most nutrient-dense foods from all food groups.

▌ Consume fewer and smaller portions of foods and beverages that contain solid fats.

▌ Check the Nutrition Facts label to choose foods with little or no saturated fat and no *trans* fat.

Breads and Cereals

▌ Select whole-grain breads, cereals, and crackers that are low in saturated and *trans* fat (for example, bagels instead of croissants).

▌ Prepare pasta with a tomato sauce instead of a cheese or cream sauce.

▌ Limit intake of cookies, doughnuts, pastries, and croissants.

Vegetables and Fruits

▌ Enjoy the natural flavor of steamed vegetables (without butter) for dinner and fruits for dessert.

▌ Eat at least two vegetables (in addition to a salad) with dinner.

▌ Snack on raw vegetables or fruits instead of high-fat items like potato chips.

▌ Buy frozen vegetables without sauce.

Milk and Milk Products

▌ Switch from whole milk to reduced-fat, from reduced-fat to low-fat, and from low-fat to fat-free (nonfat).

▌ Use fat-free and low-fat cheeses (such as part-skim ricotta and low-fat mozzarella) instead of regular cheeses.

▌ Use fat-free or low-fat yogurt or sour cream instead of regular sour cream.

▌ Use evaporated fat-free milk instead of cream.

▌ Enjoy fat-free frozen yogurt, sherbet, or ice milk instead of ice cream.

Protein Foods

▌ Fat adds up quickly, even with lean meat; limit intake to about 6 ounces (cooked weight) daily.

▌ Eat at least two servings of fish per week (particularly fish such as mackerel, lake trout, herring, sardines, and salmon).

▌ Choose fish, poultry, or lean cuts of pork or beef; look for unmarbled cuts named *round* or *loin* (eye of round, top round, bottom round, round tip, tenderloin, sirloin, center loin, and top loin).

▌ Trim the fat from pork and beef; remove the skin from poultry.

▌ Grill, roast, broil, bake, stir-fry, stew, or braise meats; don't fry. When possible, place food on a rack so that fat can drain.

▌ Use lean ground turkey or lean ground beef in recipes; brown ground meats without added fat, then drain off fat.

▌ Select tuna, sardines, and other canned meats packed in water; rinse oil-packed items with hot water to remove much of the fat.

▌ Fill kabob skewers with lots of vegetables and slivers of meat; create main dishes and casseroles by combining a little meat, fish, or poultry with whole-grain pasta or brown rice and generous amounts of vegetables.

▌ Use legumes often.

▌ Eat a meatless meal or two daily.

▌ Use egg substitutes in recipes instead of whole eggs, or use two egg whites in place of each whole egg.

Fats and Oils

▌ Use small amounts of vegetable oils in place of solid fats.

▌ Use butter or stick margarine sparingly; select soft margarines instead of hard margarines.

▌ Use fruit butters, reduced-kcalorie margarines, or butter replacers instead of butter.

▌ Use low-fat or fat-free mayonnaise and salad dressing instead of regular.

▌ Limit use of lard and meat fat.

▌ Limit use of products made with coconut oil, palm kernel oil, and palm oil (read labels on bakery goods, processed foods, microwave popcorn, and nondairy creamers).

▌ Reduce use of hydrogenated shortenings and stick margarines and products that contain them (read labels on crackers, cookies, and other commercially prepared baked goods); use vegetable oils instead.

Miscellaneous

▌ Use a nonstick pan, or coat the pan lightly with vegetable oil.

▌ Refrigerate soups and stews; when the fat solidifies, remove it before reheating.

▌ Use wine; lemon, orange, or tomato juice; herbs; spices; fruits; or broth instead of butter or margarine when cooking.

▌ Stir-fry in a small amount of oil; add moisture and flavor with broth, tomato juice, or wine.

▌ Use variety to enhance enjoyment of the meal: vary colors, textures, and temperatures—hot, cooked versus cool, raw foods—and use garnishes to complement food.

▌ Omit high-fat meat gravies and cheese sauces.

▌ Order pizzas with lots of vegetables, a little lean meat, and half the cheese.

Pork chop with fat (290 kcal, 24 g fat, 9 g saturated fat)

Potato with 1 tbs butter and 1 tbs sour cream (315 kcal, 14 g fat, 9 g saturated fat)

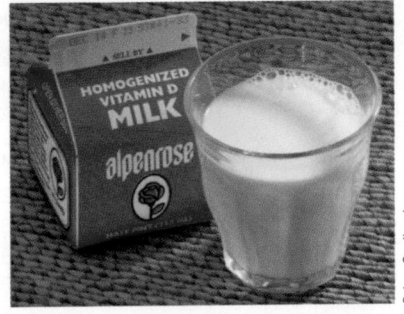

Whole milk, 1 c (150 kcal, 8 g fat, 5 g saturated fat)

Pork chop with fat trimmed off (174 kcal, 8 g fat, 3 g saturated fat)

Savings:
116 kcal, 16 g fat, 6 g saturated fat

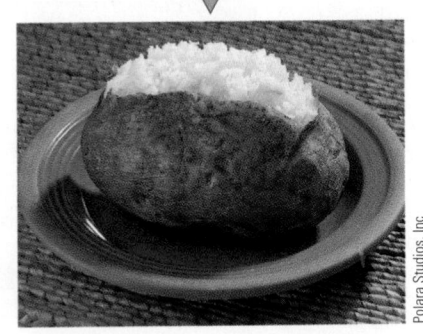

Plain potato (188 kcal, <1 g fat, 0 g saturated fat)

Savings:
127 kcal, 13 g fat, 9 g saturated fat

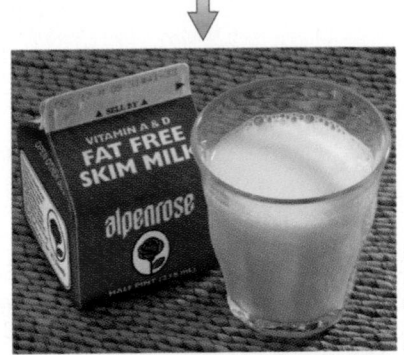

Fat-free milk, 1 c (90 kcal, <1 g fat, <1 g saturated fat)

Savings:
60 kcal, 7 g fat, 4 g saturated fat

FIGURE 3-5 Cutting Fat Cuts kCalories—and Saturated Fat

Fats and kCalories Removing fat from food also removes energy, as Figure 3-5 shows. A pork chop with the fat trimmed to within a half-inch of the lean provides 290 kcalories; with the fat trimmed off completely, it supplies 174 kcalories. A baked potato with butter and sour cream (1 tablespoon each) has 315 kcalories; a plain baked potato has 188 kcalories. The single most effective step you can take to reduce the energy value of a food is to eat it with less fat.

Choosing Unsaturated Fats When a person does eat fats, those to choose are the unsaturated ones. Remember, the softer a fat is, the more unsaturated it is. Generally speaking, vegetable and fish oils are rich in polyunsaturates, olive oil and canola oil are rich in monounsaturates, and the harder fats—animal fats—are more saturated (see Figure 3-6 on p. 76). Remember, however, that vegetable fat or vegetable oil doesn't always mean unsaturated fat. Both coconut oil and palm oil, for example, which are often used in nondairy creamers, are saturated fats, and both raise blood cholesterol.

Don't Overdo Fat Restriction Some people actually manage to eat too *little* fat—to their detriment. Among them are young women and men with eating disorders, described in Nutrition in Practice 6. As a practical guideline, it is wise to include the equivalent of at least a teaspoon of fat in every meal.

Fat Replacers Today, consumers can choose from thousands of fat-reduced products. Many bakery goods, lunch meats, cheeses, spreads, frozen desserts, and other products made with **fat replacers** offer less than half a gram of fat, saturated fat, and

At room temperature, unsaturated fats (such as those found in oil), are usually liquid, whereas saturated fats (such as those found in butter) are solid.

fat replacers: ingredients that replace some or all of the functions of fat in foods and may or may not provide energy.

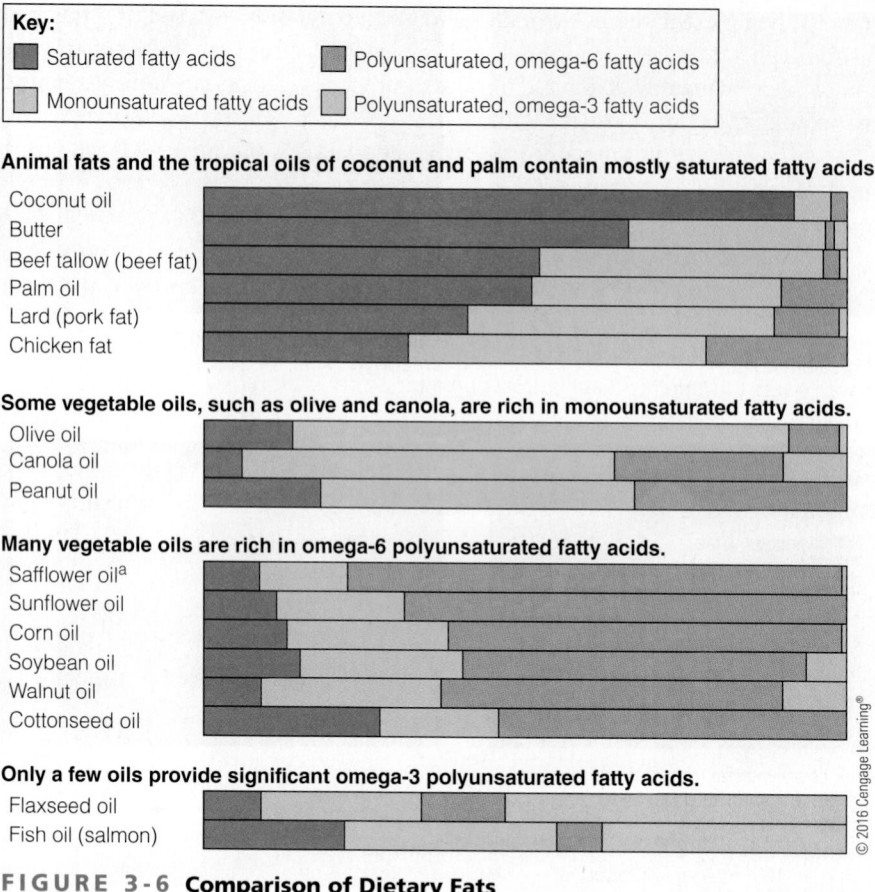

Key:
- Saturated fatty acids
- Monounsaturated fatty acids
- Polyunsaturated, omega-6 fatty acids
- Polyunsaturated, omega-3 fatty acids

Animal fats and the tropical oils of coconut and palm contain mostly saturated fatty acids.
- Coconut oil
- Butter
- Beef tallow (beef fat)
- Palm oil
- Lard (pork fat)
- Chicken fat

Some vegetable oils, such as olive and canola, are rich in monounsaturated fatty acids.
- Olive oil
- Canola oil
- Peanut oil

Many vegetable oils are rich in omega-6 polyunsaturated fatty acids.
- Safflower oil[a]
- Sunflower oil
- Corn oil
- Soybean oil
- Walnut oil
- Cottonseed oil

Only a few oils provide significant omega-3 polyunsaturated fatty acids.
- Flaxseed oil
- Fish oil (salmon)

© 2016 Cengage Learning®

FIGURE 3-6 Comparison of Dietary Fats
Most fats are a mixture of saturated, monounsaturated, and polyunsaturated fatty acids.
[a]Salad or cooking type over 70% linoleic acid.

trans fat in a serving. Some of these products contain **artificial fats,** and others use conventional ingredients in unconventional ways to reduce fats and kcalories. Among the latter, manufacturers can:

- Add water or whip air into foods.
- Add fat-free milk to creamy foods.
- Use lean meats and soy protein to replace high-fat meats.
- Bake foods instead of frying them.

Common food ingredients such as fibers, sugars, or proteins can also take the place of fats in some foods. Products made from sugars or proteins still provide kcalories but far fewer kcalories from fats. Manufactured fat replacers consist of chemical derivatives of carbohydrate, protein, or fat, or modified versions of foods rich in those constituents.

A familiar example of an artificial fat that has been approved for use in snack foods such as potato chips, crackers, and tortilla chips is **olestra.** Olestra's chemical structure is similar to that of a regular fat (a triglyceride) but with important differences. A triglyceride is composed of a glycerol molecule with three fatty acids attached, whereas olestra is made of a sucrose molecule with six to eight fatty acids attached. Enzymes in the digestive tract cannot break the bonds of olestra, so unlike sucrose or fatty acids, olestra passes through the system unabsorbed.

The FDA's evaluation of olestra's safety addressed two questions. First, is olestra toxic? Research on both animals and humans supports the safety of olestra as a partial replacement for dietary fats and oils, with no reports of cancer or birth defects. Second, does olestra affect either nutrient absorption or the health of the digestive

artificial fats: zero-energy fat replacers that are chemically synthesized to mimic the sensory and cooking qualities of naturally occurring fats but are totally or partially resistant to digestion.

olestra: a synthetic fat made from sucrose and fatty acids that provides zero kcalories per gram; also known as *sucrose polyester.*

76

tract? When olestra passes through the digestive tract unabsorbed, it binds with the fat-soluble vitamins A, D, E, and K and carries them out of the body, robbing the person of these valuable nutrients. To compensate for these losses, the FDA requires the manufacturer to fortify olestra with vitamins A, D, E, and K. Saturating olestra with these vitamins does not make the product a good source of vitamins, but it does block olestra's ability to bind with the vitamins from other foods. An asterisk in the ingredients list informs consumers that these added vitamins are "dietarily insignificant."

Consumers need to keep in mind that low-fat and fat-free foods still deliver kcalories. Decades ago, consumers hailed the arrival of artificial sweeteners as a weight-loss wonder, but in reality, kcalories saved by using artificial sweeteners were readily replaced by kcalories from other foods. Alternatives to fat can help to lower energy intake and support weight loss only when they actually *replace* fat and energy in the diet.

Read Food Labels Labels list total fat, saturated fat, *trans* fat, and cholesterol contents of foods. Because each package provides information for a single serving, and serving sizes are standardized, consumers can easily compare similar products.

IN SUMMARY

▌ Fats in foods contribute to sensory appeal—enhancing the flavor, aroma, and texture of foods.

▌ Fats in foods deliver fat-soluble vitamins, energy, and essential fatty acids.

▌ While some fat in the diet is necessary, the *Dietary Guidelines for Americans* recommend limiting intakes of saturated fat and *trans* fat.

▌ Fats added to foods during preparation or at the table are a major source of fat in the diet.

▌ The choice between whole and fat-free milk products can make a big difference to the fat, saturated fat, and cholesterol content of a diet.

▌ Meats account for a large proportion of hidden solid fats in many people's diets.

▌ Most people consume more meat than is recommended.

▌ Most vegetables and fruits naturally contain little or no fat.

▌ Grain products such as croissants and biscuits can be high in saturated fat, so consumers need to read food labels to learn which foods in this group contain fats.

▌ Consumers today can choose from an array of fat-reduced products, and many bakery goods and other foods made with fat replacers offer less than a half a gram of fat, saturated fat, and *trans* fat in a serving.

▌ Some products use artificial fats such as olestra, while others use conventional ingredients such as water or fat-free milk to reduce fat and kcalories.

▌ Food labels list total fat, saturated fat, cholesterol, and *trans* fat.

Chapters 2 and 3 have looked briefly at the two major energy fuels in the body—carbohydrate and fat. When used for energy, each has desirable characteristics. The glucose derived from carbohydrate is needed by the brain and nerve tissues and is easily used for energy in other cells. Fat is a particularly useful fuel because the body stores it efficiently and in generous amounts. Chapter 4 looks at protein, a nutrient that can be used as fuel, but whose primary role is to provide machinery for getting things done.

Your Diet

Lipids

To maintain good health, eat enough fat—but not too much—and select the right kinds of fats. For example, moderate intakes of foods rich in polyunsaturated and monounsaturated fatty acids such as olive oil, nuts, and fish lower the risk of heart disease. Conversely, diets high in saturated fats and *trans* fats increase the risk of heart disease. Table NP3-1 (p. 84) in the Nutrition in Practice that follows this chapter lists food sources of healthful and harmful fatty acids. As Chapter 3 describes, the major sources of saturated fats in most people's diets are whole milk and whole milk products such as cheese and ice cream, fatty cuts of beef and pork, processed meats such as bacon and sausage, and products that contain tropical oils (coconut oil, palm kernel oil, and palm oil) such as cookies, pastries, and doughnuts. Major sources of *trans* fats include fast foods, chips, baked goods, and other commercially prepared foods.

■ Make a list of all the fast foods and packaged foods such as chips and cookies that you ate today, or that you might typically eat in a day.

■ Use Appendix A or the restaurant's website to look up the saturated fat contents of the fast foods you ate and add this information to your list of foods.

■ Check the labels of the packaged foods you ate and write down their saturated and *trans* fat contents.

■ The recommended saturated fat intake is less than 10 percent of total kcalories per day. The recommendation for *trans* fat is to keep it as low as possible. Thus, for a 2,000-kcalorie diet, the recommended saturated fat intake is 22 grams or less. (Recall that 1 gram of fat is equal to 9 kcalories.)

Example:

$$2000 \text{ kcal} \times 0.10 = 200 \text{ kcal}$$
$$200 \text{ kcal} \div 9 \text{ kcal/gram fat} = 22 \text{ grams saturated fat}$$

■ Based on your own estimated kcalorie needs (see Table 1-5 on p. 18), is your saturated fat intake 10 percent or less of total kcalories?

Estimated kcalorie need: _____ kcalories

Saturated fat recommendation: _____ grams

Your saturated fat intake: _____ grams

■ If not, list several foods you consumed that supplied large amounts of saturated fat and suggest alternative foods in the same food group that contain less.

■ If your food choices included packaged or fast foods that contain significant amounts of *trans* fats, suggest alternative foods in the same food group that contain minimal amounts.

Clinical Applications

1. The connection between the overconsumption of saturated and *trans* fats and chronic diseases (obesity, diabetes, cancer, and cardiovascular disease) underscores the importance of being alert to a client's fat intake. What advice would you offer a client who reports the following?

   ■ Eats more than 12 ounces of meat each day.

   ■ Drinks whole milk and eats regular cheddar cheese each day.

   ■ Eats the following breads and cereals each day: a bagel with cream cheese for breakfast, a bologna sandwich on white bread for lunch, and biscuits or cornbread with butter to accompany dinner.

   ■ Eats less than the equivalent of a cup of fruit each day and eats vegetables only on occasion.

2. Make a list of foods, beverages, and seasonings that your client can substitute for foods high in saturated fat.

Self Check

1. Three classes of lipids in the body are:
   a. triglycerides, fatty acids, and cholesterol.
   b. triglycerides, phospholipids, and sterols.
   c. fatty acids, phospholipids, and cholesterol.
   d. glycerol, fatty acids, and triglycerides.

2. A triglyceride consists of:
   a. three glycerols attached to a lipid.
   b. three fatty acids attached to a glucose.
   c. three fatty acids attached to a glycerol.
   d. three phospholipids attached to a cholesterol.

3. A fatty acid that has the maximum possible number of hydrogen atoms is known as a(n):
   a. saturated fatty acid.
   b. monounsaturated fatty acid.
   c. PUFA.
   d. essential fatty acid.

4. The difference between *cis*- and *trans*-fatty acids is:
   a. the number of double bonds.
   b. the length of their carbon chains.
   c. the location of the first double bond.
   d. the configuration around the double bond.

5. Essential fatty acids:
   a. are used to make substances that regulate blood pressure, among other functions.
   b. can be made from carbohydrates.
   c. include lecithin and cholesterol.
   d. cannot be found in commonly eaten foods.

6. Lecithins and other phospholipids in the body function as:
   a. emulsifiers.
   b. enzymes.
   c. temperature regulators.
   d. shock absorbers.

7. To minimize saturated fat intake and lower the risk of heart disease, most people need to:
   a. eat less meat.
   b. select fat-free milk.
   c. use nonhydrogenated margarines and cooking oils such as olive oil or canola oil.
   d. All of the above

8. To include omega-3 fatty acids in the diet, the *Dietary Guidelines for Americans* recommend eating:
   a. cholesterol-free margarine.
   b. fish oil supplements.
   c. hydrogenated margarine.
   d. 8 to 12 ounces of seafood per week.

9. Some examples of foods with hidden solid fats are:
   a. cheese, lettuce, and fruit juices.
   b. fried foods, sauces, dips, and lunch meats.
   c. fish, rice, and nuts.
   d. baked potatoes, vegetables, and fruits.

10. Generally speaking, vegetable and fish oils are rich in:
    a. polyunsaturated fat.
    b. saturated fat.
    c. cholesterol.
    d. *trans*-fatty acids.

Answers to these questions are found in Appendix H.

Notes

1. H. Cao, Adipocytokines in obesity and metabolic disease, *Journal of Endocrinology* 220 (2014): T47–T59; C. Stryjecki and D. M. Mutch, Fatty acid–gene interactions, adipokines, and obesity, *European Journal of Clinical Nutrition* 65 (2011): 285–297; N. Ouchi and coauthors, Adipokines in inflammation and metabolic disease, *Nature Reviews, Immunology* 11 (2011): 85–97; Y. Deng and P. E. Scherer, Adipokines as novel biomarkers and regulators of the metabolic syndrome, *Annals of the New York Academy of Sciences* 1212 (2010): E1–E19.

2. Position of the Academy of Nutrition and Dietetics: Dietary fatty acids for healthy adults, *Journal of the Academy of Nutrition and Dietetics* 114 (2014): 136–153; A. S. Go and coauthors, Heart disease and stroke statistics—2014 update: A report from the American Heart Association, *Circulation* 129 (2014): e28–e292; D. Mozaffarian, J. Lawrence, and L. Van Horn, Recent advances in preventive cardiology and lifestyle medicine, *Circulation* 123 (2011): 2870–2891; V. Remig and coauthors, *Trans* fats in America: A review of their use, consumption, health implications, and regulation, *Journal of the American Dietetic Association* 110 (2010): 585–592.

3. E. Lacroix and coauthors, Randomized controlled study of the effect of a butter naturally enriched in *trans* fatty acids on blood lipids in healthy women, *American Journal of Clinical Nutrition* 95 (2012): 318–325; S. Gebauer and coauthors, Effects of ruminant trans fatty acids on cardiovascular disease and cancer: A comprehensive review of epidemiological, clinical, and mechanistic studies, *Advances in Nutrition* 2 (2011): 332–354; I. A. Brouwer, A. J. Wanders, and M. B. Katan, Effect of animal and industrial trans fatty acids on HDL and LDL cholesterol levels in humans—A quantitative review, *PLoS ONE* 5 (2010): e9434.

4. S. W. Ing and M. A. Belury, Impact of conjugated linoleic acid on bone physiology: Proposed mechanism involving inhibition of adipogenesis, *Nutrition Reviews* 69 (2011): 123–131; L. A. Smit, A. Baylin, and H. Campos, Conjugated linoleic acid in adipose tissue and risk of myocardial infarction, *American Journal of Clinical Nutrition* 92 (2010): 34–40.

5. Position of the Academy of Nutrition and Dietetics, Dietary fatty acids for healthy adults, 2014; G. H. Johnson and K. Fritsche, Effect of dietary linoleic acid on markers of inflammation in healthy persons: A systematic review of randomized controlled trials, *Journal of the Academy of Nutrition and Dietetics* 112 (2012): 1029–1041; R. J. Deckelbaum and C. Torrejon, The omega-3 fatty acid nutritional landscape: Health benefits and sources, *Journal of Nutrition* 142 (2012): 587S–591S.

6. N. G. Bazan, M. F. Molina, and W. C. Gordon, Docosahexaenoic acid signalolipidomics in nutrition: Significance in aging, neuroinflammation, macular degeneration, Alzheimer's, and other neurodegenerative diseases, *Annual Review of Nutrition* 31 (2011): 321–351; R. K. McNamara and coauthors, Docosahexaenoic acid supplementation increases prefrontal cortex activation during sustained attention in healthy boys: A placebo-controlled, dose-ranging, functional magnetic resonance imaging study, *American Journal of Clinical Nutrition* 91 (2010): 1060–1067.

7. Bazan, Molina, and Gordon, 2011; E. E. Birch and coauthors, The DIAMOND (DHA Intake and Measurement of Neural Development) Study: A double-masked, randomized controlled clinical trial of the maturation of infant visual acuity as a function of the dietary level of docosahexaenoic acid, *American Journal of Clinical Nutrition* 91 (2010): 848–859.

8. D. Mozaffarian and J. H. Y. Wu, Omega-3 fatty acids and cardiovascular disease: Effects on risk factors, molecular pathways, and clinical events, *Journal of the American College of Cardiology* 58 (2011): 2047–2067; M. N. Di Minno and coauthors, Exploring newer cardioprotective strategies: ω-3 fatty acids in perspective, *Thrombosis and Haemostasis* 104 (2010): 664–680.

9. A. M. Ismail and coauthors, Extra virgin olive oil potentiates the effects of aromatase inhibitors via glutathione depletion in estrogen receptor-positive human breast cancer (MCF-7) cells, *Food and Chemical Toxicology* 62 (2013): 817–824; T. Psaltopoulou and coauthors, Olive oil intake is inversely related to cancer prevalence: A systematic review and a meta-analysis of 13800 patients and 23340 controls in 19 observational studies, *Lipids in Health and Disease* 10 (2011): 127–143; M. Solanas and coauthors, Dietary olive oil and corn oil differentially affect experimental breast cancer through distinct modulation of the p21 Ras signaling and the proliferation-apoptosis balance, *Carcinogenesis* 31 (2010): 871–879.

10. J. Sheng Zheng and coauthors, Intake of fish and marine n-3 polyunsaturated fatty acids and risk of breast cancer: Meta-analysis of data from 21 independent prospective cohort studies, *BMJ* 346 (2013): f3706; S. Wu and coauthors, Fish consumption and colorectal cancer risk in humans: A systematic review and meta-analysis, *The American Journal of Medicine* 125 (2012): 551–559;T. M. Brasky and coauthors, Specialty supplements and breast cancer risk in the VITamins And Lifestyle (VITAL) Cohort, *Cancer Epidemiology, Biomarkers, and Prevention* 19 (2010); 1696–1708.

11. G. A. Bray, Is dietary fat important? *American Journal of Clinical Nutrition* 93 (2011): 481–482.

12. M. Miller and coauthors, Triglycerides and cardiovascular disease: A scientific statement from the American Heart Association, *Circulation* 123 (2011): 2292–2333.

13. Go and coauthors, 2014; J. Heineckem, HDL and cardiovascular-disease risk: Time for a new approach? *New England Journal of Medicine* 364 (2011): 170–171.

14. S. J. Baum and coauthors, Fatty acids in cardiovascular health and disease: A comprehensive update, *Journal of Clinical Lipidology* 6 (2012): 216–234; A. Astrup, The role of reducing intakes

of saturated fats in the prevention of cardiovascular disease: Where does the evidence stand in 2010? *American Journal of Clinical Nutrition* 93 (2011): 684-688.

15. U.S. Department of Agriculture, U.S. Department of Health and Human Services, *Dietary Guidelines for Americans 2010*, available at www .dietaryguidelines.gov.

16. Baum and coauthors, 2012; K. Zelman, The great fat debate: A closer look at the controversy—Questioning the validity of age-old dietary guidance, *Journal of the American Dietetic Association* 111 (2011): 655–658.

17. Position of the American Academy of Nutrition and Dietetics, Dietary fatty for healthy adults, 2014; P. Nestel, Trans fatty acids: Are its cardiovascular risks fully appreciated? *Clinical Therapeutics* 36 (2014): 315–321; Brouwer, Wanders, and Katan, 2010.

18. U.S. Department of Agriculture, U.S. Department of Health and Human Services, *Dietary Guidelines for Americans 2010*, available at www .dietaryguidelines.gov.

19. F. O. Otite and coauthors, Trends in trans fatty acids reformulations of US supermarket brand-name foods from 2007 through 2011, *Preventing Chronic Disease* 10 (2013): E85; V. Bemig and coauthors, *Trans* fats in America; A review of their use, consumption, health implications, and regulation, *Journal of the American Dietetic Association* 110 (2010): 585–592.

20. D. J. McNamara, Dietary cholesterol, heart disease risk and cognitive dissonance, *Proceedings of the Nutrition Society* 73 (2014): 161-166; A. M. Brownawell and M. C. Falk, Where science and public health policy intersect, *Nutrition Reviews* 68 (2010): 355–364; M. L. Fernandez and M. Calle, Revisiting dietary cholesterol recommendations: Does the evidence support a limit of 300 mg/d, *Current Atherosclerosis Reports* 12 (2010): 377–383.

21. U.S. Department of Agriculture, U.S. Department of Health and Human Services, *Dietary Guidelines for Americans 2010*, available at www .dietaryguidelines.gov.

22. J. Y. Shin and coauthors, Egg consumption in relation to risk of cardiovascular disease and diabetes: A systematic review and meta-analysis, *American Journal of Clinical Nutrition* 98 (2013): 146–159; M. R. Flock and P. M. Kris-Etherton, Dietary Guidelines for Americans 2010: Implications for cardiovascular disease, *Current Atherosclerosis Reports* 13 (2011): 499–507.

23. O. Castañer and coauthors, Protection of LDL from oxidation by olive oil polyphenols is associated with a downregulation of CD40-ligand expression and its downstream products in vivo in humans, *American Journal of Clinical Nutrition* 95 (2012): 1238–1244; S. Cicerale, L. J. Lucas, and R. S. Keast, Antimicrobial, antioxidant and anti-inflammatory phenolic activities in extra virgin olive oil, *Current Opinion in Biotechnology* 23 (2012): 129–135; C. Samieri and coauthors, Olive oil consumption, plasma oleic acid, and stroke incidence: The Three-City Study, *Neurology* 77 (2011): 418–425.

24. Castañer and coauthors, 2012; Cicerale, Lucas, and Keast, 2012.

25. Baum and coauthors, 2012; Flock and Kris-Etherton, 2011; Mozaffarian and Wu, 2011.

26. U.S. Department of Agriculture, U.S. Department of Health and Human Services, *Dietary Guidelines for Americans 2010*, available at www .dietaryguidelines.gov.

27. R. J. Belin and coauthors, Fish intake and the risk of incident heart failure: The Women's Health Initiative, *Circulation Heart Failure* 4 (2011): 404–413.

28. P. C. Calder, Mechanisms of action of (n-3) fatty acids, *Journal of Nutrition* 142 (2012): 592S–599S; S. M. Kwak and coauthors, Efficacy of omega-3 fatty acid supplements (eicosapentaenoic acid and docosahexaenoic acid) in the secondary prevention of cardiovascular disease: a meta-analysis of randomized, double-blind, placebo-controlled trials, *Archives of Internal Medicine,* 172 (2012): 686–694; V. A. Andreeva and coauthors, B vitamin and/or ω-3 fatty acid supplementation and cancer, *Archives of Internal Medicine* 172 (2012): 540–547; Flock and Kris-Etherton, 2011.

29. American Heart Association, Fish 101, www.heart.org/HEARTORG/GettingHealthy /NutritionCenter/Fish-101_UCM_305986_Article .jsp, updated February 21, 2014.

30. U.S. Department of Agriculture, U.S. Department of Health and Human Services, *Dietary Guidelines for Americans 2010*, available at www .dietaryguidelines.gov.

31. U.S. Department of Agriculture, U.S. Department of Health and Human Services, *Dietary Guidelines for Americans 2010*, available at www .dietaryguidelines.gov.

LO 3.5 Identify which fats support health and which may impair it.

To consumers, advice about dietary fat appears to change almost daily. "Eat less fat." "Eat more fatty fish." "Give up butter—use margarine instead." "Give up margarine—replace it with olive oil." "Steer clear of saturated fats." "Seek out omega-3." "Stay away from *trans* fats." "Stick with mono- and polyunsaturated fats." No wonder some people feel confused about dietary fat. This Nutrition in Practice begins with a look at the dietary guidelines for fat intake. It continues by identifying which foods provide which fats. It closes with strategies to help consumers choose the right amounts of the right kinds of fats for a healthy diet.

Why do today's fat messages seem to change constantly and become more confusing?

The confusion stems in part from the complexities of fat and in part from the nature of recommendations. As Chapter 3 explained, "dietary fat" refers to several kinds of fats; some fats support health, whereas others damage it, and foods typically provide a mixture of fats in varying proportions. It has taken researchers decades to sort through the relationships among the various kinds of fat and their roles in supporting or harming health. Translating these research findings into dietary recommendations is a challenging process. Too little information can mislead consumers, but too much detail can overwhelm them. As scientific understanding has grown, recommendations have evolved to become less general and more specific. Recommendations may seem to "change constantly and become more confusing," but in fact they are becoming more meaningful.

How exactly have dietary recommendations for fat changed to become more meaningful for consumers?

Dietary recommendations for fat have shifted away from reducing total fat, in general, to limiting saturated and *trans* fats, specifically, along with a greater emphasis on kcalorie control to maintain a healthy body weight.[1] For decades, health experts urged consumers to limit total fat intake to 30 percent or less of energy intake. This advice was straightforward—cut the fat and improve your health. Health experts recognized that saturated fats and *trans* fats were the ones that raise blood cholesterol, but they reasoned that when total fat was limited, saturated and *trans* fat intake would decline as well. People were simply advised to cut back on all fat so that they would cut back on saturated and *trans* fat. Such advice may have oversimplified the message and unnecessarily restricted total fat.

But low-fat diets have been recommended for years to help people manage weight and reduce the risk of heart disease. Are you saying that low-fat diets are no longer recommended?

Low-fat diets remain a key recommendation in treatment plans for people with elevated blood lipids or heart disease and,

therefore, they are important in nutrition.[2] As for healthy people, evidence from around the world has led researchers to change population-wide recommendations from a "low-fat" to a "wise-fat" approach. Several problems accompany low-fat diets. For one, many people find low-fat diets difficult to maintain over time. For another, low-fat diets are not necessarily low-kcalorie diets; if energy intake exceeds energy needs, weight gain follows, and obesity brings a host of health problems, including heart disease. For another, diets high in refined carbohydrates, even if low in fat, can cause blood triglycerides to rise and HDL to fall, a deleterious combination for heart health.[3] Finally, taken to the extreme, a low-fat diet may exclude fatty fish, nuts, seeds, and vegetable oils—all valuable sources of many essential fatty acids, phytochemicals, vitamins, and minerals. The fats from these sources protect against heart disease, as later sections explain.

How have today's recommendations for fat been revised?

Today, health experts have revised dietary recommendations to acknowledge that not all fats have damaging health consequences.[4] In fact, higher intakes of some kinds of fats (for example, the omega-3 fatty acids) support good health. Instead of urging people to cut back on all fats, current recommendations suggest carefully replacing the "bad" saturated and *trans* fats with the "good" unsaturated fats and enjoying these fats within kcalorie limits.[5] The goal is to create an overall eating pattern moderate in kcalories that provides enough of the fats that support good health, but not too much of those that harm health. (Turn to pp. 68–70 for a review of the health consequences of each type of fat.)

With these findings and goals in mind, the committee writing the *Dietary Guidelines for Americans 2010* concluded that a diet containing up to 35 percent of total kcalories from fat, but reduced in saturated fat and *trans* fat and moderate in energy, is compatible with low rates of heart disease, diabetes, obesity, and cancer.[6]

How can people distinguish between the fats in foods that support health and those that might harm it?

Asking consumers to limit their total fat intake was less than perfect advice, but it was straightforward—find the fat and cut back. Asking consumers to keep their intakes of saturated fats, *trans* fats, and cholesterol low and to use monounsaturated and polyunsaturated fats instead may be more on target with heart health, but it also makes diet planning more complicated. To make appropriate selections, consumers must first learn which foods contain which fats. For example, avocados, bacon, walnuts, potato chips, and mackerel are all high-fat foods, yet some of these foods have detrimental effects on heart health when consumed in excess, and others seem neutral or even beneficial.

Is there evidence to clarify why some high-fat foods are compatible with a heart-healthy diet and others are not?

Yes. The traditional diets of Greece and other countries in the Mediterranean region are exemplary in their use of "good" fats, especially olives and olive oil. A classic study of the world's people, the Seven Countries Study, found that death rates from heart disease were strongly associated with diets high in saturated fats, but only weakly linked with total fat.[7] In fact, the two countries with the highest fat intakes, Finland and the Greek island of Crete, had the highest (Finland) and lowest (Crete) rates of heart disease deaths. In both countries, the people consumed 40 percent or more of their kcalories from fat. Clearly, a high-fat diet was not the primary problem.[8] When researchers refocused their attention on the *type* of fat, they found that the Cretes ate diets high in olive oil but low in saturated fat (less than 10 percent of kcalories), a pattern they linked with relatively low disease risks. Many studies that followed yielded similar results—people who follow "Mediterranean-type" eating patterns have low rates of heart disease, some cancers, and other chronic diseases, and their life expectancy is high.[9] Unfortunately, many busy Mediterranean people today, especially the young, are trading labor-intensive traditional diets for convenient and fast Western-style foods. At the same time, their health advantages are rapidly disappearing.[10]

When olive oil replaces saturated fats, such as those of butter, coconut oil or palm oil, hydrogenated stick margarine, lard, or shortening, it may offer numerous health benefits.[11] Olive oil helps to protect against heart disease by:

▪ Lowering total and LDL cholesterol and not lowering HDL cholesterol or raising triglycerides.[12]

▪ Reducing blood-clotting factors.[13]

▪ Providing antioxidant phytochemicals that may reduce LDL cholesterol's vulnerability to oxidation (see Nutrition in Practice 8).[14]

▪ Lowering blood pressure.[15]

▪ Interfering with the inflammatory process related to disease progression.[16]

The phytochemicals of olives captured in extra virgin olive oil, and not its monounsaturated fatty acids, seem responsible for these potential effects.[17] When processors lighten olive oils to make them more appealing to consumers, they strip away the intensely flavored phytochemicals of the olives, thus diminishing not only the bitter flavor of the oils, but also their potential for protecting the health of the heart.

It is important to recognize that olive oil is not a magic potion; drizzling it on foods does not make them healthier. Like other fats, olive oil delivers 9 kcalories per gram, which can contribute to weight gain in people who fail to balance their energy intake with their energy output. Its role in a healthy diet is to *replace* the saturated fats.

Other vegetable oils, such as canola oil or safflower oil, in their liquid unhydrogenated states, are also generally low in saturated fats and high in unsaturated fats. Such oils, when they replace solid, saturated fats in the diet, may help to preserve heart health.

Olives and their oil may benefit heart health.

So olive oil may help protect against heart disease; are there other food fats that may also be protective?

Possibly so. People who eat an ounce of nuts two or more days a week appear to have lower risks of sudden death from heart events than those consuming no nuts.[18] Even in people with diabetes, whose risks are high, nuts are associated with reduced heart disease risk.[19]

The nuts under study are those commonly eaten in the United States: almonds, Brazil nuts, cashews, hazelnuts, macadamia nuts, pecans, pistachios, walnuts, and even peanuts.[20] On average, these nuts contain mostly monounsaturated fat (59 percent), some polyunsaturated fat (27 percent), and little saturated fat (14 percent).

Research has shown a benefit from walnuts and almonds in particular. In study after study, walnuts, when substituted for other fats in the diet, produce favorable effects on blood lipids—even in people with elevated total and LDL cholesterol.[21] Results are similar for almonds.[22]

Studies on peanuts, macadamia nuts, pecans, and pistachios follow suit, indicating that including nuts may be a wise strategy against heart disease. Nuts may protect against heart disease because they provide:

▪ Monounsaturated and polyunsaturated fats in abundance, but few saturated fats.

▪ Fiber, vegetable protein, essential fatty acids, and other valuable nutrients, including the antioxidant vitamin E.

▪ Phytochemicals that act as antioxidants (see Nutrition in Practice 8).

▪ Plant sterols.

Tree nuts and peanuts once had no place in a low-fat or low-kcalorie diet—and for good reason. Nuts provide up to 80 percent of their kcalories from fat, and a quarter cup (about an ounce) of mixed nuts provides more than 200 kcalories. Despite this, people who regularly eat nuts tend to be leaner, not fatter, and generally have smaller waistlines than others.[23] No one can yet say, however, whether nut eaters owe their leaner physiques to an

Stay mindful of kcalories when snacking on nuts.

overall health-conscious lifestyle or to an extra-satiating effect of nuts that reduces food and kcalorie intake at other meals.[24] In any case, replacing potato chips or chocolate candy snacks with nuts certainly improves nutrition by reducing intakes of saturated fats and increasing intakes of vitamin E and other nutrients.[25]

When designing a test diet, researchers must carefully use nuts *instead of,* not in addition to, other fat sources (such as meat, potato chips, or oil) to keep kcalories constant. If you decide to snack on nuts, you should probably do the same thing and use them to replace other fats in your diet. Remember that nuts, although not associated with obesity or weight gain in research, provide substantially more kcalories per bite than crunchy raw vegetables, for example.

What about fish? I have a friend whose doctor told her that eating fish is good for the heart. Is this true?

Yes. The preceding chapter made clear that fish oils hold the potential to improve health, and particularly the health of the heart. Research studies have provided strong evidence that increasing omega-3 fatty acids in the diet supports heart health and lowers the risk of death from heart disease.[26] For this reason, the American Heart Association and other authorities recommend including at least two 3.5-ounce servings of fish (see Table 3-3 on p. 69) per week in a heart-healthy diet. People who eat some fish each week can lower their risks of heart attack and stroke.

Fish is the best source of EPA and DHA in the diet, but it is also a major source of mercury and other environmental contaminants. Most fish contain at least trace amounts of mercury, but tilefish, swordfish, king mackerel, and shark have especially high levels. Freshwater fish may contain PCBs and other pollutants, so local advisories warn sport fishers of species that can pose problems. The chapter listed safer species of fish. To minimize risks while obtaining fish benefits, vary your choices among fatty fish species often.

If olive oil, nuts, and fatty fish are protective against heart disease, which fats are harmful?

A main dietary determinant of LDL cholesterol is saturated fat. Emerging evidence suggests, however, that the effects of reduced saturated fat consumption on heart health vary based on which nutrients or foods replace it in the diet.[27] As noted in Chapter 3,

Fish is a good source of the omega-3 fatty acids.

replacing dietary saturated fat with added sugars and refined starches can be detrimental to heart health. Replacing dietary saturated fat with fiber-rich carbohydrate foods such as whole grains, legumes, vegetables, and fruits, along with foods rich in polyunsaturated fatty acids such as fish, nuts, and vegetable oils, reduces the risk of heart disease.[28] *Trans* fats, of course, also raise heart disease risk by elevating LDL cholesterol.

Which foods are highest in saturated and *trans* fats?

The major sources of saturated fats in the U.S. diet are fatty meats, whole-milk products, tropical oils, and products made from any of these foods. To limit saturated fat intake, consumers must choose carefully among these high-fat foods. More than a third of the fat in most meats is saturated. Similarly, more than half of the fat is saturated in whole milk and other high-fat dairy products, such as cheese, butter, cream, half-and-half, cream cheese, sour cream, and ice cream. Consumers rarely use the tropical oils of palm, palm kernel, and coconut in the kitchen, but these oils are used heavily by food manufacturers and are therefore commonly found in many commercially prepared foods.

When choosing meats, milk products, and commercially prepared foods, look for those lowest in saturated fat. Labels provide a useful guide for comparing products in this regard, and Appendix A lists the saturated fat in several thousand foods.

TABLE NP3-1 Food Sources of Various Fatty Acids

Potentially Healthful Fatty Acids

Monounsaturated	Omega-6 Polyunsaturated	Omega-3 Polyunsaturated
▪ Avocado	▪ Margarine (nonhydrogenated)	▪ Fatty fish (herring, mackerel, salmon, tuna)
▪ Oils (canola, olive, peanut, sesame)	▪ Oils (corn, cottonseed, safflower, soybean)	▪ Flaxseed
▪ Nuts (almonds, cashews, filberts, hazelnuts, macadamia nuts, peanuts, pecans, pistachios)	▪ Nuts (pine nuts, walnuts)	▪ Nuts (walnuts)
▪ Olives	▪ Mayonnaise	
▪ Peanut butter	▪ Salad dressing	
▪ Seeds (sesame)	▪ Seeds (pumpkin, sunflower)	

Potentially Harmful Fatty Acids

Saturated	Trans
▪ Bacon, butter, lard	▪ Fried foods (hydrogenated shortening)
▪ Cheese, whole milk products	▪ Margarine (hydrogenated or partially hydrogenated)
▪ Chocolate, coconut	▪ Nondairy creamers
▪ Cream, half-and-half, cream cheese, sour cream	▪ Many fast foods
▪ Meats	▪ Shortening
▪ Oil (coconut, palm, palm kernel)	▪ Commercial baked goods (including doughnuts, cakes, cookies)
▪ Shortening	▪ Many snack foods (including microwave popcorn, chips, crackers)

FIGURE NP3-1 Two Meals Compared: Replacing Saturated Fat with Unsaturated Fat
Examples of ways to replace saturated fats with unsaturated fats include sautéing vegetables in olive oil instead of butter, garnishing salads with avocado and sunflower seeds instead of bacon and blue cheese, and eating salmon instead of steak. Each of these meals provides roughly the same number of kcalories and grams of fat, but the one on the left has almost four times as much saturated fat and only half as many omega-3 fatty acids.

Even with careful selections, a nutritionally adequate diet will provide some saturated fat. Zero saturated fat is not possible even when experts design menus with the mission to minimize saturated fat. Eating patterns based on fruits, vegetables, legumes, nuts, soy products, and whole grains can, and often do, deliver less saturated fat than diets that depend heavily on animal-derived foods, however.

As for *trans* fats, Chapter 3 explained that solid shortening and margarine are made from vegetable oil that has been hardened through hydrogenation. This process both saturates some of the unsaturated fatty acids and introduces *trans*-fatty acids. Many convenience foods contain *trans* fats. Table NP3-1 summarizes which foods provide which fats. Substituting unsaturated fats for saturated fats at each meal and snack can help protect against heart disease. Figure NP3-1 compares two meals and shows how such substitutions can lower saturated fat and raise unsaturated fat—even when total fat and kcalories remain the same.

So it seems that some fats are "good" and others are "bad" from the body's point of view. Is that right?

The saturated and *trans* fats do indeed seem mostly bad for the health of the heart. Aside from providing energy, which unsaturated fats can do equally well, saturated and *trans* fats bring no indispensable benefits to the body. Furthermore, no harm can come from consuming diets low in them.

In contrast, the unsaturated fats are mostly good for the health of the heart when consumed in moderation. To date, their one proven fault seems to be that they, like all fats, provide abundant energy to the body and so may promote obesity if they drive kcalorie intakes higher than energy needs. Obesity, in turn, often begets many body ills, as Chapter 6 makes clear.

When judging foods by their fatty acids, keep in mind that the fat in foods is a mixture of "good" and "bad," providing both saturated and unsaturated fatty acids. Even predominantly monounsaturated olive oil delivers some saturated fat. Consequently, even when a person chooses foods with mostly unsaturated fats, saturated fat can still add up if total fat is high. For this reason, fat must be kept below 35 percent of total kcalories if the diet is to be moderate in saturated fat.

Additionally, food manufacturers may come to the assistance of consumers wishing to avoid the health threats from saturated and *trans* fats. Some companies now make margarine without *trans* fats, and many snack manufacturers have reduced the saturated and *trans* fats in some products and offer snack foods in 100-kcalorie packages. Other companies are likely to follow if consumers respond favorably.

Eating a balanced diet based on vegetables, fruits, and legumes is a good idea, as is *replacing* saturated fats such as butter, shortening, and meat fat with unsaturated fats like olive oil and the oils from nuts and fish. These foods provide vitamins, minerals, and phytochemicals—all valuable in protecting the body's health. To further protect health, you may want to reduce fats from convenience foods and fast foods; choose small portions of meats, fish, and poultry; and include fresh foods from all the groups each day. Take care to select portion sizes that will best meet your energy needs. Also, be physically active each day.

Notes

1. A. Astrup and coauthors, The role of reducing intakes of saturated fat in the prevention of cardiovascular disease: Where does the evidence stand in 2010? *American Journal of Clinical Nutrition* 93 (2011): 684–688; U.S. Department of Agriculture and U.S. Department of Health and Human Services, *Dietary Guidelines for Americans 2010,* available at www.dietaryguidelines.gov.

2. R. H. Eckel and coauthors, 2013 AHA/ACC guidelines on lifestyle management to reduce cardiovascular risk: A report of the American College of Cardiology/American Health Association Task Force on Practice Guidelines, *Circulation,* http://circ.ahajournals.org/content/early/2013/11/11/01 .cir.000437740.48606.dl.citation; M. R. Flock and P. M. Kris-Etherton, Dietary Guidelines for Americans 2010: Implications for cardiovascular disease, *Current Atherosclerosis Reports* 13 (2011): 499–507.

3. D. Mozaffarian, L. J. Appel, and L. Van Horn, Recent advances in preventive cardiology and lifestyle medicine, *Circulation* 123 (2011): 2870–2891.

4. Eckel and coauthors, 2013; S. E. Chiuve and coauthors, Dietary fat quality and risk of sudden cardiac death in women, *American Journal of Clinical Nutrition* 96 (2012): 498–507; Flock and Kris-Etherton, 2011.

5. Mozaffarian, Appel, and Van Horn, 2011; Flock and Kris-Etherton, 2011; U.S. Department of Agriculture and U.S. Department of Health and Human Services, *Dietary Guidelines for Americans 2010,* available at www.dietaryguidelines.gov.

6. U.S. Department of Agriculture and U.S. Department of Health and Human Services, *Dietary Guidelines for Americans 2010,* available at www.dietaryguidelines.gov.

7. A. Keys, *Seven Countries: A Multivariate Analysis of Death and Coronary Heart Disease* (Cambridge, MA: Harvard University Press, 1980).

8. W. C. Willett, The great fat debate: Total fat and health, *Journal of the American Dietetic Association* 111 (2011): 660–662.

9. E. Lopez-Garcia and coauthors, The Mediterranean-style dietary pattern and mortality among men and women with cardiovascular disease, *American Journal of Clinical Nutrition* 99 (2014): 172–180; M. L. Bertoia and coauthors, Mediterranean and Dietary Approaches to Stop Hypertension dietary patterns and risk of sudden cardiac death in postmenopausal women, *American Journal of Clinical Nutrition* 99 (2014): 344–351; R. Estruch and coauthors, Primary prevention of cardiovascular disease with a Mediterranean diet, *New England Journal of Medicine* 368 (2013): 1279–1290; G. Buckland and coauthors, Olive oil intake and mortality within the Spanish population (EPIC-Spain), *American Journal of Clinical Nutrition* 96 (2012): 142–149; H. Gardener and coauthors, Mediterranean-style diet and risk of ischemic stroke, myocardial infarction, and vascular death: the Northern Manhattan Study, *American Journal of Clinical Nutrition* 94 (2011): 1458–1464.

10. L. M. León-Muñoz and coauthors, Adherence to the Mediterranean Diet Pattern has declined in Spanish adults, *Journal of Nutrition* 142 (2012): 1843–1850.

11. O. Castañer and coauthors, Protection of LDL from oxidation by olive oil polyphenols is associated with a downregulation of CD40-ligand expression and its downstream products *in vivo* in humans, *American Journal of Clinical Nutrition* 95 (2012): 1238–1244; S. Cicerale, L. J. Lucas, and R. S. Keast, Antimicrobial, antioxidant and anti-inflammatory phenolic activities in extra virgin olive oil, *Current Opinion in Biotechnology* 23 (2012): 129–135; C. Samieri and coauthors, Olive oil consumption, plasma oleic acid, and stroke incidence: The Three-City Study, *Neurology* 77 (2011): 418–425.

12. N. R. Damasceno and coauthors, Crossover study of diets enriched with virgin olive oil, walnuts, or almonds: Effects on lipids and other cardiovascular risk markers, *Nutrition, Metabolism, and Cardiovascular Diseases* 21 (2011): S14–S20; S. Cicerale, L. Lucas, and R. Keast, Biological activities of phenolic compounds present in virgin olive oil, *International Journal of Molecular Sciences* 11 (2010): 458–479.

13. S. Granados-Principal and coauthors, Hydroxytyrosol: From laboratory investigations to future clinical trials, *Nutrition Reviews* 68 (2010): 191–206.

14. Cicerale, Lucas, and Keast, 2012.

15. R. Moreno-Luna and coauthors, Olive oil polyphenols decrease blood pressure and improve endothelial function in young women with mild hypertension, *American Journal of Hypertension* 25 (2012): 1299–1304; R. Estruch, Anti-inflammatory effects of the Mediterranean diet: The experience of the PREDIMED study, *Proceedings of the Nutrition Society* 69 (2010): 333–340.

16. Castañer and coauthors, 2012; L. Lucas, A. Russell, and R. Keast, Molecular mechanisms of inflammation. Anti-inflammatory benefits of virgin olive oil and the phenolic compound oleocanthal, *Current Pharmacological Design* 17 (2011): 754–768; Cicerale, Lucas, and Keast, 2010.

17. C. Degirolamo and L. L. Rudel, Dietary monounsaturated fatty acids appear not to provide cardioprotection, *Current Atherosclerosis Reports* 12 (2010): 391–396; Cicerale, Lucas, and Keast, 2010.

18. C. Luo and coauthors, Nut consumption and risk of type 2 diabetes, cardiovascular disease, and all-cause mortality: A systematic review and meta-analysis, *American Journal of Clinical Nutrition* 100 (2014): 256–269; E. Ros, Health benefits of nut consumption, *Nutrients* 2 (2010): 652–682.

19. S. C. Li and coauthors, Almond consumption improved glycemic control and lipid profiles in patients with type 2 diabetes mellitus, *Metabolism* 60 (2011): 474–479.

20. A. Kamil and C. Y. Chen, Health benefits of almonds beyond cholesterol reduction, *Journal of Agriculture and Food Chemistry* 27 (2012): 6694–6702; M. L. Dreher, Pistachio nuts: Composition and potential health benefits, *Nutrition Reviews* 70 (2012): 234–240.

21. P. M. Kris-Etherton, Walnuts decrease risk of cardiovascular disease: A summary of efficacy and biologic mechanisms, *Journal of Nutrition* 144 (2014): 547S–554S; C. E. Berryman and coauthors, Acute consumption of walnuts and walnut components differentially affect postprandial lipemia, endothelial function, oxidative stress, and cholesterol efflux in humans with mild hypercholesterolemia, *Journal of Nutrition* 143 (2013): 788–794; K. N. Aronis and coauthors, Short-term walnut consumption increases circulating total adiponectin and apolipoprotein A concentrations, but does not affect markers of inflammation or vascular injury in obese humans with the metabolic syndrome: Data from a double-blinded, randomized, placebo-controlled study, *Metabolism* 61 (2012): 445–449; Damasceno and coauthors, 2011.

22. C. E. Berryman and coauthors, Effects of almond consumption on the reduction; of LDL-cholesterol: A discussion of potential mechanisms and future research directions, *Nutrition Reviews* 69 (2011): 171–185; Li and coauthors, 2011.

23. C. L. Jackson and F. B. Hu, Long-term associations of nut consumption with body weight and obesity, *American Journal of Clinical Nutrition* 100 (2014): 408S–411S; G. Flores-Mateo and coauthors, Nut intake and adiposity: Meta-analysis of clinical trials, *American Journal of Clinical Nutrition* 97 (2013): 1346–1355; M. A. Martinez-Gonzalez and M. Bes-Rastrollo, Nut consumption, weight gain, and obesity: Epidemiological evidence, *Nutrition, Metabolism, and Cardiovascular Diseases* 21 (2011): S40–S45; P. Casa-Agustench and coauthors, Cross-sectional association of nut intake with adiposity in a Mediterranean population, *Nutrition, Metabolism, and Cardiovascular Diseases* 21 (2011): 518–525.

24. S. Y. Tan, J. Dhillon, and R. D. Mattes, A review of the effects of nuts on appetite, food intake, metabolism, and body weight, *American Journal of Clinical Nutrition* 100 (2014): 412S–422S; Casa-Agustench and coauthors, 2011.

25. S. L. Tey and coauthors, Nuts improve diet quality compared to other energy-dense snacks while maintaining body weight, *Journal of Nutrition and Metabolism* 2011, doi: 10.1155/2011/357350.

26. D. Kromhout and J. de Goede, Update on cardiometabolic health effects of ω-3 fatty acids, *Current Opinion in Lipidology* 25 (2014): 85–90; D. Mozaffarian and J. H. Y. Wu, Omega-3 fatty acids and cardiovascular disease, *Journal of the American College of Cardiology* 58 (2011): 2047–2067.

27. Position of the Academy of Nutrition and Dietetics, Dietary fatty acids for healthy adults, *Journal of the Academy of Nutrition and Dietetics* 114 (2014): 136–153; Mozaffarian, Appel, and Van Horn, 2011.

28. Mozaffarian, Appel, and Van Horn, 2011.

4

Protein

4.1 The Chemist's View of Proteins

LO 4.1 Describe the chemical structure of proteins and the difference between nonessential and essential amino acids.

4.2 Protein Turnover and Nitrogen Balance

LO 4.2 Explain the process of protein turnover and describe nitrogen balance.

4.3 Roles of Body Proteins

LO 4.3 Identify some of the roles of body proteins.

4.4 Protein and Health

LO 4.4 Describe the health effects of protein deficiency and excess, some of the people who may be harmed by

taking amino acid supplements, and the assumptions underlying the protein RDA.

4.5 Protein in Foods

LO 4.5 Explain the differences between high-quality and low-quality proteins, including notable food sources of each.

4.6 Nutrition in Practice: Vegetarian Diets

LO 4.6 Develop a well-balanced vegetarian eating pattern.

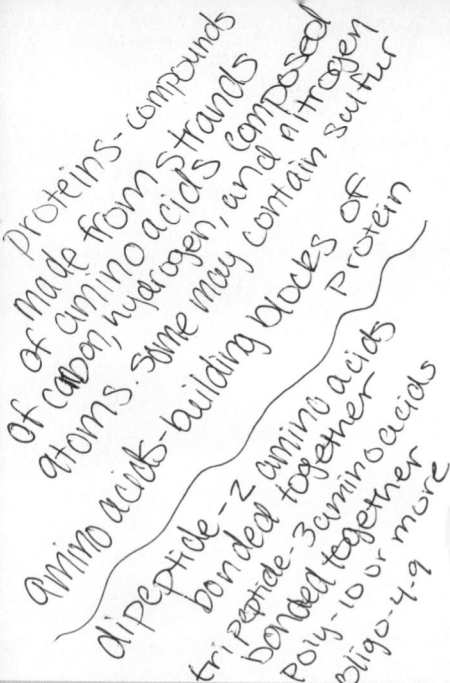

Handwritten margin notes: Proteins- compounds made from strands of amino acids composed of carbon, hydrogen, and nitrogen atoms. Some may contain sulfur. amino acids-building blocks of protein. dipeptide - 2 amino acids bonded together. tripeptide-3 amino acids bonded together. poly-10 or more. oligo-4-9

The versatility of proteins in the body is remarkable. Proteins help your muscles to contract, your blood to clot, and your eyes to see. They keep you alive and well by facilitating chemical reactions and defending against infections. Without them, your bones, skin, and hair would have no structure. No new living tissue can be built without them. No wonder they were named *proteins*, meaning "of prime importance."

4.1 The Chemist's View of Proteins

LO 4.1 Describe the chemical structure of proteins and the difference between nonessential and essential amino acids.

Proteins are chemical compounds that contain the same atoms as carbohydrates and lipids—carbon (C), hydrogen (H), and oxygen (O)—but proteins are different in that they also contain nitrogen (N) atoms. These nitrogen atoms give the name *amino* (nitrogen containing) to the amino acids that form the links in the chains we call proteins.

The Structure of Proteins

About 20 different **amino acids** may appear in proteins.* All amino acids share a common chemical "backbone," and it is these backbones that are linked together to form proteins. Each amino acid also carries a side group, which varies from one amino acid to another (see Figure 4-1). The side group makes the amino acids differ in size, shape, and electrical charge. The side groups on amino acids are what make proteins so varied in comparison with either carbohydrates or lipids.

Protein Chains The 20 amino acids can be linked end to end in a virtually infinite variety of sequences to form proteins. When two amino acids bond together, the resulting structure is known as a **dipeptide.** Three amino acids bonded together form a **tripeptide.** As additional amino acids join the chain, the structure becomes a **polypeptide.** Most proteins are a few dozen to several hundred amino acids long.

Protein Shapes Polypeptide chains twist into complex shapes. Each amino acid has special characteristics that attract it to, or repel it from, the surrounding fluids and other amino acids. Because of these interactions, polypeptide chains fold and intertwine into intricate coils (see Figure 4-2) and other shapes. The amino acid sequence of a protein determines the specific way the chain will fold.

Protein Functions The dramatically different shapes of proteins enable them to perform different tasks in the body. Some, such as hemoglobin in the blood (see Figure 4-3), are globular in shape; some are hollow balls that can carry and store materials within them; and some, such as those that form tendons, are more than 10 times as long as they are wide, forming stiff, sturdy, rodlike structures.

proteins: compounds made from strands of amino acids composed of carbon, hydrogen, oxygen, and nitrogen atoms. Some amino acids also contain sulfur atoms.

amino (a-MEEN-oh) acids: building blocks of protein. Each contains an amino group, an acid group, a hydrogen atom, and a distinctive side group, all attached to a central carbon atom.

amino = containing nitrogen

dipeptide: two amino acids bonded together.

di = two

peptide = amino acid

tripeptide: three amino acids bonded together.

tri = three

polypeptide: 10 or more amino acids bonded together. An intermediate strand of between 4 and 10 amino acids is an *oligopeptide*.

poly = many

oligo = few

FIGURE 4-1 Amino Acid Structure and Examples of Amino Acids

Handwritten note: Proteins contain nitrogen unlike carbohydrates and lipids

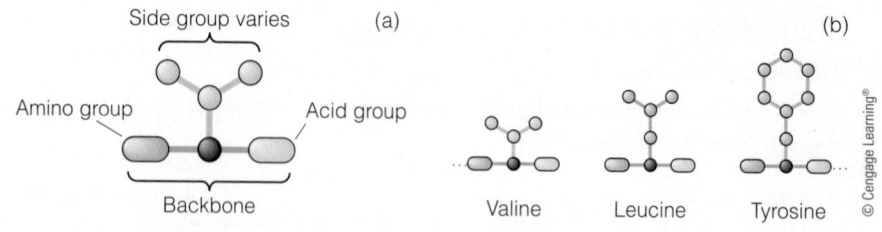

(a) All amino acids have a "backbone" made of an amino acid group (which contains nitrogen) and an acid group. The side group varies from one animo acid to the next.
(b) Note that the side group is a unique structure that differentiates one amino acid from another.

*Besides the 20 common amino acids, which can all be components of proteins, others occur individually (for example, ornithine).

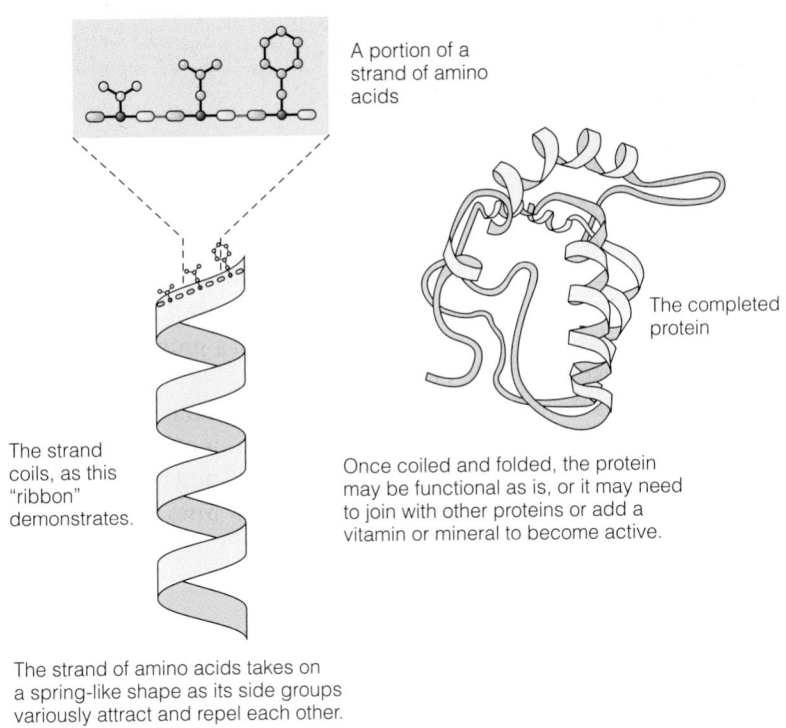

FIGURE 4-2 **The Coiling and Folding of a Protein Molecule**

A portion of a strand of amino acids

The completed protein

The strand coils, as this "ribbon" demonstrates.

Once coiled and folded, the protein may be functional as is, or it may need to join with other proteins or add a vitamin or mineral to become active.

The strand of amino acids takes on a spring-like shape as its side groups variously attract and repel each other.

essential amino acids- amino acids that must be obtained from food
nonessential amino acids- amino acids the body can make

© Cengage Learning®

Nonessential and Essential Amino Acids

More than half of the amino acids are **nonessential amino acids,** meaning that the body can make them for itself. Proteins in foods usually deliver these amino acids, but it is not essential that they do so. There are other amino acids that the body cannot make at all, however, and some that it cannot make fast enough to meet its needs. The proteins in foods must supply these nine amino acids to the body; they are therefore called **essential amino acids.** (Some researchers refer to essential amino acids as *indispensable* and to nonessential amino acids as *dispensable*.)

Under special circumstances, a nonessential amino acid can become essential. For example, the body normally makes tyrosine (a nonessential amino acid) from the essential amino acid phenylalanine. If the diet fails to supply enough phenylalanine or if the body cannot make the conversion for some reason (as happens in the inherited disease phenylketonuria), then tyrosine becomes a **conditionally essential amino acid.**

IN SUMMARY

❚ Chemically speaking, proteins are more complex than carbohydrates or lipids; proteins are made of some 20 different nitrogen-containing amino acids, 9 of which the body cannot make (they are essential).

❚ Each amino acid contains a central carbon atom with an amino group, an acid group, a hydrogen atom, and a unique side group attached to it.

❚ The distinctive sequence of amino acids in each protein determines its shape and function.

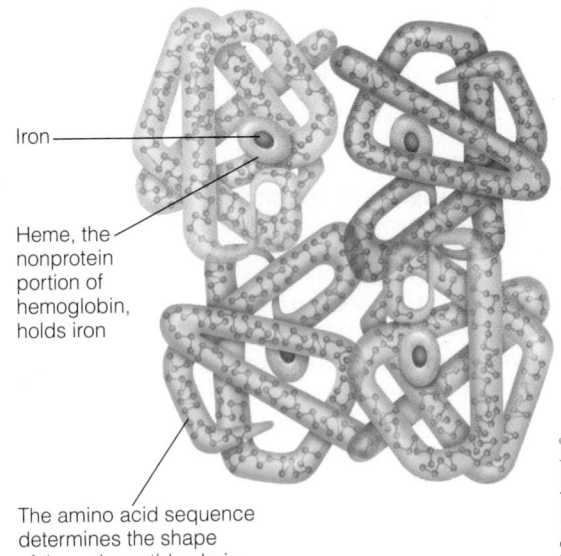

Iron

Heme, the nonprotein portion of hemoglobin, holds iron

The amino acid sequence determines the shape of the polypeptide chain

© Cengage Learning®

FIGURE 4-3 The Structure of Hemoglobin
Four highly folded polypeptide chains form the globular hemoglobin protein.

4.2 Protein Turnover and Nitrogen Balance

LO 4.2 Explain the process of protein turnover and describe nitrogen balance.

Within each cell of the body, proteins are continually being made and broken down, a process known as **protein turnover.** Amino acids must be continuously available to build the proteins of new tissues. The new tissues may be in an embryo, in the muscles of an athlete in training, in a growing child, in the scar tissue that heals wounds, or in new hair and nails.

Less obvious is the protein that helps replace worn-out cells and internal cell structures. For example, the millions of cells that line the intestinal tract live for three to five days; they are constantly being shed and must be replaced. The cells of the skin die and rub off, and new ones grow from underneath.

Protein Turnover

When proteins break down, their component amino acids are liberated within the cells or released into the bloodstream. Some of these amino acids are promptly recycled into other proteins. By reusing amino acids to build proteins, the body conserves and recycles a valuable commodity. Other amino acids are stripped of their nitrogen and used for energy. Each day, about a quarter of the body's available amino acids are irretrievably broken down and used for energy. For this reason, amino acids from food are needed each day to support the new growth and maintenance of cells.

Nitrogen Balance

Researchers use **nitrogen balance** studies to estimate protein requirements. In healthy adults, protein synthesis balances with protein degradation, and nitrogen intake from protein in food balances with nitrogen excretion in the urine, feces, and sweat. When nitrogen intake equals nitrogen output, a person is in nitrogen equilibrium, or zero nitrogen balance.

If the body synthesizes more than it degrades and adds protein, nitrogen status becomes positive. Nitrogen status is positive in growing infants, children, and adolescents; pregnant women; and people recovering from protein deficiency or illness; their nitrogen intake exceeds their nitrogen output. They are retaining protein in new tissues as they add blood, bone, skin, and muscle to their bodies.

If the body degrades more than it synthesizes and loses protein, nitrogen status becomes negative. Nitrogen status is negative in people who are starving or suffering other severe stresses such as burns, injuries, infections, and fever; their nitrogen output exceeds their nitrogen intake. During these times, the body loses nitrogen as it breaks down muscle and other body proteins for energy.

IN SUMMARY

▌ The process by which proteins are continually being made and broken down is known as protein turnover.

▌ The body needs dietary amino acids to grow new cells and to replace worn-out ones.

▌ When nitrogen intake equals nitrogen output, a person is in nitrogen equilibrium, or zero nitrogen balance.

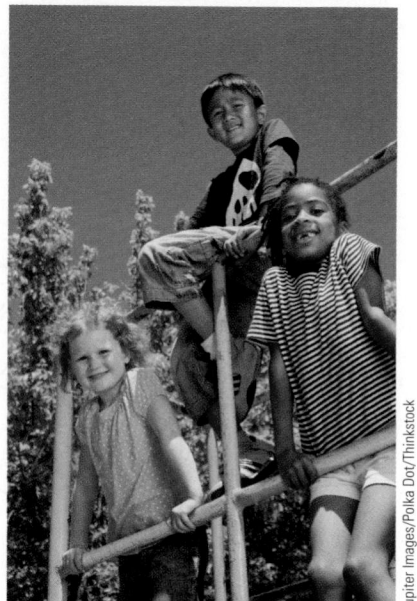

Growing children end each day with more bone, blood, muscle, and skin cells than they had at the beginning of the day.

Jupiter Images/Polka Dot/Thinkstock

nonessential amino acids: amino acids that the body can synthesize.

essential amino acids: amino acids that the body cannot synthesize in amounts sufficient to meet physiological need. Nine amino acids are known to be essential for human adults:

histidine (HISS-tuh-deen)

isoleucine (eye-so-LOO-seen)

leucine (LOO-seen)

lysine (LYE-seen)

methionine (meh-THIGH-oh-neen)

phenylalanine (fen-il-AL-uh-neen)

threonine (THREE-oh-neen)

tryptophan (TRIP-toe-fane, TRIP-toe-fan)

valine (VAY-leen)

conditionally essential amino acid: an amino acid that is normally nonessential but must be supplied by the diet in special circumstances when the need for it becomes greater than the body's ability to produce it.

protein turnover: the continuous breakdown and synthesis of body proteins involving the recycling of amino acids.

nitrogen balance: the amount of nitrogen consumed (N in) as compared with the amount of nitrogen excreted (N out) in a given period of time. The laboratory scientist can estimate the protein in a sample of food, body tissue, or excreta by measuring the nitrogen in it.`

4.3 Roles of Body Proteins

LO 4.3 Identify some of the roles of body proteins.

What distinguishes you chemically from any other human being are minute differences in your particular body proteins (enzymes, antibodies, and others). These differences are determined by your proteins' amino acid sequences, which are written into the genes you inherited from your parents and ancestors. The genes direct the making of all the body's proteins.

The human body has more than 20,000 genes that code for hundreds of thousands of proteins.[1] Relatively few proteins have been studied in detail, although this number is growing rapidly with the surge in knowledge gained from sequencing the **human genome.** Only a few of the many roles proteins play are described here, but these should serve to illustrate proteins' versatility, uniqueness, and importance.

As Structural Components A great deal of the body's protein is found in muscle tissue, which allows the body to move. The amino acids of muscle protein can also be released when the need is dire, as in starvation. These amino acids are integral parts of the muscle structure, and their loss exacts a cost in functional protein, as a later section makes clear.

Other structural proteins confer shape and strength on bones, teeth, tendons, cartilage, blood vessels, and other tissues. These proteins exist in a stable form and are more resistant to breakdown than are the proteins of muscles.

As Enzymes **Enzymes** are catalysts that are essential to all life processes. Enzymes in the cells of plants or animals put together the pairs of sugars that make disaccharides and the long strands of sugars that make starch, cellulose, and glycogen. Enzymes also dismantle these compounds to free their constituent parts and release energy. Enzymes also assemble and disassemble lipids, assemble all other compounds that the body makes, and disassemble all compounds that the body can use for building tissue and other metabolic work. Enzymes put amino acids together to make needed proteins, too. In other words, these proteins can even make other proteins. As Figure 4-4 shows, enzymes themselves are not altered by the reactions they facilitate.

The protein story moves in a circle. To follow the circle in nutrition, start with a person eating food proteins. The food proteins are broken down by digestive enzymes, proteins themselves, into amino acids. The amino acids enter the cells of the body, where other proteins (enzymes) put the amino acids together in long chains whose sequences are specified by the genes. The chains fold and twist back on themselves to form proteins, and some of these proteins become enzymes themselves. Some of these enzymes break apart compounds; others put compounds together. Day by day,

enzymes are protein. catalysts. a catalyst is a compound that facilitates chemical reactions without itself being changed in the process.

human genome (GEE-nome): the complete set of genetic material (DNA) in a human being. (Nutritional genomics is the topic of Nutrition in Practice 14.)

enzymes: protein catalysts. A catalyst is a compound that facilitates chemical reactions without itself being changed in the process.

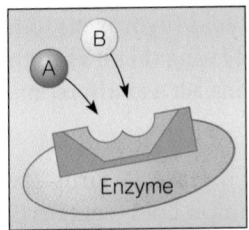

The separate compounds, A and B, are attracted to the enzyme's active site, making a reaction likely.

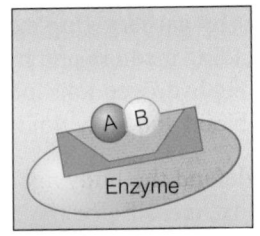

The enzyme forms a complex with A and B.

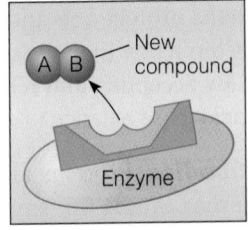

The enzyme is unchanged, but A and B have formed a new compound, AB.

© Cengage Learning®

FIGURE 4-4 **Enzyme Action**
Each enzyme facilitates a specific chemical reaction. In this diagram, an enzyme enables two compounds to make a more complex structure, but the enzyme itself remains unchanged.

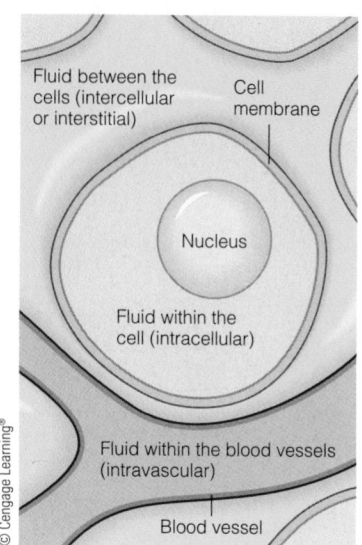

FIGURE 4-5 One Cell and Its Associated Fluids

Labels on figure:
Fluid between the cells (intercellular or interstitial)
Cell membrane
Nucleus
Fluid within the cell (intracellular)
Fluid within the blood vessels (intravascular)
Blood vessel
© Cengage Learning®

fluid and electrolyte balance: maintenance of the necessary amounts and types of fluid and minerals in each compartment of the body fluids.

edema (eh-DEEM-uh): the swelling of body tissue caused by leakage of fluid from the blood vessels and accumulation of the fluid in the interstitial spaces.

acids: compounds that release hydrogen ions in a solution.

bases: compounds that accept hydrogen ions in a solution.

acid–base balance: the balance maintained between acid and base concentrations in the blood and body fluids.

pH: the concentration of hydrogen ions. The lower the pH, the stronger the acid. Thus, pH 2 is a strong acid; pH 6 is a weak acid; pH 7 is neutral; and a pH above 7 is alkaline.

denaturation (dee-nay-cher-AY-shun): the change in a protein's shape brought about by heat, acid, or other agents. Past a certain point, denaturation is irreversible.

acidosis: acid accumulation in the blood and body fluids; depresses the central nervous system and can lead to disorientation and, eventually, coma.

alkalosis: excessive base in the blood and body fluids.

buffers: compounds that can reversibly combine with hydrogen ions to help keep a solution's acidity or alkalinity constant.

in billions of reactions, these processes repeat themselves, and life goes on. Only living systems can achieve such self-renewal. A toaster cannot produce another toaster; a car cannot fix a broken-down car. Only living creatures and the parts they are composed of—the cells—can duplicate and repair themselves.

As Transporters A large group of proteins specialize in transporting other substances, such as lipids, vitamins, and minerals, around the body. To do their jobs, those substances must move from place to place within the blood, into and out of cells, or around the cellular interiors. Two familiar examples: the protein hemoglobin transports oxygen from the lungs to the cells, and the lipoproteins transport lipids in the watery blood.

As Regulators of Fluid and Electrolyte Balance Proteins help maintain the body's **fluid and electrolyte balance.** As Figure 4-5 shows, the body's fluids are contained in three major body compartments: (1) the spaces inside the blood vessels, (2) the spaces within the cells, and (3) the spaces between the cells (the interstitial spaces outside the blood vessels). Fluids flow back and forth between these compartments, and proteins in the fluids, together with minerals, help to maintain the needed distribution of these fluids.*

Proteins are able to help determine the distribution of fluids in living systems for two reasons: first, proteins cannot pass freely across the membranes that separate the body compartments, and second, they are attracted to water. A cell that "wants" a certain amount of water in its interior space cannot move the water around directly, but it can manufacture proteins, and these proteins will hold water. Thus, the cell can use proteins to help regulate the distribution of water indirectly. Similarly, the body makes proteins for the blood and the interstitial (intercellular) spaces. These proteins help maintain the fluid volume in those spaces. Excess fluid accumulation in the interstitial spaces is called **edema.**

Not only is the quantity of the body fluids vital to life, but so is their composition. Special transport proteins in the membranes of cells continuously transfer substances into and out of cells to maintain balance. For example, sodium is concentrated outside the cells, and potassium is concentrated inside. The balance of these two minerals is critical to nerve transmission and muscle contraction. Any disturbance in this balance triggers a major medical emergency. Such imbalances can cause irregular heartbeats, kidney failure, muscular weakness, and even death.

As Regulators of Acid–Base Balance Proteins also help maintain the balance between **acids** and **bases** within the body's fluids. Normal body processes continually produce acids and bases, which must be carried by the blood to the kidneys and lungs for excretion. The blood must do this without upsetting its own **acid–base balance.** Blood **pH** is one of the most tightly controlled conditions in the body. If the blood becomes too acidic, vital proteins may undergo **denaturation,** losing their shape and ability to function. A similar situation arises when there is an excess of base. These imbalances are known as **acidosis** and **alkalosis,** respectively, and both can be fatal.

Proteins such as albumin in blood help to prevent acid–base imbalances. In a sense, the proteins protect one another by gathering up extra acid (hydrogen) ions when there are too many in the surrounding medium and by releasing them when there are too few. By accepting and releasing hydrogen ions, proteins act as **buffers,** maintaining the acid–base balance of the blood and body fluids.

As Antibodies Proteins also defend the body against disease. A virus—whether it is one that causes flu, smallpox, measles, or the common cold—enters the cells and multiplies there. One virus may produce 100 replicas of itself within an hour or so. Each replica can then burst out and invade 100 different cells, soon yielding 10,000 viruses, which invade 10,000 cells. Left free to do their worst, they will soon overwhelm the body with disease.

*Minerals are helper nutrients. The attraction of protein and mineral particles to water is due to osmotic pressure (see Chapter 9).

Fortunately, when the body detects these invading **antigens,** it manufactures **antibodies,** giant protein molecules designed specifically to combat them. The antibodies work so swiftly and efficiently that in a healthy individual, most diseases never get started. Without sufficient protein, though, the body cannot maintain its army of antibodies to resist infectious diseases.

Each antibody is designed to destroy a specific antigen. Once the body has manufactured antibodies against a particular antigen (such as the measles virus), it "remembers" how to make them. Consequently, the next time the body encounters that same antigen, it produces antibodies even more quickly. In other words, the body develops a molecular memory, known as **immunity.** (Chapter 12 describes food allergies—the immune system's response to food antigens.)

As Hormones The blood also carries messenger molecules known as **hormones,** and *some* hormones are proteins. (Recall that some hormones are sterols, members of the lipid family.) Among the proteins that act as hormones are glucagon and insulin. Hormones have many profound effects, which will become evident in subsequent chapters.

As a Source of Energy and Glucose Without energy, cells die; without glucose, the brain and nervous system falter. Even though amino acids are needed to do the work that only they can perform—build vital proteins—they will be sacrificed to provide energy and glucose during times of starvation or insufficient carbohydrate intake. When glucose or fatty acids are limited, cells are forced to use amino acids for energy and glucose. When amino acids are degraded for energy or converted into glucose, their nitrogen-containing amine groups are stripped off and used elsewhere or are incorporated by the liver into **urea** and sent to the kidneys for excretion in the urine. The fragments that remain are composed of carbon, hydrogen, and oxygen, as are carbohydrate and fat, and can be used to build glucose or fatty acids or can be metabolized like them.

The body does not make a specialized storage form of protein as it does for carbohydrate and fat. Glucose is stored as glycogen in the liver and muscles, and fat as triglycerides in the adipose tissue, but body protein is available only as the working and structural components of the tissues. When the need arises, the body dismantles its tissue proteins and uses them for energy. Thus, over time, energy deprivation (starvation) always incurs wasting of lean body tissue as well as fat loss.

IN SUMMARY

❚ The major functions of proteins are summarized in Table 4-1. This list, though by no means exhaustive, highlights the immense variety of proteins and their importance in the body.

TABLE 4-1 Summary of Protein Functions

Structural components. Proteins form integral parts of most body tissues and confer shape and strength on bones, skin, tendons, and other tissues. Structural proteins of muscles allow movement.

Enzymes. Proteins facilitate chemical reactions.

Transporters. Proteins transport substances such as lipids, vitamins, minerals, and oxygen around the body.

Fluid and electrolyte balance. Proteins help to maintain the distribution and composition of various body fluids.

Acid-base balance. Proteins help maintain the acid-base balance of body fluids by acting as buffers.

Antibodies. Proteins inactivate disease-causing agents, thus protecting the body.

Hormones. Proteins regulate body processes. Some, but not all, hormones are proteins.

Energy and glucose. Proteins provide some fuel, and glucose if needed, for the body's energy needs.

Other. The protein fibrin creates blood clots; the protein collagen forms scars; the protein opsin participates in vision.

© 2016 Cengage Learning®

[handwritten margin notes:]
hormones are chemical messengers. hormones are secreted by a variety of glands in the body in response to altered conditions.

urea— the principal nitrogen-excretion product of protein metabolism

antigens: substances that elicit the formation of antibodies or an inflammation reaction from the immune system. A bacterium, a virus, a toxin, and a protein in food that causes allergy are all examples of antigens.

antibodies: large proteins of the blood and body fluids, produced in response to invasion of the body by unfamiliar molecules (mostly proteins) called *antigens.* Antibodies inactivate the invaders and so protect the body.

anti = against

immunity: the body's ability to defend itself against diseases.

hormones: chemical messengers. Hormones are secreted by a variety of glands in the body in response to altered conditions. Each travels to one or more target tissues or organs and elicits specific responses to restore normal conditions.

urea (yoo-REE-uh): the principal nitrogen-excretion product of protein metabolism; generated mostly by removal of amine groups from unneeded amino acids or from the sacrifice of amino acids to meet a need for energy.

4.4 Protein and Health

LO 4.4 Describe the health effects of protein deficiency or excess, some of the people who may be harmed by taking amino acid supplements, and the assumptions underlying the protein RDA.

No nutrient has been more intensely scrutinized than protein. As you know by now, it is indispensable to life. And it should come as no surprise that protein deficiency can have devastating effects on people's health. But, as with the other nutrients, overconsumption of protein can be harmful, too, so this section also discusses the consequences of protein excess.

Protein Deficiency

In protein deficiency, when the diet supplies too little protein or lacks a specific essential amino acid relative to the others (a limiting amino acid), the body slows its synthesis of proteins while increasing its breakdown of body tissue protein to liberate the amino acids it needs to build other proteins of critical importance. When these proteins are not available to perform their roles, many of the body's life-sustaining activities come to a halt. The most recognizable consequences of protein deficiency include slow growth in children, impaired brain and kidney functions, weakened immune defenses, and impaired nutrient absorption from the digestive tract.

Malnutrition

In clinical settings, the term *protein-energy malnutrition* (*PEM*) has traditionally been used to describe the condition that develops when the diet delivers too little protein, too little energy, or both. PEM can be a consequence of many different conditions. PEM has been recognized in people with many chronic diseases such as cancer and AIDS (see Chapter 25) and in those experiencing severe stresses such as burns or extensive infections (see Chapter 24).

The causes and consequences of PEM are complex, but clearly, such malnutrition reflects insufficient food intake. Importantly, not only are protein and energy inadequate, but so are many, if not all, of the vitamins and minerals. For this reason, the term **severe acute malnutrition (SAM)** is now used to describe severely malnourished infants and children.

The form of malnutrition manifested in a child's condition depends partly on the nature of the food shortage. About 10 percent of the world's children suffer from SAM, which most often occurs when food suddenly becomes unavailable, such as in drought or war. These children are often underweight for their height (described as *wasting*). Each year, 6.6 million children younger than age 5 die as a result of SAM.[2] Most of them do not starve to death—they die from the diarrhea and dehydration that accompany infections.

The starving child faces this threat to life by engaging in as little activity as possible—not even crying for food. The body gathers all its forces to meet the crisis, so it cuts down on any expenditure of energy not needed for the heart, lungs, and brain to function. Digestive enzymes are in short supply, the digestive tract lining deteriorates, and absorption fails. The child cannot assimilate what little food is eaten.

A much greater number of children, 25 percent worldwide, live with **chronic malnutrition.**[3] These children have enough food to survive but not to thrive. They are short for their age—they stop growing because they chronically lack the nutrients required for normal growth (described as *stunting*). These stunted children may be no larger at age 4 than at age 2. Table 4-2 compares key features of SAM with those of chronic malnutrition. The next sections describe the symptoms of **kwashiorkor** and **marasmus,** two clinical expressions of malnutrition that can appear individually or together in a starving child.[4]

severe acute malnutrition (SAM): malnutrition caused by recent severe food restriction; characterized in children by underweight for height (wasting).

chronic malnutrition: malnutrition caused by long-term food deprivation; characterized in children by short height for age (stunting).

kwashiorkor (kwash-ee-OR-core or kwash-ee-or-CORE)**:** severe malnutrition characterized by failure to grow and develop, edema, changes in the pigmentation of the hair and skin, fatty liver, anemia, and apathy.

marasmus (ma-RAZZ-mus)**:** severe malnutrition characterized by poor growth, dramatic weight loss, loss of body fat and muscle, and apathy.

TABLE 4-2 Severe Acute Malnutrition and Chronic Malnutrition Compared

	Severe Acute Malnutrition	Chronic Malnutrition
Food deprivation	Current or recent	Long-term
Physical features	Rapid weight loss Wasting (underweight for height; small upper arm circumference) Edema	Minimal height gains Stunting (short for age)
World prevalence of children younger than age 5	5 to 15%	20 to 50%

© 2016 Cengage Learning®

Note: Vitamin and mineral deficiencies are common in both of these types of malnutrition.

Kwashiorkor *Kwashiorkor* is a Ghanaian word meaning a "sickness that infects the first child when the second child is born." When a mother who has been nursing her first child bears a second child, she weans the first child and puts the second one on the breast. The first child, suddenly switched from nutrient-dense, protein-rich breast milk to a starchy, protein-poor gruel, soon begins to sicken and die.

With too little nutritious food, concentrations of the blood protein albumin fall, causing fluids to shift out of the blood and into the tissues—edema. As the photo on top in Figure 4-6 shows, some muscle wasting may occur, but it may not be apparent because the child's face, limbs, and abdomen become swollen with edema—a distinguishing feature of kwashiorkor. Infections with parasites commonly further expand the enlarged abdomen. Other effects of too little dietary protein include loss of hair color because melanin, a dark pigment, is made from the amino acid tyrosine; in addition, patchy and scaly skin develops, often with sores that fail to heal.

Marasmus Marasmus, appropriately named from the Greek word meaning "dying away," reflects a prolonged, unrelenting deprivation of food observed in children living in impoverished nations. Children living in poverty simply do not have enough food. They subsist on diluted cereal drinks that supply scant energy and protein of low quality; such food can barely sustain life, much less support growth. Consequently, as the bottom photo in Figure 4-6 shows, marasmic children look like little old people—just skin and bones.

Without adequate nutrition, muscles, including the heart muscle, waste and weaken. Because the brain normally grows to almost its full adult size within the first 2 years of life, marasmus impairs brain development and learning ability. Reduced synthesis of key hormones leads to a metabolism so slow that body temperature drops below normal. There is little or no fat under the skin to insulate against cold. Some hospital workers find that the primary need of marasmic children is to be clothed, covered, and kept warm.

Rehabilitation Ideally, optimal breastfeeding and improved complementary feedings would prevent malnutrition and save the lives of children. Should mild to moderate malnutrition occur, it can be quickly remedied with supplemental foods in the community. SAM, on the other hand, requires hospitalization for intensive nursing care, diet, and medication.[5]

Experts assure us that we possess the knowledge, technology, and resources to end the hunger that leads to SAM. Programs that have involved the local people in the process of identifying the problem and

Stephen Dorey ABIPP/Alamy

AP Images/Farah Abdi Warsameh

FIGURE 4-6 Malnourished Children

In the top photo, the edema characteristic of kwashiorkor is apparent in the child's swollen belly. In contrast, the extreme loss of muscle and fat characteristic of marasmus is apparent in the child's matchstick arms in the bottom photo.

devising its solution have met with some success. Until those who have the food, technology, and resources make fighting hunger a priority, however, the war on hunger will not be won.

Protein Excess

While many of the world's people struggle to obtain enough food and enough protein to survive, in the developed nations protein is so abundant that problems of protein excess are observed. Overconsumption of protein offers no benefits and may pose health risks for the heart and weakened kidneys.[6]

Heart Disease Protein itself is not known to contribute to heart disease and mortality, but some of its food sources may do so.[7] Selecting too many animal-derived protein foods, such as fatty red meats, processed meats, and fat-containing milk products, adds a burden of fat kcalories and saturated fat to the diet and crowds out fruits, vegetables, legumes, and whole grains. Consequently, it is not surprising that people who eat substantial amounts of high-fat meats—particularly processed meats such as lunch meats and hot dogs—have higher body weights and a greater risk of obesity, heart disease, and diabetes than those who eat less.[8] As the Nutrition in Practice points out, people who substitute vegetable protein for animal protein lower their risk of dying from heart disease.[9]

Kidney Disease Excretion of the end products of protein metabolism depends, in part, on an adequate fluid intake and healthy kidneys. A high protein intake increases the work of the kidneys but does not appear to damage healthy kidneys or cause kidney disease.[10] In people with chronic kidney disease, however, a high-protein diet may accelerate the kidneys' decline. One of the most effective ways to slow the progression of kidney disease is to restrict dietary protein (see Chapter 23).

IN SUMMARY

- Children suffering from severe acute malnutrition (SAM) may be underweight for their height (wasting), while those experiencing chronic malnutrition are short for their age (stunting).

- Kwashiorkor and marasmus are clinical expressions of malnutrition.

- Excesses of protein offer no advantage; in fact, overconsumption of certain protein-rich foods may contribute to health problems.

Protein and Amino Acid Supplements

Why do people take protein or amino acid supplements? Athletes often take them when trying to build muscle. Dieters may take them to spare their bodies' protein while losing weight. Some women take them to strengthen their fingernails. People take individual amino acid supplements, too—to cure herpes, to improve sleep, to lose weight, and to relieve pain and depression. Do protein and amino acid supplements really do these things? Probably not. Are they safe? Not always.

Protein Supplements Though protein supplements are popular with athletes, well-fed athletes do not need them. Dietary protein is necessary for building muscle tissue, and consuming protein in conjunction with resistance exercise helps muscles build new proteins.[11] Protein supplements, however, do not improve athletic performance beyond the gains from well-timed meals of ordinary foods.

Weight-loss dieters may benefit from consistently consuming protein-rich foods because protein often satisfies the appetite. Research is ongoing to determine whether sufficient protein content of a meal may help to prolong feelings of fullness or delay the urge to eat.[12] However, extra protein from powders, pills, or beverages is unlikely to dampen the appetite further, although it contributes unneeded kcalories—the wrong effect for weight loss. Evidence does not support taking protein supplements for weight loss, and common sense opposes it.

Amino Acid Supplements Enthusiastic popular reports have led to widespread use of individual amino acids. One such amino acid is lysine, promoted to prevent or relieve the infections that cause herpes sores on the mouth or genital organs. Lysine does not cure herpes infections. Whether it reduces outbreaks or even whether it is safe is unknown because scientific studies are lacking.

Tryptophan supplements are advertised to relieve pain, depression, and insomnia. Tryptophan plays a role as a precursor for the brain neurotransmitter serotonin, an important regulator of sleep, appetite, mood, and sensory perception. The DRI committee concludes that high doses of tryptophan may induce sleepiness, but they may also cause side effects, such as nausea and skin disorders.

The body is designed to handle whole proteins best. It breaks them into manageable pieces (dipeptides and tripeptides) and then splits these, a few at a time, simultaneously releasing them into the blood. This slow bit-by-bit assimilation is ideal because groups of chemically similar amino acids compete for the carriers that absorb them into the blood. An excess of one amino acid can produce such a demand for a carrier that it limits the absorption of another amino acid, creating a temporary imbalance.

The DRI committee reviewed the available research on amino acids, but with next to no safety research in existence, the committee was unable to set Tolerable Upper Intake Levels for supplemental doses. Until research becomes available, no level of amino acid supplementation can be assumed to be safe for all people (see Table 4-3). A known side effect of these products is digestive disturbances: amino acids in concentrated supplements cause excess water to flow into the digestive tract, causing diarrhea. Anyone considering taking amino acid supplements should be cautious not to exceed levels normally found in foods.

Protein Recommendations and Intakes

The committee that established the RDA states that a generous daily protein allowance for a healthy adult is 0.8 gram per kilogram (2.2 pounds) of healthy body weight. The RDA covers the needs for replacing worn-out tissue, so it increases for larger people; it also covers the needs for building new tissue during growth, so it is slightly higher for infants, children, and pregnant and lactating women. Box 4-1 describes how to calculate your RDA for protein.

In setting the RDA, the committee assumes that the protein eaten will be of good quality, that it will be consumed together with adequate energy from carbohydrate and fat, and that other nutrients in the diet will be adequate. The committee also assumes that the RDA will be applied only to healthy individuals with no unusual alteration of protein metabolism.

Most people assume that Americans eat too much protein. Research demonstrates that a median protein intake for U.S. adult males is about 16 percent of total kcalories, an amount that falls directly within the DRI suggested range of between 10 and 35 percent of kcalories. Women, children, and some elderly people may typically take in less protein—13 to 15 percent. A small percentage of adolescent girls and elderly women consume insufficient protein or barely enough to meet their needs.

TABLE 4-3 **People Most Likely to Be Harmed by Amino Acid Supplements**
Growth or altered metabolism makes these people especially likely to be harmed by self-prescribed amino acid supplements.

- All women of childbearing age
- Pregnant or lactating women
- Infants, children, and adolescents
- Elderly people
- People with inborn errors of metabolism that affect their bodies' handling of amino acids
- Smokers
- People on low-protein diets
- People with chronic or acute mental or physical illnesses who take amino acids without medical supervision

© 2016 Cengage Learning®

How To
BOX 4-1 CALCULATE RECOMMENDED PROTEIN INTAKES

To calculate your protein RDA:

- Look up the healthy weight for a person of your height (inside back cover). If your present weight falls within that range, use it for the following calculations. If your present weight falls outside the range, use the midpoint of the healthy weight range as your reference weight.

- Convert pounds to kilograms, if necessary (pounds divided by 2.2 equals kilograms).

- Multiply kilograms by 0.8 to get your RDA in grams per day. (Teens 14 to 18 years old, multiply by 0.85.)

Example:
Weight = 150 lb
150 lb ÷ 2.2 lb/kg = 68 kg
68 kg × 0.8 g/kg = 54 g protein (rounded off)

■ Normal, healthy people do not need amino acid or protein supplements.

■ Optimally, an adult's diet will be adequate in energy from carbohydrate and fat and will deliver at least 0.8 grams of protein per kilogram of healthy body weight each day.

4.5 Protein in Foods

LO 4.5 Explain the differences between high-quality and low-quality proteins, including notable food sources of each.

In the United States and Canada, where nutritious foods are abundant, most people easily obtain enough protein to receive all the amino acids that they need. In countries where food is scarce and the people eat only marginal amounts of protein-rich foods, however, the *quality* of the protein becomes crucial.

Protein Quality

The protein quality of the diet determines, in large part, how well children grow and how well adults maintain their health. Put simply, **high-quality proteins** provide enough of all the essential amino acids needed to support the body's work, and low-quality proteins don't. Two factors influence protein quality: the protein's digestibility and its amino acid composition.

Digestibility As explained earlier, proteins must be digested before they can provide amino acids. **Protein digestibility** depends on such factors as the protein's source and the other foods eaten with it. The digestibility of most animal proteins is high (90 to 99 percent); plant proteins are less digestible (70 to 90 percent for most, but more than 90 percent for soy).

Amino Acid Composition To make proteins, cells must have all the needed amino acids available simultaneously. The liver can produce any nonessential amino acid that may be in short supply so that the cells can continue linking amino acids into protein strands. If an essential amino acid is missing, however, a cell must dismantle its own proteins to obtain it. Therefore, to prevent protein breakdown, dietary protein must supply at least the nine essential amino acids plus enough nitrogen-containing amino groups and energy for the synthesis of the others. If the diet supplies too little of any essential amino acid, protein synthesis will be limited. The body makes whole proteins only; if one amino acid is missing, the others cannot form a "partial" protein. An essential amino acid that is available in the shortest supply relative to the amount needed to support protein synthesis is called a **limiting amino acid.**

High-Quality Proteins A high-quality protein contains all the essential amino acids in amounts adequate for human use; it may or may not contain all the others. Generally, proteins derived from animal foods (meat, seafood, poultry, cheese, eggs, and milk and milk products) are high quality, although gelatin is an exception. Proteins derived from plant foods (legumes, grains, nuts, seeds, and vegetables) tend to be limiting in one or more essential amino acids. Some plant proteins, such as corn protein, are notoriously low quality. Others, such as soy protein, are high quality. As discussed in Nutrition in Practice 4, the educated vegetarian can design a diet that is adequate in protein by choosing a variety of legumes, whole grains, nuts, and vegetables. Table 4-4 lists the protein contents of foods based on the food groups

Polara Studios, Inc

Vegetarians obtain their protein from whole grains, legumes, nuts, vegetables, and, in some cases, eggs and milk products.

high-quality proteins: dietary proteins containing all the essential amino acids in relatively the same amounts that human beings require. They may also contain nonessential amino acids.

protein digestibility: a measure of the amount of amino acids absorbed from a given protein intake.

limiting amino acid: an essential amino acid that is present in dietary protein in the shortest supply relative to the amount needed for protein synthesis in the body.

TABLE 4-4 Protein-Containing Foods

Milk and Milk Products

Each of the following provides about 8 grams of protein:

- 1 c milk, buttermilk, or yogurt (choose low-fat or fat-free)
- 1 oz regular cheese (for example, cheddar or Swiss; choose low-fat)
- ¼ c cottage cheese (choose low-fat or fat-free)

Protein Foods

Each of the following provides about 7 grams of protein:

- 1 oz meat, poultry, or fish (choose lean meats to limit saturated fat intake)
- ½ c legumes (navy beans, pinto beans, black beans, lentils, soybeans, and other dried beans and peas)
- 1 egg
- ½ c tofu (soybean curd)
- 2 tbs peanut butter
- 1 to 2 oz nuts or seeds

Grains

Each of the following provides about 3 grams of protein:

- 1 slice of bread
- ½ c cooked rice, pasta, cereals, or other grain foods

Vegetables

Each of the following provides about 2 grams of protein:

- ½ c cooked vegetables
- 1 c raw vegetables

© Cengage Learning®

of the USDA Food Patterns in Chapter 1. Fruits are not included in Table 4-4 because they contribute only small amounts of protein.

Complementary Proteins If the body does not receive all the essential amino acids it needs, the supply of essential amino acids will dwindle until body organs are compromised. Obtaining enough essential amino acids presents no problem to people who regularly eat foods containing high-quality proteins, such as meat, seafood, poultry, cheese, eggs, milk, and many soybean products. The proteins of these foods contain ample amounts of all the essential amino acids. An equally sound choice is to eat two different plant-based protein foods so that each supplies the amino acids limited in the other. In this strategy, the two protein-rich foods are combined to yield **complementary proteins** (see Figure 4-7)—proteins containing all the essential amino acids in amounts sufficient to support health. The two proteins need not even be eaten together, as long as the day's meals supply them both, and the diet provides enough energy and total protein from a variety of sources.

	Ile	Lys	Met	Trp
Legumes	✓	✓		
Grains			✓	✓
Together	✓	✓	✓	✓

© Cengage Learning®

FIGURE 4-7 Complementary Proteins

In general, legumes provide plenty of isoleucine (Ile) and lysine (Lys) but fall short in methionine (Met) and tryptophan (Trp). Grains have the opposite strengths and weaknesses, making them a perfect match for legumes.

Protein Sparing

Dietary protein—no matter how high the quality—will not be used efficiently and will not support growth when energy from carbohydrate and fat is lacking. The body assigns top priority to meeting its energy need and, if necessary, will break down protein to meet this need. After stripping off and excreting the nitrogen from the amino acids, the body will use the remaining carbon skeletons in much the same way it uses those from glucose or fat. A major reason why people must have ample carbohydrate and fat in the diet is to prevent this wasting of protein. Carbohydrate and fat allow amino acids to be used to build body proteins. This is known as the *protein-sparing effect* of carbohydrate and fat.

complementary proteins: two or more proteins whose amino acid assortments complement each other in such a way that the essential amino acids limited in one are supplied by the other.

Protein on Food Labels

All food labels must state the *quantity* of protein in grams. The "percent Daily Value" for protein is not mandatory on all labels, but it is required whenever a food makes a protein claim or is intended for consumption by children younger than age four. Whenever the Daily Value percentage is declared, researchers must determine the *quality* of the protein. Thus, when a % Daily Value is stated for protein, it reflects both quantity and quality.

IN SUMMARY

▌ A diet inadequate in any of the essential amino acids limits protein synthesis.

▌ The best guarantee of amino acid adequacy is to eat foods containing high-quality proteins or combinations of foods containing complementary proteins so that each can supply the amino acids missing in the other.

▌ Vegetarians who consume no foods of animal origin can meet their protein needs by eating a variety of whole grains, legumes, seeds, nuts, and vegetables.

▌ Ample carbohydrate and fat in the diet allow amino acids to be used to build body proteins.

▌ All food labels must state the quantity of protein in grams.

Your Diet

Proteins and Amino Acids

Some people in the United States and Canada consume more protein than they need. This is not surprising, considering the abundance of food eaten and the central role meats hold in the North American diet. Foods derived from animals—meats, fish, poultry, eggs, and milk products—provide plenty of protein but are often accompanied by fat. Those derived from plants—whole grains, vegetables, and legumes—may provide less protein but also less fat.

▌ Calculate your daily protein needs: Look up the healthy weight range for a person of your height in the body mass index (BMI) table on the inside back cover of this textbook. If your present weight falls within that range, use it for the following calculations. If your present weight falls outside the range, use the midpoint of the healthy weight range as your reference weight.

▌ Convert pounds to kilograms, if necessary (pounds divided by 2.2 equals kilograms).

▌ Multiply kilograms by 0.8 to get your RDA in grams per day. (Older teens 14 to 18 years old, multiply by 0.85.)

Protein RDA: ___ grams

▌ Refer to the diet analysis reports for your 24-hour food record (from the diet exercise in Chapter 1) to determine your protein intake for that day.

Total protein intake = ___ grams

▌ Assuming this day's intake is typical, do you eat enough protein to meet your protein RDA?

▌ Next, determine whether your protein intake came mostly from plant-based foods or animal-based foods. To estimate your intake from plant-based foods, add up the grams of protein from grains, vegetables, legumes, tofu, nuts, and other plant protein sources in your intake record.

Your total protein intake from plant-based foods: ___ grams

▌ What percentage of your total protein intake derived from plant-based foods? For example, if your total protein intake for the day was 60 grams and your protein intake from plant-based foods was 20 grams:

$$20 \div 60 = 0.33 \times 100 = 33\% \text{ protein intake from plant-based foods}$$

▌ Does your diet consist of mostly plant-based or animal-based protein foods?

▌ If the majority of protein in your diet derives from animal-based foods, suggest some strategies to include more plant-based protein foods in your diet. Legumes, whole grains, vegetables, nuts, and seeds are rich in fiber and lower in saturated fat than some animal-based protein foods such as red meat, whole milk, and cheese.

Clinical Applications

1. Considering the health effects of too little dietary protein, what suggestions would you have for a teenage girl who reports the following information about her food intake?

   ▌ She never eats any meat or other animal-derived foods because she is a vegan. On a typical day, she consumes toast and juice for breakfast; chips, a soft drink, and a piece of fruit for lunch; and a small amount of plain pasta with tomato sauce or steamed vegetables for dinner, along with a glass of water or tea.

   ▌ She takes amino acid supplements because a friend told her that the only way to get amino acids if she doesn't eat meat is to take them as supplements.

2. Considering the health effects of excess dietary protein, what advice would you have for a college athlete who tells you he wants to bulk up his muscles and reports the following information about his food intake?

   ▌ He eats large portions of meat (usually red meat) at least twice a day. He drinks whole milk two or three times a day and eats eggs and bacon for breakfast almost every day.

   ▌ He avoids breads, cereals, and pasta in order to save room for protein-rich foods such as meat, milk, and eggs.

   ▌ He eats a piece of fruit once in a while but seldom eats vegetables because they are too time consuming to prepare.

Self Check

1. Proteins are chemically different from carbohydrates and fats because they also contain:
   a. iron.
   b. sodium.
   c. nitrogen.
   d. phosphorus.

2. The basic building blocks for protein are:
   a. side groups.
   b. amino acids.
   c. glucose units.
   d. saturated bonds.

3. Enzymes are proteins that, among other things:
   a. defend the body against disease.
   b. regulate fluid and electrolyte balance.
   c. facilitate chemical reactions by changing themselves.
   d. help assemble disaccharides into starch, cellulose, or glycogen.

4. Functions of proteins in the body include:
   a. supplying omega-3 fatty acids for growth, lowering serum cholesterol, and helping with weight control.
   b. supplying fiber to aid digestion, digesting cellulose, and providing the main fuel source for muscles.
   c. protecting organs against shock, helping the body use carbohydrate efficiently, and providing triglycerides.
   d. serving as structural components, supplying hormones to regulate body processes, and maintaining fluid and electrolyte balance.

5. The swelling of body tissue caused by the leakage of fluid from the blood vessels into the interstitial spaces is called:
   a. edema.
   b. anemia.
   c. acidosis.
   d. sickle-cell anemia.

6. Major proteins in the blood that protect against bacteria and other disease agents are called:
   a. acids.
   b. buffers.
   c. antigens.
   d. antibodies.

7. Marasmus can be distinguished from kwashiorkor because in marasmus:
   a. only adults are victims.
   b. the cause is usually an infection.
   c. severe wasting of body fat and muscle are evident.
   d. the limbs, face, and belly swell with edema.

8. The RDA for protein for a healthy adult is ___ gram(s) per kilogram of appropriate body weight for height.
   a. 0.5
   b. 0.8
   c. 1.1
   d. 1.4

9. Generally speaking, from which of the following foods are complete proteins derived?
   a. Milk, gelatin, and soy
   b. Rice, potatoes, and eggs
   c. Meats, fish, and poultry
   d. Vegetables, grains, and fruits

10. An incomplete protein lacks one or more:
    a. hydrogen bonds.
    b. essential fatty acids.
    c. dispensable amino acids.
    d. essential amino acids.

Answers to these questions can be found in Appendix H.

Notes

1. Position of the Academy of Nutrition and Dietetics: Nutritional genomics, *Journal of the Academy of Nutrition and Dietetics* 114 (2014): 299–312.

2. World Health Organization, 10 Facts on Child Health, www.who.int/features/factfiles/child _health2/en/index.html, updated September, 2013.

3. P. Svedberg, How many people are malnourished, *Annual Review of Nutrition* 31 (2011): 263–283.

4. T. E. Forrester and coauthors, Prenatal factors contribute to the emergence of kwashiorkor or marasmus in severe undernutrition: Evidence for the predictive adaptation model, *PLoS ONE* 7 (2012): e35907.

5. D. R. Brewster, Inpatient management of severe malnutrition: Time for a change in protocol and practice, *Annals of Tropical Paediatrics* 31 (2011): 97–107.

6. E. Kanda and coauthors, Dietary acid intake and kidney disease progression in the elderly, *American Journal of Nephrology* 39 (2014): 145–152.

7. A. Pan and coauthors, Red meat consumption and mortality: Results from 2 prospective cohort studies, *Archives of Internal Medicine* 172 (2012): 555–563; P. M. Clifton, Protein and coronary heart disease: The role of different protein sources, *Current Atherosclerosis Reports* 13 (2011): 493–498; A. M. Bernstein and coauthors, Major dietary protein sources and risk of coronary heart disease in women, *Circulation* 122 (2010): 876–883.

8. Pan and coauthors, 2012; A. M. Fretts and coauthors, Associations of processed meat and unprocessed red meat intake with incident diabetes: The Strong Heart Family Study, *American Journal of Clinical Nutrition* 95 (2012): 752–758.

9. Clifton, 2011.

10. A. Tirosh and coauthors, Renal function following three distinct weight loss dietary strategies during 2 years of a randomized controlled trial, *Diabetes Care* 36 (2013): 2225–2232.

11. W. R. Lunn and coauthors, Chocolate milk and endurance exercise recovery: Protein balance, glycogen, and performance, *Medicine and Science in Sports and Exercise* 44 (2012): 682–691; A. R. Josse and coauthors, Body composition and strength changes in women with milk and resistance exercise, *Medicine and Science in Sports and Exercise* 42 (2010): 1122–1130.

12. A. D. Blatt and coauthors, Increasing the protein content of meals and its effect on daily energy intake, *Journal of the American Dietetic Association* 111 (2011): 290–294; S. Pombo-Rodrigues and coauthors, The effects of consuming eggs for lunch on satiety and subsequent food intake, *International Journal of Food Sciences and Nutrition* 62 (2011): 593–599.

LO 4.6 Develop a well-balanced vegetarian eating pattern.

The quality of the diet depends not on whether it consists of all plant foods or centers on meat but on whether the eater's food choices are based on sound nutrition principles: adequacy of nutrient intakes, balance and variety of foods chosen, appropriate energy intake, and moderation in intakes of substances such as saturated fat, *trans* fat, added sugars, sodium, and alcohol that are harmful when consumed in excess.

The health benefits of a primarily **vegetarian diet** seem to have encouraged many people to reduce their consumption of meat and to eat more plant-based meals. The popular press sometimes refers to individuals who eat small amounts of meat, seafood, or poultry from time to time as "flexitarians."

People who choose to exclude meat and other animal-derived foods from their diets today do so for many of the same reasons the Greek philosopher Pythagoras cited in the sixth century B.C.: physical health, ecological responsibility, and philosophical concerns. Whatever their reasons, vegetarians and health professionals who work with them should be aware of the nutrition and health implications of vegetarian diets.

Vegetarian diets generally are categorized not by a person's motivation but by the foods that are excluded (see Box

---

BOX NP 4-1 GLOSSARY OF TERMS USED TO DESCRIBE VEGETARIAN DIETS

lacto-ovo vegetarian diet: an eating pattern that includes milk, milk products, eggs, vegetables, grains, legumes, fruits, and nuts; excludes meat, poultry, and seafood.

lacto-vegetarian diet: an eating pattern that includes milk, milk products, vegetables, grains, legumes, fruits, and nuts; excludes meat, poultry, seafood, and eggs.

macrobiotic diet: an eating pattern composed mostly of whole grains, beans, and certain vegetables; taken to extremes, macrobiotic diets can compromise nutrient status.

ovo-vegetarian diet: an eating pattern that includes eggs, vegetables, grains, legumes, fruits, and nuts; excludes meat, poultry, seafood, and milk and milk products.

partial vegetarian diet: a term sometimes used to describe an eating pattern that includes seafood, poultry, eggs, milk and milk products, vegetables, grains, legumes, fruits, and nuts; excludes or strictly limits certain meats, such as red meat. Also called *semi-vegetarian*.

vegan diet: an eating pattern that includes only plant-based foods: vegetables, grains, legumes, fruits, seeds, and nuts; also called *strict vegetarian*.

vegetarian diet: a general term used to describe an eating pattern that includes plant-based foods and eliminates some or all animal-derived foods.

NP4-1). Because vegetarian diets vary in both the types and the amounts of animal-derived foods they include, these differences must be considered when evaluating the health status of vegetarians.

Are vegetarian diets nutritionally sound?

The Academy of Nutrition and Dietetics takes the position that well-planned vegetarian diets offer nutrition and health benefits to adults in general.[1] Research suggests that meat-eating adults who switch to vegetarian diets reduce their risks of heart disease, hypertension, diabetes, some types of cancer, and obesity.[2] Eating patterns that include very little, if any, meat are associated with a lower rate of death from all causes.[3]

What should be my main concerns when planning a nutritionally sound vegetarian diet?

A vegetarian diet planner faces the same task as other diet planners—obtaining a variety of foods that provide all the needed nutrients within an energy allowance that maintains a healthy body weight. The challenge is to do so using at least one less food group. Because all vegetarians omit meat and some omit other animal-derived foods, protein, the nutrient that meat is famous for, merits some discussion here.

Isn't protein a problem in vegetarian diets?

No, protein is not the problem it was once thought to be in vegetarian diets. People who include animal-derived foods such as milk and eggs in their diets need not worry at all about protein deficiency. Even for those who choose a **vegan diet**—which includes only plant-based foods—protein intakes are usually satisfactory as long as energy intakes are adequate and protein sources are varied.[4] A mixture of proteins from whole grains, legumes, seeds, nuts, and vegetables can provide adequate amounts of high-quality protein. An advantage of many vegetarian sources of protein is that they are generally lower in saturated fat than meat and are often high in fiber and richer in some vitamins and minerals.

Some vegetarians may use meat replacements made of textured vegetable protein (soy protein). These foods are formulated to look and taste like meat, fish, or poultry. Many of these products are fortified to provide the vitamins and minerals found in animal sources of protein. Some products, however, may fall short of providing the nutrients of meat, and they may be high in salt, sugar, or other additives. Labels list all of the ingredients in such foods. A wise vegetarian learns to use a variety of whole, unrefined foods often and commercially prepared foods less frequently. Vegetarians may also use soybeans in other forms, such as plain tofu (soybean curd), edamame (cooked green soybeans), or soy flour, to bolster protein intake without consuming unwanted salt, sugar, or other additives.

Do vegetarian diets provide appropriate food energy?

Researchers find that vegetarians as a group are closer to a healthy body weight than nonvegetarians.[5] Because obesity impairs health in a number of ways, vegetarians therefore have a health advantage. In general, vegetarian diets tend to be nutrient-dense and consistent with the *Dietary Guidelines'* recommendations for weight management.[6]

Not all vegetarians fit the average pattern, though. Obesity can be a concern for vegetarians who include whole milk, eggs, and cheese in their diets. They can easily consume excess saturated fat and food energy and so must be careful to select fat-free and low-fat milk and milk products and to avoid relying too heavily on these foods in general.

In contrast, eating patterns that exclude all animal-derived foods (vegan diets) may not provide *enough* food energy. This is especially true for children. Vegan diets can fail to provide food energy sufficient to support the growth of a child within a bulk of food small enough for the child to eat. Frequent meals of fortified breads, cereals, or pastas with legumes, nuts, nut butters, and sources of unsaturated fats can help to meet protein and energy needs in a smaller volume at each sitting.[7] The MyPlate resources, introduced in Chapter 1, include tips for planning vegetarian diets using an adaptation of the USDA Food Patterns.

How can vegetarians and health professionals who plan vegetarian meals best utilize the USDA Food Patterns?

The recommended daily amounts from the food groups are the same for both vegetarians and nonvegetarians (see Table 1-4 on p. 18). The USDA Food Patterns are flexible enough that people who choose different types of eating patterns can use them. Selections from within the food groups may differ, of course. For example, the milk group features fortified soy milks for those who do not use milk, cheese, or yogurt. When selecting from the vegetable and fruit groups, vegetarians should emphasize particularly good sources of calcium and iron, respectively. Some green leafy vegetables, for example, provide almost five times as much calcium per serving as other vegetables. Similarly, dried fruits deserve special notice in the fruit group because they deliver six times as much iron as other fruits. The protein foods group includes eggs (for those who use them), legumes, soy products, nuts, and seeds. Table NP 4-1 provides recommended *weekly* amounts of protein foods subgroups for both vegetarians and vegans.

Most vegetarians easily obtain large quantities of the nutrients that are abundant in plant foods: carbohydrate, fiber, thiamin, folate, vitamin B_6, vitamin C, vitamin A, and vitamin E. Well-planned vegetarian eating patterns help to ensure adequate intakes of the main nutrients vegetarian diets might otherwise lack: protein, iron, zinc, calcium, vitamin B_{12}, vitamin D, and omega-3 fatty acids. Table NP4-2 presents good vegetarian sources of these key nutrients. For example, the use of vegetable oils rich in unsaturated fats provides essential omega-3 fatty acids. To ensure adequate intakes of vitamin B_{12}, vitamin D, and calcium, vegetarians need to select fortified foods or use supplements daily.

Tell me about vitamins and minerals. Does a person eating a vegetarian diet need to take vitamin supplements?

That depends on the kind of vegetarian diet. The **lacto-ovo vegetarian diet** can be adequate in all vitamins, but for those who choose a vegan diet, several vitamins may be a problem. One such vitamin is B_{12}. Because vitamin B_{12} occurs only in animal-derived foods, regular use of either vitamin B_{12}–fortified foods, such as fortified soy and rice beverages, some breakfast cereals, and meat replacements, or supplements is necessary to

TABLE NP4-1 **USDA Food Patterns: Recommended Weekly Amounts of Protein Foods for Vegetarians and Vegans**

The daily amounts for protein foods are the same for both vegetarians and nonvegetarians, but the subgroups and weekly amounts for protein foods differ. The recommended daily amounts from each of the other food groups—fruits, vegetables, grains, and milk products—are the same (see Table 1-4).

Protein Foods	1600 kcal	1800 kcal	2000 kcal	2200 kcal	2400 kcal	2600 kcal	2800 kcal	3000 kcal
Daily amounts	5 oz	5 oz	5 ½ oz	6 oz	6 ½ oz	6 ½ oz	7 oz	7 oz
Vegetarian Subgroups								
Eggs	4 oz	4 oz	4 oz	4 oz	5 oz	5 oz	5 oz	6 oz
Legumes	9 oz	9 oz	10 oz	10 oz	11 oz	11 oz	12 oz	12 oz
Soy products	11 oz	11 oz	12 oz	13 oz	14 oz	14 oz	15 oz	15 oz
Nuts and seeds	12 oz	12 oz	13 oz	15 oz	16 oz	16 oz	17 oz	17 oz
Vegan Subgroups								
Legumes	12 oz	12 oz	13 oz	15 oz	16 oz	16 oz	17 oz	17 oz
Soy products	9 oz	9 oz	10 oz	11 oz	11 oz	11 oz	12 oz	12 oz
Nuts and seeds	14 oz	14 oz	15 oz	17 oz	18 oz	18 oz	20 oz	20 oz

Note: Total recommended amounts for legumes include the sum of both the vegetables and protein foods. An ounce-equivalent of legumes in the protein foods group is ¼ cup. For a 2000-kcal vegan diet, that's 3¼ cups legumes for protein foods plus 1½ cups legumes for vegetables (see Table 1-6), or about 5 cups legumes weekly.

TABLE NP4-2 Vegetarian Sources of Key Nutrients

Nutrients	Grains	Vegetables	Fruits	Protein-Rich Foods	Milk or Soy milk	Oils
Protein	Whole grains[a]			Legumes, seeds, nuts, nut butters, soy products (tempeh, tofu, veggie burgers)[a] Eggs (for ovo-vegetarians)	Milk, cheese, yogurt (for lacto-vegetarians) Soy milk, soy yogurt, soy cheeses	
Iron	Fortified cereals, enriched and whole grains	Dark green leafy vegetables (spinach, turnip greens)	Dried fruits (apricots, prunes, raisins)	Legumes (black-eyed peas, kidney beans, lentils), soy products		
Zinc	Fortified cereals, whole grains			Legumes (garbanzo beans, kidney beans, navy beans), nuts, seeds (pumpkin seeds)	Milk, cheese, yogurt (for lacto-vegetarians) Soy milk, soy yogurt, soy cheeses	
Calcium	Fortified cereals	Dark green leafy vegetables (bok choy, broccoli, collard greens, kale, mustard greens, turnip greens, watercress)	Fortified juices, figs	Fortified soy products, nuts (almonds), seeds (sesame seeds)	Milk, cheese, yogurt (for lacto-vegetarians) Fortified soy milk, fortified soy yogurt, fortified soy cheese	
Vitamin B$_{12}$	Fortified cereals			Eggs (for ovo-vegetarians) Fortified soy products	Milk, cheese, yogurt (for lacto-vegetarians) Fortified soy milk, fortified soy yogurt, fortified soy cheese	
Vitamin D	Fortified cereals				Milk, cheese, yogurt (for lacto-vegetarians) Fortified soy milk, fortified soy yogurt, fortified soy cheese	
Omega-3 Fatty Acids		Marine algae and its oils		Flaxseed, walnuts, soybeans Fortified margarine Fortified eggs (for ovo-vegetarians)	Fortified soy milk	Flaxseed oil, walnut oil, soybean oil

Food Groups

[a]As Chapter 4 explains, many plant proteins do not contain all the essential amino acids in the amounts and proportions needed by human beings. To improve protein quality, vegetarians can eat grains and legumes together, for example, although it is not necessary if protein intake is varied and energy intake is sufficient.

prevent deficiency.[8] Women who have adhered to all-plant diets for many years are especially likely to have low vitamin B_{12} stores. Pregnant vegan women, whose needs for vitamin B_{12} are especially high, find it virtually impossible to maintain adequate vitamin B_{12} status without taking supplements or including a reliable food source of the nutrient.

People who stop eating animal-derived foods containing vitamin B_{12} may take several years to develop deficiency symptoms because the body recycles much of its vitamin B_{12}, reabsorbing it over and over again. Even when the body fails to absorb vitamin B_{12}, deficiency may take up to 3 years to develop because the body conserves its supply. For pregnant and lactating women, obtaining vitamin B_{12} is critical to prevent serious deficiency-related disorders that develop in infants who do not receive sufficient vitamin B_{12}.[9] All vegan mothers must be sure to take the appropriate supplements or to use vitamin B_{12}–fortified products.

Do vegans, who do not drink vitamin D–fortified cow's milk, get enough vitamin D?

Overall, vegetarians are similar to nonvegetarians in their vitamin D status; factors such as taking supplements, skin color, and sun exposure have a greater influence on vitamin D than diet. People who do not use vitamin D–fortified foods and do not receive enough exposure to sunlight to synthesize adequate vitamin D may need supplements to fend off bone loss. Of particular concern are infants, children, and older adults in northern climates during winter months.

So, on a vegan diet, vitamin B_{12} and vitamin D can be problems if a person is not careful. What about minerals?

For *all* vegetarians, not just the vegan, two minerals may be of concern—iron and zinc. The iron in plant foods such as legumes, dark green leafy vegetables, iron-fortified cereals, and whole-grain breads and cereals is not as absorbable as that in meat. For this reason, the iron recommendation for adult vegetarian men, premenopausal women, and adolescent girls is almost double the recommendation for meat eaters of the same gender and age.

Fortunately, the body seems to adapt to a vegetarian diet by absorbing iron more efficiently. Furthermore, iron absorption is enhanced by vitamin C, and vegetarians typically eat many vitamin C–rich fruits and vegetables. Consequently, vegetarians suffer no more iron deficiency than other people do.

Zinc is similar to iron in that meat is its richest food source, and zinc from plant sources is not as well absorbed. In addition, phytates, fiber, and calcium, which are common in vegetarian diets, interfere with zinc absorption. The zinc needs of vegetarians and the effects of mineral binders are subjects of intensive study at the present time. While research continues, vegetarians are advised to eat varied diets that include legumes such as navy beans and kidney beans, zinc-enriched cereals, and whole-grain breads well leavened with yeast, which improves the availability of their minerals.

What about calcium for the vegan?

Good thinking. Yes, calcium is of concern. The milk-drinking vegetarian is protected from deficiency, but the vegan must find other sources of calcium. Some good calcium sources are regular and ample servings of dark green leafy vegetables such as kale and collard; legumes; calcium-fortified foods such as breakfast cereals, soy milk, and orange juice; some nuts such as almonds; and certain seeds such as sesame seeds. The choices should be varied because binders in some of these foods may hinder calcium absorption. The vegan is urged to use calcium-fortified soy milk in ample quantities regularly. This is especially important for children. Infant formula based on soy is fortified with calcium and can easily be used in food preparation, even for adults.

Do vegetarian diets provide adequate amounts of the essential fatty acids?

Vegetarian diets typically provide enough of the essential fatty acids linoleic acid and linolenic acid, but they lack a dietary source of EPA and DHA. Fatty fish and DHA-fortified eggs and other products can provide EPA and DHA, but fortified sources that ultimately derive from fish are unacceptable for vegans. Alternatively, certain marine algae and their oils provide DHA, and vegans can select foods fortified with such oils, which are listed among the ingredients on a food's label. A vegetarian's daily diet should include small amounts of flaxseed, walnuts, and their oils, as well as soybeans and canola oil to provide essential fatty acids.

Are there any other health advantages to the vegetarian diet?

Yes. Vegetarian protein foods are often higher in fiber, richer in certain vitamins and minerals, and lower in fat—especially saturated fat—than meats. Vegetarians can enjoy a nutritious diet low in saturated fat provided that they limit foods such as butter, cream cheese, and sour cream. If vegetarians follow the guidelines presented here and plan carefully, they can support their health as well as, or perhaps better than, nonvegetarians.

Abundant evidence supports the idea that vegetarians may actually be healthier than meat eaters. Informed vegetarians are not only more likely to be at the desired weights for their heights, but they are also more likely to have lower blood cholesterol levels, lower rates of certain kinds of cancer, better digestive function, and more. Even among people who are health conscious, generally vegetarians experience fewer deaths from cardiovascular disease than meat eaters do. Because many vegetarians also abstain from smoking and the consumption of alcohol, dietary practices alone probably do not account for all the aspects of improved health. Clearly, however, they contribute significantly to it.

Notes

1. Position of the American Dietetic Association, Vegetarian diets, *Journal of the American Dietetic Association* 109 (2009): 1266–1282.

2. M. J. Orlich and G. E. Fraser, Vegetarian diets in the Adventist Health Study 2: A review of initial published findings, *American Journal of Clinical Nutrition* 100 (2014): 353S–358S; S. Tonstad and coauthors, Vegetarian diets and incidence of diabetes in the Adventist Health Study-2, *Nutrition, Metabolism, and Cardiovascular Diseases,* 23 (2013): 292–299; C. T. McEvoy, N. Temple, and J. V. Woodside, Vegetarian diets, low-meat diets, and health: A review,

Public Health Nutrition 15 (2012): 2287–2294; B. J. Pettersen and coauthors, Vegetarian diets and blood pressure among white subjects: Results from the Adventist Health Study-2 (AHS-2), *Public Health Nutrition* 15 (2012): 1909–1916; T. Huang and coauthors, Cardiovascular disease mortality and cancer incidence in vegetarians: A meta-analysis and systematic review, *annals of Nutrition and Metabolism* 60 (2012): 233–240; N. S. Rizzo and coauthors, Vegetarian dietary patterns are associated with a lower risk of metabolic syndrome, *Diabetes Care* 34 (2011): 1225–1227; B. Farmer and coauthors, A vegetarian dietary pattern as a nutrient-dense approach to weight management: An analysis of the national Health and Nutrition Examination Survey 1999–2004, *Journal of the American Dietetic Association* 111 (2011): 819–827; W. J. Craig, Nutrition concerns and health effects of vegetarian diets, *Nutrition in Clinical Practice* 25 (2010): 613–620.

3. M. A. Martinez-Gonzalez and coauthors, A provegetarian food pattern and reduction in total mortality in the Prevención con Dieta Mediterranea (PREDIMED) study, *American Journal of Clinical Nutrition* 100 (2014): 320S–328S; M. J. Orlich and coauthors, Vegetarian dietary patterns and mortality in Adventist Health Study 2, *JAMA Internal Medicine* 173 (2013): 1230–1238.

4. Position of the American Dietetic Association, 2009.

5. N. S. Rizzo and coauthors, Nutrient profiles of vegetarian and nonvegetarian dietary patterns, *Journal of the Academy of Nutrition and Dietetics* 113 (2013): 1610–1619; J. Sabate and M. Wien, Vegetarian diets and childhood obesity prevention, *American Journal of Clinical Nutrition* 91 (2010): 1525S–1529S.

6. Farmer and coauthors, 2011.

7. Position of the American Dietetic Association, 2009.

8. R. Pawlak and coauthors, How prevalent is vitamin B_{12} deficiency among vegetarians? *Nutrition Reviews* 71 (2013): 110–117.

9. M. R. Pepper and M. M. Black, B_{12} in fetal development, *Seminars in Cell and Developmental Biology* 22 (2011): 619–623.

Digestion and Absorption

The human body's ability to transform the foods a person eats into the nutrients that fuel the body's work is quite remarkable. Yet most people probably give little, if any, thought to what their bodies do with food once it is eaten. This chapter offers the reader the opportunity to learn how the body digests, absorbs, and transports the nutrients and how it excretes the unwanted substances in foods.

One of the beauties of the digestive tract is that it is selective. Materials that are nutritive for the body are broken down into particles that can be absorbed into the bloodstream. Most of the nonnutritive materials are left undigested and pass out the other end of the digestive tract.

5.1 Anatomy of the Digestive Tract

LO 5.1 Identify the path that food takes during digestion and describe the muscular actions of digestion.

The **gastrointestinal (GI) tract** is a flexible, muscular tube extending from the mouth to the anus. Figure 5-1 on pp. 110–111 traces the path followed by food from one end of the GI tract to the other. Box 5-1 (p. 112) defines GI anatomical terms. In a sense, the human body surrounds the GI tract. Only when a nutrient or other substance passes through the cells of the digestive tract wall does it actually enter the body.

The Digestive Organs

The process of **digestion** begins in the **mouth.** As you chew, your teeth crush and soften the food, while saliva mixes with the food mass and moistens it for comfortable swallowing. Saliva also helps dissolve the food so that you can taste it; only particles in solution can react with taste buds.

The tongue allows you not only to taste food but also to move food around the mouth, facilitating chewing and swallowing. When you swallow a mouthful of food, it passes through the **pharynx,** a short tube that is shared by both the **digestive system** and the respiratory system.

Mouth to the Esophagus Once a mouthful of food has been chewed and swallowed, it is called a **bolus.** Each bolus first slides across your **epiglottis,** bypassing the entrance to your lungs. During each swallow, the epiglottis closes off your trachea, the air passageway to the lungs, so that you do not choke.

Esophagus to the Stomach The **esophagus** has a **sphincter** muscle at each end. During a swallow, the upper **esophageal sphincter** opens. The bolus then slides down the esophagus, which conducts it through the diaphragm to the **stomach.** The lower esophageal sphincter closes behind the bolus so that it cannot slip back. The stomach retains the bolus for a while, adds juices to it (gastric juices are discussed on pp. 115-116), and transforms it into a semiliquid mass called **chyme.** Then, bit by bit, the stomach releases the chyme through another sphincter, the **pyloric sphincter,** which opens into the **small intestine** and then closes after the chyme passes through.

The Small Intestine At the beginning of the small intestine, the chyme passes by an opening from the common bile duct, which secretes digestive fluids into the small intestine from two organs outside the GI tract—the **gallbladder** and the **pancreas.** The chyme travels on down the small intestine through its three segments—the **duodenum,** the **jejunum,** and the **ileum.** Together, the segments amount to a total of about 10 feet of tubing coiled within the abdomen.* Digestion is completed within the small intestine.

*The small intestine is almost two and a half times shorter in living adults than it is at death, when muscles are relaxed and elongated.

---

gastrointestinal (GI) tract: the digestive tract. The principal organs are the stomach and intestines.
  gastro = stomach

digestion: the process by which complex food particles are broken down to smaller, absorbable particles.

digestive system: all the organs and glands associated with the ingestion and digestion of food.

bolus (BOH-lus): the portion of food swallowed at one time.

chyme (KIME): the semiliquid mass of partly digested food expelled by the stomach into the duodenum (the top portion of the small intestine).

The Large Intestine (Colon) Having traveled the length of the small intestine, what remains of the intestinal contents passes through another sphincter, the **ileocecal valve,** into the beginning of the **large intestine (colon)** in the lower right-hand side of the abdomen. Upon entering the colon, the contents pass another opening. Should any intestinal contents slip into this opening, they would end up in the **appendix,** a blind sac about the size of your little finger. Normally, the contents bypass this

FIBER	CARBOHYDRATE
Mouth and salivary glands The mechanical action of the mouth and teeth crushes and tears fiber in food and mixes it with saliva to moisten it for swallowing.	The salivary glands secrete saliva into the mouth to moisten the food. The salivary enzyme amylase begins digestion: Starch $\xrightarrow{\text{amylase}}$ small polysaccharides, maltose.
Stomach Fiber is unchanged.	Stomach acid inactivates salivary enzymes, halting starch digestion. To a small extent, stomach acid hydrolyzes maltose and sucrose.
Small intestine Fiber is unchanged.	The pancreas produces enzymes and releases them through the pancreatic duct into the small intestine: Polysaccharides $\xrightarrow{\text{pancreatic amylase}}$ disaccharides. Then enzymes on the surfaces of the small intestinal cells break disaccharides into monosaccharides, and the cells absorb them: Maltose $\xrightarrow{\text{maltase}}$ glucose + glucose. Sucrose $\xrightarrow{\text{sucrase}}$ fructose + glucose. Lactose $\xrightarrow{\text{lactase}}$ galactose + glucose.
Large intestine (colon) Most fiber passes intact through the digestive tract to the large intestine. Here, bacterial enzymes digest some fiber: Some fiber $\xrightarrow{\text{bacterial enzymes}}$ fatty acids, gas. Fiber holds water; regulates bowel activity; and binds cholesterol and some minerals, carrying them out of the body as it is excreted with feces.	

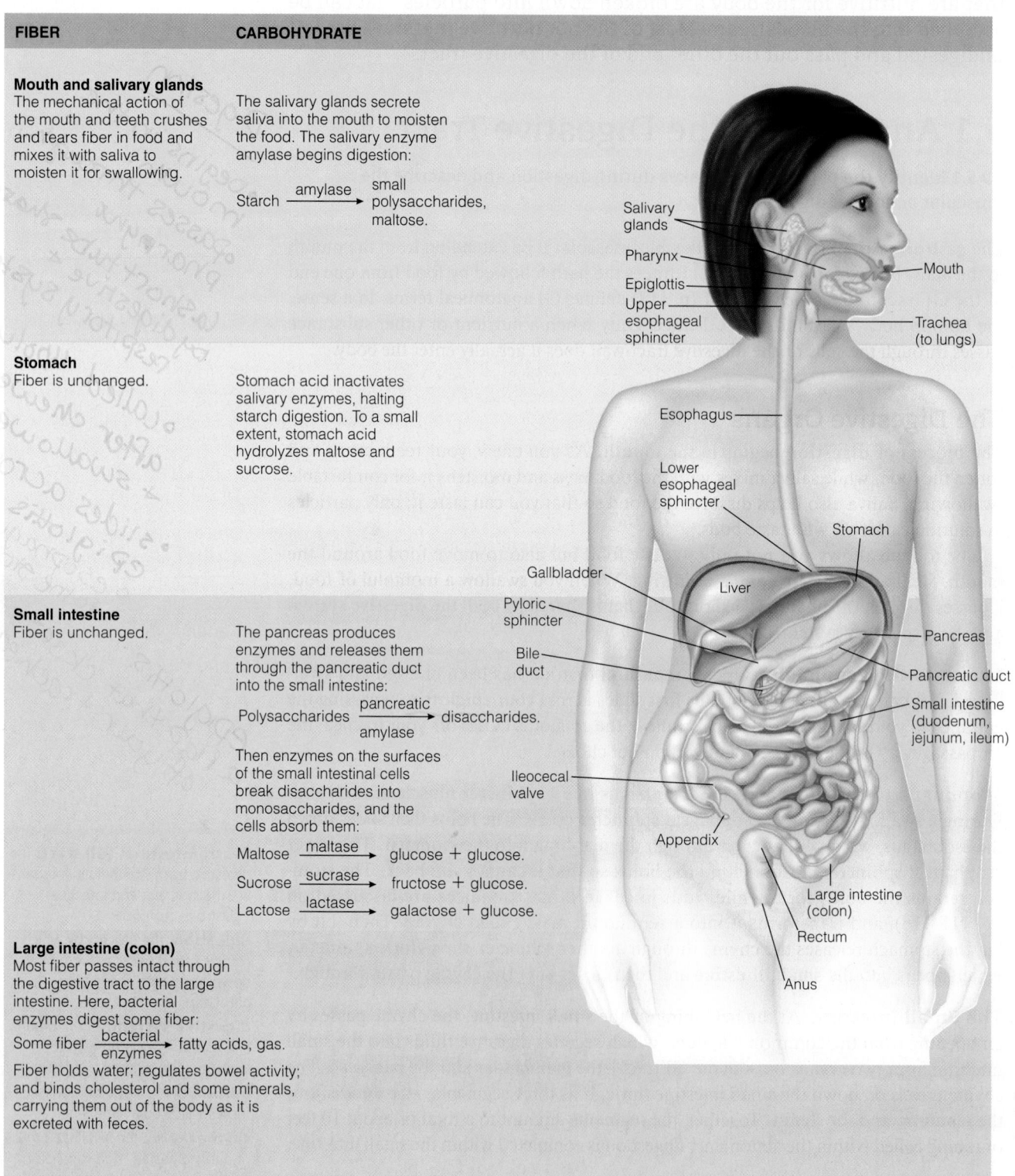

© Cengage Learning®

FIGURE 5-1 The Gastrointestinal Tract

opening, however, and travel up the right-hand side of the abdomen, across the front to the left-hand side, down to the lower left-hand side, and finally below the other folds of the intestines to the back side of the body above the **rectum.**

The Rectum   As the intestinal contents pass to the rectum, the colon withdraws water, leaving semisolid waste. The strong muscles of the rectum hold back this waste until it is time to defecate. Then the rectal muscles relax, and the last sphincter in the

FAT	PROTEIN	VITAMINS	MINERALS AND WATER
Mouth and salivary glands The sublingual salivary gland in the base of the tongue secretes a fat-digesting enzyme known as lingual lipase. Some hard fats begin to melt as they reach body temperature.	Chewing and crushing moisten protein-rich foods and mix them with saliva to be swallowed.	No action.	The salivary glands add water to disperse and carry food.
Stomach The acid-stable lingual lipase splits one bond of triglycerides to produce diglycerides and fatty acids. The degree of hydrolysis is slight for most fats but may be appreciable for milk fats. The stomach's churning action mixes fat with water and acid. A gastric lipase accesses and hydrolyzes a very small amount of fat.	Hydrochloric acid (HCL) uncoils protein strands and activates stomach enzymes: $Protein \xrightarrow[HCl]{pepsin} smaller\ polypeptides.$	Intrinsic factor (see Chapter 8) attaches to vitamin B_{12}.	Stomach acid (HCl) acts on iron to reduce it, making it more absorbable. The stomach secretes enough watery fluid to turn a moist, chewed mass of solid food into liquid chyme.
Small intestine Bile flows in from the liver and gallbladder (via the common bile duct): $Fat \xrightarrow[fat.]{bile} emulsified$ Pancreatic lipase flows in from the pancreas (via the pancreatic duct): $Emulsified\ fat \xrightarrow[lipase]{pancreatic}$ monoglycerides, glycerol, fatty acids (absorbed).	$Polypeptides \xrightarrow[\substack{and\ intestinal\\proteases}]{pancreatic} \substack{tripeptides,\\dipeptides,\\amino\ acids}$ Then enzymes on the surface of the small intestinal cells hydrolyze these peptides and the cells absorb them. $Peptides \xrightarrow[\substack{dipeptidases\\and\ tripeptidases}]{intestinal} \substack{amino\ acids\\(absorbed)}$	Bile emulsifies fat-soluble vitamins and aids in their absorption with other fats. Water-soluble vitamins are absorbed.	The small intestine, pancreas, and liver add enough fluid so that approximately 2 gallons are secreted into the intestine in a day. Many minerals are absorbed. Vitamin D aids in the absorption of calcium.
Large intestine Some fat and cholesterol, trapped in fiber, exit in feces.		Bacteria produce vitamin K, which is absorbed.	More minerals and most of the water are absorbed.

FIGURE 5-1 (continued)

DIGESTION AND ABSORPTION

BOX 5-1 GLOSSARY OF GI TERMS

These terms are listed in order from start to end of the digestive system.

mouth: the oral cavity containing the tongue and teeth.

pharynx (FAIR-inks): the passageway leading from the nose and mouth to the larynx and esophagus, respectively.

epiglottis (epp-ih-GLOTT-iss): cartilage in the throat that guards the entrance to the trachea and prevents fluid or food from entering it when a person swallows.

epi = upon (over)

glottis = back of tongue

esophagus (ee-SOFF-ah-gus): the food pipe; the conduit from the mouth to the stomach.

sphincter (SFINK-ter): a circular muscle surrounding, and able to close, a body opening. Sphincters are found at specific points along the GI tract and regulate the flow of food particles.

sphincter = band (binder)

esophageal (ee-SOF-a-GEE-al) **sphincter:** a sphincter muscle at the upper or lower end of the esophagus. The lower esophageal sphincter is also called the *cardiac sphincter.*

stomach: a muscular, elastic, saclike portion of the digestive tract that grinds and churns swallowed food, mixing it with acid and enzymes to form chyme.

pyloric (pie-LORE-ic) **sphincter:** the circular muscle that separates the stomach from the small intestine and regulates the flow of partially digested food into the small intestine; also called *pylorus* or *pyloric valve.*

pylorus = gatekeeper

small intestine: a 10-foot length of small-diameter intestine that is the major site of digestion of food and absorption of nutrients. Its segments are the duodenum, jejunum, and ileum.

duodenum (doo-oh-DEEN-um, doo-ODD-num): the top portion of the small intestine (about "12 fingers' breadth long" in ancient terminology).

duodecim = twelve

jejunum (je-JOON-um): the first two-fifths of the small intestine beyond the duodenum.

ileum (ILL-ee-um): the last segment of the small intestine.

gallbladder: the organ that stores and concentrates bile. When it receives the signal that fat is present in the duodenum, the gallbladder contracts and squirts bile through the bile duct into the duodenum.

pancreas: a gland that secretes digestive enzymes and juices into the duodenum. (The pancreas also secretes hormones into the blood that help to maintain glucose homeostasis.)

ileocecal (ill-ee-oh-SEEK-ul) **valve:** the sphincter separating the small and large intestines.

large intestine or **colon** (COAL-un): the lower portion of intestine that completes the digestive process. Its segments are the ascending colon, the transverse colon, the descending colon, and the sigmoid colon.

sigmoid = shaped like the letter S (sigma in Greek)

appendix: a narrow blind sac extending from the beginning of the colon that stores lymph cells.

rectum: the muscular terminal part of the intestine, extending from the sigmoid colon to the anus.

anus (AY-nus): the terminal outlet of the GI tract.

system, the **anus,** opens to allow the wastes to pass. Thus, food travels through the digestive tract in this order: mouth, esophagus, lower esophageal sphincter (or cardiac sphincter), stomach, pyloric sphincter, duodenum (common bile duct enters here), jejunum, ileum, ileocecal valve, large intestine (colon), rectum, and anus.

The Involuntary Muscles and the Glands

You are usually unaware of all the activity that goes on between the time you swallow and the time you defecate. As is the case with so much else that happens in the body, the muscles and **glands** of the digestive tract meet internal needs without your having to exert any conscious effort to get the work done.

People consciously chew and swallow, but even in the mouth there are some processes over which you have no control. The salivary glands secrete just enough saliva to moisten each mouthful of food so that it can pass easily down your esophagus.

Gastrointestinal Motility Once you have swallowed, materials are moved through the rest of the GI tract by involuntary muscular contractions. This motion, known as **gastrointestinal motility,** consists of two types of movement, peristalsis and segmentation (see Figure 5-2). Peristalsis propels, or pushes; segmentation mixes, with more gradual pushing.

Peristalsis Peristalsis begins when the bolus enters the esophagus. The entire GI tract is ringed with circular muscles, which are surrounded by longitudinal muscles. When the rings tighten and the long muscles relax, the tube is constricted. When the rings relax and the long muscles tighten, the tube bulges. These actions alternate

gastrointestinal motility: spontaneous motion in the digestive tract accomplished by involuntary muscular contractions.

peristalsis (peri-STALL-sis): successive waves of involuntary muscular contractions passing along the walls of the GI tract that push the contents along.

peri = around

stellein = wrap

The small intestine has two muscle layers that work together in peristalsis and segmentation.

— Circular muscles are inside.

— Longitudinal muscles are outside.

(Handwritten margin note: gastrointestinal motility — two types of movement — peristalsis & segmentation)

Peristalsis

Chyme

The inner circular muscles contract, tightening the tube and pushing the food forward in the intestine.

When the circular muscles relax, the outer longitudinal muscles contract, and the intestinal tube is loose.

As the circular and longitudinal muscles tighten and relax, the chyme moves ahead of the constriction.

Segmentation

Chyme

Circular muscles contract, creating segments within the intestine.

As each set of circular muscles relaxes and contracts, the chyme is broken up and mixed with digestive juices.

These alternating contractions, occurring 12 to 16 times per minute, continue to mix the chyme and bring the nutrients into contact with the intestinal lining for absorption.

© Cengage Learning®

FIGURE 5-2 Peristalsis and Segmentation

continually and push the intestinal contents along. If you have ever watched a bolus of food pass along the body of a snake, you have a good picture of how these muscles work. The waves of contraction ripple through the GI tract at varying rates and intensities depending on the part of the GI tract and on whether food is present. Peristalsis, aided by the sphincter muscles located at key places, keeps things moving along. However, factors such as stress, medicines, and medical conditions may interfere with normal GI tract contractions.[1]

Segmentation The intestines not only push but also periodically squeeze their contents. This motion, called **segmentation,** forces the contents back a few inches, mixing them and promoting close contact with the digestive juices and the absorbing cells of the intestinal walls before letting the contents slowly move along again.

Liquefying Process Besides forcing the intestinal contents along, the muscles of the GI tract help to liquefy them to chyme so that the digestive juices will have access to all their nutrients. The mouth initiates this liquefying process by chewing, adding

segmentation: a periodic squeezing or partitioning of the intestine by its circular muscles that both mixes and slowly pushes the contents along.

FIGURE 5-3 Stomach Muscles
The stomach has three layers of muscles.

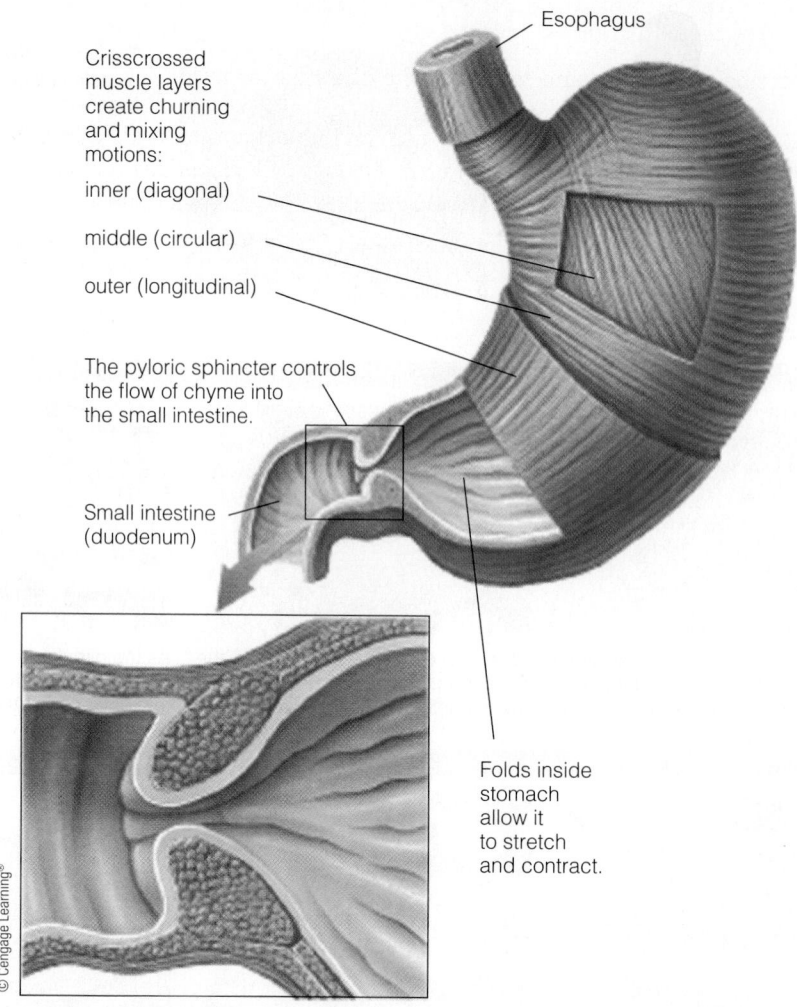

Esophagus

Crisscrossed muscle layers create churning and mixing motions:

inner (diagonal)

middle (circular)

outer (longitudinal)

The pyloric sphincter controls the flow of chyme into the small intestine.

Small intestine (duodenum)

Folds inside stomach allow it to stretch and contract.

© Cengage Learning®

saliva, and stirring with the tongue to reduce the food to a coarse mash suitable for swallowing. The stomach then further mixes and kneads the food.

Stomach Action The stomach has the thickest walls and strongest muscles of all the GI tract organs. In addition to circular and longitudinal muscles, the stomach has a third layer of diagonal muscles that also alternately contract and relax (see Figure 5-3). These three sets of muscles work to force the chyme downward, but the pyloric sphincter usually remains tightly closed, so that the stomach's contents are thoroughly mixed and squeezed before being released. Meanwhile, the gastric glands are adding juices. When the chyme is thoroughly liquefied, the pyloric sphincter opens briefly, about three times a minute, to allow small portions through. At this point, the intestinal contents no longer resemble food in the least.

IN SUMMARY

▌ As Figure 5-1 shows, food enters the mouth and travels down the esophagus and through the lower esophageal sphincter to the stomach, then through the pyloric sphincter to the small intestine, on through the ileocecal valve to the large intestine, past the appendix to the rectum, exiting through the anus.

▌ The wavelike contractions of peristalsis and the periodic squeezing of segmentation keep things moving at a reasonable pace.

5.2 The Process of Digestion

LO 5.2 Describe the actions and origins of the digestive secretions.

One person eats nothing but vegetables, fruits, and nuts; another, nothing but meat, milk, and potatoes. How is it that both people wind up with essentially the same body composition? It all comes down to the body rendering food—whatever it is to start with—into the basic units that make up carbohydrate, fat, and protein. The body absorbs these units and builds its tissues from them.

To digest food, five different body organs secrete digestive juices: the salivary glands, the stomach, the small intestine, the liver (via the gallbladder), and the pancreas. These secretions enter the GI tract at various points along the way, bringing an abundance of water and a variety of **enzymes.** Each of the juices has a turn to mix with the food and promote its breakdown to small units that can be absorbed into the body. Box 5-2 defines some of the digestive glands and their juices.

Digestion in the Mouth

Digestion of carbohydrate begins in the mouth, where the **salivary glands** secrete **saliva,** which contains water, salts, and enzymes (including salivary **amylase**) that break the bonds in the chains of starch. Saliva also protects the tooth surfaces and linings of the mouth, esophagus, and stomach from attack by molecules that might harm them. The enzymes in the mouth do not, for the most part, affect the fats, proteins, vitamins, minerals, and fiber that are present in the foods people eat (review Figure 5-1).

enzymes: protein catalysts. A catalyst is a compound that facilitates chemical reactions without itself being changed in the process.

BOX 5-2 GLOSSARY OF DIGESTIVE GLANDS AND THEIR SECRETIONS

These terms are listed in order from the beginning of the digestive tract to the end.

glands: cells or groups of cells that secrete materials for special uses in the body. Glands may be *exocrine* (EKS-oh-crin) *glands*, secreting their materials "out" (into the digestive tract or onto the surface of the skin), or *endocrine* (EN-doe-crin) *glands*, secreting their materials "in" (into the blood).

> exo = outside
> endo = inside
> krine = to separate

salivary glands: exocrine glands that secrete saliva into the mouth.

saliva: the secretion of the salivary glands. The principal enzyme is salivary amylase.

amylase (AM-uh-lace): an enzyme that splits amylose (a form of starch). Amylase is a carbohydrase. The ending *–ase* indicates an enzyme; the root tells what it digests. Other examples: protease, lipase.

gastric glands: exocrine glands in the stomach wall that secrete gastric juice into the stomach.

> gastro = stomach

gastric juice: the digestive secretion of the gastric glands containing a mixture of water, hydrochloric acid, and enzymes. The principal enzymes are pepsin (acts on proteins) and lipase (acts on emulsified fats).

hydrochloric acid (HCl): an acid composed of hydrogen and chloride atoms; normally produced by the gastric glands.

mucus (MYOO-cuss): a mucopolysaccharide (a relative of carbohydrate) secreted by cells of the stomach wall that protects the cells from exposure to digestive juices (and other destructive agents). The cellular lining of the stomach wall with its coat of mucus is known as the mucous membrane. (The noun is *mucus*; the adjective is *mucous*.)

pepsin: a protein-digesting enzyme (gastric protease) in the stomach. It circulates as a precursor, pepsinogen, and is converted to pepsin by the action of stomach acid.

intestinal juice: the secretion of the intestinal glands; contains enzymes for the digestion of carbohydrate and protein and a minor enzyme for fat digestion.

liver: the organ that manufactures bile. (The liver's other functions are described in Chapter 20.)

bile: an emulsifier that prepares fats and oils for digestion; made by the liver, stored in the gallbladder, and released into the small intestine when needed.

pancreatic (pank-ree-AT-ic) **juice:** the exocrine secretion of the pancreas, containing enzymes for the digestion of carbohydrate, fat, and protein. Juice flows from the pancreas into the small intestine through the pancreatic duct. The pancreas also has an endocrine function, the secretion of insulin and other hormones.

bicarbonate: an alkaline secretion of the pancreas; part of the pancreatic juice. (Bicarbonate also occurs widely in all cell fluids.)

Digestion in the Stomach

Gastric juice, secreted by the **gastric glands,** is composed of water, enzymes, and **hydrochloric acid.** The acid is so strong that it burns the throat if it happens to reflux into the upper esophagus and mouth. The stomach's strong acidity prevents bacterial growth and kills most bacteria that enter the body along with food. You might expect that the stomach's acid would attack the stomach itself, but the cells of the stomach wall secrete **mucus,** a thick, slimy, white polysaccharide that coats and protects the stomach's lining.

The major digestive event in the stomach is the initial breakdown of proteins. Other than being crushed and mixed with saliva in the mouth, nothing happens to protein until it comes in contact with the gastric juices in the stomach. There, the acid helps to uncoil (denature) the protein's tangled strands so that the stomach enzymes can attack the bonds. Both the enzyme **pepsin** and the stomach acid itself act as catalysts in the process. Minor events are the digestion of some fat by a gastric lipase, the digestion of sucrose (to a very small extent) by the stomach acid, and the attachment of a protein carrier to vitamin B_{12}.

The stomach enzymes work most efficiently in the stomach's strong acid, but salivary amylase, which is swallowed with food, does not work in acid this strong. Consequently, the digestion of starch gradually ceases as the acid penetrates the bolus. In fact, salivary amylase becomes just another protein to be digested. The amino acids in amylase end up being absorbed and recycled into other body proteins.

Digestion in the Small and Large Intestines

By the time food leaves the stomach, digestion of all three energy-yielding nutrients has begun, but the process gains momentum in the small intestine. There, the pancreas and the liver contribute additional digestive juices through the duct leading into the duodenum, and the small intestine adds **intestinal juice.** These juices contain digestive enzymes, bicarbonate, and bile.

Digestive Enzymes **Pancreatic juice** contributes enzymes that digest fats, proteins, and carbohydrates. Glands in the intestinal wall also secrete digestive enzymes. (Review Box 5-2 on p. 115 for details.)

Bicarbonate Pancreatic juice also contains sodium **bicarbonate,** which neutralizes the acidic chyme as it enters the small intestine. From this point on, the digestive tract contents are neutral or slightly alkaline. The enzymes of both the intestine and the pancreas work best in this environment.

Bile **Bile** is secreted continuously by the **liver** and is concentrated and stored in the gallbladder. The gallbladder squirts bile into the duodenum whenever fat arrives there. Bile is not an enzyme but an **emulsifier** that brings fats into suspension in water (see Figure 5-4).[†] After the fats are emulsified, enzymes can work on them, and they can be absorbed. Thanks to all these secretions, all three energy-yielding nutrients are digested in the small intestine.

The Rate of Digestion The rate of digestion of the energy nutrients depends on the meal contents. If the meal is high in simple sugars, digestion proceeds fairly rapidly. On the other hand, if it is rich in fat, digestion is slower.

Protective Factors The intestines contain bacteria that produce a variety of vitamins, including biotin and vitamin K (although bacteria alone cannot meet the need

emulsifier: a substance that mixes with both fat and water and that disperses the fat in the water, forming an emulsion.

[†]Mayonnaise, made from vinegar and oil, would separate as other vinegar-and-oil salad dressings do if food chemists did not blend in a third ingredient—an emulsifier. The emulsifier mixes well with the fatty oil and the watery vinegar. In the case of mayonnaise, the emulsifier is lecithin from egg yolks.

In the stomach, the fat and watery GI juices tend to separate. The enzymes are in the water and cannot get at the fat.

When fat enters the small intestine, the gallbladder secretes bile. Bile has an affinity for both fat and water, so it can bring the fat into the water.

Bile's emulsifying action converts large fat globules into small droplets that repel each other.

After emulsification, the enzymes have easy access to the fat droplets.

FIGURE 5-4 Emulsification of Fat by Bile
Like bile, detergents are emulsifiers and work the same way, which is why they are effective at removing grease spots from clothes. Molecule by molecule, the grease is dissolved out of the spot and suspended in water, where it can be rinsed away.

for these vitamins). The GI bacteria also protect people from infections. Provided that the normal **intestinal flora** are thriving, infectious bacteria have a hard time getting established and launching an attack on the system (see Nutrition in Practice 18). In addition, the small intestine and the entire GI tract manufacture and maintain a strong arsenal of defenses against foreign invaders. Several different types of defending cells are present in the GI tract, and they confer specific immunity against intestinal diseases.

The Final Stage The story of how food is broken down into nutrients that can be absorbed is now nearly complete. The three energy-yielding nutrients—carbohydrate, fat, and protein—are disassembled to basic building blocks before they are absorbed. Most of the other nutrients—vitamins, minerals, and water—are absorbed as they are. Undigested residues, such as some fibers, are not absorbed but continue through the digestive tract as a semisolid mass that stimulates the tract's muscles, helping them remain strong and able to perform peristalsis efficiently. Fiber also retains water, keeping the stools soft, and carries some bile acids, sterols, and fat out of the body. Drinking plenty of water in conjunction with eating foods high in fiber supplies fluid for the fiber to take up. This is the basis for the recommendation to drink water and eat fiber-rich foods to relieve constipation.

The process of absorbing the nutrients into the body is discussed in the next section. For the moment, let us assume that the digested nutrients simply disappear from the GI tract as they are ready. Virtually all nutrients are gone by the time the contents of the GI tract reach the end of the small intestine. Little remains but water, a few salts and body secretions, and undigested materials such as fiber. These enter the large intestine (colon).

In the colon, intestinal bacteria degrade some of the fiber to simpler compounds. The colon itself retrieves from its contents the materials that the body is designed to recycle—water and dissolved salts. The waste that is finally excreted has little or nothing of value left in it. The body has extracted all that it can use from the food.

IN SUMMARY

▪ To digest food, the salivary glands, stomach, pancreas, liver (via the gallbladder), and small intestine deliver fluids and digestive enzymes.

intestinal flora: the bacterial inhabitants of the GI tract.
flora = plant growth

5.3 The Absorptive System

LO 5.3 Describe the anatomical details of the GI tract and the features and activities of intestinal cells that facilitate nutrient absorption.

Within three or four hours after you have eaten a meal, your body must find a way to absorb millions of molecules one by one. The absorptive system is ingeniously designed to accomplish this task.

The Small Intestine

Most absorption takes place in the small intestine. The small intestine is a tube about 10 feet long and about an inch across, yet it provides a surface comparable in area to a tennis court. When nutrient molecules make contact with this surface, they are absorbed and carried off to the liver and other parts of the body.

Villi and Microvilli How does the intestine manage to provide such a large absorptive surface area? Its inner surface looks smooth, but viewed through a microscope, it turns out to be wrinkled into hundreds of folds. Each fold is covered with thousands of fingerlike projections called **villi.** The villi are as numerous as the fibers on velvet fabric. A single villus, magnified still more, turns out to be composed of several hundred cells, each covered with microscopic hairs called **microvilli** (see Figure 5-5).

The villi are in constant motion. A thin sheet of muscle lines each villus so that it can wave, squirm, and wiggle like a sea anemone's tentacles. Any nutrient molecule small enough to be absorbed is trapped among the microvilli and drawn into a cell beneath them. Some partially digested nutrients are caught in the microvilli, digested further by enzymes there, and then absorbed into the cells.

Specialization in the Intestinal Tract As you can see, the intestinal tract is beautifully designed to perform its functions. A further refinement of the system is that the cells of successive portions of the tract are specialized to absorb different nutrients. The nutrients that are ready for absorption early are absorbed near the top of the tract; those that take longer to be digested are absorbed farther down. The rate at which the nutrients travel through the GI tract is finely adjusted to maximize their availability to the appropriate absorptive segment of the tract when they are ready. The lowly "gut" turns out to be one of the most elegantly designed organ systems in the body.

The Myth of "Food Combining" Some popular fad diets advocate the idea that people should not eat certain food combinations (for example, fruit and meat) at the same meal, because the digestive system cannot handle more than one task at a time. This is a myth. The art of "food combining" (which actually emphasizes "food separating") is based on this idea, and it represents faulty logic and a gross underestimation of the body's capabilities. In fact, the opposite is often true: foods eaten together can enhance each other's use by the body. For example, vitamin C in a pineapple or citrus fruit can enhance the absorption of iron from a meal of chicken and rice or other iron-containing foods. Many other instances of mutually beneficial interactions are presented in later chapters.

Absorption of Nutrients

Once a molecule has entered a cell in a villus, the next step is to transmit it to a destination elsewhere in the body by way of the body's two transport systems—the bloodstream and the **lymphatic system.** As Figure 5-5 shows, both systems supply vessels to each villus. Through these vessels, the nutrients leave the cell and enter either the

villi (VILL-ee or VILL-eye): fingerlike projections from the folds of the small intestine. The singular form is **villus.**

villus = shaggy hair

microvilli (MY-cro-VILL-ee or MY-cro-VILL-eye): tiny, hairlike projections on each cell of every villus that can trap nutrient particles and transport them into the cells. The singular form is **microvillus.**

lymphatic system: a loosely organized system of vessels and ducts that conveys the products of digestion toward the heart.

Stomach

Small intestine

Folds with villi on them

The wall of the small intestine is wrinkled into thousands of folds and is carpeted with villi.

Muscle layers beneath folds

Between the villi are tubular glands that secrete enzyme-containing intestinal juice.

A villus

Capillaries

Lymphatic vessel

Artery

Vein

Lymphatic vessel

This is a photograph of part of an actual human intestinal cell with microvilli.

Microvilli

Three cells of a villus. Each cell is covered with microvilli.

Based on D. W. Fawcett from D. W. Fawcett, The Cell 2e, (Sanders, 1981)

FIGURE 5-5 The Small Intestinal Villi

lymph or the blood. In either case, the nutrients end up in the blood, at least for a while. The water-soluble nutrients (and the smaller products of fat digestion) are released directly into the bloodstream by way of the capillaries, but the larger fats and the fat-soluble vitamins find direct access into the capillaries impossible because these nutrients are insoluble in water (and blood is mostly water). They require some packaging before they are released.

The intestinal cells assemble the products of fat digestion into larger molecules called **triglycerides.** These triglycerides, fat-soluble vitamins (when present), and other large lipids (cholesterol and the phospholipids) are then packaged for transport. They cluster together with special proteins to form **chylomicrons,** one kind of **lipoproteins** (lipoproteins are described at the beginning on p. 121). Finally, the cells release the chylomicrons into the lymphatic system. They can then glide through the lymph vessels until they arrive at a point of entry into the bloodstream near the heart.

IN SUMMARY

▪ The many folds and villi of the small intestine dramatically increase its surface area, facilitating nutrient absorption.

▪ Nutrients pass through the cells of the villi and enter either the blood (if they are water soluble or small fat fragments) or the lymph (if they are fat soluble).

5.4 Transport of Nutrients

LO 5.4 Explain how nutrients are delivered from the GI tract to body cells by the vascular system and describe the different types of lipoproteins.

Once a nutrient has entered the bloodstream or the lymphatic system, it may be transported to any part of the body, from the tips of the toes to the roots of the hair, where it becomes available to any of the cells. The circulatory systems are arranged to deliver nutrients wherever they are needed.

The Vascular System

The vascular or blood circulatory system is a closed system of vessels through which blood flows continuously in a figure eight, with the heart serving as a pump at the crossover point. On each loop of the figure eight, blood travels a simple route: heart to arteries to capillaries to veins to heart.

The routing of blood through the digestive system is different, however. Blood is carried to the digestive system (as it is to all organs) by way of an **artery,** which (as in all organs) branches into **capillaries** to reach every cell. Blood leaving the digestive system goes by way of a **vein.** The **hepatic portal vein,** however, directs blood not back to the heart but to another organ—the liver. This vein *again* branches into a network of small blood vessels (*sinusoids*) so that every cell of the liver has access to the newly absorbed nutrients that the blood is carrying. Blood leaving the liver then *again* collects into a vein, called the **hepatic vein,** which returns the blood to the heart. The route is thus heart to arteries to capillaries (in intestines) to hepatic portal vein to sinusoids (in liver) to hepatic vein to heart.

An anatomist studying this system knows there must be a reason for this special arrangement. The liver is located in the circulation system at the point where it will have the first chance at the materials absorbed from the GI tract. In fact, the liver is the body's major metabolic organ (see Figure 5-6) and must prepare the absorbed nutrients for use by the rest of the body. Furthermore, the liver stands as a gatekeeper

lymph (LIMF)**:** the body fluid found in lymphatic vessels. Lymph consists of all the constituents of blood except red blood cells.

triglycerides (try-GLISS-er-rides)**:** one of the main classes of lipids: the chief form of fat in foods and the major storage form of fat in the body; composed of glycerol with three fatty acids attached.
  tri = three
  glyceride = a compound of glycerol

chylomicrons (kye-lo-MY-crons)**:** the lipoproteins that transport lipids from the intestinal cells into the body. The cells of the body remove the lipids they need from the chylomicrons, leaving chylomicron remnants to be picked up by the liver cells.

lipoproteins: clusters of lipids associated with proteins that serve as transport vehicles for lipids in the lymph and blood.

artery: a vessel that carries blood away from the heart.

capillaries: small vessels that branch from an artery. Capillaries connect arteries to veins. Oxygen, nutrients, and waste materials are exchanged across capillary walls.

vein: a vessel that carries blood back to the heart.

hepatic portal vein: the vein that collects blood from the GI tract and conducts it to capillaries in the liver.
  portal = gateway

hepatic vein: the vein that collects blood from the liver capillaries and returns it to the heart.
  hepatic = liver

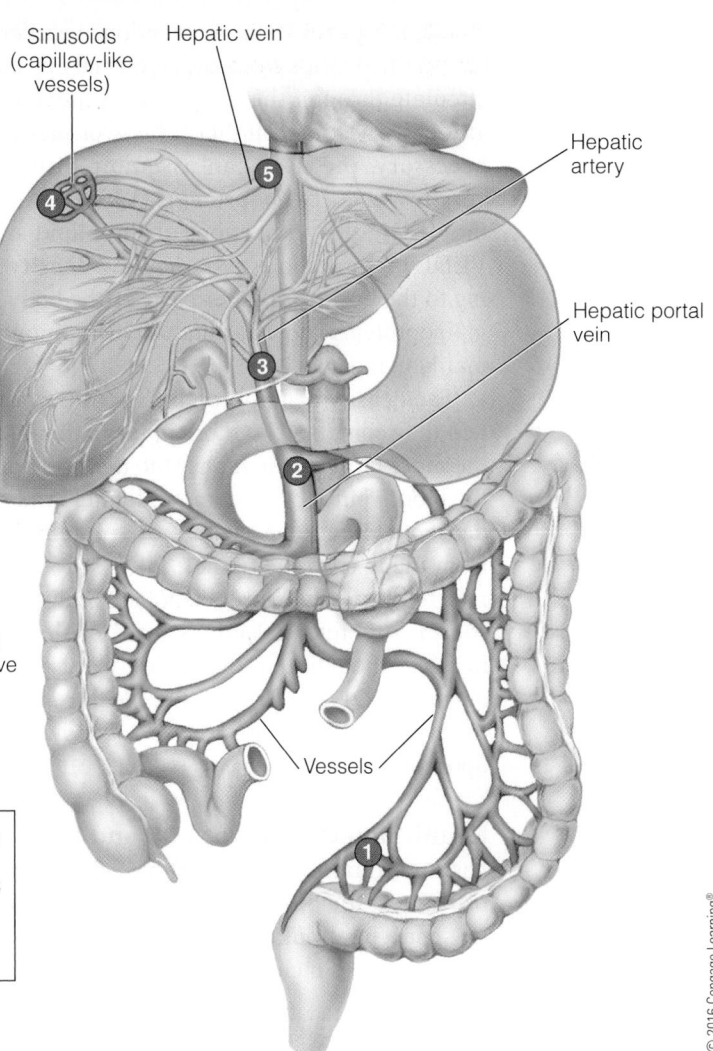

1. Vessels gather up nutrients and reabsorbed water and salts from all over the digestive tract.

Not shown here:
Parallel to these vessels (veins) are other vessels (arteries) that carry oxygen-rich blood from the heart to the intestines.

2. The vessels merge into the hepatic portal vein, which conducts all absorbed materials to the liver.

3. The hepatic artery brings a supply of freshly oxygenated blood (not loaded with nutrients) from the lungs to supply oxygen to the liver's own cells.

4. Capillary-like vessels (sinusoids) branch all over the liver, making nutrients and oxygen available to all its cells and giving the cells access to blood from the digestive system.

5. The hepatic vein gathers up blood in the liver and returns it to the heart.

In contrast, nutrients absorbed into lymph do not go to the liver first. They go to the heart, which pumps them to all the body's cells. The cells remove the nutrients they need, and the liver then has to deal only with the remnants.

Sinusoids (capillary-like vessels)

Hepatic vein

Hepatic artery

Hepatic portal vein

Vessels

FIGURE 5-6 **The Liver and Its Circulatory System**

to waylay intruders that might otherwise harm the heart or brain. Chapter 20 offers more information about this crucial organ.

The Lymphatic System

The lymphatic system is a one-way route for fluids to travel from tissue spaces into the blood. The lymphatic system has no pump; instead, lymph is squeezed from one portion of the body to another like water in a sponge, as muscles contract and create pressure here and there. Ultimately, the lymph flows into the thoracic duct, a large duct behind the heart. This duct terminates in the subclavian vein, which conducts the lymph into the right upper chamber of the heart. In this way, fat-soluble nutrients absorbed into the lymphatic system from the GI tract finally enter the bloodstream.

Transport of Lipids: Lipoproteins

Within the circulatory system, lipids always travel from place to place bundled with protein, that is, as lipoproteins. When physicians measure a person's blood lipid profile, they are interested in both the types of fat present (such as triglycerides and cholesterol) and the types of lipoproteins that carry them.

VLDL, LDL, and HDL As mentioned earlier, chylomicrons transport newly absorbed (*diet-derived*) lipids from the intestinal cells to the rest of the body. As chylomicrons circulate through the body, cells remove their lipid contents, so the chylomicrons gradually become smaller. The liver picks up these chylomicron remnants. When necessary, the liver can assemble different lipoproteins, which are known as **very-low-density lipoproteins (VLDL).** As the body's cells remove triglycerides from the VLDL, the proportions of their lipid and protein contents shift. As this occurs, VLDL become cholesterol-rich **low-density lipoproteins (LDL).** Cholesterol returning to the liver from other parts of the body for metabolism or excretion is packaged in lipoproteins known as **high-density lipoproteins (HDL).** HDL are synthesized primarily in the liver.

The density of lipoproteins varies according to the proportion of lipids and protein they contain. The more lipids in the lipoprotein molecule, the lower the density; the more protein, the higher the density. Both LDL and HDL carry lipids around in the blood, but LDL are larger, lighter, and filled with more lipid; HDL are smaller, denser, and packaged with more protein. LDL deliver cholesterol and triglycerides from the liver to the tissues; HDL scavenge excess cholesterol from the tissues and return it to the liver for metabolism or disposal. These different functions explain why some people refer to LDL as "bad" cholesterol and HDL as "good" cholesterol. Keep in mind, though, that there is only *one* kind of cholesterol molecule; the differences between LDL and HDL reflect *proportions* of lipids and proteins within them—not the type of cholesterol. Figure 5-7 shows the relative sizes and compositions of the lipoproteins.

Health Implications of LDL and HDL The distinction between LDL and HDL has implications for the health of the heart and blood vessels. High concentrations of LDL in the blood are associated with an increased risk of heart disease, as are low concentrations of HDL.[2] Factors that lower LDL concentrations and raise HDL concentrations include:

- Weight management (see Chapter 7).

- Polyunsaturated or monounsaturated, instead of saturated, fatty acids in the diet (see Chapter 3).

- Soluble fibers (see Chapter 2).

- Physical activity (see Chapter 10).

Lipoproteins and heart disease are discussed in Chapter 22.

IN SUMMARY

- Nutrients leaving the digestive system via the blood are routed directly to the liver before being transported to the body's cells. Those leaving via the lymphatic system eventually enter the vascular system, but they bypass the liver at first.

- Within the circulatory system, lipids travel bundled with proteins as lipoproteins. Different types of lipoproteins include chylomicrons, very-low-density lipoproteins (VLDL), low-density lipoproteins (LDL), and high-density lipoproteins (HDL).

- Elevated blood concentrations of LDL are associated with a high risk of heart disease, as are low levels of HDL.

very-low-density lipoproteins (VLDL): the type of lipoproteins made primarily by liver cells to transport lipids to various tissues in the body; composed primarily of triglycerides.

low-density lipoproteins (LDL): the type of lipoproteins derived from VLDL as cells remove triglycerides from them. LDL carry cholesterol and triglycerides from the liver to the cells of the body and are composed primarily of cholesterol.

high-density lipoproteins (HDL): the type of lipoproteins that transport cholesterol back to the liver from peripheral cells; composed primarily of protein.

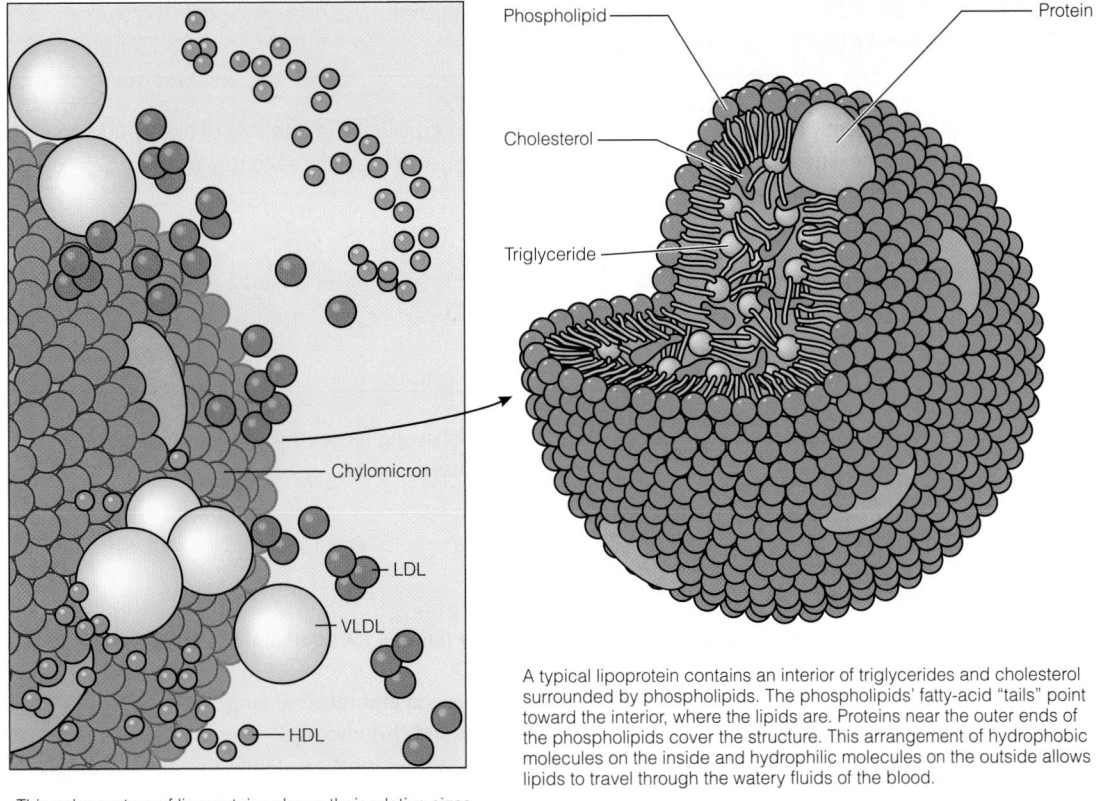

Phospholipid
Cholesterol
Triglyceride
Protein

Chylomicron

LDL

VLDL

HDL

A typical lipoprotein contains an interior of triglycerides and cholesterol surrounded by phospholipids. The phospholipids' fatty-acid "tails" point toward the interior, where the lipids are. Proteins near the outer ends of the phospholipids cover the structure. This arrangement of hydrophobic molecules on the inside and hydrophilic molecules on the outside allows lipids to travel through the watery fluids of the blood.

This solar system of lipoproteins shows their relative sizes. Notice how large the fat-filled chylomicron is compared with the others and how the others get progressively smaller as their proportion of fat declines and protein increases.

Chylomicrons contain so little protein and so much triglyceride that they are the lowest in density.

Very-low-density lipoproteins (VLDL) are half triglycerides, accounting for their low density.

Low-density lipoproteins (LDL) are half cholesterol, accounting for their implication in heart disease.

High-density lipoproteins (HDL) are half protein, accounting for their high density.

© Cengage Learning®

FIGURE 5-7 The Lipoproteins

The System at Its Best

The GI tract is the first organ in the body to deal with the nutrients that will ultimately maintain the health and nutrition status of the whole body. Its intricate architecture makes it sensitive and responsive to conditions in its environment. One condition indispensable to the GI tract's performance is its own good health. Such lifestyle factors as sleep, physical activity, state of mind, and nutrition affect GI tract health. Adequate sleep allows for repair and maintenance of tissue. Physical activity promotes healthy muscle tone and may protect against cancer of the colon.[3] Mental state profoundly affects digestion and absorption through the activity of nerves and hormones that help regulate these processes. A relaxed, peaceful attitude during a meal enhances digestion and absorption.

Clinical Applications

1. People who experience malabsorption frequently have the most difficulty digesting fat. Considering the differences in fat, carbohydrate, and protein digestion and absorption, can you offer an explanation?

2. How might you explain the importance of dietary fiber to a client who frequently experiences constipation?

Self Check

1. Once food is swallowed, it travels through the digestive tract in this order:
   a. esophagus, stomach, large intestine, liver.
   b. esophagus, stomach, small intestine, large intestine.
   c. small intestine, stomach, esophagus, large intestine.
   d. small intestine, large intestine, stomach, esophagus.

2. Once chyme travels the length of the small intestine, it passes through the ileocecal valve at the beginning of the:
   a. large intestine.
   b. stomach.
   c. esophagus.
   d. jejunum.

3. The periodic squeezing or partitioning of the intestine by its circular muscles that both mixes and slowly pushes the contents along is known as:
   a. secretion.
   b. absorption.
   c. peristalsis.
   d. segmentation.

4. An enzyme in saliva begins the digestion of:
   a. starch.
   b. vitamins.
   c. protein.
   d. minerals.

5. Bile is:
   a. an enzyme that splits starch.
   b. an alkaline secretion of the pancreas.
   c. an emulsifier made by the liver that prepares fats and oils for digestion.
   d. a stomach secretion containing water, hydrochloric acid, and the enzymes pepsin and lipase.

6. Which of the following passes through the large intestine mostly unabsorbed?
   a. Fiber
   b. Vitamins
   c. Minerals
   d. Starch

7. The two major nutrient transport systems in the body are:
   a. LDL and HDL.
   b. the digestive and absorptive systems.
   c. lipoproteins and chylomicrons.
   d. the vascular and lymphatic systems.

8. Within the circulatory system, lipids travel from place to place bundled with proteins as:
   a. microvilli.
   b. chylomicrons.
   c. lipoproteins.
   d. phospholipids.

9. Elevated LDL concentrations in the blood are associated with:
   a. a high-protein diet.
   b. a low risk of diabetes.
   c. regular physical activity.
   d. a high risk of heart disease.

10. Three factors that lower the concentration of LDL and raise the concentration of HDL in the blood are:
    a. polyunsaturated fat, rest, and dietary HDL.
    b. antioxidants, insoluble fibers, and dietary HDL.
    c. saturated fat, antioxidants, and insoluble fibers.
    d. weight control, soluble fibers, and physical activity.

Answers to these questions can be found in Appendix H.

Notes

1. P. C. Konturek, T. Brzozowski and S. J. Konturek, Stress and the gut: Pathophysiology, clinical consequences, diagnostic approach and treatment options, *Journal of Physiology and Pharmacology* 62 (2011): 591–599.

2. A. S. Go and coauthors, Heart disease and stroke statistics—2014 update: A report from the American Heart Association, *Circulation* 129 (2014): e28–e292.

3. L. H. Kushi and coauthors, American Cancer Society guidelines on nutrition and physical activity for cancer prevention, *CA Cancer Journal for Clinicians* 62 (2012): 30–67.

Nutrition in Practice

LO 5.5 Describe how foodborne illnesses can be prevented.

The Food and Drug Administration (FDA) lists **foodborne illness** as the leading food safety concern in the United States because **outbreaks** of food poisoning far outnumber episodes of any other kind of food contamination. The **CDC (Centers for Disease Control and Prevention)** estimates that 48 million cases of foodborne illnesses occur each year in the United States.[1] More than 100,000 people become so sick as to need hospitalization. For some 3000 people each year, the symptoms (Table NP5-1) are so severe as to cause death. Most vulnerable are pregnant women; very young, very old, sick, or malnourished people; and those with a weakened immune system (as in AIDS).[2] By taking the proper precautions, people can minimize their chances of contracting foodborne illnesses. Box NP5-1 defines related terms.

What is foodborne illness?

Foodborne illness can be caused by either an infection or an intoxication. Table NP5-2 (p. 126) summarizes the **pathogens** responsible for 90 percent of foodborne illnesses, related hospitalizations, and deaths, along with food sources, general symptoms, and prevention methods.

What is the difference between foodborne infections and food intoxications?

Foodborne infections are caused by eating foods contaminated by infectious microbes. Among foodborne infections, norovirus and *Salmonella* are the leading causes of hospitalizations and deaths.[3] Pathogens commonly enter the GI tract in contaminated foods such as undercooked poultry and unpasteurized milk. Symptoms generally include abdominal cramps, fever, vomiting, and diarrhea.

TABLE NP5-1 Symptoms of Foodborne Illness

Get medical help when these symptoms occur:

- Bloody diarrhea
- Diarrhea lasting more than three days
- Prolonged vomiting that prevents keeping liquids down and can lead to dehydration
- Difficulty breathing
- Difficulty swallowing
- Double vision
- Fever lasting more than 24 hours
- Headache accompanied by muscle stiffness and fever
- Numbness, muscle weakness, and tingling sensations in the skin
- Rapid heart rate, fainting, and dizziness

© Cengage Learning®

BOX NP 5-1 GLOSSARY

CDC (Centers for Disease Control and Prevention): a branch of the Department of Health and Human Services that is responsible for, among other things, monitoring foodborne diseases (*www.cdc.gov*).

cross-contamination: the contamination of food by bacteria that occurs when the food comes into contact with surfaces previously touched by raw meat, poultry, or seafood.

foodborne illness: illness transmitted to human beings through food and water, caused by either an infectious agent (foodborne infection) or a poisonous substance (foodborne intoxication); commonly known as **food poisoning.**

Hazard Analysis Critical Control Points (HACCP): a systematic plan to identify and correct potential microbial hazards in the manufacturing, distribution, and commercial use of food products; commonly referred to as "HASS-ip."

outbreaks: two or more cases of a similar illness resulting from the ingestion of a common food.

pasteurization: heat processing of food that inactivates some, but not all, microorganisms in the food; not a sterilization process. Bacteria that cause spoilage are still present.

pathogens (PATH-oh-jens): microorganisms capable of producing disease.

sushi: vinegar-flavored rice and seafood, typically wrapped in seaweed and stuffed with colorful vegetables. Some sushi is stuffed with raw fish; other varieties contain cooked seafood.

traveler's diarrhea: nausea, vomiting, and diarrhea caused by consuming food or water contaminated by any of several organisms, most commonly, *E. coli*, *Shigella*, *Campylobacter jejuni*, and *Salmonella*.

Norovirus illustrates the importance of personal hygiene.[4] Norovirus is passed in the stool and vomit of infected people. Thus, infected people who do not wash their hands adequately can pass the virus directly to other people, or they can pass it indirectly by way of contaminated food or water. Outbreaks in the United States are often linked to food touched by infected food handlers or to person-to-person contact in day care centers, in nursing homes, and on cruise ships. People can also be infected with norovirus by eating raw shellfish such as oysters and clams that are grown in sewage-contaminated waters.

Food intoxications are caused by eating foods containing natural toxins or, more likely, microbes that produce toxins. The most common food toxin is produced by *Staphylococcus aureus;* it affects more than 1 million people each year. Less common, but more infamous, is *Clostridium botulinum,* an organism that produces a deadly toxin in anaerobic conditions such as improperly canned (especially home-canned) foods and homemade garlic or herb-flavored oils stored at room temperature. The botulism toxin paralyzes muscles, making it difficult to see, speak, swallow,

TABLE NP5-2 The Major Microbes of Foodborne Illness

Organism Name	Most Frequent Food Sources	Onset and General Symptoms	Prevention Methods[a]
Foodborne Infections			
Campylobacter (KAM-pee-loh-BAK-ter) bacterium	Raw and undercooked poultry, unpasteurized milk, contaminated water	Onset: 2 to 5 days. Diarrhea, vomiting, abdominal cramps, fever; sometimes bloody stools; lasts 2 to 10 days.	Cook foods thoroughly; use pasteurized milk; use sanitary food-handling methods.
Escherichia (esh-uh-REK-ee-uh) *coli* (KOH-lye) bacterium (including Shiga toxin-producing strains)[b]	Undercooked ground beef, unpasteurized milk and juices, raw fruits and vegetables, contaminated water, and person-to-person contact	Onset: 1 to 8 days. Severe bloody diarrhea, abdominal cramps, vomiting; lasts 5 to 10 days.	Cook ground beef thoroughly; use pasteurized milk; use sanitary food-handling methods; use treated, boiled, or bottled water.
Norovirus	Person-to-person contact; raw foods, salads, sandwiches	Onset: 1 to 2 days. Vomiting; lasts 1 to 2 days.	Use sanitary food-handling methods.
Listeria (lis-TER-ee-AH) bacterium	Unpasteurized milk; fresh soft cheeses; luncheon meats, hot dogs	Onset: 1 to 21 days. Fever, muscle aches; nausea, vomiting, blood poisoning, complications in pregnancy, and meningitis (stiff neck, severe headache, and fever).	Use sanitary food-handling methods; cook foods thoroughly; use pasteurized milk.
Clostridium (claw-STRID-ee-um) *perfringens* (per-FRINGE-enz) bacterium	Meats and meat products stored at between 120°F and 130°F	Onset: 8 to 16 hours. Abdominal pain, diarrhea, nausea; lasts 1 to 2 days.	Use sanitary food-handling methods; use pasteurized milk; cook foods thoroughly; refrigerate foods promptly and properly.
Salmonella (sal-moh-NEL-ah) bacteria (>2300 types)	Raw or undercooked eggs, meats, poultry, raw milk and other dairy products, shrimp, frog legs, yeast, coconut, pasta, and chocolate	Onset: 1 to 3 days. Fever, vomiting, abdominal cramps, diarrhea; lasts 4 to 7 days; can be fatal.	Use sanitary food-handling methods; use pasteurized milk; cook foods thoroughly; refrigerate foods promptly and properly.
Toxoplasma (TOK-so-PLAZ-ma) *gondii* parasite	Raw or undercooked meat; contaminated water; unpasteurized goat's milk; contact with infected cat feces	Onset: 7 to 21 days. Swollen glands, fever, headache, muscle pain, stiff neck.	Use sanitary food-handling methods; cook foods thoroughly.
Foodborne Intoxications			
Clostridium (claw-STRID-ee-um) *botulinum* (bot-chew-LINE-um) bacterium produces botulin toxin, responsible for causing botulism	Anaerobic environment of low acidity (canned corn, peppers, green beans, soups, beets, asparagus, mushrooms, ripe olives, spinach, tuna, chicken, chicken liver, liver pâté, luncheon meats, ham, sausage, stuffed eggplant, lobster, and smoked and salted fish)	Onset: 4 to 36 hours. Nervous system symptoms, including double vision, inability to swallow, speech difficulty, and progressive paralysis of the respiratory system; often fatal; leaves prolonged symptoms in survivors.	Use proper canning methods for low-acid foods; refrigerate homemade garlic and herb oils; avoid commercially prepared foods with leaky seals or with bent, bulging, or broken cans. Do not give infants honey because it may contain spores of *Clostridium botulinum*, which is a common source of infection for infants.
Staphylococcus (STAF-il-oh-KOK-us) *aureus* bacterium produces staphylococcal toxin	Toxin produced in improperly refrigerated meats; egg, tuna, potato, and macaroni salads; cream-filled pastries	Onset: 1 to 6 hours. Diarrhea, nausea, vomiting, abdominal cramps, fever; lasts 1 to 2 days.	Use sanitary food-handling methods; cook food thoroughly; refrigerate foods promptly and properly; use proper home-canning methods.

Note: Travelers' diarrhea is most commonly caused by *E. coli*, *Campylobacter jejuni*, *Shigella*, and *Salmonella*.

[a] Table NP5-3 on pp. 129–130 provides more details on the proper handling, cooking, and refrigeration of foods.
[b] O157, O145, and other Shiga toxin-producing strains.

© Cengage Learning®

and breathe. Because death can occur within 24 hours of onset, botulism demands immediate medical attention. Even then, survivors may suffer the effects for months or years.

How do people get foodborne illness?

Transmission of foodborne illness has changed as our food supply and lifestyles have changed.[5] In the past, foodborne illness was caused by one person's error in a small setting, such as improperly refrigerated egg salad at a family picnic, and affected only a few victims. Today, we are eating more foods prepared and packaged by others. Consequently, when a food manufacturer or restaurant chef makes an error, foodborne illness can quickly affect many people. An estimated 80 percent of reported foodborne illnesses are caused by errors in a commercial setting, such as the improper **pasteurization** of milk at a large dairy.

In 2009, *Salmonella* was found in peanut butter that had been used in more than 2100 products made by more than 200 companies; another *Salmonella* outbreak in 2010 led to the recall of 500 million eggs from two farms. In 2011, a cantaloupe farm had to recall more than 300,000 cases of fruit when *Listeria* poisoning killed 29 people and made 139 others sick. These incidents and others focus the national spotlight on two important safety issues: disease-causing organisms are commonly found in foods, and safe food-handling practices can minimize harm from most of these foodborne pathogens.

What kinds of programs are in place to help keep foods safe?

To improve the safety of the U.S. food supply, the Food Safety Modernization Act (FSMA) was signed into law in 2011. It has been called "historic" because it shifts the focus of FDA activities from reacting *after* people become ill to preventing foodborne illness in the first place.[6] The new law stresses prevention at food-processing facilities; provides the FDA with greater enforcement, inspection, and recall authorities; and affords the FDA greater oversight of imported foods.

In addition, the U.S. Department of Agriculture (USDA), the FDA, and the food-processing industries have developed and implemented programs to control foodborne illness.* For example, USDA inspectors examine meat-processing plants every day to ensure that these facilities meet government standards. Seafood, egg, produce, and processed food facilities are inspected less often, but all food producers must use a **Hazard Analysis Critical Control Points (HACCP)** plan to help prevent foodborne illnesses at their source. Each slaughterhouse, packer, distributor, and transporter of susceptible foods must identify "critical control points" that pose a risk of contamination and implement verifiable procedures to eliminate or minimize the risk. The HACCP system has proved a remarkable success for domestic products, but such programs do not apply to imported foods.

An estimated $2 trillion worth of products are imported into the United States from more than 150 countries each year. Many countries cooperate with the FDA and have adopted many of the safe food-handling practices used in the United States, but some imported foods come from countries with little or no regulatory

*In addition to HACCP, other programs initiated under the Food Safety Initiative include FoodNet, PulseNet, the Environmental Health Specialists Network (EHS-Net), and Fight BAC!

oversight. To help consumers distinguish between imported and domestic foods, certain foods—including fish, shellfish, meats, fruits, vegetables, and some nuts—must display a Country of Origin Label specifying where they were produced.[7]

Importantly, the implementation of the FSMA strengthens the FDA's ability to safeguard imported foods.[8] Under the FSMA, the FDA is permitted to inspect foreign facilities. If a food producer in another country does not allow the FDA to inspect its facility, the FDA can refuse to allow food from that facility into the United States. The FSMA also requires importers to verify the food safety practices of their suppliers and adds new checks on imported foods.

Are foods bought in grocery stores and foods eaten in restaurants safe?

Canned and packaged foods sold in grocery stores are easily controlled, but rare accidents do happen. Batch numbering makes it possible to recall contaminated foods through public announcements via the Internet, newspapers, television, and radio. In the grocery store, consumers can buy items before the "sell by" date and inspect the safety seals and wrappers of packages. A broken seal, bulging can lid, or mangled package fails to protect the consumer against microbes, insects, spoilage, or even vandalism.

State and local health regulations provide guidelines on the cleanliness of facilities and the safe preparation of foods for restaurants, cafeterias, and fast-food establishments. Even so, consumers should take these actions to help prevent foodborne illnesses when dining out:

▪ Wash hands with hot, soapy water before meals.

▪ Expect clean tabletops, dinnerware, utensils, and food preparation areas.

▪ Expect cooked foods to be served piping hot and salads to be fresh and cold.

▪ Refrigerate take-home items within two hours and use leftovers within three to four days.

Improper handling of foods can occur anywhere along the line from commercial manufacturers to large supermarkets to small restaurants to private homes. Maintaining a safe food supply requires everyone's efforts.

What can people do to protect themselves from foodborne illness?

Whether microbes multiply and cause illness depends, in part, on a few key food-handling behaviors in the kitchen—whether the kitchen is in your home, a school cafeteria, a gourmet restaurant, or a canned goods manufacturer. Figure NP5-1 (p. 128) summarizes the four simple things that can help most to prevent foodborne illness:

▪ *Clean.* Keep a clean, safe kitchen by washing hands and surfaces often. Wash countertops, cutting boards, sponges, and utensils in hot, soapy water before and after each step of food preparation. To reduce bacterial contamination on hands, wash hands with soap and warm water; if soap and water are not available, use an alcohol-based sanitizing gel.[9]

▪ *Separate.* Avoid cross-contamination by keeping raw eggs, meat, poultry, and seafood separate from other foods. Wash

FIGURE NP5-1 Fight Bac!
Four ways to keep food safe. The Fight Bac! website is at *www.fightbac.org*.

PhotoDisc/Getty Images

Wash your hands with warm water and soap for at least 20 seconds before preparing or eating food to reduce the chance of microbial contamination.

all utensils and surfaces (such as cutting boards or platters) that have been in contact with these foods with hot, soapy water before using them again. Bacteria inevitably left on the surfaces from the raw meat can recontaminate the cooked meat or other foods—a problem known as **cross-contamination.** Washing raw eggs, meat, and poultry is not recommended as the extra handling increases the risk of cross-contamination.

▪ *Cook.* Keep hot foods hot by cooking to proper temperatures. Foods need to cook long enough to reach internal temperatures

that will kill microbes, and maintain adequate temperatures to prevent bacterial growth until the foods are served.

▪ *Chill.* Keep cold foods cold by refrigerating promptly. Go directly home upon leaving the grocery store and immediately unpack foods into the refrigerator or freezer upon arrival. After a meal, refrigerate any leftovers immediately.

Unfortunately, consumers commonly fail to follow these simple food-handling recommendations. See Table NP5-3 for additional food safety tips.

What precautions need to be taken when preparing meat and poultry?

Figure NP5-2 (p. 130) presents label instructions for the safe handling of meat and poultry and two types of USDA seals. Meats and poultry contain bacteria and provide a moist, nutrient-rich environment that favors microbial growth. Ground meat is especially susceptible because it receives more handling than other kinds of meat and has more surface exposed to bacterial contamination. Consumers cannot detect the harmful bacteria in or on meat. For safety's sake, cook meat thoroughly, using a thermometer to test the internal temperature (see Figure NP5-3 on p. 131).

How can a person enjoy seafood safely?

Most seafood available in the United States and Canada is safe, but eating it undercooked or raw can cause severe illnesses—hepatitis, worms, parasites, viral intestinal disorders, and other diseases.[†] Rumor has it that freezing fish will make it safe to eat raw, but this is only partly true. Commercial freezing will kill mature parasitic worms, but only cooking can kill all worm eggs and other microorganisms that can cause illness. For safety's sake, all seafood should be cooked until it is opaque. Even **sushi** can be safe to eat when chefs combine cooked seafood and other ingredients into delicacies.

Eating raw oysters can be dangerous for anyone, but people with liver disease and weakened immune systems are most vulnerable. At least 10 species of bacteria found in raw oysters can cause serious illness and even death. Raw oysters may also carry the hepatitis A virus, which can cause liver disease. Some hot sauces can kill many of these bacteria but not the virus; alcohol may also protect some people against some oyster-borne illnesses but not enough to guarantee protection (or to recommend drinking alcohol). Pasteurization of raw oysters—holding them at a specified temperature for a specified time—holds promise for killing bacteria without cooking the oyster or altering its texture or flavor.

As population density increases along the shores of seafood-harvesting waters, pollution inevitably invades the sea life there. Preventing seafood-borne illness is in large part a task of controlling water pollution. To help ensure a safe seafood market, the FDA requires processors to adopt food safety practices based on the HACCP system mentioned earlier.

Chemical pollution and microbial contamination lurk not only in the water but also in the boats and warehouses where seafood is cleaned, prepared, and refrigerated. Seafood is one of the most

[†]Diseases caused by toxins from the sea include ciguatera poisoning, scombroid poisoning, and paralytic and neurotoxic shellfish poisoning.

TABLE NP5-3 Strategies to Prevent Foodborne Illness

Most foodborne illnesses can be prevented by following four simple rules: clean, separate, cook, and chill.

Clean

- Wash fruits and vegetables in a clean sink with a scrub brush and warm water; store washed and unwashed produce separately.
- Use hot, soapy water to wash hands, utensils, dishes, nonporous cutting boards, and countertops before handling food and between tasks when working with different foods. Use a bleach solution on cutting boards (one capful per gallon of water).
- Cover cuts with clean bandages before food preparation; dirty bandages carry harmful microorganisms.
- Mix foods with utensils, not hands; keep hands and utensils away from mouth, nose, and hair.
- Anyone may be a carrier of bacteria and should avoid coughing or sneezing over food. A person with a skin infection or infectious disease should not prepare food.
- Wash or replace sponges and towels regularly.
- Clean up food spills and crumb-filled crevices.

Separate

- Wash all surfaces that have been in contact with raw meats, poultry, eggs, fish, and shellfish before reusing.
- Serve cooked foods on a clean plate with a clean utensil. Separate raw foods from those that have been cooked.
- Don't use marinade that was in contact with raw meat for basting or sauces.

Cook

- When cooking meats or poultry, use a thermometer to test the internal temperature. Insert the thermometer between the thigh and the body of a turkey or into the thickest part of other meats, making sure the tip of the thermometer is not in contact with bone or the pan. Cook to the temperature indicated for that particular meat (see Figure NP5-3 on p. 131); cook hamburgers to at least medium well done. If you have safety questions, call the USDA Meat and Poultry Hotline: (800) 535-4555.
- Cook stuffing separately, or stuff poultry just prior to cooking.
- Do not cook large cuts of meat or turkey in a microwave oven; it leaves some parts undercooked while overcooking others.
- Cook eggs before eating them (soft-boiled for at least 3 ½ minutes; scrambled until set, not runny; fried for at least 3 minutes on one side and 1 minute on the other).
- Cook seafood thoroughly. If you have safety questions about seafood, call the FDA hotline: (800) FDA-4010.
- When serving foods, maintain temperatures at 140°F or higher.
- Heat leftovers thoroughly to at least 165°F.

Chill

- When running errands, stop at the grocery store last. When you get home, refrigerate the perishable groceries (such as meats and dairy products) immediately. Do not leave perishables in the car any longer than it takes for ice cream to melt.
- Put packages of raw meat, fish, or poultry on a plate before refrigerating to prevent juices from dripping on food stored below.
- Buy only foods that are solidly frozen in store freezers.
- Keep cold foods at 40°F or less; keep frozen foods at 0°F or less (keep a thermometer in the refrigerator).
- Marinate meats in the refrigerator, not on the counter.
- Look for "Keep Refrigerated" or "Refrigerate After Opening" on food labels.
- Refrigerate leftovers promptly; use shallow containers to cool foods faster; use leftovers within 3 to 4 days.
- Thaw meats or poultry in the refrigerator, not at room temperature. If you must hasten thawing, use cool water (changed every 30 minutes) or a microwave oven.
- Freeze meat, fish, or poultry immediately if not planning to use within a few days.

In General

- Do not reuse disposable containers; use nondisposable containers or recycle instead.
- Do not taste food that is suspect. "If in doubt, throw it out."
- Throw out foods with danger-signaling odors. Be aware, though, that most food-poisoning bacteria are odorless, colorless, and tasteless.
- Do not buy or use items that have broken seals or mangled packaging; such containers cannot protect against microbes, insects, spoilage, or even vandalism. Check safety seals, buttons, and expiration dates.
- Follow label instructions for storing and preparing packaged and frozen foods; throw out foods that have been thawed or refrozen.
- Discard foods that are discolored, moldy, or decayed or that have been contaminated by insects or rodents.

continued

For Specific Food Items

- *Canned goods.* Carefully discard food from cans that leak or bulge so that other people and animals will not accidentally ingest it; before canning, seek professional advice from the USDA National Institute of Food and Agriculture (check your phone book under U.S. government listings, or go online: *www.csrees.usda.gov*).

- *Milk and cheeses.* Use only pasteurized milk and milk products. Aged cheeses, such as cheddar and Swiss, do well for an hour or two without refrigeration, but they should be refrigerated or stored in an ice chest for longer periods.

- *Eggs.* Use clean eggs with intact shells. Do not eat eggs, even pasteurized eggs, raw; raw eggs are commonly found in Caesar salad dressing, eggnog, cookie dough, hollandaise sauce, and key lime pie. Cook eggs until whites are firmly set and yolks begin to thicken.

- *Honey.* Honey may contain dormant bacterial spores, which can awaken in the human body to produce botulism. In adults, this poses little hazard, but infants younger than 1 year of age should never be fed honey. Honey can accumulate enough toxin to kill an infant; it has been implicated in several cases of sudden infant death. (Honey can also be contaminated with environmental pollutants picked up by the bees.)

- *Mayonnaise.* Commercial mayonnaise may actually help a food to resist spoilage because of the acid content. Still, keep it refrigerated after opening.

- *Mixed salads.* Mixed salads of chopped ingredients spoil easily because they have extensive surface area for bacteria to invade, and they have been in contact with cutting boards, hands, and kitchen utensils that easily transmit bacteria to food (regardless of their mayonnaise content). Chill them well before, during, and after serving.

- *Picnic foods.* Choose foods that last without refrigeration, such as fresh fruits and vegetables, breads and crackers, and canned spreads and cheeses that can be opened and used immediately. Pack foods cold, layer ice between foods, and keep foods out of water.

- *Seafood.* Buy only fresh seafood that has been properly refrigerated or iced. Cooked seafood should be stored separately from raw seafood to avoid cross-contamination.

FIGURE NP5-2 Meat and Poultry Safety, Grading, and Inspection Seals

Inspection is mandatory; grading is voluntary. Neither guarantees that the product will not cause foodborne illnesses, but consumers can help to prevent foodborne illnesses by following the safe handling instructions.

The voluntary "Graded by USDA" seal indicates that the product has been graded for tenderness, juiciness, and flavor. Beef is graded Prime (abundant marbling of the meat muscle), Choice (less marbling), and Select (lean). Similarly, poultry is graded A, B, and C.

The mandatory "Inspected and Passed by the USDA" seal ensures that meat and poultry products are safe, wholesome, and correctly labeled. Inspection does not guarantee that the meat is free of potentially harmful bacteria.

Safe Handling Instructions

THIS PRODUCT WAS PREPARED FROM INSPECTED AND PASSED MEAT AND/OR POULTRY. SOME FOOD PRODUCTS MAY CONTAIN BACTERIA THAT CAN CAUSE ILLNESS IF THE PRODUCT IS MISHANDLED OR COOKED IMPROPERLY. FOR YOUR PROTECTION, FOLLOW THESE SAFE HANDLING INSTRUCTIONS.

KEEP REFRIGERATED OR FROZEN. THAW IN REFRIGERATOR OR MICROWAVE.

KEEP RAW MEAT AND POULTRY SEPARATE FROM OTHER FOODS. WASH WORKING SURFACES (INCLUDING CUTTING BOARDS), UTENSILS, AND HANDS AFTER TOUCHING RAW MEAT OR POULTRY.

COOK THOROUGHLY.

KEEP HOT FOODS HOT. REFRIGERATE LEFTOVERS IMMEDIATELY OR DISCARD.

The USDA requires that safe handling instructions appear on all packages of meat and poultry.

perishable foods: time and temperature are critical to its freshness and flavor. To keep seafood as fresh as possible, people in the industry "keep it cold, keep it clean, and keep it moving." Wise consumers eat it cooked.

Do foods that are unsafe to eat smell bad?

Fresh food generally smells fresh. Not all types of food poisoning are detectable by odor, but some bacterial wastes produce "off" odors. Food with an abnormal odor is spoiled. Throw it out or, if it was recently purchased, return it to the grocery store. Do not taste it. Table NP5-4 lists safe refrigerator storage times for selected foods.

Local health departments and the USDA Extension Service can provide additional information about food safety. Should precautions fail and mild foodborne illness develop, drink clear liquids to replace fluids lost through vomiting and diarrhea.

Well-done meats

Stuffing, all poultry, including ground chicken and turkey; reheat leftovers

170° — Medium-done meats, raw eggs, egg dishes, ground meats (beef, veal, lamb, pork)
165°
160° — Beef, pork, lamb, and veal (steaks, roasts, and chops): Allow to rest at least 3 minutes. During the 3 minutes after meat is removed from the heat source, its temperature remains constant or continues to rise, which destroys pathogens.
145°
140° — Hold hot foods

DANGER ZONE: Do not keep foods between 40°F and 140°F for more than 2 hours or for more than 1 hour when the air temperature is greater than 90°F.

40° — Refrigerator temperatures
0° — Freezer temperatures

© 2016 Cengage Learning®

FIGURE NP5-3 **Recommended Safe Temperatures (Fahrenheit)**

Bacteria multiply rapidly at temperatures between 40°F and 140°F. Cook foods to the temperatures shown on this thermometer and hold them at 140°F or higher.

Charles Stirling/Alamy

Cook hamburgers to 160°F; color alone cannot determine doneness. Some burgers will turn brown before reaching 160°F, whereas others may retain some pink color, even when cooked to 175°F.

David Chasey/Photodisc/Getty Images

Eating raw seafood is a risky proposition.

TABLE NP5-4 **Safe Refrigerator Storage Times (≤40°F)**

1 to 2 Days: Raw ground meats, breakfast or other raw sausages, raw fish or poultry; gravies

3 to 5 Days: Raw steaks, roasts, or chops; cooked meats, poultry, vegetables, and mixed dishes; lunchmeats (packages opened); mayonnaise salads (chicken, egg, pasta, tuna); fresh vegetables (spinach, green beans, tomatoes)

1 Week: Hard-cooked eggs, bacon or hot dogs (opened packages); smoked sausages or seafood; milk, cottage cheese

1 to 2 Weeks: Yogurt; carrots, celery, lettuce

2 to 4 Weeks: Fresh eggs (in shells); lunchmeats, bacon, or hot dogs (packages unopened); dry sausages (pepperoni, hard salami); most aged and processed cheeses (Swiss, brick)

2 Months: Mayonnaise (opened jar); most dry cheeses (Parmesan, Romano)

© Cengage Learning®

If serious foodborne illness is suspected, first call a physician. Then wrap the remainder of the suspected food and label the container so that the food cannot be mistakenly eaten, place it in the refrigerator, and hold it for possible inspection by health authorities.

How can a person defend against foodborne illness when traveling to foreign countries?

People who travel to other countries have a 50-50 chance of contracting a foodborne illness, commonly described as **traveler's diarrhea.** Like many other foodborne illnesses, traveler's diarrhea is a sometimes serious, always annoying bacterial infection of the digestive tract. The risk is high because some countries' cleanliness standards for food and water may be lower than those in the United States and Canada. Also, every region's microbes are different, and while people are immune to those in their own neighborhoods, they have had no chance to develop immunity to the pathogens in places they are visiting for the first time. In addition to the food safety tips outlined on pp. 129–130, precautions while traveling include:

- Wash hands frequently with soap and hot water, especially before handling food or eating. Use sanitizing gel or hand wipes regularly.

- Eat only well-cooked and hot or canned foods. Eat raw fruits or vegetables only if washed in purified water and peeled with clean hands.

- Use purified, bottled water for drinking, making ice cubes, and brushing teeth. Alternatively, use disinfecting tablets or boil water.

- Refuse dairy products that have not been pasteurized and refrigerated properly.

- Travel with antidiarrheal medication in case efforts to avoid illness fail.

To sum up these recommendations, "Boil it, cook it, peel it, or forget it."

131

Notes

1. M. T. Osterholm, Foodborne disease in 2011—The rest of the story, *New England Journal of Medicine* 364 (2011): 889–891; Centers for Disease Control and Prevention, CDC estimates of foodborne illness in the United States, CDC 2011 Estimates: Findings, www.cdc.gov/foodborneburden/2011-foodborne -estimates.html. Updated June 21, 2013.

2. B. M. Lund and S. J. O'Brien, The occurrence and prevention of foodborne disease in vulnerable people, *Foodborne Pathogens and Disease* 8 (2011): 961–973.

3. L. H. Gould and coauthors, Surveillance for foodborne disease outbreaks—United States, 2009-2010, *Morbidity and Mortality Weekly Report* 62 (2013): 41–47.

4. A. J. Hall and coauthors, Centers for Disease Control and Prevention, Updated norovirus outbreak management and disease prevention guidelines, *Morbidity and Mortality Weekly Report* 60 (2011): 1–15.

5. Position of the American Dietetic Association: Food and water safety, *Journal of the American Dietetic Association* 109 (2009): 1449–1460.

6. K. Stewart and L. O. Gostin, Food and Drug Administration regulation of food safety, *Journal of the American Medical Association* 306 (2011): 88–89.

7. Department of Agriculture, Mandatory Country of Origin Labeling of beef, pork, lamb, chicken, goat meat, wild and farm-raised fish and shellfish, perishable agricultural commodities, peanuts, pecans, ginseng, and macadamia nuts, *Federal Register* 74 (2009): 2658–2707.

8. Stewart and Gostin, 2011.

9. Centers for Disease Control and Prevention, Handwashing: Clean hands save lives, www.cdc.gov/handwashing. Updated December 11, 2013.

6

Metabolism, Energy Balance, and Body Composition

Blend Images/SuperStock

6.1 The Organs and Their Metabolic Roles

LO 6.1 List the principal organs of metabolism, describe their primary roles in metabolism, and explain how the body maintains its constant normal temperature of 98.6°F, as well as the difference between anabolic and catabolic reactions in the body.

6.2 The Body's Use of Fuels

LO 6.2 Identify the nutrients involved in energy metabolism and the high-energy compound that captures the energy released during their breakdown, and summarize the main steps in the metabolism of glucose, glycerol, fatty acids, and amino acids.

6.3 Energy Imbalance

LO 6.3 Explain how an excess of any of the three energy-yielding nutrients contributes to body fat and how an inadequate intake of any of them shifts metabolism.

6.4 Energy Balance

LO 6.4 Describe energy balance and identify the components of energy expenditure, the factors that affect a person's BMR, and the factors that influence a person's energy expenditure.

6.5 Body Weight and Body Composition

LO 6.5 Describe the differences between body weight and body composition, including methods to assess them and health implications.

6.6 Health Risks of Underweight and Obesity

LO 6.6 Identify relationships between body weight and the risk of health problems and summarize the guidelines for identifying and evaluating the risks to health from overweight and obesity.

6.7 Nutrition in Practice: Eating Disorders

LO 6.7 Compare the criteria for diagnosis, characteristics, and treatments of the different eating disorders.

133

Every organ, every tissue, and every cell of the body engages in **metabolism**, the chemical reactions involved in releasing energy, breaking down compounds, and making new compounds. Much like a factory, the body works efficiently to manufacture needed products and dispose of wastes. All these processes are regulated by hormonal signals that coordinate supply and demand.

In disease, metabolic processes can become disturbed, and some diseases are caused by metabolic disturbances. This chapter introduces the principal organs and their metabolic roles, the metabolism of the energy nutrients, energy balance, body composition, and the health risks associated with too much or too little body fat. The next chapter offers strategies toward solving the problems of too much or too little body fat.

6.1 The Organs and Their Metabolic Roles

LO 6.1 List the principal organs of metabolism, describe their primary roles in metabolism, and explain how the body maintains its constant normal temperature of 98.6°F, as well as the difference between anabolic and catabolic reactions in the body.

The metabolic reactions of every organ contribute to the body's ability to function normally and maintain health. Metabolic reactions also use or release energy and therefore affect body weight, with consequences for health.

The Principal Organs

Of particular concern to metabolism are the digestive organs, liver, pancreas, circulatory system, and kidneys. Together, they perform much of the work of breaking down compounds, making new ones, transporting nutrients and oxygen throughout the body, and removing the wastes generated by metabolic processes.

The Digestive Organs As Chapter 5 describes, the digestive system transports foods through the gastrointestinal (GI) tract, produces digestive juices and enzymes, absorbs nutrients, provides transport proteins to carry lipids and vitamins to other sites in the body, and reabsorbs salts and fluids. The digestive system also possesses the body's most rapidly multiplying cells: when healthy, they replace themselves every few days. Disorders affecting the GI tract interfere with the ingestion, digestion, absorption, and metabolism of nutrients, as described in Chapters 17 and 18.

The Liver Nutrients absorbed into the bloodstream are taken first to the liver, as described in Chapter 5. The liver is one of the body's most active metabolic factories. It receives nutrients and metabolizes, packages, stores, or ships them out for use by other organs. It manufactures bile, which the body uses to emulsify fat for digestion and absorption. It metabolizes and detoxifies drugs, prepares waste products for excretion, and participates in iron recycling and blood cell manufacture. It also makes many proteins necessary for health, including immune factors, transport proteins, and clotting factors. When liver disorders disrupt metabolism, they profoundly affect both nutrition and health status, as described in Chapter 20.

The Pancreas The pancreas not only contributes digestive juices to the GI tract, but also has another metabolic function: it produces the hormones insulin and glucagon that regulate the body's use of glucose. After a meal, as blood glucose rises, the pancreas secretes insulin. Insulin prompts cells to take up glucose and use it as fuel; insulin also prompts liver cells to store glucose as glycogen. When blood glucose falls (as occurs between meals), the pancreas responds by secreting glucagon into the blood.

metabolism—the chemical reactions involved in releasing energy, breaking down compounds (catabolism), and making new compounds (anabolism)

metabolism: the sum total of all the chemical reactions that go on in living cells.

Glucagon raises blood glucose by signaling the liver to dismantle its glycogen stores and release glucose into the blood for use by all the other body cells. Glucose is an indispensable fuel for brain cells, nerve cells, and red blood cells. Its availability is therefore crucial to normal nervous system activity and blood chemistry. Abnormalities associated with the digestive functions of the pancreas are described in Chapter 19, and those associated with its hormonal functions are described in Chapter 21.

The Heart and Blood Vessels The heart and blood vessels conduct blood, with its cargo of nutrients and oxygen, to all the other body cells and carry wastes away from them. Diseases of the heart and arteries therefore affect the health of the whole body. Metabolic reactions that affect the heart and blood vessels include, most importantly, the making and transport of lipoproteins, which are the carriers of cholesterol and other lipids from the liver to the tissues and back again. High blood levels of low-density lipoproteins (LDL) and very-low-density lipoproteins (VLDL) promote atherosclerosis, which increases the risk of disability or death from heart attacks and strokes. Chapter 22 is devoted to these conditions.

The Kidneys The kidneys are also active metabolic organs. Unceasingly, for 24 hours of every day, they filter waste products from the blood to be excreted in the urine and reabsorb needed nutrients, thereby maintaining the blood's delicate chemical balances. The kidneys' cells also produce compounds that help to regulate blood pressure and convert a precursor compound to active vitamin D, thereby helping to maintain the bones. Thus, disorders of the kidneys nearly always involve the heart and the skeleton. Kidney disorders are the subject of Chapter 23.

The Body's Metabolic Work

The metabolic work that the body's cells do, like all work, requires energy, and foods supply that energy. Foods, in turn, get their energy from the sun, either directly (in the case of photosynthesizing plants that make carbohydrate) or indirectly (in the case of animals that eat plants). When chemical reactions in cells release stored energy from energy-yielding nutrients, that energy becomes available to do the cells' work.

Heat Energy and Body Temperature The cells of each organ conduct metabolic activities specific to that organ. In addition, all cells must maintain themselves, and many must reproduce. To do this, they must have all the essential nutrients available to them: energy nutrients, vitamins, and minerals, as well as water. As cells do their metabolic work, the chemical reactions that are involved release heat, and this heat keeps the body warm. By regulating the rates at which these metabolic reactions release heat energy, the body maintains its constant normal temperature of about 98.6°F.

Accelerated Metabolism During severe stress to the body, metabolism speeds up. Fever sometimes develops. An accelerated metabolism signifies that fuels are being used at a rate more rapid than normal; this may lead to wasting of body organs and loss of weight, including loss of vital lean tissue. Chapters 24 and 25 describe the metabolic consequences of severe stress and the wasting syndrome, respectively.

Building Up and Breaking Down Compounds When not needed by the cells for energy, the basic units of the energy-yielding nutrients are used to build body compounds. The building up of body compounds is known as **anabolism;** this book represents anabolic reactions, wherever possible, by "up" arrows in chemical diagrams (such as those shown in Figure 6-1 on p. 136). Glucose units can be strung together to make glycogen chains. Glycerol and fatty acids can be assembled into triglycerides. Amino acids can be linked together to make proteins. These anabolic reactions, in which simple compounds are put together to form larger, more complex structures, involve doing work and so require the energy provided by the high-energy compound, ATP.

the building up of body compounds is known as anabolism

anabolic reactions require energy

anabolism (an-AB-o-lism): reactions in which small molecules are put together to build larger ones. Anabolic reactions require energy.
 ana = up

Anabolic reactions include the making of glycogen, triglycerides, and protein; these reactions require differing amounts of energy.

CATABOLIC REACTIONS

Catabolic reactions include the breakdown of glycogen, triglycerides, and protein; the further catabolism of glucose, glycerol, fatty acids, and amino acids releases differing amounts of energy. Much of the energy released is captured in the bonds of adenosine triphosphate (ATP).

© Cengage Learning®

FIGURE 6-1 Anabolic and Catabolic Reactions Compared

The breaking down of body compounds is known as **catabolism.** Catabolic reactions usually release energy and are represented, wherever possible, by "down" arrows in chemical diagrams (review Figure 6-1). Glycogen can be broken down to glucose, triglycerides to fatty acids and glycerol, and protein to amino acids.

IN SUMMARY

▌ The digestive organs, the liver, the pancreas, the circulatory system, and the kidneys perform much of the metabolic work of the body.

▌ Metabolism occurs throughout the body, all the time, and supports normal health. Foods supply the energy required for the metabolic work of the body.

▌ When not needed for energy, the basic units of the energy-yielding nutrients are used by the body's cells to build body compounds (anabolism).

▌ When the body needs energy, the cells break the basic units of the energy-yielding nutrients down further to release energy (catabolism).

6.2 The Body's Use of Fuels

LO 6.2 Identify the nutrients involved in energy metabolism and the high-energy compound that captures the energy released during their breakdown, and summarize the main steps in the metabolism of glucose, glycerol, fatty acids, and amino acids.

How does your body get the energy needed to maintain all of its cellular activities from the foods you eat? The answer to this question lies in an understanding of metabolism, the chemical reactions that occur in all living cells.

catabolism (ca-TAB-o-lism)**:** reactions in which large molecules are broken down to smaller ones. Catabolic reactions release energy.
 kata = down

Energy Metabolism

Although every aspect of our lives depends on energy, the concept of energy can be difficult to grasp because it cannot be seen or touched, and it manifests in various forms, including heat, mechanical, electrical, and chemical energy. In the body, heat energy maintains a constant body temperature, and electrical energy sends nerve impulses, for example. Energy is stored in foods and in the body as chemical energy. **Energy metabolism** is the sum total of all the chemical reactions that the body uses to obtain or expend energy from foods. Earlier chapters described how the energy-yielding nutrients—carbohydrate, fat, and protein—are broken down into basic units that are absorbed into the blood:

▪ From carbohydrates: glucose

▪ From fat (triglycerides): glycerol and fatty acids

▪ From proteins: amino acids

This section picks up from there, describing what becomes of these nutrients.

The high-energy compound **ATP (adenosine triphosphate)** is able to transfer small amounts of usable energy to move our muscles and supply our enzymes with the energy they need to catalyze chemical reactions. Figure 6-2 illustrates how ATP does this. When ATP breaks down and releases one of its phosphate groups, a small amount of energy is released and used in the body to build compounds. With the loss of the phosphate group, the ATP becomes ADP (adenosine diphosphate). During energy metabolism, ATP is re-created by attaching a phosphate group to ADP. ATP is produced continuously throughout the day, using the energy from the breakdown of the energy-yielding nutrients.

Breaking Down Nutrients for Energy To produce ATP, the body breaks down any or all of the four basic units—glucose, fatty acids, glycerol, and amino acids—into even smaller units. Each of these nutrients travels down a different pathway, but all can eventually become acetyl CoA, enter the TCA cycle, and provide hydrogens for the electron transport chain. Details follow.

The breakdown of glucose (a 6-carbon compound) into two molecules of **pyruvate** (a 3-carbon compound) is called **glycolysis,** and it produces just two usable ATP. As the carbons in glucose are broken apart to produce pyruvate, the hydrogen atoms attached to the carbons are transferred by **coenzymes** to the electron transport chain.* Thus, the reactions of glycolysis produce a small amount of ATP, pyruvate, and hydrogen-rich coenzymes that are used later in energy metabolism. After glycolysis,

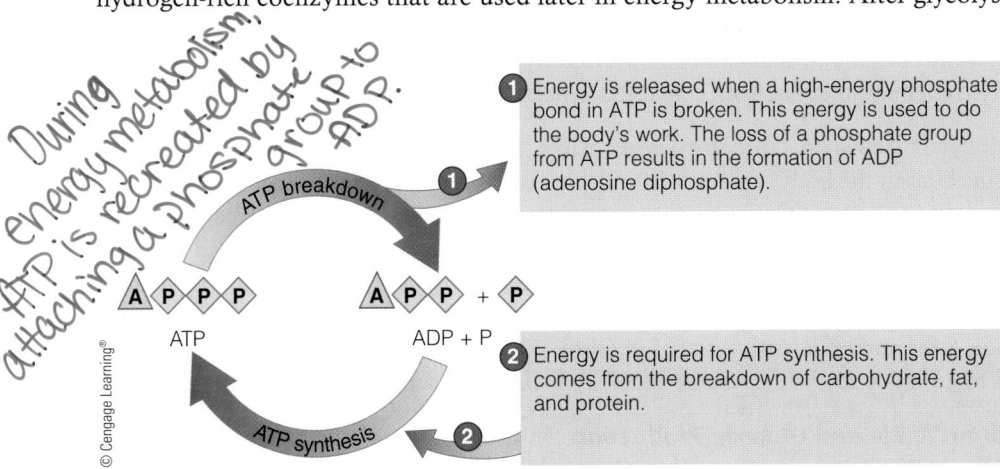

1. Energy is released when a high-energy phosphate bond in ATP is broken. This energy is used to do the body's work. The loss of a phosphate group from ATP results in the formation of ADP (adenosine diphosphate).

2. Energy is required for ATP synthesis. This energy comes from the breakdown of carbohydrate, fat, and protein.

ATP breakdown

ATP synthesis

ATP   ADP + P

FIGURE 6-2 ATP

*The coenzymes used in energy metabolism contain B vitamins; hence, B vitamins play critical roles in ATP production.

energy metabolism: all the reactions by which the body obtains and expends the energy from food.

ATP or adenosine (ah-DEN-ohseen) **triphosphate** (tri-FOS-fate)**:** a common high-energy compound that contains three phosphate groups. The bonds between the phosphate groups are often described as "high-energy" because of their readiness to release energy.

pyruvate (PIE-roo-vate)**:** a 3-carbon compound that plays a key role in energy metabolism.

glycolysis (gligh-COLL-ih-sis)**:** the metabolic breakdown of glucose to pyruvate.
glyco = glucose
lysis = breakdown

coenzymes (co-EN-zime)**:** small molecules that work with enzymes to facilitate the enzymes' activity. Most coenzymes have B vitamins as part of their structures.

pyruvate is converted to **acetyl CoA,** which consists of a 2-carbon fragment and a coenzyme called **CoA.**

Acetyl CoA can be produced not only from pyruvate, but also from the other energy-yielding nutrients. Fatty acids can be broken down into 2-carbon fragments that combine with CoA to form acetyl CoA. As the carbons in fatty acids are broken apart to produce acetyl CoA, hydrogen atoms are released to coenzymes that transfer them to the electron transport chain. Glycerol can easily be converted to pyruvate and therefore can also produce acetyl CoA. The amino acids have various pathways; some can be converted to pyruvate, others can be converted to acetyl CoA, and a few can enter the TCA cycle directly.

TCA Cycle The breakdown of energy nutrients continues in the **TCA cycle (tricarboxylic acid cycle),** as enzymes break down acetyl CoA molecules. With each turn of the TCA cycle, hydrogen atoms are carried by coenzymes to the electron transport chain. The waste product of these reactions is carbon dioxide, which is eventually exhaled.

Electron Transport Chain The final step in energy metabolism occurs at the **electron transport chain.** In this process, enzymes attach a phosphate group to ADP, creating ATP (review Figure 6-2). The hydrogen atoms that were collected by coenzymes during glycolysis, fat breakdown, and the TCA cycles provide the chemical energy that drives ATP production. Finally, the same hydrogen atoms are linked with oxygen to produce water. Figure 6-3 summarizes the metabolic pathways just described.

Aerobic and Anaerobic Metabolism The production of ATP via the electron transport chain requires oxygen in the final step and is called *aerobic* metabolism. Glycolysis produces ATP without oxygen and is therefore called *anaerobic* metabolism. When exercise intensity requires more ATP than can be provided by the electron transport chain (due to limited oxygen or other factors), ATP production from glycolysis is stepped up, making glucose a critical fuel for the exercising muscles. Chapter 10 provides information about anaerobic and aerobic activities and their effects on fuel use.

Glucose Production

When glucose levels drop, glucose can be produced from several other compounds in a process called **gluconeogenesis.** In Figure 6-3, you can see two-way arrows between glucose and pyruvate, but only a one-way arrow between pyruvate and acetyl CoA. The arrows show that pyruvate can be reconverted to glucose, but that acetyl CoA cannot. Any compound that can be converted to pyruvate can be used to make glucose. Any compound that has been converted to acetyl CoA cannot be used to make glucose.

Triglycerides and Glucose Production Recall that triglycerides (the primary form of fat in the body) consist of three fatty acids and a glycerol. Because fatty acids break down to acetyl CoA, they cannot be used to make glucose. The glycerol portion of a triglyceride, however, can be converted to pyruvate and thus can yield glucose. Because glycerol represents only about 5 percent of the weight of a triglyceride molecule, about 95 percent of a triglyceride cannot be converted to glucose at all. Thus, fat is an inefficient source of glucose.[†] The task of serving as a glucose source is left to amino acids, which are obtained by breaking down the body's proteins.

Amino Acids and Glucose Production As Chapter 4 explains, the primary role of amino acids is to maintain supplies of needed body proteins. If amino acids are needed

acetyl CoA (ASS-eh-teel, or ah-SEET-il, coh-AY)**:** a 2-carbon compound (acetate, or acetic acid) with a molecule of CoA attached to it.

CoA (coh-AY)**:** coenzyme A; the coenzyme derived from the B vitamin pantothenic acid and central to energy metabolism.

TCA cycle or tricarboxylic (trycar-box-ILL-ick) **acid cycle:** a series of metabolic reactions that break down molecules of acetyl CoA to carbon dioxide and hydrogen atoms; also called the Krebs cycle after the biochemist who elucidated its reactions.

electron transport chain: the final pathway in energy metabolism that transports electrons from hydrogen to oxygen and captures the energy released in the bonds of a high-energy compound, ATP.

gluconeogenesis (gloo-conee-oh-GEN-ih-sis)**:** the making of glucose from a noncarbohydrate source.

[†]Figure 3-2 in Chapter 3 showed that glycerol (3 carbons) plus 3 fatty acids (most often 16 to 18 carbons) equals a triglyceride. Thus the small glycerol molecule represents only 3 of the 50 or so carbons in the triglyceride.

Amino acids

Carbohydrates

Fats (Triglycerides)

Glucose

Most amino acids can be converted to pyruvate and glucose; they are glucogenic.

Energy released

Pyruvate

CoA

Carbon dioxide

CoA

Glycerol

Fatty acid

Some amino acids can be converted to acetyl CoA; they are ketogenic.

C—C—CoA

Acetyl CoA

CoA

Energy released

2-carbon fragments combine with CoA

Some amino acids can enter the TCA cycle directly.

TCA Cycle

Carbon dioxide

Carbon dioxide

Electron transport chain[a] ➝ **Energy, water, carbon dioxide**

[a] Coenzymes carry hydrogens from the breakdown of the energy nutrients to the electron transport chain.

FIGURE 6-3 The Central Pathways of Energy Metabolism

for energy or if they are consumed in excess, they first undergo **deamination,** a reaction in which they are stripped of their nitrogen. The nitrogen can be used to make other compounds, including the nonessential amino acids, or it can be excreted. The principal nitrogen-excretion product of metabolism is **urea.** With nitrogen removed, most of the amino acids can be converted to pyruvate and can therefore provide glucose. Several of the amino acids can only be converted to acetyl CoA and therefore cannot supply glucose. Thus protein, unlike fat, is a fairly efficient source of glucose when carbohydrate is not available.

IN SUMMARY

▌ ATP provides chemical energy for our bodies' cells and is produced by breaking down the energy-yielding nutrients.

▌ The chemical pathways that produce ATP are glycolysis, the TCA cycle, and the electron transport chain.

deamination: removal of the amino group (NH_2) from a compound such as an amino acid.

urea (yoo-REE-uh)**:** the principal nitrogen-excretion product of protein metabolism.

- Glycolysis breaks down glucose to pyruvate, which can be converted to acetyl CoA. Fatty acids can be broken down to acetyl CoA, as can many amino acids.

- The TCA cycle breaks down acetyl CoA molecules, producing carbon dioxide as waste and releasing hydrogen atoms to coenzymes that deliver them to the electron transport chain.

- When the hydrogen atoms that originate from energy-yielding nutrients enter the electron transport chain, ATP is made.

- Glucose can be produced from compounds that can be converted to pyruvate, including glycerol and most amino acids. Fatty acids can be used only for energy and cannot make glucose.

6.3 Energy Imbalance

LO 6.3 Explain how an excess of any of the three energy-yielding nutrients contributes to body fat and how an inadequate intake of any of them shifts metabolism.

The average person takes in and expends close to a million kcalories a year while maintaining a stable weight for years on end. In other words, the body's energy is in balance. Many people, however, eat too much or exercise too little and get fat; others eat too little or exercise too much and get thin. This section examines the two extremes of energy imbalance—feasting and fasting.

Feasting

When people consume more energy than they expend, much of the excess is stored as body fat. Fat can be made from an excess of any energy-yielding nutrient. In addition, excess energy from alcohol is also stored as fat. Alcohol has also been shown to slow down the body's use of fat for fuel, causing more fat to be stored, much of it as abdominal fat tissue.[1] Alcohol therefore is fattening, both through the kcalories it provides and through its effects on fat metabolism. The fat cells of the adipose tissue enlarge as they fill with fat, as Figure 6-4 shows.

Excess Carbohydrate Surplus carbohydrate (glucose) is first stored as glycogen in the liver and muscles, but the glycogen-storing cells have a limited capacity. Once glycogen stores are filled, most of the additional carbohydrate is burned for energy, displacing the body's use of fat for energy and allowing body fat to accumulate. Thus, excess carbohydrate can contribute to obesity.

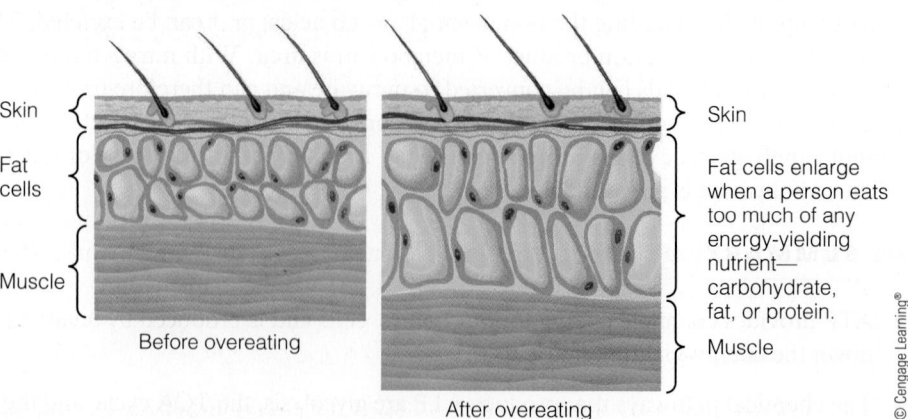

FIGURE 6-4 Fat Cell Enlargement

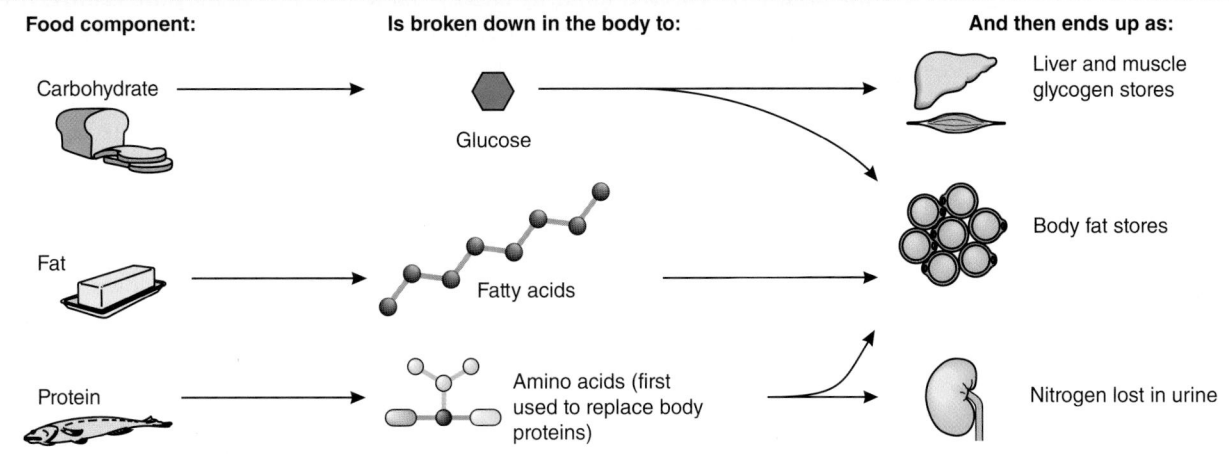

Food component: **Is broken down in the body to:**   **And then ends up as:**

Carbohydrate → Glucose → Liver and muscle glycogen stores

Fat → Fatty acids → Body fat stores

Protein → Amino acids (first used to replace body proteins) → Nitrogen lost in urine

© Cengage Learning®

FIGURE 6-5 Feasting
When people overeat, they store energy.

Excess Fat Surplus dietary fat contributes more directly to the body's fat stores. After a meal, fat is routed to the body's adipose tissue, where it is stored until needed for energy. Thus, excess fat from food easily adds to body fat.

Excess Protein Surplus protein may also contribute to body fat. If not needed to build body protein (as in response to physical activity) or to meet energy needs, amino acids will lose their nitrogens and be converted, through intermediates, to triglycerides. These, too, swell the fat cells and add to body weight. Figure 6-5 shows the metabolic events of feasting.

IN SUMMARY

- Too much food, too little physical activity, or both encourage body fat accumulation.

- A net excess of energy is almost all stored in the body as fat in adipose (fat) tissue.

- Alcohol both delivers kcalories and encourages storage of body fat.

- Once glycogen stores are filled, excess carbohydrate is used for energy, displacing the body's use of fat for energy and allowing fat to accumulate.

- Fat from food is particularly easy for the body to store as adipose tissue.

- If not needed to build body protein or to meet energy needs, excess protein can be converted to fat.

- In short, excess energy intake from carbohydrate, fat, protein, and alcohol leads to storage of body fat.

The Economics of Fasting

The body expends energy all the time. Even when a person is asleep and totally relaxed, the cells of many organs are hard at work. In fact, this cellular work, which maintains all life processes, represents about two-thirds of the total energy a sedentary person expends in a day. (The other one-third is the work that a person's muscles do voluntarily during waking hours.)

Energy Deficit The body's top priority is to meet the energy needs for this ongoing cellular activity. Its normal way of doing so is by periodic refueling, that is, by eating several times a day. When food is not available, the body uses fuel reserves from its own tissues. If people voluntarily choose not to eat, we say they are fasting; if they have no choice (as in a famine), we say they are starving. The body, however, makes no distinction between the two—metabolically, fasting and starving are identical. In either case, the body is forced to switch to a wasting metabolism, drawing on its stores of carbohydrate and fat and, within a day or so, on its vital protein tissues as well.

Glycogen Used First As fasting begins, glucose from the liver's glycogen stores and fatty acids from the body's adipose tissue flow into the cells to fuel their work. Within a day, liver glycogen is exhausted, and most of the glucose is used up. Low blood glucose concentrations serve as a signal to promote further fat breakdown.

Glucose Needed for the Brain At this point, a few hours into a fast, most cells depend on fatty acids to continue providing fuel. But the nervous system (brain and nerves) and red blood cells cannot use fatty acids; they still need glucose. Even if other energy sources are available, glucose has to be present to permit the brain's energy-metabolizing machinery to work. Normally, the nervous system consumes a little more than half of the total glucose used each day—about 400 to 600 kcalories' worth.

Protein Breakdown and Ketosis Because fat stores cannot provide the glucose needed by the brain and nerves, body protein tissues (such as liver and muscle) always break down to some extent during fasting. In the first few days of a fast, body protein provides about 90 percent of the needed glucose, and glycerol provides about 10 percent. If body protein losses were to continue at this rate, death would ensue within about three weeks. As the fast continues, however, the body finds a way to use its fat to fuel the brain. It adapts by condensing together fragments derived from fatty acids to produce **ketone bodies,** which can serve as fuel for some brain cells. Ketone body production rises until, after several weeks of fasting, it is meeting much of the nervous system's energy needs. Still, many areas of the brain rely exclusively on glucose, and body protein continues to be sacrificed to produce it. Thus, in fasting, muscle and lean tissues give up protein to supply amino acids for conversion to glucose. This glucose, with ketone bodies produced from fat, fuels the brain's activities. Figure 6-6 shows the metabolic events that occur during fasting.

Slowed Metabolism As fasting continues and the nervous system shifts to partial dependence on ketone bodies for energy, the body simultaneously reduces its energy output (metabolic rate) and conserves both fat and lean tissue. Because of the slowed metabolism, energy use falls to a bare minimum.

Hazards of Fasting The body's adaptations to fasting are sufficient to maintain life for a long period. Mental alertness need not be diminished. Even physical energy may remain unimpaired for a surprisingly long time. Still, fasting is not without its hazards. Among the many changes that take place in the body are:

| Wasting of lean tissues.

| Impairment of disease resistance.

| Lowering of body temperature.

| Disturbances of the body's fluid and electrolyte balances.

For the person who wants to lose weight, fasting is not the best way to go. The body's lean tissue continues to be degraded, sometimes amounting to as much as 50 percent of the weight lost over the first week. Over the long term, a diet only moderately restricted in energy promotes primarily *fat* loss and the retention of more lean tissue than a severely restrictive fast.

Handwritten margin notes:
- carbohydrate metabolism
- ATP + H_2O + CO_2
- "metabolism"
- Protein Breakdown
- ATP + H_2O + CO_2 + urea
- Fat/Lipid Breakdown "metabolism"
- ATP + H_2O + CO_2 + ketones

ketone bodies: acidic, water-soluble compounds produced by the liver during the breakdown of fat when carbohydrate is not available. Small amounts of ketone bodies are normally produced during energy metabolism, but when their blood concentration rises, they spill into the urine. The combination of a high blood concentration of ketone bodies (*ketonemia*) and ketone bodies in the urine (*ketonuria*) is called *ketosis*.

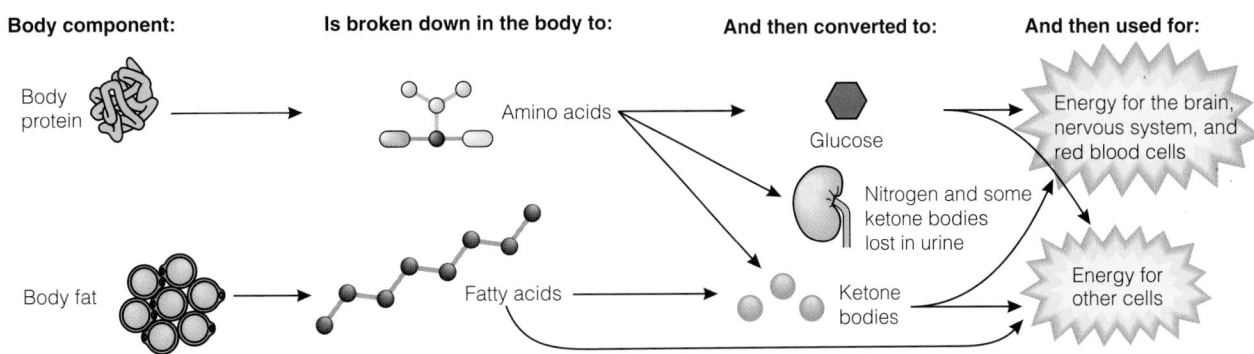

FIGURE 6-6 Fasting
When people are fasting, they draw on stored energy.

IN SUMMARY

▌ When fasting, the body makes a number of adaptations: increasing the breakdown of fat to provide energy for most of the cells, using glycerol and amino acids to make glucose for the red blood cells and central nervous system, producing ketones to fuel the brain, and slowing metabolism.

▌ All of these measures conserve energy and minimize losses.

▌ Over the long term, a diet moderately restricted in energy promotes primarily fat loss and the retention of lean tissue.

6.4 Energy Balance

LO 6.4 Describe energy balance and identify the components of energy expenditure, the factors that affect a person's BMR, and the factors that influence a person's energy expenditure.

If a person maintains a healthy weight over time, the person is in energy balance. Food energy intake equals energy expenditure: deposits of fat made at one time have been compensated for by withdrawals made at another. In other words, the body uses fat as a savings account for energy. But, unlike money, having more fat is not better; there is an optimum.

A day's energy balance can be stated like this: change in energy stores equals the food energy taken in (kcalories) minus the energy spent on metabolism and physical activities (kcalories). More simply:

Change in energy stores = energy in (kcalories) − energy out (kcalories).

METABOLISM, ENERGY BALANCE, AND BODY COMPOSITION

FIGURE 6-7 Components of Energy Expenditure
The amount of energy expended in a day differs for each individual, but, in general, basal metabolism is the largest component of energy expenditure, and the thermic effect of food is the smallest. The amount expended in voluntary physical activities has the greatest variability, depending on a person's activity patterns. For a sedentary person, physical activities may account for less than half as much energy as basal metabolism, whereas an extremely active person may expend as much on activity as for basal metabolism.

basal metabolism: the energy needed to maintain life when a person is at complete digestive, physical, and emotional rest. Basal metabolism is normally the largest part of a person's daily energy expenditure.

voluntary activities: the component of a person's daily energy expenditure that involves conscious and deliberate muscular work—walking, lifting, climbing, and other physical activities. Voluntary activities normally require less energy in a day than basal metabolism does.

basal metabolic rate (BMR): the rate of energy use for metabolism under specified conditions: after a 12-hour fast and restful sleep, without any physical activity or emotional excitement, and in a comfortable setting. It is usually expressed as kcalories per kilogram of body weight per hour.

resting metabolic rate (RMR): a measure of the energy use of a person at rest in a comfortable setting—similar to the BMR but with less stringent criteria for recent food intake and physical activity. Consequently, the RMR is slightly higher than the BMR.

Energy In

The energy in food and beverages is the only contributor to the "energy in" side of the energy balance equation. Before you can decide how much food will supply the energy you or one of your clients needs in a day, you must first become familiar with the amounts of energy in foods and beverages. One way to do so is to look up the kcalories provided by various foods and beverages in the Table of Food Composition (Appendix A). Alternatively, computer programs can readily provide this information.

Food composition data would reveal that an apple provides about 70 kcalories from carbohydrate and a candy bar supplies about 250 kcalories, mostly from fat and carbohydrate. You may have heard that for each 3500 kcalories you eat in excess of expenditures, you store 1 pound of body fat—a general rule that has previously been used for mathematical estimations. Keep in mind, however, that this number can vary widely with individual metabolic tendencies and efficiencies of nutrient digestion and absorption. Currently, the dynamics of energy storage is a topic of intense scientific investigation.[2] The fat stores of even a healthy-weight adult represent an ample reserve of energy—50,000 to 200,000 kcalories.

Energy Out

The body expends energy in two major ways: to fuel its **basal metabolism** and to fuel its **voluntary activities.** People can change their voluntary activities to expend more or less energy in a day, and over time they can also change their basal metabolism by building up the body's metabolically active lean tissue, as explained in Chapter 7.

Basal Metabolism Basal metabolism supports the body's work that goes on all the time without the person's conscious awareness. The beating of the heart, the inhaling and exhaling of air, the maintenance of body temperature, and the transmission of nerve and hormonal messages to direct these activities are the basal processes that maintain life. As Figure 6-7 shows, basal metabolism represents about two-thirds of the total energy a sedentary person expends in a day. In practical terms, a person whose total energy needs are 2000 kcalories per day may expend 1000 to 1300 of them to support basal metabolism.

The **basal metabolic rate (BMR)** is the rate at which the body expends energy for these life-sustaining activities. This rate varies from person to person and may vary for an individual with a change in circumstance or physical condition. The rate is slowest when a person is sleeping undisturbed, but it is usually measured when the person is awake, but lying still, in a room with a comfortable temperature after a restful sleep and an overnight (12- to 14-hour) fast. A similar measure of energy output—called the **resting metabolic rate (RMR)**—is slightly higher than the BMR because its criteria for recent food intake and physical activity are not as strict.

Table 6-1 summarizes the factors that raise and lower the BMR. For the most part, the BMR is highest in people who are growing (children, adolescents, and pregnant women) and in those with considerable lean body mass (physically fit people and males). One way to increase the BMR, then, is to maximize lean body tissue by participating regularly in endurance and strength-building activities. The BMR is also fast in people who are tall and so have a large surface area for their weight, in people with fever or under stress, in people taking certain medications, and in people with highly active thyroid glands. The BMR slows down with a loss of lean body mass and during fasting and malnutrition.

Energy for Physical Activities The number of kcalories spent on voluntary activities depends on three factors: muscle mass, body weight, and activity. The larger the muscle mass required for the activity and the heavier the weight of the body part being moved, the more kcalories are spent. The activity's duration, frequency, and intensity also influence energy costs: the longer, the more frequent, and the more intense the activity, the more kcalories are expended. Table 6-2 gives average energy expenditures for various activities.

TABLE 6-1 Factors That Affect the BMR

Factor	Effect on BMR
Age	Lean body mass diminishes with age, slowing the BMR.[a]
Height	In tall, thin people, the BMR is higher.[b]
Growth	In children and pregnant women, the BMR is higher.
Body composition (gender)	The more lean tissue, the higher the BMR (which is why males usually have a higher BMR than females). The more fat tissue, the lower the BMR.
Fever	Fever raises the BMR.[c]
Stresses	Stresses (including many diseases and certain drugs) raise the BMR.
Environmental temperature	Both heat and cold raise the BMR.
Fasting/starvation	Fasting/starvation lowers the BMR.[d]
Malnutrition	Malnutrition lowers the BMR.
Hormones (gender)	The thyroid hormone thyroxin, for example, can speed up or slow down the BMR.[e] Premenstrual hormones slightly raise the BMR.
Smoking	Nicotine increases energy expenditure.
Caffeine	Caffeine increases energy expenditure.
Sleep	BMR is lowest when sleeping.

© Cengage Learning®

[a]The BMR begins to decrease in early adulthood (after growth and development cease) at a rate of about 2 percent a decade. A reduction in voluntary activity as well brings the total decline in energy expenditure to 5 percent a decade.
[b]If two people weigh the same, the taller, thinner person will have the faster metabolic rate, reflecting the greater skin surface, through which heat is lost by radiation, in proportion to the body's volume.
[c]Fever raises the BMR by 7 percent for each degree Fahrenheit.
[d]Prolonged starvation reduces the total amount of metabolically active lean tissue in the body, although the decline occurs sooner and to a greater extent than body losses alone can explain. More likely, the neural and hormonal changes that accompany fasting are responsible for changes in the BMR.
[e]The thyroid gland releases hormones that travel to the cells and influence cellular metabolism. Thyroid hormone activity can speed up or slow down the rate of metabolism by as much as 50 percent.

TABLE 6-2 Energy Spent on Various Activities

The values listed in this table reflect both the energy spent in physical activity and the amount used for BMR.

Activity	kcal/lb/min[a]	Activity	kcal/lb/min[a]	Activity	kcal/lb/min[a]
Aerobic dance (vigorous)	0.062	Horseback riding (trot)	0.052	Table tennis (skilled)	0.045
Basketball (vigorous, full court)	0.097	Rowing (vigorous)	0.097	Tennis (beginner)	0.032
Bicycling		Running		Walking (brisk pace)	
13 mph	0.045	5 mph	0.061	3.5 mph	0.035
15 mph	0.049	6 mph	0.074	4.5 mph	0.048
17 mph	0.057	7.5 mph	0.094	Weight lifting	
19 mph	0.076	9 mph	0.103	light-to-moderate effort	0.024
21 mph	0.090	10 mph	0.114	vigorous effort	0.048
23 mph	0.109	11 mph	0.131	Wheelchair basketball	0.084
25 mph	0.139	Soccer (vigorous)	0.097	Wheeling self in wheelchair	0.030
Canoeing, flat water, moderate pace	0.045	Studying	0.011	Wii games	
		Swimming			
Cross-country skiing		20 yd/min	0.032	bowling	0.021
8 mph	0.104	45 yd/min	0.058	boxing	0.021
Golf (carrying clubs)	0.045	50 yd/min	0.070	tennis	0.022
Handball	0.078				

© Cengage Learning®

[a]To calculate kcalories spent per minute of activity for your own body weight, multiply kcal/lb/min by your exact weight and then multiply that number by the number of minutes spent in the activity. For example, if you weigh 142 pounds, and you want to know how many kcalories you spent doing 30 minutes of vigorous aerobic dance: 0.062 × 142 = 8.8 kcalories per minute; 8.8 × 30 (minutes) = 264 total kcalories spent.

METABOLISM, ENERGY BALANCE, AND BODY COMPOSITION

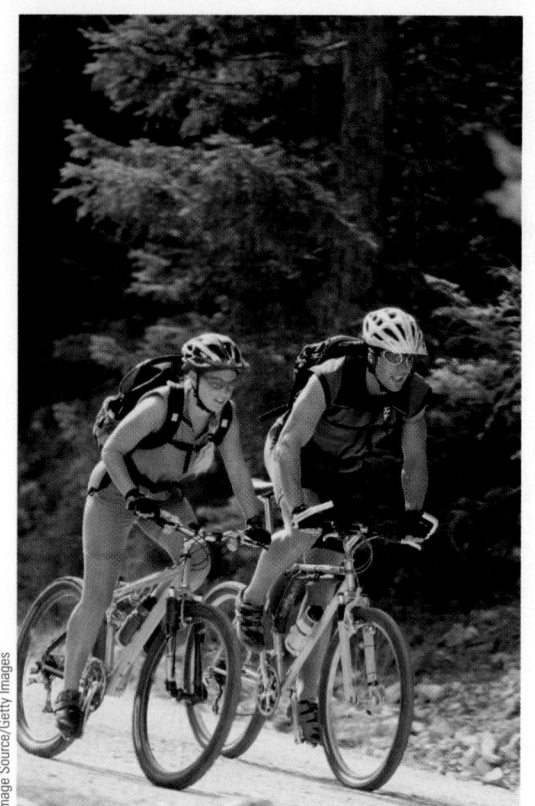

Physical activity expends energy and benefits health in many ways.

Energy to Manage Food When food is taken into the body, many cells that have been dormant become active. The muscles that move the food through the intestinal tract speed up their rhythmic contractions, and the cells that manufacture and secrete digestive juices begin their tasks. All these and other cells need extra energy as they participate in the digestion, absorption, and metabolism of food. This cellular activity produces heat and is known as the **thermic effect of food.** The thermic effect of food is generally thought to represent about 10 percent of the total food energy taken in. For purposes of rough estimates, though, the thermic effect of food is not always included.

Estimating Energy Requirements

In estimating energy requirements, the DRI committee developed equations that consider how the following factors influence energy expenditure:[‡]

- *Gender.* Women generally have a lower BMR than men, in large part because men typically have more lean body mass. In addition, menstrual hormones influence the BMR in women, raising it just prior to menstruation. Two sets of energy equations—one for men and one for women—were developed to accommodate the influence of gender on energy expenditure.

- *Growth.* The BMR is high in people who are growing. For this reason, pregnant and lactating women, infants, children, and adolescents have their own sets of energy equations.

- *Age.* The BMR declines during adulthood as lean body mass diminishes. Physical activities tend to decline as well, bringing the average reduction in energy expenditure to about 5 percent per decade. The decline in the BMR that occurs when a person becomes less active reflects the loss of lean body mass and may be prevented with ongoing physical activity. Because age influences energy expenditure, it is also factored into the energy equations.

- *Physical activity.* Using individual values for various physical activities (as in Table 6-2) is time consuming and impractical for estimating the energy needs of a population. Instead, various activities are clustered according to the typical intensity of a day's efforts (Appendix D provides details).

- *Body composition and body size.* The BMR is high in people who are tall and so have a large surface area. Similarly, the more a person weighs, the more energy is expended on basal metabolism. For these reasons, the energy equations include a factor for both height and weight.

As just explained, energy needs vary among individuals depending on such factors as gender, growth, age, physical activity, and body composition. Even when two people are similarly matched, however, their energy needs will still differ because of genetic differences. Perhaps one day genetic research will reveal how to estimate requirements for each individual. For now, Box 6-1 provides instructions on calculating estimated energy requirements using the DRI equations and physical activity factors.[§] Appendix D presents tables that provide a shortcut to estimating total energy expenditure.

thermic effect of food: an estimation of the energy required to process food (digest, absorb, transport, metabolize, and store ingested nutrients).

[‡]Note that Table 6-1 (p. 145) listed these factors among those that influence BMR and, consequently, energy expenditure.

[§]For *most* people, the energy requirement falls within these ranges: (Men) EER ±200 kcal; (Women) EER ±160 kcal. For almost all people, the actual energy requirement falls within these larger ranges: (Men) EER ±400 kcal; (Women) EER ±320 kcal.

To determine your estimated energy requirements (EER), use the appropriate equation (of the two options below), inserting your age in years, weight (wt) in kilograms, height (ht) in meters, and physical activity (PA) factor from the accompanying table. (To convert pounds to kilograms, divide by 2.2; to convert inches to meters, divide by 39.37.)

▌ For men 19 years and older:

EER = [662 − (9.53 × age)] + PA × [(15.91 × wt) + (539.6 × ht)]

▌ For women 19 years and older:

EER = [354 − (6.91 × age)] + PA × [(9.36 × wt) + (726 × ht)]

For example, consider an active 30-year-old male who is 5 feet 11 inches tall and weighs 178 pounds. First, he converts his weight from pounds to kilograms and his height from inches to meters, if necessary:

$$178 \text{ lb} \div 2.2 = 80.9 \text{ kg}$$
$$71 \text{ in} \div 39.37 = 1.8 \text{ m}$$

Next, he considers his level of daily physical activity and selects the appropriate PA factor from the accompanying table (in this example, 1.25 for an active male). Then, he inserts his age, PA factor, weight, and height into the appropriate equation:

EER = [662 − (9.53 × 30)] + 1.25 × [(15.91 × 80.9) + (539.6 × 1.8)]

(A reminder: do calculations within the parentheses first, and multiply before adding or subtracting.) He calculates:

EER = [662 − (9.53 × 30)] + 1.25 × (1287 + 971)
EER = [662 − (9.53 × 30)] + (1.25 + 2258)
EER = 662 − 286 + 2823
EER = 3199

The estimated energy requirement for an active 30-year-old male who is 5 feet 11 inches tall and weighs 178 pounds is about 3200 kcalories/day. His actual requirement probably falls within a range of 200 kcalories above and below this estimate.

Physical Activity (PA) Factors for EER Equations

	Men	Women	Physical Activity
Sedentary	1.0	1.0	Typical daily living activities
Low active	1.11	1.12	Plus 30 to 60 minutes moderate activity
Active	1.25	1.27	Plus ≥60 minutes moderate activity
Very active	1.48	1.45	Plus ≥60 minutes moderate activity and 60 minutes vigorous activity or 120 minutes moderate activity

Note: Moderate activity is equivalent to walking at 3½ to 4½ miles per hour.

IN SUMMARY

▌ A person takes in energy from food and, on average, expends most of it on basal metabolic activities, some of it on physical activities, and about 10 percent on the thermic effect of food.

▌ Because energy requirements vary from person to person, such factors as age, gender, and weight must be considered when calculating energy expended on basal metabolism, and the intensity and duration of the activity must be taken into account when calculating expenditures on physical activities.

6.5 Body Weight and Body Composition

LO 6.5 Describe the differences between body weight and body composition, including methods to assess them and health implications.

The body's weight reflects its composition—the proportions of its bone, muscle, fat, fluid, and other tissue. All of these body components can vary in quantity and quality: the bones can be dense or porous, the muscles can be well developed or under-developed, fat can be abundant or scarce, and so on. By far the most variable tissue, though, is body fat. For health's sake, weight management efforts should focus on eating and activity habits to improve body composition.

Defining Healthy Body Weight

How much should a person weigh? How can a person know if her weight is appropriate for her height and age? How can a person know if his weight is jeopardizing his health? Questions such as these seem so simple, yet the answers can be complex—and different depending on whom you ask.

The Criterion of Fashion When asking the question, "What is an ideal body weight?" people often mistakenly turn to fashion for the answer. Without a doubt, our society sets unrealistic ideals for body weight, especially for women.[3] Magazines, movies, and television all convey the message that to be thin is to be beautiful and happy. As a result, the media have a great influence on the weight concerns and dieting patterns of people of all ages but most tragically on young, impressionable children and adolescents.

Importantly, perceived body image has little to do with actual body weight or size. People of all shapes, sizes, and ages—including extremely thin fashion models with anorexia nervosa and fitness instructors with ideal body composition—have learned to be unhappy with their "overweight" bodies. Such dissatisfaction can lead to damaging behaviors, such as starvation diets, diet pill abuse, and failure to seek health care. The first step toward making healthy changes may be self-acceptance. Keep in mind that fashion is fickle; the body shapes that our society values change with time and, furthermore, differ from those valued by other societies. The standards defining "ideal" are subjective and frequently have little in common with health. Table 6-3 offers some tips for adopting health as an ideal.

The Criterion of Health Even if our society were to accept fat as beautiful, obesity would still be a major risk factor for several life-threatening diseases, as discussed later in the chapter. For this reason, the most important criterion for determining how much a person should weigh and how much body fat a person needs is not appearance but good health and longevity. A range of healthy body weights has been identified using a common measure of weight and height—the body mass index.

Body Mass Index The **body mass index (BMI)** describes relative weight for height:

$$\text{BMI} = \frac{\text{weight (kg)}}{\text{height (m)}^2} \quad \text{or} \quad \frac{\text{weight (lb)}}{\text{height (in)}^2} \times 703$$

To convert pounds to kilograms, divide by 2.2. To convert inches to meters, divide by 39.37.

Weight classifications based on BMI are presented in the table on the inside back cover. Notice that a healthy weight falls between a BMI of 18.5 and 24.9, with **underweight** below 18.5, **overweight** above 25, and **obese** above 30. Most people with a BMI within the healthy weight range have few of the health risks typically associated with

body mass index (BMI): an index of a person's weight in relation to height; determined by dividing the weight (in kilograms) by the square of the height (in meters).

underweight: body weight lower than the weight range that is considered healthy; BMI below 18.5.

overweight: body weight greater than the weight range that is considered healthy; BMI 25.0 to 29.9.

obese: having too much body fat with adverse health effects; BMI 30 or more.

TABLE 6-3 Tips for Accepting a Healthy Body Weight

- Value yourself and others for human attributes other than body weight. Realize that prejudging people by weight is as harmful as prejudging them by race, religion, or gender.
- Use positive, nonjudgmental descriptions of your body.
- Accept positive comments from others.
- Focus on your whole self, including your intelligence, social grace, and professional and scholastic achievements.
- Accept that no magic diet exists.
- Stop dieting to lose weight. Adopt a lifestyle of healthy eating and physical activity permanently.
- Follow the USDA Food Patterns. Never restrict food intake below the minimum levels that meet nutrient needs.
- Become physically active, not because it will help you get thin but because it will make you feel good and enhance your health.
- Seek support from loved ones. Tell them of your plan for a healthy life in the body you have been given.
- Seek professional counseling, not from a weight-loss counselor but from someone who can help you make gains in self-esteem without weight as a factor.

© Cengage Learning®

too-low or too-high body weight. Risks increase as BMI falls below 18.5 or rises above 24.9 (see Figure 6-8), reflecting the reality that both underweight and overweight impair health status.

The BMI values are most accurate in assessing degrees of obesity and are less useful for evaluating nonobese people's body fatness. BMI values fail to provide two valuable pieces of information used in assessing disease risk: they don't reveal how much of the weight is fat, and they don't indicate where the fat is located. To obtain these data, measures of body composition are needed.

Body Composition

For many people, being overweight compared with the standard means that they are over-*fat*. This is not the case, though, for athletes with dense bones and well-developed muscles; they may be over*weight* but carry little body fat. Conversely, inactive people may seem to have acceptable weights but still carry too much body fat. In addition, among some racial and ethnic groups, BMI values may not precisely identify overweight and obesity. African American people of all ages may have more lean tissue per pound of body weight than Asians or Caucasians, for example.[4] Thus, a diagnosis of obesity or overweight requires a BMI value *plus* some measure of body composition and fat distribution.

Central Obesity The distribution of fat on the body may influence health as much as, or more than, the total fat alone. **Visceral fat** that is stored deep within the central abdominal area of the body is referred to as **central obesity** or upper body fat (see Figure 6-9). Much research supports the widely held belief that central obesity—significantly and independently of BMI—contributes to heart disease, cancers, diabetes, and related deaths.[5]

FIGURE 6-8 Body Mass Index and Mortality

This J-shaped curve describes the relationship between body mass index (BMI) and mortality and shows that both underweight and overweight present risks of a premature death.

In healthy-weight people, some fat is stored around the organs of the abdomen.

In overweight people, excess abdominal fat increases the risks of diseases.

FIGURE 6-9 Abdominal Fat

visceral fat: fat stored within the abdominal cavity in association with the internal abdominal organs, as opposed to fat stored directly under the skin (subcutaneous fat); also called *intra-abdominal fat*.

central obesity: excess fat around the trunk of the body; also called *abdominal fat* or *upper-body fat*.

Upper-body fat is more common in men than in women and is closely associated with heart disease, stroke, diabetes, hypertension, and some types of cancer.

Lower-body fat is more common in women than in men and is not usually associated with chronic diseases.

© Cengage Learning®

FIGURE 6-10 *"Apple" and "Pear" Body Shapes Compared*
Popular articles sometimes call bodies with upper-body fat "apples" and those with lower-body fat "pears."

adipokines (AD-ih-poh-kynz): protein hormones made and released by adipose tissue (fat) cells.

inflammation: an immunological response to cellular injury characterized by an increase in white blood cells.

subcutaneous fat: fat stored directly under the skin.
- *sub* = beneath
- *cutaneous* = skin

waist circumference: a measurement used to assess a person's abdominal fat.

skinfold measure: a clinical estimate of total body fatness in which the thickness of a fold of skin on the back of the arm (over the triceps muscle), below the shoulder blade (subscapular), or in other places is measured with a caliper.

One possible explanation for why fat in the abdomen may increase the risk of disease involves **adipokines,** hormones released by adipose tissue. Adipokines help to regulate **inflammation** and energy metabolism in the tissues.[6] The inflammatory response is described in detail in Chapter 24.

In central obesity, a shift occurs in the balance of adipokines, favoring those that increase both inflammation and insulin resistance of tissues.[7] The resulting chronic inflammation and insulin resistance contribute to diabetes, atherosclerosis (a cause of heart disease), and other chronic diseases. Insulin resistance is a central feature of the metabolic syndrome, which is discussed in Nutrition in Practice 21.

Visceral fat creates the "apple" profile of central obesity. **Subcutaneous fat** around the hips and thighs creates more of a "pear" profile (see Figure 6-10). Visceral fat is common in women past menopause and even more common in men. Even when total body fat is similar, men have more visceral fat than either premenopausal or postmenopausal women. For those women with visceral fat, the risks of cardiovascular disease and mortality are increased, just as they are for men. Interestingly, smokers tend to have more visceral fat than nonsmokers even though they typically have a lower BMI.[8] Two other factors that may affect body fat distribution are intakes of alcohol and physical activity. Moderate-to-high alcohol consumption may favor central obesity. In contrast, regular physical activity seems to prevent abdominal fat accumulation.[9]

Waist Circumference A person's **waist circumference** is a good indicator of fat distribution and central obesity (see Appendix E). In general, women with a waist circumference greater than 35 inches and men with a waist circumference greater than 40 inches have a high risk of central obesity–related health problems.

Skinfold Measures Skinfold measurements provide an accurate estimate of total body fat and a fair assessment of the fat's location. About half of the fat in the body lies directly beneath the skin, so the thickness of this subcutaneous fat is assumed to reflect total body fat. Measures taken from central-body sites (around the abdomen) better reflect changes in fatness than those taken from upper sites (arm and back). A skilled assessor can obtain an accurate **skinfold measure** and then compare the measurement with standards (see Appendix E).

How Much Body Fat Is Too Much?

People often ask exactly how much fat is too fat for health. Ideally, a person has enough fat to meet basic needs but not so much as to incur health risks. The ideal amount of body fat depends partly on the person. A man with a BMI within the recommended range may have between 18 and 24 percent body fat; a woman, because of her greater quantity of essential fat, 23 to 31 percent.

Many athletes have a lower percentage of body fat—just enough fat to provide fuel, insulate and protect the body, assist in nerve impulse transmissions, and support normal hormone activity, but not so much as to burden the muscles. For athletes, then, body fat might be 5 to 10 percent for men and 15 to 20 percent for women.

For an Alaskan fisherman, a higher-than-average percentage of body fat is probably beneficial because fat helps prevent heat loss in cold weather. A woman starting a pregnancy needs sufficient body fat to support conception and fetal growth. Below a certain threshold for body fat, individuals may become infertile, develop depression, experience abnormal hunger regulation, or be unable to keep warm. These thresholds differ for each function and for each individual; much remains to be learned about them.

- Clearly, the most important criterion of appropriate fatness is health.

- Current standards for body weight are based on the body mass index (BMI), which describes a person's weight in relation to height.

- Health risks increase with a BMI below 18.5 or above 24.9.

- Central obesity, in which excess fat is distributed around the trunk of the body, may present greater health risks than excess fat distributed on the lower body.

- Researchers use a number of techniques to assess body composition, including waist circumference and skinfold measures.

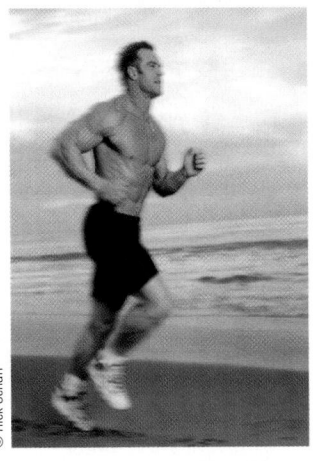

At 6 feet 4 inches tall and 250 pounds, this runner would be considered overweight by most standards. Yet he is clearly not overfat.

6.6 Health Risks of Underweight and Obesity

LO 6.6 Identify relationships between body weight and the risk of health problems and summarize the guidelines for identifying and evaluating the risks to health from overweight and obesity.

As mentioned earlier and shown in Figure 6-8 (p. 149), health risks increase as BMI falls below 18.5 or rises above 24.9. People who are extremely underweight or extremely obese carry higher risks of early death than those whose weights fall within the healthy, or even the slightly overweight, range.[10] These mortality risks decline with age. Independently of BMI, factors such as smoking habits raise health risks, and physical fitness lowers them.

Health Risks of Underweight Some underweight people enjoy an active, healthy life, but others are underweight because of malnutrition, smoking habits, substance abuse, or illnesses. Weight and fat measures alone would not reveal these underlying causes, but a complete assessment that includes a diet and medical history, physical examination, and biochemical analysis would.

Underweight people, especially older adults, may be unable to preserve lean tissue when fighting a wasting disease such as cancer. Overly thin people are also at a disadvantage in the hospital, where nutrient status can easily deteriorate if they have to go without food for an extended time while undergoing tests or surgery. Underweight women often develop menstrual irregularities and become infertile. Underweight and significant weight loss are also associated with osteoporosis and bone fractures. For all these reasons, underweight people may benefit from enough of a weight gain to provide an energy reserve and protective amounts of all the nutrients that can be stored.

An extreme underweight condition known as anorexia nervosa is sometimes seen in young people who exercise unreasonable self-denial in order to control their weight. Anorexia nervosa is a major eating disorder seen in our society today. Eating disorders are the subject of Nutrition in Practice 6.

Health Risks of Overweight and Obesity Despite our nation's preoccupation with body image and weight loss, the prevalence of overweight and obesity continues to rise dramatically (see Figure 6-11 on p. 152).[11] During the previous three decades, obesity increased in every state, in both genders, and across all ages, races, and education levels. Today, 68 percent of U.S. adults are overweight (BMI of 25 or greater) or dangerously obese (BMI of 30 or greater).[12] Obesity rates are expected to continue rising into the foreseeable future, although at a somewhat slower rate than in the past.[13] The problem reaches around the globe, in urban and rural areas alike.[14] In short, obesity is a major public health problem that is becoming more prevalent.

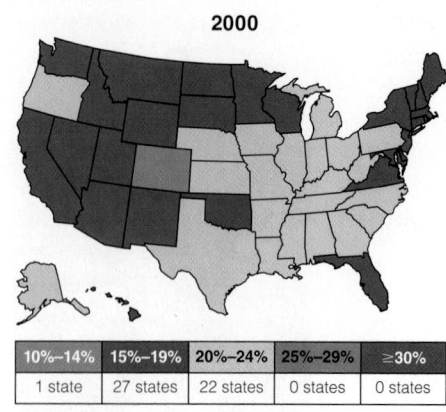

2000

10%–14%	15%–19%	20%–24%	25%–29%	≥30%
1 state	27 states	22 states	0 states	0 states

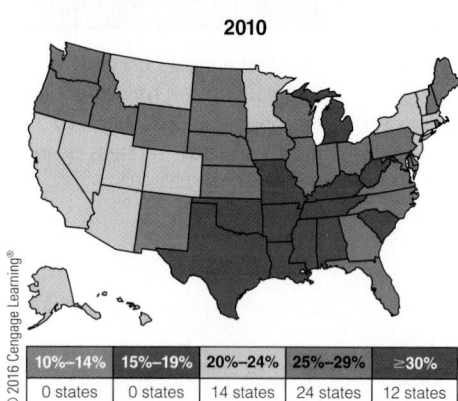

2010

10%–14%	15%–19%	20%–24%	25%–29%	≥30%
0 states	0 states	14 states	24 states	12 states

© 2016 Cengage Learning®

FIGURE 6-11 The Increasing Prevalence of Obesity among U.S. Adults by State

insulin resistance: the condition in which a normal amount of insulin produces a subnormal effect in muscle, adipose, and liver cells, resulting in an elevated fasting glucose; a metabolic consequence of obesity that precedes type 2 diabetes.

The growing prevalence of overweight and obesity is a matter of concern because both conditions present risks to health. Indeed, the health risks of obesity are so numerous that it has been declared a disease. Excess weight contributes to up to half of all cases of hypertension, thereby increasing the risk of heart attack and stroke. Obesity raises blood pressure in part by altering kidney function, increasing blood volume, and promoting blood vessel damage through insulin resistance.[15] Often weight loss alone can normalize the blood pressure of an overweight person.

Excess body weight also increases the risk of type 2 diabetes. Most adults with type 2 diabetes are overweight or obese, and obesity itself can directly cause some degree of **insulin resistance.**[16] Diabetes (type 2) is three times more likely to develop in an obese person than in a nonobese person. Furthermore, the person with type 2 diabetes often has central obesity.[17] Central-body fat cells appear to be larger and more insulin resistant than lower-body fat cells.

In addition to diabetes and hypertension, other risks threaten obese adults. Among them are high blood lipids, cardiovascular disease, sleep apnea (abnormal cessation of breathing during sleep), osteoarthritis, abdominal hernias, some cancers, varicose veins, gout, gallbladder disease, kidney stones, respiratory problems (including Pickwickian syndrome, a breathing blockage linked with sudden death), nonalcoholic fatty liver disease, complications in pregnancy and surgery, flat feet, and even a high accident rate.[18] Each year these obesity-related illnesses cost our nation billions of dollars. The cost in terms of lives is also great. People with lifelong obesity are twice as likely to die prematurely as others. In the United States, obesity is second only to tobacco use as the most significant cause of preventable death.[19]

Some overweight people, however, remain healthy and live long lives despite their body fatness. Genetic inheritance, smoking habits, and level of physical activity may help to explain why some overweight individuals stay well while others become ill. Overweight but fit people have lower risks than normal-weight, unfit ones, for example.[20] To help in identifying those most at risk, obesity experts have developed guidelines for health practitioners, described next.

Guidelines for Identifying Those at Risk from Obesity The guidelines for identifying and evaluating the risks to health from overweight and obesity rely on three indicators. The first indicator is a person's BMI. As a general guideline, overweight for adults is defined as BMI of 25.0 through 29.9, and obesity is defined as BMI equal to or greater than 30.

The second indicator is waist circumference, which, as discussed earlier, reflects the degree of abdominal fatness in proportion to body fatness. Women with a waist circumference greater than 35 inches and men with a waist circumference greater than 40 inches are at greater risk of type 2 diabetes, hypertension, and cardiovascular disease than women or men with waist circumferences equal to, or below, these measures. In other words, waist circumference is an independent predictor of disease risk.

The third indicator is the person's disease risk profile. The disease risk profile takes into account life-threatening diseases, family history, and risk factors for heart disease (such as blood lipid profile). The higher the BMI, the greater the waist circumference, and the more risk factors, the greater the urgency to treat obesity. People who are obese or those who are overweight and have one or more indicators of increased risk of heart disease (diabetes, prediabetes, hypertension, abnormal lipid profile, or elevated waist circumference), have a high risk for disease complications and mortality that requires treatment to manage the disease or modify the risk factors.[21]

Other Risks of Obesity Although some obese people seem to escape health problems, few in our society can avoid the social and economic handicaps. Our society places enormous value on thinness. Obese people are less sought after for romance, less often hired, and less often admitted to college. They pay higher insurance premiums and more for clothing. This is especially true for women. In contrast, people with other chronic conditions such as asthma, diabetes, and epilepsy do not differ socially or economically from healthy nonoverweight people.

Prejudice defines people by their appearance rather than by their abilities and characters. Obese people suffer emotional pain when others treat them with insensitivity, hostility, and contempt, and they may internalize a sense of guilt and self-deprecation. Health-care professionals, even dietitians, can be among the offenders without realizing it. To free our society of its obsession with body fatness and prejudice against obese people, activists are promoting respect for individuals of all body weights.

IN SUMMARY

▋ The health risks of underweight include infertility (women), bone loss, and inability to preserve lean tissue when fighting a wasting disease such as cancer; risks of obesity include chronic diseases such as hypertension, type 2 diabetes, and heart disease. Both underweight and obesity increase the risk of premature death.

▋ Guidelines for identifying the health risks of overweight and obesity are based on a person's BMI, waist circumference, and disease risk profile.

▋ Obesity also incurs social, economic, and psychological risks.

Clinical Applications

1. Compare the energy a person might spend on various physical activities. Refer to Table 6-2 on p. 145, and compute how much energy a person who weighs 142 pounds would spend doing each of the following activities. An example using aerobic dance has been provided for you. You may want to compare various activities based on your own weight.

   30 minutes of vigorous aerobic dance:

   0.062 kcal/lb/min × 142 lb = 8.8 kcal/min.
       8.8 kcal/min × 30 min = 264 kcal.

   a. 2 hours of golf, carrying clubs.
   b. 20 minutes running at 9 mph.
   c. 45 minutes of swimming at 20 yd/min.
   d. 1 hour of walking at 3.5 mph.

2. Using Box 6-1 on p. 147 as a guide, determine your Estimated Energy Requirement (EER).

Answers

1. (a) 0.045 kcal/lb/min × 142 lb = 6.4 kcal/min, 6.4 kcal/min × 120 min = 768 kcal; (b) 0.103 kcal/lb/min × 142 lb = 14.6 kcal/min, 14.6 kcal/min × 20 min = 292 kcal; (c) 0.032 kcal/lb/min × 142 lb = 4.5 kcal/min, 4.5 kcal/min × 45 = 202.5 kcal; (d) 0.035 kcal/lb/min × 142 lb = 5 kcal/min 5 kcal/min × 60 min = 300 kcal.

Self Check

1. Before entering the TCA cycle, each of the energy-yielding nutrients is broken down to:
   a. ammonia.
   b. pyruvate.
   c. electrons.
   d. acetyl CoA.

2. As carbohydrate and fat stores are depleted during fasting or starvation, the body then uses ___ as its fuel source.
   a. alcohol
   b. protein
   c. glucose
   d. triglycerides

3. When carbohydrate is not available to provide energy for the brain, as in starvation, the body produces ketone bodies from:
   a. glucose.
   b. glycerol.
   c. fatty acid fragments.
   d. amino acids.

4. Two activities that contribute to the basal metabolic rate are:
   a. walking and running.
   b. maintenance of heartbeat and running.
   c. maintenance of body temperature and walking.
   d. maintenance of heartbeat and body temperature.

5. Three factors that affect the body's basal metabolic rate are:
   a. height, weight, and energy intake.
   b. age, body composition, and sodium intake.
   c. fever, body composition, and altitude.
   d. weight, fever, and environmental temperature.

6. The largest component of energy expenditure is:
   a. basal metabolism.
   b. physical activity.
   c. indirect calorimetry.
   d. thermic effect of food.

7. Which of the following reflects height and weight?
   a. Body mass index
   b. Central obesity
   c. Waist circumference
   d. Body composition

8. The BMI range that correlates with the fewest health risks is:
   a. 16.5 to 20.9.
   b. 18.5 to 24.9.
   c. 25.5 to 30.9.
   d. 30.5 to 34.9.

9. The profile of central obesity is sometimes referred to as a(n):
   a. beer.
   b. pear.
   c. apple.
   d. potato.

10. Which of the following health risks is *not* associated with being overweight?
    a. Hypertension
    b. Heart disease
    c. Type 1 diabetes
    d. Gallbladder disease

Answers to these questions can be found in Appendix H.

Notes

1. M. M. Bergmann and coauthors, The association of lifetime alcohol use with measures of abdominal and general adiposity in a large-scale European cohort, *European Journal of Clinical Nutrition* 65 (2011): 1079–1087.

2. S. B. Hymsfield and coauthors, Energy content of weight loss: Kinetic features during voluntary caloric restriction, *Metabolism* 61 (2012): 937–943; K. D. Hall and coauthors, Energy balance and its components: Implications for body weight regulation, *American Journal of Clinical Nutrition* 95 (2012): 989–994; K. D. Hall and coauthors, Quantification of the effect energy imbalance on bodyweight, *Lancet* 378 (2011): 826–837.

3. J. B. Martin, The development of ideal body image perceptions in the United States, *Nutrition Today* 45 (2010): 98–110.

4. M. Heo and coauthors, Percentage of body fat cutoffs by sex, age, and race-ethnicity in the US adult population from NHANES 1999–2004, *American Journal of Clinical Nutrition* 95 (2012): 594–602; H. R. Hull and coauthors, Fat-free mass index: Changes and race/ethnic differences in adulthood, *International Journal of Obesity (London)* 35 (2011): 121–127; N. Farah and coauthors, Comparison in maternal body composition between Caucasian Irish and Indian women, *Journal of Obstetrics and Gynecology* 31 (2011): 483–485; A. Liu and coauthors, Ethnic differences in the relationship between body mass index and percentage of body fat among Asian children from different backgrounds, *British Journal of Nutrition* 106 (2011): 1390–1397.

5. K. A. Britton and coauthors, Body fat distribution, incident cardiovascular disease, cancer, and all-cause mortality, *Journal of the American College of Cardiology* 62 (2013): 921–925; M.J. Lee, Y. Wu, and S. K. Fried, Adipose tissue heterogeneity: Implication of depot differences in adipose tissue for obesity complications, *Molecualr Aspects of Medicine* 344 (2013): 1–11; M. Al-Daghri and coauthors, Visceral adiposity index is highly associated with adiponectin values and glycaemic disturbances, *European Journal of Clinical Investigation* 43 (2013): 183–189; A. M. Sironi and coauthors, Impact of increased visceral and cardiac fat on cardiometabolic risk and disease, *Diabetic Medicine* 29 (2012): 622–627; M. A. Cornier and coauthors, Assessing adiposity: A scientific statement from the American Heart Association, *Circulation* 124 (2011): 1996–2019; B. J. Arsenault and coauthors, Physical inactivity, abdominal obesity and risk of coronary heart disease in apparently healthy men and women, *International Journal of Obesity* 34 (2010): 340–347; E. J. Jacobs and coauthors, Waist circumference and all-cause mortality in a large US cohort, *Archives of Internal Medicine* 170 (2010): 1293–1301.

6. J. M. Northcott and coauthors, Adipokines and the cardiovascular system: Mechanisms mediating health and disease, *Canadian Journal of Physiology and Pharmacology* 90 (2012): 1029–1059; Cornier and coauthors, 2011; Y. Deng and P. E. Scherer, Adipokines as novel biomarkers and regulators of the metabolic syndrome, *Annals of the New York Academy of Sciences* 1212 (2010): E1–E19.

7. Cornier and coauthors, 2011.

8. E. W. Demerath, Causes and consequences of human variation in visceral adiposity, *American Journal of Clinical Nutrition* 91 (2010): 1–2.

9. U. Ekelund and coauthors, Physical activity and gain in abdominal adiposity and body weight: Prospective cohort study in 288,498 men and women, *American Journal of Clinical Nutrition* 93 (2011): 826–835; Arsenault and coauthors, 2010.

10. D. W. Gord and coauthors, Body mass index, poor diet quality, and health-related quality of life are associated with mortality in rural older adults, *Journal of Nutrition in Gerontology and Geriatrics* 33 (2014): 23–34; K. M. Flegal and coauthors, Association of all-cause mortality with overweight and obesity using standard body mass index categories: A systematic review and meta-analysis, *Journal of the American Medical Association* 309 (2013): 71–82.

11. C. L. Ogden, M. D. Carroll, and K. M. Flegal, Prevalence of childhood and adult obesity in the United States, 2011–2012, *Journal of the American Medical Association* 311 (2014): 806–814; S. A. Cunningham, M. R. Kramer, and K. M. Venkat Narayan, Incidence of childhood obesity in the United States, *New England Journal of Medicine* 370 (2014): 403–411.

12. Ogden, Carroll, and Flegal, 2014.

13. E. A. Finkelstein and coauthors, Obesity and severe obesity forecasts through 2030, *American Journal of Preventive Medicine* 42 (2012): 563–570.

14. B. M. Popkin, L. S. Adair, and S. W. Ng, Global nutrition transition and pandemic of obesity in developing countries, *Nutrition Reviews* 70 (2012): 3–21; B. A. Swinburn and coauthors, The global obesity pandemic: Shaped by global drivers and local environments, *Lancet* 378 (2011):

804–814; B. M. Popkin, Recent dynamics suggest selected countries catching up to U.S. obesity, *American Journal of Clinical Nutrition* 91 (2010): 284S–288S.

15. L. Landsberg and coauthors, Obesity-related hypertension: Pathogenesis, cardiovascular risk, and treatment: A position paper of The Obesity Society and the American Society of Hypertension, *The Journal of Clinical Hypertension* 15 (2013): 14–33; C. W. Mende, Obesity and hypertension: A common coexistence, *Journal of Clinical* Hypertension 14 (2012): 137–138.

16. Position statement: Diagnosis and classification of diabetes mellitus, *Diabetes Care* 37 (2014): S81–S90; M. L. Biggs and coauthors, Association between adiposity in midlife and older age and risk of diabetes in older adults, *Journal.of the American Medical Association* 303 (2010): 2504–2512.

17. The InterAct Consortium, Long-term risk of incident type 2 diabetes and measures of overall and regional obesity: The EPIC-InterAct Case-Cohort Study, *PLos Medicine* 9 (2012): e1001230, doi:10.1371/journal.pmed.1001230.

18. A. S. Go and coauthors, Heart disease and stroke statistics—2014 update: A report from the American Heart Association, *Circulation* 129 (2014): e28–e292; H. E. Bays and coauthors, Obesity, adiposity, and dyslipidemia: A consensus statement from the National Lipid Association, *Journal of Clinical Lipidology* 7 (2013): 304–383; B. G. Nordestgaard and coauthors, The effect of elevated body mass index on ischemic heart disease risk: Causal estimates from a Mendelian randomization approach, *PLoS Medicine* 9 (2012): e1001212; C. Eheman and coauthors, Annual Report to the Nation on the status of cancer, 1975–2008, featuring cancers associated with excess weight and lack of sufficient physical activity, *Cancer* 118 (2012): 2338–2366; World Cancer Research Fund/American Institute for Cancer Research, Continuous Update Project, Colorectal Cancer Report 2010 Summary, *Food, Nutrition, Physical Activity, and the Prevention of Colorectal Cancer* (Washington, D.C.: American Institute of Cancer Research, 2011); K. L. Kopec, Nonalcoholic fatty liver disease, *Nutrition in Clinical Practice* 26 (2011): 565–576.

19. H. Jia and E. I. Lubetkin, Trends in quality-adjusted life-years lost contributed by smoking and obesity, *American Journal of Preventive Medicine* 38 (2010): 138–144.

20. M. Hamer and E. Stamatakis, Metabolically healthy obesity and risk of all-cause and cardiovascular disease mortality, *Journal of Clinical Endocrinology and Metabolism* 97 (2012): 2482–2488; D. Lee and coauthors, Long-term effects of changes in cardiorespiratory fitness and body mass index on all-cause and cardiovascular disease mortality in men, *Circulation* 124 (2011): 2483–2490; D. E. Larson-Meyer and coauthors, Caloric restriction with or without exercise: The fitness versus fatness debate, *Medicine and Science in Sports and Exercise* 42 (2010): 152–159.

21. M. D. Jensen and coauthors, 2013 AHA/ACC/TOS guidelines for the management of overweight and obesity in adults: A report of the American College of Cardiology/American Heart Association Task Force on Practice Guidelines and The Obesity Society, *Circulation,* http://circ.ahajournals.org/content/early/2013/11/11/01.cir.0000437739.71477.ee.citation.

LO 6.7 Compare the criteria for diagnosis, characteristics, and treatments of the different eating disorders.

The exact number of people in the United States afflicted with some form of eating disorder (see Box NP6-1 for the relevant terms) is unknown because many cases are never reported.[1] An estimated 6 percent of females and 3 percent of males have **anorexia nervosa, bulimia nervosa,** or **binge eating disorder.** Many more suffer from other unspecified eating disorders that do not meet the strict diagnostic criteria for anorexia nervosa, bulimia nervosa, or binge eating disorder but still imperil a person's well-being. Characteristics of **disordered eating,** such as restrained eating, binge eating, purging, fear of fatness, and distortion of body image, are common, especially among young middle-class girls. The incidence and prevalence of eating disorders in young people has increased steadily since the 1950s.[2] Most alarming is the rising prevalence of eating disorders at progressively younger ages. In most other societies, these behaviors and attitudes are much less prevalent.

Why do so many young people in our society suffer from eating disorders?

Most experts agree that the causes are multifactorial: sociocultural, psychological, genetic, and probably also neurochemical.[3] However, excessive pressure to be thin in our society is at least partly to blame. When low body weight becomes an important goal, people begin to view normal, healthy body weight as too fat. Healthy people then take unhealthy actions to lose weight. Severe restriction of food intake can create intense stress and extreme hunger that leads to binges.[4] Research confirms this theory, showing that unhealthy or dangerous diets often precede binge eating in adolescent girls.[5] Energy restriction followed by bingeing can set in motion a pattern of **weight cycling,** which may make weight loss and maintenance more difficult over time. Importantly, healthful dieting and physical activity in overweight adolescents do not appear to trigger eating disorders.

People who attempt extreme weight loss are dissatisfied with their bodies to begin with; they may also be depressed or suffer social anxiety.[6] As weight loss becomes increasingly difficult, psychological problems worsen, and the likelihood of developing full-blown eating disorders increases.

People with anorexia nervosa suffer from an extreme preoccupation with weight loss that seriously endangers their health and even their lives. People with bulimia engage in episodes of binge eating alternating with periods of severe dieting or self-starvation. Some bulimics also follow binge eating with self-induced vomiting, laxative abuse, or diuretic abuse in an attempt to undo the perceived damage caused by the binge.

BOX NP 6-1 GLOSSARY

amenorrhea (ay-MEN-oh-RE-ah): the absence of or cessation of menstruation. Primary amenorrhea is menarche delayed beyond 16 years of age. Secondary amenorrhea is the absence of three to six consecutive menstrual cycles.

anorexia nervosa: an eating disorder characterized by a refusal to maintain a minimally normal body weight, self-starvation to the extreme, and a disturbed perception of body weight and shape; seen (usually) in adolescent girls and young women.

  anorexia = without appetite
  nervosa = of nervous origin

binge eating disorder: an eating disorder characterized by recurring episodes of eating a significant amount of food in a short period of time with marked feelings of lack of control.

bulimia (byoo-LEM-ee-uh) **nervosa:** recurring episodes of binge eating combined with a morbid fear of becoming fat, usually followed by self-induced vomiting or purging.

cathartic: a strong laxative.

cognitive therapy: psychological therapy aimed at changing undesirable behaviors by changing underlying thought processes contributing to these behaviors. In anorexia nervosa, a goal is to replace false beliefs about body weight, eating, and self-worth with health-promoting beliefs.

disordered eating: eating behaviors that are neither normal nor healthy, including restrained eating, fasting, binge eating, and purging.

eating disorder: a disturbance in eating behavior that jeopardizes a person's physical and psychological health.

emetic (em-ET-ic): an agent that causes vomiting.

RED-S (relative energy deficiency in sport): a syndrome of impaired physiological function including, but not limited to, metabolic rate, menstrual function, bone health, immunity, protein synthesis, and cardiovascular health caused by relative energy deficiency.

stress fractures: bone damage or breaks caused by stress on bone surfaces during exercise.

weight cycling: repeated rounds of weight loss and subsequent regain, with reduced ability to lose weight with each attempt; also called *yo-yo dieting.*

Are there other groups, besides girls and young women, who are vulnerable to anorexia nervosa and bulimia nervosa?

Yes. Athletes and dancers are at special risk for eating disorders.[7] They may severely restrict energy intakes in an attempt to enhance performance or appearance or to meet weight guidelines of a sport. In reality, severe energy restriction causes a loss of lean tissue that impairs physical performance and imposes a risk of eating disorders. Risk factors for eating disorders among athletes include:

- Young age (adolescence)

- Pressure to excel in a sport

- Focus on achieving or maintaining an "ideal" body weight or body fat percentage

- Participation in sports or competitions that judge performance on aesthetic appeal such as gymnastics, figure skating, or dance

- Unhealthy, unsupervised weight-loss dieting at an early age

Female athletes are most vulnerable, but males—especially dancers, swimmers, divers, wrestlers, skaters, jockeys, and gymnasts—suffer from eating disorders, too, and their numbers may be increasing.[8]

Male athletes and dancers with eating disorders often deny having them because they mistakenly believe that such disorders afflict only women. Under the same pressures as female athletes, males may also develop eating disorders. They skip meals, restrict fluids, practice in plastic suits, or train in heated rooms to lose a quick 4 to 7 pounds.[9] Wrestlers, especially, must "make weight" to compete in the lowest possible weight class to face smaller opponents. Conversely, male athletes may suffer weight-*gain* problems. When young men with low self-esteem internalize unrealistically bulky male body images, they can become dissatisfied with their own healthy bodies and practice unhealthy behaviors, even steroid drug abuse.

Even among athletes, however, women are most susceptible to developing eating disorders, and the term "female athlete triad" has thus been used in the past to refer to the syndrome characterized by disordered eating, **amenorrhea** (the absence of three or more consecutive menstrual cycles), and osteoporosis observed in these women. Recognizing that some male athletes are susceptible to eating disorders, however, and that this syndrome encompasses more than these three components, the International Olympic Committee (IOC) has introduced a more comprehensive term to describe the overall syndrome: **relative energy deficiency in sport (RED-S)**.[10]

How does RED-S develop?

The underlying problem of RED-S is an energy deficiency—too little energy intake for the energy expenditure needed to support health and the activities of daily living, growth, and sporting activities. This energy imbalance disrupts the body's normal hormonal, metabolic, and functional activities. Disordered eating underlies many cases of RED-S, but other situations such as rapid, unsupervised weight loss or failure to eat enough during times of extreme exercise may also play a part.

Many athletic women and men engage in self-destructive eating behaviors (disordered eating) because they and their coaches have adopted unsuitable weight standards. An athlete's body must be heavier for height than a nonathlete's body because the athlete's bones and muscles are denser. Weight standards that may be appropriate for others are inappropriate for athletes. Techniques such as skinfold measures yield more useful information about body composition.

As for amenorrhea, its prevalence among premenopausal women in the United States is about 2 to 5 percent overall, but among female athletes it may be as high as 66 percent. Amenorrhea is *not* a normal adaptation to strenuous physical training: it is a symptom of something going wrong. Amenorrhea is characterized by low blood estrogen, infertility, and often bone mineral losses.

In general, weight-bearing physical activity, dietary calcium, and the hormone estrogen protect against the bone loss of osteoporosis, but in women with disordered eating and amenorrhea, strenuous activity may impair bone health.[11] As noted above, vigorous training combined with low food energy intakes disrupts metabolic

and hormonal balances. These disturbances compromise bone health, greatly increasing the risks of **stress fractures.**[12] Stress fractures, a serious form of bone injury, commonly occur among dancers and other competitive athletes with amenorrhea, low calcium intakes, and disordered eating. Many underweight young athletes have bones like those of postmenopausal women, and they may never recover their lost bone even after diagnosis and treatment—which makes prevention critical. Young athletes should be encouraged to consume at least 1300 milligrams of calcium each day, to eat nutrient-dense foods, and to obtain enough food energy to support weight gain and the energy expended in physical activity. Nutrition is critical to bone recovery.

What can be done to prevent eating disorders in athletes and dancers?

To prevent eating disorders in athletes and dancers, both the performers and their coaches must be educated about links between inappropriate body weight ideals, improper weight-loss techniques, eating disorder development, adequate nutrition, and safe weight-management strategies. Coaches and dance instructors should never encourage unhealthy weight loss to qualify for competition or to conform with distorted artistic ideals. Frequent weighings can push young people who are striving to lose weight into a cycle of starving to confront the scale and then bingeing uncontrollably afterward. The erosion of self-esteem that accompanies these events can interfere with the normal psychological development of the teen years and set the stage for serious problems later on.

Table NP6-1 provides some suggestions to help athletes and dancers protect themselves against developing eating disorders. The next sections describe eating disorders that anyone, athlete or nonathlete, may experience.

TABLE NP6-1 Strategies to Combat Eating Disorders

The following guidelines may be useful in combating eating disorders:

- Never restrict food intakes to below the amounts suggested for adequacy by the USDA Food Patterns.

- Eat frequently. People often do not eat frequent meals because of time constraints, but eating can be incorporated into other activities, such as snacking while studying or commuting. The person who eats frequently never gets so hungry as to allow hunger to dictate food choices.

- If not at a healthy weight, establish a reasonable weight goal based on a healthy body composition.

- Allow a reasonable time to achieve the goal. A reasonable loss of excess fat can be achieved at the rate of about 1 percent of body weight per week.

- Learn to recognize media image biases, and reject ultra-thin standards for beauty. Shift focus to health, competencies, and human interactions; bring behaviors in line with those beliefs.

Specific guidelines for athletes and dancers:

- Replace weight-based goals with performance-based goals.

- Remember that eating disorders impair physical performance. Seek confidential help in obtaining treatment if needed.

- Restrict weight-loss activities to the off-season.

- Focus on proper nutrition as an important facet of your training—as important as proper technique.

Who is at risk for anorexia nervosa?

Most anorexia nervosa victims are females who come from middle- or upper-class families. The person with anorexia nervosa is often a perfectionist who works hard to please her parents. She may identify so strongly with her parents' ideals and goals for her that she sometimes feels she has no identity of her own. She is respectful of authority but sometimes feels like a robot, and she may act that way, too: polite but controlled, rigid, and unspontaneous. She earnestly desires to control her own destiny, but she feels controlled by others. When she does not eat, she gains control.

How does a person know when dieting is going too far?

When a person loses weight to well below the average for her height, becoming too slim, and still doesn't stop, she has gone too far. Regardless of how thin she is, she looks in the mirror and sees herself as fat. Specific criteria for the diagnosis of anorexia nervosa include significantly low body weight caused by persistent restriction of energy intake; an intense fear of gaining weight or becoming fat, or persistent behaviors that interfere with weight gains; and a disturbance in self-perceived weight or shape.[13] Central to the diagnosis of anorexia nervosa is a distorted body image that overestimates body fatness. Anorexia nervosa resembles an addiction. The characteristic behavior is obsessive and compulsive. Before drawing conclusions about someone who is extremely thin or who eats very little, remember that diagnosis of anorexia nervosa requires professional assessment.

© Sniegirova Mariia/Shutterstock.com

People with anorexia nervosa see themselves as fat, even when they are dangerously underweight.

What is the harm in being very thin?

Anorexia nervosa damages the body much as starvation does. In young people, growth ceases, and normal development falters. They lose so much lean tissue that basal metabolic rate slows. Bones weaken, too—osteoporosis develops in about a third of those with anorexia nervosa.[14] Additionally, the heart pumps inefficiently and irregularly, the heart muscle becomes weak and thin, the heart chambers diminish in size, and the blood pressure falls. Minerals that help to regulate the heartbeat become unbalanced. Many deaths in people with anorexia nervosa are due to heart failure. The kidneys often fail as well.[15]

Starvation brings other physical consequences: loss of brain tissue, impaired immune response, anemia, and a loss of digestive function that worsens malnutrition. Digestive functioning becomes sluggish, the stomach empties slowly, and the lining of the intestinal tract shrinks. The ailing digestive tract fails to sufficiently digest any food the victim may eat. The pancreas slows its production of digestive enzymes. The person may suffer from diarrhea, further worsening malnutrition.

What kind of treatment helps people with anorexia nervosa?

Treatment of anorexia nervosa requires a multidisciplinary approach that addresses two sets of issues and behaviors: those relating to food and weight, and those involving relationships with oneself and others. Teams of physicians, nurses, psychiatrists, family therapists, and dietitians work together to treat people with anorexia nervosa. The expertise of a registered dietitian nutritionist is essential because an appropriate, individually crafted diet is crucial for normalizing body weight, and dietary counseling is indispensable.[16] Seldom are clients willing to eat for themselves, but if they are, chances are they can recover without other interventions.

Professionals classify clients based on the risks posed by the degree of malnutrition present.* Clients with low risks may benefit from family counseling, **cognitive therapy,** behavior modification, and nutrition guidance; those with greater risks may also need other forms of psychotherapy and supplemental formulas to provide extra nutrients and energy.

Sometimes, intensive behavior management treatment in a live-in facility can help to normalize food intake and exercise. When starvation leads to severe underweight (less than 75 percent of ideal body weight), high medical risks ensue, and patients require hospitalization. They must be stabilized and carefully fed to forestall death. However, involuntary feeding through a tube can cause psychological trauma and may not be necessary in all cases. Antidepressants and other drugs are commonly prescribed but are often ineffective in anorexia nervosa.

Stopping weight loss is a first goal; establishing regular eating patterns is next. Because body weight is low and fear of weight gain is high, initial food intake may be small—1200 kcalories per day can be an achievement. A variety of high-energy foods and beverages can help deliver needed kcalories and nutrients. Even

*Indicators of malnutrition include a low percentage of body fat, low blood proteins, and impaired immune response.

after recovery, however, energy intakes and eating behaviors may not fully return to normal.

Almost half of women who are treated can successfully maintain their body weight at just below a healthy weight; at that weight, many of them begin menstruating again. The other half have poor or fair treatment outcomes, relapse into abnormal eating behaviors, or die. Anorexia nervosa has one of the highest mortality rates among psychiatric disorders—most commonly from cardiac complications or by suicide.[17]

How does bulimia nervosa differ from anorexia nervosa?

Bulimia nervosa is distinct from anorexia nervosa and is more prevalent. More men suffer from bulimia nervosa than from anorexia, but bulimia is still more common in women. The secretive nature of bulimic behaviors makes recognition of the problem difficult, but once it is recognized, diagnosis is based on such criteria as number and frequency of binge eating episodes, inappropriate compensatory behaviors to prevent weight gain (such as self-induced vomiting or misuse of laxatives), and self-evaluation that is unduly influenced by body shape and weight.[18]

The typical person with bulimia is well educated, in her early twenties, and close to ideal body weight. She is a high achiever but emotionally insecure. She experiences considerable social anxiety and has difficulty establishing personal relationships. She is sometimes depressed and often exhibits impulsive behavior.

Like the person with anorexia nervosa, the person with bulimia spends much time thinking about her body weight and food. Her preoccupation with food manifests itself in secretive binge eating episodes followed by self-induced vomiting, fasting, or the use of laxatives or diuretics. Such behaviors typically begin in late adolescence after a long series of various unsuccessful weight-reduction diets. People with bulimia commonly follow a pattern of restrictive dieting interspersed with bulimic behaviors and experience weight fluctuations of more than 10 pounds over short periods of time.

Unlike the person with anorexia nervosa, the person with bulimia is aware of the consequences of her behavior, feels that it is abnormal, and is deeply ashamed of it. She feels inadequate and unable to control her eating, so she tends to be passive and to look to others for confirmation of her sense of self-worth. When she is rejected, either in reality or in her imagination, her bulimia becomes worse. If her depression deepens, she may seek solace in drug or alcohol abuse or other addictive behaviors. Clinical depression is common in people with bulimia nervosa, and the rates of substance abuse are high.

What exactly is binge eating?

Binge eating is unlike normal eating, and the food is not consumed for its nutritional value. The binge eater has a compulsion to eat. A typical binge occurs periodically, is done in secret, usually at night, and lasts an hour or more. A binge frequently follows a period of rigid dieting, so the binge eating is accelerated by hunger. During a binge, the person with bulimia may consume a thousand kcalories or more. The food typically contains little fiber or water, has a smooth texture, and is high in sugar and fat, so it is easy to consume vast amounts rapidly with little chewing.

What are the consequences of binge eating and purging?

After a binge, the person may use a **cathartic**—a strong laxative that can injure the lower intestinal tract. Or the person may induce vomiting, using an **emetic**—a drug intended as first aid for poisoning.

On first glance, purging seems to offer a quick and easy solution to the problems of unwanted kcalories and body weight. Many people perceive such behavior as neutral or even positive, when, in fact, bingeing and purging have serious physical consequences. Fluid and electrolyte imbalances caused by vomiting or diarrhea can lead to abnormal heart rhythms and injury to the kidneys. Vomiting causes irritation and infection of the pharynx, esophagus, and salivary glands; erosion of the teeth; and dental caries. The esophagus may rupture or tear, as may the stomach. Overuse of emetics depletes potassium concentrations and can lead to death by heart failure.

What is the treatment for bulimia nervosa?

As for people with anorexia nervosa, a team approach provides the most effective treatment for people with bulimia nervosa. Bulimia nervosa is easier to treat than anorexia nervosa in many respects because it seems to be more of a chosen behavior. People with bulimia know that their behavior is abnormal, and many are willing to try to cooperate.

The goal of the dietary plan to treat bulimia is to help the client gain control, establish regular eating patterns, and restore nutritional health. Energy intake should not be severely restricted—hunger can be a trigger for a binge. The person needs to learn to eat a quantity of nutritious food sufficient to nourish her body and to satisfy hunger (at least 1600 kcalories per day). Table NP6-2 offers some ways

TABLE NP6-2 Strategies to Combat Bulimia Nervosa

Planning Principles

- Plan meals and snacks; record plans in a food diary prior to eating.
- Plan meals and snacks that require eating at the table and using utensils.
- Refrain from finger foods.
- Refrain from fasting or skipping meals.

Nutrition Principles

- Eat a well-balanced diet and regularly timed meals consisting of a variety of foods.
- Include raw vegetables, salad, or raw fruit at meals to prolong eating times.
- Choose whole-grain, high-fiber breads, pasta, rice, and cereals to increase bulk.
- Consume adequate fluid, particularly water.

Other Tips

- Choose foods that provide protein and fat for satiety and bulky, fiber-rich carbohydrates for immediate feelings of fullness.
- Try including soups and other water-rich foods for satiety.
- Choose portions that are appropriate for your energy needs according to the USDA Food Patterns (pp. 16–17).
- For convenience (and to reduce temptation) select foods that naturally divide into portions. Select one potato, rather than rice or pasta that can be overloaded onto the plate; purchase yogurt and cottage cheese in individual containers; look for small packages of precut steak or chicken; choose frozen dinners with measured portions.
- Include 30 minutes of physical activity every day—exercise may be an important tool in defeating bulimia.

to begin correcting bulimia nervosa. Most people diagnosed with bulimia nervosa recover within 5 to 10 years, with or without treatment, but treatment probably speeds the recovery process.

Anorexia nervosa and bulimia nervosa are distinct eating disorders, yet they sometimes overlap. Anorexia victims may purge, and victims of both conditions share an overconcern with body weight and the tendency to drastically undereat. The two disorders can also appear in the same person, or one can lead to the other. Other people have eating disorders that fall short of anorexia nervosa or bulimia nervosa but share some of their features, such as fear of body fatness. One such condition is binge eating disorder.

How does binge eating disorder differ from bulimia nervosa?

Up to half of all people who restrict eating to lose weight periodically binge without purging, including about one-third of obese people. Obesity itself, however, does not constitute an eating disorder.

Clinicians note differences between people with bulimia nervosa and those with binge eating disorder. People with binge eating disorder consume less during a binge, rarely purge, and exert less restraint during times of dieting. Similarities also exist, including feeling out of control, disgusted, depressed, embarrassed, or guilty because of their self-perceived gluttony. Binge eating behavior responds more readily to treatment than other eating disorders, and resolving such behaviors can be a first step to authentic weight control. Successful treatment also improves physical health, mental health, and the chances of breaking the cycle of rapid weight losses and gains.

Chapter 6 describes how our society sets unrealistic ideals for body weight, especially in women, and devalues those who do not conform to them. Anorexia nervosa and bulimia nervosa are not a form of rebellion against these unreasonable expectations but rather the exaggerated acceptance of them. Body dissatisfaction is a primary factor in the development of eating disorders. Perhaps a person's best defense against these disorders is to learn to appreciate his or her own uniqueness.

Notes

1. Position of the American Dietetic Association, Nutrition intervention in the treatment of eating disorders, *Journal of the American Dietetic Association* 111 (2011): 1236–1241.

2. D. S. Rosen and the Committee on Adolescence, Clinical report—Identification and management of eating disorders in children and adolescents, *Pediatrics* 126 (2010): 1240–1253.

3. T. K. Clarke, A. R. Weiss, and W. H. Berrettini, The genetics of anorexia nervosa, *Clinical Pharmacology and Therapeutics* 91 (2012): 181–188; R. Calati and coauthors, The 5-HTTLPR polymorphism and eating disorders: A meta-analysis, *International Journal of Eating Disorders* 44 (2011): 191–199; Position of the American Dietetic Association, 2011.

4. K. D. Carr, Food scarcity, neuroadaptations, and the pathogenic potential of dieting in an unnatural ecology: Binge eating and drug abuse, *Psychology and Behavior* 104 (2011): 515–524.

5. D. Neumark-Sztainer and coauthors, Dieting and disordered eating behaviors from adolescence to young adulthood: Findings from a 10-year longitudinal study, *Journal of the American Dietetic Association* 111 (2011): 1004–1011.

6. U. Pauli-Pott and coauthors, Links between psychopathological symptoms and disordered eating behaviors in overweight/obese youths, *International Journal of Eating Disorders* 46 (2013): 156–163; M. L. Norris and coauthors, An examination of medical and psychological morbidity in adolescent males with eating disorders, *Eating Disorders* 20 (2012): 405–415; R. D. Grave, Eating disorders: Progress and challenges, *European Journal of Internal Medicine* 22 (2011): 153–160.

7. M. Martinsen and J. Sundgot-Borgen, Higher prevalence of eating disorders among adolescent elite athletes than controls, *Medicine and Science in Sports and Exercise* 45 (2013): 1188–1197; C. A. Hincapie and J. D. Cassidy, Disordered eating, menstrual disturbances, and low bone mineral density in dancers: A systematic review, *Archives of Physical Medicine and Rehabilitation* 91 (2010): 1777–1789.

8. A. Melin and coauthors, Disordered eating and eating disorders in aquatic sports, International Journal of *Sport Nutrition and Exercise Metabolism*, March 25, 2014, epub ahead of print; S. Bratland-Sanda and J. Sundgot-Borgen, Eating disorders in athletes: Overview of prevalence, risk factors, and recommendations for prevention and treatment, *European Journal of Sport Science* 13 (2013): 499–508; J. B. Martin, The development of ideal body image perceptions in the United States, *Nutrition Today* 45 (2010): 98–110.

9. G. G. Artioli and coauthors, Prevalence, magnitude, and methods of rapid weight loss among judo competitors, *Medicine and Science in Sports and Exercise* 42 (2010): 436–442.

10. M. Mountjoy and coauthors, Consensus statement: The IOC consensus statement: Beyond the female athlete triad—relative energy deficiency in sport (RED-S), *British Journal of Sports Medicine* 48 (2014): 491–497.

11. M. T. Barrack and coauthors, Physiologic and behavioral indicators of energy deficiency in female adolescent runners with elevated bone turnover, *American Journal of Clinical Nutrition* 92 (2010): 652–659; Position of the American Dietetic Association, Dietitians of Canada, and the American College of Sports Medicine, Nutrition and Athletic Performance, *Journal of the American Dietetic Association* 109 (2009): 509–527.

12. C. Rosenbloom, Stress fractures in athletes, *Nutrition Today* 48 (2013): 81–87.

13. American Psychiatric Association, *Diagnostic and Statistical Manual of Mental Disorders* (Washington, D.C.: American Psychiatric Publishing, 2013).

14. A. P. Winston, The clinical biochemistry of anorexia nervosa, *Annals of Clinical Biochemistry* 49 (2012): 132–143; P. S. Mehler, B. S. Cleary, and J. L. Gaudiani, Osteoporosis in anorexia nervosa, *Eating Disorders* 19 (2011): 194–202.

15. Winston, 2012.

16. Position of the American Dietetic Association, 2011.

17. Grave, 2011.

18. American Psychiatric Association, *Diagnostic and Statistical Manual of Mental Disorders* (Washington, D.C.: American Psychiatric Publishing, 2013).

7

Weight Management

Are you pleased with your body weight? If you answered yes, you are a rare individual. Nearly all people in our society think they should weigh more or less (mostly less) than they do. Usually, their primary reason is appearance, but they often perceive, correctly, that their weight is also related to physical health. Chapter 6 addressed the health risks of being overweight or underweight.

Overweight and underweight both result from energy imbalance. The simple picture is as follows. Overweight people have consumed more food energy than they have expended and have banked the surplus in their body fat. To reduce body fat, overweight people need to expend more energy than they take in from food. In contrast, underweight people have consumed too little food energy to support their activities and so have depleted their bodies' fat stores and possibly some of their lean tissues as well. To gain weight, they need to take in more food energy than they expend.

This chapter's missions are to present strategies for solving the problems of excessive and deficient body fatness and to point out how appropriate body composition, once achieved, can be maintained. The chapter emphasizes overweight and obesity, partly because they have been more intensively studied and partly because they represent a major health problem in the United States and a growing concern worldwide.

7.1 Causes of Obesity

LO 7.1 Discuss the genetic and environmental causes of obesity.

Henceforth, this chapter will use the term *obesity* to refer to excess body fat. Excess body fat accumulates when people take in more food energy than they expend. Why do they do this? Is it genetic? Metabolic? Psychological? Behavioral? All of these? Most likely, obesity has many interrelated causes. This section reviews the two major contributing and interacting factors—genetics and the environment.[1]

Genetics and Weight

A person's genetic makeup influences the body's tendency to consume or store too much energy or to expend too little.[2] Evidence that genes influence eating behavior and body composition comes from family, twin, and adoption studies. Adopted children tend to be more similar in weight to their biological parents than to their adoptive parents.[3] Studies of twins yield similar findings: compared with fraternal twins, identical twins are far more likely to weigh the same.[4] Genes clearly influence a person's tendency to gain weight or stay lean.[5] The risk of obesity is two to three times higher for a person with a family history of obesity than for a person without such history. Despite such findings, however, only 1 to 5 percent of obesity cases can be explained by a single gene mutation.[6] Furthermore, although genomics researchers have identified hundreds of genes with possible roles in obesity development, they have not yet identified genetic causes of common obesity.[7]

Exceptionally complex relationships exist among the many genes related to energy metabolism and obesity, and they each interact with environmental factors, too. Although an individual's genetic inheritance may make obesity likely, it will not necessarily develop unless given a push by environmental factors that encourage energy consumption and discourage energy expenditure.[8] High-fat diets, sugar-sweetened beverages, and low physical activity, for example, can accentuate the genetic influences on obesity.[9] Likewise, physical activity can minimize the genetic influences on BMI.[10] The following sections describe research involving proteins that might help explain appetite control, energy regulation, and obesity development.

Lipoprotein Lipase Some of the research investigating genetic influence on obesity focuses on the enzyme **lipoprotein lipase (LPL),** which promotes fat storage in fat cells and muscle cells.[11] People with high LPL activity are especially efficient at storing fat. Obese people generally have much more LPL activity in their fat cells than lean people do (their muscle cell LPL activity is similar, though). This high LPL activity makes fat storage especially efficient. Consequently, even modest excesses in energy intake have a more dramatic impact on obese people than on lean people.

Leptin Researchers have identified a gene in humans called the obesity (*ob*) gene. The obesity gene codes for the protein **leptin.** Leptin is a hormone primarily produced and secreted by the fat cells in proportion to the amount of fat stored. A gain in body fatness stimulates the production of leptin, which, by way of the **hypothalamus,** suppresses the appetite, increases energy expenditure, and produces fat loss.[12] Fat loss produces the opposite effect—suppression of leptin production, increased appetite, and decreased energy expenditure. As Figure 7-1 shows, mice with a defective obesity gene do not produce leptin and can weigh up to three times as much as normal mice. When injected with leptin, the mice lose weight. (Because leptin is a protein, it would be destroyed during digestion if given orally; consequently, it must be given by injection.)

Although it is extremely rare, researchers have identified a genetic deficiency of leptin in human beings as well. An error in the gene that codes for leptin was discovered in two extremely obese children whose blood levels of leptin were barely detectable. Without leptin, the children had little appetite control; they were constantly hungry and ate considerably more than their siblings or peers. Given daily injections of leptin, these children lost a substantial amount of weight, confirming leptin's role in regulating appetite and body weight.

Most obese people do not have leptin deficiency, however. In fact, most obese people produce plenty of leptin, but they fail to respond to it, a condition called *leptin resistance.*[13] Researchers speculate that blood leptin rises in an effort to suppress appetite and inhibit fat storage when fat cells are ample. Obese people with elevated leptin concentrations may be resistant to its satiating effect. The absence of or resistance to leptin in obesity parallels the scenario of insulin in diabetes: some people have an insulin deficiency (type 1), whereas many others have elevated insulin but are resistant to its glucose-storing effect (type 2).

Ghrelin Another protein known as **ghrelin** works in the opposite direction of leptin. Ghrelin is synthesized and secreted primarily by the stomach cells but works in the hypothalamus to promote a positive energy balance by increasing smell sensitivity, stimulating appetite and promoting efficient energy storage.[14] The role ghrelin plays in regulating food intake and body weight is the subject of much intense research.[15] Pharmaceutical companies are eager to develop products that mimic ghrelin to treat wasting conditions, as well as products that oppose ghrelin's action to treat obesity.[16]

Ghrelin powerfully triggers the desire to eat. Blood levels of ghrelin typically rise before and fall after a meal—reflecting the hunger and satiety that precede and follow eating. In general, fasting blood levels correlate inversely with body weight: lean people have high ghrelin levels and obese people have low levels.

Ghrelin fights to maintain a stable body weight. On average, ghrelin levels are high whenever the body is in negative energy balance, as occurs during low-kcalorie diets, for example. This response may help explain why weight loss is so difficult to maintain. Ghrelin levels decline again whenever the body is in positive energy balance, as occurs with weight gains.

Fat Cell Development When "energy in" exceeds "energy out," much of the excess energy is stored in the fat cells of adipose tissue. The amount of fat in adipose tissue reflects both the *number* and the *size* of the fat cells.* Thus, obesity develops when

*Obesity due to an increase in the *number* of fat cells is *hyperplastic obesity.* Obesity due to an increase in the *size* of fat cells is *hypertrophic obesity.*

FIGURE 7-1

The mouse on the left is genetically obese—it lacks the gene for producing leptin. The mouse on the right is *also* genetically obese, but because it receives leptin, it eats less, expends more energy, and is less obese than it would be had it not received the leptin.

lipoprotein lipase (LPL): an enzyme mounted on the surface of fat cells (and other cells) that hydrolyzes triglycerides in the blood into fatty acids and glycerol for absorption into the cells. There they are metabolized or reassembled for storage.

leptin: a hormone produced by fat cells under the direction of the (*ob*) gene. It decreases appetite and increases energy expenditure.

leptos = thin

hypothalamus (high-po-THAL-ah-mus): a brain center that controls activities such as maintenance of water balance, regulation of body temperature, and control of appetite.

ghrelin (GRELL-in): a hormone produced primarily by the stomach cells. It signals the hypothalamus of the brain to stimulate appetite and food intake.

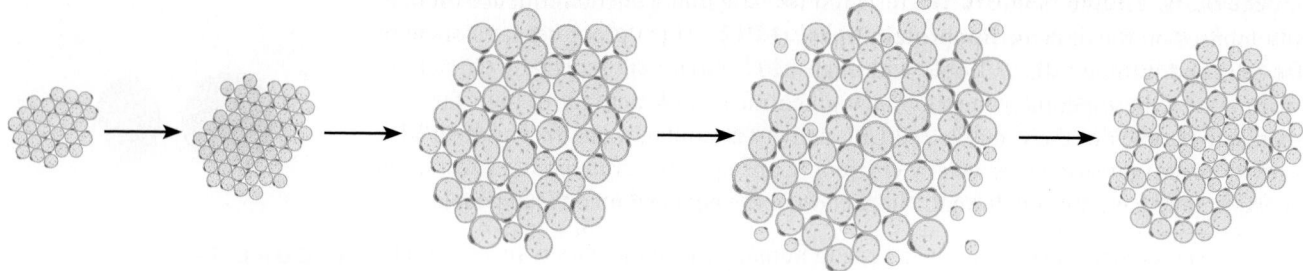

During growth, fat cells increase in number.

When energy intake exceeds expenditure, fat cells increase in size.

When fat cells have enlarged and energy intake continues to exceed energy expenditure, fat cells increase in number again.

With fat loss, the size of the fat cells shrinks, but not the number.

© Cengage Learning®

FIGURE 7-2 Fat Cell Development
Fat cells are capable of increasing their size by 20-fold and their number by several thousand-fold.

a person's fat cells increase in number, in size, or quite often both. The number of fat cells increases most rapidly during the growing years of late childhood and early puberty. After growth ceases, fat cell number may continue to increase whenever energy balance is positive.[17] Fat cells can also expand in size. After they reach their maximum size, more cells can develop to store more fat. Obese people have more fat cells than healthy-weight people; their fat cells are also larger. Figure 7-2 illustrates fat cell development.

With fat loss, the size of the fat cells shrinks, but their number cannot. For this reason, people with extra fat cells may tend to regain lost weight rapidly. Prevention of obesity is most critical, then, during the growing years of childhood and adolescence when fat cells increase in number most profoundly.

As mentioned, excess fat first fills the body's natural storage site—adipose tissue. If fat is still abundant, the excess is deposited in organs such as the heart and liver and plays a key role in the development of heart failure and fatty liver, respectively.[18] As adipose tissue produces adipokines, metabolic changes that indicate disease risk— such as insulin resistance—become apparent and chronic inflammation develops.[19]

Set-Point Theory One popular theory of why a person may store too much fat is the **set-point theory.** The set-point theory proposes that body weight, like body temperature, is physiologically regulated.[20] Researchers have noted that many people who lose weight quickly regain it all. This suggests that somehow the body chooses a preferred weight and defends that weight by regulating eating behaviors and hormonal actions. After weight losses, the body reduces its metabolic rate. The decrease in metabolic rate after weight loss is greater than would be expected based on body composition alone.[21] This adaptation helps to explain why it can be difficult for an overweight person to maintain weight losses. While set point answers some questions regarding the biology of energy balance, it fails to explain the many other influences contributing to the population's obesity epidemic.[22]

Environmental Stimuli

As discussed earlier, genetic factors play a partial role in determining a person's susceptibility to obesity, but they do not fully explain obesity. Obesity rates have risen dramatically during recent decades, but the human gene pool has remained unchanged. The environment must therefore play a role as well. Obesity reflects the interaction between genes and the environment.[23] An **obesogenic environment** includes all of the circumstances that people encounter daily that push them toward fatness. Over the past four decades, the demand for physical activity has decreased as the abundance of food has increased.

set-point theory: the theory that the body tends to maintain a certain weight by means of its own internal controls.

obesogenic (oh- BES-oh-JEN-ick) **environment:** all the factors surrounding a person that promote weight gain, such as an increased food intake—especially of unhealthy choices—and decreased physical activity.

Overeating People may overeat in response to stimuli in their surroundings—primarily, the availability of many delectable foods. Most people in the United States find high-kcalorie foods readily available, relatively inexpensive, heavily advertised, and reasonably tasty—thanks largely to fast food. With around-the-clock access to rich palatable foods, we eat more and more often than in decades past—and energy intakes have risen accordingly.[24]

Most alarming are the extraordinarily large serving sizes and ready-to-go meals offered in supersize combinations. Eating large portion sizes multiple times a day accounts for much of the weight increase seen over the decades.[25] People buy the large sizes and combinations, perceiving them to be a good value, but then they eat more than they need. Research shows that people eat more if they're served more.[26] "Portion distortion" is a term used to describe the perception that large portions are the appropriate amounts to eat at a single sitting.[27] And portion sizes of virtually all foods and beverages (and even sizes of plates, glasses, and utensils) have increased markedly in the past several decades, most notably at fast-food restaurants. The increase in portion sizes parallels the growing prevalence of overweight and obesity in the United States, beginning in the 1970s, rising sharply in the 1980s, and continuing today.

Research suggests that fast-food consumption contributes significantly to the development of obesity.[28] Fast food is often energy-dense food, which increases energy intake, BMI, and body fatness. The combination of large portions and energy-dense foods strikes a double blow. Reducing portion sizes is helpful, but the real kcalorie savings come from lowering the energy density. Satisfying portions of foods with low energy density such as fruits and vegetables can help with weight loss.

Consumers' health would benefit from restaurants providing appropriate portion sizes and offering more fruits, vegetables, legumes, and whole grains. In an effort to help consumers make healthier choices, national legislation now requires restaurants with 20 or more locations to provide menu listings of an item's kcalories, grams of saturated fat, and milligrams of sodium.[29] Once such information displays become standard throughout the country, perhaps restaurants will have greater incentives to offer healthier choices.

Learned Behavior Psychological stimuli also trigger inappropriate eating behaviors in some people. Appropriate eating behavior is a response to **hunger.** Hunger is a drive programmed into people by their heredity. **Appetite,** in contrast, is learned and can lead people to ignore hunger or to over-respond to it. Hunger is physiological, whereas appetite is psychological, and the two do not always coincide.

During the course of a meal, as food enters the GI tract and hunger diminishes, **satiation** occurs. As receptors in the stomach stretch and hormones become active, the person begins to feel full. The response is satiation, which prompts the person to stop eating.

After a meal, the feeling of **satiety** continues to suppress hunger and allow a person to not eat again for a while. Whereas *satiation* tells us to "stop eating," *satiety* reminds us to "not start eating again." As mentioned above, people can override these signals, especially when presented with favorite foods or stressful situations.

Food behavior is intimately connected to deep emotional needs such as the primitive fear of starvation. Yearnings, cravings, and addictions with profound psychological significance can express themselves in people's eating behavior. An emotionally insecure person might eat rather than call a friend and risk rejection. Another person might eat to relieve boredom or to ward off depression.

Physical Inactivity The possible causes of obesity mentioned so far all relate to the input side of the energy equation. What about output? People may be obese, not because they eat too much, but because they move too little—both in purposeful exercise and in the activities of daily life.[30] Obese people observed closely are often seen to eat less than lean people, but they are sometimes so extraordinarily inactive that they still manage to accumulate an energy surplus. Reducing their food intake further would jeopardize health and incur nutrient deficiencies. Physical activity, then, is a

hunger: the physiological need to eat, experienced as a drive to obtain food; an unpleasant sensation that demands relief.

appetite: the psychological desire to eat; a learned motivation that is experienced as a pleasant sensation that accompanies the sight, smell, or thought of appealing foods.

satiation (say-she-AY-shun): the feeling of satisfaction and fullness that occurs during a meal and halts eating. Satiation determines how much food is consumed during a meal.

satiety: the feeling of fullness and satisfaction that occurs after a meal and inhibits eating until the next meal. Satiety determines how much time passes between meals.

Lack of physical activity fosters obesity.

necessary component of nutritional health. People must be physically active if they are to eat enough food to deliver all the nutrients needed without unhealthy weight gain.

Our environment, however, fosters inactivity.[31] In turn, inactivity contributes to obesity and poor health.[32] Sedentary **screen time** has all but replaced outdoor activity for many people. In addition, most people work at sedentary jobs. One hundred years ago, 30 percent of the energy used in farm and factory work came from muscle power; today, only 1 percent does. Modern technology has replaced physical activity at home, at work, at school, and in transportation. The more time spent sitting still, the higher the risk of dying from heart disease and other causes.[33]

Health experts urge people to "take the stairs instead of the elevator" or "walk or bike to work." These are excellent suggestions: climbing stairs provides an impromptu workout, and people who walk or ride a bicycle for transportation most often meet their needs for physical activity. Physical activity strategies for weight loss and weight maintenance are offered in a later section of this chapter.

Neighborhood Obstacles to Physical Activity and Healthy Foods Some aspects of the **built environment,** including buildings, sidewalks, and transportation opportunities, can discourage physical activity. For example, most stairwells of modern buildings are inconvenient, isolated, and unsafe. Roadways often lack sidewalks, crosswalks, or lanes marked for bicycles. The air on roadways can be dangerously high in carbon monoxide gas and other pollutants from gasoline engine emissions. Hot and cold weather also pose hazards for outdoor commuters. In contrast, those with access to health-promoting foods and built environments more easily make healthy choices.[34] Safe, affordable biking and walking areas and public exercise facilities help maintain health and body leanness.

In addition, residents of many low-income urban and rural areas lack access to even a single supermarket.[35] Often overweight and lacking transportation, residents of these so-called **food deserts** have limited access to the affordable, fresh, nutrient-dense foods they need.[36] Instead, they shop at local convenience stores and fast-food places, where they can purchase mostly refined packaged sweets and starches, sugary soft drinks, fatty canned meats, or fast foods, and they often have an eating pattern that predicts nutrient deficiencies and excesses along with high rates of obesity and type 2 diabetes.[37]

In truth, in most neighborhoods across the United States, the most accessible, affordable, and tempting foods and beverages are high-kcalorie, good-tasting, inexpensive fare from fast-food restaurants, and it takes a great deal of attention, planning, and time to "go against the flow" to keep kcalorie intakes reasonable. Today, only about a third of the population succeeds in doing so. The prestigious National Academies' Institute of Medicine has put forth the national goals in Table 7-1 as most likely to slow or reverse the obesity epidemic and improve the nation's health.[38] Accomplishing any one of these goals on its own might speed up progress in preventing obesity, but if all these goals are realized, their effects will be powerful allies in the nationwide struggle to regain control over weight and health. Such changes require leaders at all levels and citizenry across all sectors of society to work toward one goal: improving the health of the nation.

Until these changes occur, the best way for most people to attain a healthy body composition boils down to overcoming obstacles to making dietary changes and increasing physical activity. Later sections focus on these areas, while the next section delves into the details of obesity treatment.

IN SUMMARY

▪ Genetics, fat cell development, set point, overeating, and inactivity all offer possible, but still incomplete, explanations of obesity.

▪ Most likely, obesity has not one cause but different causes and combinations of causes in different people.

TABLE 7-1 National Goals to Combat Obesity

▪ Make physical activity an integral and routine part of American life.

▪ Make healthy foods and beverages available everywhere—create food and beverage environments to make healthy food and beverage choices the routine, easy choice.

▪ Advertise and market what matters for a healthy life.

▪ Activate employers and health-care professionals.

▪ Strengthen schools as the heart of health.

Source: Adapted from: Institute of Medicine (U.S.) Committee on Accelerating Progress in Obesity Prevention, *Accelerating Progress in Obesity Prevention: Solving the Weight of the Nation* (Washington, D.C.: National Academies Press, 2012), available at www.nap.edu.

screen time: sedentary time spent using an electronic device, such as a television, computer, or video game player.

built environment: the buildings, roads, utilities, homes, fixtures, parks, and all other manufactured entities that form the physical characteristics of a community.

food deserts: urban and rural low-income areas with limited access to affordable and nutritious foods.

- The easy availability of large portions of energy-dense foods is a major environmental factor thought to be contributing to the obesity epidemic.

- Built environments that lack opportunities for safe physical activity and access to fresh, nutrient-dense foods are also linked with obesity.

7.2 Obesity Treatment: Who Should Lose?

LO 7.2 Explain why weight-loss advice does not apply equally to all overweight people.

Millions of U.S. adults are trying to lose weight at any given time. Some of these people do not even need to lose weight. Others may benefit from weight loss but are not successful. Relatively few people succeed in losing weight, and even fewer succeed permanently.

Many people assume that every overweight person can achieve slenderness and should pursue that goal. Consider, however, that most overweight people cannot become slender. People vary in their weight tendencies just as they vary in their potentials for height and degrees of health. The question of whether a person should lose weight depends on many factors: the extent of overweight, age, health, and genetics, to name a few. Weight-loss advice, then, does not apply equally to all overweight people. Some people may risk more in the process of losing weight than in remaining overweight. Others may reap significant health benefits with even modest weight loss.

IN SUMMARY

- Weight-loss advice does not apply equally to all overweight people.

- Some people may risk more through misguided efforts to lose weight than by remaining overweight, whereas others may benefit from even a modest weight loss.

7.3 Inappropriate Obesity Treatments

LO 7.3 Describe some of the dangers of over-the-counter weight-loss products.

The risks people incur in attempting to lose weight often depend on how they go about it. Weight-loss plans and obesity treatments abound—some are adequate, but many are ineffective and possibly dangerous. Fad diets are the topic of Nutrition in Practice 7. This section addresses other inappropriate obesity interventions. Aggressive treatment approaches for obese people who face high risks of medical problems and must lose weight rapidly are discussed in the next section. Reasonable approaches to overweight for those seeking safe, gradual weight losses are saved for the last part of the obesity treatment discussion.

Over-the-Counter Weight-Loss Products

Millions of people in the United States use over-the-counter (OTC) weight-loss products, believing them to be safe. Most of the people who use such products are women, especially young overweight women, but almost 10 percent are of normal weight. Promoters and marketers of weight-loss products make all kinds of claims for their products with only one intention—profit. Such claims as "eat all you want and lose weight," "take three pills before bedtime and watch the fat disappear," "blocks carbs," "blocks fat," and many more lure people into believing that maybe this time a product will really work.

In an investigation of OTC weight-loss pills, powders, and other "dietary supplements," the FDA found that an alarming number of products illegally contained prescription medications. Strong diuretics, unproven experimental drugs, psychotropic drugs used to treat mental illnesses, and even drugs deemed unsafe and so banned from U.S. markets were among those discovered, and all pose serious health risks.[39]

In their search for weight-loss magic, some consumers turn to "natural" herbal products and dietary supplements, even though few have proved to be effective.[40] People mistakenly believe that "natural" herbs are not harmful to the body, but many herbs contain toxins. Belladonna and hemlock are infamous examples, but many lesser-known herbs, such as sassafras, contain toxins as well. Furthermore, because herbs are marketed as "dietary supplements," manufacturers need not present scientific evidence of their safety or effectiveness to the FDA before marketing them. Evidence about their safety is gathered only through reports of consumers who sicken or die after using the remedies.

A now familiar example is ephedra (also called *ma huang*), an herb that showed promise as a weight-loss drug in preliminary studies. Immediately, ephedra-containing products for dieters and athletes flooded the market. Many consumers of these products reported ill effects including cardiac arrest, abnormal heartbeats, hypertension, strokes, and seizures; the supplements have been linked to some deaths as well. For this reason, the FDA has banned the sale of dietary supplements containing ephedra and its active constituent, ephedrine.*

OTC weight-loss pills, powders, herbs, and other "dietary supplements" are not associated with successful weight loss and maintenance.[41] Nutrition in Practice 15 explores the possible benefits and potential dangers of herbal products and other alternative therapies. Anyone using dietary supplements for weight loss should first consult a physician.

Other Gimmicks

Other gimmicks don't help with weight loss either. Hot baths do not speed up metabolism so that pounds can be lost in hours. Steam and sauna baths do not melt the fat off the body, although they may dehydrate people so that they lose water weight. Brushes, sponges, wraps, creams, and massages intended to move, burn, or break up fat do nothing of the kind.

IN SUMMARY

▌ Efforts to lose weight via unwise techniques, such as use of over-the-counter supplements and herbal products, can be physically and psychologically damaging.

7.4 Aggressive Treatments of Obesity

LO 7.4 Explain the risks and benefits, if any, of drugs and surgery used to treat obesity.

For some obese people, the medical problems caused by obesity demand treatment approaches that may, themselves, incur some risks. The health benefits to be gained by weight loss, however, may make these risks worth taking.

Obesity Drugs

Several prescription medications for weight loss have been tried over the years. When used as part of a long-term, comprehensive weight-loss program, medications can

---

*Ephedrine is an amphetamine-like substance extracted from the Chinese herb *ma huang*. Ma huang (ephedrine) is illegal in Canada.

TABLE 7-2 FDA-Approved Drugs for Weight Loss

Product	Action	Side Effects
Orlistat (OR-leh-stat), trade names: Alli, Xenical	Inhibits pancreatic lipase activity in the GI tract, thus blocking digestion and absorption of dietary fat and limiting energy intake	Cramping, diarrhea, gas, frequent bowel movements, reduced absorption of fat-soluble vitamins; rare cases of liver injury
Phentermine (FEN-ter-mean), diethylpropion (DYE-eth-ill-PRO-pee-on), phendimetrazine (FEN-dye-MEH-tra-zeen)	Enhances the release of the neurotransmitter norepinephrine, which suppresses appetite	Increased blood pressure and heart rate, insomnia, nervousness, dizziness, headache
Lorcaserin hydrochloride, trade name: Belviq (BELL-veek)	Interacts with brain serotonin receptors to increase satiety	Headache, dizziness, fatigue, nausea, dry mouth, and constipation; low blood glucose in people with diabetes; serotonin syndrome, including agitation, confusion, fever, loss of coordination, rapid or irregular heart rate, shivering, seizures, and unconsciousness; cannot be safely used by pregnant or lactating women or people with heart valve problems; high doses cause hallucinations
Phentermine (an appetite suppressant) and topiramate (a seizure/migraine medication) combination, trade name: Qsymia (kyoo-sim-EE-uh)	Enhances the release of the neurotransmitter norepinephrine, which suppresses appetite, and increases feelings of fullness, making foods taste less appealing	Increased heart rate; can cause birth defects if taken in the first weeks or months of pregnancy; may worsen glaucoma or hyperthyroidism; may interact with other medications

Note: Weight-loss drugs are most effective when taken as directed and used in combination with a reduced-kcalorie diet and increased physical activity.

help with modest weight loss.[42] Drugs may be an option for people who are unable to achieve adequate weight loss with diet and exercise; have a BMI ≥30 (or ≥27 with weight-related health problems); and have no medical contraindications. Because weight regain commonly occurs with the discontinuation of drug therapy, treatment is long term—and the long-term use of medications poses risks. Medical experts do not yet know whether a person would benefit more from maintaining a 50-pound excess or from taking a medication for a decade to keep the 50 pounds off.

The challenge, then, is to develop an effective drug—or more likely, a combination of drugs—that can be used over time without adverse side effects or the potential for abuse. Weight-loss drugs should be prescribed in tandem with a healthy diet and physical activity program. Table 7-2 presents the drugs to treat obesity that meet the FDA mandate that "benefits must exceed risks."[43]

Surgery

The prevalence of **clinically severe obesity** is increasing at an incredibly rapid rate.[44] At this level of obesity, lifestyle changes and modest weight losses can improve disease risks a little, but the most effective treatment is surgery.[45] Two procedures, **gastric bypass** and **gastric banding**, have gained wide acceptance. Both procedures limit food intake by effectively reducing the capacity of the stomach. In addition, gastric bypass suppresses hunger by changing production of gastrointestinal hormones.[46] The results are significant: depending on the type of surgery, nearly 50 percent of the excess weight remains lost after 15 years.[47] More long-term studies are needed, but surgery with weight loss often brings immediate and lasting improvements in blood lipids, diabetes, sleep apnea, heart disease, and hypertension.[48]

Laparoscopic weight-loss surgery techniques are now used to perform gastric bypass and other weight-loss surgeries. Laparoscopic weight-loss surgery produces significant, long-term weight loss, shortens recovery, and is less invasive than open surgery.

clinically severe obesity: a BMI of 40 or greater, or a BMI of 35 or greater with one or more serious conditions such as hypertension. Another term used to describe the same condition is *morbid obesity.*

gastric bypass: surgery that restricts stomach size and reroutes food from the stomach to the lower part of the small intestine; creates a chronic, lifelong state of malabsorption by preventing normal digestion and absorption of nutrients.

gastric banding: a surgical means of producing weight loss by restricting stomach size with a constricting band.

laparoscopic weight-loss surgery: a weight-loss surgery procedure in which surgeons gain access to the abdomen via several small incisions. A tiny video camera is inserted through one of the incisions and surgical instruments through the others. The surgeons watch their work on a large-screen monitor.

Because the long-term safety and effectiveness of gastric surgery depend, in large part, on compliance with dietary instructions, nutrition care plays an important role in follow-up treatment.[49] Common immediate postsurgical complications include infections, nausea, vomiting, and dehydration; in the long term, vitamin and mineral deficiencies and psychological problems are common. Lifelong medical supervision is necessary for those who choose the surgical route, but in suitable candidates, the health benefits of weight loss may prove worth the risks.

IN SUMMARY

▌ Obese people with high risks of medical problems may need aggressive treatment, including drugs or surgery.

7.5 Reasonable Strategies for Weight Loss

LO 7.5 Outline reasonable strategies for achieving and maintaining a healthy body weight.

Efforts to combat obesity must integrate healthy eating patterns, physical activities, supportive environments, and psychosocial support.[50] Successful weight-loss strategies embrace small changes, moderate, sustained losses, and reasonable goals. People who consistently choose nutrient-dense foods and engage in regular physical activity can reap substantial health benefits. In keeping with this philosophy, the *Dietary Guidelines for Americans* advise those who need to lose weight to "consume fewer kcalories from foods and beverages, increase physical activity, and reduce time spent in sedentary behaviors." A modest, sustained weight loss of 3 to 5 percent, even when a person is still overweight, can reduce blood glucose and improve control of diabetes as well as reduce the risk of heart disease by lowering blood triglycerides.[51] Greater weight loss reduces blood pressure, improves levels of low-density and high-density lipoproteins, and further reduces levels of blood triglycerides and blood glucose.

Of course, the same eating and activity habits that improve health often lead to a healthier body weight and composition as well. Successful weight loss, then, is defined not by pounds lost but by health gained. People less concerned with disease risks may prefer to set goals for personal fitness, such as being able to play with children or climb stairs without becoming short of breath.

Whether the goal is health or fitness, weight-loss expectations need to be reasonable. Unreachable targets ensure frustration and failure. Setting reasonable goals helps to achieve the desired result in managing weight. For example, obese people who must reduce their weight to lower their disease risks might set three broad goals:

1. Reduce body weight by about 5 to 10 percent over half a year's time.
2. Maintain a lower body weight over the long term.
3. At a minimum, prevent further weight gain.

Such goals may be achieved or even exceeded, providing a sense of accomplishment instead of disappointment.

After all, excess weight takes years to accumulate. Losing excess body fat also takes time, along with patience and perseverance. The person must adopt healthy eating patterns, engage in physical activity, create a supportive environment, and seek out behavioral and social support. These behaviors must be continued for at least 6 months for initial weight loss, and then for a lifetime to maintain the losses.[52] Setbacks are a given, and according to recent evidence, the size of the kcalorie deficit required to lose a pound of weight initially may be smaller than that required later on. In other words, weight loss is hard at first, and then it may get harder.[53]

A healthy body contains enough lean tissue to support health and the right amount of fat to meet body needs.

A Healthful Eating Plan

Contrary to the claims of many fad diets, no particular eating plan is magical, and no specific food must be either included or avoided for weight management. In designing an eating pattern, people need only consider foods that they like or can learn to like, that are available, and that are within their means.

A Realistic Energy Intake The main characteristic of a weight-loss diet is that it provides less energy than the person needs to maintain present body weight. If food energy is restricted too severely, dieters may not receive sufficient nutrients and may lose lean tissue. Rapid weight loss usually means excessive loss of lean tissue, a lower BMR, and a rapid weight regain to follow. Restrictive eating may also set in motion the unhealthy behaviors of eating disorders (described in Nutrition in Practice 6).

Obesity experts from the American Heart Association and the American College of Cardiology recommend that reductions in energy intake should be based on a person's BMI.[54] Overweight (BMI of 25 or greater) and obese (BMI of 30 or greater) people are encouraged to reduce their usual daily kcalorie intakes by about 500 to 750 kcalories. Based on the assumption that a 3,500-calorie deficit will consistently produce a pound of weight loss, these recommendations are predicted to produce a weight loss of about 1 to 1½ pounds per week while retaining lean tissue.[55] However, this assumption has been called into question.[56]

Recent research suggests that the kcalorie deficit required to lose a pound of weight may increase as weight loss progresses.[57] Weight loss may proceed rapidly for some weeks or months but will eventually slow down. The following factors contribute to a decline in the rate of loss:

- Metabolism may slow in response to a lower kcalorie intake and loss of metabolically active lean tissue.

- Less energy may be expended in physical activity as body weight diminishes.

In addition, the composition of weight loss itself may affect the rate of loss. Body weight lost early in dieting may be composed of a greater percentage of water and lean tissue, which contains fewer kcalories per pound as compared with later losses that appear to be composed mostly of fat.[58] This may mean that dieters should expect a slowdown in weight loss as they progress past the initial phase.

Most people can lose weight safely on an eating pattern providing approximately 1200 to 1500 kcalories per day for women and 1500 to 1800 kcalories per day for men.[59] Table 7-3 suggests daily food amounts from which to build balanced 1200- to 1800-kcalorie diets.

Some people skip meals, typically breakfast, in an effort to reduce energy intake and lose weight. Research does not support such a causal relationship between breakfast and body weight, but it does suggest some interesting associations.[60] Breakfast frequency is inversely associated with obesity and its risk factors—that is, people who frequently eat breakfast have lower BMI values and lower blood pressure and blood

TABLE 7-3 **Daily Amounts from Each Food Group for 1200- to 1800-kCalorie Diets**

Food Group	1200 kCalories	1400 kCalories	1600 kCalories	1800 kCalories
Fruit	1 c	1 ½ c	1 ½ c	1 ½ c
Vegetables	1 ½ c	1 ½ c	2 c	2 ½ c
Grains	4 oz	5 oz	5 oz	6 oz
Protein foods	3 oz	4 oz	5 oz	5 oz
Milk	2 ½ c	2 ½ c	3 c	3 c
Oils	4 tsp	4 tsp	5 tsp	5 tsp

© Cengage Learning®

cholesterol levels than those who tend to skip breakfast.[61] Furthermore, eating breakfast, especially a protein-rich breakfast, improves satiety and diet quality—two factors that support healthy body weight.[62]

Nutritional Adequacy Nutritional adequacy is difficult to achieve on fewer than 1200 kcalories a day, and most healthy adults need never consume any less than that. A plan that provides an adequate intake supports a healthier and more successful weight loss than a restrictive plan that creates feelings of starvation and deprivation, which can lead to an irresistible urge to binge.

Take a look at the 1200-kcalorie diet in Table 7-3. Such an intake would allow most people to lose weight and still meet their nutrient needs with careful, low-kcalorie, nutrient-dense food selections. Healthy eating patterns for weight loss should provide all of the needed nutrients in the form of fresh fruits and vegetables; low-fat milk products or substitutes; legumes; small amounts of lean protein foods; nuts; and whole grains.[63] These foods are necessary for adequate protein, carbohydrate, fiber, vitamins, and minerals and are generally associated with leanness. They are also best for managing weight.

Wholesome, high-fiber, unprocessed or lightly processed foods offer bulk and satiety for fewer kcalories than smooth, quickly consumed refined foods. Thus, choosing whole grains and fiber-rich vegetables in place of most refined grains and added sugars benefits both weight and nutrition.

Choose fats sensibly by avoiding most solid fats and including enough unsaturated oils (details in Nutrition in Practice 3) to support health but not so much as to over-supply kcalories. Nuts provide unsaturated fat and protein, and people who regularly eat nuts often maintain a healthy body weight.[64] Lean meats or other low-fat protein sources also play important roles in weight loss and provide satiety. Sufficient protein foods may also help to preserve lean tissue, including muscle tissue, during weight loss.[65]

A dietary supplement providing vitamins and minerals—especially iron and calcium for women—at or below 100 percent of the Daily Values can help people following low-kcalorie eating patterns to achieve nutrient adequacy. A person who plans resolutely to include all of the foods from each group needed each day will be satisfied, be well-nourished, and have little appetite left for high-kcalorie treats.

Small Portions As mentioned earlier, large portion sizes increase energy intakes, and the huge helpings served by restaurants and sold in packages are the enemies of people striving to manage their weight. Similarly, big bowls, plates, utensils, and drinking glasses encourage people to take and consume larger portions. Small plates and bowls, tall and thin drinking glasses, and luncheon-sized plates have the opposite effect.

For health's sake, overweight people may need to learn to eat less food at each meal—one piece of chicken for dinner instead of two, a teaspoon of butter on the vegetables instead of a tablespoon, and one cookie for dessert instead of six. Chew foods slowly and thoroughly. The goal is to eat enough food for energy, nutrients, and pleasure, but not more. This amount should leave a person feeling satisfied—not necessarily full. Keep in mind that even fat-free and low-fat foods can deliver a lot of kcalories when a person eats large quantities.

People who have difficulty making low-kcalorie selections or controlling portion sizes may find it easier to use prepared meal plans. Prepared meals that provide low-kcalorie, nutritious meals or snacks can support weight loss while easing the task of diet planning.[66] Ideally, those using a prepared meal plan will also receive counsel from a registered dietitian nutritionist to learn how to select appropriately from conventional food choices as well.

Lower Energy Density As discussed earlier, to lower energy intake, people can choose smaller portion sizes, or they can reduce the energy density of the foods they eat. Research shows that eating satisfying portions of foods that are low in energy density (such as fruits, vegetables, and broth-based soups) maintains satiety while reducing energy intake.[67] Foods containing substantial water or fiber and those low in fat

Selecting grapes with their high water content instead of raisins increases the volume and cuts the energy intake in half.

Even at the same weight and similar serving sizes, the fiber-rich broccoli delivers twice the fiber of the potatoes for about one-fourth the energy.

By selecting the water-packed tuna (on the right) instead of the oil-packed tuna, a person can enjoy the same amount for fewer kcalories.

FIGURE 7-3 Energy Density

Decreasing the energy density (kcal/g) of foods allows a person to eat satisfying portions while still reducing energy intake. To lower energy density, select foods high in water or fiber and low in fat.

help to lower a meal's energy density (see Figure 7-3). The Clinical Applications feature at the end of this chapter describes how to calculate the energy density of foods.

Sugar and Alcohol A person trying to achieve or maintain a healthy weight needs to limit intakes of added sugars and alcohol, as well as fat. Including them for pleasure on occasion is compatible with health as long as most daily choices are of nutrient-dense foods.

Meal Spacing Three meals a day is standard in our society, but no law says you can't have four or five—just be sure they are smaller, of course. People who eat small, frequent meals can be as successful at weight loss and maintenance as those who eat three. Make sure that mild hunger, not appetite, is prompting you to eat. Eat regularly, and eat before you become extremely hungry.

Adequate Water Learn to satisfy thirst with water. Water helps with weight management in several ways. For one, foods with high water content (such as broth-based soups) increase fullness, reduce hunger, and consequently reduce energy intake. For another, drinking a large glass of water before a meal may ease hunger, fill the stomach, and reduce energy intake.[68] Importantly, water adds no kcalories. The average U.S. diet delivers an estimated 75 to 150 kcalories a day from sweetened beverages. Simply replacing nutrient-poor, energy-dense beverages with water could save a person up to 15 pounds a year. Water also helps the GI tract adapt to a high-fiber diet.

Physical Activity

The best approach to weight management includes physical activity.[69] Either energy restriction or physical activity alone can produce some weight loss. Clearly, however, the combination is most effective.[70] People who combine diet and physical activity are more likely to lose more fat, retain more muscle, and regain less weight than those who only diet. The *Physical Activity Guidelines for Americans, 2008* (available at www.health.gov/PAGuidelines/) specify the minimum amount of physical activity people need to gain general *health* benefits. Table 7-4 (p. 174) presents physical activity strategies from the American College of Sports Medicine developed specifically to prevent weight gain and promote at least modest weight loss.[71]

Even without weight loss, physical activity may also help counteract some of the negative effects of excess body weight on health.[72] For example, physical activity reduces abdominal obesity, and this change improves blood pressure, insulin resistance, and fitness of the heart and lungs, even without weight loss.[73]

Energy Expenditure Physical activity directly increases energy output by the muscles and cardiovascular system. Table 6-2 in Chapter 6 (p. 145) shows how much

Being active—even if overweight—is healthier than being sedentary. Weight loss itself, however, best reduces disease risks.

TABLE 7-4 Physical Activity Strategies for Weight Management

A negative energy balance incurred through physical activity will result in weight loss, and the larger the negative energy balance, the greater the weight loss.

▮ Weight gain prevention and augmented weight loss occur with at least 2 hours and 30 minutes (150 minutes) per week of at least moderate-intensity physical activity.

▮ Greater weight loss and improved weight maintenance after weight loss occur with more than 4 hours and 10 minutes (>250 minutes) per week of at least moderate-intensity physical activity.

▮ Both aerobic (endurance) and muscle-strengthening (resistance) physical activities are beneficial, but kcalorie restriction must accompany resistance training to achieve weight loss.

Source: American College of Sports Medicine, Position stand: Appropriate physical activity intervention strategies for weight loss and prevention of weight regain for adults, *Medicine and Science in Sports and Exercise* 41 (2009): 459–471.

energy each of several activities uses. The number of kcalories spent in an activity depends on body weight, intensity, and duration. For example, a 150-pound person who walks 3.5 miles in 60 minutes expends about 315 kcalories. That same person running 3 miles in 30 minutes uses a similar amount. By comparison, a 200-pound person running 3 miles in 30 minutes expends an additional 125 kcalories or so (about 444 kcalories total). The goal is to expend as much energy as time allows. The greater the energy deficit created by physical activity, the greater the fat loss. A word of caution, however: people who reward themselves with high-kcalorie foods for "good behavior" can easily negate any kcalorie deficits incurred with physical activity.

Basal Metabolic Rate (BMR) The BMR is elevated in the hours after vigorous physical activity, but this effect requires a sustained high-intensity workout beyond the level achievable by most weight-loss seekers.[74] Over the long term, however, a person who engages in daily vigorous activity gradually develops more lean tissue, which is more active metabolically than fat tissue. Metabolic rate rises accordingly, and this makes a contribution toward continued weight loss or maintenance.

Appetite Control Physical activity also helps to control appetite. Some people think that being active will make them want to eat, but research does not show that exercise causes overeating; in fact, when sedentary people participate in an ongoing activity program, they reduce their energy intakes.[75] Active people do have healthy appetites, but appetite is suppressed immediately after an aerobic workout and satiation during meals is heightened.[76] The reasons are unclear, but physical activity may help to control appetite by altering the levels of appetite-regulating hormones.[77]

Psychological Benefits Physical activity helps especially to curb the inappropriate appetite that prompts a person to eat when bored, anxious, or depressed. Weight-management programs encourage people to go out and be active when they're tempted to eat but are not really hungry.

Physical activity also helps to reduce stress. Because stress itself is a trigger for inappropriate eating behavior for many people, activity can help here, too. In addition, physical activity helps to improve body image and separate the connections between body weight and self-worth.[78] A physically active person begins to look and feel healthy, and, as a result, gains self-esteem. High self-esteem tends to support a person's resolve to persist in a weight-control effort, rounding out a beneficial cycle. Table 7-5 and Chapter 10 present the benefits of physical activity.

Choosing Activities What kind of physical activity is best? For health, a combination of moderate to vigorous aerobic physical activity along with **resistance training** at a safe level provides benefits.[79] However, any physical activity is better than being sedentary.

People seeking to lose weight should choose activities that they enjoy and are willing to do regularly. Health care professionals frequently advise people who want to manage their body weight and lose fat to engage in activities of low-to-moderate

TABLE 7-5 Benefits of Physical Activity in a Weight-Management Program

▮ Improved body composition

▮ Favorable effects on disease risks

▮ Short-term increase in energy expenditure (from exercise and from a slight rise in BMR)

▮ Long-term increase (slight) in BMR (from an increase in lean tissue)

▮ Appetite control

▮ Stress reduction and control of stress eating

▮ Physical, and therefore psychological, well-being

▮ Improved self-esteem

© 2016 Cengage Learning®

resistance training: the use of free weights or weight machines to provide resistance for developing muscle strength, power, and endurance; also called *weight training*. A person's own body weight may also be used to provide resistance as when a person does push-ups, pull-ups, or abdominal crunches.

intensity for a long duration, such as an hour-long fast-paced walk. The reasoning behind such advice is that people exercising at low to moderate intensity are likely to stick with their activity for longer times and are less likely to injure themselves. People who regularly engage in more *vigorous* physical activities (fast bicycling or endurance running, for example), however, have less body fat than those who engage in moderately intense activities. The conditioned body that is adapted to strenuous and prolonged aerobic activity uses more fat all day long, not just during activity. The bottom line on physical activity and weight and/or fat loss seems to be that total energy expenditure is the main factor, regardless of how a person does it.

In addition to activities such as walking or cycling, there are hundreds of ways to incorporate energy-expending activities into daily routines: take the stairs instead of the elevator, walk to the neighbor's apartment instead of making a phone call, and rake the leaves instead of using a blower. These activities burn only a few kcalories each, but over a year's time they become significant.

Spot Reducing People sometimes ask about "spot reducing." Unfortunately, no one part of the body gives up fat in preference to another. Fat cells all over the body release fat in response to demand, and the fat is then used by whatever muscles are active. No exercise can remove the fat from any one particular area—and, incidentally, neither can a massage machine that claims to break up fat on trouble spots.

Physical activity can help with trouble spots in another way, though. Strengthening muscles in a trouble area can help to improve their tone; stretching to gain flexibility can help with posture problems. Thus, cardiorespiratory endurance, strength, and flexibility workouts all have a place in fitness programs.

Behavior and Attitude

Behavior-modification therapy provides ways to overcome barriers to making dietary changes and increasing physical activity. Behavior-modification therapy does more than help people decide which behaviors to change: it also teaches them how to change. Behavior and attitude are important supporting factors in achieving and maintaining appropriate body weight and composition. Changing the behaviors of overeating and underexercising that lead to, and perpetuate, obesity requires time and effort. A person must commit to take action.

Becoming Aware of Behaviors A person who is aware of all the behaviors that create a problem has a head start on developing a solution. First, the person needs to establish a baseline (a record of present eating and physical activity behaviors) against which to measure future progress.[80] It is best to keep a diary (see Figure 7-4 on p. 176) that includes the time and place of meals and snacks, the type and amount of foods eaten, the persons present when food is eaten, and a description of the individual's feelings when eating. The diary should also record physical activities: the kind, the intensity level, the duration, and the person's feelings about them. These entries will help the individual identify possible behaviors to change.

Many companies have developed weight-loss applications for smartphones and other mobile devices to help users manage their daily food and physical activity behaviors.* Applications include diet analysis tools that can track eating habits, scanning devices that can quickly enter food data, customized activity and meal plans that can be sent to users, and support programs that deliver encouraging messages and helpful tips. Social media sites allow users to upload progress reports and receive texts. Using these applications can help a person become more aware of behaviors that lead to weight gains and losses.

Making Small Changes Behavior modification strategies focus on learning desired eating and exercise behaviors and eliminating unwanted behaviors. With so many

behavior modification: the changing of behavior by the manipulation of *antecedents* (cues or environmental factors that trigger behavior), the behavior itself, and *consequences* (the penalties or rewards attached to behavior).

*Reliable reviews of food and nutrition apps are available at *www.eatright.org/appreviews*.

FIGURE 7-4 **Food and Activity Diary**

Time	Place	Activity or food eaten	People present	Mood
10:30– 10:40	School vending machine	6 peanut butter crackers and 12 oz. cola	by myself	Starved
12:15– 12:30	Restaurant	Sub sandwich and 12 oz. cola	friends	relaxed & friendly
3:00– 3:45	Gym	Weight training	workout partner	tired
4:00– 4:10	Snack bar	Small frozen yogurt	by myself	OK

© Cengage Learning®

possible behavior changes, a person can feel overwhelmed. Start with small time-specific goals for each behavior—for example, "I'm going to take a 30-minute walk after dinner every evening" instead of "I'm going to run a marathon someday." Practice desired behaviors until they become routine. Using a reward system seems to effectively support weight-loss efforts. Box 7-1 describes behavioral strategies to support weight

How To BOX 7-1 APPLY BEHAVIOR MODIFICATION TO MANAGE BODY FATNESS

1. Eliminate inappropriate cues:
   ▌ Do not buy problem foods.
   ▌ Eat only in one room at the designated time.
   ▌ Shop when not hungry.
   ▌ Replace large plates, cups, and utensils with smaller ones.
   ▌ Avoid vending machines, fast-food restaurants, and convenience stores.
   ▌ Turn off television, video games, and computers or measure out appropriate food portions to eat during entertainment.

2. Suppress the cues you cannot eliminate:
   ▌ Serve individual plates; do not serve "family style."
   ▌ Remove food from the table after eating a meal to enjoy company and ambience without excess food to trigger overeating.
   ▌ Create obstacles to consuming problem foods—wrap them and freeze them, making them less quickly accessible.
   ▌ Control deprivation; plan and eat regular meals.
   ▌ Plan the time spent in sedentary activities, such as watching television or using a computer—do not use these activities just to fill time.

3. Strengthen cues to appropriate behaviors:
   ▌ Choose to dine with companions who make appropriate food choices.
   ▌ Store appropriate foods in convenient spots in the refrigerator.
   ▌ Learn appropriate portion sizes.
   ▌ Plan appropriate snacks.
   ▌ Keep sports and play equipment by the door.

4. Repeat desired behaviors:
   ▌ Slow down eating—put down utensils between bites.
   ▌ Always use utensils.
   ▌ Leave some food on your plate.
   ▌ Move more—shake a leg, pace, stretch often.
   ▌ Join groups of active people and participate.

5. Arrange negative consequences for negative behavior:
   ▌ Ask that others respond neutrally to your deviations (make no comments—even negative attention is a reward).
   ▌ If you slip, do not punish yourself.

6. Reward yourself personally and immediately for positive behaviors:
   ▌ Buy tickets to sports events, movies, concerts, or other nonfood amusement.
   ▌ Indulge in a new small purchase.
   ▌ Get a massage; buy some flowers.
   ▌ Take a hot bath; read a good book.
   ▌ Treat yourself to a lesson in a new active pursuit such as horseback riding, handball, or tennis.
   ▌ Praise yourself; visit friends.
   ▌ Nap; relax.

management. A particularly attractive feature of these strategies is that they do not involve blaming oneself or putting oneself down—an important element in fostering self-esteem.

Cognitive Skills Behavior therapists often teach **cognitive skills,** or new ways of thinking, to help overweight people solve problems and correct false thinking that can undermine healthy eating behaviors. Thinking habits are as important for achieving a healthy body weight as eating and activity habits, and they can be changed.[81] A paradox of making a change is that it takes belief in oneself and honoring of oneself to lay the foundation for changing that self. That is, self-acceptance predicts success, while self-loathing predicts failure. "Positive self-talk" is a concept worth cultivating—many people succeed because their mental dialogue supports, rather than degrades, their efforts. Negative thoughts ("I'm not getting thin anyway, so what is the use of continuing?") should be viewed in light of empirical evidence ("my starting weight: 174 pounds; today's weight: 163 pounds").

Take credit for new behaviors; be aware of any physical improvements, too, such as lower blood pressure, or less painful knees, even without a noticeable change in pant size. Finally, remember to enjoy your emerging fit and healthy self.

Personal Attitude For many people, overeating and being overweight may have become an integral part of their identity. Changing diet and activity behaviors without attention to a person's self-concept invites failure.

Many people overeat to cope with the stresses of life. To break out of that pattern, they must first identify the particular stressors that trigger their urges to overeat. Then, when faced with these situations, they must learn to practice problem-solving skills. When the problems that trigger the urge to overeat are dealt with in alternative ways, people may find that they eat less. The message is that sound emotional health supports the ability to take care of health in all ways—including nutrition, weight management, and fitness.

Weight Maintenance

Finally, be aware that it can be hard to maintain weight loss. Millions of people have experienced the frustration of achieving a desired change in weight only to see their hard work visibly slip away in a seemingly never-ending cycle of weight loss and weight regain. Disappointment, frustration, and self-condemnation are common in people who have slipped back to their original weight or even higher.

A key to weight maintenance is accepting it as a lifelong endeavor and not a goal to be achieved and then forgotten. People who maintain their weight loss continue to employ the behaviors that reduced their weight in the first place (see Table 7-6). They cultivate habits of people who maintain a healthy weight, such as eating low-kcalorie

TABLE 7-6 Behaviors to Maintain Weight Loss

Those who maintain weight losses over time:

- Believe they have the ability to control their weight, an attribute known as **self-efficacy.**
- Eat breakfast every day.
- Average about one hour of physical activity per day.
- Monitor body weight about once a week.
- Maintain consistent lower-kcalorie eating patterns.
- Quickly address small **lapses** to prevent small gains from turning into major ones.
- Watch less than 10 hours of television per week.
- Eat high-fiber food, particularly whole grains, vegetables, and fruit, and consume sufficient water each day.
- Cultivate and honor realistic expectations regarding body size and shape.

© 2016 Cengage Learning®

cognitive skills: as taught in behavior therapy, changes to conscious thoughts with the goal of improving adherence to lifestyle modifications; examples are problem-solving skills or the correction of false negative thoughts, termed *cognitive restructuring*.

self-efficacy: a person's belief in his or her ability to succeed in an undertaking.

lapses: periods of returning to old habits.

TABLE 7-7 Weight-Loss Strategies

Food

- To maintain weight, consume foods and drinks to meet, not exceed, kcalorie needs. To lose weight, energy out should exceed energy in by about 500 kcalories/day.
- Emphasize foods with a low energy density and a high nutrient density; make legumes, whole grains, vegetables, and fruits central to your eating pattern.
- Eat slowly.
- Drink water before you eat and while you eat; drink plenty of water throughout the day.
- Track food and kcalorie intake.
- Plan ahead to make better food choices.
- Limit kcalorie intake from solid fats and added sugars.
- Reduce portions, especially of high-kcalorie foods.
- Cook and eat more meals at home, instead of eating out. When eating out, think about choosing healthy options.

Activities

- Limit screen time.
- Increase physical activity.
- Choose moderate- or vigorous-intensity physical activities.
- Avoid inactivity. Some physical activity is better than none.
- Slowly build up the amount of physical activity you choose.

meals (averaging 1800 kcalories per day) and being physically active. They must also control susceptibility to overeating regardless of the initial weight-loss method.

IN SUMMARY

- A person who adopts a lifelong "eating plan for good health" rather than a "diet for weight loss" will be more likely to keep the lost weight off. Table 7-7 offers strategies for successful weight management.

- Reducing daily energy intake, choosing foods of low energy density, and eating smaller portions are important dietary strategies for weight management.

- Physical activity should be an integral part of a weight-management program.

- Physical activity can increase energy expenditure, improve body composition, help control appetite, reduce stress and stress eating, and enhance physical and psychological well-being.

- Behavior modification provides ways to overcome barriers to successful weight management.

7.6 Strategies for Weight Gain

LO 7.6 Summarize strategies for gaining weight.

Underweight is far less prevalent than overweight, affecting about 2 percent of U.S. adults.[82] Whether the underweight person needs to gain weight is a question of health and, like weight loss, a highly individual matter. People who are healthy at their present weight may stay there; there are no compelling reasons to try to gain weight. Those who are thin because of malnourishment or illness, however, might benefit from a diet that supports weight gain. Medical advice can help make the distinction. Eating disorders are the subject of Nutrition in Practice 6.

Some people are unalterably thin by reasons of genetics or early physical influences. Those who wish to gain weight for appearance's sake or to improve athletic performance should be aware that a healthful weight can be achieved only through physical activity, particularly strength training, combined with a high energy intake. Eating many high-kcalorie foods can bring about weight gain, but it will be mostly fat, and this can be as detrimental to health as being slightly underweight. In an athlete, such a weight gain can impair performance. Therefore, in weight gain, as in weight loss, physical activity and energy intake are essential components of a sound plan.

Physical Activity to Build Muscles The person who wants to gain weight should use resistance training primarily. As activity is increased, energy intake must be increased to support that activity. Eating extra food will then support a gain of both muscle and fat.

Energy-Dense Foods Energy-dense foods (the very ones eliminated from a successful weight-loss diet) hold the key to weight gain. Pick the highest-kcalorie items from each food group—that is, milk shakes instead of fat-free milk, peanut butter instead of lean meat, avocados instead of cucumbers, and whole-wheat muffins instead of whole-wheat bread. Because fat contains more than twice as many kcalories per teaspoon as sugar does, fat adds kcalories without adding much bulk.

Be aware that health experts recommend a moderate-fat diet for the general U.S. population because the general population is overweight and at risk for heart disease. Consumption of excessive fat is not healthy for most people, of course, but may be essential for an underweight individual who needs to gain weight. An underweight person who is physically active and eating a nutritionally adequate diet can afford a few extra kcalories from fat. For health's sake, it is wise to select foods with monounsaturated and polyunsaturated fats instead of those with saturated or *trans* fats: for example, sautéing vegetables in olive oil instead of butter or hydrogenated margarine.

Three Meals Daily People wanting to gain weight should eat at least three healthy meals a day. Many people who are underweight have simply been too busy (sometimes for months) to eat enough to gain or maintain weight. Therefore, they need to make meals a priority and plan them in advance. Taking time to prepare and eat each meal can help, as can learning to eat more food within the first 20 minutes of a meal before you begin to feel full. Another suggestion is to eat meaty appetizers or the main course first and leave the soup or salad until later.

Large Portions It is also important for the underweight person to learn to eat more food at each meal: have two sandwiches for lunch instead of one, drink milk from a larger glass, and eat cereal from a larger bowl. Expect to feel full. Most underweight individuals are accustomed to small quantities of food. When they begin eating significantly more, they feel uncomfortable. This is normal and passes over time.

Extra Snacks Because a substantially higher energy intake is needed each day, in addition to eating more food at each meal, it is necessary to eat more frequently. Between-meal snacking offers a solution. For example, a student might make three sandwiches in the morning and eat them between classes in addition to the day's three regular meals.

Juice and Milk Beverages provide an easy way to increase energy intake. Consider that 6 cups of cranberry juice add almost 1000 kcalories to the day's intake. kCalories can be added to milk by mixing in powdered milk or packets of instant breakfast.

For people who are underweight due to illness, concentrated liquid formulas are often recommended because a weak person can swallow them easily. A registered dietitian nutritionist can recommend high-protein, high-kcalorie formulas to help the underweight person maintain or gain weight. Used in addition to regular meals, these formulas can help considerably.

TABLE 7-8 Weight-Gain Strategies

In General:

- Eat enough to store more energy than you expend—at least 500 extra kcalories a day.
- Exercise to build muscle.
- Be patient. Weight gain takes time (1 pound per month would be reasonable).
- Choose energy-dense foods most often.
- Eat at least three meals a day, and add snacks between meals.
- Choose large portions and expect to feel full.
- Drink kcaloric fluids—juice, chocolate milk, sweet coffee drinks, sweet iced tea.

In Addition:

- Cook and bake often—delicious cooking aromas whet the appetite.
- Invite others to the table—companionship often boosts eating.
- Make meals interesting—try new vegetables and fruit, add crunchy nuts or creamy avocado, and explore the flavors of herbs and spices.
- Keep a supply of favorite snacks, such as trail mix or granola bars, handy for grabbing.
- Control stress and relax. Enjoy your food.

IN SUMMARY

- Both the incidence of underweight and the health problems associated with it are less prevalent than overweight and its associated problems.

- To gain weight, a person must train physically and increase energy intake by selecting energy-dense foods, eating regular meals, taking larger portions, and consuming extra snacks and beverages. Table 7-8 offers a summary of weight-gain strategies.

Your Diet

To enjoy good health and maintain a reasonable body weight, you need to combine sensible eating habits and regular physical activity. This exercise allows you to evaluate your current body weight and consider some lifestyle factors important for weight management.

First, check to see whether your current body weight falls within the "healthy weight" range, which usually equates to a BMI range of 18.5 to 24.9. In the BMI table at the back of this text, find your height in the left-hand column of the table and look across the row to find your weight. Alternatively, you can calculate your BMI using the equation shown on p. 148. What is your BMI? Does it fall within the healthy range?

If your BMI falls within the underweight, overweight, or obese range, you may want to gain or lose weight to improve your health. Even if your BMI is within the healthy range, you may wish to improve your eating habits or fitness level. Review Figure 7-4 (p. 176) and complete your own food and activity record (listing time, place, activity or food eaten, people present, and mood) for at least a 24-hour period.

- Make a list of the habits that support maintaining or achieving a healthy weight. For example, do you drink water rather than soda throughout the day and limit the time you spend watching television or playing computer games?

- Make a list of the habits that do not support maintaining or achieving a healthy weight. For example, do you eat when you aren't hungry or regularly choose fast food or vending machine food?

- What changes would you like to make in your daily habits to improve your health and nutrition?

Clinical Applications

1. Chapter 1 discussed the nutrient density of foods—their nutrient contribution per kcalorie. Another way to evaluate foods is to consider their energy density—their energy contribution per gram:

   ▪ A carrot weighing 72 grams delivers 31 kcalories.

   ▪ To calculate the energy density, divide kcalories by grams: 31 kcalories divided by 72 grams = 0.43 kcalories per gram.

2. Do the same for french fries weighing 50 grams and contributing 167 kcalories: 167 kcalories divided by 50 grams = _____ kcalories per gram.

   ▪ The more kcalories per gram, the greater the energy density.

   ▪ Which food is more energy dense? The conclusion is no surprise, but understanding the mathematics may offer valuable insight into the concept of energy density.

   ▪ French fries are more energy dense, providing 3.34 kcalories per gram. They provide more energy per gram—and per bite.

Matthew Farruggio Photography

3. Considering a food's energy density is especially useful in planning diets for weight management. Foods with a high energy density can help with weight gain, whereas those with a low energy density can help with weight loss. Give some examples of foods that you might suggest for a client who wants to gain weight and some that might be appropriate for a client who is trying to lose weight.

Self Check

1. Two causes of obesity in humans are:
   a. set-point theory and BMI.
   b. genetics and physical inactivity.
   c. genetics and low-carbohydrate diets.
   d. mineral imbalances and fat cell imbalance.

2. The protein produced by the fat cells under the direction of the *ob* gene is called:
   a. leptin.
   b. orlistat.
   c. sibutramine.
   d. lipoprotein lipase.

3. All of the following describe the behavior of fat cells *except:*
   a. the number decreases when fat is lost from the body.
   b. the storage capacity for fat depends on both cell number and cell size.
   c. the size is larger in obese people than in normal-weight people.
   d. the number increases most rapidly during the growth years and tapers off when adult status is reached.

4. The obesity theory that suggests the body chooses to be at a specific weight is the:
   a. fat cell theory.
   b. enzyme theory.
   c. set-point theory.
   d. external cue theory.

5. The biggest problem associated with the use of prescription drugs in the treatment of obesity is:
   a. cost.
   b. the necessity for long-term use.
   c. ineffectiveness.
   d. adverse side effects.

6. A nutritionally sound weight-loss diet might restrict daily energy intake to create a:
   a. 1000-kcalorie-per-month deficit.
   b. 500-kcalorie-per-month deficit.
   c. 500-kcalorie-per-day deficit.
   d. 3500-kcalorie-per-day deficit.

7. What is the best approach to weight loss?
   a. Avoid foods containing carbohydrates.
   b. Eliminate all fats from the diet and decrease water intake.
   c. Greatly increase protein intake to prevent body protein loss.
   d. Reduce daily energy intake and increase energy expenditure.

8. Physical activity does *not* help a person to:
   a. lose weight.
   b. lose fat in trouble spots.
   c. retain muscle.
   d. maintain weight loss.

9. Which of these behaviors will best support successful weight management?
   a. Shop only when hungry.
   b. Eat in front of the television for distraction.
   c. Learn appropriate portion sizes.
   d. Eat quickly.

10. Which strategy would *not* help an underweight person to gain weight?
   a. Exercise.
   b. Drink plenty of water.
   c. Eat snacks between meals.
   d. Eat large portions of foods.

Answers to these questions can be found in Appendix H.

Notes

1. J. R. Speakman, Evolutionary perspectives on the obesity epidemic: Adaptive, maladaptive, and neutral viewpoints, *Annual Review of Nutrition* 33 (2013): 289–317; L. Dubois and coauthors, Genetic and environmental contributions to weight, height, and BMI from birth to 19 years of age: An international study of over 12,000 twin pairs, *PLoS One* 7 (2012): e30153; B. Levin, Developmental gene x environment interactions affecting systems regulating energy homeostasis and obesity, *Frontiers in Neuroendocrinology* 31 (2010): 270–283.

2. J. Cecil and coauthors, Obesity and eating behavior in children and adolescents: Contribution of common gene polymorphisms, *International Review of Psychiatry* 24 (2012): 200–210; C. E. Elks and coauthors, Adult obesity susceptibility variants are associated with greater childhood weight gain and a faster tempo of growth: The 1946 British Birth Cohort Study, *American Journal of Clinical Nutrition* 95 (2012): 1150–1156; K. E. North and coauthors, Genetic epidemiology of BMI and body mass change from adolescence to young adulthood, *Obesity (Silver Spring)* 18 (2010): 1474–1476.

3. K. Silventhoinen and coauthors, The genetic and environment influences on childhood obesity: A systematic review of twin and adoption studies, *International Journal of Obesity* 34 (2010): 29–40.

4. J. Naukkarinen and coauthors, Causes and consequences of obesity: The contribution of recent twin studies, *International Journal of Obesity* 36 (2012): 1017–1024.

5. Naukkarinen and coauthors, 2012; M. M. Hetherington and J. E. Cecil, Gene-environment interactions in obesity, *Forum of Nutrition* 63 (2010): 195–203.

6. C. Bouchard, Defining the genetic architecture of the predisposition to obesity: A challenging but not insurmountable task, *American Journal of Clinical Nutrition* 91 (2010): 5–6.

7. Li Shengxu and coauthors, Cumulative effects and predictive value of common obesity-susceptibility variants identified by genome-wide association studies, *American Journal of Clinical Nutrition* 91 (2010): 184–190.

8. Hetherington and Cecil, 2010.

9. J. Mattei and coauthors, *TCF7L2* genetic variants modulate the effect of dietary fat intake on changes in body composition during a weight-loss intervention, *American Journal of Clinical Nutrition* 96 (2012): 1129–1136; Q. Qibin and coauthors, Sugar-sweetened beverages and genetic risk of obesity, *New England Journal of Medicine* 367 (2012): 1387–1396.

10. P. T. Williams, Attenuated inheritance of body weight by running in monozygotic twins, *Medicine and Science in Sports and Exercise* 44 (2012): 98–103.

11. H. Wong and R. H. Eckel, Lipoprotein lipase in the brain and nervous system, *Annual Review of Nutrition* 32 (2012): 147–160.

12. H. Pan, J. Guo, and Z. Su, Advances in understanding the interrelations between leptin resistance and obesity, *Physiology and Behavior* April 9, 2014, epub ahead of print.

13. Pan, Guo, and Su, 2014.

14. C. Delporte, Recent advances in potential clinical application of ghrelin in obesity, *Journal of Obesity* 2012, doi: 10.1155/2012/535624; J. Tong and coauthors, Ghrelin enhances olfactory sensitivity and exploratory sniffing in rodents and humans, *Journal of Neuroscience* 31 (2011): 5841–5846; T. R. Castañeda and coauthors, Ghrelin in the regulation of body weight and metabolism, *Frontiers in Neuroendocrinology* 31 (2010): 44–60.

15. Delporte, 2012; Castañeda and coauthors, 2010.

16. E. Egecioglu and coauthors, Hedonic and incentive signals for body weight control, *Reviews in Endocrine and Metabolic Disorders,* 12 (2011): 141–151; Castañeda and coauthors, 2010.

17. Y. D. Tchoukalova and coauthors, Regional differences in cellular mechanisms of adipose tissue gain with overfeeding, *Proceedings of the National Academy of Sciences of the United States of America,* 107 (2010): 18226–18231.

18. M. A. Cornier and coauthors, AHA scientific statement: Assessing adiposity, *Circulation* 124 (2011): 1996–2019; M. Krawczyk, L. Bonfrate, and P. Portincasa, Nonalcoholic fatty liver disease, *Best Practice and Research, Clinical Gastroenterology* 24 (2010): 695–708; D. M. Muoio, Metabolism and vascular fatty acid transport, *New England Journal of Medicine* 363 (2010): 291–293; G. Tarantino, S. Savastano, and A. Colao, Hepatic steatosis, low-grade chronic inflammation and hormone/growth factor/ adipokine imbalance, *World Journal of Gastroenterology* 16 (2010): 4773–4783.

19. P. Trayhurn, C. A. Drevon, and J. Eckel, Secreted proteins from adipose tissue and skeletal muscle: Adipokines, myokines and adipose/muscle cross-talk, *Archives of Physiology and Biochemistry* 117 (2011): 47–56; N. Ouchi and coauthors, Adipokines in inflammation and metabolic disease, *Nature Reviews Immunology* 11 (2011): 85–97; C. Stryjecki and D. M. Mutch, Fatty acid-gene

interactions, adipokines, and obesity, *European Journal of Clinical Nutrition* 65 (2011): 285–297.

20. J. R. Speakman and coauthors, Set points, settling points and some alternative models: Theoretical options to understand how genes and environment combine to regulate body adiposity, *Disease Models and Mechanisms* 4 (2011): 733–745; M. M. Farias, A. M. Cuevas, and F. Rodriguez, Set-point theory and obesity, *Metabolic Syndrome and Related Disorders* 9 (2011): 85–89.

21. S. Camps, S. Verhoef, and K. R. Westerterp, Weight loss, weight maintenance, and adaptive thermogenesis, *American Journal of Clinical Nutrition* 97 (2013): 990–994.

22. Speakman and coauthors, 2011.

23. Hetherington and Cecil, 2010; D. Heber, An integrative view of obesity, *American Journal of Clinical* 91 (2010): 280S–283S.

24. B. M. Popkin and K. J. Duffey, Does hunger and satiety drive eating anymore? Increasing eating occasions and decreasing time between eating occasions in the United States, *American Journal of Clinical Nutrition* 91 (2010): 1342–1347.

25. K. J. Duffey and B. M. Popkin, Energy density, portion size, and eating occasions: Contributions to increased energy intake in the United States, 1977–2006, *PLoS Medicine* 8 (2011): e1001050.

26. B. J. Rolls, Plenary Lecture 1: Dietary strategies for the prevention and treatment of obesity, *Proceedings of the Nutrition Society* 69 (2010): 70–79.

27. Position of the American Dietetic Association, Weight management, *Journal of the American Dietetic Association* 109 (2009): 330–346.

28. I. N. Bezerra, C. Curioni, and R. Sichieri, Association between eating out of home and body weight, *Nutrition Reviews* 70 (2012): 65–79.

29. L. Marr, National restaurant menu labeling, legislation: Public nutrition education and professional opportunities, *Journal of the American Dietetic Association* 111 (2011): S7; K. Stein, A national approach to restaurant menu labeling: The Patient Protection and Affordable Health Care Act, section 4205, *Journal of the American Dietetic Association* 110 (2010): 1280–1286.

30. J. S. Schiller and coauthors, Summary health statistics for U.S. adults: National Health Interview Survey, *Vital and Health Statistics* 10 (2012): 1–217.

31. J. F. Sallis and coauthors, Role of built environments in physical activity, obesity, and cardiovascular disease, *Circulation* 125 (2012): 729–737.

32. H. Du and coauthors, Physical activity and sedentary leisure time and their associations with BMI, waist circumference, and percentage body fat in 0.5 million adults: The China Kadoorie Biobank Study, *American Journal of Clinical Nutrition* 97 (2013): 487–496; B. G. Nordestgaard and coauthors, The effect of elevated body mass index on ischemic heart disease risk: Causal estimates form a Mendelian randomization approach, *PLOS Medicine,* May 1, 2012, doi: 10.1371/journal.pmed.1001212; J. Sattelmair and coauthors, Dose response between physical activity and risk of coronary heart disease: A meta-analysis, *Circulation* 124 (2011): 789–795.

33. L. M. Leon-Munoz and coauthors, Continued sedentariness, change in sitting and mortality in older adults, *Medicine and Science in Sports and Exercise* 45 (2013): 1501–1507; H. P. van der Ploeg and coauthors, Sitting time and all-cause mortality risk in 222,497 Australian adults, *Archives of Internal Medicine* 172 (2012): 494–500.

34. Sallis and coauthors, 2012; D. Ding and coauthors, Neighborhood environment and physical activity among youth: A review, *American Journal of Preventive Medicine* 41 (2011): 442–455.

35. C. Larson and coauthors, Development of a community-sensitive strategy to increase availability of fresh fruits and vegetables in Nashville's urban food deserts, 2010–2012, *Preventing Chronic Disease* 10 (2013): e125.

36. J. L. Blitstein, J. Snider, and W. D. Evans, Perceptions of the food shopping environment are associated with greater consumption of fruits and vegetables, *Public Health Nutrition* 21 (2012): 1–6.

37. Bezerra, Curioni, and Sichieri, 2012; A. M. Fretts and coauthors, Associations of processed meat and unprocessed red meat intake with incident diabetes: The Strong Heart Family Study, *American Journal of Clinical Nutrition* 95 (2012): 752–758; H. J. Song and coauthors, Understanding a key feature of urban food stores to develop nutrition intervention, *Journal of Hunger & Environmental Nutrition* 7 (2012): 77–90.

38. Institute of Medicine (U.S.) Committee on Accelerating Progress in Obesity Prevention, *Accelerating Progress in Obesity Prevention: Solving the Weight of the Nation* (Washington, D.C.: National Academies Press, 2012), available at www.nap.edu.

39. A. Bendich, Prescription and over-the-counter options for weight loss, *Nutrition Today* 48 (2013): 76–78; U.S. Food and Drug Administration, Questions and answers about FDA's initiative against contaminated weight loss products, http://www.fda.gov/Drugs/ResourcesForYou/Consumers/QuestionsAnswers/ucm136187.htm, updated September 3, 2013.

40. K. Poddar and coauthors, Nutraceutical supplements for weight loss: A systematic review, *Nutrition in Clinical Practice* 26 (2011): 539–552.

41. J. M. Nicklas and coauthors, Successful weight loss among obese U.S. adults, *American Journal of Preventive Medicine* 42 (2012): 481–485; D. Laddu and coauthors, A review of evidence-based strategies to treat obesity in adults, *Nutrition in Clinical Practice* 26 (2011): 512–525.

42. Laddu and coauthors, 2011.

43. E. H. Morrato and D. B. Allison, FDA approval of obesity drugs: A difference in risk-benefit perceptions, *Journal of the American Medical Association* 308 (2012): 1097–1098; E. Colman and coauthors, The FDA's assessment of two drugs for chronic weight management, *New England Journal of Medicine* 367 (2012): 1577–1579.

44. E. A. Finkelstein and coauthors, Obesity and severe obesity forecasts through 2030, *American Journal of Preventive Medicine* 42 (2012): 563–570.

45. R. Padwal and coauthors, Bariatric surgery: A systematic review of the clinical and economic evidence, *Journal of Internal Medicine* 26 (2011): 1183–1194; A. Nagle, Bariatric surgery—A surgeon's perspective, *Journal of the American Dietetic Association* 110 (2010): 520–523; G. L. Blackburn, S. Wollner, and S. B. Heymsfield, Lifestyle interventions for the treatment of class III obesity: A primary target for nutrition medicine in the obesity epidemic, *American Journal of Clinical Nutrition* 91 (2010): 289S–292S.

46. B. Laferrère, Diabetes remission after bariatric surgery: Is it just the incretins? *International Journal of Obesity* 35 (2011): S22–S25.

47. P. E. O'Brien and coauthors, Long-term outcomes after bariatric surgery: Fifteen-year follow-up of adjustable gastric banding and a systematic review of the bariatric surgical literature, *Annals of Surgery* 257 (2013): 87–94.

48. T. D. Adams, Health benefits of gastric bypass surgery after 6 years, *Journal of the American Medical Association* 308 (2012): 1122–1131; G. Mingrone and coauthors, Bariatric surgery versus conventional medical therapy for type 2 diabetes, *New England Journal of Medicine* 366 (2012): 1577–1585; M. Attiah and coauthors, Durability of Roux-en-Y gastric bypass surgery: A meta-regression study, *Annals of Surgery* 256 (2012): 251–254; L. Sjöström and coauthors, Bariatric surgery and long-term cardiovascular events, *Journal of the American Medical Association* 307 (2012): 56–65; P. R. Schauer and coauthors, Bariatric surgery versus intensive medical therapy in obese patients with diabetes, *New England Journal of Medicine* 366 (2012): 1567–1576; D. Sandoval, Bariatric surgeries: Beyond restriction and malabsorption, *International Journal of Obesity* 35 (2011): S45–S49.

49. L. Beckman and C. Earthman, Nutritional implications of bariatric surgery and the role of registered dietitians, *Journal of the Academy of Nutrition and Dietetics* 113 (2013): 398–399.

50. Laddu and coauthors, 2011; Heber, 2010.

51. M. D. Jensen and coauthors, 2013 AHA/ACC/TOS guideline for the management of overweight and obesity in adults: A report of the American College of Caridology/American Heart Association Task Force on Practice Guidelines and The Obesity Society, *Circulation* http://circ.ahajournals.org/content/early/2013/11/11/01.cir0000437739.71477.ee.citation.

52. S.F. Kirk and coauthors, Effective weight management practice; A review of the lifestyle intervention evidence, *International Journal of Obesity* 36 (2012): 178–185.

53. S. B. Heymsfield and coauthors, Energy content of weight loss: Kinetic features during voluntary caloric restriction, *Metabolism* 61 (2012): 937–943.

54. Jensen and coauthors, 2013.

55. Position of the American Dietetic Association, 2009.

56. K. D. Hall and coauthors, Energy balance and its components: Implications for body weight regulation, *American Journal of Clinical Nutrition* 95 (2012): 989–995.

57. Heymsfield and coauthors, 2012.

58. Heymsfield and coauthors, 2012.

59. Jensen and coauthors, 2013.

60. A. W. Brown, M. M. B. Brown, and D. B. Allison, Belief beyond the evidence: Using the proposed effect of breakfast on obesity to show 2 practices that distort scientific evidence, *American Journal of Clinical Nutrition* 98 (2013): 1298–1308.

61. P. Deshmukh-Taskar and coauthors, The relationship of breakfast skipping and type of breakfast consumed with overweight/obesity, abdominal obesity, other cardiometabolic risk factors and the metabolic syndrome in young adults. The National Health and Nutrition Examination Survey (NHANES): 1999–2006, *Public Health Nutrition* 16 (2013): 2073–2082; S. P. P. Tin and coauthors, Breakfast skipping and change in body mass index in young children, *International Journal of Obesity* 35 (2011): 899–906; K. J. Smith and coauthors, Skipping breakfast: Longitudinal associations with cardiometabolic risk factors in the Childhood Determinants of Adult Health Study, *American Journal of Clinical Nutrition* 92 (2010): 1316–1325.

62. C H. J. Leidy and coauthors, Beneficial effects of a higher-protein breakfast on the appetitive, hormonal, and neural signals controlling energy intake regulation in overweight/obese, "breakfast skipping," late-adolescent girls, *American Journal of Clinical Nutrition* 97 (2013): 677–688; P. R. Deshmukh-Taskar and coauthors, The relationship of breakfast skipping and type of breakfast consumption with nutrient intake and weight status in children and adolescents: The National Health and Nutrition Examination Survey 1999–2006, *Journal of the American Dietetic Association* 110 (2010): 869–878.

63. M. Shay and coauthors, Food and nutrient intakes and their associations with lower BMI in middle-aged US adults: The International Study of Macro-/Micronutrients and Blood Pressure, *American Journal of Clinical Nutrition* 96 (2012): 483–491; M. Kristensen and coauthors, Whole grain compared with refined wheat decreases the percentage of body fat following a 12-week, energy restricted dietary intervention in postmenopausal women, *Journal of Nutrition* 142 (2012): 710–716.

64. G. Flores-Mateo and coauthors, Nut intake and adiposity: Meta-analysis of clinical trials, *American Journal of Clinical Nutrition* 97 (2013): 1346–1355; M. A. Martinez-Gonzalez and M. Bes-Rastrollo, Nut consumption, weight gain, and obesity: Epidemiological evidence, *Nutrition, Metabolism, and Cardiovascular Diseases* 21 (2011): S40–S45; P. Casa-Agustench and coauthors, Cross-sectional association of nut intake with adiposity in a Mediterranean population, *Nutrition, Metabolism, and Cardiovascular Diseases* 21 (2011): 518–525.

65. J. W. Carbone, J. P. McClung, and S. M. Pasiakos, Skeletal muscle responses to negative energy balance: Effects of dietary protein, *Advances in Nutrition* 3 (2012): 119–126.

66. C. L. Rock and coauthors, Effect of a free prepared meal and incentivized weight loss program on weight loss and weight loss maintenance in obese and overweight women: A randomized controlled trial, *Journal of the American Medical*

Association 304 (2010): 1803–1810; Position of the American Dietetic Association, 2009.

67. R. A. Williams, L. S. Roe, and B. J. Rolls, Comparison of three methods to reduce energy density: Effects on daily energy intake, *Appetite* 66 (2013): 75–83; R. Pérez-Escamilla and coauthors, Dietary energy density and body weight in adults and children: A systematic review, *Journal of the Academy of Nutrition and Dietetics* 112 (2012): 671–684; H. A. Raynor and coauthors, The effects of an energy density prescription on diet quality and weight loss: A pilot randomized controlled trial, *Journal of the Academy of Nutrition and Dietetics* 112 (2012): 1397–1402.

68. M. C. Daniels and B. M. Popkin, Impact of water intake on energy intake and weight status: A systematic review, *Nutrition Reviews* 68 (2010): 505–521.

69. Nicklas and coauthors, 2012; B. H. Goodpaster and coauthors, Effects of diet and physical activity interventions on weight loss and cardiometabolic risk factors in severely obese adults: A randomized study, *Journal of the American Medical Association* 304 (2010): 1795–1802; A. L. Hankinson and coauthors, Maintaining a high physical activity level over 20 years and weight gain, *Journal of the American Medical Association* 304 (2010): 2603–2610; D. E. Larson-Meyer and coauthors, Caloric restriction with or without exercise: The fitness versus fatness debate, *Medicine and Science in Sports and Exercise* 42 (2010): 152–159; J. E. Donnelly and coauthors, American College of Sports Medicine Position Stand: Appropriate physical activity intervention strategies for weight loss and prevention of weight regain for adults, *Medicine and Science in Sports and*

Exercise 41 (2009): 459–471; American Dietetic Association, 2009.

70. A. E. Field and coauthors, Weight control behaviors and subsequent weight change among adolescents and young adult females, *American Journal of Clinical Nutrition* 91 (2010): 147–153; Donnelly and coauthors, 2009.

71. Donnelly and coauthors, 2009.

72. U. Ekelund and coauthors, Physical activity and gain in abdominal adiposity and body weight: Prospective cohort study in 288, 498 men and women, *American Journal of Clinical Nutrition* 93 (2011): 826–835; Larson-Meyer and coauthors, 2010.

73. M. Hamer and G. O'Donovan, Cardiorespiratory fitness and metabolic risk factors in obesity, *Current Opinion in Lipidology* 21 (2010): 1–7.

74. A. M. Knab and coauthors, A 45-minute vigorous exercise bout increases metabolic rate for 14 hours, *Medicine and Science in Sports and Exercise* 43 (2011): 1642–1648.

75. C. W. Bales and coauthors, Aerobic and resistance training effects on energy intake: The STRRIDE-AT/RT Study, *Medicine and Science in Sports and Exercise* 44 (2012): 2033–2039; D. Stensel, Exercise, appetite and appetite-regulating hormones: Implications for food intake and weight control, *Annals of Nutrition and Metabolism* 57 (2010): 36–42; J. A. King and coauthors, Influence of brisk walking appetite, energy intake, and plasma acylated ghrelin, *Medicine and Science in Sports and Exercise* 42 (2010): 485–492.

76. K. J. Guelfi, C. E. Conges, and R. Duffield, Beneficial effects of 12 weeks of aerobic compared with

resistance exercise training on perceived appetite in previously sedentary overweight and obese men, *Metabolism: Clinical and Experimental* 62 (2013): 235–243; K. Deighton, J. C. Zahra, and D. J. Stensel, Appetite, energy intake and resting metabolic responses to 60 min treadmill running performed in a fasted versus a postprandial state, *Appetite* 58 (2012): 946–954.

77. Stensel, 2010.

78. E. V. Carraca and coauthors, Physical activity predicts changes in body image during obesity treatment in women, *Medicine and Science in Sports and Exercise* 44 (2012): 1604–1612.

79. S. S. Ho and coauthors, The effect of 12 weeks of aerobic, resistance or combination exercise training on cardiovascular risk factors in the overweight and obese in a randomized trial, *BMC Public Health* 12 (2012): 704.

80. L. E. Burke, J. Wang, and M. A. Sevick, Self-monitoring in weight loss: A systematic review of the literature, *Journal of the American Dietetic Association* 111 (2011): 92–102.

81. N. R. Reyes and coauthors, Similarities and differences between weight loss maintainers and regainers: A qualitative analysis, *Journal of the Academy of Nutrition and Dietetics* 112 (2012): 499–505.

82. C. D. Fryar and C. L. Ogden, Prevalence of underweight among adults aged 20 and over; United States, 1960–1962 through 2007–2010, 2012, www.cdc.gov/nchs/data/hestat/underweight_adult_07_08/underweight_adult_07_08.htm.

LO 7.7 Describe several popular fad diets and explain how to evaluate weight-loss diets based on sound nutrition.

To paraphrase William Shakespeare, "a fad diet by any other name would still be a fad diet." Year after year, "new and improved" diets appear on bookstore shelves and circulate among friends.* People of all sizes eagerly try the best diet ever on the market, hoping that this one will really work. Sometimes the diets seem to work for a while, but more often than not, their success is short-lived. Then another fad diet takes the spotlight. Here's how Dr. K. Brownell, an obesity researcher, describes this phenomenon: "When I get calls about the latest diet fad, I imagine a trick birthday cake candle that keeps lighting up and we have to keep blowing it out."

Why don't health professionals speak out against the relentless promotion of fad diets?

Realizing that many fad diets do not offer a safe and effective plan for weight loss, health professionals speak out, but they never get the candle blown out permanently. New fad diets can keep making outrageous claims because no one requires their advocates to prove what they say. Fad diet promoters do not have to conduct credible research on the benefits or dangers of their diets. They can simply make recommendations and then later, if questioned, search for bits and pieces of research that support the conclusions they have already reached. That's backward. Diet and health recommendations should *follow* years of sound research that has been reviewed by panels of scientists *before* being offered to the public.

How can the promoters of fad diets get away with exaggerated claims?

Because anyone can publish anything—in books or on the Internet—peddlers of fad diets can make unsubstantiated

AP Images/Evan Vucci

*The Academy of Nutrition and Dietetics offers evaluations of popular diets for your review. Look for reviews of popular diets at their website, *www.eatright.org/dietreviews*.

statements that fall far short of the truth but sound impressive to the uninformed. They often offer distorted bits of legitimate research. They may start with one or more actual facts but then leap from one erroneous conclusion to the next. Anyone who wants to believe these claims has to wonder how the thousands of scientists working on obesity research over the past century could possibly have missed such obvious connections.

Each popular diet features a unique way to make losing weight fast and easy. Which one works best?

Fad diets come in almost as many shapes and sizes as the people who search them out. Some restrict fats or carbohydrates, some limit portion sizes, some focus on food combinations, and some claim that a person's genetic type or blood type determines the foods best suited to manage weight and prevent disease. A lack of scientific evidence just doesn't seem to stop the advertised claims made for fad diets.[1] Despite claims that each new diet is "unique" in its approach to weight loss, most fad diets are designed to ensure a low energy intake. The "magic feature" that best supports weight loss is to limit energy intake to less than energy expenditure. Most of the sample menu plans, especially in the early stages, deliver an average of 1200 kcalories per day. Total kcalories tend to be low simply because food intake is so limited. Table NP7-1 (p. 186) compares some of today's more popular diets.

What is the appeal of fad diets?

Probably the greatest appeal of some fad diets is that they tend to ignore current diet recommendations. Foods such as meats and milk products that need to be selected carefully to limit saturated fat can now be eaten with abandon. Whole grains, legumes, vegetables, and fruits that should be eaten in abundance can now be bypassed. For some people, this is a dream come true: steaks without the potatoes, ribs without the coleslaw, and meatballs without the pasta. Who can resist the promise of weight loss while eating freely from a list of favorite foods?

Dieters are also lured into fad diets by sophisticated—yet often erroneous—explanations of the metabolic consequences of eating certain foods. Terms such as *eicosanoids* or *adipokines* are scattered about, often intimidating readers into believing that the authors must be right given their brilliance in understanding the body.

With over half of our nation's adults overweight and many more concerned about their weight, weight-loss books and products are a $33 billion-a-year business. Even a plan that offers only minimal weight-loss success easily attracts a following.

Are fad diets adequate?

When food choices are limited, nutrient intakes may be inadequate. To help shore up some of these inadequacies, fad diets often recommend a dietary supplement. Conveniently, many of the companies selling fad diets also sell these supplements,

TABLE NP7-1 Popular Diets Compared

Diet	Claim(s)	Strong Point(s)	Weak Point(s)
The 4-Hour Body	■ Small, simple changes produce big, long-lasting results. ■ The Slow-Carb diet supports a 20-pound weight loss in 30 days without exercise.	■ Encourages lean proteins, legumes, and vegetables. ■ Organized format provides simple plan.	■ Excludes fruit, whole grains, and milk (except cottage cheese), which may lead to nutrient deficiencies. ■ Lacks variety.
The 17 Day Diet	■ Changing the way you eat every few days creates "body confusion," which prevents metabolism from settling into homeostasis. ■ You can boost metabolism by "eating clean," which means no sugar, no processed food, and no fried foods.	■ Prevents boredom by alternating between cycles. ■ Fairly well-balanced diet promotes healthy eating.	■ Lacks scientific evidence that changing the diet creates "body confusion." ■ Does not provide individualized kcalorie goals. ■ Promotes its own processed foods.
The 100	■ Restricting sugar consumption to 100 kcalories a day will reduce insulin levels (the weight-gaining hormone), speed weight loss, improve health, and boost metabolism. ■ The real problem causing weight gains is hidden sugars in healthy foods such as yogurt and fruit.	■ Limits processed foods. ■ Encourages consumption of vegetables and fiber-rich foods.	■ Focuses on very basic food choices and lacks variety. ■ Limits important food groups such as low-fat dairy, legumes, and fruits, which may lead to nutrient deficiencies.
Biggest Loser Diet	■ Lose weight, gain health, feel young, and take control of your life by using portion control, progressively lowering energy intake, and following a customized food pyramid.	■ Provides motivation and promotes selecting low-fat foods and drinking water. ■ Stresses the importance of exercise.	■ Recommends energy intakes below the recommended minimum of 1200 kcalories a day, which may lead to nutrient deficiencies.
Cinch!	■ A nutrient-dense diet composed mainly of plant-based foods will help you lose weight and lower the risk of disease.	■ Recommends a plant-based, nutrient-dense diet. ■ Stresses the importance of exercise.	■ A little confusing and dense with facts.
The Dukan Diet	■ A high-protein, low-kcalorie diet promotes rapid and permanent weight loss.	■ Encourages daily exercise, moderate salt intake, and life-long weight management. ■ Provides a highly structured plan.	■ Restricts carbohydrates to induce ketosis, which can cause nausea, light-headedness, and fatigue and can worsen medical problems such as kidney disease. ■ Not suited for vegetarians and others who prefer not to emphasize animal proteins.
The Fast Diet	■ Lose weight by eating "normally" for five days while choosing two non-consecutive days to "fast"—limiting kcalories to 500 for women and 600 for men.	■ Focuses only on two days of the week. ■ Promotes lean protein and low glycemic foods on "fast" days.	■ Little research supporting the health benefits of intermittent fasting diets. ■ Fasting can cause irritability, sleeplessness or sleepiness, and dehydration.
New Sonoma Diet	■ Enjoying portion-controlled Coastal California style foods supports weight loss and promotes good health.	■ Emphasizes nutrient-dense foods. ■ Limits processed foods.	■ No individualized kcalorie plan.
Wheat Belly	■ Lose weight and reverse health problems by eliminating all forms of wheat.	■ Creates a low-kcalorie diet.	■ Restrictive diet would likely be low in B vitamins, calcium, and vitamin D.
The Zen Diet Revolution	■ Combine spiritual wisdom and dietary adjustments to reduce fat cells without counting kcalories. ■ Visualization, meditation, and mindfulness can change mental, dietary, lifestyle, and activity habits.	■ Offers a basic nutrition approach that does no harm. ■ Reminds you to make food meaningful and treat your body with respect.	■ Recommendations to use fat-burning herbs, supplements, and green tea to decrease fat cells are unsubstantiated and expensive.

Source: Adapted from Academy of Nutrition and Dietetics, *Consumer Diet and Lifestyle Book Reviews,* www.eatright.org/dietreviews, accessed November 2013.

often at an inflated price. As Nutrition in Practice 9 explains, however, foods offer many more health benefits than any supplement can provide. Quite simply, if the diet is inadequate, it needs to be improved, not supplemented.

Are the diets effective?

If fad diets were entirely ineffective, consumers would eventually stop pursuing them. Obviously, this is not the case. Similarly, if the diets were especially effective, then consumers who tried them would lose weight, and the obesity problem would be solved. Clearly, this is not happening either. As mentioned earlier, most fad diets succeed in contriving ways to limit kcalorie intakes, and so produce weight loss (at least in the short term). Studies demonstrate, however, that fad diets are particularly ineffective for weight-loss maintenance—people may drop some weight, but they quickly gain it back.[2] Straightforward kcalorie deficit is the real key to weight loss—not the elimination of protein, carbohydrate, or fat, or the still unidentified metabolic mechanisms proposed by many fad diets.[3]

For example, diet promoters make much of research showing that high-protein, low-carbohydrate diets produce a little more weight loss than balanced diets over the first few months of dieting. However, in the long run, any low-kcalorie diet produces about the same degree of loss.[4] In addition, most people cannot sustain such a diet and they quickly return to their original or an even higher weight.[5]

Protein nutrition during kcalorie restriction deserves attention, however. A meal with too little protein may not produce enough satiety, the satisfaction of feeling full after a meal, to prevent between-meal hunger.[6] Diets providing more than 35 percent of total kcalories as protein (the upper end of the DRI range), however, are no more effective for producing long-term weight loss than more balanced kcalorie-controlled diets.[7] Eating the normal amount of lean protein-rich foods while reducing carbohydrate- and fat-containing foods automatically reduces kcalories and shifts the balance towards a higher percentage of energy from protein.[8]

Many people seem confused about what kinds of dietary changes they need to make to lose weight. Isn't it helpful to follow a plan?

Yes. Most people need specific instructions and examples to make dietary changes. Popular diets offer dieters a plan. The user doesn't have to decide what foods to eat, how to prepare them, or how much to eat. Unfortunately, these instructions serve short-term weight-loss needs only. Over the long run, people tire of the monotony of diet plans, and most revert to their previous patterns.

By now you can see that the major drawback of most fad weight-loss schemes is that they fail to create lifestyle changes needed to support long-term weight maintenance and improve health. For that, people must do the hard work of learning the facts about nutrition and weight loss, setting their own realistic goals and then devising a lifestyle plan that can achieve them. A balanced, kcalorie-restricted diet with sufficient physical activity to support it may not be the shortcut that most people wish for, but it ensures nutrient adequacy and provides the best chance of long-term success.

Some currently popular diet plans offer a sensible approach to weight loss and healthy eating. The challenge is sorting the fad diets from the healthy options. Table NP7-2 presents some tips for identifying fad diets and weight-loss scams.

Chapter 7 describes reasonable approaches to weight management and concludes that the ideal diet is one you can live with for the rest of your life. Keep that criterion in mind when you evaluate the next "latest and greatest weight-loss diet" that comes along.

TABLE NP7-2 **Tips for Identifying Fad Diets and Weight-Loss Scams**

It may be a fad diet or weight-loss scam if it:

- Sounds too good to be true.
- Recommends using a single food consistently as the key to the program's success.
- Promises quick and easy weight loss with no effort. "Lose weight while you sleep!"
- Eliminates an entire food group such as grains or milk and milk products.
- Guarantees an unrealistic outcome in an unreasonable time period. "Lose 10 pounds in 2 days!"
- Bases evidence for its effectiveness on anecdotal stories.
- Requires that you buy special products that are not readily available in the marketplace at affordable prices.
- Specifies a proportion for the energy nutrients that falls outside the recommended ranges—carbohydrate, 45 to 65 percent; fat, 20 to 35 percent; and protein, 10 to 35 percent.
- Claims to alter your genetic code or reset your metabolism.
- Fails to mention potential risks or additional costs.
- Promotes products or procedures that have not been proven safe and effective.
- Neglects plans for weight maintenance following weight loss.

© 2016 Cengage Learning®

Notes

1. L. Cusack and coauthors, Blood type diets lack supporting evidence: A systematic review, *American Journal of Clinical Nutrition* 98 (2013): 99–104.

2. J. M. Nicklas and coauthors, Successful weight loss among obese U. S, adults, *American Journal of Preventive Medicine* 42 (2012): 481–485.

3. W. S. Yancy and coauthors, A randomized trial of a low-carbohydrate diet vs orlistat plus a low-fat diet for weight loss, *Archives of Internal Medicine* 170 (2010): 136–145

4. R. J. de Souza and coauthors, Effects of 4 weight-loss diets differing in fat, protein, and carbohydrate on fat mass, lean mass, visceral adipose tissue, and hepatic fat: Results from the POUNDS LOST trial, *American Journal of Clinical Nutrition* 95 (2012): 614–625.

5. de Souza and coauthors, 2012.

6. M. S. Westerterp-Plantenga, S. G. Lemmens, and K. R. Westerterp, Dietary protein: Its role in satiety, energetics, weight loss and health, *British Journal of Nutrition* 108 (2012): S105–S112.

7. The *Dietary Guidelines for Americans 2010,* www .dietaryguidelines.gov.

8. A. M. Johnstone, Safety and efficacy of high-protein diets for weight loss, *Proceedings of the Nutrition Society* 71 (2012): 339–349.

8 The Vitamins

8.1 The Vitamins—An Overview

LO 8.1 Describe how vitamins differ from the energy nutrients and how fat-soluble vitamins differ from water-soluble vitamins.

8.2 The Fat-Soluble Vitamins

LO 8.2 Identify the main roles, deficiency symptoms, toxicity symptoms, and food sources of the fat-soluble vitamins.

8.3 The Water-Soluble Vitamins

LO 8.3 Identify the main roles, deficiency symptoms, toxicity symptoms, and food sources of the water-soluble vitamins.

8.4 Nutrition in Practice: Phytochemicals and Functional Foods

LO 8.4 Describe phytochemicals and functional foods and explain how they might defend against chronic diseases.

Exactostock/SuperStock

Earlier chapters focused primarily on the energy-yielding nutrients—carbohydrate, fat, and protein. This chapter and the next one discuss the nutrients everyone thinks of when nutrition is mentioned—the vitamins and minerals.

8.1 The Vitamins—An Overview

LO 8.1 Describe how vitamins differ from the energy nutrients and how fat-soluble vitamins differ from water-soluble vitamins.

The **vitamins** occur in foods in much smaller quantities than do the energy-yielding nutrients, and they themselves contribute no energy to the body. Instead, they serve mostly as facilitators of body processes. They are a powerful group of substances, as their absence attests: Vitamin A deficiency can cause blindness, a lack of niacin can cause dementia, and a lack of vitamin D can retard bone growth. The consequences of deficiencies are so dire and the effects of restoring the needed nutrients so dramatic that people spend billions of dollars each year on **dietary supplements** to cure many different ailments. Vitamins certainly contribute to sound nutritional health, but supplements do not cure all ills. Furthermore, vitamin supplements do not offer the many benefits that come from vitamin-rich foods. The only disease a vitamin will *cure* is the one caused by a deficiency of that vitamin. The vitamins' roles in supporting optimal health extend far beyond preventing deficiency diseases, however. Emerging evidence supports the role of vitamin-rich *foods*, but not vitamin supplements, as protective against cancer and heart disease.[1]

A child once defined vitamins as "what, if you don't eat, you get sick." The description is both insightful and accurate. A more prosaic definition is that vitamins are potent, essential, nonkaloric, organic nutrients needed from foods in trace amounts to perform specific functions that promote growth, reproduction, and the maintenance of health and life. The vitamins differ from carbohydrates, fats, and proteins in the following ways:

- *Structure.* Vitamins are individual units; they are not linked together (as are molecules of glucose or amino acids).

- *Function.* Vitamins do not yield energy when metabolized; many of them do, however, assist the enzymes that participate in the release of energy from carbohydrate, fat, and proteins.

- *Dietary intakes.* The amounts of vitamins people ingest daily from foods and the amounts they require are measured in *micrograms* (µg) or *milligrams* (mg), rather than grams (g).

The vitamins are similar to the energy-yielding nutrients, though, in that they are vital to life, organic, and available from foods.

As the individual vitamins were discovered, they were named or given letters, numbers, or both. This led to the confusion that still exists today. This chapter uses the names shown in Table 8-1; alternative names are given in Tables 8-4 and 8-5, which appear later in the chapter.

Bioavailability The amount of vitamins available from foods depends on two factors: the quantity provided by a food and the amount absorbed and used by the body (the vitamin's **bioavailability**). Researchers analyze foods to determine their vitamin contents and publish the results in tables of food composition such as Appendix A. Determining the bioavailability of a vitamin is more difficult because it depends on many factors, including:

- Efficiency of digestion and time of transit through the GI tract.

- Previous nutrient intake and nutrition status.

TABLE 8-1 Vitamin Names

Fat-Soluble Vitamins

Vitamin A
Vitamin D
Vitamin E
Vitamin K

Water-Soluble Vitamins

B vitamins
  Thiamin
  Riboflavin
  Niacin
  Pantothenic acid
  Biotin
  Vitamin B_6
  Folate
  Vitamin B_{12}
Vitamin C

© Cengage Learning®

vitamins: essential, nonkaloric, organic nutrients needed in tiny amounts in the diet.

dietary supplements: products that are added to the diet and contain any of the following ingredients: a vitamin, a mineral, an herb or other botanical, an amino acid, a metabolite, a constituent, or an extract.

bioavailability: the rate and extent to which a nutrient is absorbed and used.

TABLE 8-2 Minimizing Nutrient Losses

Each of these tactics saves a small percentage of the vitamins in foods, but repeated each day this can add up to significant amounts in a year's time.

Prevent Enzymatic Destruction

▪ Refrigerate most fruits, vegetables, and juices to slow breakdown of vitamins.

Protect from Light and Air

▪ Store milk and enriched grain products in opaque containers to protect riboflavin.

▪ Store cut fruits and vegetables in the refrigerator in airtight wrappers; reseal opened juice containers before refrigerating.

Prevent Heat Destruction or Losses in Water

▪ Wash intact fruits and vegetables before cutting or peeling to prevent vitamin losses during washing.

▪ Cook fruits and vegetables in a microwave oven, or quickly stir-fry, or steam them over a small amount of water to preserve heat-sensitive vitamins and to prevent vitamin loss in cooking water. Recapture dissolved vitamins by using cooking water for soups, stews, or gravies.

▪ Avoid high temperatures and long cooking times.

▪ Other foods consumed at the same time.

▪ The method of food preparation (raw or cooked, for example).

▪ Source of the nutrient (naturally occurring, synthetic, or fortified).

This chapter and the next describe factors that inhibit or enhance the absorption of individual vitamins and minerals. Experts consider these factors when estimating recommended intakes.

Precursors Some of the vitamins are available from foods in inactive forms known as **precursors,** or provitamins. Once inside the body, the precursor is converted to the active form of the vitamin. Thus, in measuring a person's vitamin intake, it is important to count both the amount of the actual vitamin and the potential amount available from its precursors. Tables 8-4 and 8-5 later in the chapter specify which vitamins have precursors.

Organic Nature Fresh foods naturally contain vitamins, but because they are organic, vitamins can be readily destroyed during processing. Therefore, processed foods should be used sparingly, and fresh foods must be handled with care during storage and in cooking. Prolonged heating may destroy much of the thiamin in food. Because riboflavin can be destroyed by the ultraviolet rays of the sun or by fluorescent light, foods stored in transparent glass containers are most likely to lose riboflavin. Oxygen destroys vitamin C, so losses occur when foods are cut, processed, and stored. Table 8-2 summarizes ways to minimize nutrient losses in the kitchen.

Solubility Vitamins fall naturally into two classes—fat soluble and water soluble. The water-soluble vitamins are the B vitamins and vitamin C; the fat-soluble ones are vitamins A, D, E, and K. The solubility of a vitamin confers on it many characteristics and determines how it is absorbed, transported, stored, and excreted (see Table 8-3). This discussion of vitamins begins with the fat-soluble vitamins.

IN SUMMARY

▪ Vitamins are essential, nonkcaloric, organic nutrients that are needed in trace amounts in the diet to help facilitate body processes.

▪ The amount of vitamins available from foods depends on the quantity provided by a food and the amount absorbed and used by the body—the vitamins' bioavailability.

precursors: compounds that can be converted into other compounds; with regard to vitamins, compounds that can be converted into active vitamins; also known as *provitamins*.

TABLE 8-3 Fat-Soluble and Water-Soluble Vitamins Compared

While each vitamin has unique functions and features, a few generalizations about the fat-soluble and water-soluble vitamins can aid understanding.

Feature	Fat-Soluble Vitamins: Vitamins A, D, E, and K	Water-Soluble Vitamins: B Vitamins and Vitamin C
Absorption	Absorbed like fats, first into the lymph and then into the blood.	Absorbed directly into the blood.
Transport and storage	Must travel with protein carriers in watery body fluids; stored in the liver or fatty tissues.	Travel freely in watery fluids; most are not stored in the body.
Excretion	Not readily excreted; tend to build up in the tissues.	Readily excreted in the urine.
Toxicity	Toxicities are likely from supplements but occur rarely from food.	Toxicities are unlikely but possible with high doses from supplements.
Requirement	Needed in periodic doses (perhaps weekly or even monthly) because the body can draw on its stores.	Needed in frequent doses (perhaps every 1 to 3 days) because the body does not store most of them to any extent.

- Vitamin precursors in foods are converted into active vitamins in the body.

- Vitamins can be readily destroyed during processing.

- The water-soluble vitamins are the B vitamins and vitamin C; the fat-soluble vitamins are vitamins A, D, E, and K.

8.2 The Fat-Soluble Vitamins

LO 8.2 Identify the main roles, deficiency symptoms, toxicity symptoms, and food sources of the fat-soluble vitamins.

The fat-soluble vitamins—A, D, E, and K—usually occur together in the fats and oils of foods, and the body absorbs them in the same way it absorbs lipids. Therefore, any condition that interferes with fat absorption can precipitate a deficiency of the fat-soluble vitamins. Once absorbed, fat-soluble vitamins are stored in the liver and fatty tissues until the body needs them. They are not readily excreted, and, unlike most of the water-soluble vitamins, they can build up to toxic concentrations.

The capacity to store fat-soluble vitamins affords a person some flexibility in dietary intake. When blood concentrations begin to decline, the body can retrieve the vitamins from storage. Thus, a person need not eat a day's allowance of each fat-soluble vitamin every day but need only make sure that, over time, average daily intakes approximate recommended intakes. In contrast, most water-soluble vitamins must be consumed more regularly because the body does not store them to any great extent.

Vitamin A and Beta-Carotene

Vitamin A has the distinction of being the first fat-soluble vitamin to be recognized. More than a century later, vitamin A and its plant-derived precursor, **beta-carotene,** continue to intrigue researchers with their diverse roles and profound effects on health.

Vitamin A is a versatile vitamin, with roles in gene expression, vision, cell differentiation (thereby maintaining the health of body linings and skin), immunity, and reproduction and growth.[2] Three different forms of vitamin A are active in the body: retinol, retinal, and retinoic acid. Each form of vitamin A performs specific tasks. Retinol supports reproduction and is the major transport and storage form of the vitamin; the cells convert retinol to retinal or retinoic acid as needed. Retinal is active in vision, and retinoic acid acts as a hormone, regulating cell differentiation, growth, and embryonic development. A special transport protein, **retinol-binding protein (RBP),** picks up retinol from the liver, where it is stored, and carries it in the blood.

Vitamin A's Role in Gene Expression Vitamin A exerts considerable influence on an array of body functions through its interaction with genes—hundreds of genes are regulated by the retinoic acid form of the vitamin.[3] Genes direct the synthesis of proteins, including enzymes, and enzymes perform the metabolic work of the tissues (see Chapter 4). Hence, factors that influence gene expression also affect the metabolic activities of the tissues and the health of the body.

Researchers have long known that simply possessing the genetic equipment needed to make a particular protein does not guarantee that the protein will be produced, any more than owning a car guarantees you a trip across town. To make the journey, you must also use the right key to trigger the events that start up its engine or turn it off at the appropriate time. Some dietary components, including the retinoic acid form of vitamin A, are now known to be such keys—they help to activate or deactivate certain genes and thus affect the production of specific proteins.[4]

vitamin A: a fat-soluble vitamin with three chemical forms: *retinol* (the alcohol form), *retinal* (the aldehyde form), and *retinoic acid* (the acid form).

beta-carotene: a vitamin A precursor made by plants and stored in human fat tissue; an orange pigment.

retinol-binding protein (RBP): the specific protein responsible for transporting retinol. Measurement of the blood concentration of RBP is a sensitive test of vitamin A status.

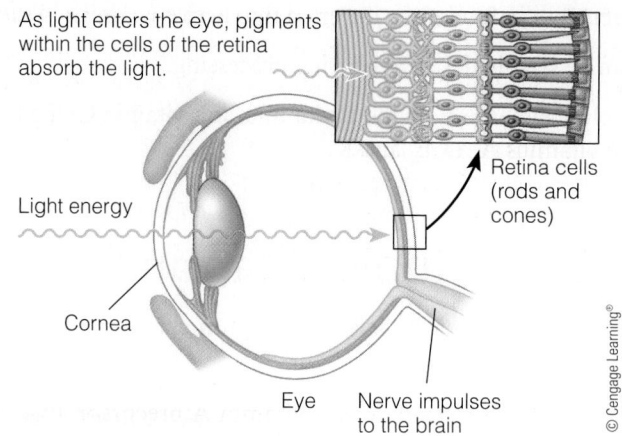

As light enters the eye, pigments within the cells of the retina absorb the light.

Retina cells (rods and cones)

Light energy

Cornea

Eye

Nerve impulses to the brain

© Cengage Learning®

FIGURE 8-1 **Vitamin A's Role in Vision**

Vitamin A's Role in Vision Vitamin A plays two indispensable roles in the eye. It helps maintain a healthy, crystal-clear outer window, the **cornea;** and it participates in light detection at the **retina.** Some of the photosensitive cells of the retina contain **pigment** molecules called **rhodopsin;** each rhodopsin molecule is composed of a protein called **opsin** bonded to a molecule of retinal, which plays a central role in vision.[5] When light passes through the cornea of the eye and strikes the retina, rhodopsin responds by changing shape and becoming bleached. In turn, this initiates the signal that conveys the sensation of sight to the optic center in the brain. Figure 8-1 shows vitamin A's site of action inside the eye.

When vitamin A is lacking, the eye has difficulty adapting to changing light levels. At night, after the eye has adapted to darkness, a flash of bright light is followed by a brief delay before the eye can see again. This lag in the recovery of night vision is known as **night blindness.** Because night blindness is easy to test, it aids in the diagnosis of vitamin A deficiency. Night blindness is only a symptom, however, and may indicate a condition other than vitamin A deficiency.

Vitamin A's Role in Protein Synthesis and Cell Differentiation The role that vitamin A plays in vision is undeniably important, but only one-thousandth of the body's vitamin A is in the retina. Much more is in the skin and the linings of organs, where it works behind the scenes at the genetic level to promote protein synthesis and cell **differentiation.** The process of cell differentiation allows each type of cell to mature so that it is capable of performing a specific function.

All body surfaces, both inside and out, are covered by layers of cells known as **epithelial cells.** The **epithelial tissue** on the outside of the body is, of course, the skin—and vitamin A and beta-carotene help to protect against skin damage from the sunlight.[6] In the eye, epithelial tissue covers the outermost layer of the cornea, where it blocks the passage of foreign materials such as dust, water, and bacteria. The epithelial tissues inside the body include the linings of the mouth, stomach, and intestines; the linings of the lungs and the passages leading to them; the lining of the bladder; the linings of the uterus and vagina; and the linings of the eyelids and sinus passageways. The epithelial tissues on the inside of the body must be kept smooth. To ensure that they are, the epithelial cells on their surfaces secrete a smooth, slippery substance (mucus) that coats the tissues and protects them from invasive microorganisms and other harmful particles. The **mucous membrane** that lines the stomach also shields its cells from digestion by gastric juices. Vitamin A, by way of its role in cell differentiation, helps to maintain the integrity of the epithelial cells.

Vitamin A's Role in Immunity Vitamin A has gained a reputation as an "anti-infective" vitamin because so many of the body's defenses against infection depend on

cornea (KOR-nee-uh): the hard, transparent membrane covering the outside of the eye.

retina (RET-in-uh): the layer of light-sensitive nerve cells lining the back of the inside of the eye; consists of rods and cones.

pigment: a molecule capable of absorbing certain wavelengths of light so that it reflects only those that we perceive as a certain color.

rhodopsin (ro-DOP-sin): a light-sensitive pigment of the retina; contains the retinal form of vitamin A and the protein opsin.
  rhod = red (pigment)
  opsin = visual protein

opsin (OP-sin): the protein portion of the visual pigment molecule.

night blindness: the slow recovery of vision after exposure to flashes of bright light at night; an early symptom of vitamin A deficiency.

differentiation: the development of specific functions different from those of the original.

epithelial (ep-i-THEE-lee-ul) **cells:** cells on the surface of the skin and mucous membranes.

epithelial tissue: tissue composing the layers of the body that serve as selective barriers between the body's interior and the environment (examples are the cornea, the skin, the respiratory lining, and the lining of the digestive tract).

mucous membrane: membrane composed of mucus-secreting cells that lines the surfaces of body tissues. (Reminder: *Mucus* is the smooth, slippery substance secreted by these cells.)

an adequate supply.[7] Much research supports the need for vitamin A in the regulation of the genes involved in immunity. Without sufficient vitamin A, these genetic interactions produce an altered response to infection that weakens the body's defenses.

Vitamin A's Role in Reproduction, Growth, and Development Vitamin A is crucial to normal reproduction and growth. In men, vitamin A participates in sperm development, and, in women, vitamin A promotes normal fetal growth and development.[8] During pregnancy, vitamin A is transferred to the fetus and is essential to the development of the nervous system, lungs, heart, kidneys, skeleton, eyes, and ears. (Nutrition during pregnancy is discussed in Chapter 11.)

Beta-Carotene's Role as an Antioxidant For many years scientists believed beta-carotene to be of interest solely as a vitamin A precursor. Eventually, though, researchers began to recognize that beta-carotene is an extremely effective **antioxidant** in the body. Antioxidants are compounds that protect other compounds (such as lipids in cell membranes) from attack by oxygen. Oxygen triggers the formation of compounds known as **free radicals** that can start chain reactions in cell membranes. If left uncontrolled, these chain reactions can damage cell structures and impair cell functions. Oxidative and free-radical damage to cells is suspected of instigating some early stages of cancer and heart disease.[9] Research has identified links between oxidative damage and the development of many other diseases, including age-related blindness, Alzheimer's disease, arthritis, cataracts, diabetes, and kidney disease.[10]

Studies of populations suggest that people whose diets are low in foods rich in beta-carotene have higher incidences of certain types of cancer than those whose diets contain generous amounts of such foods. Based on findings that beta-carotene in foods may protect against cancer, researchers designed a study to determine the effects of beta-carotene *supplements* on the incidence of lung cancer among smokers. The researchers expected to see a beneficial effect, but instead they found that smokers taking the beta-carotene supplements suffered a *greater* incidence of lung cancer than those taking placebos. Beta-carotene is one of many **dietary antioxidants** present in foods—others include vitamin E, vitamin C, the mineral selenium, and many phytochemicals. Dietary antioxidants are just one class of a complex array of constituents in whole foods that seem to benefit health synergistically. Until more is known, eating beta-carotene–rich foods, not supplements, is in the best interests of health. Based on research so far, the DRI committee has not established a recommended intake value for beta-carotene.

Vitamin A Deficiency Up to a year's supply of vitamin A can be stored in the body, 90 percent of it in the liver. If a healthy adult were to stop eating vitamin A–rich foods, deficiency symptoms would not begin to appear until after stores were depleted, which would take 1 to 2 years. Then, however, the consequences would be profound and severe. Table 8-4, later in this chapter, lists some of them.

In vitamin A deficiency, cell differentiation and maturation are impaired. The epithelial cells flatten and begin to produce **keratin**—the hard, inflexible protein of hair and nails. In the eye, this process leads to drying and hardening of the cornea, which may progress to permanent blindness. Vitamin A deficiency is the major cause of preventable blindness in children worldwide, causing as many as half a million children to lose their sight every year.[11] Blindness due to vitamin A deficiency, known as **xerophthalmia,** develops in stages. At first, the cornea becomes dry and hard because of inadequate mucus production—a condition known as **xerosis.** Then xerosis quickly progresses to **keratomalacia,** the softening of the cornea that leads to irreversible blindness. Many children worldwide endure less severe forms of vitamin A deficiency, making them vulnerable to infectious diseases. Routine vitamin A supplementation and food fortification can be life-saving interventions.[12]

antioxidant (anti-OX-ih-dant): a compound that protects other compounds from oxygen by itself reacting with oxygen. *Oxidation* is a potentially damaging effect of normal cell chemistry involving oxygen.
anti = against
oxy = oxygen

free radicals: highly reactive chemical forms that can cause destructive changes in nearby compounds, sometimes setting up a chain reaction.

dietary antioxidants: compounds typically found in plant foods that significantly decrease the adverse effects of oxidation on living tissues. The major antioxidant vitamins are vitamin E, vitamin C, and beta-carotene.

keratin (KERR-uh-tin): a water-insoluble protein; the normal protein of hair and nails. Keratin-producing cells may replace mucus-producing cells in vitamin A deficiency.

xerophthalmia (zer-off-THAL-mee-uh): progressive blindness caused by inadequate mucus production due to severe vitamin A deficiency.
xero = dry
ophthalm = eye

xerosis (zee-ROW-sis): abnormal drying of the skin and mucous membranes; a sign of vitamin A deficiency

keratomalacia (KARE-ah-toe-ma-LAY-shuh): softening of the cornea that leads to irreversible blindness; a sign of severe vitamin A deficiency.

All body surfaces, both inside and out, maintain their integrity with the help of vitamin A. When vitamin A is lacking, cells of the skin harden and flatten, making it dry, rough, scaly, and hard. An accumulation of keratin makes a lump around each hair **follicle** (keratinization).

In the mouth, a vitamin A deficiency results in drying and hardening of the salivary glands, making them susceptible to infection. Secretions of mucus in the stomach and intestines are reduced, hindering normal digestion and absorption of nutrients. Infections of other mucous membranes also become likely.

Vitamin A's role in maintaining the body's defensive barriers may partially explain the relationship between vitamin A deficiency and susceptibility to infection. In developing countries around the world, measles is a devastating infectious disease, killing 430 children each day.[13] Deaths are usually due to related infections such as pneumonia and severe diarrhea. Providing large doses of vitamin A reduces the risk of dying from these infections.

The evidence that vitamin A reduces the severity of measles and measles-related infections and diarrhea has prompted the World Health Organization (WHO) and the United Nations International Children's Emergency Fund (UNICEF) to make control of vitamin A deficiency a major goal in their quest to improve child survival throughout the developing world. They recommend routine vitamin A supplementation for all children with measles in areas where vitamin A deficiency is a problem or where the measles death rate is high. The American Academy of Pediatrics recommends vitamin A supplementation for certain groups of measles-infected infants and children in the United States.

Vitamin A Toxicity Vitamin A toxicity is a real possibility when people consume concentrated amounts of **preformed vitamin A** in foods derived from animals, fortified foods, or supplements. Plant foods contain the vitamin only as beta-carotene, its inactive precursor form. The precursor does not convert to active vitamin A rapidly enough to cause toxicity.

Overdoses of vitamin A damage the same body systems that exhibit symptoms in vitamin A deficiency (see Table 8-4 later in the chapter). Children are most vulnerable to vitamin A toxicity because they need less vitamin A and are more sensitive to overdoses. The availability of breakfast cereals, instant meals, fortified milk, and chewable candy-like vitamins, each containing 100 percent or more of the recommended daily intake of vitamin A, makes it possible for a well-meaning parent to provide several times the daily allowance of the vitamin to a child within a few hours.

Excessive vitamin A also poses a **teratogenic** risk. Excessive vitamin A during pregnancy can injure the spinal cord and other tissues of the developing fetus, increasing the risk of birth defects.[14] The Tolerable Upper Intake Level of 3000 micrograms for women of childbearing age is based on the teratogenic effect of vitamin A.

Excessive amounts of vitamin A over the years may weaken the bones and contribute to fractures and osteoporosis (see the later discussion of vitamin D for more on osteoporosis).[15] More research is needed to clarify the relationship between vitamin A intake and bone health, but such findings suggest that most people should not take vitamin A supplements. Even multivitamin supplements typically provide 1500 micrograms—much more vitamin A than most people need. For perspective, the RDA for vitamin A is 700 micrograms for women and 900 micrograms for men.

Certain vitamin A relatives are available by prescription as acne treatments. When applied directly to the skin surface, these preparations help relieve the symptoms of acne. Taking massive doses of vitamin A internally will *not* cure acne, however, and may cause the symptoms itemized in Table 8-4, later in the chapter. In most cases, foods are a better choice than supplements for needed nutrients. The best way to ensure a safe vitamin A intake is to eat generous servings of vitamin A–rich foods.

follicle (FOLL-i-cul)**:** a group of cells in the skin from which a hair grows.

preformed vitamin A: vitamin A in its active form.

teratogenic (ter-AT-oh-jen-ik)**:** causing abnormal fetal development and birth defects.
  terato = monster
  genic = to produce

Beta-Carotene Conversion and Toxicity Nutrition scientists do not use micrograms to specify the quantity of beta-carotene in foods. Instead, they use a value known as **retinol activity equivalents (RAE),** which express the amount of retinol the body actually derives from a plant food after conversion. One microgram of retinol counts as 1 RAE, as does 12 micrograms of dietary beta-carotene. This difference recognizes that beta-carotene's absorption and conversion are significantly less efficient than those of the retinoids.

As mentioned earlier, beta-carotene from plant foods is not converted to the active form of vitamin A rapidly enough to be hazardous. It has, however, been known to turn people bright yellow if they eat too much. Beta-carotene builds up in the fat just beneath the skin and imparts a yellowish cast (see Figure 8-2). Additionally, as discussed earlier, overconsumption of beta-carotene from *supplements* may be harmful, especially to smokers.

Vitamin A in Foods Preformed vitamin A is found only in foods of animal origin. The richest sources of vitamin A are liver and fish oil, but milk, cheese, and fortified cereals are also good sources. Healthy people can eat vitamin A–rich foods—with the possible exception of liver—in large amounts without risking toxicity. Eating liver once every week or so is enough. Butter and eggs also provide some vitamin A to the diet.

Because vitamin A is fat soluble, it is lost when milk is skimmed. To compensate, reduced-fat, low-fat, and fat-free milks are often fortified with vitamin A. Margarine is also usually fortified so as to provide the same amount of vitamin A as butter. Figure 8-3 shows a sampling of the richest food sources of both preformed vitamin A and beta-carotene.

Fast-food meals often lack vitamin A. When fast-food restaurants offer salads with cheese, carrots, and other vitamin A–rich foods, the nutritional quality of their meals greatly improves.

[handwritten margin note: the richest sources of vitamin A are liver + fish oil, but milk, cheese + fortified cereals are also a good source]

FIGURE 8-2 Symptom of Beta-Carotene Excess—Discoloration of the Skin
The hand on the right shows the skin discoloration that occurs when blood levels of beta-carotene rise in response to a low-kcalorie diet that features carrots, pumpkins, and orange juice. (The hand on the left belongs to someone else and is shown here for comparison.)

James Stevenson/Science Source

> **retinol activity equivalents (RAE):** a measure of vitamin A activity; the amount of retinol that the body will derive from a food containing preformed retinol or its precursor beta-carotene.

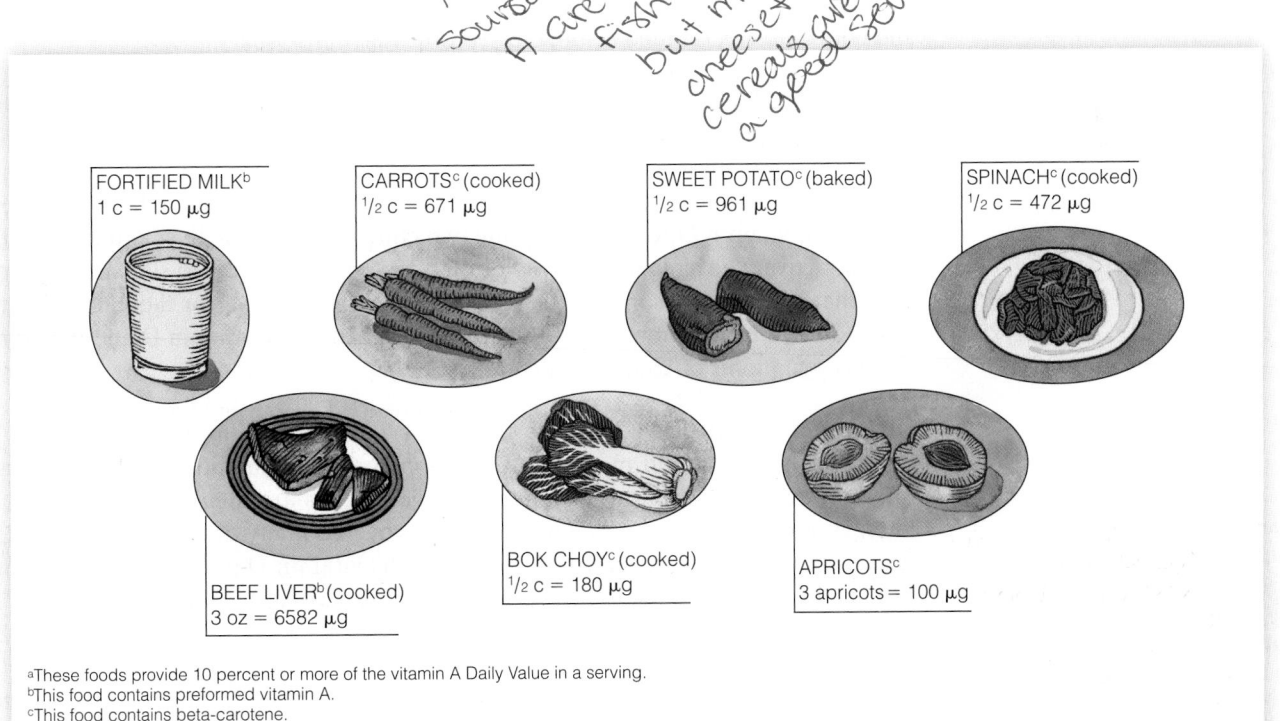

FORTIFIED MILK[b]
1 c = 150 μg

CARROTS[c] (cooked)
1/2 c = 671 μg

SWEET POTATO[c] (baked)
1/2 c = 961 μg

SPINACH[c] (cooked)
1/2 c = 472 μg

BEEF LIVER[b] (cooked)
3 oz = 6582 μg

BOK CHOY[c] (cooked)
1/2 c = 180 μg

APRICOTS[c]
3 apricots = 100 μg

[a]These foods provide 10 percent or more of the vitamin A Daily Value in a serving.
[b]This food contains preformed vitamin A.
[c]This food contains beta-carotene.

© 2016 Cengage Learning®

FIGURE 8-3 Good Sources of Vitamin A and Beta-Carotene[a]

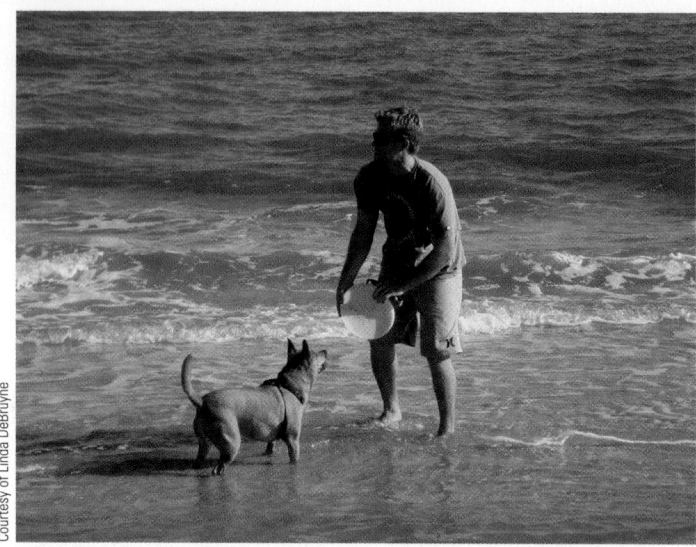

Sunlight promotes vitamin D synthesis in the skin. Exposure to the sun should be moderate; however, excessive exposure may cause skin cancer.

Beta-Carotene in Foods Many foods from plants contain beta-carotene, the orange pigment responsible for the bold colors of many fruits and vegetables. Carrots, sweet potatoes, pumpkins, cantaloupe, and apricots are all rich sources, and their bright orange color enhances the eye appeal of the plate. Another colorful group, *dark* green vegetables, such as spinach, other greens, and broccoli, owe their color to both chlorophyll and beta-carotene. The orange and green pigments together impart a deep, murky green color to the vegetables. Other colorful vegetables, such as iceberg lettuce, beets, and sweet corn, can fool you into thinking they contain beta-carotene, but these foods derive their color from other pigments and are poor sources of beta-carotene. As for "white" plant foods such as rice and potatoes, they have little or none. Recommendations to eat *dark* green or *deep* orange vegetables and fruits at least every other day help people to meet their vitamin A needs.

Vitamin D

Vitamin D is different from all the other nutrients in that the body can synthesize it in significant quantities with the help of sunlight. Therefore, in a sense, vitamin D is not an essential nutrient. Given enough sun, people need no vitamin D from foods.

Also known as **calciferol,** vitamin D comes in two major forms.[16] **Vitamin D$_2$** derives primarily from plant foods in the diet. **Vitamin D$_3$** derives from animal foods in the diet and from synthesis in the skin. These two forms of vitamin D are similar and both must be activated before they become fully functional.

Vitamin D's Metabolic Conversions The liver manufactures a vitamin D precursor, which migrates to the skin, where it is converted to a second precursor with the help of the sun's ultraviolet rays. Next, the liver and then the kidneys alter the second precursor to produce the active vitamin. Whether made from sunlight or obtained from food, vitamin D requires the same two conversions by the liver and kidneys to become active. The biological activity of the active vitamin is 500- to 1000-fold greater than that of its precursor. Diseases that affect either the liver or the kidneys may impair the transformations of precursor vitamin D to active vitamin D and therefore produce symptoms of vitamin D deficiency.

Vitamin D's Actions Although known as a vitamin, vitamin D is actually a hormone—a compound manufactured by one organ of the body that has effects on another. The best-known vitamin D target organs are the small intestine, the kidneys, and the bones, but scientists have discovered many other vitamin D target tissues. In the brain and nerve cells, for example, vitamin D protects against cognitive decline and slows the progression of Parkinson disease.[17] Vitamin D in muscle cells encourages growth in children and preserves strength in adults.[18] Vitamin D signals cells of the immune system to defend against infectious diseases.[19] Vitamin D may also regulate the cells of the adipose tissue in ways that might contribute to obesity.[20] In many cases, vitamin D enhances or suppresses the activity of genes that regulate cell growth. As such, it may be valuable in treating a number of diseases.

calciferol (kal-SIF-er-ol)**:** vitamin D

vitamin D$_2$: vitamin D derived from plants in the diet; also called *ergocalciferol* (ER-go-kal-SIF-er-ol).

vitamin D$_3$: vitamin D derived from animals in the diet or made in the skin from 7-dehydrocholesterol, a precursor of cholesterol, with the help of sunlight; also called *cholecalciferol* (KO-lee-kal-SIF-er-ol).

Research suggests that a deficit of vitamin D is associated with an increased risk of high blood pressure; type 2 diabetes, cardiovascular diseases; some common cancers; infections such as tuberculosis; inflammatory conditions; autoimmune diseases such as type 1 diabetes, rheumatoid arthritis, and multiple sclerosis; and even premature death.[21] Even so, evidence does not support taking vitamin D supplements to prevent diseases (except those caused by deficiency), and experts recommend against it.[22] The well-established vitamin D roles, however, concern calcium balance and the bones during growth and throughout life, and these form the basis of the recommended intakes for vitamin D, discussed in a later section.

Vitamin D's Roles in Bone Growth Vitamin D is a member of a large, cooperative bone-making and maintenance team composed of nutrients and other compounds, including vitamins A, C, and K; the hormones parathormone (parathyroid hormone) and calcitonin; the protein collagen; and the minerals calcium, phosphorus, magnesium, and fluoride. Many of their interactions take place at the genetic level in ways that are under investigation. Vitamin D's special role in bone health is to assist in the absorption of calcium and phosphorus, thus helping to maintain blood concentrations of these minerals.[23] The bones grow denser and stronger as they absorb and deposit these minerals. Details of calcium balance and mineral deposition appear in Chapter 9.

Vitamin D raises blood concentrations of bone minerals in three ways. When the diet is sufficient, vitamin D enhances their absorption from the GI tract. When the diet is insufficient, vitamin D provides the needed minerals from other sources: reabsorption by the kidneys and mobilization from the bones into the blood. The vitamin may work alone, as it does in the GI tract, or in combination with parathyroid hormone, as it does in the bones and kidneys.

Vitamin D Deficiency Overt signs of vitamin D deficiency are relatively rare, but vitamin D insufficiency is remarkably common.[24] Almost 10 percent of the U.S. population is deficient, and another 25 percent is marginal.[25] Factors that contribute to vitamin D deficiency include dark skin, breastfeeding without supplementation, lack of sunlight, and not using fortified milk.

Worldwide, the prevalence of the vitamin D–deficiency disease **rickets** is extremely high, affecting more than half of the children in countries such as China and Mongolia, and regions such as sub-Saharan Africa, the Middle East, and Latin America.[26] In the United States, rickets is not common, but when it occurs, black children and adolescents—especially females and overweight teens—are most likely to be affected.[27] To prevent rickets and support optimal bone health, the DRI committee recommends that all infants, children, and adolescents consume the recommended 15 micrograms of vitamin D each day.[28] In rickets, the bones fail to calcify normally, causing growth retardation and skeletal abnormalities. The bones become so weak that they bend when they have to support the body's weight (see Figure 8-4). A child with rickets who is old enough to walk characteristically develops bowed legs, often the most obvious sign of the disease. Another sign is the beaded ribs that result from the poorly formed attachments of the bones to the cartilage.

Adolescents, who often abandon vitamin D–fortified milk in favor of soft drinks, may also prefer indoor pastimes such as computer games to outdoor activities during daylight hours. Such teens often lack vitamin D and so fail to develop the bone density needed to prevent bone loss in later life.

In adults, the poor mineralization of bone results in the painful bone disease **osteomalacia**. Any failure to synthesize adequate vitamin D or obtain enough from foods sets the stage for a loss of calcium from the bones, which can result in fractures secondary to **osteoporosis** (reduced bone density). The simple act of taking a vitamin D supplement could easily save the life of an elderly person who might otherwise suffer dangerous bone fractures and falls.[29]

Bowed legs. In rickets, the poorly formed long bones of the legs bend outward as weight-bearing activities such as walking begin.

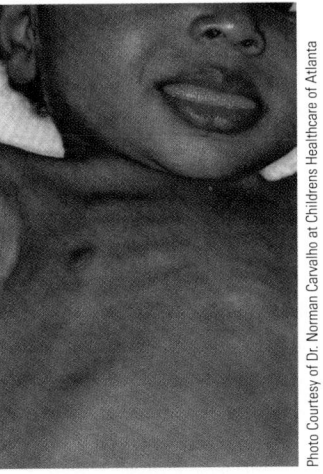

Beaded ribs. In rickets, a series of "beads" develop where the cartilages and bones attach.

rickets: the vitamin D–deficiency disease in children.

osteomalacia (os-tee-oh-mal-AY-shuh)**:** a bone disease characterized by softening of the bones. Symptoms include bending of the spine and bowing of the legs. The disease occurs most often in adults with renal failure or malabsorption disorders.

osteo = bone
mal = bad (soft)

osteoporosis: (os-tee-oh-pore-OH-sis)**:** literally, porous bones; reduced density of the bones, also known as *adult bone loss*.

Vitamin D Toxicity Vitamin D clearly illustrates how optimal amounts of nutrients support health, but both inadequacies and excesses cause harm. Vitamin D is among the vitamins most likely to have toxic effects when consumed in excess. Excess vitamin D raises the concentration of blood calcium. Excess blood calcium tends to precipitate in the soft tissues and form stones, especially in the kidneys, where calcium is concentrated in an effort to excrete it. Calcification may also harden the blood vessels and is especially dangerous in the major arteries of the brain, heart, and lungs, where it can cause death.

The amounts of vitamin D made by the skin and found in foods are well within safe limits, but supplements containing the vitamin in concentrated form should be kept out of the reach of children and used cautiously, if at all, by adults. The DRI committee has set a Tolerable Upper Intake Level for vitamin D at 50 micrograms per day (2000 International Units [IU] on supplement labels).

Vitamin D from the Sun Most of the world's population relies on natural exposure to sunlight to maintain adequate vitamin D nutrition. The sun imposes no risk of vitamin D toxicity. Prolonged exposure to sunlight degrades the vitamin D precursor in the skin, preventing its conversion to the active vitamin.

Prolonged exposure to sunlight has other undesirable consequences, however, such as premature wrinkling of the skin and skin cancers. Sunscreens help reduce the risks of these outcomes, but sunscreens with sun protection factors (SPF) of 8 and above also retard vitamin D synthesis. Still, even with an SPF 15–30 sunscreen, sufficient vitamin D synthesis can be obtained in 10 to 20 minutes of sun exposure. A strategy to avoid this dilemma is to apply sunscreen after enough time has elapsed to provide sufficient vitamin D. For most people, exposing hands, face, and arms on a clear summer day for 5 to 10 minutes, a few times a week, should be sufficient to maintain vitamin D nutrition. Dark-skinned people require longer exposure than light-skinned people, but by three hours, vitamin D synthesis in heavily pigmented skin arrives at the same plateau as in fair skin after 30 minutes.

Latitude, season, and time of day also have dramatic effects on vitamin D synthesis and status. Heavy cloud cover, smoke, or smog block the ultraviolet (UV) rays of the sun that promote vitamin D synthesis. Differences in skin pigmentation, latitude, and smog may account for the finding that African Americans, especially those in northern, smoggy cities, are most likely to be vitamin D deficient and develop rickets. Vitamin D deficiency is especially prevalent in the winter and in the Arctic and Antarctic regions of the world.[30] To ensure an adequate vitamin D status, supplements may be needed. The body's vitamin D supplies from summer synthesis alone are insufficient to meet winter needs.

The ultraviolet rays from tanning lamps and tanning booths may also stimulate vitamin D synthesis, but the hazards outweigh any possible benefits. The Food and Drug Administration (FDA) warns that, if the lamps are not properly filtered, people using tanning booths risk burns, damage to the eyes and blood vessels, and skin cancer.

Vitamin D in Foods Only a few animal foods—notably, eggs, liver, butter, some fatty fish, and fortified milk—supply significant amounts of vitamin D. For those who use margarine in place of butter, fortified margarine is a significant source. Infant formulas are fortified with vitamin D in amounts adequate for daily intake as long as infants consume at least one liter (1000 milliliters) or one quart (32 ounces) of formula. Breast milk is low in vitamin D, so vitamin D supplements (10 micrograms daily) are recommended for infants who are breastfed exclusively and for those who do not receive at least 1000 milliliters of vitamin D–fortified formula per day. These sources, plus any exposure to the sun, provide infants with more than enough of this vitamin.

The fortification of milk with vitamin D is the best guarantee that children will meet their vitamin D needs and underscores the importance of milk in children's diets. Unlike milk, cheese and yogurt are not fortified with vitamin D. Vegans, and especially their children, may have low vitamin D intakes because few fortified plant sources exist. Exceptions include margarine and some soy milks. In the United States, breakfast cereals may be fortified with vitamin D, as their labels indicate.

Vitamin D Recommendations In setting the recently revised dietary recommendations, the DRI Committee assumed that no vitamin D was available from skin synthesis.[31] Advancing age increases the risk of vitamin D deficiency, so intake recommendations increase with age (see the inside front cover).

Vitamin E

Almost a century ago, researchers discovered a compound in vegetable oils necessary for reproduction in rats. The compound was named **tocopherol,** which means "offspring." Eventually, the compound was named vitamin E. When chemists isolated four tocopherol compounds, they designated them by the first four letters of the Greek alphabet: alpha, beta, gamma, and delta. Of these, alpha-tocopherol is the gold standard for vitamin E activity; recommended intakes are based on it. Four additional forms of vitamin E have also been identified and are of interest to researchers for potential roles in health.*[32] Table 8-4 later in the chapter summarizes important information about vitamin E.

Vitamin E as an Antioxidant Like beta-carotene, vitamin E is a fat-soluble antioxidant. It protects other substances from oxidation by being oxidized itself. If there is plenty of vitamin E in the membranes of cells exposed to an oxidant, chances are this vitamin will take the brunt of any oxidative attack, protecting the lipids and other vulnerable components of the membranes. Vitamin E is especially effective in preventing the oxidation of the polyunsaturated fatty acids (PUFA), but it protects all other lipids (for example, vitamin A) as well.

Vitamin E exerts an especially important antioxidant effect in the lungs, where the cells are exposed to high concentrations of oxygen. Vitamin E also protects the lungs from air pollutants that are strong oxidants.

Vitamin E may also offer protection against heart disease by protecting low-density lipoproteins (LDL) from oxidation and reducing inflammation.[33] The oxidation of LDL encourages the development of atherosclerosis; thus, in theory, halting LDL oxidation should reduce atherosclerosis. The results of controlled clinical studies in which human beings were given vitamin E supplements, however, have been disappointing.[34] Several leading vitamin E researchers point out that clinical trials of vitamin E supplementation differ in many important ways, such as the selection of subjects, the source of the vitamin, the dose of the vitamin, and the outcomes studied. Such differences may partly explain the inconsistent findings. Further research that addresses such issues may clarify the relationship between vitamin E and heart disease. In the mean time, the American Heart Association supports the consumption of antioxidant-rich fruits and vegetables, as well as whole grains and nuts, to reduce the risk of heart disease.[35]

Vitamin E Deficiency When blood concentrations of vitamin E fall below a certain critical level, the red blood cells tend to break open and spill their contents, probably because the PUFA in their membranes oxidize. This classic vitamin E–deficiency symptom, known as **erythrocyte hemolysis,** is seen in premature infants born before the transfer of vitamin E from the mother to the fetus that takes place in the last weeks of pregnancy. Vitamin E treatment corrects **hemolytic anemia.**

The few symptoms of vitamin E deficiency that have been observed in adults include loss of muscle coordination and reflexes with impaired movement, vision, and speech. Vitamin E treatment corrects all of these symptoms.

In adults, vitamin E deficiency is usually associated with diseases, notably those that cause malabsorption of fat. These include diseases of the liver, gallbladder, and pancreas, as well as various hereditary diseases involving digestion and use of nutrients

---

tocopherol (tuh-KOFF-er-ol)**:** a general term for several chemically related compounds, one of which has vitamin E activity.

erythrocyte (er-REETH-ro-cite) **hemolysis** (he-MOLL-uh-sis)**:** rupture of the red blood cells, caused by vitamin E deficiency.
> erythro = red
> cyte = cell
> hemo = blood
> lysis = breaking

hemolytic (HE-moh-LIT-ick) **anemia:** the condition of having too few red blood cells as a result of erythrocyte hemolysis.

---

*The other forms of vitamin E are tocotrienols: alpha, beta, gamma, and delta.

FIGURE 8-5 **Good Sources of Vitamin E**

Vegetable oils, some nuts and seeds such as almonds and sunflower seeds, and wheat germ are rich in vitamin E.

vitamin E in foods (handwritten note)

(see Chapters 18, 19, and 20). On rare occasions, vitamin E deficiencies develop in people without diseases. Most likely, such deficiencies occur after years of eating diets extremely low in fat; using fat substitutes, such as diet margarines and salad dressings, as the only sources of fat; or consuming diets composed of highly processed or "convenience" foods. Extensive heating in the processing of foods destroys vitamin E.

Vitamin E Toxicity Vitamin E in foods is safe to consume. Reports of vitamin E toxicity symptoms are rare across a broad range of intakes. Vitamin E supplement use has increased in recent years, however, as its antioxidant action against disease has been recognized. As a result, signs of toxicity are now known or suspected, although vitamin E toxicity is not nearly as common, and its effects are not as serious, as vitamin A or vitamin D toxicity. Extremely high doses of vitamin E interfere with the blood-clotting action of vitamin K and enhance the action of anticoagulant medications, leading to hemorrhage. The UL (1000 milligrams) for vitamin E is more than 65 times greater than the recommended intake for adults (15 milligrams).

Vitamin E in Foods Vitamin E is widespread in foods. Much of the vitamin E in the diet comes from vegetable oils and the products made from them, such as margarine, salad dressings, and shortenings (Figure 8-5). Wheat germ oil is especially rich in vitamin E. Other sources of the vitamin include whole grains, fruits, vegetables, and nuts. Because vitamin E is readily destroyed by heat processing and oxidation, fresh foods are the best sources of this vitamin.

Vitamin K

Vitamin K has long been known for its role in blood clotting, where its presence can make the difference between life and death. Vitamin K appropriately gets its name from the Danish word *koagulation* (coagulation, or "clotting"). The vitamin also participates in the synthesis of several bone proteins. Without vitamin K, the bones produce an abnormal protein that cannot effectively bind to the minerals that normally form bones.[36] An adequate intake of vitamin K helps to decrease bone turnover and protect against fractures. Vitamin K supplements seem ineffective against bone loss, however, and more research is needed to clarify the links between vitamin K and bone health.[37]

Blood Clotting At least 13 different proteins and the mineral calcium are involved in making blood clots. Vitamin K is essential for the activation of several of these proteins, among them prothrombin, the precursor of the enzyme thrombin (see Figure 8-6).

FIGURE 8-6 **Blood-Clotting Process**

When blood is exposed to air, to foreign substances, or to secretions from injured tissues, platelets (small, cell-like structures in the blood) release a phospholipid known as thromboplastin. Thromboplastin catalyzes the conversion of the inactive protein prothrombin to the active enzyme thrombin. Thrombin then catalyzes the conversion of the precursor protein fibrinogen to the active protein fibrin that forms the clot.

When any of the blood-clotting factors is lacking, **hemorrhagic disease** results. If an artery or vein is cut or broken, bleeding goes unchecked. Note, though, that hemorrhaging is not always caused by a vitamin K deficiency.

Intestinal Synthesis Like vitamin D, vitamin K can be obtained from a nonfood source. Bacteria in the intestinal tract synthesize vitamin K that the body can absorb, but people cannot depend on this source alone for their vitamin K.

Vitamin K Deficiency Vitamin K deficiency is rare, but it may occur in two circumstances. First, it may arise in conditions of fat malabsorption. Second, some medications interfere with vitamin K's synthesis and action in the body: antibiotics kill the vitamin K–producing bacteria in the intestine, and anticoagulant medications interfere with vitamin K metabolism and activity. When vitamin K deficiency does occur, it can be fatal.

Vitamin K for Newborns Newborn infants present a unique case of vitamin K nutrition. An infant is born with a **sterile** digestive tract, and some weeks pass before the vitamin K–producing bacteria become fully established in the infant's intestines. At the same time, plasma prothrombin concentrations are low (this helps prevent blood clotting during the stress of birth, which might otherwise be fatal). A single dose of vitamin K, usually in a water-soluble form, is given at birth to prevent hemorrhagic disease in the newborn.[38]

Vitamin K Toxicity Vitamin K toxicity is rare, and no adverse effects have been reported with high intakes. Therefore, a Tolerable Upper Intake Level has not been established. High doses of vitamin K can reduce the effectiveness of anticoagulant medications used to prevent blood clotting. People taking these medications should eat vitamin K–rich foods in moderation and keep their intakes consistent from day to day.

Vitamin K in Foods Many foods contain ample amounts of vitamin K, notably, green leafy vegetables, members of the cabbage family, and some vegetable oils (Figure 8-7). Other vegetables such as iceberg lettuce and green beans provide smaller amounts.

FIGURE 8-7 Good Sources of Vitamin K
Notable food sources of vitamin K include green vegetables such as collards, spinach, Bibb lettuce, brussels sprouts, and cabbage and vegetable oils such as soybean oil and canola oil.

IN SUMMARY

- The fat-soluble vitamins are vitamins A, D, E, and K.

- Vitamin A is essential to gene expression, vision, cell differentiation and integrity of epithelial tissues, immunity, and reproduction and growth.

- Vitamin A deficiency can cause blindness, sickness, and death and is a major problem worldwide.

- Overdoses of vitamin A are possible and dangerous.

- Vitamin D raises calcium and phosphorus levels in the blood. A deficiency can cause rickets in children or osteomalacia in adults.

- Vitamin D is the most toxic of all the vitamins.

- People exposed to the sun make vitamin D in their skin; fortified milk is an important food source.

- Vitamin E acts as an antioxidant in cell membranes and is especially important in the lungs, where cells are exposed to high concentrations of oxygen.

- Vitamin E may protect against heart disease, but the evidence is not conclusive yet.

- Vitamin E deficiency is rare in healthy human beings. The vitamin is widely distributed in plant foods.

- Vitamin K is necessary for blood to clot and for bone health.

hemorrhagic (hem-oh-RAJ-ik) **disease:** the vitamin K–deficiency disease in which blood fails to clot.

sterile: free of microorganisms such as bacteria.

TABLE 8-4 The Fat-Soluble Vitamins—A Summary

Vitamin Name	Chief Functions	Deficiency Symptoms	Toxicity Symptoms	Significant Sources
Vitamin A (Retinol, retinal, retinoic acid; main precursor is beta-carotene)	Vision, maintenance of cornea, epithelial cells, mucous membranes, skin; bone and tooth growth; reproduction; regulation of gene expression; immunity	Infectious diseases, night blindness, blindness (xerophthalmia), keratinization	*Chronic:* reduced bone mineral density, liver abnormalities, birth defects *Acute (single large dose or short-term):* blurred vision, nausea, vomiting, vertigo; increase of pressure inside skull; headache; muscle incoordination	*Retinol:* milk and milk products; eggs; liver *Beta-carotene:* spinach and other dark, leafy greens; broccoli; deep orange fruits (apricots, cantaloupe) and vegetables (carrots, winter squashes, sweet potatoes, pumpkin)
Vitamin D (Calciferol, cholecalciferol, dihydroxy vitamin D; precursor is cholesterol)	Mineralization of bones (raises blood calcium and phosphorus by increasing absorption from digestive tract, withdrawing calcium from bones, stimulating retention by kidneys)	Rickets, osteomalacia	Calcium imbalance (calcification of soft tissues and formation of stones)	Synthesized in the body with the help of sunshine; fortified milk, margarine, butter, and cereals; eggs; liver; fatty fish (salmon, sardines)
Vitamin E (Alpha-tocopherol, tocopherol)	Antioxidant (stabilization of cell membranes, regulation of oxidation reactions, protection of polyunsaturated fatty acids [PUFA] and vitamin A)	Erythrocyte hemolysis, nerve damage	Hemorrhagic effects	Polyunsaturated plant oils (margarine, salad dressings, shortenings), green and leafy vegetables, wheat germ, whole-grain products, nuts, seeds
Vitamin K (Phylloquinone, menaquinone)	Synthesis of blood-clotting proteins and bone proteins	Hemorrhage	None known	Synthesized in the body by GI bacteria; green, leafy vegetables; cabbage-type vegetables; vegetable oils

- The bacterial inhabitants of the digestive tract produce vitamin K, but people need vitamin K from foods as well.

- Dark green, leafy vegetables are good sources of vitamin K.

Table 8-4 offers a complete summary of the fat-soluble vitamins.

8.3 The Water-Soluble Vitamins

LO 8.3 Identify the main roles, deficiency symptoms, toxicity symptoms, and food sources of the water-soluble vitamins.

The B vitamins and vitamin C are the water-soluble vitamins. These vitamins, found in the watery compartments of foods, are distributed into water-filled compartments of the body. They are easily absorbed into the bloodstream and are just as easily excreted if their blood concentrations rise too high. Thus, the water-soluble vitamins are less likely to reach toxic concentrations in the body than are the fat-soluble vitamins. Foods never deliver excessive amounts of the water-soluble vitamins, but the large doses concentrated in vitamin supplements can reach toxic levels.

The B Vitamins

Despite advertisements that claim otherwise, the B vitamins do not give people energy. Carbohydrate, fat, and protein—the *energy-yielding* nutrients—are used for fuel. The B vitamins *help* the body use that fuel but do not serve as fuel themselves.

Coenzymes The eight B vitamins were listed in Table 8-1. Each is part of an enzyme helper known as a **coenzyme.** Some B vitamins have other important functions in the body as well, but the roles these vitamins play as parts of coenzymes are the best understood. A coenzyme is a small molecule that combines with an enzyme to make it active. With the coenzyme in place, a substance is attracted to the enzyme, and the reaction proceeds instantaneously. Figure 8-8 illustrates coenzyme action.

Active forms of five of the B vitamins—thiamin, riboflavin, niacin, pantothenic acid, and biotin—participate in the release of energy from carbohydrate, fat, and protein. A coenzyme containing vitamin B_6 assists enzymes that metabolize amino acids. Folate and vitamin B_{12} help cells to multiply. Among these cells are the red blood cells and the cells lining the GI tract—cells that deliver energy to all the others.

The eight B vitamins play many specific roles in helping the enzymes to perform thousands of different molecular conversions in the body. They must be present in every cell continuously for the cells to function as they should. As for vitamin C, its primary role, discussed later, is as an antioxidant.

B Vitamin Deficiencies In academic and clinical discussions of the vitamins, different sets of deficiency symptoms are ascribed to each individual vitamin. Such clear-cut symptoms, however, are found only in laboratory animals that have been fed contrived diets that lack just one nutrient. In reality, a deficiency of any single B vitamin seldom shows up in isolation because people do not eat nutrients one by one; they eat foods containing mixtures of many nutrients. If a major class of foods is missing from the diet, all of the nutrients delivered by those foods will be lacking to various extents.

In only two cases have dietary deficiencies associated with single B vitamins been observed on a large scale in human populations. Diseases have been named for these deficiency states. One of them, **beriberi,** was first observed in Southeast Asia when the custom of polishing rice became widespread. Rice contributed 80 percent of the energy intake of the people in these areas, and rice bran was their principal source of thiamin. When the bran was removed to make the rice whiter, beriberi spread like wildfire.

The niacin-deficiency disease, **pellagra,** became widespread in the southern United States in the early part of the 20th century among people who subsisted on a low-protein diet with corn as a staple grain. This diet was unusual in that it supplied neither enough niacin nor enough tryptophan, its amino acid precursor, to make the niacin intake adequate.

Even in the cases of beriberi and pellagra, the deficiencies were probably not pure. When foods were provided containing the one vitamin known to be needed, other vitamins that may have been in short supply came as part of the package.

Major deficiency diseases such as pellagra and beriberi no longer occur in the United States and Canada, but more subtle deficiencies of nutrients, including the B vitamins, are sometimes observed. When they do occur, it is usually in people whose food choices are poor because of poverty, ignorance, illness, or poor health habits such as alcohol abuse.

Interdependent Systems Table 8-5, at the end of this chapter, sums up a few of the better-established facts about B vitamin deficiencies. A look at the table will make another generalization possible. Different body systems depend on these vitamins to different extents. Processes in nerves and in their responding tissues, the muscles, depend heavily on glucose metabolism and hence on thiamin, so paralysis sets in when this vitamin is lacking. But thiamin is important in all cells, not just in nerves and muscles. Similarly, because the red blood cells and GI tract cells divide the most rapidly, two of the first symptoms of a deficiency of folate are a type of anemia and GI tract deterioration—but again, all systems depend on folate, not just these. The list of symptoms in Table 8-5, later in the chapter, is far from complete.

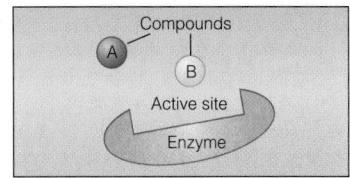

Without the coenzyme, compounds A and B do not respond to the enzyme.

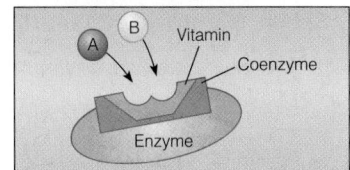

With the coenzyme in place, compounds A and B are attracted to the active site on the enzyme, and they react.

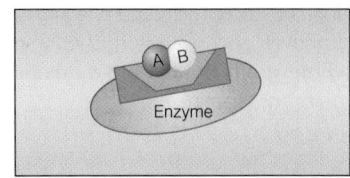

The reaction is completed with the formation of a new product. In this case, the product is AB.

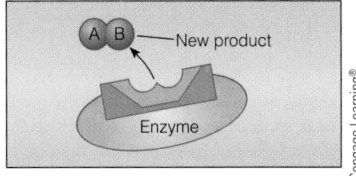

The product AB is released.

© Cengage Learning®

FIGURE 8-8 Coenzyme Action

coenzyme (co-EN-zime): a small molecule that works with an enzyme to promote the enzyme's activity. Many coenzymes contain B vitamins as part of their structure.
  co = with

beriberi: the thiamin-deficiency disease; characterized by loss of sensation in the hands and feet, muscular weakness, advancing paralysis, and abnormal heart action.

pellagra (pell-AY-gra)**:** the niacin-deficiency disease. Symptoms include the "4 Ds": diarrhea, dermatitis, dementia, and, ultimately, death.
  pellis = skin
  agra = seizure

Polara Studios, Inc

FIGURE 8-9 Good Sources of Thiamin
Nutritious foods such as pork, legumes, sunflower seeds, and enriched and whole-grain breads are valuable sources of thiamin.

refined grain: a product from which the bran, germ, and husk have been removed, leaving only the endosperm.

fortification: the addition to a food of nutrients that were either not originally present or present in insignificant amounts. Fortification can be used to correct or prevent a widespread nutrient deficiency, to balance the total nutrient profile of a food, or to restore nutrients lost in processing. The terms *fortified* and *enriched* may be used interchangeably.

enrichment: the addition to a food of nutrients to meet a specified standard. In the case of refined bread or cereal, five nutrients have been added: thiamin, riboflavin, niacin, and folate in amounts approximately equivalent to, or higher than, those originally present and iron in amounts to alleviate the prevalence of iron-deficiency anemia.

Wernicke-Korsakoff syndrome: severe thiamin deficiency in alcohol abusers; symptoms include disorientation, loss of short-term memory, jerky eye movements, and staggering gait.

B Vitamin Enrichment of Foods If the staple food of a region is made from **refined grain,** vitamin B deficiencies are especially likely. One way to protect people from deficiencies is to add nutrients to their staple food, a process known as **fortification** or **enrichment.** The enrichment of refined breads and cereals has drastically reduced the incidence of iron and B vitamin deficiencies.

The preceding discussion has shown both the great importance of the B vitamins in promoting normal, healthy functioning of all body systems and the severe consequences of deficiency. Now you may want to know how to be sure you and your clients are getting enough of these vital nutrients. The next sections present information on each B vitamin. While reading further, keep in mind that *foods* can provide all the needed nutrients and that supplements are a poor second choice. Some supplements are absurdly costly, but even if they are inexpensive, most people don't need them. Nutrition in Practice 9 discusses uses and choices of supplements in more detail.

Thiamin

All cells use thiamin, which plays a critical role in their energy metabolism. Thiamin also occupies a special site on nerve cell membranes. Consequently, as mentioned earlier, thiamin is critical to the normal functioning of the nerves and muscles.

Thiamin Deficiency and Toxicity People who fail to eat enough food to meet energy needs risk nutrient deficiencies, including thiamin deficiency. Inadequate thiamin intakes have been reported among the nation's malnourished and homeless people. Similarly, people risk thiamin deficiency when they derive most of their energy from empty-kcalorie foods and beverages. Alcohol is a good example. It contributes energy but provides few, if any, nutrients and often displaces food. In addition, alcohol impairs thiamin absorption and enhances thiamin excretion in the urine, doubling the risk of deficiency. Many alcoholics are thiamin deficient; some develop **Wernicke-Korsakoff syndrome.** No adverse effects have been associated with excesses of thiamin, and no UL has been determined.

Thiamin in Foods Thiamin occurs in small quantities in virtually all nutritious foods, but it is concentrated in only a few foods, of which pork is the most commonly eaten (Figure 8-9). Generally, thiamin needs will be met if a person keeps empty-kcalorie foods to a minimum and eats enough nutritious foods to meet energy needs. Foods chosen from the bread and cereal group should be either whole grain or enriched. Thiamin is not stored in the body to any great extent, so daily intake is important.

Riboflavin

Like thiamin, riboflavin serves as a coenzyme in many reactions, most notably in energy metabolism. Women who are carrying more than one fetus or breastfeeding more than one infant may have increased needs for riboflavin. Individuals who are extremely physically active may also have increased riboflavin needs.

Riboflavin Deficiency and Toxicity When thiamin is deficient, riboflavin may be lacking too, but its deficiency symptoms, such as cracks at the corners of the mouth and sore throat, may go undetected because those of thiamin are more severe. A diet that remedies riboflavin deficiency invariably contains some thiamin and so clears up both deficiencies. Excesses of riboflavin appear to cause no harm, and no UL has been established.

Riboflavin in Foods Unlike thiamin, riboflavin is not evenly distributed among the food groups. The major contributors of riboflavin to people's diets are milk and milk products, followed by enriched breads, cereals, and other grain products (Figure 8-10). Green vegetables (broccoli, turnip greens, asparagus, and spinach) and meats are also contributors. The riboflavin richness of milk and milk products is a good reason to include these foods in every day's meals. No other commonly eaten food can make such a substantial contribution. People who omit milk and milk products from their diets can substitute generous servings of dark green, leafy vegetables. Among the meats, liver and heart are the richest sources, but all lean meats, as well as eggs, offer some riboflavin.

Effects of Light Riboflavin is light sensitive; the ultraviolet rays of the sun or of fluorescent lamps can destroy it, as can irradiation. For this reason, milk is often sold in cardboard or opaque plastic containers to protect the riboflavin in the milk from light. In contrast, riboflavin is heat stable, so ordinary cooking does not destroy it.

Niacin

Like thiamin and riboflavin, niacin participates in the energy metabolism of every body cell. Niacin is unique among the B vitamins in that the body can make it from protein. The amino acid tryptophan can be converted to niacin in the body: 60 milligrams of tryptophan yield 1 milligram of niacin. Recommended intakes are therefore stated in **niacin equivalents (NE).** A food containing 1 mg of niacin and 60 mg of tryptophan contains the niacin equivalent of 2 mg, or 2 mg NE.

Naturally occurring niacin from foods causes no harm. Certain forms of niacin supplements taken in doses three to four times the dietary recommendation or larger cause "niacin flush," a dilation of the capillaries of the skin with perceptible tingling that, if intense, can be painful.[39] The Tolerable Upper Intake Level (35 milligrams NE) is based on flushing as the critical adverse effect.

Niacin Used as a Medication A normal dose of a nutrient that clears up a deficiency condition exerts a *physiological* effect, whereas a large dose of a nutrient that overwhelms a body system (like a drug) exerts a *pharmacological* one. Physicians sometimes use diet and large doses of a form of niacin (nicotinic acid) to lower blood cholesterol in the treatment of atherosclerosis. When used this way, niacin becomes a pharmacological agent, a drug. As with any medication, self-dosing with niacin is ill advised; large doses may injure the liver and produce some symptoms of diabetes.[40]

Niacin in Foods Meat, poultry, fish, legumes, and enriched and whole grains contribute about half the niacin equivalents most people consume (Figure 8-11). Among the vegetables, mushrooms, asparagus, and potatoes are the richest niacin sources. Niacin is less vulnerable to losses during food preparation and storage than other water-soluble vitamins. Being fairly heat resistant, niacin can withstand reasonable cooking times, but like other water-soluble vitamins, it will leach into cooking water.

Pantothenic Acid and Biotin

Two other B vitamins—pantothenic acid and biotin—are also important in energy metabolism. Pantothenic acid was first recognized as a substance that stimulates growth. It is a component of a key enzyme that makes possible the release of energy from the energy nutrients. Pantothenic acid is involved in more than 100 different steps in the synthesis of lipids, neurotransmitters, steroid hormones, and hemoglobin. Biotin plays an important role in metabolism as a coenzyme that carries carbon dioxide. Emerging evidence indicates that biotin participates in other processes such as gene expression and cell signaling and in the structure of DNA-binding proteins in the cell nucleus.[41]

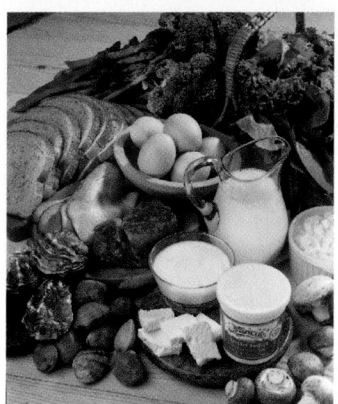

FIGURE 8-10 Good Sources of Riboflavin
Milk and milk products supply much (about 50 percent) of the riboflavin in people's diets, but meats, eggs, green vegetables, and enriched and whole-grain breads and cereals are good sources, too.

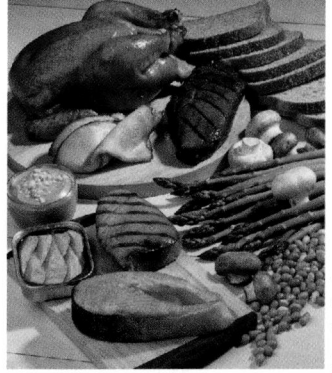

FIGURE 8-11 Good Sources of Niacin
Niacin-rich foods include meat, fish, poultry, and peanut butter, as well as enriched breads and cereals and a few vegetables.

niacin equivalents (NE): the amount of niacin present in food, including the niacin that can theoretically be made from tryptophan, its precursor, present in the food.

Pantothenic Acid and Biotin in Foods Both pantothenic acid and biotin are more widespread in foods than the other vitamins discussed so far. There seems to be no danger that people who consume a variety of foods will suffer deficiencies. Claims that pantothenic acid and biotin are needed in pill form to prevent or cure disease conditions are at best unfounded and at worst intentionally misleading.

Biotin Deficiency Biotin deficiencies are rare but have been reported in adults fed artificially by vein without biotin supplementation. Researchers can induce biotin deficiency in animals or human beings by feeding them raw egg whites, which contain the protein avidin, which binds biotin and prevents its absorption.

Vitamin B$_6$

A surge of research interest in the past several decades has not only revealed new knowledge about vitamin B$_6$ but has also raised new questions. Most recently, research interest has centered on a possible role for vitamin B$_6$ in the treatment of disease.[42]

Metabolic Roles of Vitamin B$_6$ Vitamin B$_6$ has long been known to play roles in carbohydrate, fatty acid, and protein and amino acid metabolism.[43] In the cells, vitamin B$_6$ helps convert one kind of amino acid, which the cells have in abundance, to other nonessential amino acids that the cells lack. It also aids in the conversion of the amino acid tryptophan to niacin and plays important roles in the synthesis of hemoglobin and neurotransmitters, the communication molecules of the brain. Vitamin B$_6$ also assists in releasing stored glucose from glycogen and thus contributes to the regulation of blood glucose.

Vitamin B$_6$ Deficiency Vitamin B$_6$ deficiency is expressed in general symptoms, such as weakness, depression, confusion, and irritability. Other symptoms include a greasy, flaky dermatitis; anemia; and, in advanced cases, convulsions. A shortage of vitamin B$_6$ may also weaken the immune response. Some evidence links low vitamin B$_6$ intakes with increased risk of some cancers and cardiovascular disease; more research is needed to clarify these associations.[44]

Vitamin B$_6$ Toxicity For years it was believed that vitamin B$_6$, like other water-soluble vitamins, could not reach toxic concentrations in the body. Toxic effects of vitamin B$_6$ became known when a physician reported them in women who had been taking more than 2 *grams* of vitamin B$_6$ daily (20 times the current UL of 100 *milligrams*) for 2 months or more, attempting to cure premenstrual syndrome. The first symptom of toxicity was numb feet; then the women lost sensation in their hands; then they became unable to walk. The women recovered after they discontinued the supplements.

Vitamin B$_6$ Recommendations The RDA for vitamin B$_6$ is based on the amounts needed to maintain adequate levels of its coenzymes. Unlike other water-soluble vitamins, vitamin B$_6$ is stored extensively in muscle tissue. Research does not support claims that large doses of vitamin B$_6$ enhance muscle strength or physical endurance.

Vitamin B$_6$ in Foods The richest food sources of vitamin B$_6$ are protein-rich meat, fish, and poultry (Figure 8-12). Potatoes, a few other vegetables, and some fruits are good sources, too. Foods lose vitamin B$_6$ when heated.

Folate

The term *folate* refers to two forms of the B vitamin: the naturally occurring folates in foods and folic acid, which is the form used in dietary supplements and fortified foods. Folate is active in cell division. During periods of rapid growth and cell division, such as pregnancy and adolescence, folate needs increase, and deficiency is especially likely. When a deficiency occurs, the replacement of the rapidly dividing cells of the blood and

Polara Studios, Inc.

FIGURE 8-12 Good Sources of Vitamin B$_6$
Most protein-rich foods such as meat, fish, and poultry provide ample vitamin B$_6$; some vegetables and fruits are good sources, too.

the GI tract falters. Not surprisingly, then, two of the first symptoms of a folate deficiency are a type of anemia and GI tract deterioration (see Table 8-5 later in the chapter).

Folate, Alcohol, and Drugs Of all the vitamins, folate appears to be the most vulnerable to interactions with alcohol and other drugs. As Nutrition in Practice 20 describes, alcohol-addicted people risk folate deficiency because alcohol impairs folate's absorption and increases its excretion. Furthermore, as people's alcohol intakes rise, their folate intakes decline. Many medications, including aspirin, oral contraceptives, and anticonvulsants, also impair folate status. Smoking exerts a negative effect on folate status as well.

Folate and Neural Tube Defects Research studies confirm the importance of folate in preventing **neural tube defects (NTD).** The brain and spinal cord develop from the neural tube, and defects in its orderly formation during the early weeks of pregnancy may result in various central nervous system disorders and death. Folate supplements taken before conception and continued throughout the first trimester of pregnancy can prevent NTD. For this reason, all women of childbearing age who are capable of becoming pregnant should consume 400 micrograms (0.4 milligrams) of folic acid daily from supplements, fortified foods, or both, *in addition* to eating folate-rich foods. Chapter 11 includes a figure of a neural tube defect and further discussion.

Folate status improves more with supplementation or fortification than with a dietary intake that meets recommendations. NTDs arise early in pregnancy before most women realize they are pregnant, and most women eat too few fruits and vegetables to supply even half the folate needed to prevent NTD.[45] For these reasons, the FDA mandated that enriched grain products (flour, cornmeal, pasta, and rice) be fortified with folic acid, which is an especially absorbable synthetic form of folate. Bread products, flour, corn grits, and pasta must be fortified with 140 µg folate per 100 g of food (about ½ c cooked food or 1 slice of bread).

Fortification has improved folate status in women of childbearing age and lowered the number of NTDs that occur each year.[46] Folate fortification also raises safety concerns, however. High doses of folate can complicate the diagnosis of vitamin B_{12} deficiency, as discussed later. Other suspected but unconfirmed potential harms from high blood folic acid levels include suppression of normal immune functioning and increased cancer risks.[47] The DRI committee set a Tolerable Upper Intake Level of 1000 micrograms per day from fortified foods or supplements. Except for individuals who take supplements with more than 400 micrograms of folic acid, few people (less than 3 percent of the U.S. population) exceed the Tolerable Upper Intake Level for folic acid.[48] Thus, researchers conclude that the current level of fortification of the food supply appears to be safe.

Folate in Foods As Figure 8-13 (on p. 208) shows, the best food sources of folate are liver, legumes, beets, and leafy green vegetables (the vitamin's name suggests the word *foliage*). Among the fruits, oranges, orange juice, and cantaloupe are the best sources. With fortification, grain products are good sources of folate, too. Heat and oxidation during cooking and storage can destroy up to half of the folate in foods.

The difference in absorption between naturally occurring food folate and synthetic folate that enriches foods and is added to supplements must be considered when establishing folate recommendations. **Dietary folate equivalents (DFE)** convert all forms of folate into units that are equivalent to the folate in foods. Box 8-1 (on p. 208) describes how to estimate dietary folate equivalents.

Vitamin B_{12}

Vitamin B_{12} and folate share a special relationship: vitamin B_{12} assists folate in cell division. Their roles intertwine, but each performs a specific task that the other cannot accomplish.

neural tube defects (NTD): malformations of the brain, spinal cord, or both that occur during embryonic development. The two main types of neural tube defects are *spina bifida* (literally, "split spine") and *anencephaly* ("no brain").

dietary folate equivalents (DFE): the amount of folate available to the body from naturally occurring sources, fortified foods, and supplements, accounting for differences in bioavailability from each source.

BEEF LIVER (cooked)
3 oz = 221 μg DFE

PINTO BEANS (cooked)
$^1/_2$ c = 146 μg DFE

ASPARAGUS
$^1/_2$ c = 134 μg DFE

AVOCADO
$^1/_2$ cubed = 61 μg DFE

LENTILS (cooked)
$^1/_2$ c = 179 μg DFE

SPINACH (raw)
1 c = 58 μg DFE

ENRICHED CEREAL
(ready-to-eat)[b]
$^3/_4$ c = 676 μg DFE

BEETS
$^1/_2$ c = 68 μg DFE

© 2016 Cengage Learning®

[a]Folate recommendations are expressed in dietary folate equivalents (DFE). Note that for natural folate sources, 1 microgram equals 1 DFE; for enriched sources, 1 microgram equals 1.7 DFE. These foods provide 10 percent or more of the folate Daily Value in a serving. For a 2000-kcalorie diet, the DV is 400 micrograms per day.
[b]Some highly enriched cereals may provide 400 or more micrograms DFE in a serving.

FIGURE 8-13 Good Sources of Folate[a]

How To   BOX 8-1 ESTIMATE DIETARY FOLATE EQUIVALENTS

Folate is expressed in terms of dietary folate equivalents (DFE) because synthetic folate from supplements and fortified foods is absorbed at almost twice (1.7 times) the rate of naturally occurring folate from other foods. Use the following equation to calculate:

DFE = μg food folate + (1.7 × μg synthetic folate)

Consider, for example, a pregnant woman who takes a supplement and eats a bowl of fortified corn flakes, two slices of fortified bread, and one cup of fortified pasta. From the supplement and fortified foods, she obtains synthetic folate:

Supplement	100 μg folate
Fortified corn flakes	100 μg folate
Fortified bread	40 μg folate
Fortified pasta	60 μg folate
	300 μg folate

To calculate the DFE, multiply the amount of synthetic folate by 1.7:

300 μg × 1.7 = 510 μg DFE

Now add the naturally occurring folate from the other foods in her diet—in this example, another 90 micrograms of folate.

510 μg DFE + 90 μg = 600 mg DFE

Notice that if we had not converted synthetic folate from supplements and fortified foods to DFE, this woman's intake would appear to fall short of the 600 micrograms recommended for pregnancy (300 μg + 90 μg = 390 μg). But as this example shows, her intake does meet the recommendation. At this time, supplement and fortified food labels list folate in micrograms only, not micrograms DFE, making such calculations necessary.

Vitamin B$_{12}$, Folate, and Cell Division Vitamin B$_{12}$ (in coenzyme form) stands by to accept carbon groups from folate as folate removes them from other compounds. The passing of these carbon groups from folate to vitamin B$_{12}$ regenerates the active form of folate so that it can continue its dismantling tasks. In the absence of vitamin B$_{12}$, folate is trapped in its inactive, metabolically useless form, unable to do its job. When folate is either trapped due to a vitamin B$_{12}$ deficiency or unavailable due to a deficiency of folate itself, cells that are growing most rapidly—notably, the blood cells—are the first to be affected. Thus, a deficiency of either nutrient—vitamin B$_{12}$ or folate—impairs maturation of the blood cells and produces **macrocytic anemia**. The anemia is identifiable by microscopic examination of the blood, which reveals many large, immature red blood cells. Either vitamin B$_{12}$ or folate will clear up the anemia.

macrocytic anemia: large-cell anemia; also known as *megaloblastic anemia.*

Vitamin B$_{12}$ and the Nervous System Although either vitamin will reverse the anemia caused by vitamin B$_{12}$ deficiency, providing folate when vitamin B$_{12}$ is needed is disastrous to the nervous system. The reason: vitamin B$_{12}$ also helps maintain nerve fibers. A vitamin B$_{12}$ deficiency can ultimately result in devastating neurological symptoms, undetectable by a blood test. A deceptive folate "cure" of the anemia in vitamin B$_{12}$ deficiency allows the nerve deterioration to progress, leading to paralysis and permanent nerve damage. Evidence is mounting to suggest that even a marginal vitamin B$_{12}$ deficiency may impair mental functioning in the elderly, worsening dementia.[49] This interaction between folate and vitamin B$_{12}$ raises safety concerns about the use of folate supplements and fortification of foods. In an effort to prevent excessive folate intakes that could mask symptoms of a vitamin B$_{12}$ deficiency, the FDA specifies the exact amounts of folic acid that can be added to enriched foods.

The way folate masks vitamin B$_{12}$ deficiency underlines a point already made several times: it takes a skilled diagnostician to make a correct diagnosis. A person who self-diagnoses on the basis of a single observed symptom takes a serious risk.

Vitamin B$_{12}$ Absorption Absorption of vitamin B$_{12}$ requires **intrinsic factor,** a compound made by the stomach with instructions from the genes. With the help of the stomach's acid to liberate vitamin B$_{12}$ from the food proteins that bind it, intrinsic factor attaches to the vitamin and the complex is absorbed into the bloodstream.

A few people have an inherited defect in the gene for intrinsic factor, which makes vitamin B$_{12}$ absorption abnormal beginning in mid-adulthood. Many others lose the ability to produce enough stomach acid and intrinsic factor to allow efficient absorption of vitamin B$_{12}$ in later life due to **atrophic gastritis.** In these cases, vitamin B$_{12}$ must be supplied by injection to bypass the defective absorptive system. The anemia of the vitamin B$_{12}$ deficiency caused by lack of intrinsic factor is known as **pernicious anemia.**

Vitamin B$_{12}$ in Foods A unique characteristic of vitamin B$_{12}$ is that it is found almost exclusively in foods derived from animals. People who eat meat are guaranteed an adequate intake, and lacto-ovo vegetarians (who consume milk, cheese, and eggs) are also protected from deficiency. It is a myth, however, that fermented soy products, such as miso (a soybean paste), or sea algae, such as spirulina, provide vitamin B$_{12}$ in its active form. Extensive research shows that the amounts of vitamin B$_{12}$ listed on the labels of these plant products are inaccurate and misleading because the vitamin B$_{12}$ in these products occurs in an inactive, unavailable form. Vegans need a reliable source such as vitamin B$_{12}$-fortified soy milk or vitamin B$_{12}$ supplements. Some loss of vitamin B$_{12}$ occurs when foods are heated in microwave ovens.

Vitamin B$_{12}$ Deficiency in Vegans Vegans are at special risk for undetected vitamin B$_{12}$ deficiency for two reasons: first, they receive none in their diets, and second, they consume large amounts of folate in the vegetables they eat. Because the body can store many times the amount of vitamin B$_{12}$ used each day, a deficiency may take years to develop in a new vegetarian. When a deficiency does develop, though, it may progress to a dangerous extreme because the deficiency of vitamin B$_{12}$ may be masked by the high folate intake.

Worldwide, vitamin B$_{12}$ deficiency among vegetarians is a growing problem.[50] A pregnant or lactating vegetarian woman who eats no foods of animal origin should be aware that her infant can develop a vitamin B$_{12}$ deficiency, even if the mother appears healthy. Breastfed infants born to vegan mothers with low concentrations of vitamin B$_{12}$ in their breast milk can develop severe neurological symptoms such as seizures and cognitive problems.

Non–B Vitamins

Other compounds are sometimes inappropriately called B vitamins because, like the true B vitamins, they serve as coenzymes in metabolism. Even if they were essential, however, supplements would be unnecessary because these compounds are abundant in foods.

intrinsic factor: a substance secreted by the stomach cells that binds with vitamin B$_{12}$ in the small intestine to aid in the absorption of vitamin B$_{12}$. Anemia that reflects a vitamin B$_{12}$ deficiency caused by lack of intrinsic factor is known as *pernicious anemia.*

intrinsic = on the inside

atrophic gastritis (a-TROH-fik gas-TRY-tis)**:** a chronic inflammation of the stomach accompanied by a diminished size and functioning of the stomach's mucous membrane and glands.

pernicious (per-NISH-us) **anemia:** a blood disorder that reflects a vitamin B$_{12}$ deficiency caused by lack of intrinsic factor and characterized by large, immature red blood cells and damage to the nervous system (*pernicious* means "highly injurious or destructive").

Inositol, Choline, and Carnitine Among the non–B vitamins are a trio of substances known as inositol, choline, and carnitine. Researchers are exploring the possibility that these substances may be essential. Thus far, only choline has been assigned an Adequate Intake value.

Other Non–B Vitamins Other substances have also been mistaken for essential nutrients. They include para-aminobenzoic acid (PABA), bioflavonoids (vitamin P or hesperidin), and ubiquinone. Other names you may hear are "vitamin B_{15}" (a hoax) and "vitamin B_{17}" (laetrile, a fake cancer-curing drug and not a vitamin by any stretch of the imagination). There is, however, one other water-soluble vitamin of great interest and importance—vitamin C.

Vitamin C

More than 300 years ago, any man who joined the crew of a seagoing ship knew he had only half a chance of returning alive—not because he might be slain by pirates or die in a storm, but because he might contract the dread disease **scurvy.** Then, a physician with the British navy found that citrus fruits could cure the disease, and thereafter, all ships were required to carry lime juice for every sailor. (This is why British sailors are still called "limeys" today.) In the 1930s, the antiscurvy factor in citrus fruits was isolated from lemon juice and named **ascorbic acid.** Today, hundreds of millions of vitamin C pills are produced in pharmaceutical laboratories.

Metabolic Roles of Vitamin C Vitamin C's action defies a simple, tidy description. It plays many important roles in the body, and its modes of action differ in different situations.

Vitamin C's Role in Collagen Formation The best-understood action of vitamin C is its role in helping to form **collagen,** the single most important protein of connective tissue. Collagen serves as the matrix on which bone is formed, the material of scars, and an important part of the "glue" that attaches one cell to another. This latter function is especially important in the artery walls, which must expand and contract with each beat of the heart, and in the walls of the capillaries, which are thin and fragile.

Vitamin C as an Antioxidant Vitamin C is also an important antioxidant.[51] Recall that the antioxidants beta-carotene and vitamin E protect fat-soluble substances from oxidizing agents; vitamin C protects water-soluble substances the same way. By being oxidized itself, vitamin C regenerates already-oxidized substances such as iron and copper to their original, active form. In the intestines, it protects iron from oxidation and so enhances iron absorption. In the cells and body fluids, it helps to protect other molecules, including the fat-soluble compounds vitamin A, vitamin E, and the polyunsaturated fatty acids.

Vitamin C in Amino Acid Metabolism Vitamin C is also involved in the metabolism of several amino acids. Some of these amino acids end up being used to make substances of great importance in body functioning, among them the neurotransmitter norepinephrine and the hormone thyroxine. Vitamin C also plays a role in the production of carnitine, important for transporting fatty acids within cells.

Role of Stress During stress, the adrenal glands release large quantities of vitamin C together with the stress hormones epinephrine and norepinephrine. The vitamin's exact role in the stress reaction remains unclear, but physical stresses (described in a later section) raise vitamin C needs.

Vitamin C as a Possible Antihistamine Newspaper headlines touting vitamin C as a cure for colds have appeared frequently over the years. Some research suggests

scurvy: the vitamin C–deficiency disease.

ascorbic acid: one of the two active forms of vitamin C. Many people refer to vitamin C by this name.
  a = without
  scorbic = having scurvy

collagen: the characteristic protein of connective tissue.
  kolla = glue
  gennan = produce

that vitamin C (2 g per day for two weeks) may reduce the severity and duration of cold and allergy symptoms by reducing blood histamine concentrations. In other words, vitamin C acts as an antihistamine. If further research confirms vitamin C's antihistamine effect, its use may permit people to rely less heavily on antihistamine drugs when suffering from cold and allergy symptoms.

Vitamin C's Role in Cancer Prevention and Treatment The role of vitamin C in the prevention and treatment of cancer is still being studied.[52] Evidence to date indicates that foods containing vitamin C probably protect against cancer of the esophagus. The correlation may reflect not just an association with vitamin C but the broader benefits of a diet rich in fruits and vegetables and low in fat. It does not support the taking of vitamin C supplements to prevent or treat cancer.

Vitamin C Deficiency When intake of vitamin C is inadequate, the body's vitamin C pool dwindles, and the blood vessels show the first deficiency signs. The gums around the teeth begin to bleed easily, and capillaries under the skin break spontaneously, producing pinpoint hemorrhages. As vitamin C concentrations continue to fall, the symptoms of scurvy appear. Muscles, including the heart muscle, may degenerate. The skin becomes rough, brown, scaly, and dry. Wounds fail to heal because scar tissue will not form without collagen. Bone rebuilding falters; the ends of the long bones become softened, malformed, and painful; and fractures occur. The teeth may become loose in the jawbone and fall out. Anemia and infections are common. Sudden death is likely, perhaps because of massive bleeding into the joints and body cavities.

It takes only 10 or so milligrams of vitamin C a day to prevent scurvy, and not much more than that to cure it. Once diagnosed, scurvy is readily reversible with moderate doses, in the neighborhood of 100 milligrams per day. Such an intake is easily achieved by including vitamin C–rich foods in the diet.

Vitamin C Toxicity The easy availability of vitamin C in pill form and the publication of books recommending vitamin C to prevent everything from the common cold to life-threatening cancer have led thousands of people to take large doses of vitamin C. Not surprisingly, instances of vitamin C causing harm have surfaced. The Tolerable Upper Intake Level for vitamin C is 2000 milligrams per day.

Some of the suspected toxic effects of excess vitamin C have not been confirmed, but others have been seen often enough to warrant concern. Nausea, abdominal cramps, and diarrhea are often reported. Several instances of interference with medical regimens are known. Large amounts of vitamin C excreted in the urine obscure the results of tests used to detect diabetes. People taking anticoagulants may unwittingly counteract the effect of these medications if they also take massive doses of vitamin C. Large doses of vitamin C can also enhance iron absorption too much, resulting in iron overload (see Chapter 9).

People with sickle-cell anemia may be especially vulnerable to excessive intakes of vitamin C. Those who have a tendency toward **gout,** as well as those who have a genetic abnormality that alters the way they metabolize vitamin C, are more prone to forming kidney stones if they take large doses of vitamin C.

Recommended Intakes of Vitamin C The vitamin C RDA is 90 milligrams for men and 75 milligrams for women. These amounts are far higher than the 10 milligrams per day needed to prevent the symptoms of scurvy. In fact, they are close to the amount at which the body's pool of vitamin C is full to overflowing: about 100 milligrams per day.

Special Needs for Vitamin C As is true of all nutrients, unusual circumstances may raise vitamin C needs. Among the stresses known to do so are infections; burns; surgery; extremely high or low temperatures; toxic doses of heavy metals, such as

gout (GOWT): a metabolic disease in which crystals of uric acid precipitate in the joints.

SWEET RED PEPPER
(chopped, raw)
1/2 c = 95 mg

BRUSSELS SPROUTS
(cooked)
1/2 c = 48 mg

GRAPEFRUIT
1/2 c = 43 mg

SWEET POTATO
1/2 c = 20 mg

ORANGE JUICE
1/2 c = 62 mg

GREEN PEPPERS
(chopped, raw)
1/2 c = 60 mg

BROCCOLI (cooked)
1/2 c = 51 mg

STRAWBERRIES
1/2 c = 43 mg

BOK CHOY
1/2 c = 22 mg

© 2016 Cengage Learning®

aThese foods provide 10 percent or more of the vitamin C Daily Value in a serving.

FIGURE 8-14 Good Sources of Vitamin Cª

lead, mercury, and cadmium; and the chronic use of certain medications, including aspirin, barbiturates, and oral contraceptives. Smoking, too, has adverse effects on vitamin C status. Cigarette smoke contains oxidants, which deplete this potent antioxidant. Accordingly, the vitamin C recommendation for smokers is set high, at 125 milligrams for men and 110 milligrams for women.

Safe Limits Few instances warrant the taking of more than 100 to 300 milligrams of vitamin C a day. The risks may not be great for adults who dose themselves with 1 to 2 grams a day, but those taking more than 2 grams, and especially those taking more than 3 grams per day, should be aware of the distinct possibility of harm.

Vitamin C in Foods The inclusion of intelligently selected fruits and vegetables in the daily diet guarantees a generous intake of vitamin C. Even those who wish to ingest amounts well above the RDA can easily meet their goals by eating certain foods (see Figure 8-14). Citrus fruits are rightly famous for their vitamin C contents. Certain other fruits and vegetables are also rich sources: cantaloupe, strawberries, broccoli, and brussels sprouts. No animal foods other than organ meats, such as chicken liver and kidneys, contain vitamin C. The humble potato is an important source of vitamin C in Western countries, where potatoes are eaten so frequently that they make substantial contributions overall: about 20 percent of the vitamin C in the average diet. Vitamin C in foods is easily oxidized, so store cut produce and juices in airtight containers.

Vitamin C and Iron Absorption Eating foods containing vitamin C at the same meal with foods containing iron can double or triple the absorption of iron from those foods. This strategy is highly recommended for women and children, whose energy intakes are not large enough to guarantee that they will get enough iron from the foods they eat. Iron is discussed in Chapter 9.

IN SUMMARY

▪ The B vitamins and vitamin C are the water-soluble vitamins.

▪ Each B vitamin is part of an enzyme helper known as a coenzyme.

- As parts of coenzymes, the B vitamins assist in the release of energy from glucose, amino acids, and fats and help in many other body processes.

- Folate and vitamin B_{12} are important in cell division.

- Vitamin C's primary role is as an antioxidant.

- Historically, famous B vitamin–deficiency diseases are beriberi (thiamin) and pellagra (niacin). The vitamin C–deficiency disease is known as scurvy.

Table 8-5 summarizes functions, deficiency and toxicity symptoms, and food sources of the water-soluble vitamins.

TABLE 8-5 The Water-Soluble Vitamins—A Summary

Vitamin Name	Chief Functions	Deficiency Symptoms	Toxicity Symptoms	Significant Sources
Thiamin (Vitamin B_1)	Part of a coenzyme used in energy metabolism	Beriberi (edema or muscle wasting), anorexia and weight loss, neurological disturbances, muscular weakness, heart enlargement and failure	None reported	Enriched, fortified, or whole-grain products; pork
Riboflavin (Vitamin B_2)	Part of coenzymes used in energy metabolism	Inflammation of the mouth, skin, and eyelids; sensitivity to light; sore throat	None reported	Milk products; enriched, fortified, or whole-grain products; liver
Niacin (Nicotinic acid, nicotinamide, niacinamide, vitamin B_3; precursor is dietary tryptophan, an amino acid)	Part of coenzymes used in energy metabolism	Pellagra (diarrhea, dermatitis, and dementia)	Niacin flush, liver damage, impaired glucose tolerance	Milk, eggs, meat, poultry, fish, whole-grain and enriched breads and cereals, nuts, and all protein-containing foods
Biotin	Part of a coenzyme used in energy metabolism	Skin rash, hair loss, neurological disturbances	None reported	Widespread in foods; GI bacteria synthesis
Pantothenic acid	Part of a coenzyme used in energy metabolism	Digestive and neurological disturbances	None reported	Widespread in foods
Vitamin B_6 (Pyridoxine, pyridoxal, pyridoxamine)	Part of coenzymes used in amino acid and fatty acid metabolism	Scaly dermatitis, depression, confusion, convulsions, anemia	Nerve degeneration, skin lesions	Meats, fish, poultry, potatoes, legumes, noncitrus fruits, fortified cereals, liver, soy products
Folate (Folic acid, folacin, pteroylglutamic acid)	Activates vitamin B_{12}; helps synthesize DNA for new cell growth	Anemia; smooth, red tongue; mental confusion; elevated homocysteine	Masks vitamin B_{12} deficiency	Fortified grains, leafy green vegetables, legumes, seeds, liver
Vitamin B_{12} (Cobalamin)	Activates folate; helps synthesize DNA for new cell growth; protects nerve cells	Anemia; nerve damage and paralysis	None reported	Animal-derived foods (meat, fish, poultry, shellfish, milk, cheese, eggs), fortified cereals
Vitamin C (Ascorbic acid)	Synthesis of collagen, carnitine, hormones, neurotransmitters; antioxidant	Scurvy (bleeding gums, pinpoint hemorrhages, abnormal bone growth, and joint pain)	Diarrhea, GI distress	Citrus fruits, cabbage-type and dark green vegetables, cantaloupe, strawberries, lettuce, tomatoes, potatoes, papayas, mangoes

Your Diet

Vitamins

A diet that supplies nutrient-dense foods from each food group can provide ample vitamins. Complete this activity to learn whether your food choices include good sources of vitamins.

- Review the nutrient analysis reports for your 24-hour food intake from the Chapter 1 Your Diet exercise (or another 24-hour period that you have recorded and entered into an online diet analysis tool). How do your vitamin intakes for that day compare to your RDA/AI?

Remember that vitamin intakes over time are much more important than whether you meet the DRI on any one day. Consider both the amounts of each food group you ate during your 24-hour intake (refer to the appropriate reports) and your typical eating pattern over a week's time and respond to these questions.

- Do you eat an adequate amount of fruits (see Table 1-4 on p. 15)? Citrus fruits offer abundant vitamin C and some folate.

Some deep orange fruits such as cantaloupe (not oranges) supply vitamin A.

- Do you choose whole or enriched grains often? These choices supply substantial amounts of thiamin, riboflavin, niacin, and folate.
- Do you consume vitamin A- and D-fortified milk products regularly? Milk products supply riboflavin and vitamins A, D, and B_{12}.
- Do you make frequent choices from the vegetable subgroups (see Table 1-6 on p. 18)? Most dark green vegetables provide significant folate and vitamins A and E. Many deep orange vegetables supply vitamin A. Legumes supply substantial folate.
- If you take supplements, list the vitamin content of each supplement. Then compare your intake with the UL for vitamins listed at the front of this book.

Clinical Applications

1. How might a vitamin deficiency weaken a client's resistance to disease?
2. Pull together information from Chapter 1 about the different food groups and the significant sources of vitamins shown in the figures throughout this chapter. Consider which vitamins might be lacking in the diet of a client who reports the following:

- Dislikes leafy, green vegetables
- Never uses milk, milk products, or cheese
- Follows a very low-fat diet
- Eats a fruit or vegetable once a day

What additional information would help you pinpoint problems with vitamin intake?

Self Check

1. Which of the following vitamins are fat soluble?
   a. Vitamins B, C, and E
   b. Vitamins B, C, D, and E
   c. Vitamins A, C, E, and K
   d. Vitamins A, D, E, and K

2. Which of the following describes fat-soluble vitamins?
   a. They include thiamin, vitamin A, and vitamin K.
   b. They cannot be stored to any great extent and so must be consumed daily.
   c. Toxic levels can be reached by consuming deep orange and dark green vegetables.
   d. They can be stored in the liver and fatty tissues and can reach toxic concentrations.

3. Night blindness and susceptibility to infection result from a deficiency of which vitamin?
   a. Niacin
   b. Vitamin C
   c. Vitamin A
   d. Vitamin B_{12}

4. Good sources of vitamin D include:
   a. eggs, fortified milk, and sunlight.
   b. citrus fruits, sweet potatoes, and spinach.
   c. leafy green vegetables, cabbage, and liver.
   d. breast milk, polyunsaturated plant oils, and citrus fruits.

5. Which of the following describes water-soluble vitamins?
   a. They all play key roles in bone maintenance.
   b. They are frequently toxic.
   c. They are stored extensively in tissues.
   d. They are easily absorbed and excreted.

6. A coenzyme is:
   a. a fat-soluble vitamin.
   b. a molecule cells use to communicate.
   c. a connective tissue protein.
   d. a molecule that combines with an enzyme to make it active.

7. Good food sources of folate include:
   a. citrus fruits, dairy products, and eggs.
   b. liver, legumes, and leafy green vegetables.
   c. dark green vegetables, corn, and cabbage.
   d. potatoes, broccoli, and whole-wheat bread.

8. Which vitamin is present only in foods of animal origin?
   a. Riboflavin
   b. Pantothenic acid
   c. Vitamin B$_{12}$
   d. The inactive form of vitamin A

9. Which of the following nutrients is an antioxidant that protects water-soluble substances from oxidizing agents?
   a. Beta-carotene   c. Vitamin C
   b. Thiamin   d. Vitamin D

10. Eating foods containing vitamin C at the same meal can increase the absorption of which mineral?
    a. Iron   c. Magnesium
    b. Calcium   d. Folate

Answers to these questions appear in Appendix H.

Notes

1. S. T. Mayne, L. M. Ferrucci, and B. Cartmel, Lessons learned from randomized clinical trials of micronutrient supplementation for cancer prevention, *Annual Review of Nutrition* 32 (2012): 369–390; L. Franzini and coauthors, Food selection based on high total antioxidant capacity improves endothelial function in a low cardiovascular risk population, *Nutrition, Metabolism, and Cardiovascular Diseases* 22 (2012): 50–57.

2. J. C. Saari, Vitamin A metabolism in rod and cone visual cycles, *Annual Review of Nutrition* 32 (2012): 125–145; A. C. Ross, Vitamin A and retinoic acid in T cell-related immunity, *American Journal of Clinical Nutrition* 96 (2012): 1166S–1172S; M. Clagett-Dame and D. Knutson, Vitamin A in reproduction and development, *Nutrients* 3 (2011): 385–428; J. von Lintig, Colors with functions: Elucidating the biochemical and molecular basis of carotenoid metabolism, *Annual Review of Nutrition* 30 (2010): 35–56; N. Noy, Between death and survival: Retinoic acid in regulation of apoptosis, *Annual Review of Nutrition* 30 (2010): 201–217.

3. A. S. Kato and R. Fujiki, Transcriptional controls by nuclear fat-soluble vitamin receptors through chromatin reorganization, *Bioscience, Biotechnology, and Biochemistry* 75 (2011): 410–413; A. C. Ross and R. Zolfaghari, Cytochrome P450s in the regulation of cellular retinoic acid metabolism, *Annual Review of Nutrition* 31 (2011): 65–87.

4. Z. Zhou and coauthors, TRIM14 is a mitochondrial adaptor that facilitates retinoic acid-inducible gene-I-like receptor-mediated innate immune response, *Proceedings of the National Academy of Sciences of the United States of American* 111 (2014): E245–E254; Noy, 2010.

5. Saari, 2012; J. von Lintig, Metabolism of carotenoids and retinoids related to vision, *Journal of Biological Chemistry* 287 (2012): 1627–1634.

6. W. Stahl and H. Sies, β-Carotene and other carotenoids in protection from sunlight, *American Journal of Clinical Nutrition* 96 (2012): 1179S–1184S.

7. Ross, 2012; Y. Yang and coauthors, Effects of vitamin A deficiency on mucosal immunity and response to intestinal infection in rats, *Nutrition* 27 (2011): 227–232.

8. Clagett-Dame and Knutson, 2011.

9. Franzini and coauthors, 2012; M. Goodman and coauthors, Clinical trials of antioxidants as cancer prevention agents: Past, present, and future, *Free Radical Biology and Medicine* 51 (2011): 1068–1084.

10. M. Ramamoorthy and coauthors, Sporadic Alzheimer Disease fibroblasts display an oxidative stress phenotype, *Free Radical Biology and Medicine* 53 (2012): 1371–1380; L. Ho and coauthors, Reducing the genetic risk of age-related macular degeneration with dietary antioxidants, zinc, and ω-3 fatty acids, *Archives of Ophthalmology* 129 (2011): 758–766.

11. World Health Organization, Micronutrient deficiencies: Vitamin A deficiency, available at www.who.int/nutrition/topics/vad/en, 2014.

12. E. Mayo-Wilson and coauthors, Vitamin A supplements for preventing mortality, illness, and blindness in children aged under 5: Systematic review and meta-analysis, *British Medical Journal* 343 (2011): d5094.

13. World Health Organization, Measles fact sheet, February 2013, www.who.int/mediacentre/factsheets/fs286/en/index.html.

14. M. M. G. Ackermans and coauthors, Vitamin A and clefting: Putative biological mechanisms, *Nutrition Reviews* 69 (2011): 613–624.

15. S. A. Tanumihardjo, Vitamin A and bone health: The balancing act, *Journal of Clinical Densitometry* 16 (2013): 414–419; H. Ahmadieh and A. Arabi, Vitamins and bone health: Beyond calcium and vitamin D, *Nutrition Reviews* 69 (2011): 584–598.

16. G. Jones, Extrarenal vitamin D activation and interactions between vitamin D$_2$, vitamin D$_3$, and vitamin D analogs, *Annual Review of Nutrition* 33 (2013): 23–44.

17. X. Cui and coauthors, Low vitamin D concentration exacerbates adult brain dysfunction, *American Journal of Clinical Nutrition* 97 (2013): 907–908; D. J. Llewellyn and coauthors, Vitamin D and risk of cognitive decline in elderly persons, *Archives of Internal Medicine* 170 (2010): 1135–1141.

18. A. S. Grimaldi and coauthors, 25(OH) Vitamin D is associated with greater muscle strength in healthy men and women, *Medicine and Science in Sports and Exercise* 45 (2013): 157–162; T. J. Hazell, J. R. DeGuire, and H. A. Weiler, Vitamin D: An overview of its role in skeletal muscle physiology in children and adolescents, *Nutrition Reviews* 70 (2012): 520–533.

19. I. Laaksi, Vitamins, infectious and chronic disease during adulthood and aging: Vitamin D and respiratory infection in adults, *Proceedings of the Nutrition Society* 71 (2012): 90–97; M. E. Sundaram and L. A. Coleman, Vitamin D and influenza, *Advances in Nutrition: An International Review Journal* 3 (2012): 517–525; M. Hewison, Vitamin D and innate and adaptive immunity, *Vitamins and Hormones* 86 (2011): 23–62; F. Baeke and coauthors, Human T lymphocytes are direct targets of 1,25-dihydroxyvitamin D3 in the immune system, *Journal of Steroid Biochemistry and Molecular Biology* 121 (2010): 221–227.

20. C. P. Earthman and coauthors, The link between obesity and low circulating 25-hydroxy vitamin D concentrations: Considerations and implications, *International Journal of Obesity* 36 (2012): 387–396; C. Ding and coauthors, Vitamin D signalling in adipose tissue, *British Journal of Nutrition* 108 (2012): 1915–1923.

21. E. Kassi and coauthors, Role of vitamin D in atherosclerosis, *Circulation* 128 (2013): 2517–2531; S. Lim and coauthors, Association of vitamin D deficiency with incidence of type 2 diabetes in high-risk Asian subjects, *American Journal of Clinical Nutrition* 97 (2013): 524–530; T. D. Cheng and coauthors, Vitamin D intake and lung cancer risk in the Women's Health Initiative, *American Journal of Clinical Nutrition* 98 (2013): 1002–1011; F. M. Yousef and coauthors, Vitamin D status and breast cancer in Saudi Arabian women: Case-control study, *American Journal of Clinical Nutrition* 98 (2013): 105–110; R. E. Stubbins, A. Hakeem, and N. P. Núñez, Using components of the vitamin D pathway to prevent and treat colon cancer, *Nutrition Reviews* 70 (2012): 721–729; G. J. Fung and coauthors, Vitamin D intake is inversely related to risk of developing metabolic syndrome in African American and white men and women over 20 y: The Coronary Artery Risk Development in Young Adults Study, *American Journal of Clinical Nutrition* 96 (2012): 24–29; I. Laaski, Vitamin D and respiratory infections in adults, *Proceedings of the Nutrition Society* 71 (2012): 90–97; Y. Liss and W. H. Frishman, Vitamin D: A cardioprotective agent? *Cardiology in Review* 20 (2012): 38–44; A. Zittermann and coauthors, Vitamin D deficiency and mortality risk in the general population: A meta-analysis of prospective cohort studies, *American Journal of Clinical Nutrition* 95 (2012): 91–100; C. D. Davis and J. A. Milner, Nutrigenomics, vitamin D and cancer prevention, *Journal of Nutrigenetics and Nutrigenomics* 4 (2011): 1–11; R. Jorde and G. Grimnes, Vitamin D and metabolic health with

special reference to the effect of vitamin D on serum lipids, *Progress in Lipid Research* 50 (2011): 303–312; Hewison, 2011; E. M. Mowry, Vitamin D: Evidence for its role as a prognostic factor in multiple sclerosis, *Journal of Neurological Science* 311 (2011): 19–22; M. H. Hopkins and coauthors, Effects of supplemental vitamin D and calcium on biomarkers of inflammation in colorectal adenoma patients: A randomized, controlled clinical trial, *Cancer Prevention Research* 4 (2011): 1645–1654; K. Luong and L. T. Nguyen, Impact of vitamin D in the treatment of tuberculosis, *American Journal of Medical Sciences* 341 (2011): 493–498; A. E. Millen and coauthors, Vitamin D status and early age-related macular degeneration in postmenopausal women, *Archives of Ophthalmology* 129 (2011): 481–489; N. Parekh, Protective role of vitamin D against age-related macular degeneration: A hypothesis, *Topics in Clinical Nutrition* 25 (2010): 290–301; A. G. Pittas and coauthors, Systematic review: Vitamin D and cardiometabolic outcomes, *Annals of Internal Medicine* 152 (2010): 307–314; S. Cheng and coauthors, Adiposity, cardiometabolic risk, and vitamin status: The Framingham heart study, *Diabetes* 59 (2010): 242–248.

22. U. S. Preventive Services Task Force, Vitamin D and calcium supplementation to prevent cancer and osteoporotic fractures, Draft recommendations, August 2012, available at www .uspreventiveservicestaskforce.org/uspstf12 /vitamind/vitdart.htm; M. Chung and coauthors, Vitamin D with or without calcium supplementation for prevention of cancer and fractures preventive services task force, *Annals of Internal Medicine* 155 (2011): 827–838; C. McGreevy and coauthors, New insights about vitamin D and cardiovascular disease, *Annals of Internal Medicine* 155 (2011): 820–826.

23. Committee on Dietary Reference Intakes, *Dietary Reference Intakes for Calcium and Vitamin D* (Washington, D.C.: National Academies Press, 2011), pp. 75–124.

24. C. J. Rosen, Vitamin D insufficiency, *New England Journal of Medicine* 364 (2011): 248–254.

25. A. C. Looker and coauthors, Vitamin D status: United States, 2001–2006, *NCHS Data Brief* 59 (2011): 1–8.

26. A. Arabi, R. El Rassi, G. El-Hajj Fuleihan, Hypovitaminosis D in developing countries—prevalence, risk factors and outcomes, *Nature Reviews: Endocrinology* 6 (2010): 550–561.

27. L. E. Au and coauthors, Associations of vitamin D intake with 25-hydroxyvitamin D in overweight and racially/ethnically diverse US children, *Journal of the Academy of Nutrition and Dietetics* 113 (2013): 1511–1516.

28. Committee on Dietary Reference Intakes, 2011, pp. 362–402.

29. U. S. Preventive Services Task Force, Vitamin D and calcium supplementation to prevent cancer and osteoporotic fractures, Draft recommendations, 2012; V. A. Moyer and the U. S. Preventive Services Task Force, Prevention of falls in community-dwelling older adults: U. S. Preventive Services Task Force Recommendation Statement, *Annals of Internal Medicine* 157 (2012): 197–204; H. A. Bischoff-Ferrari and coauthors, A pooled analysis of vitamin D dose requirements for fracture prevention, *New England Journal of Medicine* 367 (2012): 40–49; P. Lips and coauthors, Once-weekly dose of 8400 IU vitamin D₃ compared with placebo: Effects on neuromuscular function and tolerability in older adults with vitamin D insufficiency, *American Journal of Clinical Nutrition* 91 (2010): 985–991.

30. S. Sharma and coauthors, Vitamin D deficiency and disease risk among aboriginal Arctic populations, *Nutrition Reviews* 69 (2011): 468–478; L. M. Hall and coauthors, Vitamin D intake needed to maintain target serum 25-hydroxyvitamin D concentrations in participants with low sun exposure and dark skin pigmentation is substantially higher than current recommendations, *Journal of Nutrition* 140 (2010): 542–550.

31. Committee on Dietary Reference Intakes, 2011, pp. 362–402.

32. Q. Jiang, Natural forms of vitamin E: Metabolism, antioxidant, and anti-inflammatory acitvities and their role in disease prevention and therapy, *Free Radical Biology and Medicine,* April 3, 2014, doi: 10.1016/j.freeradbiomed.2014.03.035, epub ahead of print; R. S. Y. Wong and A. K. Radhakrishnan, Tocotrienol research: Past into present, *Nutrition Reviews* 70 (2012): 483–490; P. W. Sylvester and coauthors, The value of tocotrienols in the prevention and treatment of cancer, *Journal of the American College of Nutrition* 29 (2010): 324S–333S; B. B. Aggarwal and coauthors, Tocotrienols, the vitamin E of the 21st century: Its potential against cancer and other chronic disease, *Biochemical Pharmacology* 80 (2010): 1613–1631.

33. M. G. Traber and J. F. Stevens, Vitamins C and E: Beneficial effects from a mechanistic perspective, *Free Radical Biology and Medicine* 51 (2011): 1000–1013.

34. G. Riccioni and coauthors, Carotenoids and vitamins C and E in the prevention of cardiovascular disease, *International Journal for Vitamin and Nutrition Research* 82 (2012): 15–26.

35. R. H. Eckel and coauthors, 2013 AHA/ACC Guideline on Lifestyle management to reduce cardiovascular risk: A Report of the American College of Cardiology/American Heart Association Task Force on Practice Guidelines, *Circulation,* http:// circ.ahajournals.org/content/early/2013/11/11/01 .cir.0000437740.48606.dl.citation

36. H. Ahmadieh and A. Arabi, Vitamins and bone health: Beyond calcium and vitamin D, *Nutrition Reviews* 69 (2011): 584–598.

37. C. M. Gundberg, J. B. Lian, and S. L. Booth, Vitamin K-dependent carboxylation of osteocalcin; Friend or foe? *Advances in Nutrition* 3 (2012): 149–157.

38. G. Lippi and M. Franchini, Vitamin K in neonates: Facts and myths, *Blood Transfusion* 9 (2011): 4–9.

39. D. MacKay, J. Hathcock, and E. Guarneri, Niacin: Chemical forms, bioavailability, and health effects, *Nutrition Reviews* 70 (2012): 357–366.

40. MacKay, Hathcock, and Guarneri, 2012.

41. C. A. Perry and M. A. Caudill, Biotin: Critical for fetal growth and development yet often overlooked, *Nutrition Today* 47 (2012): 79–85.

42. L. Paul, P. M. Ueland, and J. Selhub, Mechanistic perspective on the relationship between pyridoxal 5′–phosphate and inflammation, *Nutrition Reviews* 71 (2013): 239–244; J. Shen and coauthors, Association of vitamin B-6 status with inflammation, oxidative stress, and chronic inflammatory conditions: The Boston Puerto Rican Health Study, *American Journal of Clinical Nutrition* 91 (2010): 337–342.

43. F. G. Bowling, Pyridoxine supply in human development, *Seminars in Cell and Developmental Biology* 22 (2011): 611–618.

44. L. Sharp and coauthors, Intakes of dietary folate and other B vitamins are associated with risks of esophageal adenocarcinoma, Barrett's esophagus, and reflux esophagitis, *Journal of Nutrition* 143 (2013): 1966–1973; S. C. Larsson, N. Orsini, and A. Wolk, Vitamin B₆ and risk of colorectal cancer: A meta-analysis of prospective studies, *Journal of the American Medical Association* 303 (2010): 1077–1083; J. Shen and coauthors, 2010.

45. R. L. Bailey and coauthors, Total folate and folic acid intake from foods and dietary supplements in the United States: 2003–2006, *American Journal of Clinical Nutrition* 91 (2010): 231–237.

46. Centers for Disease Control and Prevention, Folic acid data and statistics, available at www .cdc.gov/ncbddd/folicacid/data.html, updated July 7, 2010.

47. J. B. Mason, Folate consumption and cancer risk: A confirmation and some reassurance, but we're not out of the woods quite yet, *American Journal of Clinical Nutrition* 94 (2011): 965–966.

48. Bailey and coauthors, 2010; Q. Yang and coauthors, Folic acid source, usual intake, and folate and vitamin B-12 status in US adults: National Health and Nutrition Examination Survey (NHANES) 2003–2006, *American Journal of Clinical Nutrition* 91 (2010): 64–72.

49. J. G. Walker and coauthors, Oral folic acid and vitamin B-12 supplementation to prevent cognitive decline in community-dwelling older adults with depressive symptoms—The Beyond Ageing Project: A randomized controlled trial, *American Journal of Clinical Nutrition* 95 (2012): 194–203; E. Moore and coauthors, Cognitive impairment and vitamin B₁₂: A review, *International Psychogeriatrics* 24 (2012): 541–556; Y. Minn and coauthors, Sequential involvement of the nervous system in subacute combined degeneration, *Yonsei Medical Journal* 53 (2012): 276–278.

50. R. Pawlak, S. E. Lester, and T. Babatunde, The prevalence of cobalamin deficiency among vegetarians assessed by serum vitamin B₁₂: A review of literature, *European Journal of Clinical Nutrition* 68 (2014): 541–548; R. Pawlak and coauthors, How prevalent is vitamin B(12) deficiency among vegetarians? *Nutrition Reviews* 71 (2013): 110–117.

51. M. F. Garcia-Saura and coauthors, Nitroso-redox status and vascular function in marginal and severe ascorbate deficiency, *Antioxidants and Redox Signaling* 17 (2012): 937–950.

52. A. C. Mamede and coauthors, Cytotoxicity of ascorbic acid in a human colorectal adenocarcinoma cell line (WiDr): In vitro and in vivo studies, *Nutrition and Cancer* 64 (2012): 1049–1057; Traber and Stevens, 2011.

LO 8.4 Describe phytochemicals and functional foods and explain how they might defend against chronic diseases.

The wisdom of the familiar advice, "Eat your vegetables; they're good for you," stands on firmer scientific ground today than ever before as population studies around the world suggest that diets rich in vegetables and fruits protect against heart disease, cancer, and other chronic diseases.[1] We now know that the "goodness" of vegetables, fruits, and other whole foods such as legumes and grains comes not only from the nutrients they contain but also from the **phytochemicals** that they offer.[2] Phytochemicals often act as **bioactive food components,** food constituents with the ability to alter body processes. (Terms are defined in Table NP8-1.)

Vegetables, fruits, and other whole foods are the simplest examples of foods now known as **functional foods.** Functional foods provide health benefits beyond basic nutrition by altering one or more physiological processes. Foods that have been fortified, enriched, or enhanced with nutrients, phytochemicals, herbs, or other food components are also functional foods.[3] Functional foods that fit this description include orange juice fortified with calcium, folate-enriched cereal, beverages with herbal additives, and margarine enhanced with **plant sterols.** This Nutrition in Practice begins with a look at the evidence concerning the effectiveness and safety of a few selected phytochemicals in the simplest of functional foods—vegetables, fruits, and other whole foods. Then, the discussion turns to examine the most controversial of functional foods—novel foods to which phytochemicals have been added to promote health. How these foods fit into a healthy diet is still unclear.

What are phytochemicals, and what do they do?

Phytochemicals are bioactive compounds found in plants. In foods, phytochemicals impart tastes, aromas, colors, and other characteristics. They give hot peppers their burning sensation, garlic and onions their pungent flavor, chocolate its bitter tang, and tomatoes their dark red color. In the body, phytochemicals can have profound physiological effects—acting as antioxidants, mimicking hormones, stimulating or inhibiting enzymes, interfering with

TABLE NP8-1 Phytochemical and Functional Food Terms

antioxidants (anti-OX-ih-dants): compounds that protect other compounds from damaging reactions involving oxygen by themselves reacting with oxygen (*anti* means "against"; *oxy* means "oxygen"); *oxidation* is a potentially damaging effect of normal cell chemistry involving oxygen.

bioactive food components: compounds in foods, either nutrients or phytochemicals, that alter physiological processes in the body.

carotenoids (kah-ROT-eh-noyds): pigments commonly found in plants and animals, some of which have vitamin A activity. The carotenoid with the greatest vitamin A activity is beta-carotene.

flavonoids (FLAY-von-oyds): a common and widespread group of phytochemicals, with more than 6000 identified members; physiologic effects may include antioxidant, antiviral, anticancer, and other activities. Flavonoids are yellow pigments in foods; *flavus* means "yellow."

flaxseed: small brown seed of the flax plant; used in baking, cereals, and other foods. Valued in nutrition as a source of fiber, lignans, and the omega-3 fatty acid linolenic acid.

functional foods: whole, fortified, enriched, or enhanced foods that have a potentially beneficial effect on health when consumed as part of a varied diet on a regular basis at effective levels.

genistein (GEN-ih-steen): a phytoestrogen found primarily in soybeans that both mimics and blocks the action of estrogen in the body.

lignans: phytochemicals present in flaxseed, but not flaxseed oil, that are converted to phytoestrogens by intestinal bacteria and are under study as possible anticancer agents.

lutein (LO-teen): a plant pigment of yellow hue; a phytochemical believed to play roles in eye functioning and health.

lycopene (LYE-koh-peen): a pigment responsible for the red color of tomatoes and other red-hued vegetables; a phytochemical that may act as an antioxidant in the body.

organosulfur compounds: a large group of phytochemicals containing the mineral sulfur. Organosulfur phytochemicals are responsible for the pungent flavors and aromas of foods belonging to the onion, leek, chive, shallot, and garlic family and are thought to stimulate cancer defenses in the body.

phytochemicals (FIGH-toe-CHEM-ih-cals): compounds in plants that confer color, taste, and other characteristics. Some phytochemicals are bioactive food components in functional foods.

phytoestrogens (FIGHT-toe-ESS-troh-gens): phytochemicals structurally similar to human estrogen. Phytoestrogens weakly mimic or modulate estrogen in the body.

plant sterols: phytochemicals that resemble cholesterol in structure but that lower blood cholesterol by interfering with cholesterol absorption in the intestine. Plant sterols include sterol esters and stanol esters. Formerly called *phytosterols.*

resveratrol (rez-VER-ah-trol): a phytochemical of grapes under study for potential health benefits.

tofu: white curd made of soybeans, popular in Asian cuisines, and considered to be a functional food.

DNA replication, destroying bacteria, and binding physically to cell walls. Any of these actions may suppress the development of diseases, depending in part on how genetic factors interact with the phytochemicals.[4] Notably, cancer and heart disease are linked to processes involving oxygen compounds in the body, and **antioxidants** are thought to oppose these actions.[5] Table NP8-2 introduces the names, possible physiological effects, and food sources of some of the better-known phytochemicals.

TABLE NP8-2 Phytochemicals—Possible Health Effects and Food Sources

Chemical Name	Possible Effects	Food Sources
Alkylresorcinols (phenolic lipids)	May contribute to the protective effect of grains in reducing the risks of diabetes, heart disease, and some cancers	Whole-grain wheat and rye
Allicin (organosulfur compound)	Antimicrobial that may reduce ulcers; may lower blood cholesterol	Chives, garlic, leeks, onions
Capsaicin	Modulates blood clotting, possibly reducing the risk of fatal clots in heart and artery disease	Hot peppers
Carotenoids (include beta-carotene, lycopene, lutein, and hundreds of related compounds)	Act as antioxidants, possibly reducing risks of cancer and other diseases	Deeply pigmented fruits and vegetables (apricots, broccoli, cantaloupe, carrots, pumpkin, spinach, sweet potatoes, tomatoes)
Curcumin	Acts as an antioxidant and anti-inflammatory agent; may reduce blood clot formation; may inhibit enzymes that activate carcinogens	Tumeric, a yellow-colored spice
Flavonoids (include flavones, flavonols, isoflavones, catechins, and others)	Act as antioxidants; scavenge carcinogens; bind to nitrates in the stomach, preventing conversion to nitrosamines; inhibit cell proliferation	Berries, black tea, celery, citrus fruits, green tea, olives, onions, oregano, grapes, purple grape juice, soybeans and soy products, vegetables, whole wheat and other grains, wine
Genistein and daidzein (isoflavones)	Phytoestrogens that inhibit cell replication in GI tract; may reduce or elevate risk of breast, colon, ovarian, prostate, and other estrogen-sensitive cancers; may reduce cancer cell survival; may reduce risk of osteoporosis	Soybeans, soy flour, soy milk, tofu, textured vegetable protein, other legume products
Indoles (organosulfur compounds)	May trigger production of enzymes that block DNA damage from carcinogens; may inhibit estrogen action	Cruciferous vegetables such as broccoli, brussels sprouts, cabbage, cauliflower; horseradish, mustard greens, kale
Isothiocyanates (organosulfur compounds that include sulforaphane)	Act as antioxidants; inhibit enzymes that activate carcinogens; activate enzymes that detoxify carcinogens; may reduce risk of breast cancer, prostate cancer	Cruciferous vegetables such as broccoli, brussels sprouts, cabbage, cauliflower; horseradish, mustard greens, kale
Lignans	Phytoestrogens that block estrogen activity in cells, possibly reducing the risk of cancer of the breast, colon, ovaries, and prostate	Flaxseed, whole grains
Monoterpenes (including limonene)	May trigger enzyme production to detoxify carcinogens; inhibit cancer promotion and cell proliferation	Citrus fruit peels and oils
Phenolic acids	May trigger enzyme production to make carcinogens water soluble, facilitating excretion	Coffee beans, fruits (apples, blueberries, cherries, grapes, oranges, pears, prunes), oats, potatoes, soybeans
Phytic acid	Binds to minerals, preventing free-radical formation, possibly reducing cancer risk	Whole grains
Resveratrol	Acts as antioxidant; may inhibit cancer growth; reduces inflammation, LDL oxidation, and blood clot formation	Red wine, peanuts, grapes, raspberries
Saponins (glucosides)	May interfere with DNA replication, preventing cancer cells from multiplying; stimulate immune response	Alfalfa sprouts, other sprouts, green vegetables, potatoes, tomatoes
Tannins	Act as antioxidants; may inhibit carcinogen activation and cancer promotion	Black-eyed peas, grapes, lentils, red and white wine, tea

Why are phytochemicals receiving so much attention these days, and what are some examples of those in the spotlight?

Diets rich in whole grains, legumes, vegetables, and fruits seem to be protective against heart disease and cancer, but identifying *the* specific foods or components of foods that are responsible is difficult. Scientists are conducting extensive research studies to discover phytochemical connections to disease prevention, but, so far, solid evidence is generally lacking. Some of the likeliest candidates include **flavonoids** and **carotenoids** (including **lycopene**).

What are flavonoids, and in which foods are they found?

Flavonoids, a large group of phytochemicals known for their health-promoting qualities, are found in whole grains, soy, vegetables, fruits, herbs, spices, teas, chocolate, nuts, olive oil, and red wine. Flavonoids are powerful antioxidants that may help to protect LDL against oxidation, minimize inflammation, and reduce blood platelet stickiness, thereby slowing the progression of atherosclerosis and making blood clots less likely.[6] Whereas an abundance of flavonoid-containing *foods* in the diet may lower the risks of chronic diseases, no claims can be made for flavonoids themselves as the protective factor, particularly when they are extracted from foods and sold as supplements. In fact, purified flavonoids may even be harmful.[7]

Flavonoids impart a bitter taste to foods, so manufacturers often refine away the natural flavonoids to please consumers, who usually prefer milder flavors. For example, for white grape juice or white wine, manufacturers remove the red, flavonoid-rich grape skins to lighten the flavor and color of the product, while greatly reducing its beneficial flavonoid content. One such flavonoid in purple grape juice and red wine, **resveratrol,** seems to hold promise as a disease fighter, but the amount present in wine or a serving of grape juice may be too small to benefit human health.[8]

What about carotenoids?

In addition to flavonoids, fruits and vegetables are rich in carotenoids—the red and yellow pigments of plants. Some carotenoids, such as beta-carotene, are vitamin A precursors. Some research suggests that a diet rich in carotenoids is associated with a lower risk of hypertension and heart disease.[9] Among the carotenoids that may defend against heart disease as well as stroke is lycopene, although findings are somewhat inconsistent.[10] Lycopene may also protect against certain types of cancer.[11]

What is lycopene, and what foods contain it?

Lycopene is a red pigment with powerful antioxidant activity found in guava, papaya, pink grapefruit, tomatoes (especially cooked tomatoes and tomato products), and watermelon. More than 80 percent of the lycopene consumed in the United States comes from tomato products such as tomato sauce, tomato juice, and ketchup. Around the world, people who eat five or more tomato-containing meals per week are less likely to suffer from cancers of the esophagus, prostate, or stomach than those who avoid tomatoes. Lycopene is a leading candidate for this protective effect.

Theoretically, the potent antioxidant capability of lycopene may play a role in its action against cancer, but research suggests that several other mechanisms may underlie lycopene's possible anticancer activity.[12] The Food and Drug Administration (FDA) concludes that no or very little solid evidence links lycopene or tomato consumption with reduced cancer risks. Tomatoes contain many other phytochemicals and nutrients that may contribute to the beneficial health effects of eating tomatoes and tomato products.

Do foods contain other phytochemicals that may help to protect people from cancer or other diseases?

Foods contain thousands of different phytochemicals, and so far only a few have been researched at all. There are still many questions about the phytochemicals that have been studied and only tentative answers about their roles in human health. For example, compared with people in the West, Asians living in Asia consume far more soybeans and soy products such as **tofu,** and they suffer less frequently from heart disease and certain cancers.* Women in Asia also suffer less from problems arising in menopause, the midlife drop in blood estrogen and cessation of menstruation, such as sensations of heat ("hot flashes") and loss of minerals from the bones. When Asians living in the United States adopt Western diets and habits, however, they experience diseases and symptoms at the same rates as native Westerners.[13]

In research, evidence concerning soy and heart health seems promising.[14] Soy's cholesterol-like plant sterols theoretically could inhibit cholesterol absorption in the intestine, and thus lower blood cholesterol.[15] A meta-analysis revealed a significant blood cholesterol–lowering effect from soy foods, attributable partly to soy's metabolic effects on the body and partly to the replacement of saturated fat–rich meats and dairy foods with soy foods in the diet.[16]

Cancers of the breast, colon, and prostate can be estrogen-sensitive—meaning that they grow when exposed to estrogen.[17] In addition to plant sterols, soy contains **phytoestrogens,** chemical relatives of human estrogen that may mimic or oppose its effects.[18] Phytoestrogens also have antioxidant activity that appears to slow the growth of some cancers. Soy foods appear to be most effective when consumed in moderation early and throughout life.[19] A study of women in China suggests a somewhat better outcome for breast cancer among soy consumers.[20] Studies that include U.S. women report no effect or mixed results.[21] Clearly, more research is needed before conclusions may be drawn about soy intake and cancer risk.

As for menopause, no consistent findings indicate that soy phytoestrogens can eliminate hot flashes, and in some studies, soy intake accompanied a greater incidence.[22] Some evidence does suggest that soy foods may help to preserve bone density after menopause, but supplements of isolated soy phytoestrogens fail to do so.[23]

Low doses of one soy phytoestrogen, **genistein,** appear to speed up division of breast cancer cells in laboratory cultures and in mice, whereas high doses seem to do the opposite.[24] It seems unlikely, however, that moderate intakes of soy foods cause harm.

*Among the cancers occurring less often in Asia are breast, colon, and prostate cancers.

The opposing actions of phytoestrogens should raise a red flag against taking supplements, especially by people who have had cancer or have close relatives with cancer. The American Cancer Society recommends that breast cancer survivors and those under treatment for breast cancer should consume only moderate amounts of soy foods as part of a healthy plant-based diet and should not intentionally ingest very high levels of soy products.

Other foods under study for potential health benefits include **flaxseed,** found as a whole seed, ground meal, or flaxseed oil. Flaxseed is of interest for its possible benefits to heart health because it is a good source of soluble fiber, and it is the richest known source of both the omega-3 fatty acid linolenic acid and **lignans.**[25] Lignans are converted into biologically active phytoestrogens by bacteria that normally reside in the human intestine.[26] Flaxseed oil, though rich in linolenic acid, does not contain fiber or lignans. Large quantities of flaxseed can cause digestive distress, and severe allergic reactions to flaxseed have been reported.

What about other phytochemical supplements?

Even when people don't make healthy food choices, taking supplements of purified phytochemicals is not the way to go. Phytochemicals can alter body functions, sometimes powerfully. Researchers are just beginning to understand how a handful of phytochemicals work, and what is current today may change tomorrow. Foods deliver thousands of bioactive food components, all within a food matrix that maximizes their availability and effectiveness. The body is equipped to handle phytochemicals in diluted form, mixed with all of the other constituents of foods, but it does not adapt well to phytochemicals in concentrated form.[27] The best way to reap the benefits of phytochemicals is by eating foods, not taking supplements (see Figure NP8-1).

FIGURE NP8-1 An Array of Phytochemicals in a Variety of Fruits and Vegetables

Broccoli and broccoli sprouts contain an abundance of the cancer-fighting phytochemical sulforaphane.

An apple a day—rich in flavonoids—may protect against lung cancer.

The phytoestrogens of soybeans seem to starve cancer cells and inhibit tumor growth; the phytosterols may lower blood cholesterol and protect cardiac arteries.

Garlic, with its abundant organosulfur compounds, may lower blood cholesterol and protect against stomach cancer.

The phytochemical resveratrol found in grapes (and nuts) protects against cancer by inhibiting cell growth and against heart disease by limiting clot formation and inflammation.

The ellagic acid of strawberries may inhibit certain types of cancer.

Tomatoes, with their abundant lycopene, may defend against cancer by protecting DNA from oxidative damage.

The monoterpenes of citrus fruits (and cherries) may inhibit cancer growth.

The flavonoids in black tea may protect against heart disease, whereas those in green tea may defend against cancer.

The flavonoids in cocoa and chocolate defend against oxidation and reduce the tendency of blood to clot.

Spinach and other colorful vegetables contain the carotenoids lutein and zeaxanthin, which help protect the eyes against macular degeneration.

Flaxseed, the richest source of lignans, may prevent the spread of cancer.

Blueberries, a rich source of flavonoids, improve memory in animals.

How do whole foods compare with processed foods that have been enriched with phytochemicals?

Good question. The American food supply is being transformed by a proliferation of functional foods—foods claimed to provide health benefits beyond those of the traditional nutrients. Virtually all whole foods have some special value in supporting health and are therefore functional foods. Cranberries may protect against urinary tract infections because cranberries contain a phytochemical that dislodges bacteria from the tract.[28] Cooked tomatoes, as mentioned, provide lycopene, along with **lutein** (an antioxidant associated with healthy eye function), vitamin C (an antioxidant vitamin), and many other healthful attributes. This has not stopped food manufacturers from trying to create functional foods as well. As consumer demand for healthful foods continues to grow, so will the development of functional foods.[29]

What are some examples of manufactured functional foods?

Many processed foods become functional foods when they are fortified with nutrients (calcium-fortified orange juice to support bone health, for example). In other cases, processed foods are enhanced with bioactive food components (margarine blended with a plant sterol to lower cholesterol, for example). The creation of some novel manufactured functional foods raises the question—is it a food or a drug?

Isn't the distinction between a food and a drug pretty clear?

Not long ago, most of us could agree on what was a food and what was a drug. Today, functional foods blur the distinctions. They have characteristics similar to both foods and drugs but do not fit neatly into either category. Consider the margarine example above.

Eating nonhydrogenated margarine sparingly instead of butter generously may lower blood cholesterol slightly over several months and clearly falls into the food category. Taking a statin drug, on the other hand, lowers blood cholesterol significantly within weeks and clearly falls into the drug category. But margarine enhanced with a plant sterol that lowers blood cholesterol is in a gray area between the two.[†] The margarine looks and tastes like a food, but it acts like a drug.

What are the health advantages and disadvantages of eating manufactured functional foods?

To achieve a desired health effect, which is the better choice: to eat a food designed to affect some body function or simply to adjust the diet? Does it make more sense to use a margarine enhanced with a plant sterol that lowers blood cholesterol or simply to limit the amount of butter eaten? Is it smarter to eat eggs enriched with omega-3 fatty acids or to restrict egg consumption?

[†]Margarine products that lower blood cholesterol contain either sterol esters—from vegetable oils, soybeans, and corn—or stanol esters from wood pulp.

Might functional foods offer a sensible solution for improving our nation's health—if done correctly? Perhaps so, but there is a problem with functional foods: the food industry is moving too fast for either scientists or the FDA to keep up. Consumers were able to buy soup with St. John's wort that claimed to enhance mood and fruit juice with echinacea that was supposed to fight colds while scientists were still conducting their studies on these ingredients. Research to determine the safety and effectiveness of these substances is still in progress. Until this work is complete, consumers are on their own in finding the answers to the following questions:

▪ *Does it work?* Research is generally lacking, and findings are often inconclusive.

▪ *How much does it contain?* Food labels are not required to list the quantities of added phytochemicals. Even if they were, consumers have no standard for comparison and cannot deduce whether the amounts listed are a little or a lot. Most importantly, until research is complete, food manufacturers do not know what amounts (if any) are most effective—or most toxic.

▪ *Is it safe?* Functional foods can act like drugs. They contain ingredients that can alter body functions and cause allergies, drug interactions, drowsiness, and other side effects. Yet, unlike drug labels, food labels do not provide instructions for the dosage, frequency, or duration of treatment.

▪ *Has the FDA issued warnings about any of the ingredients?* Check the FDA's website (www.fda.gov) to find out.

▪ *Is it healthy?* Adding phytochemicals to a food does not magically make it a healthy choice. A candy bar may be fortified with phytochemicals, but it is still made mostly of sugar and fat.

Critics suggest that the designation "functional foods" may be nothing more than a marketing tool. After all, even the most experienced researchers cannot yet identify the perfect combination of nutrients and phytochemicals to support optimal health. Yet manufacturers are freely experimenting with various concoctions as if they possessed that knowledge. Is it okay for them to sprinkle phytochemicals on fried snack foods and label them "functional," thus implying health benefits?

Functional foods currently on the market promise to "enhance mood," "promote relaxation and good karma," "increase alertness," and "improve memory," among other claims.

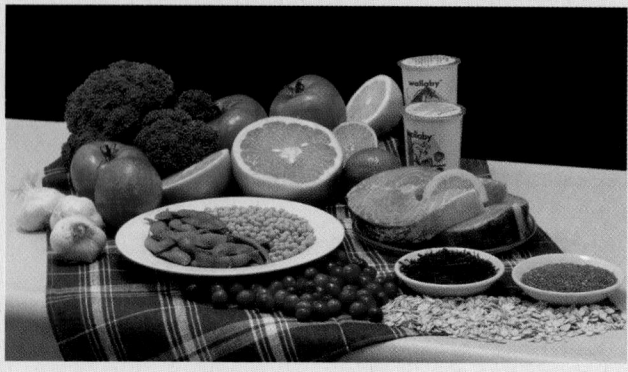

Nature offers a variety of functional foods that provide us with many health benefits.

What is the final word regarding phytochemicals and functional foods?

Nature has elegantly designed foods to provide us with a complex array of dozens of nutrients and thousands of additional compounds that may benefit health—most of which we have yet to identify or understand. Over the years, we have taken those foods and first deconstructed them and then reconstructed them in an effort to "improve" them. With new scientific understandings of how nutrients—and the myriad of other compounds in foods—interact with genes, we may someday be able to design *specific* eating patterns to meet the *exact* health needs of *each* individual. Indeed, our knowledge of the human genome and of human nutrition may well merge to allow specific recommendations for individuals based on their predisposition to diet-related diseases.

If the present trend continues, then someday physicians may be able to prescribe the perfect foods to enhance a person's health, and farmers will be able to grow them. In the mean time, however, it seems clear that a moderate approach to phytochemicals and functional foods is warranted. People who eat the recommended amounts of a variety of fruits and vegetables may cut their risk of many diseases by as much as half. Replacing some meat with soy foods and other legumes may also lower heart disease and cancer risks. Beneficial constituents are widespread among foods. Take a no-nonsense approach where your health is concerned: choose a wide variety of whole grains, legumes, fruits, and vegetables in the context of an adequate, balanced, and varied diet, and receive all of the health benefits that these foods offer. Table NP8-3 offers some tips for consuming the whole foods known to provide phytochemicals.

Notes

1. D. Aune and coauthors, Fruits, vegetables and breast cancer risk: A systematic review and meta-analysis of prospective studies, *Breast Cancer Research and Treatment* 134 (2012): 479–493; L. M. Oude Griep, and coauthors, Colors of fruit and vegetables and 10-year incidence of stroke, *Stroke* 42 (2011):3190-3195; F. L. Crowe and coauthors, Fruit and vegetable intake and mortality from ischaemic heart disease: Results from the European Prospective Investigation into

TABLE NP8-3 Tips for Consuming Phytochemicals

- *Eat more fruit.* The average U.S. diet provides little more than ½ cup fruit per day. Remember to choose juices and raw, dried, or cooked fruits and vegetables at mealtimes as well as for snacks. Choose dried fruit in place of candy.

- *Increase vegetable portions to meet recommendations.* Choose 1 cup of cut-up raw or cooked vegetables, or 2 cups of raw, leafy greens.

- *Use herbs and spices.* Cookbooks offer ways to include parsley, basil, garlic, hot peppers, oregano, and other beneficial seasonings.

- *Replace some meat with grains, legumes, and vegetables.* Oatmeal, soy meat replacer, or grated carrots mixed with ground meat and seasonings make a luscious, nutritious meatloaf, for example.

- *Add grated vegetables.* Carrots in chili or meatballs and celery, mushrooms, and squash in spaghetti sauce or other sauces add phytochemicals without greatly changing the taste of the food.

- *Try new foods.* Try a new fruit, vegetable, or whole grain each week. Walk through vegetable aisles and visit farmers' markets.

- *Read recipes.* Try tofu, fortified soy milk, or soybeans in cooking.

Cancer and Nutrition (EPIC)-Heart study, *European Heart Journal* 32 (2011): 1235–1243; T. J. Key, Fruit and vegetables and cancer risk, *British Journal of Cancer* (2010), doi:10.1038/sj.bjc.6606032.

2. M. M. Murphy and coauthors, Phytonutrient intake by adults in the United States in relation to fruit and vegetable consumption, *Journal of the Academy of Nutrition and Dietetics* 112 (2012): 222–2; J. M. Matés and coauthors, Anticancer antioxidant regulatory functions of phytochemicals, *Current Medicinal Chemistry* 18 (2011): 2315–2338; 29; N. P. Gullett and coauthors, Cancer prevention with natural compounds, *Seminars in Oncology* 37 (2010): 258–281; B. B. Aggarwal, Targeting inflammation-induced obesity and metabolic diseases by curcumin and other nutraceuticals, *Annual Review of Nutrition* 30 (2010): 173–199.

3. Position of the Academy of Nutrition and Dietetics: Functional foods, *Journal of the Academy of Nutrition and Dietetics* 113 (2013): 1096–1103.

4. G. Supic, M. Jagodic, and Z. Magic, Epigenetics: A new link between nutrition and cancer, *Nutrition and Cancer* 65 (2013): 781–792.

5. L. Franzini and coauthors, Food selection based on high total antioxidant capacity improves endothelial function in a low cardiovascular risk population, *Nutrition Metabolism and Cardiovascular Diseases* 22 (2012): 50–57.

6. M. L. McCullough and coauthors, Flavonoid intake and cardiovascular disease mortality in a prospective cohort of US adults, *American Journal of Clinical Nutrition* 95 (2012): 454–464; G. Chiva-Blanch and coauthors, Differential effects of polyphenols and alcohol of red wine on the expression of adhesion molecules and inflammatory cytokines

related to atherosclerosis: A randomized clinical trial, *American Journal of Clinical Nutrition* 95 (2012): 326–334; A. Jennings and coauthors, Higher anthocyanin intake is associated with lower arterial stiffness and central blood pressure in women, *American Journal of Clinical Nutrition* 96 (2012): 781–788; A. Basu, M. Rhone, and T. J. Lyons, Berries: Emerging impact on cardiovascular health, *Nutrition Reviews* 68 (2010): 168–177.

7. S. Egert and G. Rimbach, Which sources of flavonoids: Complex diets or dietary supplements? *Advances in Nutrition* 2 (2011): 8–14.

8. J. K. Aluyen and coauthors, Resveratrol: Potential as anticancer agent, *Journal of Dietary Supplements* 9 (2012): 45–56; J. M. Smoliga, J. A. Baur, and H. A. Hausenblas, Resveratrol and health—A comprehensive review of human clinical trials, *Molecular Nutrition and Food Research* 55 (2011): 1129–1141; Y. Shukla and R. Singh, Resveratrol and cellular mechanisms of cancer prevention, *Annals of the New York Academy of Sciences*, 1215 (2011): 1–8; J. M. Wu, T. C. Hsieh, and Z. Wang, Cardioprotection by resveratrol: A review of effects/targets in cultured cells and animal tissues, *American Journal of Cardiovascular Disease* 1 (2011): 38–47.

9. J. Karppi and coauthors, Low serum lycopene and β-carotene increase risk of acute myocardial infarction in men, *European Journal of Public Health*, 22 (2012): 835-840; C. Li and coauthors, Serum alpha-carotene concentrations and risk of death among US adults, *Archives of Internal Medicine* 171 (2011): 507–515.

10. F. Thies and coauthors, Effect of a tomato-rich diet on markers of cardiovascular disease risk in moderately overweight, disease-free, middle-aged adults: A randomized controlled trial, *American Journal of Clinical Nutrition* 95 (2012): 1013–1022; J. Karppi and coauthors, Serum lycopene decreases the risk of stroke in men, *Neurology* 79 (2012): 1540–1547; A. Mordente and coauthors, Lycopene and cardiovascular diseases: An update, *Current Medicinal Chemistry* 18 (2011): 1146–1163.

11. A. J. Teodoro and coauthors, Effect of lycopene on cell viability and cell cycle progression in human cancer cell lines, *Cancer Cell International* 12 (2012): 36; Y. Sharoni and coauthors, The role of lycopene and its derivatives in the regulation of transcription systems: Implications for cancer prevention, *American Journal of Clinical Nutrition* 96 (2012): 1173S-1178S; J. Talvas and coauthors, Differential effects of lycopene consumed in tomato paste and lycopene in the form of a purified extract on target genes of cancer prostatic cells, *American Journal of Clinical Nutrition* 91 (2010): 1716–1724.

12. Teodoro and coauthors, 2012; Sharoni and coauthors, 2012; Talvas and coauthors, 2010.

13. N. Mehrotra, S. Gaur, and A. Petrova, Health care practices of the foreign born Asian Indians in the United States. A community based survey, *Journal of Community Health* 37 (2012): 328–334.

14. M. Messina, Soy foods, isoflavones, and the health of postmenopausal women, *American Journal of Clinical Nutrition* 100 (2014): 423S–430S; D. J. Jenkins and coauthors, Soy protein reduces serum cholesterol by both intrinsic and food displacement mechanisms, *Journal of Nutrition* 140 (2010): 2302S–2311S.

15. S. B. Racette and coauthors, Dose effects of dietary plant sterols on cholesterol metabolism: A controlled feeding study, *American Journal of Clinical Nutrition* 91 (2010): 32–38.

16. Jenkins and coauthors, 2010.

17. P. Dey and coauthors, Insight into the mechanisms of action of estrogen receptor β in the breast, prostate, colon, and CNS, *Journal of Molecular Endocrinology* 51 (2013): T61–74; P. L. de Souza and coauthors, Clinical pharmacology of isoflavones and its relevance for potential prevention of prostate cancer, *Nutrition Reviews* 68 (2010): 542–555.

18. G. Leclercq and Y. Jacquot, Interactions of isoflavones and other plant derived estrogens with estrogen receptors for prevention and treatment of breast cancer—Considerations concerning related efficacy and safety, *Journal of Steroid Biochemistry and Molecular Biology* 139 (2014): 237–244.

19. Messina, 2014; L. Hilakivi-Clarke, J. E. Andrade, and W. Helferich, Is soy consumption good or bad for the breast? *Journal of Nutrition* 140 (2010): 2326S–2334S.

20. X.O. Liu and coauthors, Association between dietary factors and breast cancer risk among Chinese females: Systematic review and meta-analysis, *Asian Pacific Journal of Cancer Prevention* 15 (2014): 1291–1298.

21. S. J. Nechuta and coauthors, Soy food intake after diagnosis of breast cancer and survival: An in-depth analysis of combined evidence from cohort studies of U.S. and Chinese women, *American Journal of Clinical Nutrition* 96 (2012): 123–132; S. A. Khan and coauthors, Soy isoflavones supplementation for breast cancer risk reduction: A randomized phase II trial, *Cancer Prevention Research* 5 (2012): 309–319.

22. S. Levis and coauthors, Soy isoflavones in the prevention of menopausal bone loss and menopausal symptoms, *Archives of Internal Medicine* 171 (2011): 1363–1369; North American Menopause Society, The role of soy isoflavones in menopausal health: Report of the North American Menopause Society/Wulf H. Utian Translational Science Symposium in Chicago, IL (October 2010), *Menopause* 18 (2011): 732–753.

23. D. L. Alekel and coauthors, The Soy Isoflavones for Reducing Bone Loss (SIRBL) Study: A 3-y randomized controlled trial in postmenopausal women, *American Journal of Clinical Nutrition* 91 (2010): 218–230.

24. R. Bosviel and coauthors, Can soy phytoestrogens decrease DNA methylation in BRCA1 and BRCA2 oncosuppressor genes in breast cancer? *Omics* 16 (2012): 235–244; T. T. Rajah and coauthors, Physiological concentrations of genistein and

17β-estradiol inhibit MDA-MB231 breast cancer cell growth by increasing BAX/BC1-2 and reducing pERK 1/2, *Anticancer Research* 32 (2012): 1181–1191.

25. R. U. Almario and S. E. Daradas, Lignan content of the flaxseed influences its biological effects in healthy men and women, *Journal of the American College of Nutrition* 32 (2013): 194–199; D. Rodriquez-Leyva and coauthros, Potent antihypertensive action of dietary flaxseed in hypertensive patients, *Hypertension* 62 (2013): 1081–1089.

26. A. During and coauthors, Among plant lignans, pinoresinol has the strongest anti-inflammatory properties in human intestinal Caco-2 cells, *Journal of Nutrition* 142 (2012): 1798–1805.

27. Egert and Rimbach, 2011.

28. C. Wang and coauthors, Cranberry-containing products for prevention of urinary tract infections in susceptible populations, *Archives of Internal Medicine* 172 (2012): 988–996; H. Shmuely and coauthors, Cranberry components for the therapy of infectious disease, *Current Opinion in Biotechnology* 23 (2012): 148–152.

29. Position of the Academy of Nutrition and Dietetics, 2013.

9

Water and the Minerals

9.1 Water and Body Fluids

LO 9.1 List the functions of water in body fluids and explain how the body regulates fluid, electrolyte, and acid-base balance.

9.2 The Major Minerals

LO 9.2 Identify the main roles, deficiency and toxicity symptoms, and food sources for each of the major minerals (sodium, chloride, potassium, calcium, phosphorus, magnesium, sulfate).

9.3 The Trace Minerals

LO 9.3 Identify the main roles, deficiency and toxicity symptoms, and food sources for each of the trace minerals (iron, zinc, selenium, iodine, copper, manganese, fluoride, chromium, and molybdenum).

9.4 Nutrition in Practice: Vitamin and Mineral Supplements

LO 9.4 Present arguments for and against the use of dietary supplements.

BananaStock/SuperStock

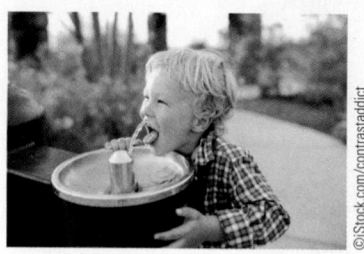

Water is the most indispensable nutrient of all.

TABLE 9-1 Signs of Mild and Severe Dehydration

Mild Dehydration (Loss of <5% Body Weight)

- Thirst
- Sudden weight loss
- Rough, dry skin
- Dry mouth, throat, body linings
- Rapid pulse
- Low blood pressure
- Lack of energy; weakness
- Impaired kidney function
- Reduced quantity of urine; concentrated urine
- Decreased mental functioning
- Decreased muscular work and athletic performance
- Fever or increased internal temperature
- Fainting

Severe Dehydration (Loss of >5% Body Weight)

- Pale skin
- Bluish lips and fingertips
- Confusion; disorientation
- Rapid, shallow breathing
- Weak, rapid, irregular pulse
- Thickening of blood
- Shock; seizures
- Coma; death

Source: Based on Standing Committee on the Scientific Evaluation of Dietary Reference Intakes, Food and Nutrition Board, Institute of Medicine, *Dietary Reference Intakes: Water, Potassium, Sodium, Chloride, and Sulfate* (Washington, DC: National Academies Press, 2005), pp. 90–122.

water balance: the balance between water intake and water excretion that keeps the body's water content constant.

dehydration: the loss of water from the body that occurs when water output exceeds water input. The symptoms progress rapidly from thirst, to weakness, to exhaustion and delirium, and end in death if not corrected.

The body's water cannot be considered separately from the minerals dissolved in it. A person can drink pure water, but in the body, water mingles with minerals to become fluids in which all life processes take place. This chapter begins by discussing the body's fluids and their chief minerals. The focus then shifts to other functions of the minerals.

9.1 Water and Body Fluids

LO 9.1 List the functions of water in body fluids and explain how the body regulates fluid, electrolyte, and acid-base balance.

Water constitutes about 60 percent of an adult's body weight and a higher percentage of a child's. Every cell in the body is bathed in a fluid of the exact composition that is best for that cell. The body fluids bring to each cell the ingredients it requires and carry away the end products of the life-sustaining reactions that take place within the cell's boundaries. Without water, cells quickly die. The water in the body fluids:

- Carries nutrients and waste products throughout the body.

- Maintains the structure of large molecules such as proteins and glycogen.

- Participates in metabolic reactions.

- Serves as the solvent for minerals, vitamins, amino acids, glucose, and many other small molecules so that they can participate in metabolic activities.

- Maintains blood volume.

- Aids in the regulation of normal body temperature, as the evaporation of sweat from the skin removes excess heat from the body.

- Acts as a lubricant and cushion around joints and inside the eyes, spinal cord, and amniotic sac surrounding a fetus in the womb.

To support these and other vital functions, the body actively regulates its **water balance.**

Water Balance

The cells themselves regulate the composition and amounts of fluids within and surrounding them. The entire system of cells and fluids remains in a delicate but firmly maintained state of dynamic equilibrium. Imbalances such as **dehydration** (see Table 9-1) and **water intoxication** can occur, but the body quickly restores the balance to normal if it can. The body controls both water intake and water excretion to maintain water equilibrium.

Water Intake Regulation The body can survive for only a few days without water. In healthy people, thirst and satiety govern water intake.[1] When the blood becomes too concentrated (having lost water but not salt and other dissolved substances), the mouth becomes dry, and the brain center known as the **hypothalamus** initiates drinking behavior.

Thirst lags behind the lack of water. A water deficiency that develops slowly can switch on drinking behavior in time to prevent serious dehydration, but a deficiency that develops quickly may not. Also, thirst itself does not remedy a water deficiency; a person must respond to the thirst signal by drinking. With aging, thirst sensations may diminish.[2] Dehydration can threaten elderly people who do not develop the habit of drinking water regularly.

Water intoxication, on the other hand, is rare but can occur with excessive water consumption and kidney disorders that reduce urine production. The symptoms may include severe headache, confusion, convulsions, and even death in extreme cases. Excessive water ingestion (several gallons) within a few hours dilutes the sodium concentration of the blood and contributes to a dangerous condition known as **hyponatremia.**

TABLE 9-2 Water Balance

Water Sources	Amount (mL)	Water Losses	Amount (mL)
Liquids	550 to 1500	Kidneys (urine)	500 to 1400
Foods	700 to 1000	Skin (sweat)	450 to 900
Metabolic water	200 to 300	Lungs (breath)	350
		GI tract (feces)	150
Total	1450 to 2800	Total	1450 to 2800

© Cengage Learning®

[handwritten note, top right:] water balance— the balance between water intake & water excretion to keep the water balance constant.

Water Excretion Regulation Water excretion is regulated by the brain and the kidneys. The cells of the brain's hypothalamus, which monitor blood salts, stimulate the **pituitary gland** to release **antidiuretic hormone (ADH)** whenever the salts are too concentrated, or the blood volume or blood pressure is too low. ADH stimulates the kidneys to reabsorb water rather than excrete it. Thus, the more water you need, the less you excrete.

If too much water is lost from the body, blood volume and blood pressure fall. Cells in the kidneys respond to the low blood pressure by releasing **renin.** Through a complex series of events involving the hormone **aldosterone,** this enzyme also causes the kidneys to retain more water. Again, the effect is that, when more water is needed, less is excreted.

Minimum Water Needed These mechanisms can maintain water balance only if a person drinks enough water. The body must excrete a minimum of about 500 milliliters (about ½ quart) each day as urine—enough to carry away the waste products generated by a day's metabolic activities. Above this amount, excretion adjusts to balance intake, so the more a person drinks, the more dilute the urine becomes. In addition to urine, some water is lost from the lungs as vapor, some is excreted in feces, and some evaporates from the skin. A person's water losses from all of these routes total about 2½ liters (about 2½ quarts) a day on the average. Table 9-2 shows how fluid intake and output naturally balance out.

Water Recommendations and Sources Water needs vary greatly depending on the foods a person eats, the environmental temperature and humidity, the person's activity level, and other factors. Accordingly, a general water requirement is difficult to establish. In the past, recommendations for adults were expressed in proportion to the amount of energy expended under normal environmental conditions. For the person who expends about 2000 kcalories a day, this works out to 2 to 3 liters, or about 8 to 12 cups. This recommendation is in line with the Adequate Intake (AI) for *total* water (3.7 liters for men and 2.7 liters for women) set by the DRI committee. Total water includes not only drinking water but also water in other beverages and in foods.

Because a wide range of water intakes will prevent dehydration and its harmful consequences, the AI is based on average intakes. Strenuous physical activity and heat stress can increase water needs considerably, however.[3] In general, you can tell from the color of the urine whether a person needs more water. Pale yellow urine reflects appropriate dilution.

The obvious dietary sources of water are water itself and other beverages, but nearly all foods also contain water. Water constitutes up to 95 percent of the volume of most fruits and vegetables and at least 50 percent of many meats and cheeses (see Table 9-3 on p. 228). The energy nutrients in foods also give up water during metabolism.

Which beverages are best? Any beverage can readily meet the body's fluid needs, but those with few or no kcalories do so without contributing to weight gain. Given that obesity is a major health problem and that beverages contribute more than 20 percent of the total energy intake in the United States, water is the best choice for most people.[4] Other choices include tea, coffee, nonfat and low-fat milk and soy milk, artificially sweetened beverages, fruit and vegetable juices, sports drinks, and, lastly, sweetened nutrient-poor beverages. Carbonated soft drinks are chosen most often but this choice crowds more nutritious beverages out of the diet, and the regular sugar-sweetened varieties provide many empty kcalories from added sugars.

[handwritten note, right margin:] water needs vary greatly depending on the food a person eats, temp & humidity, activity level, etc.

water intoxication: the rare condition in which body water contents are too high. The symptoms may include confusion, convulsion, coma, and even death in extreme cases.

hypothalamus (high-poh-THAL-ah-mus)**:** a brain center that controls activities such as maintenance of water balance, regulation of body temperature, and control of appetite.

hyponatremia (HIGH-po-na-TREE-me-ah)**:** a decreased concentration of sodium in the blood.

pituitary (pit-TOO-ih-tary) **gland:** in the brain, the "king gland" that regulates the operation of many other glands.

antidiuretic hormone (ADH): a hormone released by the pituitary gland in response to high salt concentrations in the blood. The kidneys respond by reabsorbing water. ADH elevates blood pressure and so is also called *vasopressin* (VAS-oh-PRES-in).

- *vaso* = vessel
- *press* = press

renin (REN-in)**:** an enzyme released by the kidneys in response to low blood pressure that helps them retain water through the renin-angiotensin mechanism.

aldosterone (al-DOS-ter-own)**:** a hormone secreted by the adrenal glands that stimulates the reabsorption of sodium by the kidneys; also regulates chloride and potassium concentrations.

Water follows salt. Notice the beads of "sweat," formed on the right-hand slices of eggplant, which were sprinkled with salt. Cellular water moves across each cell's membrane (water-permeable divider) toward the higher concentration of salt (dissolved particles) on the surface.

TABLE 9-3 **Percentage of Water in Selected Foods**

- 100%: Water, diet soft drinks, plain tea
- 90–99%: Fat-free milk, black coffee, Gatorade, strawberries, watermelon, grapefruit, tomato, lettuce, celery, spinach, broccoli
- 80–89%: Fruit juice, regular soft drinks, whole milk, yogurt, apples, grapes, oranges, carrots
- 70–79%: Shrimp, bananas, potatoes, avocados, ricotta cheese
- 60–69%: Pasta, cooked rice, legumes, salmon, chicken breast, ice cream
- 50–59%: Ground beef, pork chop, hot dogs, feta cheese
- 40–49%: Pizza, cheeseburger
- 30–39%: Cheddar cheese, bagels, bread
- 20–29%: Pepperoni sausage, cake, biscuits
- 10–19%: Butter, margarine, raisins
- 1–9%: Crackers, ready-to-eat cereals, peanut butter, nuts
- 0%: Oils, white sugar, meat fats, shortening

salts: compounds composed of charged particles (ions). An example of a salt is potassium chloride (K^+Cl^-).

electrolyte: a salt that dissolves in water and dissociates into charged particles called ions.

electrolyte solutions: solutions that can conduct electricity.

People often ask whether caffeine-containing beverages such as coffee, tea, or soda can help to meet water needs. People who drink caffeinated beverages lose a little more fluid than when they drink water because caffeine acts as a mild diuretic. The DRI committee considered such findings in making its recommendations for water intake and concluded that "caffeinated beverages contribute to the daily total water intake similar to that contributed by non-caffeinated beverages."[5] In other words, it doesn't seem to matter whether people rely on caffeine-containing beverages or other beverages to meet their fluid needs.

In contrast, alcohol should probably not be used to meet fluid needs. As Nutrition in Practice 20 explains, alcohol acts as a diuretic, and it has many adverse effects on health and nutrition status.

Fluid and Electrolyte Balance

When mineral **salts** dissolve in water, they separate (dissociate) into charged particles known as ions, which can conduct electricity. For this reason, a salt that dissociates in water is known as an **electrolyte.*** The body fluids, which contain water and partly dissociated salts, are **electrolyte solutions.**

The body's electrolytes are vital to the life of the cells and therefore must be closely regulated to help maintain the appropriate distribution of body fluids. The major minerals form salts that dissolve in the body fluids; the cells direct where these salts go; and the movement of the salts determines where the fluids flow because water follows salt. Cells use this force, called *osmosis*, to move fluids back and forth across their membranes. Thanks to the electrolytes, water can be held in compartments where it is needed.

Proteins in the cell membranes move ions into or out of the cells. These protein pumps tend to concentrate sodium and chloride outside cells and potassium and other ions inside. By maintaining specific amounts of sodium outside and potassium inside, cells can regulate the exact amounts of water inside and outside their boundaries.

Healthy kidneys regulate the body's sodium, as well as its water, with remarkable precision. The intestinal tract absorbs sodium readily, and it travels freely in the blood, but the kidneys excrete unneeded amounts. The kidneys actually filter all of the sodium out of the blood; then they return to the bloodstream the exact amount the body needs to retain. Thus, the body's total electrolytes remain constant, while the urinary electrolytes fluctuate according to what is eaten.

In some cases, the body's mechanisms for maintaining fluid and electrolyte balances cannot compensate for a sudden loss of large amounts of fluid and electrolytes. Vomiting, diarrhea, heavy sweating, fever, burns, wounds, and the like may incur great fluid and electrolyte losses, precipitating an emergency that demands medical intervention. The body's responses to severe stress and trauma are discussed in Chapter 24.

Acid–Base Balance

The body uses ions not only to help maintain water balance but also to regulate the acidity (pH) of its fluids. Like proteins, electrolyte mixtures in the body fluids protect the body against changes in acidity by acting as **buffers**—substances that can accommodate excess acids or bases.

The body's buffer systems serve as a first line of defense against changes in the fluids' acid–base balance. The lungs, skin, gastrointestinal (GI) tract, and kidneys provide other defenses. Of these organ systems, the kidneys play the primary role in maintaining acid–base balance. Thus, disorders of the kidneys impair the body's ability to regulate its acid–base balance, as well as its fluid and electrolyte balances.

*Exceptions: A compound in which the positive ions are hydrogen ions (H^+) is an acid (example: hydrochloric acid, or H^+Cl^-); a compound in which the negative ions are hydroxyl ions (OH^-) is a base (example: potassium hydroxide, or K^+OH^-).

CHAPTER NINE

IN SUMMARY

■ Water makes up about 60 percent of the body's weight.

■ Water helps transport nutrients and waste products throughout the body, participates in metabolic reactions, acts as a solvent, assists in maintaining blood volume and body temperature, acts as a lubricant and cushion around joints, and serves as a shock absorber.

■ To maintain water balance, intake from liquids, foods, and metabolism must equal losses from the kidneys, skin, lungs, and feces.

■ Electrolytes help maintain the appropriate distribution of body fluids and acid–base balance.

9.2 The Major Minerals

LO 9.2 Identify the main roles, deficiency and toxicity symptoms, and food sources for each of the major minerals (sodium, chloride, potassium, calcium, phosphorus, magnesium, sulfate).

Table 9-4 lists the major minerals and the nine essential trace minerals. Other trace minerals are recognized as essential nutrients for some animals but have not been proved to be required for human beings. Figure 9-1 shows the amounts of the major minerals found in the body, and for comparison, some of the trace minerals. As you can see, the most prevalent minerals are calcium and phosphorus, the chief minerals of bone. The distinction between the **major minerals** and the **trace minerals** does not mean that one group is more important than the other. A deficiency of the few micrograms of iodine needed daily is just as serious as a deficiency of the several hundred milligrams of calcium. The major minerals are so named because they are present, and needed, in larger amounts in the body than the trace minerals.

Although all the major minerals influence the body's fluid balance, sodium, chloride, and potassium are most noted for that role. For this reason, these three minerals are discussed first. Each major mineral also plays other specific roles in the body. Sodium, potassium, calcium, and magnesium are critical to nerve transmission and muscle contractions. Phosphorus and magnesium are involved in energy metabolism.

TABLE 9-4 The Major and Trace Minerals

Major Minerals	Trace Minerals
Calcium	Chromium
Chloride	Copper
Magnesium	Fluoride
Phosphorus	Iodine
Potassium	Iron
Sodium	Manganese
Sulfur	Molybdenum
	Selenium
	Zinc

© Cengage Learning®

Calcium	1150
Phosphorus	600
Potassium	210
Sulfur	150
Sodium	90
Chloride	90
Magnesium	30
Iron	2.4
Zinc	2.0
Copper	0.09
Manganese	0.02
Iodine	0.02
Selenium	0.02

MAJOR MINERALS
The major minerals are those present in amounts larger than 5 g (a teaspoon). A pound is about 454 g; thus only calcium and phosphorus appear in amounts larger than one pound.

TRACE MINERALS
There are more than one dozen trace minerals, although only six are shown here.

Amount (g): 0 100 200 300 400 500 600 700 800 900 1000 1100 1200

© Cengage Learning®

FIGURE 9-1 Amounts of Minerals in a 60-kilogram (132-pound) Human Body
Not only are the major minerals present in the body in larger amounts than the trace minerals, but they are also needed by the body in large amounts. Recommended intakes for the major minerals are stated in hundreds of milligrams or grams, whereas those for the trace minerals are listed in tens of milligrams or even micrograms.

buffers: compounds that can reversibly combine with hydrogen ions to help keep a solution's acidity or alkalinity constant.

major minerals: essential mineral nutrients required in the adult diet in amounts greater than 100 milligrams per day.

trace minerals: essential mineral nutrients required in the adult diet in amounts less than 100 milligrams per day.

Calcium, phosphorus, and magnesium contribute to the structure of the bones. Sulfur helps determine the shape of proteins. Table 9-8, shown later in the chapter, provides a summary of information about the major minerals.

Sodium

Sodium is the principal electrolyte in the **extracellular fluid** (the fluid outside the cells) and the primary regulator of the extracellular fluid volume. When the blood concentration of sodium rises, as when a person eats salted foods, thirst prompts the person to drink water until the appropriate sodium-to-water ratio is restored. Sodium also helps maintain acid–base balance and is essential to muscle contraction and nerve transmission. Too much sodium, however, can contribute to high blood pressure (hypertension).

Sodium Recommendations and Food Sources Diets rarely lack sodium, and even when intakes are low, the body adapts by reducing sodium losses in urine and sweat, thus making deficiencies unlikely. Sodium recommendations (see the inside front cover) are set low enough to protect against high blood pressure but high enough to allow an adequate intake of other nutrients. Because high sodium intakes correlate with high blood pressure, the Tolerable Upper Intake Level (UL) for adults is set at 2300 milligrams per day—equivalent to about 1 teaspoon of salt (sodium chloride). Three groups of people encompassing the majority of U.S. adults—all those age 51 and older, all African Americans, and everyone with hypertension, diabetes, or chronic kidney disease—are urged to limit their sodium intakes to no more than 1500 milligrams per day for the sake of their blood pressure and heart health.[6]

Today, the average U.S. sodium intake is more than 3200 mg per day, an amount that far exceeds the UL.[7] People who eat mostly processed and fast foods have the highest sodium intakes, whereas those who eat mostly whole, unprocessed foods, such as fresh fruits and vegetables, have the lowest intakes. In fact, about three-fourths of the sodium in people's diets comes from salt added to foods by manufacturers. Figure 9-2 shows that processed foods contain not only more sodium but also less potassium than their less processed counterparts.

extracellular fluid: fluid residing outside the cells; includes the fluid between the cells (*interstitial fluid*), plasma, and the water of structures such as the skin and bones. Extracellular fluid accounts for about one-third of the body's water.

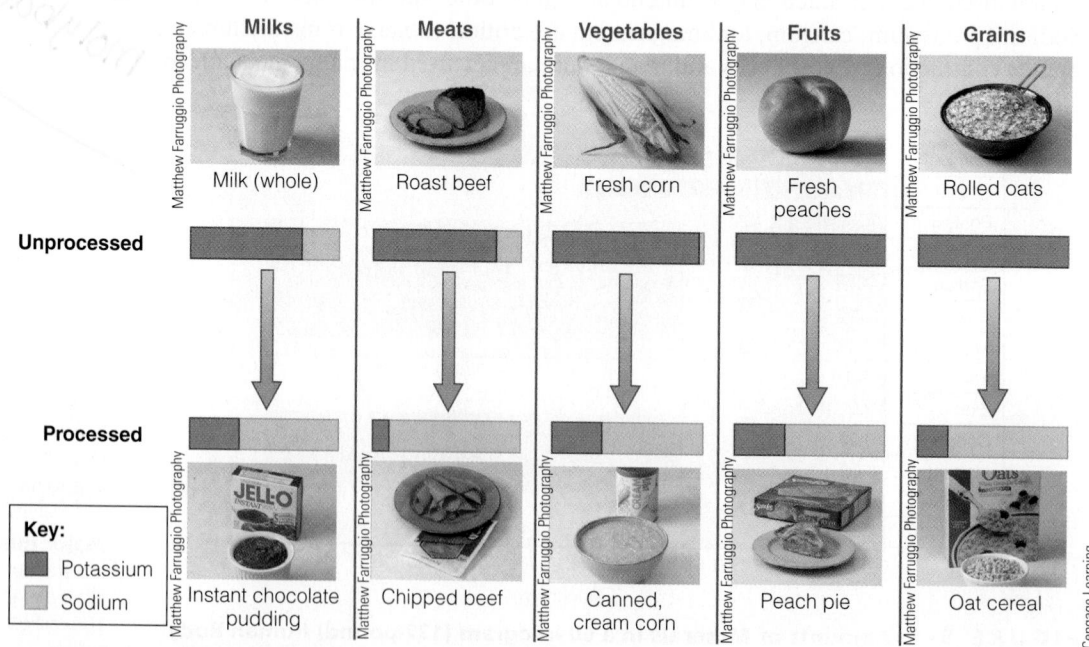

FIGURE 9-2 What Processing Does to the Sodium and Potassium Contents of Foods
People who eat foods high in salt often happen to be eating fewer potassium-containing foods at the same time. Notice how potassium is lost and sodium is gained as foods become more processed, causing the potassium-to-sodium ratio to fall dramatically. Even when potassium is not lost, the addition of sodium still lowers the potassium-to-sodium ratio.

[Handwritten margin note: Sodium–principle electrolyte in the extracellular fluid.]

230

Many experts today are calling for reductions of sodium in the food supply to give consumers more low-salt options to choose from.[8] Reducing the sodium content in processed foods could prevent an estimated 100,000 deaths and save up to $24 billion in health care costs in the United States annually.[9] Table 9-5 lists the top 10 sodium sources.[10]

Sodium and Blood Pressure High intakes of salt among a population correlate with high rates of **hypertension,** heart disease, and stroke.[11] Over time, a high-salt diet may damage the linings of blood vessels in ways that make hypertension likely to develop.[12] In many people, the relationship between salt intake and blood pressure is direct—as chronic sodium intakes increase, blood pressure rises with them in a stepwise fashion.[13] Once hypertension sets in, the risk of death from stroke and heart disease climbs steeply. Nearly one-third of U.S. adults have hypertension and the rate among African American adults is one of the highest in the world—42 percent.[14] An additional 36 percent of U.S. adults have **prehypertension.**

Because reducing salt intake diminishes the risk of hypertension and heart disease, the *Dietary Guidelines for Americans* advise limiting daily sodium intakes to less than 2300 milligrams (or <1500 mg for the at-risk groups mentioned above). Higher intakes seem to be well tolerated in most healthy people, however. Box 9-1 offers strategies for cutting salt (and, therefore, sodium) intake.

An eating pattern proven to help people to reduce sodium and increase potassium intakes, and thereby often reduce their blood pressure, is DASH (Dietary Approaches to Stop Hypertension).[15] The DASH approach emphasizes potassium-rich fruits and vegetables and fat-free or low-fat milk products; includes whole grains, nuts, poultry, and fish; and calls for reduced intakes of red and processed meats, sweets, and sugar-containing beverages. The DASH diet in combination with a reduced sodium intake is even more effective at lowering blood pressure than either strategy alone (see Chapter 22). Incorporating physical activity provides further benefits because regular moderate exercise reliably lowers blood pressure.

Chloride

The chloride ion is the major negative ion of the extracellular fluids, where it occurs primarily in association with sodium. Like sodium, chloride is critical to maintaining fluid, electrolyte, and acid–base balances in the body. In the stomach,

TABLE 9-5 Top Contributors of Sodium in the Diet

- Breads and rolls
- Cold cuts and cured meats
- Pizza
- Fresh and processed poultry
- Soups
- Sandwiches (including cheeseburgers)
- Cheese
- Pasta dishes
- Meat mixtures (including meatloaf)
- Salty snacks (including popcorn, chips, and pretzels)

© 2016 Cengage Learning®

hypertension: high blood pressure.
prehypertension: blood pressure values that predict hypertension.

How To BOX 9-1 CUT SALT INTAKE

Strategies to cut salt intake include:
- Select fresh, unprocessed foods.
- Cook with little or no added salt.
- Prepare foods with sodium-free spices such as basil, bay leaves, curry, garlic, ginger, mint, oregano, pepper, rosemary, and thyme; lemon juice; vinegar; or wine.
- Add little or no salt at the table; taste foods before adding salt.
- Read labels with an eye open for sodium. (See Table 1-9 on p. 25 for terms used to describe the sodium contents of foods on labels.)
- Select low-salt or salt-free products when available.

Use these foods sparingly:
- Foods prepared in brine, such as pickles, olives, and sauerkraut.
- Salty or smoked meats, such as bologna, corned or chipped beef, bacon, frankfurters, ham, lunch meats, salt pork, sausage, and smoked tongue.
- Salty or smoked fish, such as anchovies, caviar, salted and dried cod, herring, sardines, and smoked salmon.
- Snack items such as potato chips, pretzels, salted popcorn, salted nuts, and crackers.
- Condiments such as bouillon cubes; seasoned salts; MSG; soy, teriyaki, Worcestershire, and barbeque sauces; prepared horseradish, catsup, and mustard.
- Cheeses, especially processed types.
- Canned and instant soups.

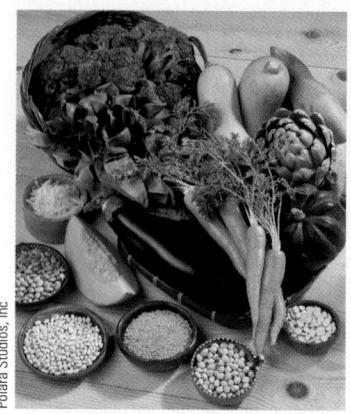

FIGURE 9-3 Good Food Sources of Potassium
Fresh fruits and vegetables provide potassium in abundance.

the chloride ion is part of hydrochloric acid, which maintains the strong acidity of the gastric fluids.

Salt is a major food source of chloride, and, as with sodium, processed foods are a major contributor of this mineral to people's diets. Because salt contains a higher proportion of chloride (by weight) than sodium, chloride recommendations are slightly higher than, but still equivalent to, those of sodium. In other words, ¾ teaspoon of salt will deliver some sodium and more chloride, and still meet the AI for both.

Potassium

Outside the body's cells, sodium is the principle positively charged ion. *Inside* the cells, potassium takes the role of the principal positively charged ion. Potassium plays a major role in maintaining fluid and electrolyte balance and cell integrity. During nerve impulse transmission and muscle contraction, potassium and sodium briefly trade places across the cell membrane. The cell then quickly pumps them back into place. Controlling potassium distribution is a high priority for the body because it affects many aspects of homeostasis, including maintaining a steady heartbeat. The sudden deaths that occur with fasting, eating disorders, severe diarrhea, or severe malnutrition in children may be due to heart failure caused by potassium loss.

Potassium Deficiency and Toxicity Potassium deficiency is characterized by an increase in blood pressure, kidney stones, and bone turnover. As deficiency progresses, symptoms include irregular heartbeats, muscle weakness, and glucose intolerance. Potassium deficiency results more often from excessive losses than from deficient intakes. Deficiency arises in abnormal conditions such as diabetic acidosis, dehydration, or prolonged vomiting or diarrhea; potassium deficiency can also result from the regular use of certain medications, including **diuretics, steroids,** and **cathartics.**

Potassium toxicity does not result from overeating foods high in potassium; therefore, a UL was not set. Toxicity can result from overconsumption of potassium salts or supplements and from certain diseases or medications. Given more potassium than the body needs, the kidneys accelerate their excretion. If the GI tract is bypassed, however, and potassium is injected directly into a vein, it can stop the heart.

Potassium Recommendations and Food Sources In healthy people, almost any reasonable diet provides enough potassium to prevent the dangerously low blood potassium that indicates a severe deficiency. Potassium is abundant inside all living cells, both plant and animal, and because cells remain intact until foods are processed, the richest sources of potassium are *fresh* foods of all kinds—especially fruits and vegetables (see Figure 9-3). A typical U.S. eating pattern, however, is low in fruits and vegetables and provides far less potassium than the recommended intake.[16] Although blood potassium may remain normal on such a diet, chronic diseases are more likely to occur.

Potassium and Hypertension Low potassium intakes, especially when combined with high sodium intakes, raise blood pressure and increase the risk of death from heart disease and stroke.[17] In contrast, eating patterns with ample potassium, particularly when low in sodium, appear to both prevent and correct hypertension. This effect earns potassium its status as a *Dietary Guidelines* nutrient of concern.[18] Recall that the DASH eating pattern described earlier emphasizes potassium-rich foods such as fruits and vegetables.

Calcium

Calcium occupies more space in this chapter than any other major mineral. Other minerals with key roles in heart disease and kidney disease are revisited later in this book, but calcium deserves emphasis here because an adequate intake of calcium early in life helps grow a healthy skeleton and prevent bone disease in later life.

diuretics (dye-yoo-RET-ics): medications that promote the excretion of water through the kidneys. Some diuretics increase the urinary loss of potassium; others, called potassium-sparing diuretics, are less likely to result in a potassium deficiency (see Chapter 22).

steroids (STARE-oids): medications used to reduce tissue inflammation, to suppress the immune response, or to replace certain steroid hormones in people who cannot synthesize them.

cathartics (ca-THART-ics): strong laxatives.

CHAPTER NINE

Calcium Roles in the Body Calcium is the most abundant mineral in the body. Ninety-nine percent of the body's calcium is stored in the bones (and teeth), where it plays two important roles. First, it is an integral part of bone structure. Second, it serves as a calcium bank available to the body fluids should a drop in blood calcium occur.

Calcium in Bone As bones begin to form, calcium salts form crystals on a matrix of the protein collagen. As the crystals become denser, they give strength and rigidity to the maturing bones. As a result, the long leg bones of children can support their weight by the time they have learned to walk. Figure 9-4 shows the lacy network of calcium-containing crystals in the bone.

Many people have the idea that bones are inert, like rocks. Not so. Bones continuously gain and lose minerals in an ongoing process of remodeling. Growing children gain more bone than they lose, and healthy adults maintain a reasonable balance. When withdrawals substantially exceed deposits, however, problems such as osteoporosis develop.

From birth to approximately age 20, the bones are actively growing by modifying their length, width, and shape (see Figure 9-5). This rapid growth phase overlaps with the next period of peak bone mass development, which occurs between the ages of 12 and 30. During this period, skeletal mass increases. Bones grow thicker and denser by remodeling, a maintenance and repair process involving the loss of existing bone and the deposition of new bone. In the final phase, which begins between 30 and 40 years of age and continues throughout the remainder of life, bone loss exceeds new bone formation.

Calcium in Body Fluids The 1 percent of the body's calcium that circulates in the fluids as ionized calcium is vital to life. It plays these major roles:

▮ Regulates the transport of ions across cell membranes and is particularly important in nerve transmission.

▮ Helps maintain normal blood pressure.

▮ Plays an essential role in the clotting of blood.

▮ Is essential for muscle contraction and therefore for the heartbeat.

▮ Allows secretion of hormones, digestive enzymes, and neurotransmitters.

▮ Activates cellular enzymes that regulate many processes.

Because of its importance, blood calcium is tightly controlled.

Calcium Balance Whenever blood calcium rises too high, a system of hormones, including vitamin D, promotes its deposit into bone.* Whenever blood calcium falls too low, the regulatory system acts in three locations to raise it: (1) the small intestine absorbs more calcium; (2) the bones release more calcium into the blood; and (3) the kidneys excrete less calcium. Thus, blood calcium rises to normal.

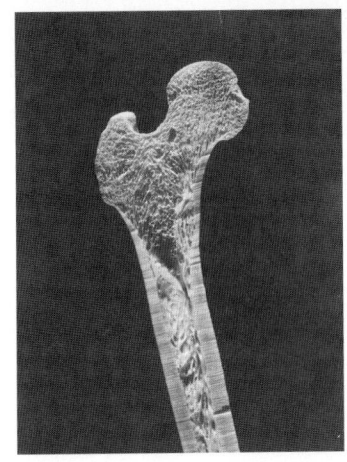

FIGURE 9-4 Cross-Section of Bone
The lacy structural elements are trabeculae (tra-BECK-you-lee), which can be drawn on to replenish blood calcium.

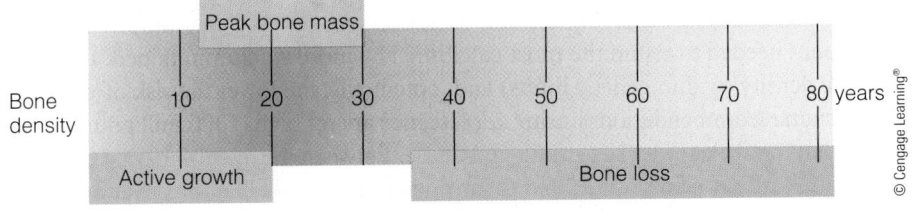

FIGURE 9-5 Phases of Bone Development throughout Life
The active growth phase occurs from birth to approximately age 20. The next phase of peak bone mass development occurs between the ages of 12 and 30. The final phase, when bone resorption exceeds formation, begins between the ages of 30 and 40 and continues through the remainder of life.

*The regulators are hormones from the thyroid and parathyroid glands, as well as vitamin D. One hormone, parathormone, raises blood calcium. Another hormone, calcitonin, lowers blood calcium by inhibiting release of calcium from bone.

TABLE 9-6 Risk Factors for Osteoporosis

Nonmodifiable

- Female gender
- Older age
- Small frame
- Caucasian, Asian, or Hispanic/Latino heritage
- Family history of osteoporosis or fractures
- Personal history of fractures
- Estrogen deficiency in women (amenorrhea or menopause, especially early or surgically induced); testosterone deficiency in men

Modifiable

- Sedentary lifestyle
- Diet inadequate in calcium and vitamin D
- Diet excessive in sodium, caffeine
- Cigarette smoking
- Alcohol abuse
- Low body weight
- Certain medications, such as glucocorticoids and anticonvulsants

© 2016 Cengage Learning®

The calcium stored in bone provides a nearly inexhaustible source of calcium for the blood. Even in a calcium deficiency, blood calcium remains normal. Blood calcium changes only in response to abnormal regulatory control. Thus, a chronic deficiency of calcium due to a low dietary intake or poor absorption does not change blood calcium, but does deplete the calcium in the bones. To restate: it is the bones, not the blood, that are robbed by calcium deficiency.

Calcium and Osteoporosis As mentioned earlier, bone mass peaks at the time of skeletal maturity (about age 30), and a high peak bone mass is the best protection against later age-related bone loss and fracture. Adequate calcium nutrition during the growing years is essential to achieving optimal peak bone mass.[19] Following menopause, women may lose up to 20 percent of their bone mass, as may middle-aged and older men. When bone loss has reached such an extreme that bones fracture under even common, everyday stresses, the condition is known as **osteoporosis.** An estimated 52 million people in the United States, most of them women older than 50, have or are developing osteoporosis.[20] Men, however, are not immune to osteoporosis. Each year, 1.5 million people—30 percent of them men—break a hip, leg, arm, hand, ankle, or other bone as a result of osteoporosis.

Both genetic and environmental factors contribute to osteoporosis; Table 9-6 summarizes these risk factors. Osteoporosis is more prevalent in women than men for several reasons. First, women consume less dietary calcium than men do. Second, at all ages, women's bone mass is lower than men's because women generally have smaller bodies. Finally, women often lose more bone, particularly in the 6 to 8 years following menopause when the hormone estrogen diminishes.[21]

In addition to calcium, many other minerals and vitamins, including phosphorus, magnesium, fluoride, and vitamin D, help to form and stabilize the structure of bones. Any or all of these elements are needed to prevent bone loss. The first, most obvious lines of defense, however, are to maintain a lifelong adequate intake of calcium and to "exercise it into place." Physical activity supports bone growth during adolescence and may protect the bones later on.[22] Weight-bearing physical activity, such as walking, running, dancing, and weight training, prompts the bones to deposit minerals. It has long been known that, when people are confined to bed, both their muscles and their bones lose strength. Muscle strength and bone strength go together: when muscles work, they pull on the bones, and both are stimulated to grow stronger.

Calcium and Disease Prevention Other roles for calcium are emerging as well. Calcium may protect against hypertension.[23] The blood pressure-lowering DASH diet is not particularly low in sodium, but it is rich in calcium, as well as in potassium and magnesium. Calcium-rich foods may play a role in reducing body fat, protecting lean tissue, and maintaining a healthy body weight.[24]

Calcium Recommendations As mentioned earlier, blood calcium concentration does not reflect calcium status. Calcium recommendations are therefore based on balance studies, which measure daily intake and excretion. An optimal calcium intake reflects the amount needed to retain the most calcium. The more calcium retained, the greater the bone density (within genetic limits) and, potentially, the lower the risk of osteoporosis. Calcium recommendations during adolescence are set high (1300 milligrams) to help ensure that the skeleton will be strong and dense. Between the ages of 19 and 50, recommendations are lowered slightly, and for women over 50 and all adults over age 70, recommendations are raised again to minimize bone loss. Many people in the United States have calcium intakes below current recommendations.[25] Findings about the effectiveness of calcium supplements in reducing fractures in older women, however, are inconclusive or negative.[26] Because adverse effects such as kidney stone formation are possible with high supplemental doses, a UL has been established (see inside front cover).

Calcium in Foods Calcium is found most abundantly in a single food group—milk and milk products. For this reason, dietary recommendations advise daily

osteoporosis (os-tee-oh-pore-OH-sis): literally, porous bones; reduced density of the bones, also known as *adult bone loss*.

consumption of low-fat or fat-free milk products. A cup of milk offers about 300 milligrams of calcium, so an adult who drinks 3 cups of milk a day (or eats the equivalent in yogurt) is well on the way to meeting daily calcium needs (see Table 9-7). The other dairy food that contains comparable amounts of calcium is cheese. One slice of cheese (1 ounce) contains about two-thirds as much calcium as a cup of milk. Cottage cheese, however, contains much less. Figure 9-6 shows foods that are rich in calcium, and Box 9-2 on p. 236 suggests ways of adding calcium to meals.

Some foods offer large amounts of calcium because of fortification. Calcium-fortified juice, high-calcium milk (milk with extra calcium added), and calcium-fortified cereals are examples. Some calcium-rich mineral waters may also be a useful source, providing calcium that may be as absorbable as that from milk but accompanied by zero kcalories.

Among the vegetables, beet greens, bok choy (a Chinese cabbage), broccoli, kale, mustard greens, rutabaga, and turnip greens provide some available calcium. So do collard greens, green cabbage, kohlrabi, parsley, and watercress. Some dark green, leafy vegetables—notably, spinach and Swiss chard—appear to be calcium rich but actually provide very little, if any, calcium to the body. These foods contain **binders** that prevent calcium absorption.

Aided by vitamin D, the body is able to regulate its absorption of calcium by altering its production of the calcium-binding protein. More of this protein is made if more calcium is needed. Infants and children absorb up to 60 percent of the calcium they ingest, and pregnant women, about 50 percent. Other adults, who are not growing, absorb about 25 to 30 percent.[27]

People may think that taking a calcium supplement is preferable to getting calcium from food, but foods offer important fringe benefits. For example, drinking 3 cups of milk fortified with vitamins A and D will supply substantial amounts of other nutrients. Furthermore, the vitamin D and possibly other nutrients in the milk enhance calcium absorption. Some people absorb calcium better from milk and milk products than from even the most absorbable supplements. The National Institutes of Health concludes that foods are the best sources of calcium and recommends supplements only when intake from food is insufficient.

Phosphorus

Phosphorus is the second most abundant mineral in the body. About 85 percent of it is found combined with calcium in the crystals of the bones and teeth. As part of one of the body's buffer systems (phosphoric acid), phosphorus is also found in all body tissues. Phosphorus is a part of DNA and RNA, the genetic material present in every cell. Thus, phosphorus is necessary for all growth. Phosphorus also plays many key roles in

TABLE 9-7 **Suggested Minimum Daily Fluid Milk Intakes**

Young children (4 to 8 years of age)	2½ cups
Older children and adolescents	3 cups
Adults	3 cups
Pregnant or lactating women	3 cups
Women past menopause	3 cups

© Cengage Learning®

binders: chemical compounds in foods that combine with nutrients (especially minerals) to form complexes the body cannot absorb. Examples include *phytates* and *oxalates*.

SARDINES (with bones) 3 oz = 325 mg

MILK 1 c = 300 mg

TOFU (calcium set) ½ c = 250 mg

CHEDDAR CHEESE 1½ oz = 300 mg

TURNIP GREENS (cooked) 1 c = 198 mg

WAFFLE (whole grain) 1 waffle = 196 mg

BOK CHOY[b] (cooked) 1 c = 158 mg

Cengage Learning

[a] These foods provide 10 percent or more of the calcium Daily Value in a serving.
[b] Broccoli, bok choy, kale, and some other cooked green leafy vegetables are important sources of bioavailable calcium. Almonds also supply calcium. Other greens, such as spinach and chard, contain calcium in an unabsorbable form. Some calcium-rich mineral waters may also be good sources.

FIGURE 9-6 **Good Sources of Calcium**[a]

Those who tolerate milk can slip extra calcium into meals by sprinkling a tablespoon or two of fat-free dry milk into almost everything. The added kcalorie value is small, and changes to the taste and texture of the dish are practically nil. Yet each 2 tablespoons adds about 100 extra milligrams of calcium and moves people closer to meeting the recommendation to obtain 3 cups of milk each day. Here are some more tips for including calcium-rich foods in your meals.

At Breakfast

- Choose calcium-fortified orange or vegetable juice.
- Serve tea or coffee, hot or iced, with milk.
- Choose cereals, hot or cold, with milk.
- Cook hot cereals with milk instead of water; then mix in 2 tablespoons of fat-free dry milk.
- Make muffins or quick breads with milk and extra fat-free powdered milk.
- Add milk to scrambled eggs.
- Moisten cereals with flavored yogurt.

At Lunch

- Add low-fat cheeses to sandwiches, burgers, or salads.
- Use a variety of green vegetables, such as watercress or kale, in salads and on sandwiches.
- Drink fat-free milk or calcium-fortified soy milk as a beverage or in a smoothie.

- Drink calcium-rich mineral water as a beverage (studies suggest significant calcium absorption).
- Marinate cabbage shreds or broccoli spears in low-fat Italian dressing for an interesting salad that provides calcium.
- Choose coleslaw over potato and macaroni salads.
- Mix the mashed bones of canned salmon into salmon salad or patties.
- Eat sardines with their bones.
- Stuff potatoes with broccoli and low-fat cheese.
- Try pasta such as ravioli stuffed with low-fat ricotta cheese instead of meat.
- Sprinkle Parmesan cheese on pasta salads.

At Supper

- Toss a handful of thinly sliced green vegetables, such as kale or young turnip greens, with hot pasta; the greens wilt pleasingly in the steam of the freshly cooked pasta.
- Serve a green vegetable every night and try new ones—how about kohlrabi? It tastes delicious when cooked like broccoli.
- Learn to stir-fry Chinese cabbage and other Asian foods.
- Try tofu (the calcium-set kind); this versatile food has inspired whole cookbooks devoted to its creative uses.
- Add fat-free powdered milk to almost anything—meatloaf, sauces, gravies, soups, stuffings, casseroles, blended beverages, puddings, quick breads, cookies, brownies. Be creative.
- Choose frozen yogurt, ice milk, or custards for dessert.

the transfer of energy that occurs during cellular metabolism. Phosphorus-containing lipids (phospholipids) help transport other lipids in the blood. Phospholipids are also principal components of cell membranes.

Animal protein is the best source of phosphorus because the mineral is so abundant in the cells of animals. Milk and cheese are also rich sources. Diets that provide adequate energy and protein also supply adequate phosphorus. Dietary deficiencies are rare. A summary of facts about phosphorus appears in Table 9-8 later in the chapter.

Magnesium

Magnesium barely qualifies as a major mineral. Only about 1 ounce of magnesium is present in the body of a 130-pound person, more than half of it in the bones. Most of the rest is in the muscles, heart, liver, and other soft tissues, with only 1 percent in the body fluids. Bone magnesium seems to be a reservoir to ensure that some will be on hand for vital reactions regardless of recent dietary intake.

Magnesium is critical to the operation of hundreds of enzymes and other cellular functions.[28] It acts in all the cells of the soft tissues, where it forms part of the protein-making machinery and is necessary for the release of energy. Magnesium and calcium work together for proper functioning of the muscles: calcium promotes contraction, and magnesium helps relax the muscles afterward. Magnesium is also critical to normal heart function.[29] Like many other nutrients, magnesium supports the normal functioning of the immune system and inflammatory response.[30]

Magnesium Deficiency Magnesium deficiency can result from inadequate intake, vomiting, diarrhea, alcohol abuse, or malnutrition; in people who have been fed nutritionally incomplete fluids intravenously for too long after surgery; or in people using diuretics. Magnesium deficiency symptoms include a low blood calcium level, muscle cramps, and seizures. Magnesium deficiency is thought to cause the hallucinations commonly experienced during withdrawal from alcohol intoxication. In addition, magnesium deficiency may worsen inflammation associated with many chronic diseases and may increase the risk of stroke and sudden death by heart failure, even in otherwise healthy people.[31] Low intakes of magnesium may have adverse effects on bone metabolism and increase the risk for osteoporosis as well.[32]

Magnesium Toxicity Magnesium toxicity is rare, but it can be fatal. Toxicity occurs only with high intakes from nonfood sources such as supplements or magnesium salts. Accidental poisonings may occur in children with access to medicine cabinets and in older adults who abuse magnesium-containing laxatives, antacids, and other medications. The consequences include diarrhea, abdominal cramps, and, in severe cases, acid–base imbalance and potassium depletion.

Magnesium Intakes and Food Sources Although average magnesium intakes typically fall below recommendations, deficiency symptoms are rare in healthy people. In some areas of the country, the water naturally contains both calcium and magnesium. This so-called "hard" water can contribute significantly to magnesium intakes.

Magnesium-rich food sources include dark green, leafy vegetables; nuts; legumes; whole-grain breads and cereals; seafood; chocolate; and cocoa (see Figure 9-7). Magnesium is easily lost from foods during processing, so unprocessed foods are the best choices.

Sulfate

Sulfate is the oxidized form of sulfur as it exists in foods and water. The body requires sulfate for the synthesis of many important sulfur-containing compounds. Sulfur-containing amino acids play an important role in helping to shape strands of protein.* The particular shape of a protein enables it to do its specific job, such as enzyme work. Skin, hair, and nails contain some of the body's more rigid proteins, which have high sulfur contents.

There is no recommended intake for sulfur, and no deficiencies are known. Only a person who lacks protein to the point of severe deficiency will lack the sulfur-containing amino acids.

SPINACH (cooked)
1/2 c = 78 mg

BLACK BEANS (cooked)
1/2 c = 60 mg

SOY MILK
1 c = 46 mg

BRAN CEREAL[b]
(ready-to-eat)
1 c = 80 mg

OYSTERS[c] (steamed)
3 oz = 42 mg

YOGURT (plain)
1 c = 43 mg

© Cengage Learning®

[a]These foods provide 10 percent or more of the magnesium Daily Value in a serving.
[b]Wheat bran provides magnesium, but refined grain products are low in magnesium.
[c]Magnesium in oysters varies.

FIGURE 9-7 Good Sources of Magnesium[a]

*The sulfur-containing amino acids are methionine and cysteine. Cysteine in one part of a protein chain can bind to cysteine in another part of the chain by way of a sulfur-sulfur bridge, thus helping to stabilize the protein structure.

IN SUMMARY

- All of the major minerals influence the body's fluid balance, but sodium, chloride, and potassium are most noted for this role.

- Excess sodium in the diet contributes to high blood pressure.

- Most of the body's calcium is in the bones, where it provides a rigid structure and a reservoir of calcium for the blood.

- Magnesium is critical to the operation of hundreds of enzymes and other cellular functions.

Table 9-8 offers a summary of the major minerals and their functions.

TABLE 9-8 The Major Minerals—A Summary

Mineral Name	Chief Functions in the Body	Deficiency Symptoms	Toxicity Symptoms	Significant Sources
Sodium	With chloride and potassium (electrolytes), maintains cells' normal fluid balance and acid–base balance in the body. Also critical to nerve impulse transmission and muscle contraction.	Muscle cramps, mental apathy, loss of appetite	Hypertension	Salt, soy sauce, processed foods
Chloride	Part of the hydrochloric acid found in the stomach and necessary for proper digestion.	Does not occur under normal circumstances	Normally harmless (the gas chlorine is a poison but evaporates from water); can cause vomiting	Salt, soy sauce; moderate quantities in whole, unprocessed foods; large amounts in processed foods
Potassium	Facilitates reactions, including the making of protein; the maintenance of fluid and electrolyte balance; the support of cell integrity; the transmission of nerve impulses; and the contraction of muscles, including the heart.	Moderate deficiency: elevated blood pressure, increased salt sensitivity, increased risk of kidney stones, increased bone turnover. Severe deficiency: cardiac arrhythmias, muscle weakness, glucose intolerance.	Causes muscular weakness; triggers vomiting; if given into a vein, can stop the heart	All whole foods: meats, milk, fruits, vegetables, grains, legumes
Calcium	The principal mineral of bones and teeth. Also acts in normal muscle contraction and relaxation, nerve functioning, blood clotting, blood pressure, and immune defenses.	Stunted growth in children; adult bone loss (osteoporosis)	Constipation; increased risk of urinary stone formation and kidney dysfunction; interference with absorption of other minerals	Milk and milk products, oysters, small fish (with bones), tofu (bean curd), greens, legumes
Phosphorus	Involved in the mineralization of bones and teeth. Important in cells' genetic material, in cell membranes as phospholipids, in energy transfer, and in buffering systems.	Phosphorus deficiency unknown	Calcification of nonskeletal tissues, particularly the kidneys	Foods from animal sources (meat, fish, poultry, eggs, milk)
Magnesium	Another factor involved in bone mineralization, the building of protein, enzyme action, normal muscular contraction, and transmission of nerve impulses.	Low blood calcium; muscle cramps; confusion; if extreme, seizures, bizarre movements, hallucinations, and difficulty in swallowing; in children, growth failure.	From nonfood sources only; diarrhea, nausea, and abdominal cramps; acid–base imbalance; potassium depletion	Nuts, legumes, whole grains, dark green vegetables, seafoods, chocolate, cocoa
Sulfate	A component of certain amino acids; part of the vitamins biotin and thiamin and the hormone insulin; stabilizes protein shape by forming sulfur–sulfur bridges.	None known; protein deficiency would occur first	Would occur only if sulfur amino acids were eaten in excess; this (in animals) depresses growth	All protein-containing foods (meats, fish, poultry, eggs, milk, legumes, nuts)

9.3 The Trace Minerals

LO 9.3 Identify the main roles, deficiency and toxicity symptoms, and food sources for each of the trace minerals (iron, zinc, selenium, iodine, copper, manganese, fluoride, chromium, and molybdenum).

Figure 9-1, earlier in this chapter, shows how tiny the quantities of trace minerals in the human body are. If you could remove all of them from your body, you would have only a bit of dust, hardly enough to fill a teaspoon. Yet each of the trace minerals performs some vital role for which no substitute will do. A deficiency of any of them can be fatal, and an excess of many can be equally deadly. Table 9-9, at the end of the chapter, provides a summary of the trace minerals.

Iron

Every living cell—both plant and animal—contains iron. Most of the iron in the body is a component of the proteins **hemoglobin** in red blood cells and **myoglobin** in muscle cells. The iron in both hemoglobin and myoglobin helps them carry and hold oxygen and then release it. Hemoglobin in the blood carries oxygen from the lungs to tissues throughout the body. Myoglobin holds oxygen for the muscles to use when they contract. As part of many enzymes, iron is vital to the processes by which cells generate energy. Iron is also needed to make new cells, amino acids, hormones, and neurotransmitters.

The special provisions the body makes for iron's handling show that it is a precious mineral to be tightly hoarded. For example, when a red blood cell dies, the liver saves the iron and returns it to the bone marrow, which uses it to build new red blood cells. The body does lose iron from the digestive tract, in nail and hair trimmings, and in shed skin cells, but only in tiny amounts. Bleeding, however, can cause significant iron loss from the body.

Special measures are needed to maintain an appropriate iron balance in the body. Iron is a powerful oxidant that generates free-radical reactions. Free radicals increase oxidative stress and inflammation associated with diseases such as diabetes, heart disease, and cancer.[33] To ensure that enough iron is available to meet the body's needs and yet guard against excessive and damaging levels, special proteins transport and store the body's iron supply, and its absorption is tightly regulated.[34] Because the body has no active means of excreting excess iron, regulation of absorption plays a critical role in iron homeostasis.[35]

Normally, only about 10 to 15 percent of dietary iron is absorbed, but if the body's supply is diminished or if the need increases for any reason (such as pregnancy), absorption increases. The body makes several provisions for absorbing iron. A special protein in the intestinal cells captures iron and holds it in reserve for release into the body as needed; another protein transfers the iron to **transferrin,** an iron carrier in the blood. Transferrin carries the iron to tissues throughout the body. When more iron is needed, more of these proteins are produced so that more than the usual amount of iron can be absorbed and carried. If there is a surplus, iron storage proteins—ferritin and hemosiderin—in the liver, bone marrow, and other organs store it.

Researchers are discovering genes that participate in the regulation of the body's iron at an extraordinary pace.[36] Along the way, new information about how the body controls the uptake, storage, and distribution of iron is emerging. The hormone **hepcidin,** produced by the liver, is central to the regulation of iron balance.[37] Hepcidin helps to maintain blood iron within the normal range by limiting absorption from the small intestine and controlling release from the liver, spleen, and bone marrow.[38] Many details are known about this process, but simply described, hepcidin works in an elegant feedback system to control blood iron: Elevated levels of iron in the blood (and liver) trigger hepcidin secretion, which reduces iron absorption and inhibits the

hemoglobin: the oxygen-carrying protein of the red blood cells.
hemo = blood
globin = globular protein

myoglobin: the oxygen-carrying protein of the muscle cells.
myo = muscle

transferrin (trans-FERR-in): the body's iron-carrying protein.

hepcidin (HEP-sid-in): a hormone secreted by the liver in response to elevated blood iron. Hepcidin reduces iron's absorption from the intestine and its release from storage.

release of stored iron, thereby reducing the blood iron concentration. Low levels of iron in the blood suppress hepcidin secretion, which increases iron absorption and mobilizes storage iron, raising the blood iron concentrations. Thus, the body adjusts to changing iron needs and iron availability in the diet.[39]

Iron Deficiency Worldwide, **iron deficiency** is the most common nutrient deficiency, with **iron-deficiency anemia** affecting 1.5 to 2 billion people—mostly preschool children and pregnant women.[40] In the United States, iron deficiency is less prevalent, but it still affects about 10 percent of toddlers, adolescent girls, and women of childbearing age. Iron deficiency is also relatively common among those who are overweight.[41] The association between iron deficiency and obesity has yet to be explained, but researchers are currently examining the relationships between the inflammation that develops with excess body fat and reduced iron absorption.[42]

Some stages of life demand more iron but provide less, making deficiency likely.[43] Women are especially prone to iron deficiency during their reproductive years because of blood losses during menstruation. Pregnancy places further iron demands on women: iron is needed to support the added blood volume, the growth of the fetus, and blood loss during childbirth. Infants (6 months or older) and young children receive little iron from their high-milk diets, yet they need extra iron to support their rapid growth and brain development. The rapid growth of adolescence, especially for males, and the blood losses of menstruation for females also demand extra iron that a typical teen diet may not provide. To summarize, an adequate iron intake is especially important for women in their reproductive years, pregnant women, infants, toddlers, and adolescents.

Causes of Iron Deficiency The cause of iron deficiency is usually inadequate intake resulting from iron-poor food choices or a sheer lack of food altogether. In the Western world, high sugar and fat intakes are often associated with low iron intakes. Blood loss is the primary nonnutritional cause, especially in poor regions of the world where parasitic infections of the GI tract may lead to blood loss.

Assessment of Iron Deficiency Iron deficiency develops in three stages that can be identified using laboratory tests (Appendix E provides more details). In the first stage of iron deficiency both iron stores and ferritin levels diminish. Measures of serum ferritin (in the blood) reflect iron stores and are most valuable in assessing iron status at this earliest stage.

The second stage of iron deficiency is characterized by a decrease in transport iron: levels of serum iron fall, and levels of the iron-carrying protein transferrin *increase* (an adaptation that enhances iron absorption). Together, these two measures can determine the severity of the deficiency—the more transferrin and the less iron in the blood, the more advanced the deficiency is. Transferrin saturation—the percentage of transferrin that is saturated with iron—decreases as iron stores decline.

The third stage of iron deficiency occurs when the lack of iron limits hemoglobin production. Now the hemoglobin precursor, **erythrocyte protoporphyrin,** begins to accumulate as hemoglobin and **hematocrit** values decline.

Hemoglobin and hematocrit tests are easy, quick, and inexpensive, so they are the tests most commonly used in evaluating iron status. Their usefulness is limited, however, because they are late indicators of iron deficiency. Furthermore, other nutrient deficiencies and medical conditions can influence their values.

Iron Deficiency and Anemia Iron deficiency and iron-deficiency anemia are not the same: people may be iron deficient without being anemic. The term *iron deficiency* refers to depleted body iron stores without regard to the degree of depletion or to the presence of anemia. The term *iron-deficiency anemia* refers to the severe depletion of iron stores that results in a low hemoglobin concentration. In iron-deficiency anemia,

iron deficiency: the condition of having depleted iron stores.

iron-deficiency anemia: a blood iron deficiency characterized by small, pale red blood cells; also called *microcytic hypochromic anemia*.

micro = small
cytic = cells
hypo = too little
chrom = color

erythrocyte protoporphyrin (PRO-toh-PORE-fe-rin)**:** a precursor to hemoglobin.

hematocrit (hee-MAT-oh-crit)**:** measurement of the volume of the red blood cells packed by centrifuge in a given volume of blood.

red blood cells are pale and small (see Figure 9-8). They can't carry enough oxygen from the lungs to the tissues. Without adequate iron, energy metabolism in the cells falters. The result is fatigue, weakness, headaches, apathy, pallor, and poor resistance to cold temperatures. Because hemoglobin is the bright red pigment of the blood, the skin of a fair person who is anemic may become noticeably pale. In a dark-skinned person, the tongue and eye lining, normally pink, will be very pale.

The fatigue that accompanies iron-deficiency anemia differs from the tiredness a person experiences from a simple lack of sleep. People with anemia feel fatigue only when they exert themselves. Iron supplementation can, over time, relieve the fatigue and improve the body's response to physical activity.

Less severe iron deficiency produces symptoms, too. Long before the red blood cells are affected and anemia is diagnosed, a developing iron deficiency affects behavior.[44] Even at slightly lowered iron levels, energy metabolism is impaired and neurotransmitter synthesis is altered, reducing physical work capacity and mental productivity.[45] Without the physical energy and mental alertness to work, plan, think, play, sing, or learn, people simply do these things less. They have no obvious deficiency signs; they just appear unmotivated, apathetic, and less physically fit. Children deprived of iron become irritable, restless, and unable to pay attention (see Chapter 12). These symptoms are among the first to appear when the body's iron begins to fall and among the first to disappear when iron status is restored.

Iron Deficiency and Pica A curious behavior seen in some iron-deficient (and sometimes zinc-deficient) people, especially in women and children of low-income groups, is **pica**—the craving for and consumption of ice, chalk, starch, and other non-food substances. These substances contain no iron and cannot remedy a deficiency; in fact, clay actually inhibits iron absorption, which may explain the iron deficiency that accompanies such behavior. Pica is poorly understood. Its cause is unknown, but researchers hypothesize that it may be motivated by hunger, nutrient deficiencies, or an attempt to protect against toxins or microbes.[46]

Caution on Self-Diagnosis Low hemoglobin may reflect an inadequate iron intake, and, if it does, the physician may prescribe iron supplements. Any nutrient deficiency, disease, or agent that interferes with hemoglobin synthesis, disrupts hemoglobin function, or causes a loss of red blood cells can precipitate anemia, however. Thus, feeling fatigued, weak, and apathetic is a sign that something is wrong and that a person should consult a physician, not an indication that he or she should take supplements. In fact, iron supplements can mask a serious medical condition, such as hidden bleeding from cancer or an ulcer. Furthermore, a person can waste precious time by not seeking treatment. Remember, don't self-diagnose.

Iron Overload As mentioned earlier, because too much iron can be toxic, its levels in the body are closely regulated and absorption normally decreases when iron stores are full.[47] Even a diet that includes fortified foods usually poses no risk for most people, but some people are vulnerable to excess iron. Once considered rare, **iron overload** has emerged as an important disorder of iron metabolism and regulation.

Iron overload, known as **hemochromatosis,** is usually caused by a genetic failure to prevent unneeded iron in the diet from being absorbed.[48] Research suggests that just as insulin supports normal glucose homeostasis, and its absence or ineffectiveness causes diabetes, the hormone hepcidin supports iron homeostasis and a deficiency of or (rarely) resistance to it causes hemochromatosis.[49] Other causes of iron overload include repeated blood transfusions, massive doses of supplementary iron, and other rare metabolic disorders.

Some of the signs and symptoms of iron overload are similar to those of iron deficiency: apathy, lethargy, and fatigue. Therefore, taking iron supplements before assessing iron status is clearly unwise; hemoglobin tests alone would fail to make the distinction because excess iron accumulates in storage. Iron overload assessment tests measure transferrin saturation and serum ferritin.

Normal red blood cells. Both size and color are normal.

Blood cells in iron-deficiency anemia. These cells are small and pale because they contain less hemoglobin.

FIGURE 9-8 Normal and Anemic Blood Cells

pica (PIE-ka)**:** a craving for nonfood substances; also known as *geophagia* (jee-oh-FAY-jee-uh) when referring to clay-eating behavior.
  picus = woodpecker or magpie
  geo = earth
  phagein = to eat

iron overload: toxicity from excess iron.

hemochromatosis (heem-oh-crome-a-TOH-sis)**:** iron overload characterized by deposits of iron-containing pigment in many tissues, with tissue damage. Hemochromatosis is usually caused by a hereditary defect in iron absorption.

Iron overload is characterized by free-radical tissue damage, especially in iron-storing organs such as the liver.[50] Infections are likely because bacteria thrive on iron-rich blood.[51] Symptoms are most severe in alcohol abusers because alcohol damages the intestine, further impairing its defenses against absorbing excess iron. Untreated hemochromatosis aggravates the risk of diabetes, liver cancer, heart disease, and arthritis.

Iron overload is much more common in men than in women and is twice as prevalent among men as iron deficiency. The widespread fortification of foods with iron makes it difficult for people with hemochromatosis to follow an iron-restricted diet.

Iron Poisoning The rapid ingestion of massive amounts of iron can cause sudden death. Iron-containing supplements can easily cause accidental poisonings in young children.[52] As few as five iron tablets have caused death in a child. Keep iron-containing supplements out of children's reach. If you suspect iron poisoning, call the nearest poison center or a physician immediately.

Iron Recommendations The average eating pattern in the United States provides only about 6 to 7 milligrams of iron for every 1000 kcalories. Men need 8 milligrams of iron each day; most men easily take in more than 2000 kcalories, so a man can meet his iron needs without special effort. The recommendation for women during childbearing years, however, is 18 milligrams. Because women have higher iron needs and typically consume fewer than 2000 kcalories per day, they have trouble achieving appropriate iron intakes. On average, women receive only 12 to 13 milligrams of iron per day, not enough until after menopause. To meet their iron needs from foods, premenopausal women need to select iron-rich foods at every meal. Vegetarians, because vegetable sources of iron are poorly absorbed, should aim for 1.8 times the normal requirement (see Nutrition in Practice 4).

Iron in Foods Iron occurs in two forms in foods: heme and nonheme. Heme iron, which is up to 10 times more absorbable than nonheme iron, is bound into the iron-carrying proteins hemoglobin and myoglobin in meat, poultry, and fish. Heme iron contributes a small portion of the iron consumed by most people, but it is absorbed at a fairly constant rate of about 23 percent. Nonheme iron is found in both meats and plant foods. People absorb nonheme iron at a lower rate (2 to 20 percent); its absorption depends on several dietary factors and iron stores. Most of the iron people consume is nonheme iron from vegetables, grains, eggs, meat, fish, and poultry. Figure 9-9 shows the iron contents of several different foods.

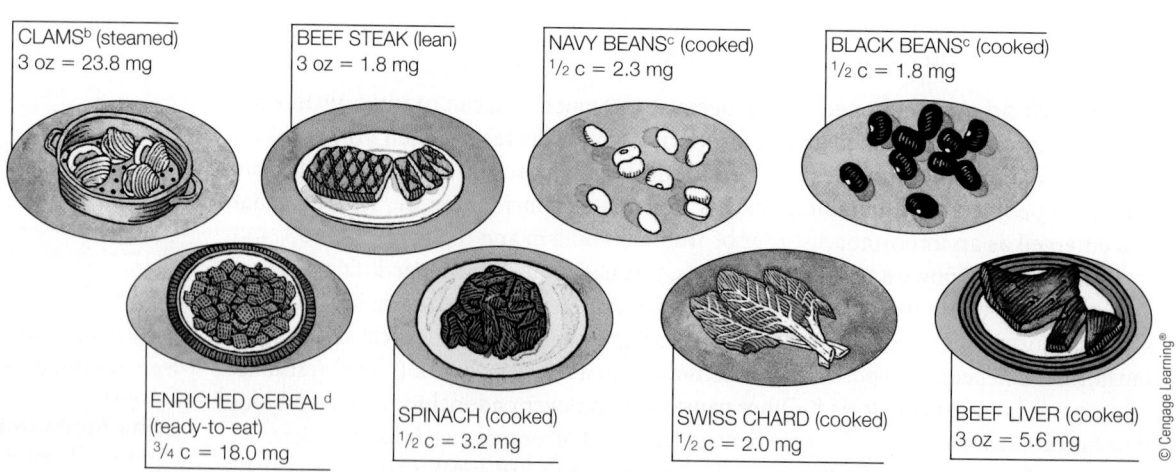

CLAMS[b] (steamed)
3 oz = 23.8 mg

BEEF STEAK (lean)
3 oz = 1.8 mg

NAVY BEANS[c] (cooked)
1/2 c = 2.3 mg

BLACK BEANS[c] (cooked)
1/2 c = 1.8 mg

ENRICHED CEREAL[d]
(ready-to-eat)
3/4 c = 18.0 mg

SPINACH (cooked)
1/2 c = 3.2 mg

SWISS CHARD (cooked)
1/2 c = 2.0 mg

BEEF LIVER (cooked)
3 oz = 5.6 mg

© Cengage Learning®

[a]These foods provide 10 percent or more of the iron Daily Value in a serving. For a 2000-kcalorie diet, the DV is 18 mg/day.
Note: Dried figs contain 0.6 mg per 1/4 cup; raisins contain 0.8 mg per 1/4 cup.
[b]Some clams may contain less, but most types are iron-rich foods.
[c]Legumes contain phytates that reduce iron absorption.
[d]Enriched cereals vary widely in iron content.

FIGURE 9-9 Good Sources of Iron[a]

The following set of guidelines can be used for planning an iron-rich diet:

- *Breads and cereals.* Use only whole-grain, enriched, and fortified products (iron is one of the enrichment nutrients).
- *Vegetables.* The dark green, leafy vegetables are good sources of vitamin C and iron. Eat vitamin C–rich vegetables often to enhance absorption of the iron from foods eaten with them.
- *Fruits.* Dried fruits, such as raisins, apricots, peaches, and prunes, are high in iron. Eat vitamin C–rich fruits often with iron-containing foods.

- *Milk and cheese.* Do not overdo foods from the milk group; they are poor sources of iron. But do not omit them, either, because they are rich in calcium. Drink fat-free milk to free kcalories to be invested in iron-rich foods.
- *Meats.* Meat, fish, and poultry are excellent iron sources.
- *Legumes.* Include legumes frequently. One cup of peas or beans can supply up to 7 milligrams of iron.

Iron absorption from foods can be maximized by two substances that enhance iron absorption: MFP factor and vitamin C. Meat, fish, and poultry contain MFP factor, a factor other than heme that promotes the absorption of iron—even nonheme iron from other foods eaten at the same time. Vitamin C eaten in the same meal also doubles or triples nonheme iron absorption. Additionally, cooking with iron skillets can contribute iron to the diet. Some substances impair iron absorption; they include the **tannins** of tea and coffee, the calcium in milk, and the **phytates** that accompany fiber in legumes and whole-grain cereals. Box 9-3 offers suggestions for obtaining adequate iron.

This chili dinner provides iron and MFP factor from meat, iron from legumes, and vitamin C from tomatoes. The combination of heme iron, nonheme iron, MFP factor, and vitamin C helps to achieve maximum iron absorption.

Zinc

Zinc is a versatile trace mineral necessary for the activation of more than 50 different enzymes.[53] These zinc-requiring enzymes perform tasks in the eyes, liver, kidneys, muscles, skin, bones, and male reproductive organs. Zinc works with the enzymes that make genetic material; manufacture heme; digest food; metabolize carbohydrate, protein, and fat; liberate vitamin A from storage in the liver; and dispose of damaging free radicals. Zinc also interacts with platelets in blood clotting, affects thyroid hormone function, assists in immune function, and affects behavior and learning performance. Zinc is needed to produce the active form of vitamin A in visual pigments and is essential to wound healing, taste perception, the making of sperm, and fetal development. When zinc deficiency occurs, it impairs all these and other functions.

The body's handling of zinc differs from that of iron but with some interesting similarities. For example, like iron, extra zinc that enters the body is held within the intestinal cells, and only the amount needed is released into the bloodstream. As with iron, zinc status influences the percentage of zinc absorbed from the diet; if more is needed, more is absorbed.

Zinc's main transport vehicle in the blood is the protein albumin. This may account for observations that serum zinc concentrations decline in conditions that lower plasma albumin concentrations—for example, pregnancy and malnutrition.

Zinc Deficiency Zinc deficiency in human beings was first reported in the 1960s in studies of growing children and male adolescents in Egypt, Iran, and Turkey. Their diets were typically low in zinc and high in fiber and phytates (which impair zinc absorption). The zinc deficiency was marked by dwarfism, or severe growth retardation, and arrested sexual maturation—symptoms that were responsive to zinc supplementation.

tannins: compounds in tea (especially black tea) and coffee that bind iron.

phytates: nonnutrient components of grains, legumes, and seeds. Phytates can bind minerals such as iron, zinc, calcium, and magnesium in insoluble complexes in the intestine, and the body excretes them unused.

Since that time, zinc deficiency has been recognized elsewhere and is known to affect more than growth. It drastically impairs immune function, causes loss of appetite, and, during pregnancy, may lead to growth and developmental disorders. In the developing world, more than 2 billion people are zinc deficient, and zinc deficiency is a substantial contributor to illness and death.[54] A detailed list of symptoms of zinc deficiency is presented later in Table 9-9.

Pronounced zinc deficiency is not widespread in developed countries, but deficiencies do occur in the most vulnerable groups of the U.S. population—pregnant women, young children, the elderly, and the poor. Even mild zinc deficiency can result in metabolic changes such as impaired immune response, abnormal taste, and abnormal dark adaptation (zinc is required to produce the active form of vitamin A, retinal, in visual pigments).

Some people are at greater risk of zinc deficiency than others. Pregnant teenagers need zinc for their own growth as well as for the developing fetus. Vegetarians whose diets emphasize whole grains, legumes, and other plant foods may also be at risk. These foods, though rich in zinc, also contain phytate, a potent inhibitor of zinc absorption.[55] Protein enhances zinc absorption, but most plant-protein foods also contain phytate. The DRI committee suggests that the dietary zinc requirement for vegetarians who exclude all animal-derived foods may be as much as 50 percent greater than the RDA, but so far evidence is insufficient to establish zinc recommendations based on the presence of other food components or nutrients. Vegetarians who include cheese, eggs, or other animal protein in their diet absorb more zinc than those who exclude these foods.

Zinc Toxicity Zinc can be toxic if consumed in large enough quantities. A high zinc intake is known to produce copper-deficiency anemia by inducing the intestinal cells to synthesize large amounts of a protein (metallothionein) that captures copper in a nonabsorbable form. Accidental consumption of high levels of zinc can cause vomiting, diarrhea, headaches, exhaustion, and other symptoms (see Table 9-9, later in the chapter). Large doses can even be fatal. The UL for zinc for adults is 40 milligrams per day.

Zinc Recommendations and Food Sources Most people in the United States have zinc intakes that approximate recommendations. Zinc is most abundant in foods high in protein, such as shellfish (especially oysters), meats, poultry, and milk products. In general, two 3-ounce servings a day of animal protein foods provide most of the zinc a healthy person needs. Legumes and whole-grain products are good sources of zinc if eaten in large quantities. For infants, breast milk is a good source of zinc, which is more efficiently absorbed from human milk than from cow's milk. Commercial infant formulas are fortified with zinc, of course. Figure 9-10 shows zinc-rich foods.

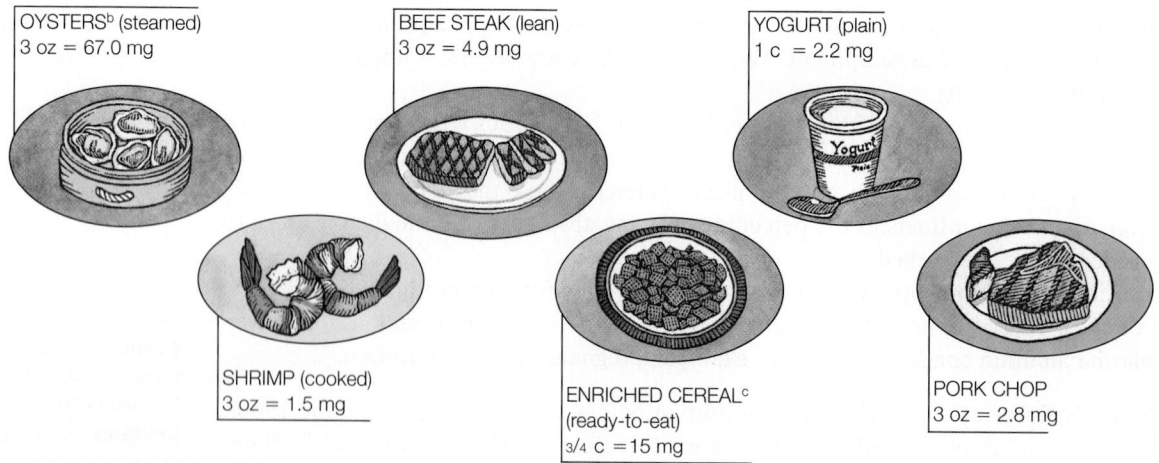

OYSTERS[b] (steamed)
3 oz = 67.0 mg

BEEF STEAK (lean)
3 oz = 4.9 mg

YOGURT (plain)
1 c = 2.2 mg

SHRIMP (cooked)
3 oz = 1.5 mg

ENRICHED CEREAL[c]
(ready-to-eat)
3/4 c = 15 mg

PORK CHOP
3 oz = 2.8 mg

[a]These foods provide 10 percent or more of the zinc Daily Value in a serving.
[b]Some oysters contain more or less than this amount, but all types are zinc-rich foods.
[c]Enriched cereals vary widely in zinc content.

FIGURE 9-10 Good Sources of Zinc[a]

Zinc supplements are not recommended unless prescribed for an accurately diagnosed zinc deficiency or as a medication to displace other ions in unusual medical circumstances. Normally, it is possible to obtain enough zinc from the diet. Zinc from cold-relief lozenges, sprays, and gels may sometimes shorten the duration of a cold, but they can upset the stomach and contribute supplemental zinc to the body.[56]

Selenium

Selenium is an essential trace mineral that functions as an antioxidant nutrient, working primarily as a part of proteins—most notably, the enzyme glutathione peroxidase.[57] Glutathione peroxidase and vitamin E work in tandem. Glutathione peroxidase prevents free-radical formation, thus blocking the damaging chain reaction before it begins; if free radicals do form, and a chain reaction starts, vitamin E halts it. Selenium-containing enzymes are necessary for the proper functioning of the iodine-containing thyroid hormones that regulate metabolism.[58]

Selenium and Cancer The question of whether selenium protects against the development of certain cancers, particularly prostate cancer, is under intense investigation.[59] Adequate *blood* selenium seems protective against cancers of the prostate, colon, and other sites.[60] Many questions remain unanswered regarding selenium status, intake, and cancer, however. For example, the range of selenium status and the levels of intakes most beneficial to reducing cancer risk have not been established.[61] Given the potential for harm from excess selenium and the lack of conclusive evidence, recommending selenium supplements to prevent cancer would be premature.

Selenium Deficiency Selenium deficiency is associated with Keshan disease—a heart disease observed in children and young women living in regions of China where the soil and foods lack selenium. Keshan disease is named for one of the provinces where it was studied. Although the primary cause of Keshan disease is probably a virus, selenium deficiency appears to predispose people to it, and adequate selenium seems to prevent it.

Selenium Toxicity Because high doses of selenium are toxic, a UL has been set (see inside front cover). Selenium toxicity causes vomiting, diarrhea, loss of hair and nails, and lesions of the skin and nervous system.[62]

Selenium Recommendations and Intakes Anyone who eats a normal diet composed mostly of unprocessed foods need not worry about meeting selenium recommendations. Selenium is widely distributed in foods such as meats and shellfish and in vegetables and grains grown on selenium-rich soil. Some regions in the United States and Canada produce crops on selenium-poor soil, but people are protected from deficiency because they eat selenium-rich meat and supermarket foods transported from other regions. Eating as few as two Brazil nuts a day effectively improves selenium status.

Iodine

Traces of the iodine ion (called iodide) are indispensible to life. In the GI tract, iodine from foods becomes iodide. This chapter uses the term *iodine* when referring to the nutrient in foods, and *iodide* when referring to it in the body. Iodide occurs in the body in minuscule amounts, but its principal role in human nutrition is well known, and the amount needed is well established. Iodide is an integral part of the thyroid hormones, which regulate body temperature, metabolic rate, reproduction, growth, the making of blood cells, nerve and muscle function, and more.

FIGURE 9-11 Iodine-Deficiency Symptom—The Enlarged Thyroid of Goiter

In iodine deficiency, the thyroid gland enlarges—a condition known as simple goiter.

Iodine Deficiency and Toxicity When the iodide concentration in the blood is low, the cells of the thyroid gland enlarge in an attempt to trap as many particles of iodide as possible. If the gland enlarges until it is visible, the swelling is called a **goiter** (see Figure 9-11). People with iodine deficiency this severe become sluggish and may gain weight. Goiter afflicts about 200 million people the world over, many of them in South America, Asia, and Africa. In most cases of goiter, the cause is iodine deficiency, but some people have goiter because they overconsume foods of the cabbage family and others that contain an antithyroid substance (**goitrogen**) whose effect is not counteracted by dietary iodine.

Goiter may be the earliest and most obvious sign of iodine deficiency, but the most tragic and prevalent damage occurs in the brain. Iodine deficiency is the most common cause of *preventable* mental retardation and brain damage in the world. Nearly one-third of the world's school-age children have iodine deficiency.[63] Children with even a mild iodine deficiency typically have goiters and perform poorly in school. With sustained treatment, however, mental performance in the classroom as well as thyroid function improves. Programs to provide iodized salt to the world's iodine-deficient areas now prevent much misery and suffering worldwide.[64]

A severe iodine deficiency during pregnancy causes the extreme and irreversible mental and physical retardation known as **cretinism.** A child with cretinism may have an IQ as low as 20 (100 is normal) and a face and body with many abnormalities. Cretinism can be averted if the pregnant woman's deficiency is detected and treated in time.

Excessive intakes of iodine can enlarge the thyroid gland, just as deficiencies can. For this reason, a UL of 1100 micrograms per day for adults has been set.

Iodine Sources and Intakes The ocean is the world's major source of iodine. In coastal areas, seafood, water, and even iodine-containing sea mist are important iodine sources.* Further inland, the amount of iodine in the diet is variable and generally reflects the amount present in the soil in which plants are grown or on which animals graze. In the United States and Canada, the use of iodized salt has largely wiped out the iodine deficiency that once was widespread. In the United States, you have to read the label to find out whether salt is iodized; in Canada, all table salt is iodized.

Average intakes in the United States are slightly above the recommended intake of 150 micrograms but still below the UL. Iodine intakes of young women, however, barely meet their need.[65]

Copper

The body contains about 100 milligrams of copper. About one-fourth is in the muscles; one-fourth is in the liver, brain, and blood; and the rest is in the bones, kidneys, and other tissues. The primary function of copper in the body is to serve as a constituent of enzymes. The copper-containing enzymes have diverse metabolic roles: they catalyze the formation of hemoglobin, help manufacture the protein collagen, inactivate histamine, degrade serotonin, assist in the healing of wounds, and help maintain the sheaths around nerve fibers. One of copper's most vital roles is to help cells use iron. Like iron, copper is needed in many reactions related to respiration and energy metabolism. The copper-dependent enzyme superoxide dismutase helps to control damage from free-radical activity in the tissues.

goiter (GOY-ter): an enlargement of the thyroid gland due to an iodine deficiency, malfunction of the gland, or overconsumption of a thyroid antagonist. Goiter caused by iodine deficiency is sometimes called *simple goiter*.

goitrogen (GOY-troh-jen): a substance that enlarges the thyroid gland and causes *toxic goiter*. Goitrogens occur naturally in such foods as cabbage, kale, brussels sprouts, cauliflower, broccoli, and kohlrabi.

cretinism (CREE-tin-ism): an iodine-deficiency disease characterized by mental and physical retardation.

*Iodine in sea mist combines with particles in the air or with water. Iodine may then enter the soil or surface water or land on plants when these particles fall to the ground or when it rains.

Copper Deficiency Copper deficiency is rare but not unknown. It has been seen in premature infants and malnourished infants. High intakes of zinc interfere with copper absorption and can lead to deficiency.

Copper Toxicity Some genetic disorders create a copper toxicity. Copper toxicity from foods, however, is unlikely. The UL for copper is set at 10,000 micrograms per day.

Copper Recommendations and Food Sources The RDA for copper is 900 micrograms per day, which is slightly below the average intake for adults in the United States. The best food sources of copper are organ meats, legumes, whole grains, seafood, nuts, and seeds.

Manganese

The human body contains a tiny 20 milligrams of manganese, mostly in the bones and metabolically active organs such as the liver, kidneys, and pancreas. Manganese is a cofactor for many enzymes, helping to facilitate dozens of different metabolic processes. Deficiencies of manganese have not been noted in people, but toxicity may be severe. Miners who inhale large quantities of manganese dust on the job over prolonged periods show many symptoms of a brain disease, along with abnormalities in appearance and behavior. The UL for manganese is 11 milligrams per day.

Manganese requirements are low, and plant foods such as nuts, whole grains, and leafy green vegetables contain significant amounts of this trace mineral. Deficiencies are therefore unlikely.

Fluoride

Fluoride's primary role in health is the prevention of dental caries throughout life.[66] Only a trace of fluoride occurs in the human body, but it is important to the mineralization of the bones and teeth. When bones and teeth become mineralized, first a crystal called hydroxyapatite forms from calcium and phosphorus. Then fluoride replaces the hydroxy portion of hydroxyapatite, forming **fluorapatite.** During development, fluorapatite enlarges crystals in bones and teeth, decreasing their susceptibility to demineralization and making the teeth more resistant to decay. Once the teeth have erupted, the topical application of fluoride by way of toothpaste or mouth rinse continues to exert a caries-reducing effect.

Fluoride Deficiency Where fluoride is lacking in the water supply, the incidence of dental decay is high. Fluoridation of water is thus recommended as an important public health measure. Those fortunate enough to have had sufficient fluoride during the tooth-forming years of infancy and childhood are protected throughout life from dental decay. Dental problems are of great concern because they can lead to a multitude of other health problems affecting the whole body. Based on the accumulated evidence of its beneficial effects, water fluoridation has been endorsed by nearly 100 national and international organizations including the National Institute of Dental Health, the Academy of Nutrition and Dietetics, the American Medical Association, the National Cancer Institute, and the Centers for Disease Control and Prevention (CDC).[67] In fact, the CDC named water fluoridation as one of the 10 most important public health measures of the 20th century. About 70 percent of the U.S. population served by public water systems receives optimal levels of fluoride (about 0.7 milligram per liter). Most bottled waters lack fluoride.

Fluoride Sources All normal diets include some fluoride, but drinking water; processed soft drinks and fruit juice made with fluoridated water; and fluoride

fluorapatite (floor-APP-uh-tite): the stabilized form of bone and tooth crystal, in which fluoride has replaced the hydroxy portion of hydroxyapatite.

FIGURE 9-12 Fluoride Toxicity Symptom—The Mottled Teeth of Fluorosis

toothpastes, gels, and oral rinses are the most common fluoride sources in the United States. Fish and tea may supply substantial amounts as well.

In some areas, the natural fluoride concentration in water is high, and too much fluoride can damage teeth, causing **fluorosis.** For this reason, a UL (10 mg per day for adults) has been established. In mild cases, the teeth develop small white specks; in severe cases, the enamel becomes pitted and permanently stained (see Figure 9-12). Fluorosis occurs only during tooth development and cannot be reversed, making its prevention during the first three years of life a high priority. To limit fluoride ingestion, take care not to swallow fluoride-containing dental products such as toothpaste and mouthwash and use fluoride supplements only as prescribed by a physician.

Chromium

Chromium is an essential mineral that participates in carbohydrate and lipid metabolism. Chromium enhances the activity of the hormone insulin.* When chromium is lacking, a diabetes-like condition with elevated blood glucose and impaired glucose tolerance, insulin response, and glucagon response may develop. Some research findings suggest that chromium supplements improve glucose or insulin responses in diabetes, but these relationships are uncertain.[68]

Chromium deficiency is unlikely, given the small amount of chromium required and its presence in a variety of foods. The more refined foods people eat, however, the less chromium they obtain from their diets. Unrefined foods such as liver, brewer's yeast, whole grains, nuts, and cheeses are the best sources.

Other Trace Minerals

An RDA has been established for one other trace mineral, molybdenum. **Molybdenum** functions as a working part of several metal-containing enzymes, some of which are giant proteins. Deficiencies or toxicities of molybdenum are unknown.

Several other trace minerals are known or suspected to contribute to the health of the body. Nickel is recognized as important for the health of many body tissues. Nickel deficiencies harm the liver and other organs. Silicon is involved in the formation of bones and collagen. Cobalt is found in the large vitamin B_{12} molecule. Boron influences the activity of many enzymes and may play a key role in bone health, brain activities, and immune response. The future may reveal that other trace minerals also play key roles. Even arsenic—famous as the deadly poison in many murder mysteries and known to be a carcinogen—may turn out to be an essential nutrient in tiny quantities.

IN SUMMARY

▌ The body requires trace minerals in tiny amounts, and they function in similar ways—assisting enzymes all over the body.

▌ Eating a diet that consists of a variety of foods is the best way to ensure an adequate intake of these important nutrients.

▌ Many dietary factors, including the trace minerals themselves, affect the absorption and availability of these nutrients.

Table 9-9 offers a summary of facts about trace minerals in the body.

fluorosis (floor-OH-sis): mottling of the tooth enamel from ingestion of too much fluoride during tooth development.

molybdenum (mo-LIB-duh-num): a trace element.

*Small organic compounds that enhance insulin's activity are called glucose tolerance factors (GTF). Some glucose tolerance factors contain chromium.

CHAPTER NINE

TABLE 9-9 The Trace Minerals—A Summary

Mineral Name	Chief Functions in the Body	Deficiency Symptoms	Toxicity Symptoms	Significant Sources
Iron	Part of the protein hemoglobin, which carries oxygen in the blood; part of the protein myoglobin in muscles, which makes oxygen available for muscle contraction; necessary for the utilization of energy	Anemia: weakness, pallor, headaches, reduced work productivity, inability to concentrate, impaired cognitive function (children), lowered cold tolerance	Iron overload: infections, liver injury, possible increased risk of heart attack, acidosis, bloody stools, shock	Red meats, fish, poultry, shellfish, eggs, legumes, dried fruits
Zinc	Part of the hormone insulin and many enzymes; involved in making genetic material and proteins, immune reactions, transport of vitamin A, taste perception, wound healing, the making of sperm, and normal fetal development	Growth retardation, delayed sexual maturation, impaired immune function, loss of taste, poor wound healing, eye and skin lesions	Loss of appetite, impaired immunity, low HDL, nausea, vomiting, diarrhea, headaches, copper and iron deficiencies	Protein-containing foods: meats, fish, shellfish, poultry, grains, vegetables
Selenium	Assists a group of enzymes that break down reactive chemicals that harm cells	Predisposition to heart disease characterized by cardiac tissue becoming fibrous (uncommon)	Nausea, abdominal pain, nail and hair changes, nerve damage	Seafoods, organ meats, other meats, whole grains and vegetables (depending on soil content)
Iodine	A component of two thyroid hormones, which help to regulate growth, development, and metabolic rate	Goiter, cretinism	Depressed thyroid activity; goiter-like thyroid enlargement	Iodized salt; seafood; bread; plants grown in most parts of the country and animals fed those plants
Copper	Necessary for the absorption and use of iron in the formation of hemoglobin; part of several enzymes	Anemia, bone abnormalities	Vomiting, diarrhea, liver damage	Organ meats, seafood, nuts, seeds, whole grains, drinking water
Manganese	Facilitator, with enzymes, of many cell processes; bone formation	Rare	Nervous system disorders	Nuts, whole grains, leafy vegetables, tea
Fluoride	An element involved in the formation of bones and teeth; helps to make teeth resistant to decay	Susceptibility to tooth decay	Fluorosis (pitting and discoloration of teeth); skeletal fluorosis (weak, malformed bones)	Drinking water (if fluoride containing or fluoridated), tea, seafood
Chromium	Enhances insulin action and may improve glucose tolerance	Diabetes-like condition marked by an inability to use glucose normally	None reported	Meats, whole grains

© Cengage Learning®

Your Diet

Minerals

The two minerals most likely to fall short in the diet are calcium and iron. Interestingly, both are found in protein-rich foods, but not in the same foods. Milk and milk products are rich in calcium but poor in iron. Conversely, meats, poultry, fish, and legumes are rich in iron but (with the exception of small fish such as canned sardines and other canned fishes prepared with their bones) poor in calcium. Including food sources of calcium and iron in the diet can help defend against osteoporosis and iron deficiency, respectively.

Review the USDA Food Pattern comparison and nutrient analysis reports you created for the Chapter 1 "Your Diet" activity.

■ For calcium, did you drink three cups of milk or eat the equivalent in yogurt, low-fat cheese, calcium-set tofu, calcium-fortified foods, or dark green vegetables such as kale, mustard greens, or broccoli? For iron, did you eat a variety of foods, including some meat, poultry, fish, legumes, eggs, iron-fortified cereals, and dark green vegetables? (Review Figures 9-6 and 9-9, which show good sources of calcium and iron, or your nutrient analysis reports.)

- List the foods that supplied substantial amounts of calcium and iron along with their calcium and iron contents. What were your estimated calcium and iron intakes for the day?

- Consult the inside front cover of this text to find the recommended calcium and iron intakes for your age and gender group. What is your calcium RDA? What is your iron RDA? What percentage of each did you consume (refer to your nutrient analysis reports)?

- Comment on your calcium and iron intakes. Are these intakes typical on a day-to-day basis?

- If your calcium and iron intakes were 80 percent or less of the recommendation, which foods were your best sources? Can you eat more of these foods to bring your intake up to the recommended level? If not, list some foods that you might eat to increase your intake.

Clinical Applications

1. Pull together information from Chapter 1 about the different food groups and the significant sources of minerals shown or discussed in this chapter. Consider which minerals might be lacking (or excessive) in the diet of a client who reports the following:

   - Relies on highly processed foods, snack foods, and fast foods as mainstays of the diet.

   - Never uses milk, milk products, or cheese.
   - Dislikes leafy green vegetables.
   - Never eats meat, fish, poultry, or even other protein foods such as legumes.

   What additional information would help you pinpoint problems with mineral intake?

Self Check

1. Which of the following body structures helps to regulate thirst?
   a. Brainstem
   b. Cerebellum
   c. Optic nerve
   d. Hypothalamus

2. Which of the following is *not* a function of water in the body?
   a. Lubricant
   b. Source of energy
   c. Maintains protein structure
   d. Participant in chemical reactions

3. Two situations in which a person may experience fluid and electrolyte imbalances are:
   a. vomiting and burns.
   b. diarrhea and cuts.
   c. broken bones and fever.
   d. heavy sweating and excessive carbohydrate intake.

4. Three-fourths of the sodium in people's diets comes from:
   a. fresh meats.
   b. home-cooked foods.
   c. frozen vegetables and meats.
   d. salt added to food by manufacturers.

5. Which mineral is critical to keeping the heartbeat steady and plays a major role in maintaining fluid and electrolyte balance?
   a. Sodium
   b. Calcium
   c. Potassium
   d. Magnesium

6. The two best ways to prevent age-related bone loss and fracture are to:
   a. take calcium supplements and estrogen.
   b. participate in aerobic activity and drink eight glasses of milk daily.
   c. eat a diet low in fat and salt and refrain from smoking.
   d. maintain a lifelong adequate calcium intake and engage in weight-bearing physical activity.

7. Three good food sources of calcium are:
   a. milk, sardines, and broccoli.
   b. spinach, yogurt, and sardines.
   c. cottage cheese, spinach, and tofu.
   d. Swiss chard, mustard greens, and broccoli.

8. Foods high in iron that help prevent or treat anemia include:
   a. green peas and cheese.
   b. dairy foods and fresh fruits.
   c. homemade breads and most fresh vegetables.
   d. meat and dark green, leafy vegetables.

9. Two groups of people who are especially at risk for zinc deficiency are:
   a. Asians and children.
   b. infants and teenagers.
   c. smokers and athletes.
   d. pregnant adolescents and vegetarians.

10. A deficiency of ___ is one of the world's most common preventable causes of mental retardation.
    a. zinc
    b. iodine
    c. selenium
    d. magnesium

Answers to these questions appear in Appendix H.

Notes

1. S. A. Kavouras, Thirst, *Nutrition Today* 48 (2013): S7–S9; B. M. Popkin, K. E. D'Anci, and I. H. Rosenberg, Water, hydration, and health, *Nutrition Reviews* 68 (2010): 439–458.

2. J. C. Mentes, The complexities of hydration issues in the elderly, *Nutrition Today* 48 (2013): S10–S12.

3. Kavouras, 2013; F. Péronnet, Healthy hydration for physical activity, *Nutrition Today* 45 (2010): S41–S44.

4. D. F. Tate and coauthors, Replacing caloric beverages with water or diet beverages for weight loss in adults: Main results of the Choose Healthy Options Consciously Everyday (CHOICE) randomized clinical trial, *American Journal of Clinical Nutrition* 95 (2012): 555–563.

5. Standing Committee on the Scientific Evaluation of Dietary Reference Intakes, *Dietary Reference Intakes for Water, Potassium, Sodium, Chloride, and Sulfate* (National Academies Press, Washington, D.C.: 2005), pp. 133–134.

6. U. S. Department of Agriculture and U. S. Department of Health and Human Services, *Dietary Guidelines for Americans 2010*, available at www.dietaryguidelines.gov.

7. Centers for Disease Control and Prevention, Vital signs: Food categories contributing the most to sodium consumption—United States, 2007–2008, *Morbidity and Mortality Weekly Report* 61 (2012): 92–98.

8. P. K. Whelton and coauthors, American Heart Association Presidential Advisory, Sodium, blood pressure, and cardiovascular disease, *Circulation* 126 (2012): 2880–2889; Centers for Disease Control and Prevention, Where's the sodium? *Vital Signs*, February 2012, available at www.cdc.gov/VitalSigns/Sodium/index.html; L. J. Appel and coauthors, The importance of population-wide sodium reduction as a means to prevent cardiovascular disease and stroke: A call to action from the American Heart Association, *Circulation* 123 (2011): 1138–1143.

9. K. Bibbins-Domingo and coauthors, Projected effect of dietary salt reductions on future cardiovascular disease, *New England Journal of Medicine* 362 (2010): 590–599; Institute of Medicine (US) Committee on Strategies to Reduce Sodium Intake, *Strategies to Reduce Sodium Intake in the United States* (Washington, D.C.: National Academies Press, 2010).

10. Centers for Disease Control and Prevention, Vital signs: Food categories contributing the most to sodium consumption—United States, 2012.

11. Whelton and coauthors, 2012; H. Gardener and coauthors, Dietary sodium and risk of stroke in the Northern Manhattan Study, *Stroke* 43 (2012): 1200–1205; R. Takachi and coauthors, Consumption of sodium and salted foods in relation to cancer and cardiovascular disease: The Japan Public Health Center-based prospective study, *American Journal of Clinical Nutrition* 91 (2010): 456–464.

12. J. P. Forman and coauthors, Association between sodium intake and change in uric acid, urine albumin excretion, and the risk of developing hypertension, *Circulation* 125 (2012): 3108–3116.

13. Forman and coauthors, 2012; Appel and coauthors, 2011.

14. A. S. Go and coauthors, Heart disease and stroke statistics—2014 update: A report from the American Heart Association, *Circulation* 129 (2014): e28–e292.

15. D. E. Epstein and coauthors, Determinants and consequences of adherence to the Dietary Approaches to Stop Hypertension Diet in African-American and white adults with high blood pressure: Results from the ENCORE Trial, *Journal of the Academy of Nutrition and Dietetics* 112 (2012): 1763–1773; J. A. Blumenthal and coauthors, Effects of the DASH diet alone and in combination with exercise and weight loss on blood pressure and cardiovascular biomarkers in men and women with high blood pressure: The ENCORE study, *Archives of Internal Medicine* 170 (2010): 126–135.

16. M. K. Hoy and J. D. Goldman, Potassium intake of the U.S. population, What We Eat in America, NHANES 2009–2010, *Food surveys Research Group Dietary Data Brief No. 10,* September 2012, available at http://ars.usda.gov/Services/docs.htm?docid=19476.

17. Gardener and coauthors, 2012; Appel and coauthors, 2011; Q. Yang and coauthors, Sodium and potassium intake and mortality among US adults: Prospective data from the third National Health and Nutrition Examination Survey, *Archives of Internal Medicine* 171 (2011): 1183–1191; M. C. Houston, The importance of potassium in managing hypertension, *Current Hypertension Reports* 13 (2011): 309–317; C. J. Rodriguez and coauthors, Association of sodium and potassium intake with left ventricular mass: Coronary artery risk development in young adults, *Hypertension* 58 (2011): 410–416.

18. U. S. Department of Agriculture and U. S. Department of Health and Human Services, 2010.

19. R. P. Heaney, Diet, osteoporosis, and fracture prevention: The totality of the evidence, in *Preventive Nutrition: A Comprehensive Guide for Health Professionals,* 4th ed., eds., A. Bendich and R. J. Deckelbaum (New York: Humana Press, 2010), pp. 443–469.

20. National Osteoporosis Foundation, www.nof.org, accessed May 14, 2014.

21. J. C. Lo, S. A. Burnett-Bowie, and J. S. Finkelstein, Bone and the perimenopause, *Obstetrics & Gynecology Clinics of North America* 38 (2011): 503–517; B. Frenkel and coauthors, Regulation of adult bone turnover by sex steroids, *Journal of Cellular Physiology* 224 (2010): 305–310.

22. S. J. Warden and coauthors, Physical activity when young provides lifelong benefits to cortical bone size and strength in men, *Proceedings of the National Academy of Sciences of the United States of America* 111 (2014): 5337–5342; K. F. Janz and coauthors, Early physical activity provides sustained bone health benefits later in childhood, *Medicine and Science in Sports and Exercise* 42 (2010): 1072–1078.

23. J. Kaluza and coauthors, Dietary calcium and magnesium intake and mortality: A prospective study of men, *American Journal of Epidemiology* 171

(2010): 801–807; I. R. Reid and coauthors, Effects of calcium supplementation on lipids, blood pressure, and body composition in healthy older men: A randomized controlled trial, *American Journal of Clinical Nutrition* 91 (2010): 131–139.

24. J. L. Rosenblum and coauthors, Calcium and vitamin D supplementation is associated with decreased abdominal visceral adipose tissue in overweight and obese adults, *American Journal of Clinical Nutrition* 95 (2012): 101–108; J. A. Gilbert and coauthors, Milk supplementation facilitates appetite control in obese women during weight loss: A randomized, single-blind, placebo-controlled trial, *British Journal of Nutrition* 105 (2011): 133–143; D. R. Shahar and coauthors, Dairy calcium intake, serum vitamin D, and successful weight loss, *American Journal of Clinical Nutrition* 92 (2010): 1017–1022.

25. A. Moshfegh and coauthors, *What We Eat in America, NHANES 2005–2006: Usual Nutrient Intakes from Food and Water Compared to 1997 Dietary Reference Intakes for Vitamin D, Calcium, Phosphorus, and Magnesium* (Beltsville, Md.: USDA, 2009).

26. M. Chung and coauthors, Vitamin D with or without calcium supplementation for prevention of cancer and fractures: An updated meta-analysis for the U.S. Preventive Services Task Force, *Annals of Internal Medicine* 155 (2011): 827–838; Committee on Dietary Reference Intakes, *Dietary Reference Intakes for Calcium and Vitamin D* (Washington, D.C.: National Academies Press, 2011), pp. 410–411.

27. Committee on Dietary Reference Intakes, *Dietary Reference Intakes for Calcium and Vitamin D,* (Washington, D.C.: National Academies Press, 2011), pp. 38–40.

28. A. M. Romani, Cellular magnesium homeostasis, *Archives of Biochemistry and Biophysics* 512 (2011): 1–23.

29. M. Shechter, Magnesium and cardiovascular system, *Magnesium Research* 23 (2010): 60–72.

30. A. Rosanoff, C. M. Weaver, and R. K. Rude, Suboptimal magnesium status in the United States: Are the health consequences underestimated? *Nutrition Reviews* 70 (2012): 153–164; J. Sugimoto and coauthors, Magnesium decreases inflammatory cytokine production: A novel innate immunomodulatory mechanism, *Journal of Immunology* 188 (2012): 6338–6346; W. B. Weglicki, Hypomagnesemia and inflammation: Clinical and basic aspects, *Annual Review of Nutrition* 32 (2012): 55–71.

31. M. M. Joosten and coauthors, Urinary and plasma magnesium and risk of ischemic heart disease, *American Journal of Clinical Nutrition* 97 (2013): 1299–1306; L. C. Del Gobbo and coauthors, Circulating and dietary magnesium and risk of cardiovascular disease: A systematic review and meta-analysis of prospective studies, *American Journal of Clinical Nutrition* 98 (2013): 160–173; S. C. Larsson, N. Orsini, and A. Wolk, Dietary magnesium intake and risk of stroke: a meta-analysis of prospective studies, *American Journal of Clinical Nutrition* 95 (2012): 362–366; S. E. Chiuve and coauthors, Plasma and dietary magnesium and risk of sudden cardiac death in women,

American Journal of Clinical Nutrition 93 (2011): 253–260; F. H. Nielsen, Magnesium, inflammation, and obesity in chronic disease, *Nutrition Reviews* 68 (2010): 333–340.

32. Rosanoff, Weaver, and Rude, 2012.

33. M. Wessling-Resnick, Iron homeostasis and the inflammatory response, *Annual Review of Nutrition* 30 (2010): 105–122.

34. G. J. Anderson and F. Wang, Essential but toxic: Controlling the flux of iron in the body, *Clinical and Experimental Pharmacology and Physiology* 39 (2012): 719–724.

35. M. D. Knutson, Iron-sensing proteins that regulate hepcidin and enteric iron absorption, *Annual Review of Nutrition* 30 (2010): 149–171.

36. M. Mastrogiannaki, P. Matak, and C. Peyssonnaux, The gut in iron homeostasis: Role of HIF-2 under normal and pathological conditions, *Blood* 122 (2013): 885–892; Wessling-Resnick, 2010; Knutson, 2010.

37. D. M. Frazer and G. J. Anderson, The regulation of iron transport, *Biofactors* 40 (2014): 206–214; T. Ganz, Systemic iron homeostasis, *Physiological Reviews* 93 (2013): 1721–1741; L. Tussing-Humphreys and coauthors, Rethinking iron regulation and assessment in iron deficiency, anemia of chronic disease, and obesity: Introducing hepcidin, *Journal of the Academy of Nutrition and Dietetics* 112 (2012): 391–400; Knutson, 2010.

38. Ganz, 2013; T. Ganz, Hepcidin and iron regulation: 10 years later, *Blood* 117 (2011): 4425–4433; Knutson, 2010.

39. Ganz, 2013; Knutson, 2010.

40. World Health Organization, 2014, Micronutrient deficiencies, available at www.who.int/nutrition /topics/ida/en; S. R. Lynch, Why nutritional iron deficiency persists as a worldwide problem, *Journal of Nutrition* 141 (2011): 763S–768S.

41. Tussing-Humphreys and coauthors, 2012; A. C. Cepeda-Lopez and coauthors, Sharply higher rates of iron deficiency in obese Mexican women and children are predicted by obesity-related inflammation rather than by differences in dietary iron intake, *American Journal of Clinical Nutrition* 93 (2011): 975–983.

42. H. L. Cheng and coauthors, Iron, hepicidin and inflammatory status of young healthy overweight and obese women in Australia, *PLoS One* 8 (2013): e68675; Tussing-Humphreys and coauthors, 2012; Wessling-Resnick, 2010.

43. N. Milman, Anemia: Still a major health problem in many parts of the world, *Annals of Hematology* 90 (2011): 369–377.

44. L. E. Murray-Kolb, Iron status and neuropsychological consequences in women of reproductive age: What do we know and where are we headed? *Journal of Nutrition* 141 (2011): 747S–755S; K. Kordas, Iron, lead, and children's behavior and cognition, *Annual Review of Nutrition* 30 (2010): 123–148.

45. B. Lozoff, Early iron deficiency has brain and behavior effects consistent with dopaminergic dysfunction, *Journal of Nutrition* 141 (2011): 740S–746S.

46. S. L. Young, Pica in pregnancy: New ideas about an old condition, *Annual Review of Nutrition* 30 (2010): 403–422.

47. Anderson and Wang, 2012.

48. N. C. Andrews, Closing the iron gate, *New England Journal of Medicine* 366 (2012): 376–377; P. Brissot and coauthors, Molecular diagnosis of genetic iron-overload disorders, *Expert Review of Molecular Diagnostics* 10 (2010): 755–763.

49. Andrews, 2012; C. Camaschella and E. Poggiali, Inherited disorders of iron metabolism, *Current Opinion in Pediatrics* 23 (2011): 14–20.

50. G. A. Ramm and R. G. Ruddell, Iron homeostasis, hepatocellular injury, and fibrogenesis in hemochromatosis: The role of inflammation in a noninflammatory liver disease, *Seminars in Liver Disease* 30 (2010): 271–287.

51. Wessling-Resnick, 2010.

52. A. C. Bronstein and coauthors, 2009 Annual Report of the American Association of Poison Control Centers' National Poison Data System (NPDS): 27th Annual Report, *Clinical Toxicology* 28 (2010): 979–1178.

53. J. C. King, Zinc: An essential but elusive nutrient, *American Journal of Clinical Nutrition* 94 (2011): 679S–684S.

54. A. S. Prasad, Discovery of human zinc deficiency: Its impact on human health and disease, *Advances in Nutrition* 4 (2013): 176–190.

55. K. M. Hambidge and coauthors, Zinc bioavailability and homeostasis, *American Journal of Clinical Nutrition* 91 (2010): 1478S–1483S.

56. M. Science and coauthors, Zinc for the treatment of the common cold: A systematic review and meta-analysis of randomized controlled trials, *Canadian Medical Association* 184 (2012): E551–E561.

57. M. P. Rayman, Selenium and human health, *Lancet* 379 (2012): 1256–1268; S. J. Fairweather-Tait and coauthors, Selenium in human health and disease, *Antioxidants and Redox Signaling* 14 (2011): 1337–1383.

58. Rayman, 2012.

59. R. Hurst and coauthors, Selenium and prostate cancer: Systematic review and meta-analysis, *American Journal of Clinical Nutrition* 96 (2012): 111–122; Rayman, 2012; C. D. Davis, R. A. Tsuji, and J. A. Milner, Selenoproteins and cancer prevention, *Annual Review of Nutrition* 32 (2012): 73–95.

60. Hurst and coauthors, 2012; Rayman, 2012; Davis, Tsuji, and Milner, 2012.

61. Hurst and coauthors, 2012.

62. B. M. Aldosary and coauthors, Case series of selenium toxicity from a nutritional supplement, *Clinical Toxicology* 50 (2012): 57–64.

63. M. Andersson, V. Karumbunathan, and M. B. Zimmerman, Global iodine status in 2011 and trends over the past decade, *Journal of Nutrition* 142 (2012): 744–750.

64. GAIN-UNICEF Universal Salt Iodization Partnership Program, available at www.gainhealth.gov /programs/usi; accessed May 16, 2014.

65. Centers for Disease Control and Prevention, *Second National Report on Biochemical Indicators of Diet and nutrition in the U.S. Population, 2012, Executive Summary*, p. 9, available at www.cdc .gov/nutritionreport.

66. Position of the Academy of Nutrition and Dietetics, The impact of fluoride on health, *Journal of the Academy of Nutrition and Dietetics* 112 (2012): 1443–1453.

67. Position of the Academy of Nutrition and Dietetics, 2012.

68. Y. Hua and coauthors, Molecular mechanisms of chromium in alleviating insulin resistance, *Journal of Nutritional Biochemistry* 23 (2012): 313–319; Z. Q. Wang and W. T. Cefalu, Current concepts about chromium supplementation in type 2 diabetes and insulin resistance, *Current Diabetes Reports* 10 (2010): 145–151.

LO 9.4 Present arguments for and against the use of dietary supplements.

At least half of U.S. adults collectively spend tens of *billions* of dollars a year on dietary supplements.[1] Most people take a daily multivitamin and mineral pill to make up for dietary shortfalls; others take single-nutrient supplements in an attempt to ward off diseases. In many cases, taking supplements is a costly but harmless practice; sometimes, it is both costly and harmful to health.[2] The truth is that most healthy people can get the nutrients they need from foods. Supplements cannot substitute for a healthy diet. For some people, however, certain nutrient supplements may be desirable, either to correct deficiencies or to reduce the risks of disease.

Tom Carter/PhotoEdit

Do foods really contain enough vitamins and minerals to supply all that most people need?

Emphatically, yes, for both healthy adults and children who choose a variety of foods. The USDA Food Patterns described in Chapter 1 are the guide to follow to achieve adequate intakes. People who meet their nutrient needs from foods, rather than supplements, have little risk of deficiency or toxicity. When a health care professional finds a person's diet inadequate, the right corrective step is to improve the person's food choices and eating patterns, not to begin supplementation.

Do some people need supplements?

Yes, some people may suffer marginal nutrient deficiencies due to illness, alcohol or drug addiction, or other conditions that limit food intake. People who may benefit from nutrient supplements in amounts consistent with the RDA include the following:

- People with specific nutrient deficiencies need specific nutrient supplements.

- People whose energy intakes are particularly low (fewer than 1600 kcalories per day) need multivitamin and mineral supplements.

- Vegetarians who eat all-plant diets (vegans) and older adults with atrophic gastritis need vitamin B_{12}.

- People who have lactose intolerance or milk allergies or who otherwise do not consume enough milk products to forestall extensive bone loss need calcium.

- People in certain stages of the life cycle who have increased nutrient requirements need specific nutrient supplements. For example, infants may need vitamin D, iron, and fluoride; women who are capable of becoming pregnant and pregnant women need folate and iron; and the elderly may benefit from some of the vitamins and minerals in a balanced supplement (they may choose poor diets, have trouble chewing, or absorb or metabolize nutrients less efficiently; see Chapter 13).

- People who have inadequate intakes of milk or milk products, limited sun exposure, or heavily pigmented skin may need vitamin D.

- People who have diseases, infections, or injuries or who have undergone surgery that interferes with the intake, absorption, metabolism, or excretion of nutrients may need specific nutrient supplements (see Chapter 24).

- People taking medications that interfere with the body's use of specific nutrients may need specific nutrient supplements.

Why do so many people take supplements?

People frequently take supplements for mistaken reasons, such as "They give me energy" or "They make me strong." Other invalid reasons why people may take supplements include:

- Their feeling of insecurity about the nutrient content of the food supply.

- Their belief that extra vitamins and minerals will help them cope with stress.

- Their belief that supplements can enhance athletic performance or build lean body tissue without physical work.

- Their desire to prevent, treat, or cure symptoms or diseases ranging from the common cold to cancer.

Study after study has found that well-nourished people are the ones who take supplements, whereas people with low nutrient intakes from food generally do not.[3] In addition, little relationship exists between the nutrients people need and the ones they take in supplements. In fact, an argument against supplements is that they may lull people into a false sense of security.

Are there other arguments against taking supplements?

Yes, there are several arguments against taking supplements. First, foods rarely cause nutrient imbalances or toxicities, but supplements can. The higher the dose, the greater the risk of harm. The Tolerable Upper Intake Levels (UL) of the DRI (see inside front cover) answer the question "How much is too much?" by defining the highest amount that appears safe for *most* healthy people. However, people's tolerances for high doses of nutrients vary, just as their risks of deficiencies do. Amounts that some can tolerate may produce toxicities in others, and no one knows who falls where along the spectrum.

Supplement users are more likely to have excessive intakes of certain nutrients—notably folate, vitamin A, vitamin B_6, vitamin C, calcium, magnesium, iron, and zinc.[4] The extent and severity of supplement toxicity remain unclear. Only a few alert health care professionals can recognize toxicity, even when it is acute. When it is chronic, with the effects developing subtly and progressing slowly, it often goes unrecognized and unreported.[5] In view of the potential hazards, some authorities believe supplements should bear warning labels, advising consumers that large doses may be toxic.

Toxic overdoses of vitamins and minerals in children are more readily recognized and, unfortunately, fairly common. Fruit-flavored, chewable vitamins shaped like cartoon characters entice young children to eat them like candy in amounts that can cause poisoning. High-potency iron supplements (30 milligrams of iron or more per tablet) are especially toxic and are the leading cause of accidental ingestion fatalities among children.

Second, some dietary supplements sold on the U.S. market are contaminated with pharmaceutical drugs, such as steroid hormones and stimulants. Toxic plant material, toxic heavy metals, bacteria, and other substances have also shown up in a wide variety of dietary supplements. Even some children's chewable vitamins have contained appreciable lead, a destructive heavy metal. Even though hazardous products are quickly removed from the market upon discovery, many others remain on store shelves because current regulations make the supplement market difficult to monitor and control. Plain multivitamin and mineral supplements from reputable sources, without herbs or add-ons, often test free from contamination.

A third argument against taking supplements arises when people who are ill come to believe that high doses of vitamins or minerals can be therapeutic. Not only can high doses be toxic, but also the person may take them instead of seeking medical help.

A final argument against taking supplements is that the body absorbs nutrients best from foods that dilute and disperse them among other substances to facilitate their absorption and use by the body. Taken in pure, concentrated form, nutrients are likely to interfere with one another's absorption or with the absorption of other nutrients from foods eaten at the same time. Such effects are particularly well known among the minerals. For example, zinc hinders copper and calcium absorption, iron hinders zinc

absorption, and calcium hinders magnesium and iron absorption. Among vitamins, vitamin C supplements *enhance* iron absorption, making iron overload likely in susceptible people. These and other interactions represent drawbacks to supplement use.

Do antioxidant supplements prevent cancer?

Again, it is better advice to eat a nutrient-dense diet. Some evidence links high intakes of antioxidant-rich fruits and vegetables with good health and disease prevention.[6] More than 200 population studies have examined the effects of fruits and vegetables on cancer risk, and many show that people who eat more of these foods are less likely to develop certain cancers. Findings from other types of studies, such as intervention studies and clinical trials, however, show weaker associations between fruit and vegetable intake and reduced risk of cancer. Some researchers speculate that fruit and vegetable intake may play a smaller role in total cancer protection than previously thought.[7] However, some fruits and vegetables do contain protective factors for specific cancers. For example, research suggests dietary fiber protects against colorectal cancer.[8] When research combines many different fruits and vegetables, specific protective factors may not stand out. Many experts agree that the antioxidant vitamins in these foods are probably important protective factors, but they also note that other constituents of fruits and vegetables (see Table NP8-2 on p. 218) certainly have not been ruled out as contributing factors.

The way to apply this information is to eat nutritious foods. Taking antioxidant supplements instead of making needed lifestyle changes may sound appealing, but evidence does not support a role for supplements against chronic diseases.[9] In some cases, supplements may even be harmful.[10]

When a person needs a vitamin-mineral supplement, what kind should be used?

Ask your health care professional for advice. A single, balanced vitamin-mineral supplement with no added extras such as herbs should suffice. Choose the kind that provides all the nutrients in amounts less than, equal to, or very close to the RDA (remember, you get some nutrients from foods). For those who require a higher dose, such as young women who need supplemental folate in the childbearing years, choose a supplement with just the needed nutrient or in combination with a reasonable dose of others. Avoid any preparations that, in a daily dose, provide more than the recommended intake of vitamin A, vitamin D, or any mineral or more than the UL for any nutrient. In addition, avoid the following:

- High doses of iron (more than 10 milligrams per day), except for menstruating women.

- "Organic" or "natural" preparations with added substances. They are no better than standard types, but they cost more.

- "High-potency" or "therapeutic dose" supplements. More is not better.

- Substances not needed in human nutrition such as inositol and carnitine. These particular ingredients won't harm you, but they reveal a marketing strategy that makes the whole mix suspect.

254

FIGURE NP9-1 USP Symbol
This symbol means that a supplement contains the nutrients stated and that it will dissolve in the digestive system—the symbol does not guarantee safety or health advantages.

Used with permission of The United States Pharmacopeial Convention

As for price, be aware that local or store brands may be just as good as or better than nationally advertised brands. They may be less expensive because the price does not have to cover the cost of national advertising. Finally, be aware that if you see a USP symbol on the label (see Figure NP9-1), it means that the manufacturer has voluntarily paid an independent laboratory to test the product and affirm that it contains the ingredients listed and will dissolve or disintegrate in the digestive tract to make the ingredients available for absorption. The symbol does not imply that the supplement has been tested for safety or effectiveness with regard to health, however.

Can supplement labels help consumers make informed choices?

Yes, to some extent. To enable consumers to make more informed choices about nutrient supplements, the FDA, with the encouragement of the Academy of Nutrition and Dietetics, published labeling regulations for supplements. The Dietary Supplement Health and Education Act subjects supplements to the same general labeling requirements that apply to foods. Specifically:

▌ Nutrition labeling for dietary supplements is required. The nutrition panel on supplements is called "Supplement Facts" (see Figure NP9-2). The Supplement Facts panel lists the quantity and the percentage of the Daily Value for each nutrient in the supplement. Ingredients that have no Daily Value—for example, sugars and gelatin—appear in a list below the Supplement Facts panel.

▌ Labels may make nutrient claims (such as "high" or "low") according to specific criteria (for example, "an excellent source of vitamin C").

▌ Labels may make health claims that are supported by significant scientific agreement and are not brand specific (for example, "folate protects against neural tube defects").

▌ Labels may claim that the lack of a nutrient can cause a deficiency disease, but if they do, they must also include the prevalence of that deficiency disease in the United States.

▌ Labels may claim to diagnose, treat, cure, or relieve common complaints such as menstrual cramps or memory loss, but they

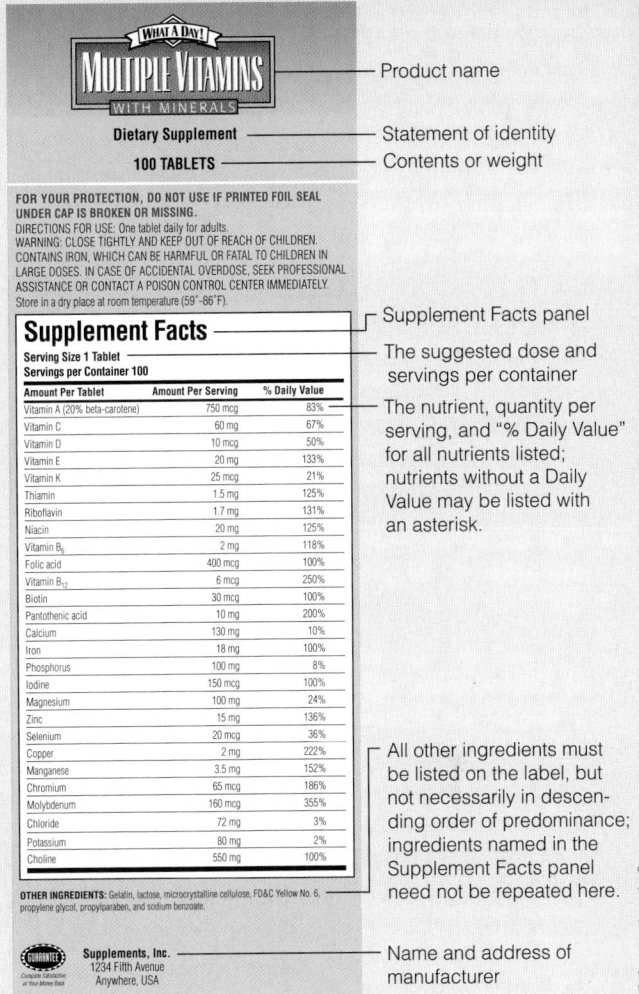

Product name
Statement of identity
Contents or weight

FOR YOUR PROTECTION, DO NOT USE IF PRINTED FOIL SEAL UNDER CAP IS BROKEN OR MISSING.
DIRECTIONS FOR USE: One tablet daily for adults.
WARNING: CLOSE TIGHTLY AND KEEP OUT OF REACH OF CHILDREN. CONTAINS IRON, WHICH CAN BE HARMFUL OR FATAL TO CHILDREN IN LARGE DOSES. IN CASE OF ACCIDENTAL OVERDOSE, SEEK PROFESSIONAL ASSISTANCE OR CONTACT A POISON CONTROL CENTER IMMEDIATELY.
Store in a dry place at room temperature (59°-86°F).

Supplement Facts panel
The suggested dose and servings per container
The nutrient, quantity per serving, and "% Daily Value" for all nutrients listed; nutrients without a Daily Value may be listed with an asterisk.

Supplement Facts
Serving Size 1 Tablet
Servings per Container 100

Amount Per Tablet	Amount Per Serving	% Daily Value
Vitamin A (20% beta-carotene)	750 mcg	83%
Vitamin C	60 mg	67%
Vitamin D	10 mcg	50%
Vitamin E	20 mg	133%
Vitamin K	25 mcg	21%
Thiamin	1.5 mg	125%
Riboflavin	1.7 mg	131%
Niacin	20 mg	125%
Vitamin B₆	2 mg	118%
Folic acid	400 mcg	100%
Vitamin B₁₂	6 mcg	250%
Biotin	30 mcg	100%
Pantothenic acid	10 mg	200%
Calcium	130 mg	10%
Iron	18 mg	100%
Phosphorus	100 mg	8%
Iodine	150 mcg	100%
Magnesium	100 mg	24%
Zinc	15 mg	136%
Selenium	20 mcg	36%
Copper	2 mg	222%
Manganese	3.5 mg	152%
Chromium	65 mcg	186%
Molybdenum	160 mcg	355%
Chloride	72 mg	3%
Potassium	80 mg	2%
Choline	550 mg	100%

OTHER INGREDIENTS: Gelatin, lactose, microcrystalline cellulose, FD&C Yellow No. 6, propylene glycol, propylparaben, and sodium benzoate.

All other ingredients must be listed on the label, but not necessarily in descending order of predominance; ingredients named in the Supplement Facts panel need not be repeated here.

GUARANTEE Complete Satisfaction or Your Money Back
Supplements, Inc.
1234 Fifth Avenue
Anywhere, USA

Name and address of manufacturer

© Cengage Learning®

FIGURE NP9-2 An Example of a Supplement Label

may *not* make claims about specific diseases (except as noted previously).

▌ Labels may make structure-function claims (see Chapter 1) about the role a nutrient plays in the body, explain how the nutrient performs its function, and indicate that consuming the nutrient is associated with general well-being. These claims must be accompanied by an FDA disclaimer statement: "This statement has not been evaluated by the Food and Drug Administration. This product is not intended to diagnose, treat, cure, or prevent any disease."

Note, however, that despite these requirements, in effect, the Dietary Supplement Health and Education Act resulted in the deregulation of the supplement industry. Under current law, the FDA is responsible only for taking action against unsafe dietary supplements already on the market. No advance registration or approval by the FDA is needed before a manufacturer can put a supplement on store shelves.[11] To act against unsafe supplements, the FDA must receive manufacturers' reports concerning serious adverse health effects reported to them by consumers. Manufacturers do list contact information on supplement labels for this purpose, but many symptoms of adverse reactions are easily mistaken for something else—stomach flu or headache or fatigue. Consumers can also report adverse reactions from supplements directly to the FDA via its hotline or website, but most people are unaware of these options.*

People in developed nations are far more likely to suffer from *overnutrition* and poor lifestyle choices than from nutrient deficiencies. People wish that swallowing vitamin pills would boost their health. The truth—that they need to improve their eating and exercise habits—is harder to swallow.

Notes

1. J. Gajcje and coauthors, Dietary supplement use among U.S. adults has increased since NHANES III (1988–1994), *National Center for Health Statistics: Data Brief* 61 (2011): 1–8; Position of the American Dietetic Association: Nutrient Supplementation, *Journal of the American Dietetic Association* 109 (2009): 2073–2085.

2. D. B. McCormick, Vitamin/mineral supplements: Of questionable benefit for the general population, *Nutrition Reviews* 68 (2010): 207–213.

3. R. L. Bailey and coauthors, Examination of vitamin intakes among US adults by dietary supplement use, *Journal of the Academy of Nutrition and Dietetics* 112 (2012): 657–663; Y. A. Shakur and coauthors, A comparison of micronutrient inadequacy and risk of high micronutrient intakes among vitamin and mineral supplement users and nonusers in Canada, *Journal of Nutrition* 142 (2012): 534–540; R. L. Bailey and coauthors, Dietary supplement use is associated with higher intakes of minerals from food sources, *American Journal of Clinical Nutrition* 94 (2011): 1376–1381; R. M. Bliss, Monitoring the population's food and supplement intakes, March 1, 2012, available at www.ars.usda.gov/is/pr/2012/120301.htm; McCormick, 2010.

4. Bailey and coauthors, 2012; Bailey and coauthors, 2011.

5. M. Cellini and coauthors, Dietary supplements: Physician knowledge and adverse event reporting, *Medicine and Science in Sports and Exercise* 45 (2013): 23–28.

6. L. H. Kushi and coauthors, American Cancer Society guidelines on nutrition and physical activity for cancer prevention: Reducing the risk of cancer with healthy food choices and physical activity, *CA: Cancer Journal for Clinicians* 62 (2012): 30–67.

7. P. Boffetta and coauthors, Fruit and vegetable intake and overall cancer risk in the European Prospective Investigation into Cancer and Nutrition (EPIC), *Journal of the National Cancer Institute* 102 (2010): 529–537; T. J. Key, Fruit and vegetables and cancer risk, *British Journal of Cancer* 104 (2010): 6–11.

8. D. Aune and coauthors, Dietary fibre, whole grains, and risk of colorectal cancer: Systematic review and dose-response meta-analysis of prospective studies, *British Medical Journal* 343 (2011): d6617; C. C. Dahm and coauthors, Dietary fiber and colorectal cancer risk: A nested case-control study using food diaries, *Journal of the National Cancer Institute* 102 (2010): 614–626.

9. M. E. Martinez and coauthors, Dietary supplements and cancer prevention: Balancing potential benefits against proven harms, *Journal of the National Cancer Institute* 104 (2012): 732–739; M. G. O'Doherty and coauthors, Effect of supplementation with B vitamins and antioxidants on levels of asymmetric dimethylarginine (ADMA) and C-reactive protein (CRP): A double-blind, randomized, factorial design, placebo-controlled trial, *European Journal of Nutrition* 49 (2010): 483–492; G. J. Hankey and VITATOPS Trial Study Group, B vitamins in patients with recent transient ischaemic attack or stroke in the VITAmins TO Prevent Stroke (VITATOPS) trial: A randomized, double-blind, parallel, placebo-controlled trial, *The Lancet Neurology* 9 (2010): 855–865.

10. M. P. Rayman, Selenium and human health, *Lancet* 379 (2012): 1256–1268; G. Bjelakovic and C. Gluud, Vitamin and mineral supplement use in relation to all-cause mortality in the Iowa Women's Health Study, *Archives of Internal Medicine* 171 (2011): 1633–1634.

11. U.S. Food and Drug Administration, Center for Food Safety and Applied Nutrition, *Dietary Supplements*, retrieved from www.fda.gov/Food/DietarySupplements/default.htm, updated May 11, 2014.

*Consumers should report suspected harm from dietary supplements to their health providers or to the FDA's MedWatch program at (800) FDA-1088 or on the Internet at *www.fda.gov/medwatch/*.

10

Fitness and Nutrition

Silverstock/Digital Vision/Getty Images

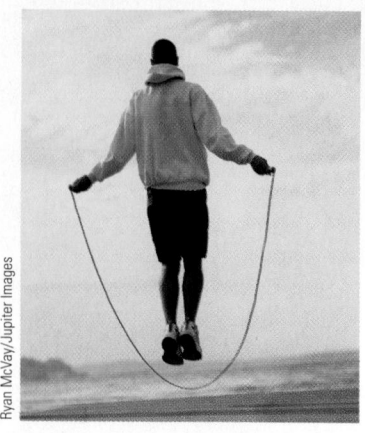

Physical activity, or lack of it, exerts a significant and pervasive influence on everyone's nutrition and overall health.

I n the body, nutrition and physical activity are interactive—each influences the other. The working body demands all three energy-yielding nutrients—carbohydrate, lipids, and protein—to fuel activity. The body also needs protein and a host of supporting nutrients to build lean tissue. Physical activity benefits the body's nutrition by helping to regulate the use of fuels, shifting body composition toward leanness, and increasing the daily kcalorie allowance. With more kcalories come more nutrients and other beneficial constituents of foods.

Those just beginning to increase **fitness** can be assured that improvement is not only possible, but also an inevitable result of becoming more active. As you improve your physical fitness, you not only *feel* better and stronger, but you also *look* better. Physically fit people walk with confidence and purpose because posture and self-image improve along with physical fitness.

If you are already physically fit, the following description applies. You move with ease and balance. You have endurance, and your energy lasts for hours. You are strong and meet daily physical challenges without strain. What is more, you are prepared to meet mental and emotional challenges because physical fitness also supports mental and emotional energy and resilience.

This chapter is written for athletes and for active people who train like athletes. Casual athletes (those who compete only with their own goals) and competitive athletes (those who compete with others) need the right foods and fluids at the right time to support their efforts. The chapter refers to "you" to make the connection between general principles and personal choices. To understand the interactions between physical activity and nutrition, you must first know a few things about fitness, its benefits, and **training** to develop fitness.

10.1 Fitness

LO 10.1 Describe the health benefits of being physically fit and explain how to develop the components of fitness.

Fitness depends on a certain minimum amount of **physical activity** or **exercise.** Both physical activity and exercise involve bodily movement, muscle contraction, and increased energy expenditure, but "exercise" is often used to describe structured, planned physical activity. This chapter focuses on how the active body uses energy nutrients—whether that body is pedaling a bike across campus or pedaling a stationary bike in a gym. Thus, for our purposes, the terms *physical activity* and *exercise* will be used interchangeably.

Benefits of Fitness

The *Dietary Guidelines for Americans 2010* emphasize the benefits of increasing physical activities and reducing **sedentary** activities.[1] Extensive evidence confirms that regular physical activity promotes health and reduces the risk of developing a number of diseases.[2] Yet, despite an increasing awareness of the health benefits that physical activity confers, only about 20 percent of adults in the United States meet physical activity guidelines.[3] Like smoking and obesity, physical inactivity is linked to the major degenerative diseases—heart disease, cancer, stroke, diabetes, and hypertension—the primary killers of adults in developed countries.[4]

fitness: the characteristics that enable the body to perform physical activity; more broadly, the ability to meet routine physical demands with enough reserve energy to rise to a physical challenge; the body's ability to withstand stress of all kinds.

training: regular practice of an activity, which leads to physical adaptations of the body with improvement in flexibility, strength, or endurance.

physical activity: bodily movement produced by muscle contractions that substantially increase energy expenditure.

exercise: planned, structured, and repetitive bodily movement that promotes or maintains physical fitness.

sedentary: physically inactive (literally "sitting down a lot").

As a person becomes physically active, the health of the entire body improves. Compared with unfit people, physically fit people enjoy:[5]

▮ *More restful sleep.* Rest and sleep occur naturally after periods of physical activity. During rest, the body repairs injuries, disposes of wastes generated during activity, and builds new physical structures.

▮ *Improved nutritional health.* Physical activity expends energy and thus allows people to eat more food. If they choose wisely, active people will consume more nutrients and be less likely to develop nutrient deficiencies.

▮ *Improved body composition.* A balanced program of physical activity limits body fat and increases or maintains lean tissue. Thus, physically active people have relatively less body fat than sedentary people at the same body weight.[6]

▮ *Improved bone density.* Weight-bearing physical activity builds bone strength and protects against osteoporosis.[7]

▮ *Enhanced resistance to colds and other infectious diseases.* Fitness enhances immunity.*[8]

▮ *Lower risks of some types of cancers.* Lifelong physical activity may help to protect against colon cancer, breast cancer, and some other cancers.[9]

▮ *Stronger circulation and lung function.* Physical activity that challenges the heart and lungs strengthens both the circulatory and the respiratory systems.

▮ *Lower risks of cardiovascular disease.* Physical activity lowers blood pressure, slows resting pulse rate, lowers total blood cholesterol, and raises HDL cholesterol, thus reducing the risks of heart attacks and strokes.[10] Some research suggests that physical activity may reduce the risk of cardiovascular disease in another way as well—by reducing intra-abdominal fat stores.[11]

▮ *Lower risks of type 2 diabetes.* Physical activity normalizes glucose tolerance.[12] Regular physical activity reduces the risk of developing type 2 diabetes and benefits those who already have the condition.

▮ *Reduced risk of gallbladder disease (women).* Regular physical activity reduces the risk of gallbladder disease—perhaps by facilitating weight control and lowering blood lipid levels.[13]

▮ *Lower incidence and severity of anxiety and depression.* Physical activity may improve mood and enhance the quality of life by reducing depression and anxiety.[14]

▮ *Stronger self-image.* The sense of achievement that comes from meeting physical challenges promotes self-confidence.

▮ *Long life and high quality of life in the later years.* Active people live longer, healthier lives than sedentary people do.[15] Even as little as 15 minutes a day of moderate-intensity activity can add years to a person's life.[16] In addition to extending longevity, physical activity supports independence and mobility in later life by reducing the risk of falls and minimizing the risk of injury should a fall occur.[17]

What does a person have to do to reap the health rewards of physical activity? To gain substantial *health* benefits, most guidelines recommend a minimum amount of time performing **aerobic physical activity.**[18] The minimum amount of time depends on whether the activity is **moderate-intensity physical activity** or **vigorous-intensity physical activity.** Table 10-1 (on p. 260) compares intensity levels. Whether moderate- or vigorous-intensity, a minimum length of 10 minutes for short bouts of aerobic physical activity is recommended.[19] Of course, more time and greater intensity bring even greater health benefits: maintaining a healthy body weight (BMI of 18.5 to 24.9) and further reducing the risk of chronic diseases.

*Moderate physical activity can stimulate immune function. Intense, vigorous, prolonged activity such as marathon running, however, may compromise immune function.

aerobic physical activity: activity in which the body's large muscles move in a rhythmic manner for a sustained period of time. Aerobic activity, also called *endurance activity,* improves cardiorespiratory fitness. Brisk walking, running, swimming, and bicycling are examples.

moderate-intensity physical activity: physical activity that requires some increase in breathing and/or heart rate and expends 3.5 to 7 kcalories per minute. Walking at a speed of 3 to 4.5 miles per hour (about 15 to 20 minutes to walk one mile) is an example.

vigorous-intensity physical activity: physical activity that requires a large increase in breathing and/or heart rate and expends more than 7 kcalories per minute. Walking at a very brisk pace (>4.5 miles per hour) or running at a pace of at least 5 miles per hour are examples.

TABLE 10-1 Levels of Physical Activity Intensity Compared

Level of Intensity	Breathing and/or Heart Rate	Perceived Exertion (on a Scale of 0 to 10)	Talk Test	Energy Expenditure	Walking Pace
Light	Little to no increase	<5	Able to sing	<3.5 kcal/min	<3 mph
Moderate	Some increase	5 or 6	Able to have a conversation	3.5 to 7 kcal/min	3 to 4.5 mph
Vigorous	Large increase	7 or 8	Conversation is difficult or "broken"	>7 kcal/min	>4.5 mph

Source: Centers for Disease Control and Prevention, www.cdc.gov/physicalactivity/everyone; updated March 30, 2011.

In addition to providing health benefits, physical activity helps to develop and maintain *fitness.* Table 10-2 presents the American College of Sports Medicine (ACSM) guidelines for physical activity.[20] Following these guidelines will help adults improve their cardiorespiratory endurance, body composition, strength, and flexibility. At this level of fitness, a person can reap still greater health benefits (further reduction of cardiovascular disease risk and improved body composition, for example).[21] Fitness and health both depend on maintaining an active lifestyle every day.

The bottom line is that any physical activity—even moderate—*beyond* activities of daily living provides some health benefits, and these benefits exhibit a dose-response relationship. In other words, some activity is better than none, and more activity is better still—up to a point. Pursued in excess, intense physical activity, especially when

TABLE 10-2 American College of Sports Medicine's Guidelines for Physical Fitness

	Cardiorespiratory	Strength	Flexibility
	Steve Cole/Photodisc/Getty Images	David Hanover Photography	David Hanover Photography
Type of Activity	Aerobic activity that uses large muscle groups and can be maintained continuously	Resistance activity that is performed at a controlled speed and through a full range of motion	Stretching activity that uses the major muscle groups
Frequency	5 to 7 days per week	2 to 3 nonconsecutive days per week	2 to 7 days per week
Intensity	Moderate (equivalent to walking at a pace of 3 to 4 miles per hour)[a]	Enough to enhance muscle strength and improve body composition	Enough to feel tightness or slight discomfort
Duration	At least 30 minutes per day	2 to 4 sets of 9 to 12 repetitions involving each major muscle group	2 to 4 repetitions of 15 to 30 seconds per muscle group
Examples	Running, cycling, dancing, swimming, inline skating, rowing, power walking, cross-country skiing, kickboxing, water aerobics, jumping rope; sports activities such as basketball, soccer, racquetball, tennis, volleyball	Pull-ups, push-ups, sit-ups, weightlifting, Pilates	Yoga

[a]For those who prefer vigorous-intensity aerobic activity such as walking at a very brisk pace (>4.5 mph) or running (≥5 mph), a minimum of 20 minutes per day, 3 days per week is recommended.

Source: American College of Sports Medicine position stand: Quantity and quality of exercise for developing and maintaining cardiorespiratory, musculoskeletal, and neuromotor fitness in apparently healthy adults—Guidance for prescribing exercise, *Medicine and Science in Sports and Exercise* 4e (2011): 1334–1359; W.L. Haskell and coauthors, Physical activity and public health: Updated recommendation for adults from the American College of Sports Medicine and the American Heart Association, *Medicine and Science in Sports and Exercise* 39 (2007): 1423–1434.

combined with poor eating habits, can undermine health, as Nutrition in Practice 6 explains (pp. 156–160).

IN SUMMARY

▪ Physical activity and fitness benefit people's physical and psychological well-being and improve their resistance to disease.

▪ Physical activity to improve physical fitness offers additional personal benefits.

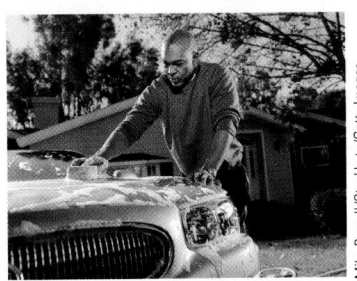

Choose an active lifestyle. Use the stairs; walk or bike to work, classes, or shops; wash and wax the car, mow the grass; rake the leaves; shovel snow; walk the dog; play with children. Be active and have fun.

Developing Fitness

A person who practices a physical activity *adapts* by becoming better able to perform it after each session. People shape their bodies by what they choose to do (and not do). Muscle cells and tissues respond to a physical activity **overload** by building, within genetic limits, the structures needed to perform it.[22]

Muscles are continually under renovation. Every day, particularly during the fasting periods between meals, a healthy body degrades a small portion of its muscle protein to amino acids and then rebuilds it with available amino acids during feeding periods.[23] This balance between protein degradation and synthesis maintains the body's muscle tissue. To *gain* muscle tissue, protein synthesis must be greater than degradation, a condition called **hypertrophy.** When protein degradation is greater than synthesis, the result is **atrophy.** Physical activity tips the balance toward muscle hypertrophy. The opposite is also true; unused muscles diminish in size and weaken over time, tipping the balance toward muscle atrophy.

The muscles adapt and build only the proteins they need to cope with the work performed.[24] Muscles engaged in activities that require strength develop more of the proteins needed for greater muscle mass; body builders have large, well-developed muscles. By comparison, those engaged in endurance activities develop more of the proteins needed to combat muscle fatigue; distance cyclists can pedal for many hours before fatigue sets in.

The Components of Fitness

To be physically fit, a person must develop enough flexibility, muscle strength and endurance, and cardiorespiratory endurance to meet the everyday demands of life with some to spare, and achieve a healthy body composition. **Flexibility** allows the joints to move freely, reducing the risk of injury. **Cardiorespiratory endurance** supports the ongoing activity of the heart and lungs. **Muscle strength** and **muscle endurance** enable

overload: an extra physical demand placed on the body; an increase in the frequency, duration, or intensity of an activity. A principle of training is that for a body system to improve, it must be worked at frequencies, durations, or intensities that increase by increments.

hypertrophy (high-PURR-tro-fee): an increase in size (for example, of a muscle) in response to use.

atrophy (AT-tro-fee): a decrease in size (for example, of a muscle) because of disuse.

flexibility: the capacity of the joints to move through a full range of motion; the ability to bend and recover without injury.

cardiorespiratory endurance: the ability to perform large-muscle dynamic exercise of moderate-to-high intensity for prolonged periods.

muscle strength: the ability of muscles to work against resistance.

muscle endurance: the ability of a muscle to contract repeatedly within a given time without becoming exhausted.

People's bodies are shaped by the activities they perform.

muscles to work harder and longer without fatigue. **Body composition** improves as physical activity supports lean body tissues and reduces excess body fat.

Although nutrition influences each component of fitness to some extent, its role in flexibility is not as apparent as for the others. For this reason, cardiorespiratory endurance and muscle strength and endurance are emphasized in the following sections. As the heart and lungs improve their capacity to sustain physical activity and the muscles become stronger and less readily fatigued, body composition improves: body fat decreases and lean body mass increases. Chapter 6 discusses body composition and the health risks of too much body fat.

IN SUMMARY

▌ The components of fitness are flexibility, muscle strength, muscle endurance, and cardiorespiratory endurance.

▌ To build fitness, a person must engage in physical activity. Muscles adapt to activities they are called upon to perform repeatedly.

Cardiorespiratory Endurance

The length of time a person can remain active with an elevated heart rate—that is, the ability of the heart, lungs, and blood to sustain a given demand—defines a person's cardiorespiratory endurance. Cardiorespiratory endurance training improves a person's ability to sustain vigorous activities such as running, brisk walking, or swimming. Such training enhances the capacity of the heart, lungs, and blood to deliver oxygen to, and remove waste from, the body's cells.[25] Cardiorespiratory training, therefore, is *aerobic*, meaning oxygen requiring. As the cardiorespiratory system gradually adapts to the demands of aerobic activity, the body delivers oxygen more efficiently. In fact, the accepted measure of a person's cardiorespiratory fitness is maximal oxygen uptake **(VO$_2$ max).** The benefits of cardiorespiratory training are not just physical, though, because all of the body's cells, including the brain cells, require oxygen to function. When the cells receive more oxygen more readily, both the body and the mind benefit.

Cardiorespiratory Conditioning **Cardiorespiratory conditioning** occurs as aerobic workouts improve heart and lung function. **Cardiac output** increases, thus enhancing oxygen delivery. The heart becomes stronger, and each beat pumps more blood. Because the heart pumps more blood with each beat, fewer beats are necessary, and the resting heart rate slows down. The average resting pulse rate for adults is around 70 beats per minute, but people who achieve cardiorespiratory conditioning may have resting pulse rates of 50 or even lower. The muscles that work the lungs become stronger, too, so breathing becomes more efficient. Circulation through the arteries and veins improves. Blood moves easily, and blood pressure falls.[26] In short, cardiorespiratory conditioning:

▐ Increases cardiac output and oxygen delivery

▐ Increases blood volume per heart beat (stroke volume)

▐ Slows resting pulse rate

▐ Increases breathing efficiency

▐ Improves circulation

▐ Reduces blood pressure

Cardiorespiratory endurance reflects the health of the heart and circulatory system, on which all other body systems depend. To improve your cardiorespiratory

body composition: the proportions of muscle, bone, fat, and other tissues that make up a person's total body weight.

VO$_2$ max: the maximum rate of oxygen consumption by an individual (measured at sea level).

cardiorespiratory conditioning: improvements in heart and lung function and increased blood volume, brought about by aerobic training.

cardiac output: the volume of blood discharged by the heart each minute.

endurance, activities must be sustained for 20 minutes or longer and use most of the large muscle groups of the body (legs, buttocks, and abdomen). The level of training must be intense enough to elevate your heart rate.

A person's own perceived effort is usually a reliable indicator of the intensity of an activity. In general, workouts should be at an intensity that raises your heart rate but still leaves you able to talk comfortably. For those who are more competitive and want to work to their limits on some days, a treadmill test can reveal the maximum heart rate. Workouts are safe at up to 85 percent of that rate. Table 10-2 (p. 260) includes the ACSM guidelines for developing and maintaining cardiorespiratory fitness.

Muscle Conditioning One of the benefits of cardiorespiratory training is that fit muscles use oxygen efficiently, reducing the heart's workload. An added bonus is that muscles that use oxygen efficiently can burn fat longer—a plus for body composition and weight control.

Muscle Strength and Endurance

Resistance training has long been recognized as a means to build and maintain muscle mass, strength, power, and endurance. Additional benefits of resistance training, however, have also emerged. Progressive resistance training helps prevent and manage several chronic diseases, including cardiovascular disease, and enhances psychological well-being.[27] Resistance training can also help to maximize and maintain bone mass.[28] Even in women past menopause (when most women are losing bone), resistance training can improve bone density, especially in combination with adequate dietary calcium and vitamin D intakes.[29]

By promoting strong muscles in the back and abdomen, resistance training can improve posture and reduce the risk of back injury. Resistance training can also help prevent the decline in physical mobility that often accompanies aging.[30] Older adults, even those in their 80s, who participate in resistance training programs not only gain muscle strength but also improve their muscle endurance, which enables them to walk longer before exhaustion. Leg strength and walking endurance are powerful indicators of an older adult's physical abilities.

Resistance training builds muscle strength, **muscle power,** and muscle endurance. To emphasize muscle strength, combine high resistance (heavy weight) with a low number of repetitions (8 to 12).[31] To emphasize muscle power, combine moderate resistance (light to medium weight) with high velocity (as fast as safely possible). To emphasize muscle endurance, combine less resistance (lighter weight) with more repetitions (15 to 20). Resistance training enhances performance in other sports too. Swimmers can develop a more efficient stroke and tennis players a more powerful serve when they train with weights, for example.

A Balanced Fitness Program

The intensity and type of physical activities that are best for one person may not be good for another. A person who has been sedentary will initially perform at a dramatically different level of intensity than a fit person.

The type of physical activity that is best for you depends, too, on what you want to achieve and what you enjoy doing. Some people love walking, whereas others prefer to dance or ride a bike. Those who want to be stronger and firmer lift weights. Keep in mind that muscle is more metabolically active than body fat, so the more muscle you have, the more energy you'll expend.

In a balanced fitness program, aerobic activity improves cardiorespiratory fitness, stretching enhances flexibility, and resistance training develops muscle strength, muscle power, and muscle endurance. Table 10-3 provides an example of a balanced fitness program.

TABLE 10-3 A Sample Balanced Fitness Program

Monday, Tuesday, Wednesday, Thursday, Friday:
- 5 minutes of warm-up activity
- 30–60 minutes of aerobic activity
- 10 minutes of cool-down activity and stretching

Tuesday, Thursday, Saturday
- 5 minutes of warm-up activity
- 30 minutes of resistance training
- 10 minutes of cool-down activity and stretching

Saturday and/or Sunday
- Sports, walking, hiking, biking, or swimming

© Cengage Learning®

resistance training: physical activity that develops muscle strength, power, endurance, and mass. Resistance can be provided by free weights, weight machines, elastic bands, or other objects. A person's own body weight may also be used to provide resistance, as when a person does push-ups, pull-ups, or sit-ups; also called *weight training*.

muscle power: the product of force generation (strength) and movement velocity (speed); the speed at which a given amount of exertion is completed.

The key to regular physical activity is finding an activity that you enjoy.

IN SUMMARY

▌ Cardiorespiratory endurance training enhances the ability of the heart and lungs to deliver oxygen to the muscles.

▌ With cardiorespiratory endurance training, the heart becomes stronger, breathing becomes more efficient, and the health of the entire body improves.

▌ Resistance training offers health and fitness benefits to adults.

▌ Resistance training reduces the risk of cardiovascular disease, improves older adults' physical mobility, and helps maximize and maintain bone mass.

The rest of this chapter describes the interactions between nutrients and physical activity. Nutrition alone cannot endow you with fitness or athletic ability, but along with the right mental attitude, it complements your effort to obtain them. Conversely, unwise food selections can stand in your way.

10.2 The Active Body's Use of Fuels

LO 10.2 Identify the factors that influence macronutrient use during and after physical activity and describe activities that depend more on glucose or fat, respectively.

The fuels that support physical activity are glucose (from carbohydrate), fatty acids (from fat), and, to a small extent, amino acids (from protein). During rest, the body derives a little more than half of its energy from fatty acids, most of the rest from glucose, and a little from amino acids. During physical activity, the body uses different mixtures of fuels. Muscles always use a mixture of fuels—never just one. How much of which fuel the muscles use during physical activity depends on an interplay among the fuels available from the diet, the intensity and duration of the activity, and the degree to which the body is conditioned to perform that activity.

In the early minutes of an activity, muscle glycogen provides the majority of energy the muscles use to go into action. As activity continues, messenger molecules, including the hormone **epinephrine,** flow into the bloodstream to signal the liver and fat cells to liberate their stored energy nutrients, primarily glucose and fatty acids.

Glucose Use During Physical Activity

Both the liver and skeletal muscles store glucose as glycogen. Glucose comes from dietary sources, but the liver can also make glucose from fragments of other nutrients. Muscles retain their glycogen stores for their own use—they do not release their glucose into the bloodstream to share with other body tissues, as the liver does. This is fortunate, since a muscle that conserves its glycogen is prepared to act quickly in emergencies because muscle glucose fuels quick action. As activity continues, glucose from the liver's stored glycogen and dietary glucose absorbed from the digestive tract also become important sources of fuel for muscle activity.

Diet Affects Glycogen Storage and Use The body constantly uses and replenishes its glycogen. The more carbohydrate a person eats, the more glycogen muscles store (up to a limit) and the longer the stores will last to support physical activity.

A classic report compared fuel use during physical activity by three groups of runners, each on a different diet. For several days before testing, one of the groups ate a normal mixed diet (55 percent of kcalories from carbohydrate), a second group ate a high-carbohydrate diet (83 percent of kcalories from carbohydrate), and the third group ate a high-fat diet (94 percent of kcalories from fat). As Figure 10-1 shows, the

epinephrine (EP-ih-NEFF-rin): the major hormone that elicits the stress response.

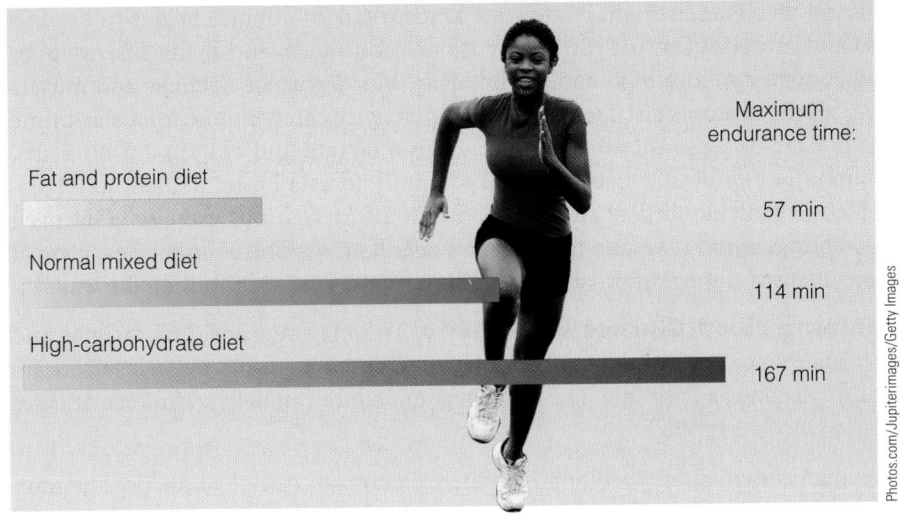

Fat and protein diet

Normal mixed diet

High-carbohydrate diet

Maximum
endurance time:

57 min

114 min

167 min

Photos.com/Jupiterimages/Getty Images

FIGURE 10-1 **The Effect of Diet on Physical Endurance**
A high-carbohydrate diet can increase an athlete's endurance. In this study, the high-fat diet provided 94 percent of kcalories from fat and 6 percent from protein; the normal mixed diet provided 55 percent of kcalories from carbohydrate; and the high-carbohydrate diet provided 83 percent of kcalories from carbohydrate.

high-carbohydrate diet enabled the athletes to work longer before exhaustion. This study and many others established that a high-carbohydrate diet enhances an athlete's endurance by ensuring ample glycogen stores.[32]

Intensity of Activity Affects Glycogen Use The body stores far less glycogen than fat. How long a person's glycogen will last during physical activity depends not only on diet but also on the intensity of the activity.

Moderate-intensity activities such as easy jogging use glycogen slowly. The lungs and circulatory system have no trouble keeping up with the muscles' need for oxygen. The individual breathes easily, and the heart beats steadily—the activity is aerobic. The muscles derive their energy from both glucose and fatty acids. By depending partly on fatty acids, moderate aerobic activity conserves glycogen stores. Joggers still use glycogen, however, and eventually they can run out of it.

Intense activities—the kind that make it difficult to catch your breath, such as a quarter-mile race—use glycogen quickly. Muscles must begin to rely more heavily on glucose, which can be partially broken down by **anaerobic** metabolism. Thus, the muscles begin drawing more heavily on their limited glycogen supply. Anaerobic breakdown of glycogen yields energy to muscle tissue when energy demands outstrip the body's ability to provide energy aerobically, but it does so by spending the muscles' glycogen reserves.

Lactate During intense activity, anaerobic breakdown of glucose produces **lactate.** Muscles release lactate formed during exercise into the blood, and it travels to the liver. There, liver enzymes convert the lactate back into glucose. Glucose can then return to the muscles to fuel additional activity. At low intensities, lactate is readily cleared from the blood by the liver, but at higher intensities, lactate accumulates. When the rate of lactate production exceeds the rate of clearance, intense activity can be maintained for only one to three minutes (as in a 400- or 800-meter race or a boxing match). Accumulation of lactate was long blamed for a type of muscle fatigue, but recent thought disputes this idea. It is true that muscles produce lactate during a type of fatigue, but the lactate does not cause the fatigue.[33]

Activity Duration Affects Glycogen Use The *duration* of a physical activity as well as its *intensity* affect glucose use. In the first 10 minutes or so of an activity, the active muscles rely almost entirely on their own stores of glycogen for glucose. Within the first 20 minutes of moderate activity, a person uses up about one-fifth of the available glycogen. As the muscles devour their own glycogen, they become ravenous for more glucose, and the liver responds by emptying out its glycogen stores.

anaerobic (AN-air-ROH-bic): not requiring oxygen. Anaerobic activity may require strength but does not work the heart and lungs very hard for a sustained period.

lactate: a compound produced during the breakdown of glucose in anaerobic metabolism.

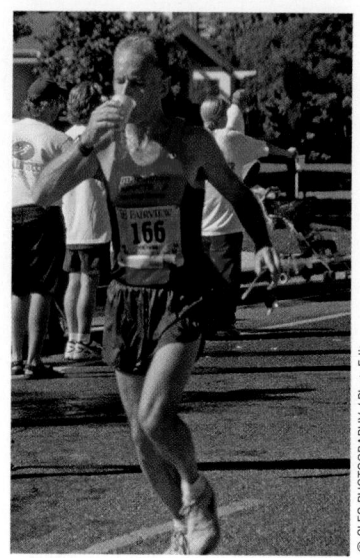

Those who compete in endurance activities require fluid and carbohydrate fuel.

A person who exercises moderately for longer than 20 minutes begins to use less glucose and more fat for fuel. Still, glucose use continues, and if the activity goes on long enough and at a high enough intensity, blood glucose declines and muscle and liver glycogen stores are depleted. Physical activity can continue for a short time thereafter only because the liver produces, from lactate and certain amino acids, the minimum amount of glucose needed to briefly forestall total depletion. Glycogen depletion generally occurs after about two hours of vigorous exercise.[†] Glycogen depletion brings nervous system function to a near halt, making continued exertion at the same intensity almost impossible. Marathon runners call this "hitting the wall."

Maintaining Blood Glucose for Activity To delay the onset of fatigue and enhance endurance performance, athletes try to maintain their blood glucose concentrations for as long as they can. The following guidelines can help endurance athletes maximize glucose supplies:

- Eat a high-carbohydrate diet (approximately 8 grams of carbohydrate per kilogram of body weight or about 70 percent of energy intake) regularly.[‡]

- Take glucose (usually in sports drinks) periodically during activities that last for one hour or more.

- Eat carbohydrate-rich foods (approximately 60 grams of carbohydrate) immediately following activity; for example, 16 ounces of sports drink and a small bagel, 16 ounces of milk and four oatmeal cookies, or 8 ounces of pineapple juice and a granola bar.

Another strategy, **carbohydrate loading,** involves training the muscles to store as much glycogen as they can, while supplying the dietary glucose to enable them to do so. This strategy benefits endurance athletes who exercise at high intensity for longer than 90 minutes and who cannot meet their carbohydrate needs during competition. Although carbohydrate-loading can increase an individual's glycogen stores, performance may or may not improve. Those who exercise for shorter times or at a slower pace are better served by a regular high-carbohydrate diet. The last section of this chapter, "Diets for Physically Active People," discusses how to design a high-carbohydrate diet for performance.

Glucose during Activity Muscles can obtain the glucose they need not only from glycogen stores but also from foods and beverages consumed during activity. Consuming carbohydrate is especially useful during exhausting endurance activities (lasting more than one hour) and during games such as soccer or hockey, which last for hours and demand repeated bursts of intense activity.[34]

Endurance athletes often run short of glucose by the end of competitive events. To insure optimal carbohydrate intake, sports nutrition experts recommend 30 to 60 grams of carbohydrate per hour during prolonged events.[35] Carbohydrate-based sports drinks offer a convenient way to meet this recommendation and also help replace water and electrolyte losses. Thus, to insure optimal hydration and carbohydrate intake, endurance athletes are advised to drink one-half to one liter of a 4 to 8 percent carbohydrate-based sports drink per hour, in small, frequent doses during activity.[36] During the last stages of an endurance competition, when glycogen is running low, glucose consumed during the event can slowly make its way from the digestive tract to the muscles and augment the body's supply of glucose enough to forestall exhaustion.

carbohydrate loading: a regimen of moderate exercise, followed by eating a high-carbohydrate diet, which enables muscles to temporarily store glycogen beyond their normal capacity; also called *glycogen loading* or *glycogen supercompensation.*

[†]Here "vigorous exercise" means exercise at 75 percent of VO_2 max.
[‡]Percentage of energy intake is meaningful only when total energy intake is known. Consider that at high energy intakes (5000 kcalories/day), even a moderate carbohydrate diet (50 percent of energy intake) supplies 625 grams of carbohydrate—enough for a 165-pound (75 kilogram) athlete in heavy training. By comparison, at a moderate energy intake (2000 kcalories/day), a high-carbohydrate intake (70 percent of energy intake) supplies 350 grams—plenty of carbohydrate for most people, but not enough for athletes in heavy training.

Some researchers have questioned whether adding protein to carbohydrate-containing sports beverages would offer a performance advantage to endurance athletes.[37] Evidence so far suggests that when carbohydrate intake is optimal, protein provides no additional performance benefit.

Glucose after Activity Muscles depleted of glycogen have greater insulin sensitivity, which enhances glucose uptake and promotes glycogen synthesis. Thus, eating high-carbohydrate foods *after* physical activity also enlarges glycogen stores. To accelerate the rate of glycogen storage, train normally; then, within two hours after physical activity, consume a high-carbohydrate meal, such as a glass of orange juice and some graham crackers, toast, or cereal.[38] After 2 hours, the rate of glycogen storage declines by almost half. This strategy is especially important to athletes who train hard more than once per day.

Nutrition in Practice 2 discusses the possible health benefits of eating a diet ranking low on the glycemic index. Such a diet may also benefit endurance performance. Some research indicates that foods with a low glycemic index enhance fatty acid availability and use during subsequent activity, thereby reducing reliance on the muscles' own lipid and glycogen stores.[39] More research is needed to confirm these findings.

Training Affects Glycogen Use Training affects glycogen use during activity in at least two ways. First, muscles that deplete their glycogen stores through work adapt to store greater amounts of glycogen to support that work. Second, trained muscles burn more fat and at higher intensities than untrained muscles, so they require less glucose to perform the same amount of work. A person attempting an activity for the first time uses up much more glucose per minute than an athlete trained to perform it.

IN SUMMARY

❚ Glucose is supplied by dietary carbohydrate or made by the liver.

❚ Glucose is stored in both liver and muscle tissue as glycogen.

❚ Total glycogen stores affect an athlete's endurance.

❚ The more intense an activity, the more glucose it demands.

❚ During anaerobic metabolism, the body spends glucose rapidly and accumulates lactate.

❚ Physical activity of long duration places demands on the body's glycogen stores.

❚ Carbohydrate ingested before and during long-duration activity may help to forestall fatigue.

❚ Carbohydrate loading is a regimen of physical activity and diet that enables an athlete's muscles to store larger-than-normal amounts of glycogen to extend endurance.

❚ Highly trained muscles use less glucose and more fat than do untrained muscles to perform the same work, so their glycogen lasts longer.

Fat Use During Activity

Sports nutrition experts recommend that athletes consume 20 to 35 percent of their energy from fat to meet nutrient and energy needs—the same recommendation as for others.[40] Athletes who restrict fat below 20 percent of total energy intake may fail to consume adequate energy and nutrients. Recommendations to include vegetable oils, nuts, olives, fatty fish, and other sources of health-promoting fats in the diet apply to athletes as well as to everyone else.

Diets high in saturated fat carry risks of heart disease. Physical activity offers some protection against cardiovascular disease, but athletes, like everyone else, can suffer heart attacks and strokes. Limiting saturated fat intake to less than 10 percent of total energy intake is another way athletes can protect themselves from heart disease.

In contrast to *dietary* fat, *body* fat stores are extremely important during physical activity, as long as the activity is not too intense. Unlike the body's glycogen stores, which are limited to less than 2000 kcalories of energy, fat stores can total 70,000 kcalories or more and can fuel hours of activity without running out. Early in activity, muscles begin to draw on fatty acids from two sources—fats stored within the working muscles and fats from fat deposits such as the fat under the skin. Areas with the most fat to spare donate the greatest amounts of fatty acids to the blood (although they may not be the areas from which one might choose to lose fat). This is why "spot reducing" does not work: muscles do not own the fat that surrounds them. Fat cells release fatty acids into the blood for all the muscles to share. Proof is found in a tennis player's arms: the fat folds measure the same in both arms, even though one arm has better-developed muscles than the other. A balanced fitness program that includes strength training, however, will tighten muscles underneath the fat, improving the overall appearance. Keep in mind that some body fat is essential to good health. (Chapter 6 discusses the health risks of too little body fat.)

Intensity and Duration Affect Fat Use The *intensity* of physical activity affects fat use. As the intensity of activity increases, fat makes less and less of a contribution to the fuel mixture. Remember that fat can be broken down for energy only by aerobic metabolism. For fat to fuel activity, oxygen must be abundantly available. If a person is breathing easily during activity, the muscles are getting all the oxygen they need and are able to use more fat in the fuel mixture.

The *duration* of activity also influences fat use. Early in an activity, as the muscles draw on fatty acids, blood levels fall. If the activity continues for more than a few minutes, the hormone epinephrine signals the fat cells to begin breaking down their stored triglycerides and liberating fatty acids into the blood. As activity continues, the blood fatty acid concentration surpasses the normal resting concentration. Thereafter, sustained, moderate activity uses body fat stores as its major fuel.

Training Affects Fat Use Training—repeated aerobic activity—produces the adaptations that permit the body to draw more heavily on fat for fuel. Aerobically trained muscles burn fat more readily than untrained muscles. With aerobic training, the heart and lungs also become stronger and better able to deliver oxygen to the muscles during high-intensity activities. In turn, this improved oxygen supply enables the muscles to burn more fat. These adaptations reward not only trained athletes, but also all active people; a person who trains by way of aerobic activities such as distance running or cycling becomes well suited to the activity.

IN SUMMARY

▌ Athletes who restrict fat below 20 percent of total energy intake may fail to consume adequate energy and nutrients.

▌ In contrast to *dietary* fat, *body* fat stores are extremely important during physical activity, as long as the activity is not too intense.

▌ The intensity and duration of activity, as well as training—repeated aerobic activity—affect fat use.

Protein Use During Activity

Athletes use protein to build and maintain muscle and other lean tissue structures and, to a small extent, to fuel activity. The body handles protein differently during activity than during rest.

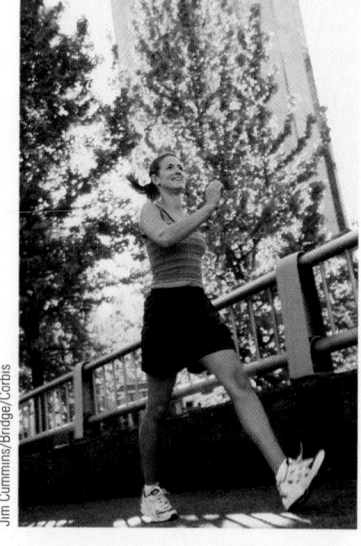

Low- to moderate-intensity aerobic exercises that can be sustained for a long time (more than 20 minutes) use some glucose but more fat for fuel.

Protein for Building Muscle Tissue In the hours of rest that follow physical activity, muscles speed up their rate of protein synthesis—they build more of the proteins they need to perform the activity. Research shows that eating high-quality protein, either by itself or together with carbohydrate, immediately following physical activity stimulates muscle protein synthesis.[41] With food intake, of course, insulin is secreted. Insulin not only stimulates muscle protein synthesis, but also greatly inhibits muscle protein breakdown.[42] Remember that the body adapts and builds the molecules, cells, and tissues it needs for the next period of activity. Whenever the body rebuilds a part of itself, it tears down old structures to make way for new ones. Repeated activity, with just a slight overload, triggers the protein-dismantling and the protein-synthesizing equipment of each muscle cell to make needed changes—that is, to adapt.

Dietary protein provides the needed amino acids for synthesis of new muscle proteins. As Chapter 4 pointed out, the true director of synthesis of muscle protein is physical activity itself.

The intensity and pattern of muscle contractions initiate signals that direct the muscles' genetic material to make particular proteins. For example, a weight lifter's workout sends the information that muscle fibers need added bulk for strength and more enzymes for making and using glycogen. A runner's workout stimulates production of proteins needed for aerobic oxidation of fat and glucose. Muscle cells are exquisitely responsive to the need for proteins, and they build them conservatively, only as needed.

Finally, after muscle cells have made all the decisions about which proteins to build and when, protein nutrition comes into play. During active muscle-building phases of training, a weight lifter might add between ¼ ounce and 1 ounce (between 7 and 28 grams) of protein to existing muscle mass each day. This extra protein comes from ordinary food.

Protein for Fuel Not only do athletes retain more protein but they also use a little more protein as fuel. Muscles speed up their use of amino acids for energy during physical activity, just as they speed up their use of glucose and fatty acids. Still, protein contributes at most about 10 percent of the total fuel used, both during activity and during rest.

Diet Affects Protein Use during Activity Diet influences how much protein is used during activity. People who consume diets adequate in energy and rich in *carbohydrate* use less protein than those who eat protein- and fat-rich diets. Recall that carbohydrates spare proteins from being broken down to make glucose when needed. Because physical activity requires glucose, a diet lacking in carbohydrate necessitates the conversion of amino acids to glucose.

Intensity and Duration Affect Protein Use during Activity The intensity and duration of the activity also modify protein use. Endurance athletes who train for more than one hour per day, engaging in aerobic activity of moderate intensity and long duration, may deplete their glycogen stores by the end of their workouts and become more dependent on body protein for energy. In contrast, anaerobic strength training does not use more protein for energy but does demand more protein to build muscle. Thus, the protein needs of both endurance and strength athletes are higher than those of sedentary people, but not as high as the protein intakes many athletes consume.

Protein Recommendations for Active People Although most athletes need somewhat more protein than do sedentary people, average protein intakes in the United States are high enough to cover those needs. Therefore, athletes in training should attend to protein needs but should back up the protein with ample carbohydrate. Otherwise, they will burn off as fuel the very protein they wish to retain in muscle.

The DRI Committee does not recommend greater-than-normal protein intakes for athletes, but other authorities do.[43] These recommendations specify different protein

For perfect functioning, every nutrient is needed.

TABLE 10-4 Recommended Protein Intakes for Athletes

	Recommendations (g/kg/day)	Protein Intakes (g/day)	
		Males	Females
RDA for adults	0.8	56	44
Recommended intake for power (strength or speed) athletes	1.2–1.7	84–119	66–94
Recommended intake for endurance athletes	1.2–1.4	84–98	66–77
U.S. average intake		102	70

Note: Daily protein intakes are based on a 70-kilogram (154-pound) man and 55-kilogram (121-pound) woman.

Sources: Position of the American Dietetic Association, Dietitians of Canada, and the American College of Sports Medicine: Nutrition and athletic performance, *Journal of the American Dietetic Association* 109 (2009): 509–527; U.S. Department of Agriculture, Agricultural Research Service, 2008, *Nutrient Intakes from Food: Mean Amounts Consumed per Individual One Day, 2005–2006.* Available at www.ars.usda.gov/ba/bhnrc/fsrg; Committee on *Dietary Reference Intakes, Dietary Reference Intakes for Energy, Carbohydrate, Fiber, Fat, Fatty Acids, Cholesterol, Protein and Amino Acids* (Washington, D.C.: National Academies Press, 2005), pp. 660–661.

intakes for athletes pursuing different activities (see Table 10-4). A later section translates protein recommendations into a diet plan and shows that no one needs protein supplements or even large servings of meat to obtain the highest recommended protein intakes.

IN SUMMARY

▌ Physical activity stimulates muscle cells to break down and synthesize protein, resulting in muscle adaptation to activity.

▌ Athletes use protein both for building muscle tissue and for energy. Diet, intensity and duration of activity, and training affect protein use during activity.

▌ Although athletes need more protein than sedentary people, a balanced, high-carbohydrate diet provides sufficient protein to cover an athlete's needs.

10.3 Vitamins and Minerals to Support Activity

LO 10.3 List the vitamin and mineral supplements athletes may need and explain why.

Many vitamins and minerals assist in releasing energy from fuels and transporting oxygen. This knowledge has led many people to believe, mistakenly, that vitamin and mineral *supplements* offer physically active people both health benefits and athletic advantages. Nutrition in Practice 9 offers a discussion of vitamin and mineral supplements and Nutrition in Practice 10 explores supplements and other products people use in the hope of enhancing athletic performance.

Supplements

Nutrient supplements do not enhance the performance of well-nourished athletes or active people. Deficiencies of vitamins and minerals, however, do impede performance. Regular, strenuous physical activity increases the demand for energy, and athletes and active people tend to eat more food. If they select nutrient-dense foods to meet those increased energy needs, they will, in most cases, also meet their vitamin and mineral needs. Remember, however, that nutrient recommendations are based on the needs of healthy people in different life stages and do not reflect the potentially greater needs of some athletes.

As Nutrition in Practice 6 mentions, athletes who struggle to meet low body-weight requirements may consume so little food that they fail to obtain all the nutrients they need.[44] The practice of "making weight" is opposed by many health and fitness organizations, but for athletes who choose this course of action, a single daily multivitamin-mineral supplement that provides no more than the DRI recommendations for nutrients can be beneficial. In addition, some athletes do not eat enough food to maintain body weight during times of intense training or competition. For these athletes, too, a daily multivitamin-mineral supplement can be helpful.

Some athletes believe that taking vitamin or mineral supplements just before competition will enhance performance. These beliefs are contrary to scientific reality. Most vitamins and minerals function as small parts of larger working units. After entering the blood, they have to wait for the cells to combine them with their appropriate other parts so that they can do their work. This takes time—hours or days. Vitamins or minerals taken right before an event do not improve performance, even if the person is actually suffering deficiencies of those nutrients.

Nutrients of Special Concern

In general, then, active people who eat well-balanced meals do not need vitamin or mineral supplements. Two nutrients, vitamin E and iron, do merit special attention, however, each for a different reason. Vitamin E is addressed because so many athletes take supplements of it. Iron is discussed because some female athletes may be unaware that they need supplements.

Vitamin E During prolonged, high-intensity physical activity, the muscles' consumption of oxygen increases tenfold or more, enhancing the production of damaging free radicals in the body.[45] Vitamin E is a potent fat-soluble antioxidant that vigorously defends cell membranes against oxidative damage.

Does vitamin E supplementation protect against exercise-induced oxidative stress? Some studies find that it does; others show no effect, and still others report enhanced oxidative stress.[46] Recent research may offer some insight into these inconsistencies. Although free radicals are usually damaging, during repeated episodes of endurance activities, they may actually be beneficial. Free radicals activate powerful antioxidant enzymes, which may enhance the athlete's tolerance to such oxidative stresses.[47] Researchers speculate that antioxidant supplements such as vitamin E interfere with this protective adaptive response. This may explain why, in some studies, athletes taking vitamin E show signs of increased oxidative stress. Clearly, more research is needed, but in the meantime, physically active people can benefit by using vegetable oils and eating generous servings of antioxidant-rich fruits and vegetables regularly. Beta-carotene and vitamin C in fruits and vegetables, as well as many of the phytochemicals in these foods, are also potent antioxidants.

Iron and Performance Physically active young women, especially those who engage in endurance activities such as distance running, are prone to iron deficiency.[48] Habitually low intakes of iron-rich foods, high iron losses through menstruation, and the high demands of muscles for the iron-containing molecules of aerobic metabolism and the muscle protein myoglobin can contribute to iron deficiency in young female athletes. In addition, endurance activities temporarily increase the release of hepicidin, which limits iron absorption (see Chapter 9).[49]

Adolescent female athletes who eat vegetarian diets may be particularly vulnerable to iron deficiency. The bioavailability of iron is often poor in plant-based diets because such diets are high in fiber and phytic acid and because the nonheme iron in plant foods is not absorbed as well as the heme iron in animal-derived foods. Vegetarian diets are usually rich in vitamin C, however, which enhances iron absorption. To protect against iron deficiency, vegetarian athletes need to pay close attention to their

Female athletes may be at special risk of iron deficiency.

intake of good dietary sources of iron (fortified cereals, legumes, nuts, and seeds) and include vitamin C-rich foods with each meal. So long as vegetarian athletes consume enough nutrient-dense foods, they can perform as well as non-vegetarians.

Iron deficiency impairs performance because iron helps deliver the muscles' oxygen. Insufficient oxygen delivery reduces aerobic work capacity, so the person tires easily. Iron deficiency without clinical signs of anemia may also impair physical performance.[50]

Early in training, athletes may develop low blood hemoglobin. This condition, sometimes called "sports anemia," is not a true iron-deficiency condition. Strenuous training promotes destruction of the more fragile, older red blood cells, and the resulting cleanup work reduces the blood's iron content temporarily. Strenuous activity also expands the blood's plasma volume, thereby reducing the red blood cell count per unit of blood. This low hematocrit looks like iron-deficiency anemia, but it is not the same. In sports anemia, the red blood cells do not diminish in size or number as in anemia, so the oxygen-carrying capacity is not hindered. Most researchers view sports anemia as an *adaptive,* temporary response to endurance training. Iron-deficiency anemia requires treatment with prescribed iron supplements, but sports anemia does not.

The best strategy for maintaining adequate iron nutrition depends on the individual. Menstruating women may border on iron deficiency even without the iron losses incurred by physical activity. Active teens of both genders have high iron needs because they are growing. Especially for women and teens, then, prescribed supplements may be needed to correct iron deficiencies. (Medical testing is needed to eliminate nondietary causes of anemia, such as internal bleeding or cancer.)

IN SUMMARY

- With the possible exception of iron, well-nourished active people and athletes do not need nutrient supplements. Athletes who do not eat enough food to maintain body weight during intense training or competition, however, may need a multivitamin-mineral supplement.

- Female athletes need to pay special attention to their iron needs.

- Iron-deficiency anemia impairs physical performance because iron is the blood's oxygen handler.

- Sports anemia is a harmless temporary adaptation to physical activity.

10.4 Fluids and Electrolytes in Physical Activity

LO 10.4 Identify the factors that influence an athlete's fluid and electrolyte needs and the symptoms of heat stroke and hypothermia, and compare water and sports drinks as fluid sources.

The body's need for water far surpasses its need for any other nutrient. If the body loses too much water, its life-supporting chemistry is compromised.

The exercising body loses water primarily via sweat; second to that, breathing uses water, exhaled as vapor. During physical activity, both routes can be significant, and dehydration is a real threat. The first symptom of dehydration is fatigue. A water loss of greater than 2 percent of body weight can reduce a person's capacity to do muscular work.[51] A person with a water loss of about 7 percent is likely to collapse. The athlete who arrives at an event even slightly dehydrated starts out at a competitive disadvantage.

Temperature Regulation

As Chapter 9 pointed out, sweat cools the body. The conversion of water to vapor uses up a great deal of heat, so as sweat evaporates, it cools the skin's surface and the blood flowing beneath it.

Hyperthermia In hot, humid weather, sweat may fail to evaporate because the surrounding air is already laden with water. In **hyperthermia,** body heat builds up and triggers maximum sweating, but without sweat evaporation, little cooling takes place. In such conditions, active people must take precautions to avoid **heat stroke.** Heat stroke is an especially dangerous accumulation of body heat with accompanying loss of body fluid. To reduce the risk of heat stroke, drink enough fluid before and during the activity, rest in the shade when tired, and wear lightweight clothing that allows sweat to evaporate. The rubber or heavy suits sold with promises of weight loss during physical activity are dangerous because they promote profuse sweating, prevent sweat evaporation, and invite heat stroke. If you experience any of the symptoms of heat stroke listed in Table 10-5 stop your activity, sip cold fluids, seek shade, and ask for help. The condition demands medical attention—it can kill.

Hypothermia In cold weather, **hypothermia,** or low body temperature, can be as serious as heat stroke is in hot weather. Inexperienced runners participating in long races on cold or wet, chilly days are especially vulnerable to hypothermia. Slow runners who produce little heat can become too cold, especially if their clothing is inadequate. Early symptoms of hypothermia include feeling cold, shivering, apathy, and social withdrawal.[52] As body temperature continues to fall, shivering stops, and disorientation, slurred speech, and change in behavior or appearance set in. People with these symptoms soon become helpless to protect themselves from further body heat losses. Even in cold weather, the body still sweats and needs fluids, but the fluids should be warm or at room temperature to help prevent hypothermia.

Fluid Needs during Physical Activity

Endurance athletes can lose 1.5 quarts or more of fluid during *each hour* of activity. To prepare for fluid losses, the athlete must hydrate before activity. To replace fluid losses, the person must rehydrate during and after activity. (Table 10-6 presents a suggested schedule of hydration for physical activity.) Even then, in hot weather, the digestive tract may not be able to absorb enough water fast enough to keep up with an athlete's

TABLE 10-5 Symptoms of Heat Stroke and Hypothermia Compared

Heat Stroke
- Clumsiness, stumbling
- Confusion, dizziness, other mental changes, loss of consciousness
- Flushed skin (skin may turn red as body temperature rises)
- Muscle cramping (early symptom)
- Nausea and vomiting
- Rapid breathing
- Rapid heart rate
- Sudden cessation of sweating (hot, dry skin)
- Throbbing headache

Hypothermia
- Clumsiness, loss of coordination
- Confusion, disorientation, other mental changes, loss of consciousness
- Drowsiness
- Shivering (early symptom)
- Cessation of shivering (late symptom)
- Slurred speech
- Slow breathing
- Slow heart rate

Source: Adapted from Centers for Disease Control and Prevention, www.cdc.gov.

TABLE 10-6 Suggested Hydration Schedule for Physical Activity

Timing	Recommended Intakes (based on body weight)	Males	Females
≥4 hours before activity	1 oz/10 lb	16 oz	12 oz
2 hours before activity, if heavy sweating is expected	Add 0.6 oz/10 lb	+9 oz	+7 oz
Every 15 minutes during activity	Drink enough to minimize loss of body weight, but don't drink too much	8 oz	4 oz
After activity	≥2 cups for each pound of body weight lost[a]		

Note: Intakes are based on a 70-kilogram (154-pound) man and a 55-kilogram (121-pound) woman.

[a]Drinking 2 cups of fluid every 20 to 30 minutes after exercise until the total amount required is consumed is more effective for rehydration than drinking the needed amount all at once. Rapid fluid replacement after exercise stimulates urine production and results in less body water retention.

Source: C.A. Rosenbloom and E.J. Coleman, eds., *Sports Nutrition: A Practice Manual for Professionals* (Chicago: Academy of Nutrition and Dietetics, 2012), p. 115; Position of the American Dietetic Association, Dietitians of Canada, and the American College of Sports Medicine: Nutrition and athletic performance, *Journal of the American Dietetic Association* 109 (2009): 509–527; American College of Sports Medicine, Position stand: Exercise and fluid replacement, *Medicine and Science in Sports and Exercise* 39 (2007): 377–390.

hyperthermia: an above-normal body temperature.

heat stroke: an acute and life-threatening reaction to heat buildup in the body.

hypothermia: a below-normal body temperature.

Active people need extra fluid, even in cold weather.

sweat losses, and some degree of dehydration may be inevitable. Athletes who know their body's **hourly sweat rate** can strive to replace the total amount of fluid lost during activity to prevent dehydration.

Athletes who are preparing for competition are often advised to drink extra fluids in the last few days of training before the event. The extra fluid is not stored in the body, but drinking extra ensures maximum tissue hydration at the start of the event. Full hydration is imperative for every athlete both in training and in competition.

Athletes who rely on thirst to govern fluid intake can easily become dehydrated. During activity thirst becomes detectable only *after* fluid stores are depleted. Do not wait to feel thirsty before drinking.

Water What is the best fluid to support physical activity? For noncompetitive, everyday active people, plain cool water is recommended for two reasons: (1) water rapidly leaves the digestive tract to enter the tissues, and (2) it cools the body from the inside out. Endurance athletes are an exception: they need more from their fluids than water alone. The first priority for endurance athletes should always be replacement of fluids to prevent life-threatening heat stroke. But endurance athletes also need carbohydrate to supplement their limited glycogen stores. A later section compares water and sports drinks as fluid sources for endurance athletes.

Electrolyte Losses and Replacement During physical activity, the body loses electrolytes—the minerals sodium, potassium, chloride, and magnesium—in sweat. Beginners lose these electrolytes to a much greater extent than do trained athletes. The body's adaptation to physical activity includes better conservation of these electrolytes. To replenish lost electrolytes, a person ordinarily needs only to eat a regular diet that meets energy and nutrient needs. In events lasting more than one hour, sports drinks may be needed to replace fluids and electrolytes. Salt tablets can worsen dehydration and impair performance; they increase potassium losses, irritate the stomach, and cause vomiting. Endurance athletes considering the use of salt tablets to replace sodium are advised to consult with a health care professional first.

Sodium Depletion When athletes compete in endurance sports lasting longer than three hours, replenishing electrolytes is crucial. If athletes sweat profusely over a long period of time and do not replace lost sodium, a dangerous condition of sodium depletion, known as **hyponatremia,** may result. The symptoms of hyponatremia are similar to, but not the same as, those of dehydration (see Table 10-7). Research shows that some athletes who sweat profusely may also lose more sodium in their sweat than others—and are prone to debilitating heat cramps.[53] These athletes lose twice as much sodium in sweat as athletes who do not cramp, making them more susceptible to hyponatremia. Depending on individual variation, exercise intensity, and changes in ambient temperature and humidity, sweat rates for these athletes can exceed 2 quarts per hour.[54]

Hyponatremia may also occur when endurance athletes drink such large amounts of water over the course of a long event that they overhydrate, diluting the body fluids to such an extent that the sodium concentration becomes extremely low. During long competitions, when athletes lose sodium through heavy sweating *and* consume excessive amounts of liquids, especially water, hyponatremia becomes likely.

Some athletes may be vulnerable to hyponatremia even when they drink sports drinks during an event. Sports drinks do contain sodium, but as a later section points out, the sodium content of sports drinks is low, and in some cases, too low to replace sweat losses. Still, sports drinks do offer more sodium than plain water.

To prevent hyponatremia, endurance athletes need to replace sodium during prolonged events by consuming sports drinks, salty pretzels, and/or other sodium sources. Some athletes may need beverages with higher sodium concentrations than commercial sports drinks. In the days before the event, especially an event in the heat, athletes should not restrict salt in their diets.

TABLE 10-7 Symptoms of Hyponatremia

- Bloating, puffiness from water retention (shoes tight, rings tight)
- Confusion
- Seizure
- Severe headache
- Vomiting

hourly sweat rate: the amount of weight lost plus fluid consumed during exercise per hour.

hyponatremia (HIGH-poh-na-TREE-mee-ah)**:** a decreased concentration of sodium in the blood (*hypo* means "below"; *natrium* means "sodium"; *emia* means "blood").

Sports Drinks

Hydration is critical to optimal performance. As stated earlier, water best meets the fluid needs of most people, yet manufacturers market many good-tasting sports drinks that deliver both fluid and carbohydrate for active people. The term *sports drink* generally refers to beverages that contain carbohydrates and electrolytes in specific concentrations, and they are the focus of this discussion.

Many sports drinks compete for their share of the multi-billion-dollar market. What do sports drinks have to offer?

Fluid Sports drinks offer fluids to help offset the loss of fluids during physical activity, but plain water can do this, too. Alternatively, diluted fruit juices or flavored water can be used if preferred to plain water.

Glucose Sports drinks offer simple sugars or **glucose polymers** that help maintain hydration and blood glucose and enhance performance as effectively as, or in some circumstances, even better than, water. Such measures are especially beneficial for strenuous endurance activities lasting longer than one hour, during intense activities, or during prolonged competitive games that demand repeated intermittent activity.[55] Either sports drinks or plain water is suitable for events lasting less than one hour.

Fluid transport to the tissues from beverages containing up to 8 percent glucose is rapid. Most sports drinks contain about 7 percent carbohydrate (about half the sugar of ordinary soft drinks, or about 5 teaspoons in each 12 ounces). Less than 6 percent may not enhance performance, and more than 8 percent may cause abdominal cramps, nausea, and diarrhea.

Although glucose does enhance endurance and performance in strenuous competitive events, it can be counterproductive for the moderate exerciser if weight loss is the goal. Glucose is sugar, and like candy, it provides only empty kcalories—no vitamins or minerals. Most sports drinks provide between 50 and 100 kcalories per 8-ounce cup.

Sodium and Other Electrolytes Sports drinks offer sodium and other electrolytes to help replace those lost during physical activity. Sodium in sports drinks also helps to increase the rate of fluid absorption from the GI tract and maintain plasma volume during activity and recovery. Most physically active people do not need to replace the minerals lost in sweat immediately; a meal eaten within hours of competition replaces these minerals soon enough. Most sports drinks are relatively low in sodium, however, so those who choose to use these beverages run little risk of excessive intake.

Good Taste Manufacturers reason that if a drink tastes good, people will drink more, thereby ensuring adequate hydration. For athletes who prefer the flavors of sports drinks over water, it may be worth paying for good taste to replace lost fluids.

For athletes who exercise for one hour or more, sports drinks provide an advantage over water. For most physically active people, though, water is the best beverage to replenish lost fluids. The most important thing to do is drink—even if you don't feel thirsty.

Enhanced Water

Another beverage often marketed to athletes and active people is **enhanced water.** Enhanced waters are lightly flavored waters with lower carbohydrate and electrolyte contents than traditional sports drinks. Marketers promote these beverages for the added vitamins, minerals, and, in some cases, protein they contain. In fact, most enhanced waters contain small amounts of only a few minerals, some of the B vitamins, and sometimes vitamin C or vitamin E. In the context of daily needs, the vitamins and minerals in these drinks do not add up to much. For example, it takes a quart of most of these beverages to provide only 10 percent of the RDA for iron or calcium. Quite simply, enhanced waters are not a substitute for eating nutrient-rich fruits and vegetables. Enhanced waters

glucose polymers: compounds that supply glucose, not as single molecules, but linked in chains somewhat like starch. The objective is to attract less water from the body into the digestive tract.

enhanced water: water that is fortified with ingredients such as vitamins, minerals, protein, oxygen, or herbs. Enhanced water is marketed as *vitamin water, sports water, oxygenated water,* and *protein water.*

may not be harmful (except maybe to the wallet), but most people do not need them. Plain water can meet fluid needs. If the flavor of enhanced waters encourages greater fluid intake, then they may offer some advantage. Serious endurance athletes need the carbohydrate-electrolyte sports drinks discussed earlier.

Other Beverages

Some beverages, such as soft drinks or the increasingly popular energy drinks, deliver caffeine along with fluid. Caffeine is a stimulant, and athletes sometime use it to enhance performance, as this chapter's Nutrition in Practice explains. Carbonated soft drinks, with or without caffeine, may not be a wise choice for athletes: bubbles make a person feel full quickly and so may limit fluid intake. Some energy drinks contain amounts of caffeine equivalent to a cup or two of coffee. When used in excess or in combination with stimulants or other unregulated substances, energy drinks can hinder performance and are potentially dangerous.[56] Another reason energy drinks should not be used for fluid replacement during athletic events is that the carbohydrate concentrations are too high for optimal fluid absorption. The caffeine contents of selected beverages (including energy drinks) and foods are listed in the table at the beginning of Appendix A.

Some athletes mistakenly believe that they can replace fluids and load up on carbohydrates by drinking beer. Beer is not carbohydrate rich. A 12-ounce beer provides 13 grams of carbohydrate—one-third the amount of carbohydrate in a glass of orange juice the same size. In addition to carbohydrate, beer also contains alcohol, of course. Energy from alcohol breakdown generates heat, but it does not fuel muscle work because alcohol is metabolized in the liver.

Beer is not rich in vitamins or minerals. Beer contains traces of some B vitamins, but it cannot compete with food sources. As for minerals, beer contains a few minerals, but to replace the minerals lost in sweat, athletes need good sources such as fruit juices or sports drinks.

Alcohol's diuretic effect impairs the body's fluid balance, making dehydration likely. After physical activity, a person needs to replace fluids, not lose them by drinking beer. Alcohol also impairs the body's ability to regulate its temperature, increasing the likelihood of hypothermia or heat stroke.

It is difficult to overstate alcohol's detrimental effects on physical activity. Alcohol alters perceptions; slows reaction time; reduces strength, power, and endurance; and hinders accuracy, balance, eye-hand coordination, and coordination in general—all opposing optimal athletic performance. In addition, it deprives people of their judgment, thereby compromising safety in sports. Many sports-related fatalities and injuries involve alcohol or other drugs.

IN SUMMARY

- Hyperthermia and heat stroke can be a threat to physically active people in hot, humid weather.

- Hypothermia threatens those who exercise in the cold.

- Physically active people lose fluids and must replace them to avoid dehydration.

- Water is the best drink for most physically active people, but endurance athletes need beverages that supply glucose as well as fluids.

- During events lasting longer than three hours, athletes need to pay special attention to replacing sodium losses to prevent hyponatremia.

- Caffeine-containing drinks within limits may not impair performance, but water and fruit juice are preferred.

- Alcohol use can impair performance in many ways and is not recommended.

10.5 Diets for Physically Active People

LO 10.5 Discuss an appropriate daily eating pattern for athletes and describe the recommended pregame or recovery meal.

No one diet best supports physical performance. Active people who choose foods within the framework of the diet-planning principles presented in Chapter 1 can design many excellent diets.

Nutrient Density A healthful diet is based on nutrient-dense foods—foods that supply adequate vitamins and minerals for the energy they provide. Active people need to eat both for nutrient adequacy and for energy—and energy needs can be extremely high. For example, during training, meals for some Olympic athletes provide as much as 12,000 kcalories a day. Still, a nutrient-rich diet remains central for adequacy's sake. Though vital, energy alone is not enough to support performance. Table 10-8 offers convenient, nutrient-dense snack ideas for athletes and active people.

Carbohydrate A diet that is high in carbohydrate (60 to 70 percent of total kcalories), moderate in fat (20 to 35 percent), and adequate in protein (10 to 20 percent) ensures full glycogen and other nutrient stores. On two occasions, however, the active person's regular high-carbohydrate, fiber-rich diet may require temporary adjustment. Both of these exceptions involve training for competition rather than for fitness in general. One special occasion is the pregame meal, when fiber-rich, bulky foods are best avoided. The pregame meal is discussed in a later section. The other occasion is during intensive training, when energy needs may be so high as to outstrip the person's capacity to eat enough food to meet them. In this case, the athlete can add concentrated carbohydrate foods, such as dried fruits, sweet potatoes, and nectars, and even high-fat foods, such as avocados and nuts.

Some athletes use commercial high-carbohydrate liquid supplements to obtain the carbohydrate and energy needed for heavy training and top performance. These supplements do not *replace* regular food; they are meant to be used in *addition* to it. Unlike the sports beverages discussed earlier, these high-carbohydrate supplements are too concentrated in carbohydrate to be used for fluid replacement.

Protein In addition to carbohydrate and some fat (and the energy they provide), physically active people need protein. Meats and milk products are rich protein sources, but recommending that active people emphasize these foods is narrow advice. As mentioned repeatedly, active people need diets rich in carbohydrate, and of course, meats have none to offer. Legumes, whole grains, and vegetables provide some protein with abundant carbohydrate. Table 10-4 (p. 270) presents recommended protein intakes.

TABLE 10-8 Nutrient-Dense Snacks for Athletes and Active People

One ounce of almonds provides protein, fiber, calcium, vitamin E, and healthy unsaturated fats. Similar choices include other nuts or trail mix consisting of dried fruit, nuts, and seeds.	Low-fat Greek yogurt contains more protein per serving than regular yogurt, but a little less calcium. A small amount of fresh fruit adds fiber and vitamins. A similar choice is low-fat cheese paired with fresh fruit.	Low-fat milk or chocolate milk together with fig bars or oatmeal-raisin cookies offer protein and fiber. A similar choice is whole-grain cereal with low-fat milk.	Popcorn offers fiber and a fruit smoothie quenches thirst and provides valuable vitamins. A similar choice is pretzels and fruit juice.

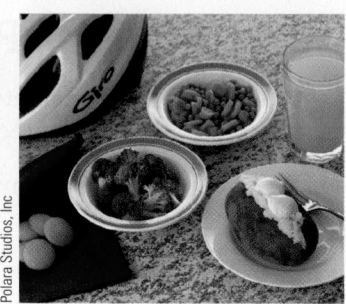

300-kcalorie meal	**500-kcalorie meal**	**750-kcalorie meal**
1 large apple	1 large whole-wheat bagel	1 large baked potato
4 saltine crackers	2 tbs jelly	2 tsp soft margarine
1½ tbs reduced-fat peanut butter	1½ c low-fat milk	1 c steamed broccoli
		1 c mixed carrots and green peas
		5 vanilla wafers
		1½ c apple or pineapple juice

FIGURE 10-2 Examples of High-Carbohydrate Pregame Meals
Pregame meals should be eaten three to four hours before the event and provide 300 to 800 kcalories, primarily from carbohydrate-rich foods. Each of these sample meals provides at least 65 percent of total kcalories from carbohydrate.

Meals before Competition Science indicates that the **pregame meal** should include plenty of fluids and be easy to digest. It should provide between 300 and 800 kcalories, primarily from carbohydrate-rich foods that are familiar to and well-tolerated by the athlete. The meal should end three to four hours before competition to allow time for the stomach to empty before exertion.

Breads, potatoes, pasta, and fruit juices—carbohydrate-rich foods low in fat, protein, and fiber—form the basis of the pregame meal (see Figure 10-2 for some examples). Bulky, fiber-rich foods such as raw vegetables and high-fiber cereals, although usually desirable, are best avoided just before competition. Such foods can cause stomach discomfort during performance.

What about drinks or sport bars claiming to provide "complete" nutrition? These mixtures of carbohydrate, protein (usually amino acids), fat, some fiber, and certain vitamins and minerals may taste good and provide additional food energy for a game or for weight gain. They fall short of providing complete nutrition, however, because they lack many of the beneficial nutrients and phytochemicals that real food offers. These products may provide one advantage for active people—they are easy to eat in the hours before competition.

Liquid meals are easy to digest, and many such meals are commercially available. Alternatively, athletes can mix fat-free milk or juice, frozen fruits, and flavorings in a blender. For example, mixing fat-free milk or apple juice with a frozen banana and cinnamon or vanilla makes a tasty, high-carbohydrate, liquid pregame meal. Do not drop a raw egg in the blender because raw eggs often carry bacteria that cause food poisoning.

Recovery Meals Athletes who perform intense practice sessions several times a day or compete for hours on consecutive days need to quickly replenish glycogen (and fluids) to be ready for the next activity. As mentioned earlier, eating high-carbohydrate foods *after* physical activity enhances glycogen storage. Including protein in recovery meals will support muscle repair and growth.[57] Because people are usually not hungry immediately following physical activity, carbohydrate-containing beverages such as sports drinks or fruit juices may be preferred. If an active person does feel hungry after an event, then foods high in carbohydrate, moderate in protein, and low in fat and fiber are the ones to choose—similar to those recommended prior to competition.

pregame meal: a meal eaten three to four hours before athletic competition.

- The person who wants to excel physically will apply accurate nutrition knowledge along with dedication to rigorous training.

- A diet that provides ample fluid and consists of a variety of nutrient-dense foods in quantities to meet energy needs will enhance not only athletic performance, but overall health as well.

- Carbohydrate-rich foods that are light and easy to digest are recommended for the pregame meal.

- Eating carbohydrate-rich foods after intense physical activity can enhance glycogen storage in preparation for the next activity. Including protein in the recovery meal will support muscle repair and growth.

Training and genetics being equal, who would win a competition—the person who habitually consumes less than the amounts of nutrients needed or the one who arrives at the event with a long history of full nutrient stores and well-met metabolic needs?

Your Diet

Fitness and Nutrition

Fitness depends on a certain minimum amount of physical activity. Ideally, the quantity and quality of the physical activity you select will improve your cardiorespiratory endurance, body composition, strength, and flexibility. Examine your activity choices by keeping an activity diary for one week. For each physical activity, be sure to record the type of activity, the level of intensity, and the duration. In addition, record the times and places of beverage consumption and the types and amounts of beverages consumed. Now compare the choices you made in your one-week activity diary to the American College of Sports Medicine's guidelines for physical fitness (Table 10-2).

- How often were you engaged in aerobic activity to improve cardiorespiratory endurance? Was the intensity of the activity moderate or vigorous? Did each session last at least 30 minutes if of moderate intensity and at least 20 minutes if of vigorous intensity?

- How often did you participate in resistance activities to develop strength? Was the intensity enough to enhance muscle strength and improve body composition? Did you perform 2 to 4 sets of 8 to 12 repetitions involving each major muscle group?

- How often did you stretch to improve your flexibility? Was the intensity enough to develop and maintain a full range of motion? Did you hold each stretch 15 to 30 seconds and repeat each stretch two to four times?

- Do you drink plenty of fluids daily, especially water, before, during, and after physical activity?

- What changes could you make to improve your fitness?

Clinical Applications

1. During her freshman year in college, Kim spent much of her free time bonding with new friends over pizzas, burgers, and fried chicken. Now in her sophomore year, she has decided that it is time to shed the "freshman 15" she gained and get fit quickly. She is replacing her pizzas and burgers with protein shakes and diet sodas; she avoids carbohydrates; and she takes vitamin supplements because she has heard they will give her energy. Kim's demanding sophomore academic load leaves little time during the week to do anything but go to class, study, and work on assignments. She has therefore decided to spend much of her weekend time running, working out with weights, swimming, and playing pick-up soccer on Sunday afternoons. After a few weeks of her new eating and fitness plan, however, Kim is feeling tired and run down much of the time, her muscles ache, and she falls asleep when she is trying to study.

    - What dietary advice would you suggest to help Kim feel healthier and more energetic?

    - What fitness strategies would you offer Kim to prevent her fatigue and sore muscles?

2. Zak, a junior in college, has been weight training four days a week for the past year to gain strength and bulk up his muscles. Along with his training, he has changed his diet from a normal mixed diet to one that emphasizes large servings of meat, eggs, and milk. Zak also takes amino acid supplements in hopes of building more muscle, faster. What advice would you offer Zak about his dietary habits? What would you tell him about the supplements he is taking?

Self Check

1. Regular physical activity helps protect against:
   a. backaches, cancer, and emphysema.
   b. cancer, diabetes, and heart disease.
   c. obesity, kidney disease, and anemia.
   d. high blood pressure, cancer, and allergies.

2. Fitness benefits health by:
   a. increasing lean body tissue and enhancing resistance to colds and other infectious diseases.
   b. lowering the risk of heart disease, decreasing muscle mass, and improving nutritional health.
   c. building bone strength, lowering the risk of some cancers, and increasing anxiety.
   d. reducing diabetes risk, compromising lung function, and promoting a strong self-image.

3. Which of the following characteristics is not a component of fitness?
   a. Muscle endurance
   b. Conditioning
   c. Flexibility
   d. Muscle strength

4. Which of the following provides most of the energy the muscles use in the early minutes of activity?
   a. Fat
   b. Protein
   c. Glycogen
   d. Vitamins

5. "Hitting the wall" is a term runners sometimes use to describe:
   a. dehydration.
   b. hyponatremia.
   c. indigestion.
   d. glucose depletion.

6. Conditioned muscles rely less on ___ and more on ___ for energy.
   a. protein; fat
   b. fat; protein
   c. glycogen; fat
   d. fat; glycogen

7. Vitamin or mineral supplements taken right before an event are useless for improving performance because the:
   a. athlete sweats the nutrients out during the event.
   b. stomach can't digest supplements during physical activity.
   c. nutrients are diluted by all the fluids the athlete drinks.
   d. body needs hours or days for the nutrients to do their work.

8. Physically active young women, especially those who are endurance athletes, are prone to:
   a. energy excess.
   b. iron deficiency.
   c. protein overload.
   d. iodine deficiency.

9. Plain, cool water is the best fluid for everyday active people because it:
   a. rapidly leaves the digestive tract to enter the tissues and cool the body.
   b. tastes good.
   c. provides carbohydrate.
   d. leaves the digestive tract slowly.

10. A recommended pregame meal includes plenty of fluids and provides between:
    a. 300 and 800 kcalories, mostly from fat-rich foods.
    b. 50 and 100 kcalories, mostly from fiber-rich foods.
    c. 1000 and 2000 kcalories, mostly from protein-rich foods.
    d. 300 and 800 kcalories, mostly from carbohydrate-rich foods.

Answers to these questions appear in Appendix H.

Notes

1. Centers for Disease Control and Prevention, www.cdc.gov/physicalactivity/everyone/health; updated February 16, 2011; US Department of Agriculture and US Department of Health and Human Services, *Dietary Guidelines for Americans*, 2010, www.dietaryguidelines.gov.

2. E. H. Bell and coauthors, Physical activity and cardiovascular disease in African Americans in Atherosclerosis Risk in Communities, *Medicine and Science in Sports and Exercise* 45 (2013): 901–907; C. R. Mikus and coauthors, Lowering physical activity impairs glycemic control in healthy volunteers, *Medicine and Science in Sports and Exercise* 44 (2012): 225–231; J. Sattelmair and coauthors, Dose response between physical activity and risk of coronary heart disease: A meta-analysis, *Circulation* 124 (2011): 789–795;

Centers for Disease Control and Prevention, 2011; M. Hamer and coauthors, Physical activity and cardiovascular mortality risk: Possible protective mechanisms, *Medicine and Science in Sports and Exercise* 44 (2012): 84–88.

3. C. D. Harris and coauthors, Adult participation in aerobic and muscle strengthening physical activities—United States, 2011, *Morbidity and Mortality Weekly Report* 62 (2013): 326–330.

4. F. L. Miller and coauthors, Exercise dose, exercise adherence, and associated health outcomes in the TIGER Study, *Medicine and Science in Sports and Exercise* 46 (2014): 69–75; P. T. Katzmarzyk and I. M. Lee, Sedentary behaviour and life expectancy in the USA: A cause-deleted life table analysis, *BMJ Open* 2 (2012): doi:10.1136;; Hamer and coauthors, 2012; H. M. Ahmed and coauthors,

Effects of physical activity on cardiovascular disease, *American Journal of Cardiology* 109 (2012): 288–295; T. Boyle and coauthors, Timing and intensity of recreational physical activity and the risk of subsite-specific colorectal cancer, *Cancer Causes and Control* 22 (2011): 1647–1658; T. Y. Warren and coauthors, Sedentary behaviors increase risk of cardiovascular disease mortality in men, *Medicine and Science in Sports and Exercise* 42 (2010): 879–885; A. V. Patel and coauthors, Leisure time spent sitting in relation to total mortality in a prospective cohort of adults, *American Journal of Epidemiology* 172 (2010): 419–429.

5. Centers for Disease Control and Prevention, 2011.

6. American College of Sports Medicine, Position paper, Appropriate physical activity intervention strategies for weight loss and prevention of

weight regain for adults, *Medicine and Science in Sports and Exercise* 41 (2009): 459–471.

7. M. T. Korhonen and coauthors, Bone density, structure and strength, and their determinants in aging sprint athletes, *Medicine and Science in Sports and Exercise* 44 (2012): 2340–2349.

8. J. Romeo and coauthors, Physical activity, immunity and infection, *Proceedings of the Nutrition Society* 69 (2010): 390–399.

9. C. Eheman and coauthors, Annual Report to the Nation on the status of cancer, 1975–2008, featuring cancers associated with excess weight and lack of sufficient physical activity, *Cancer* 118 (2012): 2338–2366; X. Sui and coauthors, Influence of cardiorespiratory fitness on lung cancer mortality, *Medicine and Science in Sports and Exercise* 42 (2010): 872–878.

10. Hamer and coauthors, 2012; N. T. Artinian and coauthors, Interventions to promote physical activity and dietary lifestyle changes for cardiovascular risk factor reduction in adults: A scientific statement from the American Heart Association, *Circulation* 122 (2010): 406–441.

11. U. Ekelund and coauthors, Physical activity and gain in abdominal adiposity and body weight: Prospective cohort study in 288,498 men and women, *American Journal of Clinical Nutrition* 93 (2011): 826–835; B. H. Goodpaster and coauthors, Effects of diet and physical activity interventions on weight loss and cardiometabolic risk factors in severely obese adults *Journal of the American Medical Association* 304 (2010): 1795–1802.

12. C. K. Roberts, J. P. Little, and J. P. Thyfault, Modification of insulin sensitivity and glycemic control by activity and exercise, *Medicine and Science in Sports and Exercise* 45 (2013): 1868–1877; M. C. Audelin and coauthors, Change of energy expenditure from physical activity is the most powerful determinant of improved insulin sensitivity in overweight patients with coronary artery disease participating in an intensive lifestyle modification program, *Metabolism* 61 (2012): 672–679; C. R. Mikus and coauthors, Lowering physical activity impairs glycemic control in healthy volunteers, *Medicine and Science in Sports and Exercise* 44 (2012): 225–231; J. Ralph and coauthors, Low-intensity exercise reduces the prevalence of hyperglycemia in type 2 diabetes, *Medicine and Science in Sports and Exercise* 42 (2010): 219–225.

13. P. J. Banim and coauthors, Physical activity reduces the risk of symptomatic gallstones: A prospective cohort study, *European Journal of Gastroenterology and Hepatology* 22 (2010): 983–988.

14. J. C. Sieverdes and coauthors, Association between leisure-time physical activity and depressive symptoms in men, *Medicine and Science in Sports and Exercise* 44 (2012), 260–265; M. O. Melancon, D. Lorrain, and I. J. Dionne, Exercise increases tryptophan availability to the brain in older men age 57–70 years, *Medicine and Science in Sports and Exercise* 44 (2012): 881–887.

15. L. M. León-Muñoz and coauthors, Continued sedentariness, change in sitting time and mortality in older adults, *Medicine and Science in Sports and Exercise* 45 (2013): 1501–1507; S. C. Moore and coauthors, Leisure time physical activity of moderate to vigorous intensity and mortality: A large pooled cohort analysis, *PLOS Medicine* 9 (2012): e1001335; B. L. Willis and coauthors, Midlife fitness and the development of chronic conditions

in later life, *Archives of Internal Medicine* 172 (2012): 1333–1340; R. Liu and coauthors, Cardiorespiratory fitness as a predictor of dementia mortality in men and women, *Medicine and Science in Sports and Exercise* 44 (2012): 253–259.

16. C. P. Wen and coauthors, Minimum amount of physical activity for reduced mortality and extended life expectancy: A prospective cohort study, *The Lancet* 378 (2011): 1244–1253.

17. M. D. Graminer and coauthors, Task-specific training reduces trip-related fall risk in women, *Medicine and Science in Sports and Exercise* 44 (2012): 2410–2414; American College of Sports Medicine position stand: Quantity and quality of exercise for developing and maintaining cardiorespiratory, musculoskeletal, and neuromotor fitness in apparently healthy adults: Guidance for prescribing exercise, *Medicine and Science in Sports and Exercise* 43 (2011): 1334–1359.

18. Centers for Disease Control and Prevention, 2011.

19. American College of Sports Medicine position stand, 2011.

20. American College of Sports Medicine position stand, 2011.

21. Centers for Disease Control and Prevention, 2011; American College of Sports Medicine position stand, 2011.

22. P. J. Atherton and K. Smith, Muscle protein synthesis in response to nutrition and exercise, *Journal of Physiology* 590.5 (2012): 1049–1047.

23. B. E. Phillips, D. S. Hill, and P. J. Atherton, Regulation of muscle protein synthesis in humans, *Current Opinion in Clinical Nutrition and Metabolic Care* 15 (2012): 58–63.

24. Atherton and Smith, 2012.

25. L. A. Bateman and coauthors, Comparison of aerobic versus resistance exercise training effects on metabolic syndrome (from the studies of a targeted risk reduction intervention through defined exercise—STRRIDEAT/RT), *American Journal of Cardiology* 108 (2011): 838–844; S. Marwood and coauthors, Faster pulmonary oxygen uptake kinetics in trained versus untrained male adolescents, *Medicine and Science in Sports and Exercise* 42 (2010): 127–134.

26. D. M. Bhammar, S. S. Angadi, and G. A. Gaesser, Effects of fractionized and continuous exercise on 24-h ambulatory blood pressure, *Medicine and Science in Sports and Exercise* 44 (2012): 2270–2276; S. Liu and coauthors, Blood pressure responses to acute and chronic exercise are related in prehypertension, *Medicine and Science in Sports and Exercise* 44 (2012): 1644–1652; D. I. Musa and C. A. Williams, Cardiorespiratory fitness, fatness, and blood pressure associations in Nigerian youth, *Medicine and Science in Sports and Exercise* 44 (2012): 1978–1985; E. G. Ciolac and coauthors, Effects of high-intensity aerobic interval training vs. moderate exercise on hemodynamic, metabolic and neuro-humoral abnormalities of young normotensive women at high familial risk for hypertension, *Hypertension Research* 33 (2010): 836–843.

27. American College of Sports Medicine position stand, 2011; American College of Sports Medicine position stand: Progression models in resistance training for healthy adults, *Medicine and Science in Sports and Exercise* 41 (2009): 687–708.

28. American College of Sports Medicine position stand, 2011.

29. E. A. Marques and coauthors, Response of bone mineral density, inflammatory cytokines, and biochemical bone markers to a 32-week combined loading exercise programme in older men and women, *Archives of Gerontology and Geriatrics* 57 (2013): 226–233; T. E. Howe and coauthors, Exercise for preventing and treating osteoporosis in postmenopausal women, *Cochrane Database of Systematic Reviews* 7 (2011): CD000333.

30. L. Krist, F. Dimeo, and T. Keil, Can progressive resistance training twice a week improve mobility, muscle strength, and quality of life in very elderly nursing-home residents with impaired mobility? A pilot study, *Clinical Interventions in Aging* 8 (2013): 443–448; L. Clemson and coauthors, Integration of balance and strength training into daily life activity to reduce rate of falls in older people (the LiFE study): randomized parallel trial, *British Medical Journal* 7 (2012): e4547.

31. American College of Sports Medicine position stand, Progression models in resistance training for healthy adults, 2009.

32. Position of the American Dietetic Association, Dietitians of Canada, and the American College of Sports Medicine: Nutrition and athletic performance, *Journal of the American Dietetic Association* 109 (2009): 509–527.

33. J. F. Moxnes and Ø. Sandbakk, The kinetics of lactate production and removal during whole-body exercise, *Theoretical Biology and Medical Modeling* 9 (2012): 7.

34. J. Temesi and coauthors, Carbohydrate ingestion during endurance exercise improves performance in adults, *Journal of Nutrition* 141 (2011): 890–897; L. M. Burke, Fueling strategies to optimize performance: Training high or training low? *Scandinavian Journal of Medicine and Science in Sports* 20 (2010): 48–58.

35. S. A. Herring and coauthors, Selected issues for nutrition and the athlete: A Team Physician Consensus Statement, *Medicine and Science in Sports and Exercise* 45 (2013): 2378–2386; C. Rosenbloom, Food and fluid guidelines before, during, and after exercise, *Nutrition Today* 47 (2012): 63–69; Position of the American Dietetic Association, Dietitians of Canada, and the American College of Sports Medicine, 2009.

36. Rosenbloom, 2012.

37. L. Breen, K. D. Tipton, and A. E. Jeukendrup, No effect of carbohydrate-protein on cycling performance and indices of recovery, *Medicine and Science in Sports and Exercise* 42 (2010): 1140–1148.

38. Position of the American Dietetic Association, Dietitians of Canada, and the American College of Sports Medicine, 2009.

39. C. M. Perry, T.L. Perry, and M.C. Rose, Glycemic index and endurance performance, *International Journal of Sport Nutrition and Exercise Metabolism* 20 (2010): 154–165.

40. Position of the American Dietetic Association, Dietitians of Canada, and the American College of Sports Medicine, 2009.

41. W. R. Lunn and coauthors, Chocolate milk and endurance exercise recovery: Protein balance, glycogen, and performance, *Medicine*

and Science in Sports and Exercise 44 (2012): 682–691; N. M. Cermack and coauthors, Protein supplementation augments the adaptive response of skeletal muscle to resistance-type exercise training: A meta-analysis, American Journal of Clinical Nutrition 96 (2012): 1454–1464; A. R. Josse and coauthors, Body composition and strength changes in women with milk and resistance exercise, Medicine and Science in Sports and Exercise 42 (2010): 1122–1130.

42. Atherton and Smith, 2012.

43. Position of the American Dietetic Association, Dietitians of Canada, and the American College of Sports Medicine, 2009.

44. Position of the American Dietetic Association: Nutrition intervention in the treatment of eating disorders, Journal of the American Dietetic Association 111 (2011): 1236–1241; Position of the Academy of Nutrition and Dietetics, Dietitians of Canada, and the American College of Sports Medicine, 2009.

45. J. E. Turner and coauthors, Prolonged depletion of antioxidant capacity after ultraendurance exercise, Medicine and Science in Sports and Exercise 43 (2011): 1770–1776; S. K. Powers, E. E. Talbert, and P. J. Adhihetty, Reactive oxygen and nitrogen species as intracellular signals in skeletal muscle, Journal of Physiology 589 (2011): 2129–2138.

46. T. T. Peternelj and J. S. Coombes, antioxidant supplementation during exercise training: Beneficial or detrimental? Sports Medicine 41 (2011): 1043–1069; N. A. Strobel and coauthors, Antioxidant supplementation reduces skeletal muscle mitochondrial biogenesis, Medicine and Science in Sports and Exercise 43 (2011): 1017–1024.

47. T. M. Farney and coauthors, Absence of blood oxidative stress in trained men after strenuous exercise, Medicine and Science in Sports and Exercise 44 (2012): 1855–1863; Peternelj and Coombes, 2011; Strobel and coauthors, 2011.

48. D. M. Dellavalle and J. D. Haas, Iron status is associated with endurance performance and training in female rowers, Medicine and Science in Sports and Exercise 44 (2012): 1552–1559.

49. M. K. Newlin and coauthors, The effects of acute exercise bouts on hepcidin in women, International Journal of Sport Nutrition and Exercise Metabolism 22 (2012): 79–88.

50. Dellavalle and Haas, 2012; D. M. DellaValle and J. D. Haas, Impact of iron depletion without anemia on performance in trained endurance athletes at the beginning of a training session: A study of female collegiate rowers, International Journal of Sport Nutrition and Exercise Metabolism 21 (2011): 501–506.

51. American College of Sports Medicine, Position stand: Exercise and fluid replacement, Medicine & Science in Sports & Exercise 39 (2007): 377–390.

52. American College of Sports Medicine, Position stand: Prevention of cold injuries during exercise, Medicine and Science in Sports and Exercise 38 (2006): 2012–2029.

53. American College of Sports Medicine, Position stand: Exercise and fluid replacement, 2007.

54. Standing Committee on the Scientific Evaluation of Dietary Reference Intakes, Food and Nutrition Board, Institute of Medicine, Dietary Reference Intakes for Water, Potassium, Sodium, Chloride, and Sulfate (Washington, DC: National Academies Press, 2005), pp. 127–132.

55. American College of Sports Medicine, Position stand: Exercise and fluid replacement, 2007.

56. C. Rosenbloom, Energy drinks, caffeine, and athletes, Nutrition Today 49 (2014): 49–54; Position of the American Dietetic Association, Dietitians of Canada, and the American College of Sports Medicine, 2009.

57. S. A. Herring and coauthors, Selected issues for nutrition and the athlete: A team physician consensus statement, Medicine and Science in Sports and Exercise 45 (2013): 2378–2386.

LO 10.6 Present arguments for and against the use of ergogenic aids.

Athletes gravitate to promises that they can enhance their performance by taking pills, powders, or potions. Unfortunately, they may often hear such promises from their coaches and peers, who advise them to use dietary supplements, take drugs, or follow procedures that claim to deliver results with little effort.[1] When such performance-enhancing aids are harmless, they are only a waste of money; when they impair performance or harm health, they waste athletic potential and cost lives.

What does ergogenic mean?

Many substances or treatments claim to be *ergogenic*, meaning work enhancing. In connection with athletic performance, **ergogenic aids** are substances or treatments that purportedly improve athletic performance above and beyond what is possible through training. For practical purposes, most ergogenic aids can be categorized as follows:[2] (1) those that perform as claimed; (2) those that may perform as claimed but for which there is insufficient evidence at this time; (3) those that do not perform as claimed; and (4) those that are dangerous, banned, or illegal, and therefore should not be used. Table NP10-1 defines several of the commonly used ergogenic aids discussed in this Nutrition in Practice.

Are any of the supplements that claim to be ergogenic effective?

For the vast majority of ergogenic aids, research findings do not support the claims made.[3] Athletes who hear that a product is ergogenic should ask who is making the claim and who will profit from the sale. Chapter 4 includes a discussion on protein powders and amino acid supplements (pp. 96–97).

Athletes should be aware that some supplements are contaminated with illegal substances such as steroids or stimulants that are not listed on the label.[4] Supplements contaminated with illegal substances pose health risks to those who use them as well as the risk of positive drug testing for athletes subject to such tests.

As of late 2013, the Food and Drug Administration (FDA) and the Centers for Disease Control and Prevention are investigating more than 50 cases of acute hepatitis and sudden liver failure in previously healthy people who used a dietary supplement for weight loss or muscle building.[5] One person died, and others await liver transplants. The FDA notified the company producing the supplement to immediately stop distribution.

What are some examples of dietary supplements that perform as claimed?

A few ergogenic aids seem to live up to the claims made for them, based on research so far. Convenient dietary supplements, caffeine, creatine, sodium bicarbonate, and beta-alanine are the examples discussed here.

TABLE NP10-1 Commonly Used Ergogenic Aids

anabolic steroids: drugs related to the male sex hormone, testosterone, that stimulate the development of lean body mass.

- *anabolic* = promoting growth
- *sterols* = compounds chemically related to cholesterol

androstenedione: *See DHEA.*

beta-alanine: a nonessential amino acid that is the rate-limiting precursor for the synthesis of the dipeptide carnosine. Carnosine acts primarily as a buffer in skeletal muscle. Beta-alanine supplements raise carnosine concentrations, which enhance the muscles' buffering capacity.

beta-hydroxymethylbutyrate (HMB): a metabolite of the amino acid leucine promoted to increase muscle mass and strength.

caffeine: a natural stimulant found in many common foods and beverages, including coffee, tea, and chocolate; may enhance endurance by stimulating fatty acid release. High doses cause headaches, trembling, rapid heart rate, and other undesirable side effects.

carnitine: a nonessential nonprotein amino acid made in the body from lysine that helps transport fatty acids across the mitochondrial membrane. As a supplement, carnitine supposedly "burns" fat and spares glycogen during endurance events, but in reality it does neither.

chromium picolinate (CROW-mee-um pick-oh-LYN-ate)**:** a trace mineral supplement; falsely promoted as building muscle, enhancing energy, and burning fat. *Picolinate* is a derivative of the amino acid tryptophan that seems to enhance chromium absorption.

convenient dietary supplements: liquid meal replacers, energy drinks, energy bars, and energy gels that athletes and active people use to replenish energy and nutrients when time is limited.

creatine (KREE-ah-tin)**:** a nitrogen-containing compound that combines with phosphate to form the high-energy compound creatine phosphate (or phosphocreatine) in muscles.

DHEA (dehydroepiandrosterone) and **androstenedione:** hormones made in the adrenal glands that serve as precursors to the male sex hormone, testosterone; falsely promoted as burning fat, building muscle, and slowing aging.

ergogenic (ER-go-JEN-ick) **aids:** substances or techniques used in an attempt to enhance physical performance.

- *ergo* = work
- *genic* = gives rise to

hGH (human growth hormone): a hormone produced by the brain's pituitary gland that regulates normal growth and development; also called *somatotropin*.

ribose: a naturally occurring 5-carbon sugar needed for the synthesis of ATP.

sodium bicarbonate (baking soda): a white crystalline powder that is used to buffer acid that accumulates in the muscles and blood during high-intensity exercise.

What are convenient dietary supplements?

Ready-to-drink supplements such as liquid meal replacers and energy drinks, energy bars, and energy gels are **convenient dietary supplements** for athletes and active people, especially when time is limited. Many such products appeal to athletes by claiming to provide "complete" nutrition. These supplements usually taste good and provide extra carbohydrate and food energy, but they fall short of providing "complete" nutrition. They can be useful as a pregame meal or a between-meal snack, but they should not replace regular meals.

Liquid meal replacers may help a nervous athlete who cannot tolerate solid food on the day of an event. A liquid meal 2 to 3 hours before competition can supply some of the fluid and carbohydrate needed in a pregame meal, but a shake of fat-free milk or juice (such as apple or papaya) and frozen fat-free yogurt or frozen fruit (such as strawberries or bananas) can do the same thing less expensively.

What about caffeine? I have heard that it can improve endurance performance.

Some research supports the use of **caffeine** to enhance endurance and, to some extent, to enhance short-term, high-intensity exercise performance.[6] Caffeine may stimulate fatty acid release during endurance activity, but in contrast to what was previously thought, caffeine does not slow muscle glycogen use.[7] Light activity before a workout also stimulates fat release, and unlike caffeine, also warms the muscles and connective tissues, making them flexible and resistant to injury.

Caffeine is a stimulant that elicits a number of physiological and psychological effects in the body. Caffeine enhances alertness and reduces fatigue.[8] The possible benefits of caffeine use must be weighed against its adverse effects—stomach upset, nervousness, irritability, headaches, and diarrhea. Caffeine-containing beverages should be used in moderation, if at all, and *in addition* to other fluids, not as a substitute for them.

Caffeine is classed as a *restricted* substance by the National Collegiate Athletic Association, which allows urine concentrations of 15 milligrams per liter or less (equivalent to about 5 cups of coffee consumed within a few hours before testing). Urine tests that detect more caffeine than this disqualify athletes from competition. (The table at the start of Appendix A provides a list of common caffeine-containing items and the doses they deliver.)

Many athletes take creatine. Why is it so popular?

Interest in—and use of—**creatine** supplements to enhance performance during intense activity has grown dramatically in the last few years. Power athletes such as weightlifters use creatine supplements to enhance stores of the high-energy compound creatine phosphate (CP) in muscles. Theoretically, the more creatine phosphate in muscles, the higher the intensity at which an athlete can train. High-intensity training stimulates the muscles to adapt, which in turn, improves performance.

Research suggests that creatine supplementation does enhance performance of short-term, repetitive, high-intensity activity such as weightlifting or sprinting.[9] Creatine may improve performance by increasing muscle strength and size, cell hydration, or glycogen loading capacity. In contrast, creatine supplementation has not been shown to benefit endurance activity.

The question of whether short-term use (up to a year) of creatine supplements (up to 5 grams per day) is safe continues to be studied, but so far, the supplements are considered safe for healthy adults.[10] More research is needed, however, to confirm the safety of larger doses and long-term use. Creatine supplementation may pose risks to athletes with kidney disease or other conditions.[11] One undisputed side effect of creatine supplementation is weight gain, which may not be desirable.

Some medical and fitness experts voice concern that creatine is being taken in huge doses (up to 30 grams per day) before evidence of its value has been ascertained. Even people who eat creatine-rich red meat do not consume nearly the amount supplements provide. (Creatine content varies, but on average, pork, chicken, and beef provide 65 to 180 *milligrams* per ounce.) Despite the uncertainties, creatine supplements are not illegal in international competition. The American Academy of Pediatrics strongly discourages the use of creatine supplements, as well as the use of any performance-enhancing substance in adolescents younger than 18 years old.

Why do some athletes take sodium bicarbonate?

During short-term, high-intensity activity, acid and carbon dioxide (CO_2) accumulate in the blood and muscles. **Sodium bicarbonate** (0.3 grams per kilogram of body weight) ingested prior to high-intensity sports performance buffers the acid and neutralizes the carbon dioxide, thereby maintaining muscle pH levels closer to normal and enhancing exercise capacity.[12] Sodium bicarbonate supplementation may cause unpleasant side effects such as diarrhea in some athletes.

What is beta-alanine?

Beta-alanine is a nonessential amino acid that is receiving a lot of attention from exercise researchers.[13] Beta-alanine is the rate-limiting precursor for the synthesis of the dipeptide carnosine. Carnosine occurs in high concentrations in skeletal muscle and is one of the primary buffering substances available in muscle. Supplementation with beta-alanine has been shown to raise muscle carnosine concentrations, which enhances muscle buffering capacity.[14] Enhanced buffering of muscle pH is especially beneficial to high-intensity exercise performance such as sprinting. One known side effect of beta-alanine supplementation is a "pins and needles" sensation that occurs with high (>800 milligrams) single doses. More research is needed to confirm the safety of beta-alanine supplementation.[15]

What are some examples of dietary supplements that may perform as claimed but for which evidence is currently insufficient?

As noted earlier, dozens of supplements are promoted to enhance performance or to improve training adaptations of athletes and active people. For some of these supplements, it is just too early to tell whether they deliver on the promises made for them because research thus far is inconclusive. Examples of supplements that may perform as claimed, but for which there is insufficient evidence of efficacy, include beta-hydroxymethylbutyrate and ribose.

What is beta-hydroxymethylbutyrate?

Beta-hydroxymethylbutyrate (HMB) is a metabolite of the amino acid leucine. Supplementing the diet with HMB during training has been shown to increase muscle mass and strength, especially among untrained individuals.[16] Additional research is needed, however, to determine whether HMB supplementation in trained athletes enhances training adaptations.

What are the claims made for ribose?

Manufacturers of ribose supplements claim that **ribose** increases ATP and improves performance. Ribose, a naturally occurring sugar, does help resynthesize muscle ATP. Based on research thus far, however, ribose supplements do not improve athletic performance.[17]

Considering the vast array of supplements promoted to athletes, there must be many that simply do not perform as claimed. What are some examples of these?

Most of the dietary supplements promoted as ergogenic aids fall into the category of "those that do not perform as claimed." Carnitine and chromium picolinate are two examples of ineffective supplements discussed here, but others include bee pollen, boron, coenzyme Q, ginseng, pyruvate, and vanadium.[18]

What is carnitine and what is it supposed to do for athletes?

In the body, **carnitine** facilitates the transfer of fatty acids across the mitochondrial membrane. Supplement manufacturers suggest that with more carnitine available, fat oxidation will be enhanced, but this does not seem to be the case. Carnitine supplements neither raise muscle carnitine concentrations nor enhance exercise performance. Milk and meat products are good sources of carnitine, and supplements are not needed.

What is chromium picolinate and why would athletes want to take supplements of it?

Chapter 9 introduces chromium as an essential trace mineral involved in carbohydrate and lipid metabolism. Claims that **chromium picolinate,** which is more easily absorbed than chromium alone, builds muscle, enhances energy, and burns fat derive from one or two early studies reporting that men who strength-trained while taking chromium picolinate supplements increased lean body mass and reduced body fat. Most subsequent studies, however, show no effects of chromium picolinate on strength, lean body mass, or body fat. Chromium-rich foods include whole grains, liver, and nuts.

What are some examples of dangerous, banned, or illegal supplements?

The dietary supplements discussed thus far may or may not help athletic performance, but in the doses commonly taken, they seem to cause little harm. The remaining discussion features hormonal supplements that are clearly damaging: anabolic steroids, DHEA (dehydroepiandrosterone), androstenedione, and hGH (human growth hormone). All of these ergogenic aids are dangerous to use and are banned by most professional sports leagues and the World Anti-Doping Agency (WADA) established by the International Olympic Committee. The American Academy of Pediatrics and the American College of Sports Medicine also condemn athletes' use of these substances.

I have heard that it is dangerous to take anabolic steroids. Is this true?

Yes. Among the most dangerous and illegal ergogenic practices is the taking of anabolic steroids. These drugs are derived from the male sex **hormone testosterone,** which promotes the development of male characteristics and lean body mass. Athletes who take steroids do so to stimulate muscle bulking.

The known toxic side effects of steroids include, but are not limited to, extreme aggression and hostility, heart disease, and liver damage. Taking these drugs is a form of cheating. Other athletes are put in the difficult position of either conceding an unfair advantage to competitors who use steroids or taking steroids and accepting the risk of harmful side effects.

The price for the potential competitive edge that steroids confer is high—sometimes it is life itself. Steroids are not simple pills that build bigger muscles. They are complex chemicals to which the body reacts in many ways, particularly when bodybuilders and other athletes take large amounts. The safest, most effective way to build muscle is to train hard and eat well.

Some manufacturers peddle specific herbs as legal substitutes for steroid drugs. They falsely claim that these herbs contain hormones, enhance the body's hormonal activity, or both. In some cases, an herb may contain plant sterols, such as gamma-oryzanol, but these compounds are poorly absorbed. Even if absorption occurs, the body cannot convert herbal compounds to anabolic steroids. None of these products has any proven anabolic steroid activity, none enhances muscle strength, and some contain natural toxins. In short, "natural" does not mean "harmless."

What are DHEA and androstenedione and why do some athletes use them?

Some athletes use **DHEA** and androstenedione as alternatives to anabolic steroids. DHEA (dehydroepiandrosterone) and androstenedione are hormones made in the adrenal glands that serve as precursors to the male hormone testosterone. Advertisements claim the hormones "burn fat," "build muscle," and "slow aging," but evidence to support such claims is lacking.

Short-term side effects of DHEA and androstenedione may include oily skin, acne, body hair growth, liver enlargement, testicular shrinkage, and aggressive behavior. Long-term effects such as serious liver damage may take years to become evident. The potential for harm from DHEA and androstenedione supplements is great, and athletes, as well as others, should avoid them.

Why do some athletes use human growth hormone?

A wide range of athletes, including weightlifters, baseball players, cyclists, and track and field participants use hGH (human growth hormone) to build lean tissue and improve athletic performance. The athletes use hGH, believing the injectable hormone will provide the benefits of anabolic steroids without the dangerous side effects.

Taken in large quantities, hGH causes the disease acromegaly, in which the body becomes huge and the organs and bones over-enlarge. Other effects include diabetes, thyroid disorder, heart disease, menstrual irregularities, diminished sexual desire, and shortened life span.

The search for a single food, nutrient, drug, or technique that will safely and effectively enhance athletic performance will no doubt continue as long as people strive to achieve excellence in sports. Improvements in athletic performance after use of an ergogenic aid can often be attributed to the placebo effect—it reflects the power of the mind over the body.

The overwhelming majority of performance-enhancing aids sold for athletes are frauds. Wishful thinking will not substitute for talent, hard training, adequate diet, and mental preparedness in competition. But don't discount the power of mind over body for a minute—it is formidable, and sports psychologists dedicate their work to harnessing it. You can use it by imagining yourself a winner and visualizing yourself excelling in your sport.

Notes

1. J. R. Hoffman and coauthors, Position stand on androgen and human growth hormone use, *Journal of Strength and Conditioning Research* 23 (2009): S1–S59.

2. Position of the American Dietetic Association, Dietetians of Canada, and the American College of Sports Medicine: Nutrition and athletic performance, *Journal of the American Dietetic Association* 109 (2009): 509–527.

3. R. B. Kreider and coauthors, ISSN exercise and sport nutrition review: Research and recommendations, *Journal of the International Society of Sports Nutrition* 7 (2010): www.jissn.com /content/7/1/7.

4. M. Dunford and E. J. Coleman, Ergogenic aids, dietary supplements, and exercise, in *Sports Nutrition: A Practice Manual for Professionals*, 5th ed., eds., C. A. Rosenbloom and E. J. Coleman (Chicago, IL: Academy of Nutrition and Dietetics, 2012), pp. 128–161.

5. U. S. Food and Drug Administration, FDA investigates acute hepatitis illnesses potentially linked to products labeled OxyElite Pro, www.fda.gov/food/recallsoutbreaks/ucm370849.htm; Centers for Disease Control and Prevention, Acute hepatitis and liver failure following the use of a dietary supplement intended for weight loss or muscle building—May–October 2013, *Morbidity and Mortality Weekly Report* 62 (2013): 817–818.

6. H. K. Stadheim and coauthors, Caffeine increases performance in cross-country double-poling time trial exercise, *Medicine and Science in Sports and Exercise* 45 (2013): 2175–2183; T. A. Astorino and coauthors, Increases in cycling performance in response to caffeine ingestion are repeatable, *Nutrition Research* 32 (2012): 78–84; Kreider and coauthors, 2010; E. R. Goldstein and coauthors, International Society of Sports Nutrition position stand: Caffeine and performance, *Journal of the International Society of Sports Nutrition* 7 (2010): www.jissn.com/content/7/1/5; G. L. Warren and coauthors, Effect of caffeine ingestion on muscular strength and endurance: A meta-analysis, *Medicine and Science in Sports and Exercise* 42 (2010): 1375–1387.

7. Dunford and Coleman, 2012.

8. Goldstein and coauthors, 2010.

9. R. Jäger and coauthors, Analysis of the efficacy, safety, and regulatory status of novel forms of creatine, *Amino Acids* 40 (2011): 1369–1383; M. A. Tarnopolsky, Caffeine and creatine use in sport, *Annals of Nutrition and Metabolism* 57 (2010): 1–8 (Supplement 2); D. H. Fukuda and coauthors, The effects of creatine loading and gender on anaerobic running capacity, *Journal of Strength and Conditioning Research* 24 (2010): 1826–1833.

10. Kreider and coauthors, 2010; Position of the American Dietetic Association, Dietitians of Canada, and the American College of Sports Medicine, 2009.

11. Position of the American Dietetic Association, Dietitians of Canada, and the American College of Sports Medicine, 2009.

12. J. C. Siegler and D. O. Gleadall-Siddall, Sodium bicarbonate ingestion and repeated swim sprint performance, *Journal of Strength and Conditioning Research* 24 (2010): 3105–3111; S. L. Cameron and coauthors, Increased blood pH but not performance in elite rugby union players, *International Journal of Sport Nutrition and Exercise Metabolism* 20 (2010): 307–321.

13. R. C. Harris and T. Stellingwerff, Effect of β-alanine supplementation on high-intensity exercise performance, *Nestle Nutrition Institute Workshop Series* 76 (2013): 61–71; C. Sale and coauthors, Carnosine: From exercise performance to health, *Amino Acids* 44 (2013): 1477–1491; W. Derave, Use of β-alanine as an ergogenic aid, *Nestle Nutrition Institute Workshop Series* 75 (2013): 99–108.

14. Derave, 2013; G. G. Artioli and coauthors, Role of β-alanine supplementation on muscle carnosine and exercise performance, *Medicine and Science in Sports and Exercise* 42 (2010): 1162–1173.

15. J. J. Quesnele and coauthors, The effects of beta alanine supplementation on performance: A systematic review of the literature, *International Journal of Sport Nutrition and Exercise Metabolism* 24 (2014): 14–27.

16. J. M. Wilson and coauthors, β-hydroxy-β-methylbutyrate free acid reduces markers of exercise-induced muscle damage and improves recovery in resistance-trained men, *British Journal of Nutrition* 110 (2013): 538–544; Kreider and coauthors, 2010.

17. Kreider and coauthors, 2010; D. Bishop, Dietary supplements and team-sport performance, *Sports Medicine* 40 (2010): 995–1017.

18. Kreider and coauthors, 2010; Position of the American Dietetic Association, Dietitians of Canada, and the American College of Sports Medicine, 2009.

11

Nutrition through the Life Span: Pregnancy and Lactation

11.1 Pregnancy: The Impact of Nutrition on the Future

LO 11.1 Explain the importance of a healthy diet and other lifestyle choices before and during a pregnancy, discuss nutrient needs of and recommended food choices for pregnant women, and identify the special nutritional needs of a pregnant teenager.

11.2 Breastfeeding

LO 11.2 Summarize the nutrient needs of women during lactation and contraindications to breastfeeding.

11.3 Nutrition in Practice: Encouraging Successful Breastfeeding

LO 11.3 Identify factors that encourage or discourage women to breastfeed their infants and describe approaches for initiating and resolving problems during breastfeeding.

Tom Grill/Iconica/Getty Images

287

All people need the same nutrients, but the amounts they need vary depending on their stage of life. This chapter focuses on nutrition in preparation for, and support of, pregnancy, lactation, and infancy. The next two chapters address the needs of children, adolescents, and older adults.

11.1 Pregnancy: The Impact of Nutrition on the Future

LO 11.1 Explain the importance of a healthy diet and other lifestyle choices before and during a pregnancy, discuss nutrient needs of and recommended food choices for pregnant women, and identify the special nutritional needs of a pregnant teenager.

The woman who enters pregnancy with full nutrient stores, sound eating habits, and a healthy body weight has done much to ensure an optimal pregnancy. Then, if she eats a variety of nutrient-dense foods during pregnancy, her own and her infant's health will benefit further.

Nutrition Prior to Pregnancy

A discussion on nutrition prior to pregnancy must, by its nature, focus mainly on women. A man's nutrition may affect his **fertility** and possibly the genetic contributions he makes to his children, but nutrition exerts its primary influence through the woman. Her body provides the environment for the growth and development of a new human being. Full nutrient stores *before* pregnancy are essential both to conception and to healthy infant development during pregnancy. In the early weeks of pregnancy, before many women are even aware that they are pregnant, significant developmental changes occur that depend on a woman's nutrient stores. In preparation for a healthy pregnancy, a woman can establish the following habits:

- *Achieve and maintain a healthy body weight.* Both underweight and overweight women, and their newborns, face increased risks of complications.

- *Choose an adequate and balanced diet.* Malnutrition reduces fertility and impairs the early development of an infant should a woman become pregnant.

- *Be physically active.* A woman who wants to be physically active *when* she is pregnant needs to become physically active *beforehand*.

- *Receive regular medical care.* Regular health care visits can help ensure a healthy start to pregnancy.

- *Avoid harmful influences.* Both maternal and paternal ingestion of, or exposure to, harmful substances (such as cigarettes, alcohol, drugs, or environmental contaminants) can cause miscarriage or abnormalities, alter genes or their expression, and interfere with fertility.[1]

Young adults who nourish and protect their bodies do so not only for their own sakes but also for future generations.

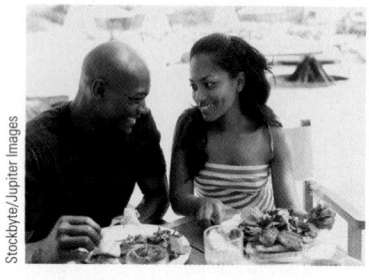

Both parents can prepare in advance for a healthy pregnancy.

Prepregnancy Weight

Appropriate weight prior to pregnancy benefits pregnancy outcome. Being either underweight or overweight (see pp. 297-298) presents medical risks during pregnancy and childbirth. Underweight women are therefore advised to gain weight before becoming pregnant and overweight women to lose excess weight.

fertility: the capacity of a woman to produce a normal ovum periodically and of a man to produce normal sperm; the ability to reproduce.

Underweight Infant birthweight correlates with prepregnancy weight and weight gain during pregnancy and is the most potent single predictor of the infant's future health and survival. An underweight woman has a high risk of having a **low-birthweight** infant, especially if she is unable to gain sufficient weight during pregnancy.[2] Compared with normal-weight infants, low-birthweight infants are more likely to contract diseases and nearly 40 times more likely to die in the first month of life. Impaired growth and development during pregnancy may have long-term health effects as well. Research suggests that, when nutrient supplies fail to meet demands, permanent adaptations take place that may make obesity or chronic diseases such as heart disease and hypertension more likely in later life.[3] Other potential problems of low birthweight may include lower adult IQ and other brain impairments, short stature, and educational disadvantages.[4] Underweight women are therefore advised to gain weight before becoming pregnant and to strive to gain adequately during pregnancy.

Nutritional deficiency, coupled with low birthweight, is the underlying cause of more than half of all the deaths worldwide of children younger than 5 years of age. In the United States, the infant mortality rate in 2010 was slightly less than 6.2 deaths per 1000 live births.[5] This rate, though higher than that of some other developed countries, has seen a significant steady decline over the past two decades and stands as a tribute to public health efforts aimed at reducing infant deaths (see Figure 11-1).

Not all cases of low birthweight reflect poor nutrition. Heredity, disease conditions, smoking, and drug use (including alcohol use) during pregnancy all contribute. Even with optimal nutrition and health during pregnancy, some women give birth to small infants for unknown reasons. But poor nutrition is the major factor in low birthweight—and an avoidable one, as later sections make clear.[6]

Overweight and Obesity Obese women are also urged to strive for healthy weights before pregnancy. Infants born to obese women are more likely to be large for gestational age, weighing more than 9 pounds.[7] Problems associated with a high birthweight include increased likelihood of a difficult labor and delivery, birth trauma, and **cesarean section**.[8] Consequently, these infants have a greater risk of poor health and death than infants of normal weight. Infants of obese mothers may also be twice as likely to be born with a neural tube defect. Folate's role has been examined, but a more likely explanation seems to be poor glycemic control.[9] Obese women themselves are likely to suffer gestational diabetes, hypertension, and complications during and infections after the birth.[10] In addition, both overweight and obese women have a greater risk of giving birth to infants with heart defects and other abnormalities.[11] An appropriate goal for the obese woman who wishes to become pregnant is to strive to attain a healthy prepregnancy body weight so as to minimize her medical risks and those of her future child.

Healthy Support Tissues

A major reason that the mother's prepregnancy nutrition is so crucial is that it determines whether her **uterus** will be able to support the growth of a healthy **placenta** during the first month of **gestation**. The placenta is both a supply depot and a waste-removal system for the fetus. If the placenta works perfectly, the fetus wants for nothing; if it doesn't, no alternative source of sustenance is available, and the fetus will fail to thrive. Figure 11-2 (on p. 290) shows the placenta, a mass of tissue in which maternal and fetal blood vessels intertwine and exchange materials. The two bloods never mix, but the barrier between them is notably thin. Across this thin barrier, nutrients and oxygen move from the mother's blood into the fetus's blood, and wastes move out of the fetal blood to be excreted by the mother. Thus, by way of the placenta, the mother's digestive tract, respiratory system, and kidneys serve the needs

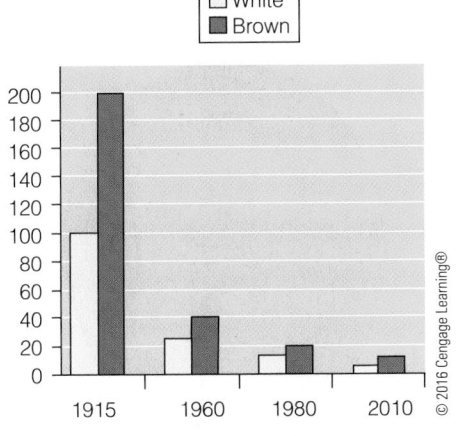

□ White
■ Brown

© 2016 Cengage Learning®

FIGURE 11-1 Infant Mortality Decline over Time
The graph shows infant deaths per 1000 live births.
Source: Data from T. J. Mathews and M. F. MacDorman, Infant mortality statistics from the 2010 period linked birth/infant death data set, National Vital Statistics Reports 62, December 18, 2013.

low birthweight (LBW): a birthweight less than 5½ lb (2500 g); indicates probable poor health in the newborn and poor nutrition status of the mother during pregnancy. Optimal birthweight for a full-term infant is 6.8 to 7.9 lb (about 3100 to 3600 g). Low-birthweight infants are of two different types. Some are **premature;** they are born early and are of a weight **appropriate for gestational age (AGA).** Others have suffered growth failure in the uterus; they may or may not be born early, but they are **small for gestational age (SGA).**

cesarean (see-ZAIR-ee-un) **section:** surgical childbirth, in which the infant is taken through an incision in the woman's abdomen.

uterus (YOO-ter-us)**:** the womb, the muscular organ within which the infant develops before birth.

placenta (pla-SEN-tuh)**:** an organ that develops inside the uterus early in pregnancy, in which maternal and fetal blood circulate in close proximity and exchange materials. The fetus receives nutrients and oxygen across the placenta; the mother's blood picks up carbon dioxide and other waste materials to be excreted via her lungs and kidneys.

gestation: the period of about 40 weeks (3 trimesters) from conception to birth; the term of a pregnancy.

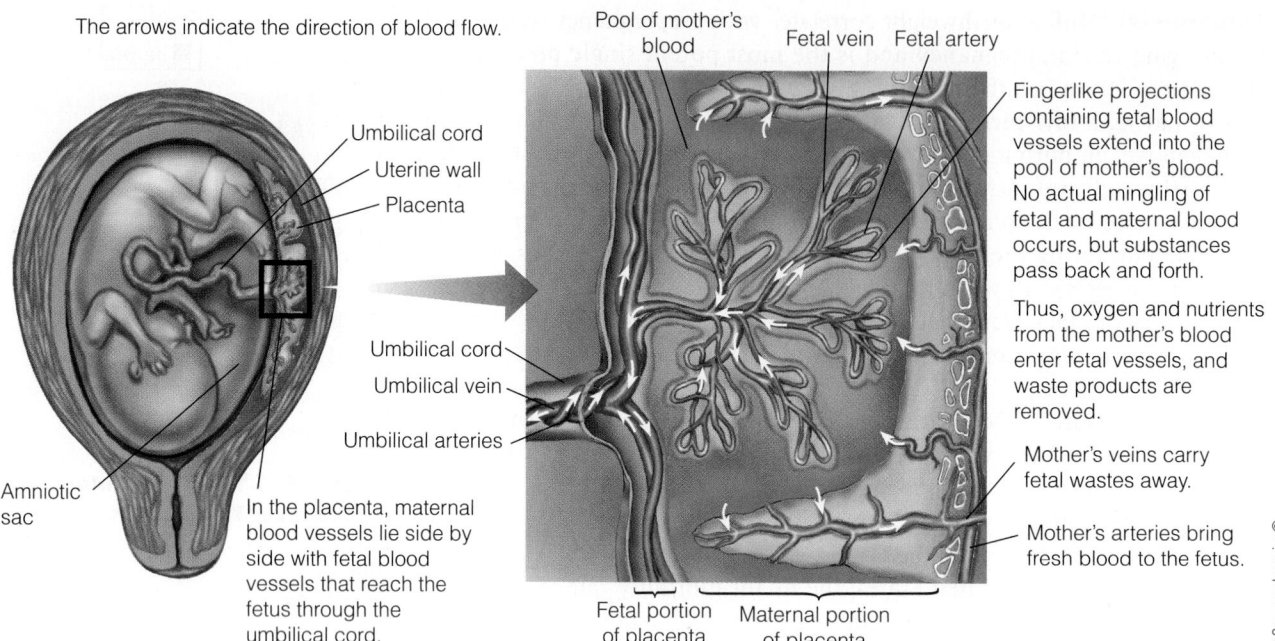

The arrows indicate the direction of blood flow.

Umbilical cord
Uterine wall
Placenta

Amniotic sac

In the placenta, maternal blood vessels lie side by side with fetal blood vessels that reach the fetus through the umbilical cord.

Umbilical cord
Umbilical vein
Umbilical arteries

Pool of mother's blood
Fetal vein   Fetal artery

Fingerlike projections containing fetal blood vessels extend into the pool of mother's blood. No actual mingling of fetal and maternal blood occurs, but substances pass back and forth.

Thus, oxygen and nutrients from the mother's blood enter fetal vessels, and waste products are removed.

Mother's veins carry fetal wastes away.

Mother's arteries bring fresh blood to the fetus.

Fetal portion of placenta   Maternal portion of placenta

© Cengage Learning®

FIGURE 11-2 The Placenta

of the fetus as well as her own. The fetus has these organ systems, but they do not yet function. The **umbilical cord** is the pipeline from the placenta to the fetus. The **amniotic sac** surrounds and cradles the fetus, cushioning it with fluids.

The placenta is an active metabolic organ with many responsibilities of its own. It actively gathers up hormones, nutrients, and protein molecules such as antibodies and transfers them into the fetal bloodstream.[12] The placenta also produces a broad range of hormones that act in many ways to maintain pregnancy and prepare the mother's breasts for **lactation.** A healthy placenta is essential for the developing fetus to attain its full potential.

IN SUMMARY

▌ Adequate nutrition before pregnancy establishes physical readiness and nutrient stores to support fetal growth.

▌ Both underweight and overweight women should strive for appropriate body weights before pregnancy.

▌ Newborns who weigh less than 5½ pounds face greater health risks than normal-weight infants.

▌ The healthy development of the placenta depends on adequate nutrition before pregnancy.

The Events of Pregnancy

The newly fertilized **ovum** is called a **zygote.** It begins as a single cell and rapidly divides to become a **blastocyst.** During the first week, the blastocyst floats down into the uterus, where it will embed itself in the inner uterine wall—a process known as **implantation.** Minimal growth in size takes place at this time, but it is a crucial period in development. Adverse influences such as smoking, drug abuse, and malnutrition at this time lead to failure to implant or to abnormalities such as neural tube defects that can cause the loss of the developing embryo, possibly before the woman knows she is pregnant.

umbilical (um-BIL-ih-cul) **cord:** the ropelike structure through which the fetus's veins and arteries reach the placenta; the route of nourishment and oxygen into the fetus and the route of waste disposal from the fetus.

amniotic (am-nee-OTT-ic) **sac:** the "bag of waters" in the uterus in which the fetus floats.

lactation: production and secretion of breast milk for the purpose of nourishing an infant.

ovum (OH-vum)**:** the female reproductive cell, capable of developing into a new organism upon fertilization; commonly referred to as an egg.

zygote (ZY-goat)**:** the product of the union of ovum and sperm; a fertilized ovum.

blastocyst (BLASS-toe-sist)**:** the developmental stage of the zygote when it is about 5 days old and ready for implantation.

implantation: the stage of development in which the blastocyst embeds itself in the wall of the uterus and begins to develop; occurs during the first 2 weeks after conception.

(1) A newly fertilized ovum is called a zygote and is about the size of the period at the end of this sentence. Less than one week after fertilization these cells have rapidly divided multiple times to become a blastocyst ready for implantation.

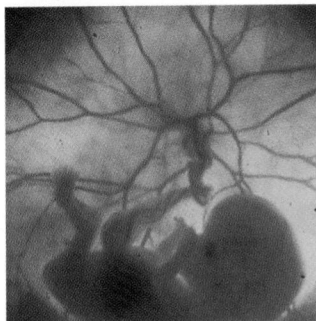

(3) A fetus after 11 weeks of development is just over an inch long. Notice the umbilical cord and blood vessels connecting the fetus with the placenta.

(2) After implantation, the placenta develops and begins to provide nourishment to the developing embryo. An embryo five weeks after fertilization is about 1/2 inch long.

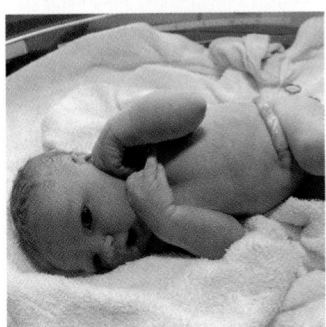

(4) A newborn infant after nine months of development measures close to 20 inches in length. The average birthweight is about 7 1/2 pounds. From eight weeks to term, this infant grew 20 times longer and 50 times heavier.

Petit Format/Nestle/Science Source

FIGURE 11-3 **Stages of Embryonic and Fetal Development**

The Embryo and Fetus During the next 6 weeks of development, the **embryo** registers astonishing physical changes (see Figure 11-3). At 8 weeks, the **fetus** has a complete central nervous system, a beating heart, a fully formed digestive system, well-defined fingers and toes, and the beginnings of facial features.

In the last 7 months of pregnancy, the fetal period, the fetus grows 50 times heavier and 20 times longer. Critical periods of cell division and development occur in organ after organ. Most successful pregnancies last 38 to 42 weeks and produce a healthy infant weighing between 6.8 and 7.9 pounds. The 40 or so weeks of pregnancy are divided into thirds, each of which is called a **trimester.**

A Note about Critical Periods Each organ and tissue type grows with its own characteristic pattern and timing. The development of each takes place only at a certain time—the **critical period.** Whatever nutrients and other environmental conditions are necessary during this period must be supplied on time if the organ is to reach its full potential. If the development of an organ is limited during a critical period, recovery is impossible. For example, the fetus's heart and brain are well developed at 14 weeks; the lungs, 10 weeks later. Therefore, early malnutrition impairs the heart and brain; later malnutrition impairs the lungs.

The effects of malnutrition during critical periods of pregnancy are seen in defects of the nervous system of the embryo (explained later), in the child's poor dental health, and in the adolescent's and adult's vulnerability to infections and possibly higher risks of diabetes, hypertension, stroke, or heart disease.[13] The effects of malnutrition during critical periods are irreversible: abundant and nourishing food, consumed after the critical time, cannot remedy harm already done.

Table 11-1 (p. 292) identifies characteristics of a **high-risk pregnancy;** the more factors that apply, the higher the risk. A woman with none of these factors is said to have a **low-risk pregnancy.** All pregnant women, especially those in high-risk categories, need prenatal medical care, including dietary advice.

embryo (EM-bree-oh): the developing infant from 2 to 8 weeks after conception.

fetus (FEET-us): the developing infant from 8 weeks after conception until its birth.

trimester: a period representing one-third of the term of gestation. A trimester is about 13 to 14 weeks.

critical period: a finite period during development in which certain events occur that will have irreversible effects on later developmental stages; usually a period of rapid cell division.

high-risk pregnancy: a pregnancy characterized by risk factors that make it likely the birth will be surrounded by problems such as premature delivery, difficult birth, retarded growth, birth defects, and early infant death.

low-risk pregnancy: a pregnancy characterized by factors that make it likely the birth will be normal and the infant healthy.

TABLE 11-1 High-Risk Pregnancy Factors

- Prepregnancy BMI either <18.5 or >25
- Insufficient or excessive pregnancy weight gain
- Nutrient deficiencies or toxicities; eating disorders
- Poverty, lack of family support, low level of education, limited food available
- Smoking, alcohol, or other drug use
- Teens, especially 15 years or younger; women 35 years or older
- Many previous pregnancies (three or more to mothers younger than age 20; four or more to mothers age 20 or older)
- Short or long intervals between pregnancies (<18 months or >59 months)
- Previous history of problems
- Twins or triplets
- Low- or high-birthweight infants
- Development of gestational hypertension
- Development of gestational diabetes
- Diabetes; hypertension; heart, respiratory, and kidney disease; certain genetic disorders; special diets and medications

IN SUMMARY

- Placental development, implantation, and early critical periods of embryonic and fetal development depend on maternal nutrition before and during pregnancy.

- The effects of malnutrition during critical periods are irreversible.

Nutrient Needs during Pregnancy

Nutrient needs during pregnancy increase more for certain nutrients than for others (see the inside front cover). Figure 11-4 shows the percentage increase in

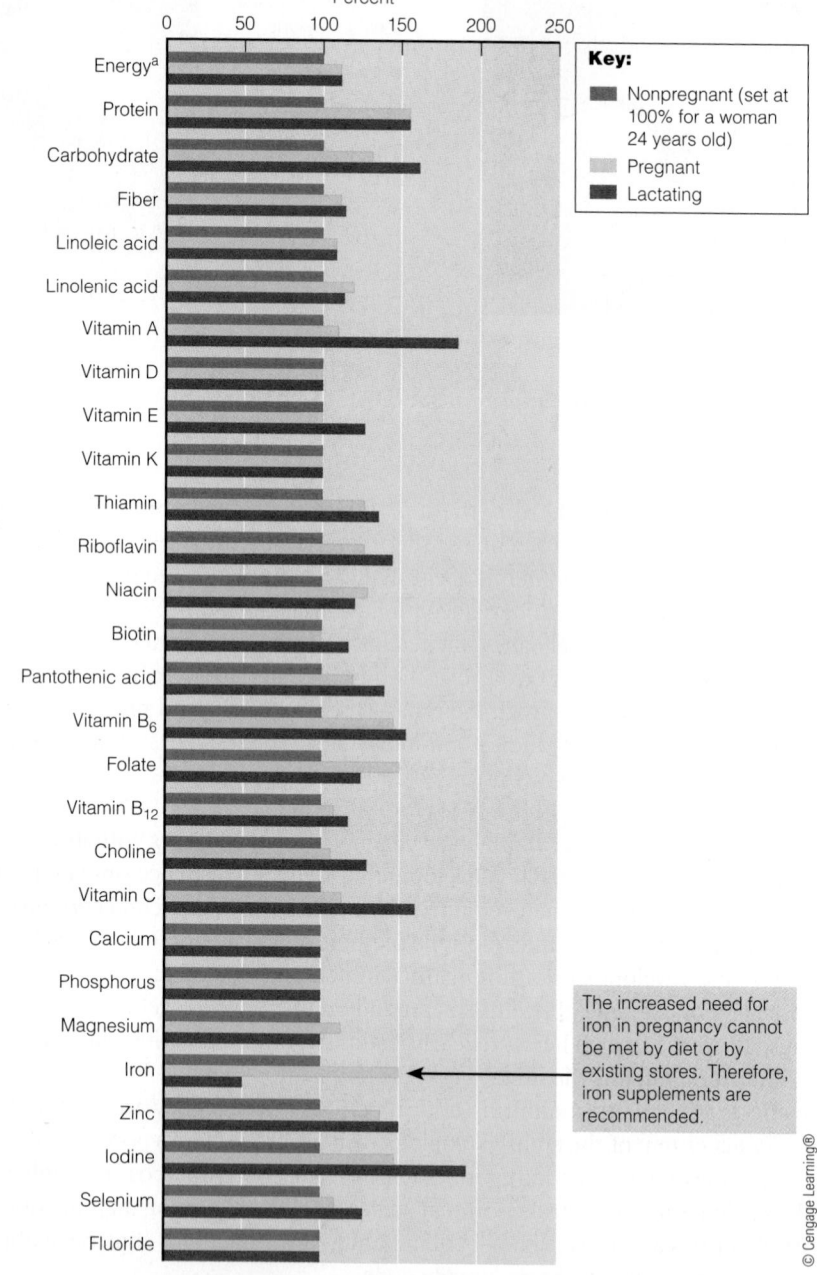

FIGURE 11-4 Comparison of Nutrient Recommendations for Nonpregnant, Pregnant, and Lactating Women

aEnergy allowance during pregnancy is for second trimester; energy allowance during the third trimester is slightly higher; no additional allowance is provided during the first trimester. Energy allowance during lactation is for the first 6 months; energy allowance during the second 6 months is slightly higher.

nutrient intakes recommended for pregnant women compared with nonpregnant women. To meet the high nutrient demands of pregnancy, a woman must make careful food choices, but her body will also do its part by maximizing nutrient absorption and minimizing losses.

Energy, Carbohydrate, Protein, and Fat Energy needs change as pregnancy progresses. In the first trimester, the pregnant woman needs no additional energy, but as pregnancy progresses, her energy needs rise. She requires an additional 340 kcalories daily during the second trimester and an extra 450 kcalories each day during the third trimester.[14] Well-nourished pregnant women meet these demands for more energy in several ways: some eat more food, some reduce their activity, and some store less of their food energy as fat.[15] A woman can easily meet the need for extra kcalories by selecting more nutrient-dense foods from the five food groups. Table 1-4 (on p. 15) provides suggested eating patterns for several kcalorie levels, and Table 11-2 offers a sample menu for pregnant and lactating women.

If a woman chooses less nutritious options such as sugary soft drinks or fatty snack foods to meet her energy needs, she will undoubtedly come up short on nutrients. The increase in the need for nutrients is even greater than that for energy, so the mother-to-be should choose nutrient-dense foods such as whole-grain breads and cereals, legumes, dark green vegetables, citrus fruits, low-fat milk and milk products, and lean meats, fish, poultry, and eggs.

Ample carbohydrate (ideally, 175 grams or more per day and certainly no less than 135 grams) is necessary to fuel the fetal brain and spare the protein needed for fetal growth. Fiber in carbohydrate-rich foods such as whole grains, vegetables, and fruit can help alleviate the constipation that many pregnant women experience.

The protein RDA for pregnancy is 25 grams per day higher than for nonpregnant women. Pregnant women can easily meet their protein needs by selecting meats, seafood, poultry, low-fat milk and milk products, and protein-containing plant foods such as legumes, tofu, whole grains, nuts, and seeds. Some vegetarian women limit or omit protein-rich meats, eggs, and milk products from their diets. For them, meeting the recommendation for food energy each day and including generous servings of protein-containing plant foods are imperative. Because use of high-protein supplements during pregnancy may be harmful to the infant's development, it is discouraged unless medically prescribed and carefully monitored to treat fetal growth problems.[16]

The high nutrient requirements of pregnancy leave little room in the diet for excess fat, especially solid fats such as fatty meats and butter. The essential fatty acids, however, are particularly important to the growth and development of the fetus.[17] The brain contains a substantial amount of lipid material and depends heavily on long-chain omega-3 and omega-6 fatty acids for its growth, function, and structure.[18] (See Table 3-3 on p. 69 for a list of good food sources of the essential fatty acids.)

IN SUMMARY

▪ The pregnant woman needs no additional energy intake during the first trimester, an increase of 340 kcalories per day during the second trimester, and an increase of 450 kcalories per day during the third trimester as compared with her nonpregnant needs.

▪ An additional 25 grams per day of protein are needed during pregnancy, but pregnant women can easily meet this need by choosing meats, poultry, seafood, eggs, low-fat milk and milk products, and plant-protein foods such as legumes, whole grains, nuts, and seeds.

▪ A balanced diet that includes more nutrient-dense foods from each of the five food groups can help to meet the increased nutrient demands of pregnancy.

TABLE 11-2 Daily Food Choices for Pregnancy (Second and Third Trimesters) and Lactation

Food Group	Amounts
Fruits	2 c
Vegetables	3 c
Grains	8 oz
Protein foods	6½ oz
Milk	3 c

Sample Menu

Breakfast

1 whole-wheat English muffin

2 tbs peanut butter

1 c low-fat vanilla yogurt

½ c fresh strawberries

1 c orange juice

Midmorning Snack

½ c cranberry juice

1 oz pretzels

Lunch

Sandwich (tuna salad on whole-wheat bread)

  ½ carrot (sticks)

  1 c low-fat milk

Dinner

Chicken cacciatore

  3 oz chicken

  ½ c stewed tomatoes

  1 c rice

  ½ c summer squash

  1½ c salad (spinach, mushrooms, carrots)

  1 tbs salad dressing

  1 slice Italian bread

  2 tsp soft margarine

  1 c low-fat milk

Note: This sample meal plan provides about 2500 kcalories (55% from carbohydrate, 20 percent from protein, and 25% from fat) and meets most of the vitamin and mineral needs of pregnant and lactating women.

FIGURE 11-5 Spina bifida—A Neural Tube Defect
Spina bifida, a common neural tube defect, occurs when the vertebrae of the spine fail to close around the spinal cord, leaving it unprotected. The B vitamin folate—consumed prior to and during pregnancy—helps prevent spina bifida and other neural tube defects.

© 2016 Cengage Learning®

Of Special Interest: Folate and Vitamin B₁₂ The vitamins famous for their roles in cell reproduction—folate and vitamin B_{12}—are needed in large amounts during pregnancy. New cells are laid down at a tremendous pace as the fetus grows and develops. At the same time, because the mother's blood volume increases, the number of her red blood cells must rise, requiring more cell division and therefore more vitamins. To accommodate these needs, the recommendation for folate during pregnancy increases from 400 to 600 micrograms a day.

As described in Chapter 8, folate plays an important role in preventing neural tube defects. To review, the early weeks of pregnancy are a critical period for the formation and closure of the **neural tube** that will later develop to form the brain and spinal cord. By the time a woman suspects she is pregnant, usually around the 6th week of pregnancy, the embryo's neural tube normally has closed. A **neural tube defect (NTD)** occurs when the tube fails to close properly. Each year in the United States, an estimated 3000 pregnancies are affected by an NTD.[19] The two most common types of NTD are anencephaly (no brain) and spina bifida (split spine).

In **anencephaly,** the upper end of the neural tube fails to close. Consequently, the brain is either missing or fails to develop. Pregnancies affected by anencephaly often end in miscarriage; infants born with anencephaly die shortly after birth.

Spina bifida is characterized by incomplete closure of the spinal cord and its bony encasement (see Figure 11-5). The membranes covering the spinal cord and sometimes the cord itself may protrude from the spine as a sac. Spina bifida often produces paralysis in varying degrees, depending on the extent of spinal cord damage. Mild cases may not be noticed. Moderate cases may involve curvature of the spine, muscle weakness, mental handicaps, and other ills, while severe cases can lead to death.

neural tube: the embryonic tissue that later forms the brain and spinal cord.

neural tube defect (NTD): a serious central nervous system birth defect that often results in lifelong disability or death.

anencephaly (AN-en-SEF-a-lee): an uncommon and always fatal type of neural tube defect; characterized by the absence of a brain.
   an = not (without)
   encephalus = brain

spina (SPY-nah) **bifida** (BIFF-ih-dah): one of the most common types of neural tube defects; characterized by the incomplete closure of the spinal cord and its bony encasement.
   spina = spine
   bifida = split

To reduce the risk of neural tube defects, women who are capable of becoming pregnant are advised to obtain 400 micrograms of folic acid daily from supplements, fortified foods, or both, *in addition* to eating folate-rich foods (see Table 11-3). The DRI committee recommends intake of synthetic folate, called folic acid, in supplements and fortified food because it is absorbed better than the folate naturally present in foods. Foods that naturally contain folate are still important, however, because they contribute to folate intakes while providing other needed vitamins, minerals, fiber, and phytochemicals.

The enrichment of grain products (cereal, grits, pasta, rice, bread, and the like) sold commercially in the United States with folic acid has improved folate status in women of childbearing age and lowered the number of neural tube defects that occur each year.[20] Researchers expect to see declines in some other birth defects (cleft lip and cleft palate) and miscarriages as well.[21] A safety concern arises, however. The pregnant woman also needs a greater amount of vitamin B_{12} to assist folate in the manufacture of new cells. Because high intakes of folate complicate the diagnosis of a vitamin B_{12} deficiency (see Chapter 8), quantities of 1 milligram or more require a prescription. Most over-the-counter multivitamin supplements contain 400 micrograms of folic acid; supplements for pregnant women usually contain at least 800 micrograms.

People who eat meat, eggs, or dairy products receive all the vitamin B_{12} they need, even for pregnancy. Those who exclude all animal-derived foods from the diet, however, need vitamin B_{12}–fortified foods or supplements.

IN SUMMARY

▌ Due to their key roles in cell reproduction, folate and vitamin B_{12} are needed in large amounts during pregnancy.

▌ Folate plays an important role in preventing neural tube defects.

Vitamin D and Calcium for Bones Vitamin D and the minerals involved in building the skeleton—calcium, phosphorus, magnesium, and fluoride—are in great demand during pregnancy. Insufficient intakes may produce abnormal fetal bone growth and tooth development.

Vitamin D plays a vital role in calcium absorption and utilization. Consequently, severe maternal vitamin D deficiency interferes with normal calcium metabolism, which, in rare cases, may cause rickets in the infant.[22] Regular exposure to sunlight and consumption of vitamin D–fortified milk are usually sufficient to provide the recommended amount of vitamin D during pregnancy (15 µg/day), which is the same as for nonpregnant women.[23] The vitamin D in **prenatal supplements** helps to protect many, but not all, pregnant women from inadequate intakes.[24]

Intestinal absorption of calcium doubles early in pregnancy, when the mother's bones store the mineral. Later, as the fetal bones begin to calcify, a dramatic shift of calcium across the placenta occurs. Whether the calcium added to the mother's bones early in pregnancy is withdrawn to build the fetus's bones later is unclear.[25] In the final weeks of pregnancy, more than 300 milligrams a day are transferred to the fetus.[26] Recommendations to ensure an adequate calcium intake during pregnancy are aimed at conserving the mother's bone mass while supplying fetal needs.

Typically, young women in the United States take in too little calcium. Of particular importance, pregnant women under age 25, whose own bones are still actively depositing minerals, should strive to meet the recommendation for calcium by increasing their intakes of milk, cheese, yogurt, and other calcium-rich foods. The USDA Food Patterns suggest consuming 3 cups per day of fat-free or low-fat milk or the equivalent in milk products. Less preferred, but still acceptable, is a daily supplement of 600 milligrams of calcium. The RDA for calcium intake is the same for nonpregnant and pregnant women in the same age group. Women who exclude milk products need

TABLE 11-3 Rich Folate Sources[a]

Natural Folate Sources

▪ Liver (3 oz): 221 µg DFE

▪ Lentils (½ c): 179 µg DFE

▪ Chickpeas or pinto beans (½ c): 145 µg DFE

▪ Asparagus (½ c): 134 µg DFE

▪ Spinach (1 c raw): 58 µg DFE

▪ Avocado (½ c): 61 µg DFE

▪ Orange juice (1 c): 74 µg DFE

▪ Beets (½ c): 68 µg DFE

Fortified Folate Sources

▪ Highly enriched ready-to-eat cereals[b] (¾ c): 680 µg DFE

▪ Pasta, cooked (1 c): 154 µg DFE (average value)

▪ Rice, cooked (1 c): 153 µg DFE

▪ Bagel (1 small whole): 156 µg DFE

▪ Waffles, frozen (2): 78 µg DFE

▪ Bread, white (1 slice): 48 µg DFE

© 2016 Cengage Learning®

[a]Folate amounts for these and 2000 other foods are listed in Appendix A.

[b]Folate in cereals varies; read the Nutrition Facts panel of the label.

prenatal supplements: nutrient supplements specifically designed to provide the nutrients needed during pregnancy, particularly folate, iron, and calcium, without excesses or unneeded constituents.

calcium-fortified foods such as soy milk, orange juice, and cereals. Read the labels: contents vary and products fortified with both calcium and vitamin D are recommended.

IN SUMMARY

▌ Maternal vitamin D deficiency interferes with calcium metabolism in the infant.

▌ All pregnant women, but especially those who are younger than 25 years of age, need to pay special attention to calcium to ensure adequate intakes.

Iron The body conserves iron especially well during pregnancy: menstruation ceases, and absorption of iron increases up to threefold due to a rise in the blood's iron-absorbing and iron-carrying protein transferrin. Still, iron needs are so high that stores dwindle during pregnancy. To help improve the iron status of women before and during pregnancy, the *Dietary Guidelines for Americans 2010* recommend that all women capable of becoming pregnant choose foods that supply heme iron (meat, seafood, and poultry), which is most readily absorbed; choose additional sources, such as iron-rich eggs, vegetables, and legumes; and consume foods that enhance iron absorption, such as vitamin C-rich fruits and vegetables.

The developing fetus draws heavily on the mother's iron stores to create stores of its own to last through the first 4 to 6 months after birth. The transfer of significant amounts of iron to the fetus is regulated by the placenta, which gives the iron needs of the fetus priority over those of the mother.[27] Even a woman with inadequate iron stores transfers a considerable amount of iron to the fetus. In addition, blood (and thus iron) losses are inevitable at birth, especially during a delivery by cesarean section.

Few women enter pregnancy with adequate iron stores, so a daily iron supplement is recommended early in pregnancy, if not before.[28] Women who enter pregnancy with iron-deficiency anemia are at increased risk of delivering low-birthweight or preterm infants.[29] When a low hemoglobin or hematocrit level is confirmed by a repeat test, more than the standard iron dose of 30 milligrams may be prescribed. To enhance iron absorption, the supplement should be taken between meals and with liquids other than milk, coffee, or tea, which inhibit iron absorption.

Zinc Zinc is required for protein synthesis and cell development during pregnancy. Typical zinc intakes of pregnant women are lower than recommendations but, fortunately, zinc absorption increases when intakes are low. Large doses of iron can interfere with zinc absorption and metabolism, but most prenatal supplements supply the right balance of these minerals for pregnancy. Zinc is abundant in protein-rich foods such as shellfish, meat, and nuts.

IN SUMMARY

▌ Iron supplements are recommended for pregnant women.

▌ Large doses of iron can interfere with zinc absorption and metabolism, but most prenatal supplements supply the right balance of these minerals.

Nutrient Supplements A healthy pregnancy and optimal infant development depend on the mother's diet. Pregnant women who make wise food choices can meet most of their nutrient needs, with the possible exception of iron. Even so, physicians often recommend daily multivitamin-mineral supplements for pregnant women. These prenatal supplements typically provide more folic acid, iron, and calcium than regular supplements. Prenatal supplements are especially beneficial for women who do not eat adequately and for those in high-risk groups: women carrying twins or triplets, cigarette smokers, and alcohol or drug abusers. For these women, prenatal supplements may be of some help in reducing the risks of preterm delivery, low infant birthweights, and birth defects.[30] Be aware, however, that supplements cannot prevent the vast majority of fetal harm from tobacco, alcohol, and drugs, which continues unopposed, as later sections explain.

IN SUMMARY

▎ Physicians often recommend daily multivitamin-mineral supplements for pregnant women.

▎ Women most likely to benefit from prenatal supplements during pregnancy include those who do not eat adequately, those carrying twins or triplets, and those who smoke cigarettes or are alcohol or drug abusers.

Food Assistance Programs

Women of limited financial means may eat diets too low in calcium, iron, vitamins A and C, and protein. Often, they and their children need help in obtaining food and benefit from nutrition counseling. At the federal level, the **Special Supplemental Nutrition Program for Women, Infants, and Children (WIC)** provides vouchers redeemable for nutritious foods, nutrition education, and referrals to health and social services to low-income pregnant and lactating women and their children.[31] WIC offers vouchers for the following nutritious foods: baby foods, eggs, dried and canned beans and peas, tuna fish, peanut butter, fruits, vegetables, and their juices, iron-fortified cereals, milk and cheese, soy-based beverages and tofu, and whole-wheat and other whole-grain products. For infants given infant formula, WIC also provides iron-fortified formula. WIC encourages mothers to breastfeed their infants, however, and offers incentives to those who do.

More than 9 million people—most of them infants and young children—receive WIC benefits each month. Participation in the WIC program benefits both the nutrient status and the growth and development of infants and children. WIC participation during pregnancy can effectively reduce iron deficiency, infant mortality, low birthweight, and maternal and newborn medical costs.

The Supplemental Nutrition Assistance Program (SNAP) provides a debit card that can also help to stretch the low-income pregnant woman's grocery dollars. In addition, many communities and organizations such as the Academy of Nutrition and Dietetics (AND) provide educational services and materials, including nutrition, food budgeting, and shopping information.

IN SUMMARY

▎ Food assistance programs such as WIC can provide nutritious food for pregnant women of limited financial means.

▎ Participation in WIC during pregnancy can reduce iron deficiency, infant mortality, low birthweight, and maternal and newborn medical costs.

Weight Gain

Women must gain weight during pregnancy—fetal and maternal well-being depend on it. Ideally, a woman will have begun her pregnancy at a healthy weight, but even more importantly, she will gain within the recommended weight range based on her prepregnancy body mass index (BMI) as shown in Table 11-4 (on p. 298). Pregnancy weight gains within the recommended ranges are associated with fewer surgical births, a greater number of healthy birthweights, and other positive outcomes for both mothers and infants, but many women do not gain within these ranges.[32] Among women in the United States, excessive weight gain during pregnancy is more prevalent than

Special Supplemental Nutrition Program for Women, Infants, and Children (WIC): a high-quality, cost-effective health care and nutrition services program administered by the U.S. Department of Agriculture for low-income women, infants, and children who are nutritionally at risk. WIC provides supplemental foods, nutrition education, and referrals to health care and other social services.

TABLE 11-4 Recommended Weight Gains Based on Prepregnancy Weight

Prepregnancy Weight	Recommended Weight Gain	
	For Single Birth	For Twin Birth
Underweight (BMI <18.5)	28 to 40 lb (12.5 to 18.0 kg)	Insufficient data to make recommendation
Healthy weight (BMI 18.5 to 24.9)	25 to 35 lb (11.5 to 16.0 kg)	37 to 54 lb (17 to 25 kg)
Overweight (BMI 25.0 to 29.9)	15 to 25 lb (7.0 to 11.5 kg)	31 to 50 lb (14 to 23 kg)
Obese (BMI ≥30)	11 to 20 lb (5 to 9 kg)	25 to 42 lb (11 to 19 kg)

© Cengage Learning®

Source: Institute of Medicine, *Weight Gain During Pregnancy: Reexamining the Guidelines.* Reprinted with permission from The National Academies Press, Copyright © 2009, National Academy of Sciences.

inadequate weight gain. To improve pregnancy outcomes, researchers and health care providers are placing greater emphasis on preventing excessive weight gains during pregnancy than in the recent past.[33]

Weight loss during pregnancy is not recommended.[34] Even obese women are advised to gain between 11 and 20 pounds for the best chance of delivering a healthy infant.[35] Ideally, overweight women will achieve a healthy body weight before becoming pregnant, avoid excessive weight gain during pregnancy, and postpone weight loss until after childbirth.

According to current recommendations, pregnant adolescents who are still growing should strive for gains at the upper end of the target range. Current concerns about obesity raise questions as to whether such recommendations are always appropriate. Compared with older mothers, for example, the risk of lifetime weight retention after pregnancy may be far greater for young adolescents.

The ideal weight gain pattern for a woman who begins pregnancy at a healthy weight is 3½ pounds during the first trimester and 1 pound per week thereafter (see the prenatal weight-gain grid in Appendix E). If a woman gains more than is recommended early in pregnancy, she should not restrict her energy intake later on in order to lose weight. A sudden, large weight gain is a danger signal, however, because it may indicate the onset of preeclampsia (discussed later in the chapter).

The weight the pregnant woman gains is nearly all lean tissue: placenta, uterus, blood, milk-producing glands, and the fetus itself (see Figure 11-6). The fat she gains is needed later for lactation. Physical activity can help a pregnant woman cope with the extra weight, as a later section explains.

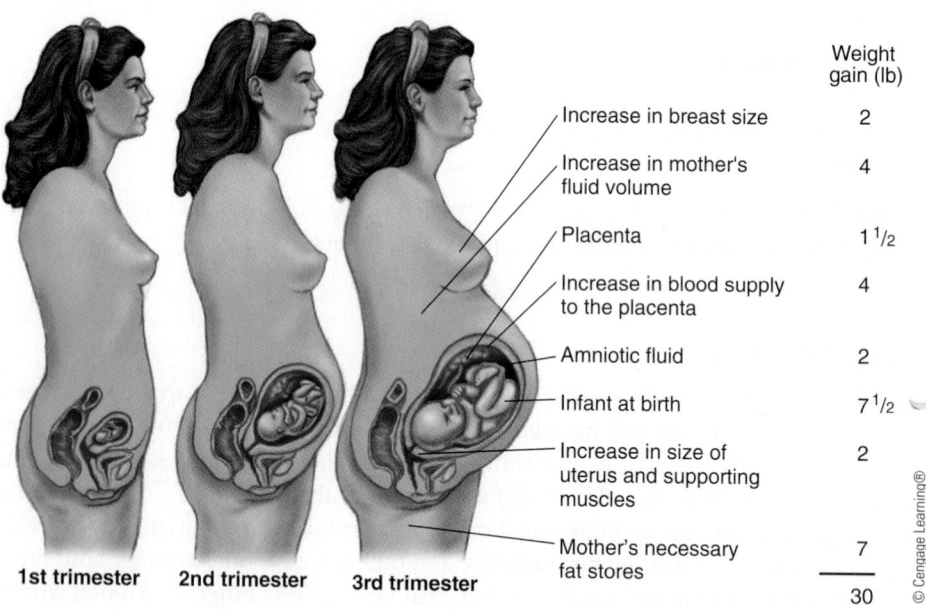

	Weight gain (lb)
Increase in breast size	2
Increase in mother's fluid volume	4
Placenta	1½
Increase in blood supply to the placenta	4
Amniotic fluid	2
Infant at birth	7½
Increase in size of uterus and supporting muscles	2
Mother's necessary fat stores	7
	30

1st trimester   2nd trimester   3rd trimester

© Cengage Learning®

FIGURE 11-6 Components of Weight Gain during Pregnancy

Weight Loss after Pregnancy

The pregnant woman loses some weight at delivery. In the following weeks, she loses more as her blood volume returns to normal and she gets rid of accumulated fluids. The typical woman does not, however, return to her prepregnancy weight. In general, the more weight a woman gains beyond the needs of pregnancy, the more she retains—mostly as body fat.[36] Even with an average weight gain during pregnancy, most women tend to retain a few pounds with each pregnancy. When those few pounds become 7 or more and BMI increases by a unit or more, complications such as diabetes and hypertension in future pregnancies as well as chronic diseases later in life can increase—even for women who are not overweight. Women who achieve a healthy weight prior to the first pregnancy and maintain it between pregnancies best avoid the cumulative weight gain that threatens health later on.

IN SUMMARY

▌ Appropriate (adequate but not excessive) weight gain is essential for a healthy pregnancy.

▌ A woman's prepregnancy BMI, her own nutrient needs, and the number of fetuses she is carrying help to determine appropriate weight gain.

Physical Activity

An active, physically fit woman experiencing a normal pregnancy can and should continue to exercise throughout pregnancy, adjusting the intensity and duration as the pregnancy progresses. Staying active during the course of a normal, healthy pregnancy improves the fitness of the mother-to-be, facilitates labor, helps to prevent or manage gestational diabetes and gestational hypertension, and reduces psychological stress.[37] Women who remain active report fewer discomforts throughout their pregnancies and retain habits that help in losing excess weight and regaining fitness after the birth.[38]

Pregnant women should choose "low-impact" activities and avoid sports in which they might fall or be hit by other people or objects. Swimming and water aerobics are particularly beneficial because they allow the body to remain cool and move freely with the water's support, thus reducing back pain.

As is true for everyone, the frequency, duration, and intensity of the activity affect the likelihood of the benefits or risks. A few guidelines are offered in Figure 11-7. Several

DO		**DON'T**
Do exercise regularly (most, if not all, days of the week).		Don't exercise vigorously after long periods of inactivity.
Do warm up with 5 to 10 minutes of light activity.		Don't exercise in hot, humid weather.
Do 30 minutes or more of moderate physical activity.		Don't exercise when sick with fever.
Do cool down with 5 to 10 minutes of slow activity and gentle stretching.		Don't exercise while lying on your back after the first trimester of pregnancy or stand motionless for prolonged periods.
Do drink water before, after, and during exercise.		Don't exercise if you experience any pain or discomfort.
Do eat enough to support the additional needs of pregnancy plus exercise.		Don't participate in activities that may harm the abdomen or involve jerky, bouncy movements.
Do rest adequately.	Pregnant women can enjoy the benefits of physical activity.	Don't scuba dive.

Tracy Frankel/The Image Bank/Getty Images

FIGURE 11-7 **Guidelines for Physical Activity during Pregnancy**

of the guidelines are aimed at preventing excessively high internal body temperatures and dehydration, both of which can harm fetal development. To this end, a pregnant woman should also stay out of saunas, steam rooms, and hot whirlpools. A pregnant woman with a medical condition or pregnancy complication should undergo a thorough evaluation by her health care provider before engaging in physical activity.

IN SUMMARY

- Physically fit women can continue physical activity throughout pregnancy but should choose activities wisely.

- Pregnant women should avoid sports in which they might fall or be hit by other people or objects and should take care not to become dehydrated or overheated.

Common Nutrition-Related Concerns of Pregnancy

Food sensitivities, nausea, heartburn, and constipation are common during pregnancy. A few simple strategies can help alleviate maternal discomforts (see Table 11-5).

Food Cravings and Aversions Some women develop cravings for, or aversions to, certain foods and beverages during pregnancy. Individual **food cravings** during pregnancy do not seem to reflect real physiological needs. In other words, a woman who craves pickles does not necessarily need salt. Similarly, cravings for ice cream are common during pregnancy but do not signify a calcium deficiency. **Food aversions** and

TABLE 11-5 Strategies to Alleviate Maternal Discomforts

To Alleviate the Nausea of Pregnancy:
▪ On waking, arise slowly.
▪ Eat dry toast or crackers.
▪ Chew gum or suck hard candies.
▪ Eat small, frequent meals whenever hunger strikes.
▪ Avoid foods with offensive odors.
▪ When nauseated, do not drink citrus juice, water, milk, coffee, or tea.
To Prevent or Alleviate Constipation:
▪ Eat foods high in fiber.
▪ Exercise daily.
▪ Drink at least 8 glasses of liquids a day.
▪ Respond promptly to the urge to defecate.
▪ Use laxatives only as prescribed by a physician; avoid mineral oil—it carries needed fat-soluble vitamins out of the body.
To Prevent or Relieve Heartburn:
▪ Relax and eat slowly.
▪ Chew food thoroughly.
▪ Eat small, frequent meals.
▪ Drink liquids between meals.
▪ Avoid spicy or greasy foods.
▪ Sit up while eating.
▪ Wait an hour after eating before lying down.
▪ Wait 2 hours after eating before exercising.

food cravings: deep longings for particular foods.

food aversions: strong desires to avoid particular foods.

cravings that arise during pregnancy are probably due to hormone-induced changes in taste and sensitivities to smells, and they quickly disappear after the birth.

Nonfood Cravings Some pregnant women develop cravings for and ingest nonfood items such as laundry starch, clay, soil, or ice—a practice known as pica.[39] Pica may be practiced for cultural reasons that reflect a society's folklore; it is especially common among African American women. Pica is often associated with iron deficiency, but whether iron deficiency leads to pica or pica leads to iron deficiency is unclear.[40] Eating clay or soil may interfere with iron absorption and displace iron-rich foods from the diet. Furthermore, if the soil or clay contains environmental contaminants such as lead or parasites, health and nutrition suffer.

Morning Sickness The nausea of "morning" (actually, anytime) sickness seems unavoidable and may even be a welcome sign of a healthy pregnancy because it arises from the hormonal changes of early pregnancy. The problem typically peaks at 9 weeks gestation and resolves within a month or two.[41] Many women complain that odors, especially cooking smells, make them sick. Thus, minimizing odors may alleviate morning sickness for some women. Traditional strategies for quelling nausea are listed in Table 11-5, but little evidence exists to support such advice.[42] Some women do best by simply eating what they desire whenever they feel hungry. Morning sickness can be persistent, however. If morning sickness interferes with normal eating for more than a week or two, the woman should seek medical advice to prevent nutrient deficiencies.

Heartburn Heartburn, a burning sensation in the lower esophagus near the heart, is common during pregnancy and is also benign. As the growing fetus puts increasing pressure on the woman's stomach, acid may back up and create a burning sensation in her throat. Tips to relieve heartburn are listed in Table 11-5.

Constipation As the hormones of pregnancy alter muscle tone and the thriving infant crowds intestinal organs, an expectant mother may complain of constipation, another harmless but annoying condition. A high-fiber diet, physical activity, and plentiful fluids will help relieve this condition. Also, responding promptly to the urge to defecate can help. Laxatives should be used only as prescribed by a physician.

IN SUMMARY

▮ Food cravings typically do not reflect physiological needs.

▮ Pica is the ingestion of nonfood items such as laundry starch, clay, soil, or ice. In some cases, pica can be harmful to health and nutrition.

▮ The nausea, heartburn, and constipation that sometimes accompany pregnancy can usually be alleviated with a few simple strategies.

Problems in Pregnancy

Just as adequate nutrition and normal weight gain support the health of the mother and growth of the fetus, maternal diseases can have an adverse effect. If discovered early, many diseases can be controlled—another reason why early prenatal care is recommended. Some nutrition measures can help alleviate the most common problems encountered during pregnancy.

Preexisting Diabetes Pregnancy presents special challenges for the management of diabetes. Insulin-induced hypoglycemia has a more rapid onset during pregnancy and is a danger to the mother, especially in those with type 1 diabetes. Women with type 2 diabetes often start pregnancy with insulin resistance and obesity, making optimal glycemic control difficult. The risks of diabetes during pregnancy depend on how well it is managed before, during, and after. Excellent glycemic control in the first trimester and throughout the pregnancy is associated with the lowest frequency of maternal, fetal, and newborn complications.[43] Without proper management, women face high infertility rates, and those who do conceive may experience episodes of severe hypoglycemia or hyperglycemia, preterm labor, and pregnancy-related hypertension. Infants may be large, suffer physical and mental abnormalities, and experience other complications such as severe hypoglycemia or respiratory distress, both of which can be fatal. Signs of fetal health problems are apparent even when maternal glucose is above normal but still below the diagnosis of diabetes. Ideally, a woman will receive the prenatal care needed to achieve glucose control before conception and continued glucose control throughout pregnancy. For optimal long-term outcomes, continuation of intensified diabetes management after pregnancy is in the best interest of the mother's health.

Gestational Diabetes Some women are prone to developing a pregnancy-related form of diabetes, **gestational diabetes.** Gestational diabetes usually resolves after the infant is born, but some women go on to develop type 2 diabetes later in life, especially if they are overweight.[44] For this reason, health care professionals strongly advise against excessive weight gain during and after pregnancy. Weight gains after pregnancy increase the risk of gestational diabetes in the next pregnancy.[45] Gestational diabetes can lead to fetal or infant sickness or death, though the risk of these outcomes falls dramatically when it is identified early and managed properly. More commonly, gestational diabetes leads to surgical birth and high infant birthweight. To ensure prompt diagnosis and treatment, physicians screen all women who are overweight (BMI ≥25) and have one or more additional risk factors for type 2 diabetes (for example, high blood pressure, family history of diabetes or heart disease, previous gestational diabetes, family background that is Hispanic/Latino American, African American, Native American, Asian American, or Pacific Islander) at the first prenatal visit. In addition, all pregnant women not previously diagnosed with diabetes are tested for glucose intolerance at 24 to 28 weeks gestation.[46] Chapter 21 provides information about medical nutrition therapy for gestational diabetes.

Hypertension Hypertension (blood pressure ≥140/90 mm Hg) complicates pregnancy and affects its outcome in different ways, depending on how severe it becomes. Hypertension during pregnancy is classified as **chronic hypertension** or **gestational hypertension.**[47] Chronic hypertension can be a preexisting condition that develops before a woman becomes pregnant. In women whose prepregnancy blood pressure is unknown, diagnosis of chronic hypertension is based on the presence of sustained hypertension before 20 weeks of gestation.[48] In contrast, gestational hypertension develops after the 20th week of gestation. In women with gestational hypertension, blood pressure usually returns to normal during the first few weeks after childbirth.

Both types of hypertension pose risks to the mother and fetus. In addition to the health risks normally imposed by hypertension (heart attack and stroke), high blood pressure increases the risks of growth restriction, preterm birth, and separation of the placenta from the wall of the uterus before the birth.[49] Both chronic hypertension and gestational hypertension also increase the risk of preeclampsia.

Preeclampsia **Preeclampsia** is a condition characterized not only by high blood pressure but also by protein in the urine.[50] Preeclampsia usually occurs with first pregnancies and almost always appears after 20 weeks' gestation.[51] Symptoms typically regress within 48 hours of delivery. Because delivery is the only known cure, preeclampsia is a leading cause of indicated preterm delivery and accounts for about 15 percent of infants who are growth restricted.[52]

Preeclampsia affects almost all of the woman's organs—the circulatory system, liver, kidneys, and brain. If it progresses, she may experience seizures; when this occurs, the condition is called **eclampsia.** Maternal mortality during pregnancy is rare in developed countries, but eclampsia is the most common cause. Preeclampsia

gestational diabetes: glucose intolerance with first onset or first recognition during pregnancy.

chronic hypertension: in pregnant women, hypertension that is present and documented before pregnancy; in women whose prepregnancy blood pressure is unknown, the presence of sustained hypertension before 20 weeks of gestation.

gestational hypertension: high blood pressure that develops in the second half of pregnancy and usually resolves after childbirth.

preeclampsia (PRE-ee-KLAMP-see-ah)**:** a condition characterized by hypertension and protein in the urine during pregnancy.

eclampsia (eh-KLAMP-see-ah)**:** a severe complication during pregnancy in which seizures occur.

demands prompt medical attention. Treatment focuses on regulating blood pressure and preventing seizures.

IN SUMMARY

▪ Conditions such as gestational diabetes, hypertension, and preeclampsia can threaten the health and life of both mother and infant.

▪ Maternal diseases require medical and nutrition treatment.

Practices to Avoid

A general guideline for the pregnant woman is to eat a normal, healthy diet and practice moderation. A woman's daily choices during pregnancy take on enormous importance. Forewarned, pregnant women can choose to abstain from or avoid potentially harmful practices.

Cigarette Smoking One practice to be avoided during pregnancy is cigarette smoking, which is associated with many complications (see Table 11-6). A surgeon general's warning states that parental smoking can kill an otherwise healthy fetus or newborn. Unfortunately, an estimated 12 percent of pregnant women in the United States smoke.[53]

Constituents of cigarette smoke, such as nicotine, carbon monoxide, arsenic, and cyanide, are toxic to a fetus. Smoking during pregnancy can cause damage to fetal chromosomes, which could lead to developmental defects or diseases such as cancer.[54] Smoking also restricts the blood supply to the growing fetus and so limits the delivery of oxygen and nutrients and the removal of wastes. It slows fetal growth, can reduce brain size, and may impair the intellectual and behavioral development of the child later in life. Smoking during pregnancy damages fetal blood vessels, an effect that is still apparent at the age of 5 years.[55] It interferes with fetal lung development and increases the risks of respiratory infections and childhood asthma.[56]

A mother who smokes is more likely to have a complicated birth and a low-birthweight infant. The more a mother smokes, the smaller her infant will be. Of all preventable causes of low birthweight in the United States, smoking has the greatest impact. Sudden infant death syndrome (SIDS), the unexplained death that sometimes occurs in an otherwise healthy infant, has also been linked to the mother's cigarette smoking during pregnancy.[57] Even in women who do not smoke, exposure to **environmental tobacco smoke** (**ETS**, or secondhand smoke) during pregnancy increases the risk of low birthweight and the likelihood of SIDS.

In addition to the harms already described, cigarette (and cigar) smoking adversely affects the pregnant woman's nutrition status and thus impairs fetal nutrition and development. Smokers tend to have lower intakes of dietary fiber, vitamin A, beta-carotene, folate, and vitamin C.

Limited research shows that vitamin C supplements taken by pregnant smokers improved newborn lung function and decreased wheezing through 1 year of age.[58] Nevertheless, any woman who uses nicotine in any form and is pregnant or considering pregnancy needs to quit. Alternatives to smoking—such as using snuff, chewing tobacco, or nicotine-replacement therapy—are not safe during pregnancy.[59]

Medicinal Drugs and Herbal Supplements Medicinal drugs taken during pregnancy can cause serious birth defects. Pregnant women should not take over-the-counter drugs or any other medications without consulting their physicians, who must weigh the benefits against the risks.

Some pregnant women mistakenly consider herbal supplements to be safe alternatives to medicinal drugs and take them to relieve nausea, promote water loss, alleviate depression, help them sleep, or for other reasons. Some herbal products may be safe,

TABLE 11-6
Complications Associated with Smoking During Pregnancy

▪ Fetal growth restriction

▪ Low birthweight

▪ Preterm birth

▪ Premature separation of the placenta

▪ Miscarriage

▪ Stillbirth

▪ Sudden infant death syndrome

▪ Congenital malformations

© 2016 Cengage Learning®

environmental tobacco smoke (ETS): the combination of exhaled smoke (mainstream smoke) and smoke from lighted cigarettes, pipes, or cigars (sidestream smoke) that enters the air and may be inhaled by other people.

TABLE 11-7 Tips to
Prevent Listeriosis

- Use only pasteurized juices and dairy products; do not eat soft cheeses such as feta, brie, Camembert, Panela, "queso blanco," "queso fresco," and blue-veined cheeses such as Roquefort; do not drink raw (unpasteurized) milk or eat foods that contain it.

- Do not eat hot dogs or luncheon or deli meats unless heated until steaming hot.

- Thoroughly cook meat, poultry, eggs, and seafood.

- Wash all fruits and vegetables.

- Do not eat refrigerated patés or meat spreads.

- Do not eat smoked seafood, or any fish labeled "nova-style," "lox," or "kippered."

© 2016 Cengage Learning®

listeriosis: a serious foodborne infection that can cause severe brain infection or death in a fetus or newborn; caused by the bacterium *Listeria monocytogenes*, which is found in soil and water.

but very few have been tested for safety or effectiveness during pregnancy. Pregnant women should stay away from herbal supplements, teas, or other products unless their safety during pregnancy has been ascertained. Nutrition in Practice 15 offers more information about herbal supplements and other alternative therapies.

Drugs of Abuse Drugs of abuse such as cocaine easily cross the placenta and impair fetal growth and development. Furthermore, such drugs are responsible for preterm births, low-birthweight infants, and sudden infant deaths. If these newborns survive, central nervous system damage is evident: their cries, sleep, and behaviors early in life are abnormal, and their cognitive development later in life is impaired.[60] They may be hypersensitive or underaroused; many suffer the symptoms of withdrawal. Delays in their growth and development persist throughout childhood and adolescence.[61]

Environmental Contaminants Infants and young children of pregnant women exposed to environmental contaminants such as lead and mercury show signs of impaired mental and psychomotor development. During pregnancy, lead readily moves across the placenta, inflicting severe damage on the developing fetal nervous system. In addition, infants exposed to even low levels of lead during gestation weigh less at birth and consequently struggle to survive. For these reasons, it is particularly important that pregnant women consume foods and beverages free of contamination. Dietary calcium can help to defend against lead toxicity by reducing its absorption.

Mercury is a contaminant of concern as well. As discussed in Chapter 3, fatty fish are a good source of omega-3 fatty acids, but some fish contain large amounts of the pollutant mercury, which can impair fetal growth and harm the developing brain and nervous system. Because the benefits of moderate seafood consumption outweigh the risks, pregnant (and lactating) women need reliable information on which fish are safe to eat.[62] The *Dietary Guidelines for Americans*, the Food and Drug Administration (FDA), and the Environmental Protection Agency (EPA) advise pregnant and lactating women to avoid shark, swordfish, king mackerel, and tilefish (also called golden snapper or golden bass). Because many pregnant women have not been consuming any fish or shellfish, the FDA and the EPA released updated recommendations encouraging pregnant and lactating women to eat *at least* 8 ounces and up to 12 ounces (cooked or canned) of seafood weekly.[63] However, the FDA and EPA continue to recommend that no more than 6 ounces (cooked or canned) of white (albacore) tuna be consumed weekly. Supplements of fish oil are not recommended because they may contain concentrated toxins and because their effects on pregnancy remain unknown.

Foodborne Illness The vomiting and diarrhea caused by many foodborne illnesses can leave a pregnant woman exhausted and dangerously dehydrated. Particularly threatening, however, is **listeriosis,** which can cause miscarriage, stillbirth, or severe brain or other infections to fetuses and newborns. Pregnant women are about 20 times more likely than other healthy adults to get listeriosis. A woman with listeriosis may develop symptoms such as fever, vomiting, and diarrhea in about 12 hours after eating a contaminated food, and serious symptoms may develop a week to 6 weeks later. A blood test can reliably detect listeriosis, and antibiotics given promptly to the pregnant sufferer can often prevent infection of the fetus or newborn. Table 11-7 presents tips to prevent listeriosis. Nutrition in Practice 5 includes precautions to minimize the risks of other common foodborne illnesses.

Large Doses of Vitamin-Mineral Supplements Many vitamins and minerals are toxic when taken in excess. Excessive vitamin A is particularly infamous for its role in fetal malformations of the cranial nervous system. Intakes before the 7th week of pregnancy appear to be the most damaging. For this reason, vitamin A supplements are not given during pregnancy, unless there is specific evidence of deficiency, which is rare.

Restrictive Dieting Restrictive dieting, even for short periods, can be hazardous during pregnancy. Low-carbohydrate diets or fasts that cause ketosis deprive the growing fetal brain of needed glucose and may impair cognitive development. Such diets are also likely to be deficient in other nutrients vital to fetal growth. Regardless of prepregnancy weight, pregnant women need an adequate diet to support healthy fetal development.

Sugar Substitutes Artificial sweeteners have been studied extensively and found to be acceptable during pregnancy if used within the FDA's guidelines (see Chapter 2).[64] Still, it would be prudent for pregnant women to use sweeteners in moderation and within an otherwise nutritious and well-balanced diet. Women with phenylketonuria should not use aspartame, as Chapter 2 explains.

Caffeine Caffeine crosses the placenta, and the fetus has only a limited ability to metabolize it. Research studies have not proved that caffeine (even in high doses) causes birth defects in human infants (as it does in animals), but limited evidence suggests that heavy use—intake equaling more than 3 cups of coffee a day—increases the risk of hypertension and miscarriage.[65] Depending on the quantities consumed and the mother's metabolism, caffeine may also interfere with fetal growth.[66] Lower doses of caffeine appear to be compatible with healthy pregnancies.[67] All things considered, it may be most sensible to limit caffeine consumption to the equivalent of one or two cups of coffee a day. The amounts of caffeine in foods and beverages are listed in Appendix A.

Alcohol Drinking alcohol during pregnancy threatens the fetus with irreversible brain damage, growth retardation, mental retardation, facial abnormalities, vision abnormalities, and many more health problems—a spectrum of symptoms known as **fetal alcohol spectrum disorders,** or **FASD.** Children at the most severe end of the spectrum (those with all of the symptoms) are defined as having **fetal alcohol syndrome (FAS),** which results in the facial abnormalities shown in Figure 11-8.[68] Less obvious is the internal harm: The fetal brain is extremely vulnerable to a glucose or oxygen deficit, and alcohol causes both by disrupting placental functioning. The lifelong mental retardation and other tragedies of FAS can be prevented by abstaining from drinking alcohol during pregnancy. Once the damage is done, however, the child remains impaired. An estimated 5 to 20 of every 10,000 children are victims of FAS, making it one of the leading known preventable causes of mental retardation in the world.[69]

Despite alcohol's potential for harm, 1 out of 13 pregnant women drinks alcohol sometime during her pregnancy, and 1 out of 71 reports binge drinking (four or more drinks on one occasion).[70] Almost half of all pregnancies are unintended, and many are conceived during a binge-drinking episode.

Women who know they are pregnant and desire to drink may wonder: How much alcohol is too much? Even one drink a day threatens neurological development and behaviors. Low birthweight is reported among infants born to women who drink 1 ounce (two drinks) of alcohol per day during pregnancy, and FAS is also known to occur with as few as two drinks a day. Birth defects have been reliably observed among the children of women who drink 2 ounces (four drinks) of alcohol daily during pregnancy. The most severe impact is likely to occur in the first 2 months, possibly before the woman is aware that she is pregnant.

Even when a child does not develop full FAS, prenatal exposure to alcohol can lead to less severe, but nonetheless serious, mental and physical problems. The cluster of mental problems is known as **alcohol-related neurodevelopmental disorder (ARND),** and the physical malformations are referred to as **alcohol-related birth defects (ARBD).** Some of these children show no outward sign of impairment, but others are short in stature or display subtle facial abnormalities. Many perform poorly in school and in social interactions and suffer a subtle form of brain damage. Mood disorders and problem behaviors, such as aggression, are common.

For every child diagnosed with full-blown FAS, many more with FASD go undiagnosed until problems develop in the preschool years. Upon reaching adulthood,

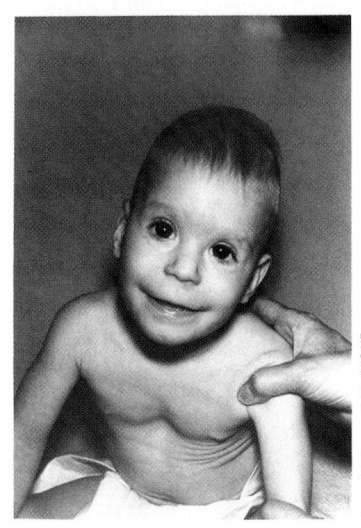

James W. Hanson, M.D./NIC HD

FIGURE 11-8 Typical Facial Characteristics of FAS
These facial traits are typical of fetal alcohol syndrome, caused by drinking alcohol during pregnancy—low nasal bridge, short eyelid opening, underdeveloped groove in the center of the upper lip, small midface, short nose, and small head circumference.

fetal alcohol spectrum disorders (FASD): a spectrum of physical, behavioral, and cognitive disabilities caused by prenatal alcohol exposure.

fetal alcohol syndrome (FAS): the cluster of symptoms seen in an infant or child whose mother consumed excessive alcohol during her pregnancy. FAS includes, but is not limited to, brain damage, growth retardation, mental retardation, and facial abnormalities.

alcohol-related neurodevelopmental disorder (ARND): a condition caused by prenatal alcohol exposure that is diagnosed when there is a confirmed history of substantial, regular maternal alcohol intake or heavy episodic drinking and behavioral, cognitive, or central nervous system abnormalities known to be associated with alcohol exposure.

alcohol-related birth defects (ARBD): a condition caused by prenatal alcohol exposure that is diagnosed when there is a history of substantial, regular maternal alcohol intake or heavy episodic drinking and birth defects known to be associated with alcohol exposure.

such children are ill equipped for employment, relationships, and the other facets of life most adults take for granted. Anyone exposed to alcohol before birth may always respond differently to it, and also to certain drugs, than if no exposure had occurred, making addictions likely.

The American Academy of Pediatrics (AAP) takes the position that women should stop drinking as soon as they *plan* to become pregnant. Researchers have looked for a "safe" alcohol intake limit during pregnancy and have found none. Their conclusion: abstinence from alcohol is the best policy for pregnant women.

For pregnant women who have already drunk alcohol, the advice is "stop now." A woman who has drunk heavily during the first two-thirds of her pregnancy can still prevent some organ damage by stopping heavy drinking during the third trimester.

IN SUMMARY

▌ Smoking during pregnancy delivers toxins to the fetus, damages DNA, restricts fetal growth, and limits delivery of oxygen and nutrients and the removal of wastes.

▌ Drinking alcohol during pregnancy threatens the fetus with irreversible brain damage, growth retardation, mental retardation, facial abnormalities, vision abnormalities, and many more health problems—a spectrum of symptoms known as fetal alcohol spectrum disorders, or FASD.

▌ Abstaining from smoking and other drugs, including alcohol, limiting intake of foods known to contain unsafe levels of contaminants such as mercury, taking precautions against foodborne illness, avoiding large doses of nutrients, refraining from restrictive dieting, using artificial sweeteners in moderation, and limiting caffeine use are recommended during pregnancy.

Adolescent Pregnancy

The number of infants born to teenage mothers has steadily declined during the last 50 years. Despite the long-term decline, however, the U.S. teen birth rate is still one of the highest among industrialized nations.[71] More than 305,000 adolescent girls give birth each year in the United States; almost 20 percent of them already have at least one child.[72]

A pregnant adolescent presents a special case of intense nutrient needs. Young teenage girls have a hard enough time meeting nutrient needs for their own rapid growth and development, let alone those of pregnancy. Many teens enter pregnancy deficient in vitamins B_{12} and D, folate, calcium, and iron, which increases the risk of impaired fetal growth. Pregnant adolescents are less likely to receive early prenatal care and are more likely to smoke during pregnancy—two factors that predict low birthweight and infant death.

The rates of stillbirths, preterm births, and low-birthweight infants are high for teenagers—both for teen moms and for teen dads. Their greatest risk, though, is death of the infant: mothers younger than 16 years of age bear more infants who die within the first year than do women in any other age group. These factors combine to make adolescent pregnancy a major public health problem.

Adequate nutrition is an indispensable component of prenatal care for adolescents and can substantially improve the outlook for both mother and infant. To support the needs of both mother and fetus, a pregnant teenager with a BMI in the normal range is encouraged to gain about 35 pounds to reduce the likelihood of a low-birthweight infant. As mentioned earlier, however, compared with older mothers, the lifetime risk of postpartum weight retention in young adolescents may be far greater.[73] Researchers agree that optimal weight gain recommendations for pregnant adolescents need focused attention. Meanwhile, pregnant and lactating adolescents would do well to follow the eating pattern presented in Table 1-4 (on p. 15) for a kcalorie level that will support adequate, but not excessive, weight gain.

IN SUMMARY

▪ Pregnant adolescents have extraordinarily high nutrient needs and an increased likelihood of problem pregnancies.

▪ Proper nutrition and adequate weight gain are especially important in reducing the risk of poor pregnancy outcome in adolescents.

11.2 Breastfeeding

LO 11.2 Summarize the nutrient needs of women during lactation and contraindications to breastfeeding.

The AAP recommends that infants receive breast milk for at least the first 12 months of life and beyond for as long as mutually desired by mother and child.[74] The Academy of Nutrition and Dietetics (AND) advocates breastfeeding for the nutritional health it confers on the infant as well as for the physiological, social, economic, and other benefits it offers the mother (see Table 11-8).[75] The AAP and the AND recognize **exclusive breastfeeding** for 6 months and breastfeeding with complementary foods for at least 12 months as an optimal feeding pattern for infants.[76] Breast milk's unique nutrient composition and protective factors promote optimal infant health and development. The only acceptable alternative to breast milk is iron-fortified

TABLE 11-8 Benefits of Breastfeeding

For Infants

▪ Provides the appropriate composition and balance of nutrients with high bioavailability

▪ Provides hormones that promote physiological development

▪ Improves cognitive development

▪ Protects against a variety of infections and illnesses

▪ May protect against some chronic diseases—such as diabetes (both types), obesity, atherosclerosis, asthma, and hypertension—later in life

▪ Protects against food allergies

▪ Supports healthy weight

▪ Reduces the risk of SIDS

For Mothers

▪ Contracts the uterus

▪ Delays the return of regular ovulation, thus lengthening birth intervals (this is not, however, a dependable method of contraception)

▪ Conserves iron stores (by prolonging amenorrhea)

▪ May protect against breast and ovarian cancer and reduce the risk of diabetes (type 2)

Other

▪ Cost and time savings from not needing medical treatment for childhood illnesses or leaving work to care for sick infants

▪ Cost and time savings from not needing to purchase and prepare formula (even after adjusting for added foods in the diet of a lactating mother)

▪ Environmental savings for society from not needing to manufacture, package, and ship formula and dispose of the packaging

exclusive breastfeeding: an infant's consumption of human milk with no supplementation of any type (no water, no juice, no nonhuman milk, and no foods) except for vitamins, minerals, and medications.

formula. Adequate nutrition of the mother supports successful lactation, and without it, lactation is likely to falter or fail. Health care professionals play an important role in providing encouragement and accurate information on breastfeeding.

Nutrition during Lactation

By continuing to eat nutrient-dense foods, not restricting weight gain unduly, and enjoying ample food and fluid at frequent intervals throughout lactation, the mother who chooses to breastfeed her infant will be nutritionally prepared to do so. An inadequate diet does not support the stamina, patience, and self-confidence that nursing an infant demands. Figure 11-4 (on p. 292) shows how a lactating woman's nutrient needs differ from those of a nonpregnant woman, and Table 11-2 (on p. 293) presents a sample menu that meets those needs.

A woman who decides to breastfeed provides her infant with a full array of nutrients and protective factors to support optimal health and development.

Energy A nursing woman produces about 25 ounces of milk a day, with considerable variation from woman to woman and in the same woman from time to time, depending primarily on the infant's demand for milk. Producing this milk costs a woman almost 500 kcalories per day above her regular need during the first 6 months of lactation. To meet this energy need, the woman is advised to eat foods providing an extra 330 kcalories each day. The other 170 kcalories can be drawn from the fat stores she accumulated during pregnancy. During the second 6 months of lactation, an additional 400 kcalories each day are recommended. The food energy consumed by the nursing mother should carry with it abundant nutrients. Severe energy restriction hinders milk production and can compromise the mother's health.

Weight Loss After the birth of the infant, many women actively try to lose the extra weight and body fat they accumulated during pregnancy. How much weight a woman retains after pregnancy depends on her gestational weight gain and the duration and intensity of breastfeeding. Many women who follow recommendations for gestational weight gain and breastfeeding can readily return to prepregnancy weight by 6 months. Neither the quality nor the quantity of breast milk is adversely affected by moderate weight loss, and infants grow normally.

Women often choose to be physically active to lose weight and improve fitness, and this is compatible with breastfeeding and infant growth.[77] A gradual weight loss (1 pound per week) is safe and does not reduce milk output. Too large an energy deficit, however, especially soon after birth, will inhibit lactation.

Vitamins and Minerals A question often raised is whether a mother's milk may lack a nutrient if she fails to get enough in her diet. The answer differs from one nutrient to the next, but, in general, nutritional deprivation of the mother reduces the *quantity,* not the *quality,* of her milk. Women can produce milk with adequate protein, carbohydrate, fat, folate, and most minerals, even when their own supplies are limited. For these nutrients, milk quality is maintained at the expense of maternal stores. This is most evident in the case of calcium: dietary calcium has no effect on the calcium concentration of breast milk, but maternal bones lose some of their density during lactation if calcium intakes are inadequate.[78] Such losses are generally made up quickly when lactation ends, and breastfeeding has no long-term harmful effects on women's bones. The nutrients in breast milk that are most likely to decline in response to prolonged inadequate intakes are the vitamins—especially vitamins B_6, B_{12}, A, and D. Vitamin supplementation of undernourished women appears to help normalize the vitamin concentrations in their milk and may be beneficial.

Water The volume of breast milk produced depends on how much milk the infant demands, not on how much fluid the mother drinks. The nursing mother is nevertheless advised to drink plenty of liquids each day (about 13 cups) to protect herself from

Ellen Cassidy is a 24-year-old woman who is 4 months pregnant. This is her first pregnancy, and she is eager to learn how to feed herself during pregnancy as well as her infant after birth. She is 5 feet 3 inches tall and currently weighs 150 pounds. Her prepregnancy weight was 148 pounds. Ellen is very concerned about her 2-pound weight gain.

1. Consult the BMI table (inside back cover), and using the "Healthy Weight" section, find a healthy weight in the middle of the range appropriate for a woman of Ellen's height.

2. Do you think that Ellen's weight at the start of her pregnancy was appropriate for her height? Why or why not? Should Ellen be concerned about her 2-pound weight gain? Why or why not?

3. What advice should you give Ellen about her weight gain during pregnancy? What other dietary advice would you give her?

4. Discuss methods of infant feeding with Ellen and describe some of the advantages breastfeeding would offer her. What advice will you give Ellen if she decides to breastfeed?

dehydration. To help themselves remember to drink enough liquid, many women make a habit of drinking a glass of milk, juice, or water each time the infant nurses as well as at mealtimes.

Particular Foods Foods with strong or spicy flavors (such as onions or garlic) may alter the flavor of breast milk. A sudden change in the taste of the milk may annoy some infants, whereas familiar flavors may enhance enjoyment. Flavors imparted to breast milk by the mother's diet can influence the infant's later food preferences.[79] A mother who is breastfeeding her infant is advised to eat whatever nutritious foods she chooses. Then, if a particular food seems to cause the infant discomfort, she can try eliminating that food from her diet for a few days and see if the problem goes away.

Current evidence does not support a major role for maternal dietary restrictions during lactation to prevent or delay the onset of food allergy in infants.[80] Generally, infants with a strong family history of food allergies benefit from breastfeeding.[81]

The case study in Box 11-1 presents a woman who is 4 months pregnant. Answering the questions offers practice in thinking through some of the issues related to pregnancy and breastfeeding.

Contraindications to Breastfeeding

Some substances impair maternal milk production or enter the breast milk and interfere with infant development. Some medical conditions prohibit breastfeeding.

Alcohol Alcohol easily enters breast milk and can adversely affect the production, volume, composition, and ejection of breast milk as well as overwhelm an infant's immature alcohol-degrading system.[82] Alcohol concentration in breast milk peaks within one hour after ingestion of even moderate amounts (equivalent to a can of beer). It may alter the taste of the milk unfavorably such that the nursing infant may, in protest, drink less milk than normal.

Tobacco and Caffeine Many women who quit smoking during pregnancy relapse after delivery. Lactating women who smoke produce less milk, and milk with a lower fat content, than do nonsmokers.[83] Consequently, infants of smokers gain less weight than infants of nonsmokers.

A lactating woman who smokes not only transfers nicotine and other chemicals to her infant via her breast milk but may also expose the infant to sidestream smoke. Infants who are "smoked over" experience a wide array of health problems—poor growth, hearing impairment, vomiting, breathing difficulties, and even unexplained death.[84] Health care professionals should actively discourage smoking by lactating women.

Excessive caffeine can make an infant jittery and wakeful. As during pregnancy, caffeine consumption during lactation should be moderate.

Medications and Illicit Drugs Many prescription medications do not reach nursing infants in sufficient quantities to affect them adversely and so have no impact on breastfeeding. Other drugs are incompatible with breastfeeding, either because they are secreted into the milk and can harm the infant or because they suppress lactation.[85] A nursing mother should consult with the prescribing physician before taking medicines or even herbal supplements—herbs may have unpredictable effects on breastfeeding infants. If a nursing mother must take medication that is secreted in breast milk and is known to affect the infant, then breastfeeding must be put off for the duration of treatment. Meanwhile, the flow of milk can be sustained by pumping the breasts and discarding the milk. Breastfeeding is also contraindicated if the mother uses illicit drugs. Breast milk can deliver such high doses of illicit drugs as to cause irritability, tremors, hallucinations, and even death in infants.

Many women wonder about using oral contraceptives during lactation. Those that combine the hormones estrogen and progestin seem to suppress milk output, lower the nitrogen content of the milk, and shorten the duration of breastfeeding. In contrast, progestin-only pills have no effect on breast milk or breastfeeding and are considered appropriate for lactating women.[86]

Maternal Illness If a woman has an ordinary cold, she can go on nursing without worry. If susceptible, the infant will catch it from her anyway, and, thanks to immunological protection, a breastfed baby may be less susceptible than a formula-fed infant would be. A woman who has active, infectious tuberculosis should not breastfeed, but she can resume or begin once she has been treated and it is documented that she is no longer infectious.[87]

The human immunodeficiency virus (HIV), responsible for causing AIDS, can be passed from an infected mother to her infant during pregnancy, at birth, or through breast milk, especially during the early months of breastfeeding. In developed countries such as the United States, where safe alternatives are available, HIV-positive women should not breastfeed their infants.[88]

Throughout the world, breastfeeding prevents millions of infant deaths each year. In developing countries, where the feeding of inappropriate or contaminated formulas causes more than 1 million infant deaths annually, breastfeeding can be critical to infant survival. Thus, the question of whether HIV-infected women in developing countries should breastfeed comes down to a delicate balance between risks and benefits. For these women, the most appropriate infant-feeding option depends on individual circumstances, including the health status of the mother and the local situation, as well as the health services, counseling, and support available. The World Health Organization (WHO) recommends exclusive breastfeeding for infants of HIV-infected women for the first 6 months of life unless replacement feeding is acceptable, feasible, affordable, sustainable, and safe for mothers and their infants before that time. Alternatively, HIV-exposed infants may be protected by receiving antiretroviral treatment while being breastfed.

IN SUMMARY

▌ The lactating woman needs enough energy and nutrients to produce about 25 ounces of milk a day. She also needs extra fluid.

▌ Alcohol, smoking, caffeine, and drugs may reduce milk production or enter breast milk and impair infant development.

▌ Some maternal illnesses are incompatible with breastfeeding.

Nutrition Assessment Checklist FOR PREGNANT AND LACTATING WOMEN

Medical History

Check the medical record for:

- Alcohol or illicit drug abuse
- Chronic diseases
- Gestational diabetes
- History of previous pregnancies (number, intervals, outcomes, multiple births, gestational age, and birth weights)
- Hypertension
- Neural tube defect in an infant born previously
- Preeclampsia

Note risk factors for complications during pregnancy, including:

- Cigarette smoking
- Food faddism
- Lactose intolerance
- Low socioeconomic status
- Significant or prolonged vomiting
- Very young or old age
- Weight-loss dieting

Note any complaints of:

- Constipation
- Heartburn
- Morning sickness

Medications

For pregnant women who are using drug therapy for medical conditions, note:

- Potential for contraindication to breastfeeding
- GI-tract side effects that might reduce food intake or change nutrient needs

Dietary Intake

For all pregnant and lactating women, especially those considered at risk nutritionally, assess the diet for:

- Total energy
- Protein
- Calcium, phosphorus, magnesium, iron, and zinc
- Folate and vitamin B_{12}
- Vitamin D

Anthropometric Data

Measure baseline height and weight:

- Prepregnancy weight

Reassess weight at each medical check-up and determine whether gains are appropriate. Note:

- Weight gain during pregnancy
- Gestational age

Laboratory Tests

Monitor the following laboratory tests for pregnant women:

- Hemoglobin, hematocrit, or other tests of iron status
- Blood glucose

Physical Signs

Blood pressure measurement is routine in physical exams but is especially important for pregnant women. Look for physical signs of:

- Iron deficiency
- Edema
- Protein-energy malnutrition
- Folate deficiency

Clinical Applications

1. Consider the different factors in a pregnant woman's history that can affect her nutrition status and the outcome of her pregnancy. Describe what steps you would take to remedy potential problems for the following clients:

   a. A 15-year-old adolescent of low socioeconomic status is in her first trimester of pregnancy. She began the pregnancy at a normal, healthy weight, but her weight gain during pregnancy so far has been less than expected. Her favorite beverages are soft drinks; her favorite foods are French fries and boxed macaroni and cheese.

   b. A lactose-intolerant, 22-year-old pregnant woman has been eating a vegan diet for the past year or so. She began the pregnancy slightly underweight (BMI = 18.4), but her weight gain has been adequate and consistent during the 4 months of her pregnancy. She complains of feeling tired all the time.

2. What information would you give to a pregnant woman who is considering breastfeeding her infant, but isn't quite sure why she should?

Self Check

1. The most important single predictor of an infant's future health and survival is:
   a. the infant's birth weight.
   b. the infant's iron status at birth.
   c. the mother's weight at delivery.
   d. the mother's prepregnancy weight.

2. A mother's prepregnancy nutrition is important to a healthy pregnancy because it determines the development of:
   a. the largest baby possible.
   b. adequate maternal iron stores.
   c. an adequate fat supply for the mother.
   d. healthy support tissues—the placenta, amniotic sac, umbilical cord, and uterus.

3. A pregnant woman needs an extra 450 calories above the allowance for nonpregnant women during which trimester(s)?
   a. First
   b. Second
   c. Third
   d. First, second, and third

4. Two nutrients needed in large amounts during pregnancy for rapid cell proliferation are:
   a. vitamin B_{12} and vitamin C.
   b. calcium and vitamin B_6.
   c. folate and vitamin B_{12}.
   d. copper and zinc.

5. For a woman who is at the appropriate weight for height and is carrying a single fetus, the recommended weight gain during pregnancy is:
   a. 40 to 60 pounds.
   b. 25 to 35 pounds.
   c. 10 to 20 pounds.
   d. 20 to 40 pounds.

6. Rewards of physical activity during pregnancy may include:
   a. weight loss.
   b. decreased incidence of pica.
   c. relief from morning sickness.
   d. reduced stress and easier labor.

7. During pregnancy, the combination of high blood pressure and protein in the urine signals:
   a. jaundice.
   b. preeclampsia.
   c. gestational diabetes.
   d. gestational hypertension.

8. Which of the following preventative measures should pregnant women take to avoid contracting listeriosis?
   a. Choose soft rather than aged cheeses.
   b. Avoid pasteurized milk.
   c. Thoroughly heat hot dogs.
   d. Avoid raw fruits and vegetables.

9. To facilitate lactation, a mother needs:
   a. about 5000 kcalories a day.
   b. adequate nutrition and fluid intake.
   c. vitamin and mineral supplements.
   d. a glass of wine or beer before each feeding.

10. A woman who breastfeeds her infant should drink plenty of water to:
    a. produce more milk.
    b. suppress lactation.
    c. prevent dehydration.
    d. dilute nutrient concentrations.

Answers to these questions can be found in Appendix H.

Notes

1. J. C. Sadeu and coauthors, Alcohol, drugs, caffeine, tobacco, and environmental contaminant exposure: Reproductive health consequences and clinical implications, *Critical Reviews in Toxicology* 40 (2010): 633–652.

2. T. A. Simas and coauthors, Prepregnancy weight, gestational weight gain, and risk of growth affected neonates, *Journal of Women's Health* 21 (2012): 410–417.

3. M. R. Skilton and coauthors, Fetal growth, omega-3 (n-3) fatty acids, and progression of subclinical atherosclerosis: Preventing fetal origins of disease? The Cardiovascular Risk in Young Finns Study, *American Journal of Clinical Nutrition* 97 (2013): 58–65; A. F. M. van Abeelen and

coauthors, Survival effects of prenatal famine exposure, *American Journal of Clinical Nutrition* 95 (2012): 179–183; J. L. Tarry-Adkins and S. E. Ozanne, Mechanisms of early life programming: Current knowledge and future directions, *American Journal of Clinical Nutrition* 94 (2011): 1765S–1771S; G. C. Burdge and K. A. Lillycrop, Nutrition, epigenetics, and developmental plasticity: Implications for understanding human disease, *Annual Review of Nutrition* 30 (2010): 315–339.

4. A. Lahat and coauthors, ADHD among young adults born at extremely low birth weight: The role of fluid intelligence in childhood, *Frontiers in Psychology* 19 (2014): 446; S. K. Berglund and coauthors, Effects of iron supplementation of LBW

infants on cognition and behavior at 3 years, *Pediatrics* 131 (2013): 47–55; P. Munck and coauthors, Stability of cognitive outcome from 2 to 5 years of age in very low birth weight children, *Pediatrics* 129 (2012): 503–508.

5. T. J. Mathews and M. F. MacDorman, Infant mortality statistics from the 2010 period linked birth/infant death data set, *National Vital Statistics Reports* 62, December 18, 2013.

6. Position of the Academy of Nutrition and Dietetics: Nutrition and lifestyle for a healthy pregnancy outcome, *Journal of the Academy of Nutrition and Dietetics* 114 (2014): 1099–1103; N. Kozuki, A. C. Lee, and J. Katz, Moderate to severe, but not mild, maternal anemia is associated with increased risk

of small-for gestational-age outcomes, *Journal of Nutrition* 142 (2012): 358–362.

7. R. Retnakaran and coauthors, Effect of maternal weight, adipokines, glucose intolerance and lipids on infant birth weight among women without gestational diabetes mellitus, *Canadian Medical Association Journal*, 184 (2012): 1353–1360.

8. A. A. Mamun and coauthors, Associations of maternal pre-pregnancy obesity and excess pregnancy weight gains with adverse pregnancy outcomes and length of hospital stay, *BMC Pregnancy and Childbirth* 11 (2011): 62.

9. Position of the American Dietetic Association and American Society for Nutrition, Obesity, reproduction, and pregnancy outcomes, *Journal of the American Dietetic Association* 109 (2009): 918–927.

10. Mamun and coauthors, 2011; Position of the American Dietetic Association and American Society for Nutrition, 2009.

11. A. Correa and J. Marcinkevage, Prepregnancy obesity and the risk of birth defects: An update, *Nutrition Reviews* 71 (2013): S68–S77; J. L. Mills and coauthors, Maternal obesity and congenital heart defects: A population-based study, *American Journal of Clinical Nutrition* 91 (2010): 1543–1549.

12. M. Desforges and C. P. Sibley, Placental nutrient supply and fetal growth, *The International Journal of Developmental Biology* 54 (2010): 377–390.

13. van Abeelen and coauthors, 2012; Tarry-Adkins and Ozanne, 2011; M. L. de Gusmão Correia and coauthors, Developmental origins of health and disease: Experimental and human evidence of fetal programming for metabolic syndrome, *Journal of Human Hypertension* 26 (2012): 405–419L. C. Schulz, The Dutch hunger winter and the developmental origins of health and disease, *Proceedings of the National Academy of Sciences* 107 (2010): 16757–16758.

14. Standing Committee on the Scientific Evaluation of Dietary Reference Intakes, Food and Nutrition Board, Institute of Medicine, *Dietary Reference Intakes for Energy, Carbohydrate, Fiber, Fat, Fatty Acids, Cholesterol, Protein, and Amino Acids* (Washington, D.C.: National Academies Press, 2005), pp. 185–194.

15. M. L. Blumfield and coauthors, Systematic review and meta-analysis of energy and macronutrient intakes during pregnancy in developed countries, *Nutrition Reviews* 70 (2012): 322–336.

16. L. D. Brown and coauthors, Maternal amino acid supplementation for intrauterine growth restriction, *Frontiers in Bioscience* 3 (2011): 428–444.

17. P. Haggarty, Fatty acid supply to the human fetus, *Annual Review of Nutrition* 30 (2010): 237–255.

18. A. S. de Souza, F. S. Fernandes, and M. Das Gracas Tavares do Carmo, Effects of maternal malnutrition and postnatal nutritional rehabilitation on brain fatty acids, learning, and memory, *Nutrition Reviews* 69 (2011): 132–144.

19. Centers for Disease Control and Prevention, Birth defects COUNT, available at www.cdc.gov/ncbddd/folicacid/global/html, updated December 23, 2013.

20. Centers for Disease Control and Prevention, available at www.cdc.gov/ncbddd/folicacid/global/html, updated December 23, 2013.

21. S. H. Blanton and coauthors, Folate pathway and nonsyndromic cleft lip and palate, *Birth Defects Research. Part A, Clinical and Molecular Teratology* 91 (2011): 50–60.

22. P. M. Brannon and M. F. Picciano, Vitamin D in Pregnancy and lactation in humans, *Annual Review of Nutrition* 31 (2011): 89–115.

23. Committee on Dietary Reference Intakes, *Dietary Reference Intakes for Calcium and Vitamin D* (Washington, D.C.: National Academies Press, 2011).

24. A. Merewood and coauthors, Widespread vitamin D deficiency in urban Massachusetts newborns and their mothers, *Pediatrics* 125 (2010): 640–647.

25. Committee on Dietary Reference Intakes, 2011, pp. 242–250.

26. A. N. Hacker, E. B. Fung, and J. C. King, Role of calcium during pregnancy: maternal and fetal needs, *Nutrition Reviews* 70 (2012): 397–409.

27. H. J. McArdle and coauthors, Role of the placenta in regulation of fetal iron status, *Nutrition Reviews* 69 (2011): S17–S22.

28. T. O. Scholl, Maternal iron status: Relation to fetal growth, length of gestation, and iron endowment of the neonate, *Nutrition Reviews* 69 (2011): S23–S29.

29. Scholl, 2011.

30. J. M. Catov and coauthors, Periconceptional multivitamin use and risk of preterm or small-for-gestational-age births in the Danish National Birth Cohort, *American Journal of Clinical Nutrition* 94 (2011): 906–912.

31. WIC, The Special Supplemental Nutrition Program for Women, Infants, and Children, available at www.fns.usda.gov/fns.

32. Position of the American Dietetic Association and American Society for Nutrition, 2009.

33. Position of the American Dietetic Association and American Society for Nutrition, 2009.

34. Position of the American Dietetic Association and American Society for Nutrition, 2009.

35. Institute of Medicine, *Weight Gain during Pregnancy: Reexamining the Guidelines* (Washington, D.C.: The National Academies Press, 2009).

36. C. K. McClure and coauthors, Associations between gestational weight gain and BMI, abdominal adiposity, and traditional measures of cardiometabolic risk in mothers 8 y postpartum, *American Journal of Clinical Nutrition* 98 (2013): 1218–1225; A. M. Siega-Riz and G. L. Gray, Gestational weight gain recommendations in the context of the obesity epidemic, *Nutrition Reviews* 71 (2013): S26–S30; A. A. Mamun and coauthors, Association of excess weight gain during pregnancy with long-term maternal overweight and obesity: Evidence from 21 y postpartum follow-up, *American Journal of Clinical Nutrition* 91 (2010): 1336–1341; Position of the American Dietetic Association and American Society for Nutrition, 2009.

37. L. M. Mudd and coauthors, Health benefits of physical activity during pregnancy: An international perspective, *Medicine and Science in Sports and Exercise* 45 (2013): 268–277; K. Melzer and coauthors, Physical activity and pregnancy: Cardiovascular adaptations, recommendations and pregnancy outcomes, *Sports Medicine* 40 (2010): 493–507.

38. S. M. Ruchat and coauthors, Nutrition and exercise reduce excessive weight gain in normal-weight pregnant women, *Medicine and Science in Sports and Exercise* 44 (2012): 1419–1426; M. F. Mottola and coauthors, Nutrition and exercise prevent excess weight gain in over-weight pregnant women, *Medicine and Science in Sports and Exercise* 42 (2010): 265–272.

39. R. W. Corbett and K. M. Kolasa, Pica and weight gain in pregnancy, *Nutrition Today* 49 (2014): 101–108; L. B. Lopez and coauthors, Characteristics of pica practice during pregnancy in a sample of Argentine women, *Journal of Obstetrics and Gynaecology* 32 (2012): 150–153; S. L. Young, Pica in pregnancy: New ideas about an old condition, *Annual Review of Nutrition* 30 (2010): 403–422.

40. Corbett and Kolasa, 2014; Young, 2010.

41. J. R. Niebyl, Nausea and vomiting in pregnancy, *New England Journal of Medicine* 363 (2010): 1544–1550.

42. A. Matthews and coauthors, Interventions for nausea and vomiting in early pregnancy, *Cochrane Database of Systemic Reviews* 8 (2010): CD007575.

43. J. L. Kitzmiller and coauthors, Preconception care for women with diabetes and prevention of major congenital malformations, *Birth Defects Research Part A: Clinical and Molecular Teratology* 88 (2010): 791–803.

44. American Diabetes Association, Position statement, Standards of medical care in diabetes—2014, *Diabetes Care* 37 (2014): S14–S80.

45. S. F. Ehrlich and coauthors, Change in body mass index between pregnancies and the risk of gestational diabetes in a second pregnancy, *Obstetrics and Gynecology* 117 (2011): 1323–1330.

46. American Diabetes Association, Position statement, 2014.

47. R. Mustafa and coauthors, A comprehensive review of hypertension in pregnancy, *Journal of Pregnancy*, 2012, doi: 10.1155/2012/105918.

48. E. W. Seely and J. Ecker, Chronic hypertension in pregnancy, *New England Journal of Medicine* 365 (2011): 439–446.

49. Seely and Ecker, 2011.

50. A. Jeyabalan, Epidemiology of preeclampsia: Impact of obesity, *Nutrition Reviews* 71 (2013): S18–S25.

51. Jeyabalan, 2013.

52. Jeyabalan, 2013.

53. V. T. Tong and coauthors, Trends in smoking before, during, and after pregnancy—Pregnancy Risk Assessment Monitoring System, United States, 40 sites, 2000–2010, *Morbidity and Mortality Weekly Report* 62 (2013): 1–19.

54. C. Metayer and coauthors, Tobacco smoke exposure and the risk of childhood acute lymphoblastic and myeloid leukemias by cytogenetic subtype, *Cancer Epidemiology, Biomarkers, and Prevention* 22 (2013): 1600–1611.

55. C. C. Geerts and coauthors, Parental smoking and vascular damage in their 5-year-old children, *Pediatrics* 129 (2010): 45–54.

56. H. Burke and coauthors, Prenatal and passive smoke exposure and incidence of asthma and

wheeze: Systematic review and meta-analysis, *Pediatrics* 129 (2012): 735–744; A. Bjerg and coauthors, A strong synergism of low birth weight and prenatal smoking on asthma in schoolchildren, *Pediatrics* 127 (2011): e905–e912.

57. J. M. Van Nguyen and H. A. Abenhaim, Sudden infant death syndrome: Review for the obstetric care provider, *American Journal of Perinatology* 30 (2013): 703–714; Tong and coauthors, 2013; F. L. Trachtenberg and coauthors, Risk factor changes for sudden infant death syndrome after initiation of back-to-sleep campaign, *Pediatrics* 129 (2012): 630–638;

58. C. T. McEvoy and coauthors, Vitamin C supplementation for pregnant smoking women and pulmonary function in their newborn infants, *Journal of the American Medical Association* 311 (2014): 2074–2082.

59. A. Gunnerbeck and coauthors, Relationship of maternal snuff use and cigarette smoking with neonatal apnea, *Pediatrics* 128 (2011): 503–509.

60. J. P. Ackerman, T. Riggings, and M. M. Black, A review of the effects of prenatal cocaine exposure among school-aged children, *Pediatrics* 125 (2010): 554–565.

61. S. Buckingham-Howes and coauthors, Systematic review of prenatal cocaine exposure and adolescent development, *Pediatrics* 131 (2013): e1917–e1936.

62. A. Bloomingdale and coauthors, A qualitative study of fish consumption during pregnancy, *American Journal of Clinical Nutrition* 92 (2010): 1234–1240.

63. United States Food and Drug Administration, New advice: Some women and young children should eat more fish, www.fda.gov/ForConsumers /ConsumerUpdates/ucm397443.htm, released June 18, 2014.

64. Position of the Academy of Nutrition and Dietetics, Use of nutritive and nonnutritive sweeteners, *Journal of the Academy of Nutrition and Dietetics* 112 (2012): 739–758.

65. R. Bakker and coauthors, Maternal caffeine intake, blood pressure, and the risk of hypertensive complications during pregnancy: The Generation R study, *American Journal of Hypertension* 24 (2011): 421–428; D. C. Greenwood and coauthors, Caffeine intake during pregnancy, late miscarriage

and stillbirth, *European Journal of Epidemiology* 25 (2010): 275–280.

66. R. Bakker and coauthors, Maternal caffeine intake from coffee and tea, fetal growth, and the risks of adverse birth outcomes: The Generation R Study, *American Journal of Clinical Nutrition* 91 (2010): 1691–1698.

67. M. Jarosz, R. Wierzejska, and M. Siuba, Maternal caffeine intake and its effect on pregnancy outcomes, *European Journal of Obstetrics and Gynecology and Reproductive Biology* 160 (2012): 156–160.

68. E. P. Riley, M. A. Infante, and K. R. Warren, Fetal alcohol spectrum disorders: An overview, *Neuropsychological Review* 21 (2011): 73–80; K. L. Jones and coauthors, Fetal alcohol spectrum disorders: Extending the range of structural defects, *American Journal of Medical Genetics* 152A (2010): 2731–2735.

69. Centers for Disease Control, *Fetal Alcohol Spectrum* Disorders, www.cdc.gov/ncbddd/fasd/data .html, updated May 23, 2014.

70. C. M. Marchetta and coauthors, Alcohol use and binge drinking among women of childbearing age—United States, 2006–2010, *Morbidity and Mortality Weekly Report* 61 (2012): 534–538.

71. B. E. Hamilton and S. J. Ventura, Birth rates for U.S. teenagers reach historic lows for all age and ethnic groups, *NCHS Data Brief*, no. 89 (Hyattsville, MD: National Center for Health statistics, 2012).

72. One in 5 teens giving birth already has a child, *Journal of the American Medical Association* 309 (2013): 1987; U.S. Department of Health and Human Services, Trends in teen pregnancy and childbearing, www.hhs.gov/ash/oah /adolescent-health-topics/reproductive-health /teen-pregnancy/trends.html, updated June 18, 2014.

73. B. E. Gould Rothberg and coauthors, Gestational weight gain and subsequent postpartum weight loss among young, low-income, ethnic minority women, *American Journal of Obstetrics and Gynecology* 204 (2011): e1–e11; M. M. Thame and coauthors, Weight retention within the puerperium in adolescents: A risk factor for obesity? *Public Health Nutrition* 13 (2010): 283–288.

74. Breastfeeding, in Committee on Nutrition, American Academy of Pediatrics, *Pediatric Nutrition,* 7th ed., ed. R. E. Kleinman (Elk Grove Village, Ill.: American Academy of Pediatrics,

2014), pp. 41–59; American Academy of Pediatrics, Policy statement: Breastfeeding and the use of human milk, *Pediatrics* 129 (2012): e827–e841, available at www.pediatrics.org/content/129/3 /e827.full.

75. Position of the American Dietetic Association: Promoting and supporting breastfeeding, *Journal of the American Dietetic Association* 109 (2009): 1926–1942.

76. American Academy of Pediatrics, 2012; Position of the American Dietetic Association: Promoting and supporting breastfeeding, 2009.

77. A. J. Daly and coauthors, Maternal exercise and growth in breastfed infants: A meta-analysis of randomized controlled trials, *Pediatrics* 130 (2012): 108–114.

78. Committee on Dietary Reference Intakes, 2011, pp. 256–257.

79. J. A. Mennella and J. C. Trabulsi, Complementary foods and flavor experiences: Setting the foundation, *Annals of Nutrition and Metabolism* 60 (2012): 40–50; G. Beauchanp and J. A. Mennella, Flavor perception in human infants: Development and functional significance, *Digestion* 83 (2011): 1–6.

80. D. M. Fleischer and coauthors, Primary prevention of allergic disease through nutritional interventions, *Journal of Allergy and Clinical Immunology: In Practice,* 1 (2013): 29–36.

81. Fleischer and coauthors, 2013.

82. American Academy of Pediatrics, 2012.

83. P. Bachour and coauthors, Effects of smoking mother's age, body mass index, and parity number on lipid, protein, and secretory immunoglobulin A concentration of human milk, *Breastfeeding Medicine,* 7 (2012): 179–188.

84. G. Liebrechts-Akkerman and coauthors, Postnatal parental smoking: An important risk factor for SIDS, *European Journal of Pediatrics* 170 (2011): 1281–1291.

85. American Academy of Pediatrics, 2012.

86. N. Kapp, K. Curtis, and K. Nanda, Progestogen-only contraceptive use among breastfeeding women: A systematic review, *Contraception* 82 (2010): 17–37.

87. American Academy of Pediatrics, 2012.

88. American Academy of Pediatrics, 2012.

LO 11.3 Identify factors that encourage or discourage women to breastfeed their infants and describe approaches for initiating and resolving problems during breastfeeding.

As discussed in Chapter 11, breastfeeding offers benefits to both mother and infant. The American Academy of Pediatrics (AAP), the Academy of Nutrition and Dietetics, and the Canadian Paediatric Society all advocate breastfeeding as the preferred means of infant feeding.[1] Promotion of breastfeeding is an integral part of the WIC program's nutrition education component. National efforts to promote breastfeeding seem to be working, at least to some extent: the percentage of infants who were ever breastfed rose from 60 percent among those born in 1994 to 77 percent among infants born in 2010.[2] Despite this encouraging trend, by 6 months, breastfeeding rates fall to 49 percent. The AAP and many other health organizations recommend exclusive breastfeeding for the first 6 months of life.[3] Exclusive breastfeeding is defined as an infant's consumption of human milk with no supplementation of any kind (no water, no other type of milk, no juice, and no other foods) except for vitamins, minerals, and medications. The AAP recommends that breastfeeding continue for at least a year and thereafter for as long as mutually desired.[4] In the United States, the prevalence of exclusive breastfeeding at 6 months is low (about 15 percent) and only about one in four infants is still breastfeeding at 1 year of age.[5] Increasing the rates of breastfeeding initiation and duration is one of the goals of *Healthy People 2020:*

> Increase the proportion of infants who are breastfed ever, at 6 months, and at 1 year. Increase the proportion of infants who are breastfed exclusively through 3 months, and through 6 months.[6]

Despite the trend toward increasing breastfeeding, the percentage of mothers choosing to breastfeed their infants and continuing to do so still falls short of goals.

Why don't more women choose to breastfeed their infants?

Many experts cite two major deterrents: infant formula manufacturers' public advertising and promotion of their products and the medical community's failure to encourage breastfeeding. Infant formula manufacturers spend millions of dollars each year marketing their products, often claiming that formula "is like breast milk." Such advertising efforts seem to be working. According to one survey, one out of four people of various ages, races, and socioeconomic backgrounds agrees with the statement "infant formula is as good as breast milk." Infant formula is an appropriate substitute for breast milk when breastfeeding is specifically contraindicated, but for most infants, the benefits of breast milk outweigh those of formula. Despite medical evidence of the benefits of breast milk, medical practice is not always supportive.[7]

As an example of the medical lack of encouragement, some hospitals routinely separate mother and infant soon after birth. The child's first feeding then comes from the bottle rather than the breast. Furthermore, many hospitals send new mothers home with free samples of infant formula. The World Health Organization opposes this practice because it sends a misleading message that medical authorities favor infant formula over breast milk for infants. Even in hospitals where women are encouraged to breastfeed and are supported in doing so, little, if any, assistance is available after hospital discharge when many breastfeeding women still need assistance. Up to half of mothers who initially breastfeed their infants stop within 3 months—seemingly due to lack of knowledge and support.

Women who receive early and repeated breastfeeding information and support breastfeed their infants longer than other women do. Information and instruction are especially important during the *prenatal* period when most women decide whether to breastfeed or to feed formula.[8] Nurses and other health care professionals can play a crucial role in encouraging successful breastfeeding by offering women adequate, accurate information about breastfeeding that permits them to make informed choices. Table NP11-1 lists tips for successful breastfeeding.

If breastfeeding is a natural process, what do mothers need to learn?

Although lactation is an automatic physiological process, breastfeeding requires some learning. This learning is most successful in a supportive environment. It begins with preparatory steps taken before the infant is born.

What are these preparatory steps?

Toward the end of pregnancy and throughout lactation, a woman who intends to breastfeed should stop using soap and lotions on her breasts. The natural secretions of the breasts themselves

---

TABLE NP11-1 Tips for Successful Breastfeeding

▪ Learn about the benefits of breastfeeding.

▪ Initiate breastfeeding within 1 hour of birth.

▪ Ask a health care professional to explain how to breastfeed and how to maintain lactation.

▪ Give newborn infants no food or drink other than breast milk, unless medically indicated.

▪ Breastfeed on demand.

▪ Give no artificial nipples or pacifiers to breastfeeding infants.[a]

▪ Find breastfeeding support groups, books, or websites to help troubleshoot breastfeeding problems.

© 2016 Cengage Learning®

[a]Compared with nonusers, infants who use pacifiers breastfeed less frequently and stop breastfeeding at a younger age.

315

lubricate the nipple area best. A woman who plans to breastfeed should also acquire at least two nursing bras before her infant is born. The bras should provide good support and have drop-flaps so that either breast can be freed for nursing.

How soon after birth should breastfeeding start?

As soon as possible. Immediately after the delivery, for a short period, the infant is intensely alert and intent on suckling. This is the ideal time for the first breastfeeding and facilitates successful lactation.

What does the new mother need to know to continue breastfeeding her infant successfully?

She needs to learn how to relax and position herself so that she and the infant will be comfortable and the infant can breathe freely while nursing. She also needs to understand that infants have a **rooting reflex** that makes them turn toward any touch on the face (see the glossary in Box NP11-1). Consequently, she should touch the infant's cheek to her nipple so that the infant will turn the right way to nurse. The mother can then place four fingers under the breast and her thumb on top to support the breast and present the nipple to the infant. The mother's fingers and thumb should be behind the areola, the colored ring around the nipple, so as not to interfere with the infant latching onto the breast (see Figure NP11-1). With the breast supported, the mother tickles the infant's lips with the breast until the infant's mouth opens wide. The mother can then gently bring the infant forward

---

BOX NP11-1 GLOSSARY OF BREASTFEEDING TERMS

engorgement: overfilling of the breasts with milk.

letdown reflex: the reflex that forces milk to the front of the breast when the infant begins to nurse.

mastitis: infection of a breast.

rooting reflex: a reflex that causes an infant to turn toward whichever cheek is touched, in search of a nipple.

© 2016 Cengage Learning®

FIGURE NP11-1 Infant's Grasp on Mother's Breast
The mother supports the breast with her fingers and thumb behind the areola to present the nipple to the infant. Once the infant latches onto the breast, the infant's lips and gums pump the areola, releasing milk from the mammary glands into the milk ducts that lie beneath the areola.

onto the breast. The nipple must rest well back on the infant's tongue so that the infant's gums will squeeze on the glands that release the milk and swallowing will be effortless. To break the suction, if necessary, the mother can slip a finger between the infant's mouth and her breast.

Does it hurt to have the infant sucking so hard on the breast?

Breastfeeding should not be painful if the infant is positioned correctly. The mother has a **letdown reflex** that forces milk to the front of her breast when the infant begins to nurse, virtually propelling the milk into the infant's mouth. Letdown is necessary for the infant to obtain milk easily, and the mother needs to relax for letdown to occur. The mother who assumes a comfortable position in an environment without interruptions will find it easiest to relax.

How long should the infant be allowed to nurse at each feeding?

Even though the infant obtains about half the milk from the breast during the first 2 or 3 minutes of suckling, and 80 to 90 percent of it within 4 minutes, the infant should be encouraged to breastfeed on the first breast for as long as he or she wishes before being offered the second breast. The suckling itself, as well as the complete removal of milk from the breast, stimulates the mammary glands to produce milk for the next nursing session. Successive sessions should start on alternate breasts to ensure that each breast is emptied regularly. This pattern maintains the same supply and demand for each breast and thus prevents either breast from overfilling.

Infants should be fed "on demand" and not be held to a rigid schedule. The breastfed infant may average 8 to 12 feedings per 24-hour period during the first month or so. Once the mother's milk supply is well established and the infant's capacity has increased, the intervals between feedings will become longer.

What if a mother wants to skip one or two feedings daily—for example, because she works outside the home?

The mother can express breast milk into a bottle ahead of time, properly store the breast milk, and, when needed, substitute the expressed breast milk for a nursing session. Breast milk can be kept refrigerated for 48 hours or frozen. Frozen milk can be kept for 1 month in a freezer attached to a refrigerator or for three to 6 months in a zero-degree deep freezer.[9]

The mother can hand express her breast milk or use one of several different breast pumps available. The bicycle-horn type of manual breast pump is difficult to keep clean and is not recommended. Cylinder-type manual pumps or electric breast pumps are safer and are also more efficient. Alternatively, a mother can substitute formula for those missed feedings and continue to breastfeed at other times.

What about problems associated with breastfeeding such as sore nipples or infection of the breast?

Most problems associated with breastfeeding can be resolved. Many mothers experience sore nipples during the initial days of breastfeeding. Sore nipples need to be treated kindly, but nursing can continue. Improper feeding position is a frequent cause of sore nipples: the mother should make sure the infant is taking the entire nipple and part of the areola onto the tongue. She should nurse on the less sore breast first to get letdown going while the infant is suckling hardest; then she can switch to the sore breast. Between times, she should expose her nipples to light and air to heal them.

Before lactation is well established, when the schedule changes, or when a feeding is missed, the breasts may become full and hard—an uncomfortable condition known as **engorgement.** The infant cannot grasp an engorged nipple and so cannot provide relief by nursing. A gentle massage or warming the breasts with a cloth soaked in warm water or in a shower helps to initiate letdown and to release some of the accumulated milk; then the mother can pump out some of her milk and allow the infant to nurse.

Infection of the breast, known as **mastitis,** is best managed by continuing to breastfeed. By drawing off the milk, the infant helps to relieve pressure in the infected area. The infant is safe because the infection is between the milk-producing glands, not inside them.

Even if everything is going smoothly, the nursing mother should ideally have enough help and support so that she can rest in bed a few hours each day for the first week or so. Successful breastfeeding requires the support of all those who care. This, plus adequate nutrition, ample fluids, fresh air, and physical activity, will do much to enhance the well-being of mother and infant.

Notes

1. Breastfeeding, in *Pediatric Nutrition,* 7th ed., ed. R. E. Kleinman (Elk Grove Village, Ill.: American Academy of Pediatrics, 2014), pp. 41–59; American Academy of Pediatrics, Policy statement: Breastfeeding and the use of human milk, *Pediatrics* 129 (2012): e827–e841, available at www.pediatrics.org /content/129/3/e827.full; Position of the American Dietetic Association: Promoting and supporting breastfeeding, *Journal of the American Dietetic Association* 109 (2009): 1926–1942.

2. Centers for Disease Control and Prevention, *Breastfeeding report card United States/2013*, available at www.cdc.gov /breastfeeding/pdf/2013breastfeedingreportcard.pdf.

3. Breastfeeding, 2014; American Academy of Pediatrics, 2012; Position of the American Dietetic Association: Promoting and supporting breastfeeding, 2009.

4. American Academy of Pediatrics, 2012.

5. J. R. Jones and coauthors, Factors associated with exclusive breastfeeding in the United States, *Pediatrics* 128 (2011): 1117–1125.

6. U. S. Department of Health and Human Services, *Healthy People, 2020* available at www.healthypeople.gov.

7. C. Perrine and coauthors, Vital signs: Hospital practices to support breastfeeding—United States, 2007 and 2009, *Morbidity and Mortality Weekly Report* 60 (2011): 1020–1025.

8. A. M. Stuebe, Enabling women to achieve their breastfeeding goals, *Obstetrics and Gynecology* 123 (2014): 643–652; A. V. Holmes, Establishing successful breastfeeding in the newborn period, *Pediatric Clinics of North America* 60 (2013): 147–166.

9. Breastfeeding beyond infancy, in *American Academy of Pediatrics, New Mother's Guide to Breastfeeding*, ed. J. Y. Meek and W. Yu (New York: Bantam Books, 2011), pp. 158–183.

12

Nutrition through the Life Span: Infancy, Childhood, and Adolescence

12.1 Nutrition of the Infant

LO 12.1 Describe the nutritional needs of infants, the beneficial components of breast milk, and the appropriate foods and feeding practices for infants.

12.2 Nutrition during Childhood

LO 12.2 Explain how children's appetites and nutrient needs reflect their stage of growth, why hunger, iron deficiency, lead poisoning, foods allergies, hyperactivity, and obesity are often concerns during childhood, and how parents and other caregivers can foster healthful eating habits and food choices in children.

12.3 Nutrition during Adolescence

LO 12.3 Describe the nutrient needs of adolescents and some of the challenges in meeting these needs.

12.4 Nutrition in Practice: Childhood Obesity and the Early Development of Chronic Diseases

LO 12.4 Describe the lifestyle factors that can help prevent childhood obesity and the development of type 2 diabetes and heart disease.

The first year of life is a time of phenomenal growth and development. After the first year, a child continues to grow and change, but more slowly. Sound nutrition throughout infancy and childhood promotes normal growth and development; facilitates academic and physical performance; and helps prevent obesity, diabetes, heart disease, cancer, and other degenerative diseases in adulthood. As children enter their teens, a foundation built by years of eating nutritious foods best prepares them to meet the upcoming demands of rapid growth. This chapter examines the special nutrient needs of infants, children, and adolescents.

12.1 Nutrition of the Infant

LO 12.1 Describe the nutritional needs of infants, the beneficial components of breast milk, and the appropriate foods and feeding practices for infants.

Early nutrition affects later development, and early feeding sets the stage for eating habits that will influence nutrition status for a lifetime. Trends change, and experts argue about the fine points, but properly nourishing an infant is relatively simple, overall. The infant initially drinks only breast milk or formula but later begins to eat some foods, as appropriate. Common sense in the selection of infant foods and a nurturing, relaxed environment go far to promote an infant's health and well-being. The remainder of this discussion is devoted to feeding the infant and identifying the nutrients most often deficient in infant diets.

Nutrient Needs during Infancy

An infant grows faster during the first year than ever again, as Figure 12-1 shows. The growth of infants and children directly reflects their nutritional well-being and is an important parameter in assessing their nutrition status. Health care professionals use growth charts to evaluate the growth and development of children from birth to 20 years of age (see Appendix E).

Nutrients to Support Growth An infant's birthweight doubles by about 5 months of age and triples by the age of 1 year, typically reaching 20 to 25 pounds. (Consider that if an adult, starting at 120 pounds, were to do this, the person's weight would increase to 360 pounds in a single year.) The infant's length changes more slowly than weight, increasing about 10 inches from birth to 1 year. By the end of the first year, the growth rate slows considerably. An infant typically gains less than 10 pounds during the second year and grows about 5 inches in height. At the age of 2, healthy children have attained approximately half of their adult height.

Not only do infants grow rapidly, but also, in proportion to body weight, their basal metabolic rate is remarkably high—about twice that of an adult. The rapid growth and metabolism of the infant demand an ample supply of all the nutrients. Of special importance during infancy are the energy nutrients and the vitamins and minerals critical to the growth process, such as vitamin A, vitamin D, and calcium.

Because they are small, infants need smaller *total* amounts of these nutrients than adults do, but as a percentage of body weight, infants need more than twice as much of most nutrients. Infants require about 100 kcalories per kilogram of body weight per day; most adults require fewer than 40 (see Table 12-1 on p. 320). Figure 12-2 (on p. 320) compares a 5-month-old infant's needs (per unit of body weight) with those of an adult man. You can see that differences in vitamin D and iodine, for instance, are extraordinary. Around 6 months of age, energy needs begin to increase less rapidly as the growth rate begins to slow, but some of the energy saved by slower growth is spent on increased activity. When their growth slows, infants spontaneously reduce their energy intakes. Parents should expect

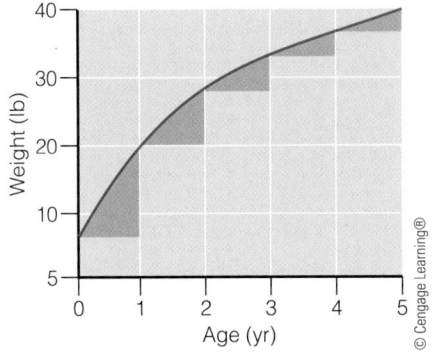

FIGURE 12-1 Weight Gain of Human Infants in Their First 5 Years of Life

In the first year, an infant's birthweight may triple, but over the following several years the rate of weight gain gradually diminishes.

TABLE 12-1 Infant and Adult Heart Rate, Respiration Rate, and Energy Needs Compared

	Infants	Adults
Heart rate (beats/minute)	120 to 140	70 to 80
Respiration rate (breaths/minute)	20 to 40	15 to 20
Energy needs (kcal/body weight)	45/lb (100/kg)	<18/lb (<40/kg)

© Cengage Learning®

their infants to adjust their food intakes downward when appropriate and should not force or coax them to eat more.

Water One of the most important nutrients for infants, as for everyone, is water. The younger a child is, the more of the child's body weight is water. Breast milk or infant formula normally provides enough water to replace fluid losses in a healthy infant. If the environmental temperature is extremely high, however, infants need supplemental water.[1] Because proportionately more of an infant's body water than an adult's is between the cells and in the vascular space, this water is easy to lose. Consequently, conditions that cause rapid fluid loss, such as vomiting or diarrhea, require an electrolyte solution designed for infants.

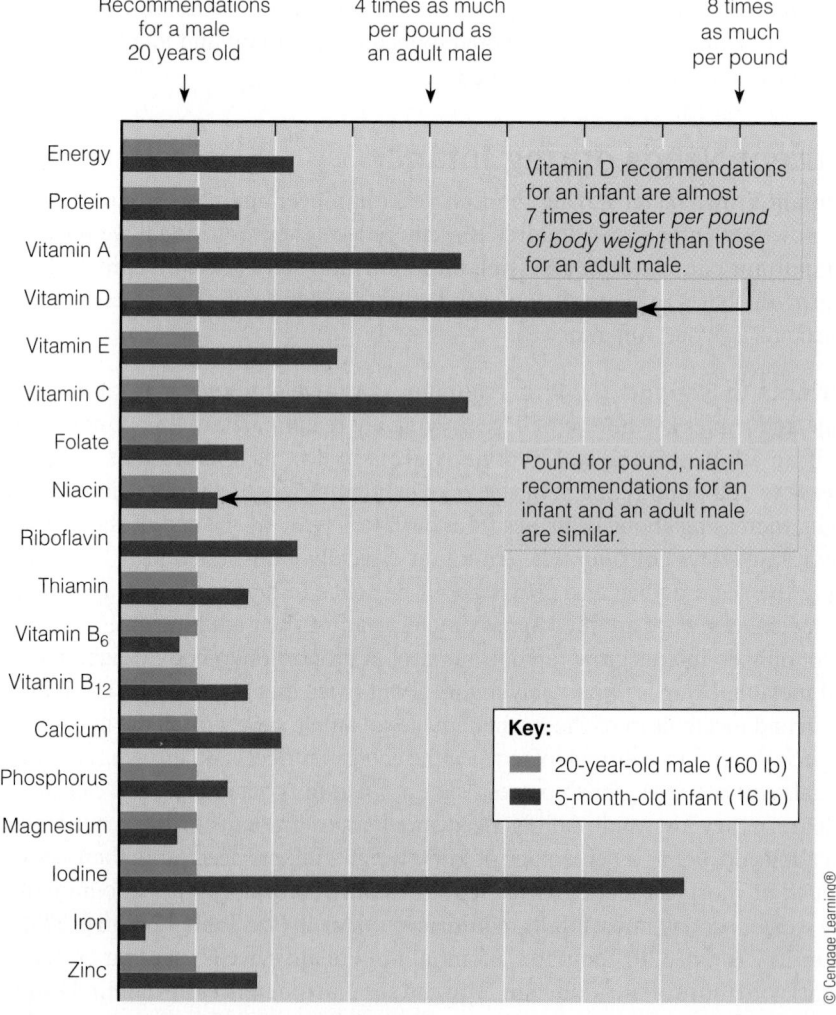

FIGURE 12-2 Nutrient Recommendations for a 5-Month-Old Infant and an Adult Male Compared on the Basis of Body Weight

Infants may be relatively small and inactive, but they use large amounts of energy and nutrients in proportion to their body size to keep all their metabolic processes going.

CHAPTER TWELVE

■ An infant's birthweight doubles by about 5 months of age and triples by 1 year.

■ Infants' rapid growth and development depend on adequate nutrient supplies, including water from breast milk and formula.

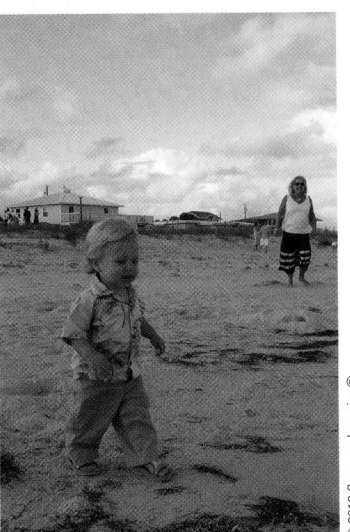

After 6 months of age, energy saved by slower growth is spent on increased activity.

Breast Milk

Breast milk excels as a source of nutrients for the young infant. With the possible exception of vitamin D (discussed later), breast milk provides all the nutrients a healthy infant needs for the first 6 months of life.[2] It provides many other health benefits as well.

Frequency and Duration of Breastfeeding Breast milk is more easily and completely digested than formula, so breastfed infants usually need to eat more frequently than formula-fed infants do. During the first few weeks, approximately 8 to 12 feedings a day—on demand, as soon as the infant shows early signs of hunger such as increased alertness, activity, or suckling motions—promote optimal milk production and infant growth. Crying is a late indicator of hunger.[3] An infant who nurses every two to three hours and sleeps contentedly between feedings is adequately nourished. As the infant gets older, stomach capacity enlarges and the mother's milk production increases, allowing for longer intervals between feedings.

Even though the infant obtains about half the milk from the breast during the first 2 or 3 minutes of suckling, the infant should be encouraged to breastfeed on the first breast for as long as he or she is actively suckling before being offered the second breast. Begin each feeding on the breast offered last. The infant's suckling, as well as the complete removal of milk from the breast, stimulates lactation.

Energy Nutrients The distribution of energy nutrients in breast milk differs dramatically from the balance recommended for adults (see Figure 12-3). Yet, for infants, breast milk is nature's most nearly perfect food, illustrating clearly that people at different stages of life have different nutrient needs.

The carbohydrate in breast milk (and standard infant formula) is lactose. In addition to being easily digested, lactose enhances calcium absorption. The carbohydrate component of breast milk also contains abundant oligosaccharides, which are present only in trace amounts in cow's milk and infant formula made from cow's milk. Human milk oligosaccharides help protect the infant from infection by preventing the binding of pathogens to the infant's intestinal cells.[4]

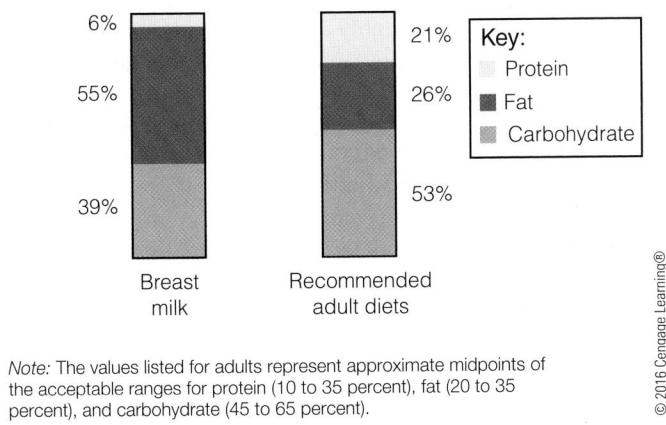

Breast milk: 6% Protein, 55% Fat, 39% Carbohydrate

Recommended adult diets: 21% Protein, 26% Fat, 53% Carbohydrate

Key:
Protein
Fat
Carbohydrate

Note: The values listed for adults represent approximate midpoints of the acceptable ranges for protein (10 to 35 percent), fat (20 to 35 percent), and carbohydrate (45 to 65 percent).

FIGURE 12-3 **Percentages of Energy-Yielding Nutrients in Breast Milk and in Recommended Adult Diets**
The proportions of energy-yielding nutrients in human breast milk differ from those recommended for adults.

Human breast milk contains less protein than cow's milk, but this is actually beneficial because less protein places less stress on the infant's immature kidneys to excrete the major end product of protein metabolism, urea. The protein in breast milk is largely **alpha-lactalbumin**, which is efficiently digested and absorbed.

The lipids in breast milk—and infant formula—provide the main source of energy in the infant's diet. Breast milk contains a generous proportion of the essential fatty acids linoleic acid and linolenic acid, as well as their longer-chain derivatives arachidonic acid and docosahexaenoic acid (DHA). Most formulas today also contain added arachidonic acid and DHA (read the label). Infants can produce some arachidonic acid and DHA from linoleic and linolenic acid, respectively, but some infants may need more than they can make.

As Chapter 3 mentioned, DHA is the most abundant fatty acid in the brain and is also present in the retina of the eye. DHA accumulation in the brain is greatest during fetal development and early infancy.[5] Research has focused on the visual and mental development of breastfed infants and infants fed standard formula with and without DHA added.[6] Results of studies for visual acuity development in term infants are mixed.[7] Factors such as the amount of DHA provided, the sources of the DHA, and the sensitivity of different measures for visual acuity may have contributed to the mixed outcomes. Some of the evidence from studies that have examined the effects of DHA status on cognitive function suggests that DHA supplementation during development can influence certain measures of cognitive function.[8] Studies that follow children beyond infancy, when more detailed tests of cognitive function can be employed, are needed to confirm the importance of DHA for optimal infant and child development.

Vitamins and Minerals With the exception of vitamin D, the vitamin content of the breast milk of a well-nourished mother is ample. Even vitamin C, for which cow's milk is a poor source, is supplied generously. The concentration of vitamin D in breast milk is low, however, and vitamin D deficiency impairs bone mineralization.[9] Vitamin D deficiency is most likely in infants who are not exposed to sunlight daily, have darkly pigmented skin, and receive breast milk without vitamin D supplementation. Reports of infants in the United States developing the vitamin D–deficiency disease rickets and recommendations by the American Academy of Pediatrics (AAP) to keep infants under 6 months of age out of direct sunlight have prompted revisions in vitamin D guidelines. The AAP currently recommends a vitamin D supplement for all infants who are breastfed exclusively and for any infants who do not receive at least 1 liter (1000 milliliters) or 1 quart (32 ounces) of vitamin D–fortified formula daily.[10] Despite such recommendations, most infants in the United States are consuming inadequate amounts of vitamin D.[11]

As for minerals, the calcium content of breast milk is ideal for infant bone growth, and the calcium is well absorbed. Breast milk is also low in sodium. The limited amount of iron in breast milk is highly absorbable, and its zinc, too, is absorbed better than from cow's milk, thanks to the presence of a zinc-binding protein.

Supplements for Infants Pediatricians may prescribe supplements containing vitamin D, iron, and fluoride (after 6 months of age). Table 12-2 offers a schedule of supplements during infancy. Vitamin K nutrition for newborns presents a unique case: the AAP recommends giving a single dose of vitamin K to infants at birth to prevent uncontrolled bleeding. (See Chapter 8 for a description of vitamin K's role in blood clotting.)

Immunological Protection In addition to its nutritional benefits, breast milk offers unsurpassed immunological protection.[12] Not only is breast milk sterile, but it also actively fights disease and protects infants from illnesses. Protective factors include antiviral agents, anti-inflammatory agents, antibacterial agents, and infection inhibitors.

During the first two or three days after delivery, the breasts produce **colostrum**, a premilk substance containing mostly serum with antibodies and white blood cells. Colostrum (like breast milk) helps protect the newborn from infections against which the mother has developed immunity—precisely those that the infant is most likely

alpha-lactalbumin (lact-AL-byoo-min): a major protein in human breast milk, as opposed to *casein* (CAY-seen), a major protein in cow's milk.

colostrum (co-LAHS-trum): a milklike secretion from the breasts, present during the first few days after delivery before milk appears; rich in protective factors.

TABLE 12-2 Supplements for Full-Term Infants

	Vitamin D[a]	Iron[b]	Fluoride[c]
Breastfed infants:			
Birth to 6 months	✓	–	–
6 months to 1 year	✓	✓	✓
Formula-fed infants:			
Birth to 6 months	–	–	–
6 months to 1 year	–	✓	✓

© 2016 Cengage Learning®

[a]Vitamin D supplements are recommended for all infants who are exclusively breastfed and for any infants who do not receive at least 1 liter (1000 milliliters) or 1 quart (32 ounces) of vitamin D–fortified formula per day.

[b]All infants 6 months of age need additional iron, preferably in the form of iron-fortified infant cereal and/or infant meats. Formula-fed infants need iron-fortified infant formula.

[c]At 6 months of age, breastfed infants and formula-fed infants who receive ready-to-use formulas (these are prepared with water low in fluoride) or formula mixed with water that contains little or no fluoride (less than 0.3 ppm) need supplements.

Source: Adapted from Committee on Nutrition, American Academy of Pediatrics, Pediatric Nutrition, 7th ed., ed. R. E. Kleinman (Elk Grove Village, IL: American Academy of Pediatrics, 2014).

to be exposed to. The maternal antibodies in colostrum and breast milk inactivate disease-causing bacteria within the infant's digestive tract before they can start infections.[13] This explains, in part, why breastfed infants have fewer intestinal infections than formula-fed infants. In addition to antibodies, colostrum and breast milk provide other powerful agents that help to fight against bacterial infection (see Table 12-3).

Breastfeeding also protects against other common illnesses of infancy such as middle ear infection and respiratory illness.[14] Breast milk offers protection against the development of allergies as well. Compared with formula-fed infants, breastfed infants have a lower incidence of allergic reactions such as asthma, wheezing, and skin rash.[15] This protection is especially noticeable among infants with a family history of allergies. Breastfeeding also reduces the risk of sudden infant death syndrome (SIDS).[16] This protective effect is stronger when breastfeeding is exclusive, but any amount of breast milk for any duration is protective against SIDS.

TABLE 12-3 Protective Factors in Breast Milk

- **Antibodies:** Offer protection in the upper respiratory tract and gastrointestinal tract, preventing adherence of pathogens to the mucosa, protecting against invasive infections; may stimulate the infant's own immune system

- **Bifidus factors:** Favor the growth of the "friendly' bacterium *Lactobacillus bifidus* in the infant's digestive tract so that other, harmful bacteria cannot become established

- **Growth factors:**
  - Epidermal growth factor: Regulates cell growth, proliferation, and differentiation
  - Transforming growth factor-beta (TGF-β): Anti-inflammatory; epithelial barrier function

- **Lactadherin:** Inhibits binding of pathogens to the intestinal mucosa

- **Lactoferrin:** Prevents bacteria from getting the iron they need to grow; helps absorb iron into the infant's bloodstream; kills some bacteria directly; antiviral effects

- **Lysozyme:** Together with lactoferrin, kills bacteria

- **Oligosaccharides:** Help to establish and maintain growth of desired bacteria in gastrointestinal tract; prevent binding of pathogens in gastrointestinal tract

© 2016 Cengage Learning®

Source: Adapted from B. Lonnerdal, Bioactive proteins in breast milk, *Journal of Paediatrics and Child Health* (Supplement S1) 49 (2013): 1–7; D. E. W. Chatterton and coauthors, Anti-inflammatory mechanisms of bioactive milk proteins in the intestine of newborns, *International Journal of biochemistry and Cell Biology* 45 (2013): 1730–1747; P. V. Jeurink and coauthors, Mechanisms underlying immune effects of dietary oligosaccharides, *American Journal of Clinical Nutrition* 98 (2013): 572S–577S; A. Walker, Breast milk as the gold standard for protective nutrients, *Journal of Pediatrics* 156 (2010): 53–57.

Clearly, breast milk is a very special substance. Nutrition in Practice 11 offers suggestions for successful breastfeeding.

Other Potential Benefits Breast milk may offer protection against the development of cardiovascular disease, but more well-conducted research, using consistent and precise definitions of breastfeeding, is needed to confirm this effect.[17] Breastfeeding may also offer some protection against excessive weight gain later, although findings are inconsistent.[18] For example, some research suggests that the longer the duration of breastfeeding, the lower the risk of overweight in childhood, while other research conflicts with such findings.[19] Researchers note that many other factors—socioeconomic status, other infant and child feeding practices, and especially the mother's weight—strongly predict a child's body weight.[20]

Many studies suggest a beneficial effect of breastfeeding on later intelligence, but when subjected to strict standards of methodology (for example, large sample size and appropriate intelligence testing), the evidence is less convincing.[21] Nevertheless, the possibility that breastfeeding may positively affect later intelligence is intriguing. It may be that some specific component of breast milk, such as DHA, contributes to brain development or that certain factors associated with the feeding process itself promote the intellect.[22] Most likely, a combination of factors is involved. More large, well-controlled studies are needed to confirm the effects, if any, of breastfeeding on later intelligence.

Infant Formula

Breastfeeding offers many benefits to both mother and infant, and it should be encouraged whenever possible. The mother who has decided to use formula, however, should be supported in her choice just as the breastfeeding mother should be. She can offer the same closeness, warmth, and stimulation during feedings as the breastfeeding mother can.

Many mothers choose to breastfeed at first but **wean** their children within the first 1 to 12 months. If infants are younger than a year of age, mothers must wean them onto *infant formula*, not onto plain cow's milk of any kind—whole, reduced-fat, low-fat, or fat-free. Infant formula is available as a powdered (least expensive option) or liquid concentrate that must be mixed with water according to label directions, and as a ready-to-feed liquid (most expensive).

Infant Formula Composition Manufacturers can prepare formulas from cow's milk in such a way that they do not differ significantly from human milk in nutrient content. Figure 12-4 illustrates the energy nutrient distributions of breast milk, infant formula, and cow's milk. Notice the higher protein concentration of cow's milk, which stresses an infant's kidneys. The AAP recommends that all formula-fed infants receive iron-fortified infant formulas.[23] Low-iron formulas have no role in infant feeding. Use of iron-fortified formulas has risen in recent decades and is credited with the decline of iron-deficiency anemia in U.S. infants.

The infant thrives on infant formula offered with affection.

©Juriah Mosin/Shutterstock.com

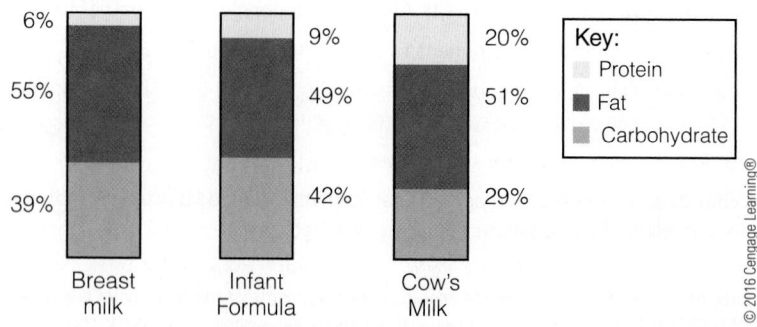

© 2016 Cengage Learning®

FIGURE 12-4 Percentages of Energy-Yielding Nutrients in Breast Milk, Infant Formula, and Cow's Milk
The average proportions of energy-yielding nutrients in human breast milk and formula differ slightly. In contrast, cow's milk provides too much protein and too little carbohydrate.

wean: to gradually replace breast milk with infant formula or other foods appropriate to an infant's diet.

Infant Formula Standards National and international standards have been set for the nutrient contents of infant formulas. U.S. standards are based on AAP recommendations, and the Food and Drug Administration (FDA) mandates quality control procedures to ensure that these standards are met. All standard formulas are therefore nutritionally similar. Small differences in nutrient content are sometimes confusing but usually unimportant. In 2014, the FDA issued new quality control procedures to further ensure that infant formulas are safe and support healthy growth.[24] These specify how and when manufacturers must inform the FDA about new formulas and changes to formulas, and require testing for contamination with harmful bacteria such as *Salmonella*.

Special Formulas Standard cow's milk–based formulas are inappropriate for some infants. Special formulas have been designed to meet the dietary needs of infants with specific conditions such as prematurity or inherited diseases. Most infants allergic to milk protein can drink formulas based on soy protein.[25] Soy formulas contain cornstarch and sucrose instead of lactose and so are recommended for infants with lactose intolerance as well. They are also useful as an alternative to milk-based formulas for vegan families. For infants who are allergic to both cow's milk protein and soy protein, special formulas based on hydrolyzed protein are available.

Risks of Formula Feeding Infant formulas contain no protective antibodies for infants, but, in general, vaccinations, purified water, and clean environments in developed countries help protect infants from infections. Formulas can be prepared safely by following the rules of proper food handling and by using water that is free of contamination. Of particular concern is lead-contaminated water, a major source of lead poisoning in infants. Because the first water drawn from the tap each day is highest in lead, a person living in a house with old, lead-soldered plumbing should let the water run a few minutes before drinking or using it to prepare formula or food.

In developing countries and in poor areas of the United States, formula may be unavailable, overdiluted in an attempt to save money, or prepared with contaminated water. Overdilution of formula can cause malnutrition and growth failure. Contaminated formula often causes infections leading to diarrhea, dehydration, and malabsorption. Wherever sanitation is poor, breastfeeding should be encouraged over feeding formula. Breast milk is sterile, and its antibodies enhance an infant's resistance to disease.

Nursing Bottle Tooth Decay Dentists advise against putting an infant to bed with a bottle. Salivary flow, which normally cleanses the mouth, diminishes as the infant falls asleep. Prolonged sucking on a bottle of formula, milk, or juice bathes the upper teeth in a carbohydrate-rich fluid that nourishes decay-producing bacteria. (The tongue covers and protects most of the lower teeth, but they, too, may be affected.) The result is extensive and rapid tooth decay (see Figure 12-5). To prevent **nursing bottle tooth decay**, no child should be put to bed with a bottle as a pacifier.

FIGURE 12-5 Nursing Bottle Tooth Decay—An Extreme Example
The upper teeth have decayed all the way to the gum line.

The Transition to Cow's Milk

The AAP advises that cow's milk is not appropriate during the first year.[26] In some infants, particularly those younger than 6 months of age, cow's milk causes intestinal bleeding, which can lead to iron deficiency.[27] Cow's milk is also a poor source of iron. Consequently, it both causes iron loss and fails to replace iron. Furthermore, the bioavailability of iron from infant cereal and other foods is reduced when cow's milk replaces breast milk or iron-fortified formula during the first year. Compared with breast milk or iron-fortified formula, cow's milk is higher in calcium and lower in vitamin C, characteristics that reduce iron absorption. In short, cow's milk is a poor choice during the first year of life; infants need breast milk or iron-fortified infant formula.

Once the infant is at least 12 months old and obtaining at least two-thirds of total daily food energy from a balanced mixture of cereals, vegetables, fruits, and other foods, reduced-fat or low-fat cow's milk (in the context of an overall diet that supplies

nursing bottle tooth decay: extensive tooth decay due to prolonged tooth contact with formula, milk, fruit juice, or other carbohydrate-rich liquid offered to an infant in a bottle.

30 percent of kcalories from fat) is an acceptable and recommended accompanying beverage.[28] After the age of 2, a transition to fat-free milk can take place, but care should be taken to avoid excessive restriction of dietary fat.

Introducing First Foods

Changes in the body organs during the first year affect the infant's readiness to accept solid foods. Until the child is several months old, the immature stomach and intestines can digest milk sugar (lactose) but not starch. This is one of the many reasons why breast milk and formula are such good foods for an infant; they provide simple, easily digested carbohydrate that supplies energy for the infant's growth and activity.

When to Introduce Solid Food The AAP supports exclusive breastfeeding for approximately 6 months but recognizes that infants are often developmentally ready to accept complementary foods between 4 and 6 months of age.[29] The main purpose of introducing solid foods is to provide needed nutrients that are no longer supplied adequately by breast milk or formula alone.[30] The foods chosen must be those that the infant is developmentally capable of handling both physically and metabolically. The exact timing depends on the individual infant's needs and developmental readiness (see Table 12-4), which vary from infant to infant because of differences in growth

TABLE 12-4 Infant Development and Recommended Foods

Age (mo)	Feeding Skills	Foods Introduced into the Diet
0–4	Turns head toward any object that brushes cheek.	Feed breast milk or infant formula.
	Initially swallows using back of tongue; gradually begins to swallow using front of tongue as well.	
	Strong reflex (extrusion) to push food out during first 2 to 3 months.	
4–6	Extrusion reflex diminishes, and the ability to swallow nonliquid foods develops.	Begin iron-fortified cereal mixed with breast milk, formula, or water.
	Indicates desire for food by opening mouth and leaning forward.	Begin pureed meats, legumes, vegetables, and fruits.
	Indicates satiety or disinterest by turning away and leaning back.	
	Sits erect with support at 6 months.	
	Begins chewing action.	
	Brings hand to mouth.	
	Grasps objects with palm of hand.	
6–8	Able to self-feed finger foods.	Begin textured vegetables and fruits.
	Develops pincher (finger to thumb) grasp.	Begin unsweetened, diluted fruit juices from cup.
	Begins to drink from cup.	
8–10	Begins to hold own bottle.	Begin breads and cereals from table.
	Reaches for and grabs food and spoon.	Begin yogurt.
	Sits unsupported.	Begin pieces of soft, cooked vegetables and fruit from table.
		Gradually begin finely cut meats, fish, casseroles, cheese, eggs, and mashed legumes.
10–12	Begins to master spoon but still spills some.	Add variety.
		Gradually increase portion sizes.[a]

© Cengage Learning®

Note: Because each stage of development builds on the previous stage, the foods from an earlier stage continue to be included in all later stages.

[a]Portion sizes for infants and young children are smaller than those for an adult. For example, a grain serving might be ½ slice of bread instead of 1 slice, or ¼ cup rice instead of ½ cup.

Source: Adapted in part from Committee on Nutrition, American Academy of Pediatrics, *Pediatric Nutrition* 7th ed., ed. R. E. Kleinman (Elk Grove Village, Ill.: American Academy of Pediatrics, 2014), pp. 123–139.

rates, activities, and environmental conditions. In short, the addition of foods to an infant's diet should be governed by three considerations: the infant's nutrient needs, the infant's physical readiness to handle different forms of foods, and the need to detect and control allergic reactions. With respect to nutrient needs, the nutrients needed earliest are iron and then vitamin C.

Foods to Provide Iron and Vitamin C Rapid growth demands iron. At about 4 to 6 months, the infant begins to need more iron than body stores plus breast milk or iron-fortified formula can provide. In addition to breast milk or iron-fortified formula, infants can receive iron from iron-fortified cereals and, once they readily accept solid foods, from meat or meat alternates such as legumes (see Figure 12-6). Iron-fortified cereals contribute a significant amount of iron to an infant's diet, but the iron's bioavailability is poor.[31] Caregivers can enhance iron absorption from iron-fortified cereals by serving vitamin C–rich foods with meals.

The best sources of vitamin C are fruits and vegetables (see p. 212 in Chapter 8). It has been suggested that infants who are introduced to fruits before vegetables may develop a preference for sweets and find the vegetables less palatable, but there is no evidence to support offering these foods in a particular order.[32] Fruit juice is a source of vitamin C, but excessive juice intake can lead to diarrhea in infants and young children.[33] Furthermore, too much fruit juice contributes excessive kcalories and displaces other nutrient-rich foods. AAP recommendations limit juice consumption for infants and young children (1 to 6 years of age) to between 4 and 6 ounces per day.[34] Fruit juices should be diluted and served in a cup, not a bottle, once the infant is 6 months of age or older.

Physical Readiness for Solid Foods The ability to swallow solid food develops at around 4 to 6 months, and food offered by spoon helps to develop swallowing ability. At 8 months to a year, an infant can sit up, can handle finger foods, and begins to teethe. At that time, hard crackers and other hard finger foods may be introduced to promote the development of manual dexterity and control of the jaw muscles. These feedings must occur under the watchful eye of an adult because the infant can also choke on such foods.

Some parents want to feed solids at an earlier age, on the theory that "stuffing the baby" at bedtime promotes sleeping through the night. There is no proof for this theory. On average, infants start to sleep through the night at about the same age (3 to 4 months) regardless of when solid foods are introduced.

Allergy-Causing Foods To prevent allergy and to facilitate its prompt identification should it occur, experts recommend introducing single-ingredient foods, one at a time, in small portions, and waiting 3 to 5 days before introducing the next new food.[35] For example, rice cereal is usually the first cereal introduced because it is the least allergenic. When it is clear that rice cereal is not causing an allergy, another grain, perhaps barley or oats, is introduced. Wheat cereal is offered last because it is the most common offender. If a cereal causes an allergic reaction such as a skin rash, digestive upset, or respiratory discomfort, it should be discontinued before introducing the next food. A later section offers more information about food allergies.

Choice of Infant Foods Infant foods should be selected to provide variety, balance, and moderation. Commercial baby foods offer a wide variety of palatable, nutritious foods in a safe and convenient form. Parents or caregivers should not feed directly from the jar—remove the infant's portion and place it in a dish so as not to contaminate the leftovers that will be stored in the jar. Homemade infant foods can be as nutritious as commercially prepared ones, as long as the cook minimizes nutrient losses during preparation. Ingredients for homemade foods should be fresh, whole foods without added salt, sugar, or seasonings. Pureed food can be frozen in ice cube trays, providing convenient-sized blocks of food that can be thawed, warmed, and fed to the infant. To guard against foodborne illnesses, hands and equipment must be kept clean.

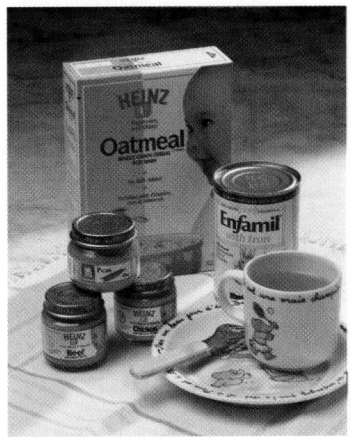

FIGURE 12-6 Iron Sources for Infants
Foods such as iron-fortified cereals and formulas, mashed legumes, and strained meats provide iron.

© Polara Studios, Inc.

TABLE 12-5 Examples of Foods and Nonfood Items Children Can Choke On

To prevent choking, do not give infants or young children:

- Gum
- Hard or gel-type candies
- Hot dog slices
- Large raw apple slices
- Marshmallows
- Nuts
- Peanut butter
- Popcorn
- Raw carrots
- Raw celery
- Sausage sticks or slices
- Whole beans
- Whole cherries
- Whole grapes

Keep these nonfood items out of their reach:

- Balloons
- Coins
- Pen tops
- Small balls and marbles
- Other items of similar size

Ideally, a 1-year-old eats many of the same healthy foods as the rest of the family.

Foods to Omit Sweets of any kind (including baby food "desserts") have no place in an infant's diet. The added food energy conveys few, if any, nutrients to support growth and contributes to obesity. Canned vegetables are also inappropriate for infants; they often contain too much sodium. Honey and corn syrup should never be fed to infants because of the risk of botulism. Infants and young children are vulnerable to foodborne illnesses. An infant's caregiver must be on guard against food poisoning and take precautions against it as described in Nutrition in Practice 5.

Infants and even young children cannot safely chew and swallow any of the foods listed in Table 12-5; they can easily choke on these foods, a risk not worth taking.[36] Non-food items of small size should always be kept out of the infant's reach to prevent choking.

Foods at 1 Year At 1 year of age, reduced-fat or low-fat cow's milk can become a primary source of most of the nutrients an infant needs; 2 to 3 cups a day meet those needs sufficiently. More milk than this displaces iron-rich foods and can lead to the iron-deficiency anemia known as milk anemia. Other foods—meat and meat alternates, iron-fortified cereals, whole-grain or enriched bread, fruits, and vegetables— should be supplied in variety and in amounts sufficient to round out total energy needs. Ideally, a 1-year-old will sit at the table, eat many of the same foods everyone else eats, and drink liquids from a cup—not a bottle. Table 12-6 shows a sample menu that meets a 1-year-old's requirements.

Looking Ahead

Probably the most important single measure to undertake during the first year is to encourage eating habits that will support continued normal weight as the child grows. This means introducing a variety of nutritious foods in an inviting way, not forcing the infant to finish the bottle or the baby food jar, avoiding concentrated sweets and empty-kcalorie foods, and encouraging physical activity. Parents should avoid teaching infants to seek food as a reward, to expect food as comfort for unhappiness, or to associate food deprivation with punishment. Normal dental development is also promoted by supplying nutritious foods, avoiding sweets, and discouraging the association of food with reward or comfort. Oral health is the subject of Nutrition in Practice 17.

Mealtimes

The nurturing of a young child involves more than nutrition. Those who care for young children are responsible for providing not only nutritious foods, milk, and water but also a safe, loving, secure environment in which the children may grow and develop. The person feeding a 1-year-old should be aware that exploring and experimenting are normal and desirable behaviors at this time in a child's life. The child is developing a sense of autonomy that, if allowed to develop, will lay the foundation for later assertiveness in choosing when and how much to eat and when to stop eating. In light of the developmental and nutrient needs of 1-year-olds, and in the face of their often contrary and willful behavior, a few feeding guidelines may be helpful:

- *Discourage unacceptable behavior (such as standing at the table or throwing food) by removing the child from the table to wait until later to eat.* Be consistent and firm, not punitive. For example, instead of saying "You make me mad when you don't sit down," say "The fruit salad tastes good—please sit down and eat some with me." The child will soon learn to sit and eat.

- *Let young children explore and enjoy food.* This may mean eating with fingers for a while. Learning to use a spoon will come in time. Children who are allowed to touch, mash, and smell their food while exploring it are more likely to accept it.

- *Don't force food on children.* Rejecting new foods is normal, and acceptance is more likely as children become familiar with new foods through repeated opportunities

328

to taste them. Instead of saying "You cannot go outside to play until you taste your carrots," say "You can try the carrots again another time."

▍ *Provide nutritious foods, and let children choose which ones, and how much, they will eat.* Gradually, they will acquire a taste for different foods.

▍ *Limit sweets.* Infants and young children have little room for empty-kcalorie foods in their daily energy allowance. Do not use sweets as a reward for eating meals.

▍ *Don t turn the dining table into a battleground.* Make mealtimes enjoyable. Teach healthy food choices and eating habits in a pleasant environment. Mealtimes are not the time to fight, argue, or scold.

These recommendations reflect a spirit of tolerance that best serves the emotional and physical interests of the infant. This attitude, carried throughout childhood, helps the child to develop a healthy relationship with food.

IN SUMMARY

▍ The primary food for infants during the first 12 months is either breast milk or iron-fortified formula.

▍ In addition to nutrients, breast milk also offers immunological protection.

▍ At about 4 to 6 months, infants should gradually begin eating solid foods.

▍ The addition of foods to an infant's diet should be governed by three considerations: the infant's nutrient needs, the infant's physical readiness to handle different forms of foods, and the need to detect and control allergic reactions.

▍ By the time infants are 1 year old, they are drinking from a cup and eating many of the same foods as the rest of the family.

12.2 Nutrition during Childhood

LO 12.2 Explain how children's appetites and nutrient needs reflect their stage of growth, why hunger, iron deficiency, lead poisoning, foods allergies, hyperactivity, and obesity are often concerns during childhood, and how parents and other caregivers can foster healthful eating habits and food choices in children.

After the age of 1, growth rate slows, but the body continues to change dramatically (see Figure 12-7). At 1, infants have just learned to stand and toddle; by 2, they walk confidently and are learning to run, jump, and climb. Nutrition and physical activity have helped them prepare for these new accomplishments by adding to the

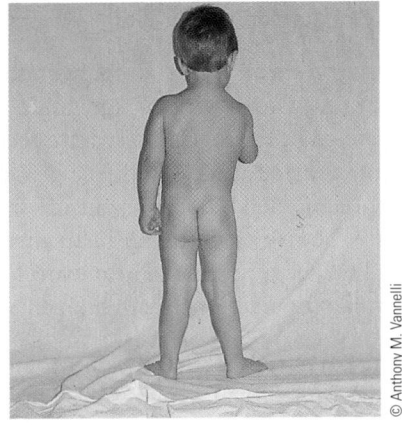

© Anthony M. Vannelli

TABLE 12-6 Sample Menu for a 1-Year-Old

Breakfast:
1 scrambled egg
1 slice whole-wheat toast
½ c reduced-fat milk

Morning Snack:
½ c yogurt
¼ c fruit[a]

Lunch:
½ grilled cheese sandwich: 1 slice whole-wheat bread with 1 slice cheese
½ c vegetables[b] (steamed carrots)
¼ c 100% fruit juice

Afternoon Snack:
½ c fruit[a]
½ c toasted oat cereal

Dinner:
1 oz chopped meat or ¼ c well-cooked mashed legumes
½ c rice or pasta
½ c vegetables[b] (chopped broccoli)
½ c reduced-fat milk

© 2016 Cengage Learning®

Note: This sample menu provides about 1000 kcalories.

[a]Include citrus fruits, melons, and berries.

[b]Include dark green, leafy, and deep yellow vegetables.

FIGURE 12-7 Body Shape of a 1-Year-Old and a 2-Year-Old Compared
The body shape of a 1-year-old (left) changes dramatically by age 2 (right). The 2-year-old has lost much of the baby fat; the muscles (especially in the back, buttocks, and legs) have firmed and strengthened; and the leg bones have lengthened.

mass and density of their bone and muscle tissue. Thereafter, their bones continue to grow longer and their muscles to gain size and strength, though unevenly and more slowly, until adolescence.

Energy and Nutrient Needs

Children's appetites begin to diminish around the first birthday, consistent with the slowed growth rate. Thereafter, the appetite fluctuates. At times children seem to be insatiable, and at other times they seem to live on air and water. Parents and other caregivers need not worry: given an ample selection of nutritious foods at regular intervals, internal appetite regulation in healthy, normal-weight children guarantees that their food energy intakes will be right for each stage of growth.

Ideally, children accumulate stores of nutrients before adolescence. Then, when they take off on the adolescent growth spurt and their nutrient intakes cannot keep pace with the demands of rapid growth, they can draw on the nutrient stores accumulated earlier. This is especially true of calcium; the denser the bones are in childhood, the better prepared they will be to support teen growth and still withstand the inevitable bone losses of later life.[37] Consequently, the way children eat influences their nutritional health during childhood, during their teen years, and for the rest of their lives.

Children's Appetites Many people mistakenly believe that they must "make" their children eat the right amounts of food, and children's erratic appetites often reinforce this belief.[38] Although children's food energy intakes vary widely from meal to meal, total daily energy intake remains remarkably constant. If children eat less at one meal, they typically eat more at the next, and vice versa.

Parents do, however, need to help children choose the right foods, and, with overweight children, they may need to help more, as described later. Overweight children may not adjust their energy intakes appropriately and may disregard appetite-regulation signals and eat in response to external cues, such as television commercials.[39]

Energy Individual children's energy needs vary widely, depending on their growth and physical activity. A 1-year-old child needs approximately 800 kcalories a day; an active 6-year-old needs twice as many. By age 10, an active child needs about 2000 kcalories a day. Total energy needs increase gradually with age, but energy needs per kilogram of body weight actually decline. Physically active children of any age need more energy because they expend more, and inactive children can become obese even when they eat less food than the average. Unfortunately, our nation's children are becoming less and less active; child care programs and schools would serve our children well by offering more activities to promote physical fitness.[40]

Some children, notably those adhering to a vegan diet, may have difficulty meeting their energy needs. Grains, vegetables, and fruits provide plenty of fiber, adding bulk, but may provide too few kcalories to support growth. Soy products, other legumes, and nut or seed butters offer more concentrated sources of energy to support optimal growth and development.[41]

Carbohydrate and Fiber Carbohydrate recommendations are based on glucose use by the brain. After 1 year of age, brain glucose use remains fairly constant and is within the adult range. Carbohydrate recommendations for children after 1 year are therefore the same as for adults (see inside front cover).[42]

Fiber recommendations (see inside front cover) derive from adult intakes shown to reduce the risk of coronary heart disease and are based on energy intakes. Consequently, fiber recommendations are lower for younger children with low energy intakes than for older ones with high energy intakes.[43]

Fat and Fatty Acids No RDA for total fat has been established, but the DRI committee recommends a fat intake of 30 to 40 percent of energy for children 1 to 3 years of age and 25 to 35 percent for children 4 to 18 years of age.[44] However, as long as children's energy intakes are adequate, fat intakes below 30 percent of total energy do not impair growth.[45] Children who eat low-fat diets, however, tend to have low intakes of some vitamins and minerals. Recommended intakes of the essential fatty acids are based on average intakes (see inside front cover).

Protein Like energy needs, total protein needs increase slightly with age but actually decline slightly per unit of body weight (see inside front cover). Protein recommendations must address the requirements for maintaining nitrogen balance, the quality of protein consumed, and the added needs of growth.

Vitamins and Minerals The vitamin and mineral needs of children increase with age (see inside front cover). A balanced diet of nutritious foods can meet children's needs for these nutrients, with the notable exception of iron and possibly vitamin D. Iron-deficiency anemia, a major problem worldwide, is prevalent among U.S. and Canadian children, especially toddlers one to 3 years of age.[46] During the second year of life, toddlers progress from a diet of iron-rich infant foods such as breast milk, iron-fortified formula, and iron-fortified infant cereal to a diet of adult foods and iron-poor cow's milk. In addition, their appetites often fluctuate—some become finicky about the foods they eat, and others prefer milk and juice to solid foods. These situations can interfere with children eating iron-rich foods at a critical time for brain growth and development.

To prevent iron deficiency, children's foods must deliver 7 to 10 milligrams of iron per day. To achieve this goal, snacks and meals should include iron-rich foods (see Table 12-7), and milk intake should be reasonable so that it will not displace lean meats, fish, poultry, eggs, legumes, and whole-grain or enriched products. That means 2½ cups of milk per day up to age eight, increasing to 3 cups per day from age nine on. After age 1, as long as the overall diet supplies 30 percent of total kcalories from fat, reduced-fat or low-fat milk can be used instead of whole milk.[47] The saved kcalories can be invested in iron-rich foods such as lean meats, fish, poultry, eggs, and legumes. Whole-grain or enriched breads and cereals also contribute iron.

The DRI committee recently revised their recommendations for vitamin D intakes for healthy Americans.[48] Children typically obtain most of their vitamin D from fortified milk (2.5 micrograms per cup) and dry cereals (1 microgram per ½ cup). Children who do not meet their RDA (15 micrograms) from these sources should receive a vitamin D supplement.[49] Remember that sunlight is also a source of vitamin D, especially in warm climates and warm seasons.

Supplements With the exception of specific recommendations for fluoride, iron, and vitamin D during infancy and childhood, the AAP and other professional groups agree that well-nourished children do not need vitamin and mineral supplements— yet many children and adolescents take them.[50] Ironically, children with poor nutrient intakes typically do not receive supplements, whereas those who do usually receive extra nutrients they do not need.[51] Furthermore, researchers are still studying the safety of supplement use by children. The Federal Trade Commission has warned parents about giving children supplements advertised to prevent or cure childhood illnesses such as colds, ear infections, or asthma. Dietary supplements on the market today include many herbal products that have not been tested for safety and effectiveness in children.

Food Patterns for Children To provide all the needed nutrients, a child's meals and snacks should include a variety of foods from each food group—in amounts suited to the child's appetite and needs. Table 12-8 (on p. 332) provides USDA Food Patterns for several kcalorie levels. (For kcalorie levels over 1800, see Table 1-4 on p. 15.) Estimated daily kcalorie needs for active and sedentary children of various ages are shown in Table 12-9 (on p. 332). MyPlate online resources for preschoolers (2 to 5 years) translate the eating patterns into messages that can help parents ensure that the foods they provide

TABLE 12-7 Iron-Rich Foods Children Like[a]

Breads, Cereals, and Grains

Cream of wheat (¼ c)

Fortified dry cereals (1 oz)[b]

Noodles, rice, or barley (½ c)

Tortillas (1 flour or whole-wheat, 2 corn)

Whole-wheat, enriched, or fortified bread (1 slice)

Vegetables

Cooked snow peas (½ c)

Cooked mushrooms (½ c)

Green peas (½ c)

Mixed vegetable juice (1 c)

Fruits

Canned plums (3 plums)

Cooked dried apricots (¼ c)

Dried peaches (4 halves)

Raisins (1 tbs)

Meats and Legumes

Bean dip (¼ c)

Lean chopped roast beef or cooked ground beef (1 oz)

Liverwurst on crackers (½ oz)

Meat casseroles (½ c)

Mild chili or other bean/meat dishes (¼ c)

Peanut butter and jelly sandwich (½ sandwich)

Sloppy joes (½ sandwich)

[a]Each serving provides at least 1 milligram of iron. Vitamin C–rich foods included with these snacks increase iron absorption.

[b]Some fortified breakfast cereals contain more than 10 milligrams of iron per half-cup serving (read the labels).

TABLE 12-8 USDA Food Patterns: Recommended Daily Amounts for Each Food Group (1000 to 1800 kCalories)

Food Group	1000 kcal	1200 kcal	1400 kcal	1600 kcal	1800 kcal
Fruit	1 c	1 c	1½ c	1½ c	1½ c
Vegetables	1 c	1½ c	1½ c	2 c	2½ c
Grains	3 oz	4 oz	5 oz	5 oz	6 oz
Protein Foods	2 oz	3 oz	4 oz	5 oz	5 oz
Milk	2 c	2½ c	2½ c	3 c	3 c

© 2016 Cengage Learning®

TABLE 12-9 Estimated Daily kCalorie Needs for Children

Children	Sedentary[a]	Active[b]
2 to 3 yr	1000	1400
Females		
4 to 8 yr	1200	1800
9 to 13 yr	1400	2200
Males		
4 to 8 yr	1200	2000
9 to 13 yr	1600	2600

© 2016 Cengage Learning®

[a]*Sedentary* describes a lifestyle that includes only the activities typical of day-to-day life.

[b]*Active* describes a lifestyle that includes at least 60 minutes per day of moderate physical activity (equivalent to walking more than 3 miles per day at 3 to 4 miles per hour) in addition to the activities of day-to-day life.

© 2016 Cengage Learning®

FIGURE 12-8 MyPlate Resources for Children
Abundant MyPlate resources for pre-school children and older children can be found at *www.choosemyplate.gov/.*

meet their child's needs. For children older than 5 (6 to 11 years), the site provides interactive nutrition games, videos, and other resources for teachers, parents, and children themselves (Figure 12-8). These guidelines and resources also stress the importance of balancing kcalorie intake with kcalorie expenditure through adequate physical activity to promote growth without excessive weight gain (as discussed later in this chapter).

Children whose diets follow the pattern presented in Table 12-8 meet their nutrient needs fully, but few children eat according to these recommendations. One analysis of the quality of children's diets found that most children (up to 88 percent) between 2 and 9 years of age have diets that need substantial improvement.[52] A comprehensive survey, called the Feeding Infants and Toddlers Study (FITS), assessed the food and nutrient intakes of more than 3000 infants and toddlers.[53] The survey found that fruit and vegetable intakes of infants and toddlers are limited, and, in fact, about 25 percent of 2- and 3-year-old children did not eat a single serving of fruits or vegetables in a day.[54] White potatoes were the most commonly consumed vegetable, often in fried form. Of great concern is the finding that more than 80 percent of preschoolers consumed one or more low-nutrient, energy-dense beverages, desserts, and snack foods in a day. Parents and caregivers of infants and toddlers thus need to offer a much greater variety of nutrient-dense vegetables and fruits at meals and snacks to help ensure adequate nutrition. Among other nutrition concerns for U.S. children are inadequate intakes of vitamin E, potassium, and fiber, and excessive intakes of sodium and saturated fat.[55]

Children's Food Choices The childhood years are the parents' best chance to influence their child's food choices.[56] Appropriate eating habits and attitudes toward food, developed in childhood, can help future adults emerge with healthy habits that reduce risks of chronic diseases in later life. The challenge is to deliver nutrients in the form of meals and snacks that are both nutritious and appealing so that children will learn to enjoy a variety of health-promoting foods.

Permitting large quantities of candy, cola, and other concentrated sweets in children's diets will result in nutrient deficiencies, obesity, or both. The *Dietary Guidelines for Americans 2010* recommend limiting intake of added sugars and solid fats to 5 to 15 percent of daily kcalories, but children and adolescents consume approximately 16 percent of total kcaloric intake from added sugars alone.[57] Children can't be trusted to choose nutritious foods on the basis of taste; the preference for sweets is innate, and children naturally gravitate to them. Overweight children, especially, need help in selecting nutrient-dense foods that will meet their nutrient needs within their energy allowances. Underweight children or active, healthy-weight children can enjoy higher-kcalorie foods, but these should still be nutritious. Examples are ice cream and pudding in the milk group and whole-grain or enriched pancakes and crackers in the bread group.

Hunger and Malnutrition in Children

Most children in the United States and Canada have access to regular meals, but hunger and malnutrition do appear in certain circumstances. Children in very low-income families, for example, are more likely to be hungry and malnourished. More

332

than 16 million U.S. children are hungry at least some of the time and are living in poverty.[58] Nutrition in Practice 13 examines the causes and consequences of hunger in the United States.

Hunger and Behavior Both short-term and long-term hunger exert negative effects on behavior and health. Short-term hunger, such as when a child misses a meal, impairs the child's ability to pay attention and to be productive. Hungry children are irritable, apathetic, and uninterested in their environment. Long-term hunger impairs growth and immune defenses. Food assistance programs such as the WIC program (discussed in Chapter 11) and the School Breakfast and National School Lunch Programs (discussed later in this chapter) are designed to protect against hunger and improve the health of children.[59]

A nutritious breakfast is a central feature of a diet that meets the needs of children and supports their healthy growth and development.[60] Children who skip breakfast typically do not make up the deficits at later meals—they simply have lower intakes of energy, vitamins, and minerals than those who eat breakfast. Malnourished children are particularly vulnerable. Children who eat no breakfast are more likely to be overweight, perform poorly in tasks requiring concentration, have shorter attention spans, and achieve lower test scores than their well-fed peers.[61] Common sense dictates that it is unreasonable to expect anyone to learn and perform without fuel. For the child who hasn't had breakfast, the morning's lessons may be lost altogether. Even if a child has eaten breakfast, discomfort from hunger may become distracting by late morning. Teachers aware of the late-morning slump in their classrooms wisely request that midmorning snacks be provided; snacks improve classroom performance all the way to lunchtime.

Iron Deficiency and Behavior Iron deficiency has well-known and widespread effects on children's behavior and intellectual performance.[62] In addition to carrying oxygen in the blood, iron transports oxygen within cells, which use it for energy metabolism. Iron is also used to make neurotransmitters—most notably, those that regulate the ability to pay attention, which is crucial to learning. Consequently, iron deficiency not only causes an energy crisis but also directly impairs attention span and learning ability.

Iron deficiency is often diagnosed by a quick, easy, inexpensive hemoglobin or hematocrit test that detects a deficit of iron in the *blood.* A child's *brain,* however, is sensitive to low iron concentrations long before the blood effects appear. Iron deficiency lowers the "motivation to persist in intellectually challenging tasks" and impairs overall intellectual performance. Anemic children perform poorly on tests and are disruptive in the classroom; iron supplementation improves learning and memory. When combined with other nutrient deficiencies, iron-deficiency anemia has synergistic effects that are especially detrimental to learning. Furthermore, children who had iron-deficiency anemia *as infants* continue to perform poorly as they grow older, even if their iron status improves.[63] The long-term damaging effects on mental development make prevention and treatment of iron deficiency during infancy and early childhood a high priority.

Other Nutrient Deficiencies A child with any of several nutrient deficiencies may be irritable, aggressive, and disagreeable, or sad and withdrawn. Such a child may be labeled "hyperactive," "depressed," or "unlikable," when in fact these traits may be due to simple, even marginal, malnutrition. Though parents

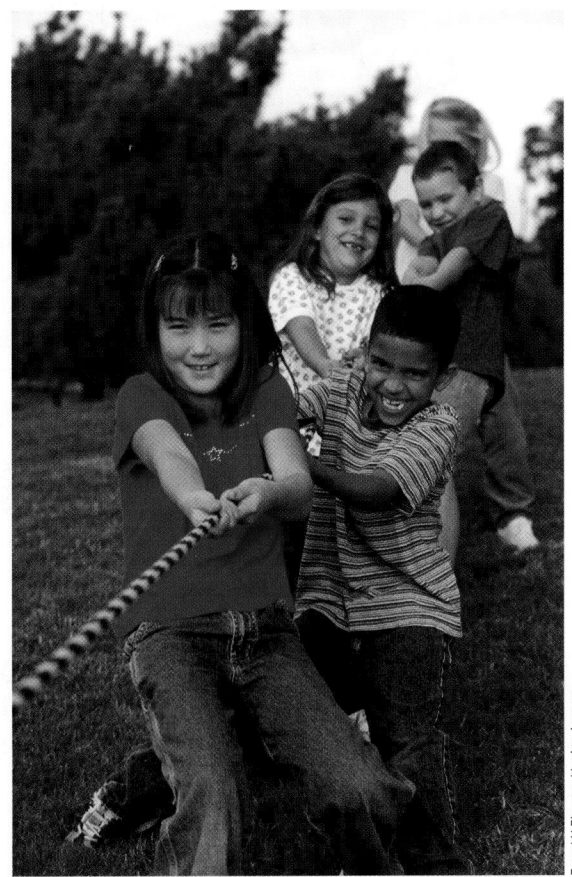

Healthy, well-nourished children are alert in the classroom and energetic at play.

Brand X Pictures/Jupiter Images

and medical practitioners often overlook this possibility, any departure from normal, healthy appearance and behavior is a sign of possible poor nutrition. In any such case, inspection of the child's diet by a registered dietitian nutritionist or other qualified health care professional is in order. Any suspicion of dietary inadequacies, *no matter what other causes may be implicated*, should prompt steps to correct those inadequacies immediately.

Lead Poisoning in Children

Children who are malnourished are vulnerable to lead poisoning. They absorb more lead if their stomachs are empty; if they have low intakes of calcium, zinc, vitamin C, or vitamin D; and, of greatest concern because it is so common, if they have an iron deficiency. Iron deficiency weakens the body's defenses against lead absorption, and lead poisoning can cause iron deficiency.[64] Circumstances associated with both iron deficiency and lead poisoning are a low socioeconomic status and a lack of immunizations against infectious diseases. Another common factor is pica—a craving for nonfood items. Many children with lead poisoning eat dirt or chips of old paint, two common sources of lead.

The anemia brought on by lead poisoning may be mistaken for a simple iron deficiency and therefore may be incorrectly treated. Like iron deficiency, mild lead toxicity has nonspecific symptoms, including diarrhea, irritability, and fatigue. Adding iron to the diet does not reverse the symptoms; exposure to lead must stop and treatment for lead poisoning must begin. With further exposure, the symptoms become more pronounced, and children develop learning disabilities and behavior problems. Still more severe lead toxicity can cause irreversible nerve damage, paralysis, mental retardation, and death.

Approximately half a million children between the ages of one and five in the United States have blood lead levels above 5 micrograms per deciliter, the level at which the Centers for Disease Control and Prevention recommend public health actions be initiated.[65] Lead toxicity in young children results from their own behaviors and activities—putting their hands in their mouths, playing in dirt and dust, and chewing on nonfood items.[66] Unfortunately, the body readily absorbs lead during times of rapid growth and hoards it possessively thereafter. Lead is not easily excreted and accumulates mainly in the bones and also in the brain, teeth, and kidneys. Because a child's neuromuscular system is maturing during these first few years of life, children with elevated lead levels experience impairment of balance, motor development, and the relaying of nerve messages to and from the brain. Deficits in intellectual development are only partially reversed when lead levels decline.

Federal laws mandating reductions in leaded gasolines, lead-based solder, and other products over the past 4 decades have helped to reduce the amounts of lead in food and in the environment in the United States. As a consequence, the prevalence of lead toxicity in children has declined dramatically for most of the nation. Nevertheless, lead exposure is still a threat in certain communities. Box 12-1 presents strategies for defending children against lead toxicity.

Tony Freeman/Photoedit,Inc

Old lead-based paint can threaten the health of an exploring child.

food allergy: an adverse reaction to food that involves an immune response; also called *food-hypersensitivity reactions.*

Food Allergy

Food allergy is frequently blamed for physical and behavioral abnormalities in children, but only 4 to 8 percent of children younger than 4 years of age are diagnosed with true food allergies.[67] Food allergies diminish with age, until in adulthood they affect less than 4 percent of the population. The prevalence of food allergy, especially peanut allergy, is on the rise, however.[68] Reasons for an increase in peanut allergy are not yet clear, but possible contributing factors include genetics, food preparation methods (roasting peanuts at very high temperatures makes them more allergenic), and exposure to medicinal skin creams containing peanut oil.

- Ask a pediatrician whether your child should be tested for lead poisoning.
- Clean floors, window frames, window sills, and other surfaces regularly. Use a mop or sponge with warm water and a general all-purpose cleaner.
- Prevent children from putting dirty or old painted objects in their mouths, and make sure children wash their hands before eating.
- Feed children balanced, timely meals with ample iron and calcium.

- Wash children's bottles, pacifiers, and toys often.
- Do not use lead-contaminated water to make infant formula.
- Have your water tested for lead. If the cold water hasn't been used for more than a few hours, let it run for 15 to 30 seconds before drinking it.
- Be aware that other countries do not have the same regulations protecting consumers against lead. Children have been poisoned by eating crayons made in China, putting toys from China in their mouths, and drinking fruit juice canned in Mexico.

A true food allergy occurs when fractions of a food protein or other large molecule are absorbed into the blood and elicit an immunologic response. (Recall that proteins are normally dismantled in the digestive tract to amino acids that are absorbed without such a reaction.) The body's immune system reacts to these large food molecules as it does to other **antigens**—by producing antibodies or other defensive agents.

Detecting Allergy Allergies may have one or two components. They always involve antibodies; they may or may not involve symptoms.* Moreover, symptoms exactly like those of an allergy may have other causes. Therefore, allergies cannot be diagnosed from symptoms alone. The National Institute of Allergy and Infectious Diseases (NIAID) has developed clinical guidelines for the diagnosis and management of food allergy.[69] The NIAID recommends that food allergy should be considered when an individual—especially a young child—experiences symptoms such as skin rash, respiratory difficulties, vomiting, diarrhea, or anaphylactic shock (described later) within minutes to hours of eating food.

Diagnosis of food allergy requires medical testing and food challenges. Once a food allergy has been diagnosed, the required treatment is strict elimination of the offending food. Children with allergies, like all children, need all their nutrients, so it is important to include other foods that offer the same nutrients as the omitted foods.[70] Nutritional counseling and growth monitoring are recommended for all children with food allergies.[71]

Immediate and Delayed Reactions Allergic reactions to food may be immediate or delayed. In either case, the antigen interacts immediately with the immune system, but symptoms may appear within minutes or after several (up to 24) hours. Identifying the food that causes an immediate allergic reaction is easy because symptoms correlate closely with the time the food is eaten. Identifying the food that caused a delayed reaction is more difficult because the symptoms may not appear until a day has passed and many foods besides the offending food have been eaten, complicating the picture.

Anaphylactic Shock The life-threatening food allergy reaction known as **anaphylactic shock** is most often caused by peanuts, tree nuts, milk, eggs, wheat, soybeans, fish, or shellfish (see Figure 12-9). Among these foods, peanuts, milk, and shellfish most often cause problems in children.[72] Children are more likely to outgrow allergies to eggs, milk, wheat, and soy than allergies to peanuts, tree nuts, fish, and shellfish.[73] Peanut allergies cause more life-threatening reactions than do all other food allergies combined. Research is currently under way to help those with peanut allergies tolerate small doses,

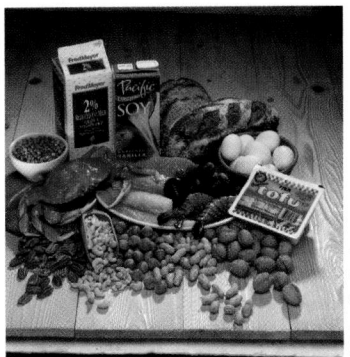

© Polara Studios, Inc.

FIGURE 12-9 Common Food Allergens
These eight normally wholesome foods—milk, shellfish, fish, peanuts, tree nuts, eggs, wheat, and soybeans (and soy products)—may cause life-threatening symptoms in people with allergies.

antigens: substances that elicit the formation of antibodies or an inflammation reaction from the immune system. A bacterium, a virus, a toxin, and a protein in food that causes allergy are all examples of antigens.

anaphylactic (AN-ah-feh-LAC-tic) shock: a life-threatening whole-body allergic reaction to an offending substance.

*A person may produce antibodies without having any symptoms (known as *asymptomatic allergy*) or may produce antibodies and have symptoms (known as *symptomatic allergy*).

TABLE 12-10
Symptoms of Impending Anaphylactic Shock

- Tingling sensation in mouth
- Swelling of the tongue and throat
- Irritated, reddened eyes
- Difficulty breathing, asthma
- Hives, swelling, rashes
- Vomiting, abdominal cramps, diarrhea
- Drop in blood pressure
- Loss of consciousness

thus saving lives and minimizing reactions.[74] Families of children with a life-threatening food allergy and school personnel who supervise those children must guard them against any exposure to the allergen. The child must learn to identify which foods pose a problem and then to use refusal skills for all foods that may contain the allergen.

Parents of allergic children can pack safe foods for lunches and snacks and ask school officials to strictly enforce a "no swapping" policy in the lunchroom. The child must be able to recognize the symptoms of impending anaphylactic shock (see Table 12-10). Any person with food allergies severe enough to cause anaphylactic shock should wear a medical alert bracelet or necklace. Finally, the responsible child and the school staff should be prepared to administer injections of **epinephrine**, which prevents anaphylaxis after exposure to the allergen.[75] Many preventable deaths occur each year when people with food allergies accidentally ingest the allergen but have no epinephrine available.

Technology may soon offer new solutions. New drugs that may interfere with the immune response that causes allergic reactions are being developed. Also, through genetic engineering, scientists may one day banish allergens from peanuts, soybeans, and other foods to make them safer.

Food Labeling Food labels must identify any common allergens present in plain language, using the names of the eight most common allergy-causing foods.[76] For example, a food containing "textured vegetable protein" must say "soy" on its label, and "casein" must be identified as "milk." Food producers must also prevent cross-contamination during production and clearly label the foods in which it is likely to occur. For example, equipment used for making peanut butter must be scrupulously clean before being used to pulverize cashew nuts for cashew butter to protect unsuspecting cashew butter consumers from peanut allergens.

Other Adverse Reactions to Foods Not all **adverse reactions** to foods are food allergies, although even physicians may describe them as such. Signs of adverse reactions to foods include stomachaches, headaches, rapid pulse rate, nausea, wheezing, hives, bronchial irritation, coughs, and other such discomforts. Among the causes may be reactions to chemicals in foods, such as the flavor enhancer monosodium glutamate (MSG), the natural laxative in prunes, or the mineral sulfur; digestive diseases, obstructions, or injuries; enzyme deficiencies, such as lactose intolerance; and even psychological aversions. These reactions involve symptoms but no antibody production. Therefore, they are **food intolerances,** not allergies.

Pesticides applied to produce in the fields may linger on foods and cause adverse reactions. Health risks from pesticide exposure may be low for healthy adults, but children are vulnerable. Therefore, government agencies have set a **tolerance level** for each pesticide by first identifying foods that children commonly eat in large amounts and then considering the effects of pesticide exposure during each developmental stage.

Food Dislikes Parents are advised to watch for signs of food dislikes and take them seriously. Children's food aversions may be the result of nature's efforts to protect them from allergic or other adverse reactions. Test for allergies, and then apply nutrition knowledge conscientiously in deciding how to alter the diet.

epinephrine: one of the stress hormones secreted whenever emergency action is needed; prescribed therapeutically to relax the bronchioles during allergy or asthma attacks.

adverse reactions: unusual responses to food (including intolerances and allergies).

food intolerances: adverse reactions to foods or food additives that do not involve the immune system.

tolerance level: the maximum amount of residue permitted in a food when a pesticide is used according to the label directions.

hyperactivity: inattentive and impulsive behavior that is more frequent and severe than is typical of others of a similar age; professionally called **attention deficit/hyperactivity disorder (ADHD)**.

Hyperactivity

Hyperactivity affects behavior and learning in about 11 percent of young school-aged children.[77] Left untreated, it can interfere with a child's social development and ability to learn. Treatment focuses on relieving the symptoms and controlling the associated problems. Physicians often manage hyperactivity through behavior modification, special educational techniques, and psychological counseling. In many cases, they prescribe medication.[78]

Research on hyperactivity has focused on several nutritional factors as possible causes or treatments.[79] Parents of hyperactive children often blame sugar as the cause

Freddie Willis is a 6-year-old boy who seldom sits still, often misbehaves, and is frequently sick. Freddie's eating habits are erratic and poor, as is his appetite. He often misses breakfast because he is too tired to get up in time to eat before school. By midmorning, Freddie is irritable and disruptive in the classroom. At lunchtime, he trades the peanut butter and banana sandwich his mother packed in his lunchbox for a piece of cake. After school, he hurries home to watch television while he eats his favorite snack—cola and potato chips. At dinnertime, Freddie picks at his food because he isn't very hungry. Later on, when it's time for bed, Freddie complains that he's hungry. His parents let him stay up to have a bowl of cereal (the kind with marshmallows) before he finally falls asleep.

1. What factors in Freddie's daily routine might be contributing to his restless behavior?

2. Discuss some changes in diet that might improve Freddie's health and disposition.

and mistakenly believe that simply eliminating candy and other sweet treats will solve the problem. Despite such speculation, which has been based on personal anecdotes, studies have consistently found no convincing evidence that sugar causes hyperactivity or worsens behavior. Restricting dietary sugar will not cure hyperactivity.

Food additives have also been blamed for hyperactivity and other behavior problems in children, but scientific evidence to substantiate the connection has been elusive.[80] Limited research suggests that food additives such as artificial colors or sodium benzoate preservative (or both) may exacerbate hyperactive symptoms such as inattention and impulsivity.[81] Additional studies are needed to confirm the findings and to determine which additives studied might be responsible for negative behaviors. An FDA review determined that evidence linking color additives to hyperactivity is lacking.[82] The FDA did not rule out the possibility that some food additives, including food colorings, may aggravate hyperactivity and other behavioral problems in some susceptible children.

Children can become excitable, rambunctious, and unruly as a result of a desire for attention, lack of sleep, overstimulation, watching too much television or playing too many computer games, too much caffeine from colas or chocolate, or a lack of physical activity. Such behaviors may suggest that more consistent care is needed. It helps to insist on regular hours of sleep, regular mealtimes, and regular outdoor activity. Box 12-2 offers an opportunity to think about these issues in relation to a specific child.

IN SUMMARY

▌ Children's appetites and nutrient needs reflect their stage of growth.

▌ Long-term hunger and malnutrition impair growth and health.

▌ Short-term hunger exerts more subtle effects on children's health and behavior—such as poor academic performance.

▌ Iron deficiency is widespread and has many physical and behavioral consequences.

▌ Lead toxicity is prevalent among young children and can have irreversible effects on health and behavior.

▌ True food allergies are somewhat rare in children, and children can outgrow some food allergies.

▌ Some allergies, however, can cause dangerous, life-threatening reactions in both children and adults.

▌ "Hyper" behavior is not caused by poor nutrition; misbehavior may reflect inconsistent care.

Childhood Obesity

The number of overweight children has increased dramatically over the past three decades. Like their parents, children in the United States are becoming fatter. An estimated 32 percent of U.S. children and adolescents 2 to 19 years of age are overweight or obese and 17 percent are obese.[83] Based on data from the BMI-for-age growth charts (see Figure E-5 in Appendix E), children and adolescents are categorized as *overweight* above the 85th percentile and as *obese* at the 95th percentile and above.[84] One exception: For older adolescents, BMI at the 95th percentile is higher than 30, the adult obesity cutoff point. Therefore, obesity in young people is defined as BMI at the 95th percentile or BMI of 30 or greater, whichever is lower. For children younger than 2 years of age, BMI values are not available. For this age group, weight-for-height values above the 95th percentile are classified as overweight.

The Expert Committee of the American Medical Association recommends a third cutoff point (99th percentile) to define severe obesity in childhood. Unfortunately, severe obesity in children is becoming more prevalent.[85] Many of these children have multiple risk factors for cardiovascular disease and a high risk of severe obesity in adulthood.[86] The special risks and treatment needs of severely obese children need to be recognized.

Obesity in children is especially troubling because overweight children may become obese adults with all the social, economic, and medical ramifications that often accompany obesity. They have additional problems, too, arising from differences in their growth, physical health, and psychological development. In trying to explain the rise in childhood obesity, researchers point to both genetic and environmental factors.

Genetic and Environmental Factors Parental obesity predicts an early increase in a young child's BMI, and it more than doubles the chances that a young child will become an obese adult.[87] Children with neither parent obese have a less than 10 percent chance of becoming obese in adulthood, whereas overweight teens with at least one obese parent have a greater than 80 percent chance of being obese adults. An obese child's risk of becoming an obese adult increases as the child grows older.[88] The link between parental and child obesity reflects both genetic and environmental factors (as described in Chapter 7).

Diet and physical inactivity are the two strongest environmental factors explaining why children are heavier today than they were 40 or so years ago. As the prevalence of childhood obesity throughout the United States has more than doubled for young children and more than tripled for children 6 to 11 years of age and adolescents, the society our children live in has changed considerably. In many families today, both parents work long hours outside the home; more emphasis is placed on convenience foods and foods eaten away from home; sedentary activities such as watching television and playing computer games occupy much of children's free time; and opportunities for physical activity and outdoor play both during and after school have declined.[89] All of these factors—and many others—influence children's eating and activity patterns.

Children learn food behaviors from their families, and research confirms the significant roles parents play in teaching their children about healthy food choices, providing nutrient-dense foods, and serving as role models.[90] When parents eat fruits and vegetables frequently, their children do, too.[91] The more fruits and vegetables children eat, the more vitamins, minerals, and fiber, and the less saturated fat, in their diets.

In children 2 to 18 years of age, about 40 percent of total energy intake comes from solid fats and added sugars—in other words, empty kcalories.[92] About half of these empty kcalories are contributed by six specific foods: soda, fruit drinks, dairy desserts (ice cream, frozen yogurt, sorbet, sherbet, pudding, and custard), grain desserts (cakes, cookies, pies, cobblers, donuts, and granola bars), pizza, and whole milk. Not surprisingly, researchers have found that children's food choices today provide more kcalories than those of 40 years ago.

As Chapter 2 discussed, as the prevalence of obesity has surged over the past four decades, so has the consumption of added sugars, especially high-fructose corn syrup—the easily consumed, energy-dense liquid sugar added to soft drinks.[93] Each

12-ounce can of soft drink provides the equivalent of about 10 teaspoons of sugar and 150 kcalories. More than half of school-age children consume at least one soft drink each day at school; adolescent males consume the most—two or more cans daily. Research shows that consumption of sugar-sweetened beverages such as soft drinks is associated with increased energy intake and body weight.[94]

No doubt, the tremendous increase in soft drink consumption plays a role, but much of the obesity epidemic can be explained by lack of physical activity. Children have become more sedentary, and sedentary children are more often overweight.[95] Television watching may contribute most to physical inactivity. Children 8 to 18 years of age spend an average of 4.5 hours per day watching television.[96] A child who spends more than an hour or two each day in front of a television, computer monitor, or other media can become overweight even while eating fewer kcalories than a more active child. Playing sedentary video games influences children's activity patterns similarly.

Children who have television sets in their bedrooms spend more time watching TV, spend less time being physically active, and are more likely to be overweight than children who do not have televisions in their rooms.[97] Children who watch a great deal of television are most likely to be overweight and least likely to eat family meals or fruits and vegetables.[98] They often snack on the nutrient-poor, energy-dense foods that are advertised.[99] The average child sees approximately 12 television food ads each day—many peddling foods high in sugar, saturated fat, and salt such as sugar-coated breakfast cereals, candy bars, chips, fast foods, and carbonated beverages.[100] More than half of all food advertisements are aimed specifically at children and market their products as fun and exciting. Not surprisingly, the more time children spend watching television, the more they request these advertised foods and beverages—and they get them about half of the time. The most popular foods and beverages are marketed to children and adolescents on the Internet as well, using "advergaming" (advertised product as part of a game), cartoon characters or "spokes-characters," and designated children's areas.[101] Food marketing to children, including TV ads and Internet ads, as well as marketing in local communities by way of store giveaways, restaurant promotions, school activities, and sporting events, has a profound effect on children's nutrition and health.[102] Despite initiatives by the food industry to answer public health concerns about child-targeted advertising, much remains to be done to reduce the marketing of unhealthy foods to children.[103]

The physically inactive time spent watching television (and playing video and computer games) is second only to time spent sleeping. These activities use no more energy than resting, displace participation in more vigorous activities, and foster snacking on high-fat foods.[104] Compared to sedentary screen-time activities, playing active video games does expend a little more energy, but not enough to count toward the daily 60 minutes of moderate-to-vigorous physical activity recommended for children.[105] Simply reducing the amount of time spent watching television (and playing video games) can improve a child's BMI. The AAP recommends no television viewing before 2 years of age and thereafter limiting television and video time to 2 hours per day as a strategy to help prevent childhood obesity.[106]

Growth Overweight children develop a characteristic set of physical traits. They typically begin puberty earlier and so grow taller than their peers at first, but then they stop growing at a shorter height. They develop greater bone and muscle mass in response to the demand of having to carry more weight—both fat and lean weight. Consequently, they appear "stocky" even when they lose their excess fat.

Physical Health Like overweight adults, overweight children display a blood lipid profile indicating that atherosclerosis is beginning to develop—high levels of total cholesterol, triglycerides, and LDL cholesterol. Overweight children also tend to have high blood pressure; in fact, obesity is a leading cause of pediatric hypertension.[107] Their risks for developing type 2 diabetes and respiratory diseases (such as asthma) are also exceptionally high.[108] These relationships between childhood obesity and chronic diseases are discussed fully in Nutrition in Practice 12.

Psychological Development In addition to the physical consequences, childhood obesity brings a host of emotional and social problems.[109] Because people frequently judge others on appearance more than on character, overweight children are often victims of prejudice. Many suffer discrimination by adults and rejection by their peers. They may have poor self-images, a sense of failure, and a passive approach to life. Television shows, which are a major influence in children's lives, often portray the fat person as the bumbling misfit. Overweight children may come to accept this negative stereotype in themselves and in others, which can lead to additional emotional and social problems. Researchers investigating children's reactions to various body types find that both normal-weight and underweight children respond unfavorably to overweight bodies.

Prevention and Treatment of Obesity Medical science has worked wonders in preventing or curing many of even the most serious childhood diseases, but obesity remains a challenge. Once excess fat has been stored, it is challenging to lose. In light of all this, parents are encouraged to make major efforts to prevent childhood obesity, starting at birth, or to begin treatment early—before adolescence. The Expert Committee of the American Medical Association recommends specific eating and physical activity behaviors to prevent obesity for all children (see Table 12-11).

Treatment of obesity must consider the many aspects of the problem and possible solutions. The main goal of obesity treatment is to improve long-term physical health through permanent healthy lifestyle habits. The most successful approach integrates diet, physical activity, psychological support, and behavioral changes.[110] As a first step, the Expert Committee recommends that overweight and obese children and their families adopt the same healthy eating and activity behaviors presented in Table 12-11 for obesity prevention. The goal for overweight and obese children is to improve BMI. If the child's BMI does not improve after several months, the Expert Committee recommends increasing the intensity of the treatment. The level of intensity depends on treatment response, age, degree of obesity, health risks, and the family's readiness to change.[111] Advanced treatment involves close follow-up monitoring by a health care provider and greater support and structure for the child.

TABLE 12-11 Recommended Eating and Physical Activity Behaviors to Prevent Obesity

The Expert Committee of the American Medical Association recommends the following healthy habits for children 2 to 18 years of age to help prevent childhood obesity:

- Limit consumption of sugar-sweetened beverages, such as soft drinks and fruit-flavored punches.
- Eat the recommended amounts of fruits and vegetables every day (2 to 4.5 cups per day based on age).
- Learn to eat age-appropriate portions of foods.
- Eat foods low in energy density such as those high in fiber and/or water and modest in fat.
- Eat a nutritious breakfast every day.
- Eat a diet rich in calcium.
- Eat a diet balanced in recommended proportions for carbohydrate, fat, and protein.
- Eat a diet high in fiber.
- Eat together as a family as often as possible.
- Limit the frequency of restaurant meals.
- Limit television watching or other screen time to no more than two hours per day, and do not have televisions or computers in sleeping areas.
- Engage in at least 60 minutes of moderate to vigorous physical activity every day.

© Cengage Learning®

Source: S. E. Barlow, Expert Committee recommendations regarding the prevention, assessment, and treatment of child and adolescent overweight and obesity: Summary report, *Pediatrics* 120 (2007): S164–S192.

Diet The initial goal for overweight children is to reduce the rate of weight gain, that is, to maintain weight as the child grows taller.[112] Continued growth will then accomplish the desired change in BMI. Weight loss is usually not recommended because diet restriction can interfere with growth and development. Intervention for some overweight children with accompanying medical conditions may warrant weight loss, but this treatment requires an individualized approach based on the degree of overweight and severity of the medical conditions.[113] Dietary strategies begin with those listed in Table 12-11 and progress to more structured family meal plans when necessary. For example, the child or the parent may be instructed to keep detailed logs of dietary intake.

Physical Activity The many benefits of physical activity are well known but often are not enough to motivate overweight people, especially children. Yet regular vigorous activity can improve a child's weight, body composition, and physical fitness.[114] Ideally, parents will limit sedentary activities and encourage at least one hour of daily physical activity to promote strong skeletal, muscular, and cardiovascular development and instill in their children the desire to be physically active throughout life. Opportunities to be physically active can include team, individual, and recreational activities (see Table 12-12). Most importantly, parents need to set a good example. Physical activity is a natural and lifelong behavior of healthy living. It can be as simple as riding a bike, playing tag, jumping rope, or doing chores. The AAP supports the efforts of schools to include more physical activity in the curriculum and encourages parents to support their children's participation.

TABLE 12-12 Examples of Aerobic, Muscle-Strengthening, and Bone-Strengthening Physical Activities for Children and Adolescents

Moderate-to-Vigorous Aerobic Activities	Muscle-Strengthening Activities	Bone-Strengthening Activities
Moderate	Games such as tug-of-war	Games such as hopscotch
Active recreation such as hiking, skateboarding, rollerblading	Modified push-ups (with knees on the floor)	Hopping, skipping, jumping
Bicycle riding[a]	Resistance exercises using body weight, free weights, or resistance bands	Jumping rope
Brisk walking	Rope or tree climbing	Running
Vigorous	Sit-ups (curl-ups or crunches)	Sports such as gymnastics, basketball, volleyball, tennis
Active games involving running and chasing, such as tag	Swinging on playground equipment/bars	
Bicycle riding[a]		
Cross-country skiing		
Jumping rope		
Martial arts		
Running		
Sports such as soccer, ice or field hockey, basketball, swimming, tennis		

[a]Some activities, such as bicycling, can be moderate or vigorous, depending on level of effort.

Behavioral Changes In contrast to traditional weight-loss programs that focus on *what* to eat, behavioral programs focus on *how* to eat. These techniques involve changing learned habits that lead a child to eat excessively. Weight-loss programs that involve parents and other caregivers in treatment report greater success than those without parental involvement. Because obesity in parents and their children tends to be positively correlated, both benefit when parents participate in a weight-loss program. Parental attitudes about food greatly influence children's eating behavior, so it is important that the influence be positive. Otherwise, eating problems may become exacerbated.

Drugs The use of weight-loss drugs to treat obesity in children merits special concern because the long-term effects of these drugs on growth and development have not been studied. The drugs may be used in addition to structured lifestyle changes for carefully selected children or adolescents who are at high risk for severe obesity in adulthood. Orlistat (see Chapter 7) is the only prescription weight-loss medication that has been approved for use in adolescents 12 years of age and older.[115] Alli, the over-the-counter version of orlistat, should not be given to anyone younger than age 18.

Surgery The efficacy of surgery as a treatment for severe obesity in adults (see Chapter 7) has created interest in its use for adolescents. Limited research shows that, after surgery, extremely obese adolescents lose significant weight and experience improvements in type 2 diabetes and cardiovascular risk factors.[116] The selection criteria for surgery to treat obesity in adolescents listed in Table 12-13 are based on recommendations of a panel of pediatricians and surgeons.[117]

Obesity is prevalent in our society. Because treatment of obesity is frequently unsuccessful, it is most important to prevent its onset. Above all, be sensible in teaching children how to maintain appropriate body weight. Children can easily get the impression that their worth is tied to their body weight. Parents and the media are most influential in shaping self-concept, weight concerns, and dieting practices.[118] Some parents fail to realize that society's ideal of slimness can be perilously close to starvation and that a child encouraged to "diet" cannot obtain the energy and nutrients required for normal growth and development. Even healthy children without diagnosable eating disorders have been observed to limit their growth through "dieting." Weight loss in truly overweight children can be managed without compromising growth, but it should be overseen by a health care professional.

TABLE 12-13 Selection Criteria for Obesity Surgery in Adolescents

- Physically mature
- BMI ≥40, or BMI >35 with significant weight-related health problems
- History of failure in a formal, 6-month weight-loss program
- Capable of adhering to the long-term lifestyle changes required after surgery

IN SUMMARY

- Childhood obesity has become a major health problem.

- Genetics, energy-dense diets, and physical inactivity play roles in childhood obesity.

- Childhood obesity can impair physical and psychological health.

- The main goal of obesity treatment in children is to improve long-term physical health through permanent healthy lifestyle habits.

Mealtimes at Home

The childhood years are the parents' last chance to influence their children's food choices. Parents who want to promote nutritious choices and healthful habits provide access to nutrient-dense, delicious foods and opportunities for active play at home. Food choices and regular physical activity can not only promote healthy growth but, as mentioned earlier, also help prevent the chronic diseases of later life. Many experts agree that early childhood is the time to put into effect practices that, until recently, were recommended only for adults.

Feeding children requires not only providing a variety of nutritious foods but also nurturing the children's self-esteem and well-being. Parents face a number of challenges in preparing meals that both appeal to their children's tastes and provide needed nutrients. Because the interactions between parents and children can set the stage for lifelong attitudes and habits, a child's preferences should be treated with respect, even when nutrient needs must take precedence.

Eating is more fun when your friends are there.

Honoring Children's Preferences Researchers attempting to explain children's food preferences encounter many contradictions. Children say they like colorful foods yet most often reject green and yellow vegetables while favoring brown peanut butter and white potatoes, apple wedges, and bread. They do like raw vegetables better than cooked ones, though, so it is wise to offer vegetables that are raw or slightly undercooked, crunchy, and bright in color. They should be warm, not hot, because a child's mouth is much more sensitive than an adult's. The flavor should be mild (a child has more taste buds), and smooth foods such as mashed potatoes or pea soup should have no lumps (a child wonders, with some disgust, what the lumps might be).

Make mealtimes fun for children. Young children like to eat at little tables and to be served little portions of food. They also love to eat with other children and have been observed to stay at the table longer and eat more food when in the company of their friends. Children are also more likely to give up their prejudices against foods when they see their peers eating them.[119] Parents who serve food in a relaxed and casual manner, without anxiety, provide an environment in which a child's negative emotions will be minimized.

Avoiding Power Struggles Problems over food often arise during the second or third year, when children begin asserting their independence. Many of these problems stem from the conflict between children's developmental stages and capabilities and parents who, in attempting to do what they think is best for their children, try to control every aspect of eating. Such conflicts can disrupt children's abilities to regulate their own food intakes or to determine their own likes and dislikes. For example, many people share the misconception that children must be persuaded or coerced to try new foods. In fact, the opposite is true. When children are forced to try new foods, especially when offered rewards for eating a particular food, they are less likely to try those foods again than are children who are left to decide for themselves. Similarly, when children are restricted from eating their favorite foods, they are more likely to want those foods. As dietitian and family therapist Ellyn Satter notes, the parent is responsible for *what* the child is offered to eat, but the child is responsible for *how much* and even *whether* to eat.

When introducing new foods at the table, parents are advised to offer them one at a time and only in small amounts at first. The more often a food is presented to a young child, the more likely the child will accept that food.[120] Between 5 and 10 exposures to a new food are necessary before a toddler shows an enhanced preference for the food. Offer the new food at the beginning of the meal, when the child is hungry, and allow the child to make the decision to accept or reject it. Parents have their own inclinations and dislikes; so do children. Never make an issue of food acceptance. Table 12-14 (on p. 344) offers tips for feeding picky eaters.

Choking Prevention Parents must always be alert to the dangers of choking. A choking child is silent, so an adult should be present whenever a child is eating. Make sure the child sits when eating; choking is more likely when a child is running or falling (see Table 12-5 for a list of foods and nonfood items most likely to cause choking).

Play First Ideally, each meal is preceded, not followed, by the activity the child looks forward to the most. A number of schools have discovered that children eat a much

TABLE 12-14 Tips for Feeding Picky Eaters

Get Them Involved

Children are more likely to feel a sense of ownership and may be more interested in trying foods when they participate in meal planning, grocery shopping, cooking, gardening, and harvesting the foods they eat.

Be Creative

▪ Try serving veggies as finger foods with dips or spreads.

▪ Use cookie cutters to cut fruits and veggies into fun shapes.

▪ Put healthy snacks in ice cube trays or muffin pans where children can easily reach them and graze on these as they play.

▪ Serve traditional meals out of order (for example, breakfast for dinner).

▪ Use healthy foods such as veggies and whole grains in craft projects to help kids become familiar with them and encourage their interest and enthusiasm for these foods.

Enhance Favorite Recipes

▪ Include sliced or shredded veggies in sauces, casseroles, pancakes, and muffins.

▪ Serve fruit over cereal, yogurt, or ice cream.

▪ Bake brownies with black beans or cookies with lentils as an ingredient.

Model and Share

▪ Be a role model to children by eating healthy foods with them. Offer to share your healthy snack with them, too.

▪ Sometimes children need to be exposed to a new food multiple times before they develop a taste for the food, so make sure healthy options are always available and don't give up on repeatedly offering foods your child might not seem interested in.

▪ Encourage your child to taste at least one bite of each food served at a meal.

Respect and Relax

▪ Remember that it is not uncommon for children to eat sporadically. They have smaller stomachs and therefore are likely to feel full faster and become hungry again not long after a snack or meal.

▪ Focus on your child's overall weekly intake of food and nutrients rather than daily consumption.

▪ If you suspect that your child might not be eating enough to support healthy growth and development, discuss your concerns with your child's doctor. It might be helpful to maintain a food log of everything your child eats over a period of three days to bring along to the doctor appointment.

Source: Based on Mayo Clinic Staff, Children's nutrition: 10 tips for picky eaters, 2011, available at www.mayoclinic.com/health/childrens-health/HQ01107.

better lunch if it is served after, rather than before, recess. Otherwise, children "hurry up and eat" so that they can go play.

Child Participation Allowing children to help plan and prepare the family's meals provides enjoyable learning experiences and encourages children to eat the foods they have prepared. Vegetables are pretty, especially when fresh, and provide opportunities for children to learn about color, growing things and their seeds, and shapes and textures—all of which are fascinating to young children. Measuring, stirring, decorating, and arranging foods are skills that even a very young child can practice with enjoyment and pride (see Table 12-15).

Snacks Parents may find that their children often snack so much that they aren't hungry at mealtimes. Instead of teaching children *not* to snack, teach them *how* to snack. Provide snacks that are as nutritious as the foods served at mealtime. Snacks can even be mealtime foods that are served individually over time, instead of all at once on one plate. When providing snacks to children, think of the food groups and

TABLE 12-15 Food Skills and Developmental Milestones of Preschool Children[a]

Age (years)	Food Skills	Developmental Milestones
1 to 2	▪ Uses a spoon ▪ Lifts and drinks from a cup ▪ Helps scrub fruits and vegetables, tear lettuce or greens, snap green beans, or dip foods ▪ Can be messy; can be easily distracted	▪ Large muscles develop ▪ Experiences slowed growth and decreased appetite ▪ Develops likes and dislikes ▪ May suddenly refuse certain foods
3	▪ Spears food with a fork ▪ Feeds self independently ▪ Helps wrap, pour, mix, shake, stir, or spread foods ▪ Follows simple instructions	▪ Medium hand muscles develop ▪ May suddenly refuse certain foods ▪ Begins to request favorite foods ▪ Makes simple either/or food choices
4	▪ Uses all utensils and napkin ▪ Helps measure dry ingredients ▪ Learns table manners	▪ Small finger muscles develop ▪ Influenced by TV, media, and peers ▪ May dislike many mixed dishes
5	▪ Measures liquids ▪ Helps grind, grate, and cut (soft foods with dull knife) ▪ Uses hand mixer with supervision	▪ Fine coordination of fingers and hands develops ▪ Usually accepts food that is available ▪ Eats with minor supervision

© 2016 Cengage Learning®

[a]These ages are approximate. Healthy, normal children develop at their own pace.

Source: Adapted from MyPlate for Preschoolers, Behavioral Milestones, available at www.choosemyplate.gov/preschoolers/healthy-habits/Milestones.pdf.

TABLE 12-16 Healthful Snack Ideas—Think Food Groups, Alone and in Combination

Selecting two or more foods from different food groups adds variety and nutrient balance to snacks. The combinations are endless, so be creative.

Grains: Grain products are filling snacks, especially when combined with other foods:

▪ Cereal with fruit and milk
▪ Crackers and cheese
▪ Whole-grain toast with peanut butter
▪ Popcorn with grated cheese
▪ Oatmeal raisin cookies with milk

Vegetables: Cut-up fresh, raw vegetables make great snacks alone or in combination with foods from other food groups:

▪ Celery with peanut butter
▪ Broccoli, cauliflower, and carrot sticks with a flavored cottage cheese dip

Fruits: Fruits are delicious snacks and can be eaten alone—fresh, dried, or juiced—or combined with other foods:

▪ Apples and cheese
▪ Bananas and peanut butter
▪ Peaches with yogurt
▪ Raisins mixed with sunflower seeds or nuts

Protein Foods: Meat, poultry, seafood, legumes, soy products, nuts, and seeds add protein to snacks:

▪ Refried beans with nachos and cheese
▪ Peanut butter, hummus, or tuna on crackers
▪ Luncheon meat on whole-grain bread

Milk and Milk Products: Milk can be used as a beverage with any snack, and many other milk products, such as yogurt and cheese, can be eaten alone or with other foods as listed above.

© 2016 Cengage Learning®

offer such snacks as pieces of cheese, sliced strawberries, cooked baby carrots, and egg salad on whole-wheat crackers (see Table 12-16). Replacing nutrient-poor, high-kcalorie snacks such as potato chips with nutrient-rich, low-kcalorie snacks such as vegetables not only reduces children's energy intakes but also improves their nutrient intakes as well.[121] Snacks that are easy to prepare should be readily available to children, especially if the children arrive home after school before their parents.

Preventing Dental Caries Children frequently snack on sticky, sugary foods that stay on the teeth and provide an ideal environment for the growth of bacteria that cause dental caries. Teach children to brush and floss after meals, to brush or rinse after eating snacks, to avoid sticky foods, and to select crisp or fibrous foods frequently.

Serving as Role Models In an effort to practice these many tips, parents may overlook perhaps the single most important influence on their children's food habits—themselves. Parents who do not eat oranges should not be surprised when their children refuse to eat oranges. Likewise, parents who dislike the smell of brussels sprouts may not be able to persuade children to try them. Children learn much through imitation. Parents, older siblings, and other caregivers set an irresistible example by sitting with younger children, eating the same foods, and having pleasant conversations during mealtime.

While serving and enjoying food, caregivers can promote both physical and emotional health at every stage of a child's life. They can help their children to develop both a positive self-concept and a positive attitude toward food. If the beginnings are right, children will grow without the conflicts and confusions over foods that lead to nutrition and health problems.

Nutrition at School

While parents are doing what they can to establish good eating habits in their children at home, others are preparing and serving foods to their children at day care centers and schools. In addition, children begin learning about food and nutrition in the classroom. Meeting the nutrition and education needs of children is critical to supporting their healthy growth and development.[122] The Academy of Nutrition and Dietetics has set nutrition standards for childcare programs (see Table 12-17).[123] In addition, childcare providers can encourage active play for children by creating opportunities for children to engage in both structured and unstructured activity throughout the day.

The U.S. government funds programs to provide nutritious, high-quality meals for children at school. Both the School Breakfast Program and the National School Lunch Program provide meals at a reasonable cost to children from families with the financial means to pay. Meals are available free or at reduced cost to children from low-income families.

School Breakfast The School Breakfast Program is available in about 90 percent of the nation's schools that offer school lunch, and nearly 13 million children participate in it.[124] Nevertheless, many children who need the School Breakfast Program either do not have access to the program or do not participate in it.[125] The majority of children who eat school breakfasts are from low-income families. As research results continue to emphasize the positive impact breakfast has on school performance and health, vigorous campaigns to expand school breakfast programs are under way.[126] The school breakfast must contain, at a minimum: one serving of fluid milk (either unflavored low-fat or flavored or unflavored fat-free); one serving of fruit or vegetable (no more than half of the servings may be 100 percent full-strength juice); and either one to two servings of whole grains or one serving of whole grains and one serving of meat or meat alternatives.

School Lunch More than 31 million children receive lunches through the National School Lunch Program—more than half of them free or at a reduced price.[127] School lunches are designed to provide at least a third of the recommendation for energy, protein, vitamin A, vitamin C, iron, and calcium. They must also

---

TABLE 12-17 Selected Academy of Nutrition and Dietetics Nutrition Standards for Childcare Programs

Meal plans should:

- Be nutritionally adequate and consistent with the *Dietary Guidelines for Americans.*

- Emphasize fresh fruit, fresh and frozen vegetables, whole grains, and low-fat milk and milk products.

- Limit foods and beverages high in energy, added sugars, solid fats, and sodium, and low in vitamins and minerals.

- Provide foods and beverages in quantities and meal patterns appropriate to ensure optimal growth and development.

- Involve parents in planning.

- Provide furniture and eating utensils that are age appropriate and developmentally suitable to encourage children to accept and enjoy mealtime.

Source: Position of the American Dietetic Association: Benchmarks for nutrition in child care, *Journal of the American Dietetic Association* 111 (2011): 607–615.

include specified numbers of servings from each food group. In an effort to help reduce disease risk, all government-funded meals served at schools must follow the *Dietary Guidelines for Americans*. Table 12-18 shows school lunch patterns for children of different ages.

The USDA Food and Nutrition Service recently updated the meal patterns and nutrition standards for school meals.[128] Changes to meals include greater availability of fruits, vegetables, whole grains, and fat-free and low-fat milk, decreased levels of sodium, saturated fat, and *trans* fat, and guidelines for meeting nutrient needs within specified kcalorie ranges based on age/grade groups for school children.

Parents often rely on school lunches to meet a significant part of their children's nutrient needs on school days. Indeed, students who regularly eat school lunches have higher intakes of many nutrients and fiber than students who do not. Children don't

TABLE 12-18 School Lunch Patterns for Different Ages

| Food Group | Amount of Food per Week (minimum per day)[a] | | |
	Elementary School Grades K to 5	Middle School Grades 6 to 8	High School Grades 9 to 12
Fruits (cups)[b]	2½ (½)	2½ (½)	5 (1)
Vegetables (cups)[b]	3¾ (¾)	3¾ (¾)	5 (1)
Dark green[c]	½	½	½
Red/orange[c]	¾	¾	1¼
Beans/peas (legumes)[c]	½	½	½
Starchy[c]	½	½	½
Other[c]	½	½	¾
Additional to reach total[d]	1	1	1½
Grains (oz eq)[e]	8–9 (1)	8–10 (1)	10–12 (2)
Meat or meat alternate (oz eq)	8–10 (1)	9–10 (1)	10–12 (2)
Milk: Fluid milk (cups)[f]	5 (1)	5 (1)	5 (1)
Other Specifications: Daily amount based on the average for a 5-day week			
kCalorie range[g, h]	550–650	600–700	750–850
Saturated fat (% of total kcalories)[h]	<10	<10	<10
Sodium (mg)[h, i]	≤1230	≤1360	≤1420
School year 2017–2018	≤935	≤1035	≤1080
School year 2022–2023	≤640	≤710	≤740
Trans fat	Nutrition label or manufacturer specifications must indicate zero grams of *trans* fat per serving.		

© 2016 Cengage Learning®

[a]Minimum creditable serving is ⅛ cup.

[b]One quarter-cup of dried fruit counts as ½ cup of fruit; 1 cup of leafy greens counts as ½ cup of vegetables. No more than half of the fruit or vegetable offerings may be in the form of juice. All juice must be 100% full-strength.

[c]Larger amounts of these vegetables may be served.

[d]Any vegetable subgroup may be offered to meet the total weekly vegetable requirement.

[e]All grains must be whole grain rich.

[f]Fluid milk must be low-fat (1% milk fat or less, unflavored) or fat-free (unflavored or flavored).

[g]The average daily amount of kcalories for a 5-day school week must be within the range (at least the minimum and no more than the maximum values).

[h]Discretionary sources of kcalories (solid fats and added sugars) may be added to the meal pattern if within the specifications for kcalories, saturated fat, *trans* fat, and sodium. Foods of minimal nutritional value and fluid milk with fat content greater than 1% milk fat are not allowed.

[i]Final sodium specifications are to be reached by school year 2022–2023 or July 1, 2022. Intermediate specifications are currently in effect and established for school year 2017–2018.

Sources: U.S. Department of Agriculture 2012; *Federal Register* 77 (2012): 4110–4111.

TABLE 12-19 **USDA Nutrition Standards for Foods Sold in Schools**

Any food sold in schools must:

- be a "whole grain-rich" grain product; or

- have a fruit, vegetable, dairy product, or protein food as the first ingredient; or

- be a combination food that contains at least ¼ cup of fruit and/or vegetable; or

- contain ≥10% of the Daily Value (DV) of one or more nutrients of concern (calcium, potassium, vitamin D, or fiber).

Foods must also limit kcalories, sodium, fat, and sugar.

All schools may sell the following beverages:

- Plain or carbonated water

- Unflavored low-fat milk

- Unflavored or flavored fat-free milk/milk alternatives

- 100% fruit or vegetable juice with no added sugars

Source: USDA's "All foods sold in schools" standards, www.fns.usda.gov/school-meals/smart-snacks-school, June 20, 2014.

always like what they are served, however, and school lunch programs must strike a balance between what children want to eat and what will nourish them and guard their health.

Competing Influences at School Serving nutritious lunches is only half the battle; students need to eat them, too. Short lunch periods and long lines prevent some students from eating a school lunch and leave others with too little time to complete their meals.[129] Nutrition efforts at schools are also undermined when students can buy what the USDA labels "competitive foods"—meals from fast-food restaurants or à la carte foods such as pizza or snack foods and carbonated beverages from snack bars, school stores, and vending machines.[130] These foods and beverages compete with nutritious school lunches. When students have access to competitive foods, participation in the school lunch program decreases, nutrient intake from lunch declines, and more food is discarded.[131]

Increasingly, school-based nutrition issues are being addressed by legislation. The USDA recently published practical, science-based nutrition standards for "all foods sold in schools," including snack foods and beverages (see Table 12-19). The standards encourage healthier snack foods while limiting junk foods.[132]

IN SUMMARY

▮ Adults at home and at school need to provide children with nutrient-dense foods and teach them how to make healthful choices. Adults also need to provide ample opportunity for children to be physically active.

▮ School-based nutrition issues are being addressed by legislation nationwide. Establishing and implementing nutrition standards for all foods available on school campuses helps to ensure that such foods comply with the *Dietary Guidelines for Americans*.

12.3 Nutrition during Adolescence

LO 12.3 Describe the nutrient needs of adolescents and some of the challenges in meeting these needs.

As children pass through **adolescence** on their way to becoming adults, they change in many ways. Their physical changes make their nutrient needs high, and their emotional, intellectual, and social changes make meeting those needs a challenge.

Teenagers make many more choices for themselves than they did as children. They are not fed; they eat. Food choices made during the teen years profoundly affect present and future health. At the same time, social pressures thrust choices at them: whether to drink alcoholic beverages and whether to develop their bodies to meet extreme ideals of slimness or athletic prowess. Their interest in nutrition—both valid information and misinformation—derives from personal, immediate experiences. They are concerned with how diet can improve their lives now—they try the latest fad diet to fit into a new bathing suit, avoid greasy foods in an effort to clear acne, or eat a plate of pasta to prepare for a big sporting event. In presenting information on the nutrition and health of adolescents, this chapter includes topics of interest to teens.

Growth and Development during Adolescence

With the onset of adolescence, the steady growth of childhood speeds up abruptly and dramatically, and the growth patterns of females and males become distinct. Hormones direct the intensity and duration of the adolescent growth spurt, profoundly affecting

adolescence: the period of growth from the beginning of puberty until full maturity. Timing of adolescence varies from person to person.

every organ of the body, including the brain. After 2 to 3 years of intense growth and a few more at a slower pace, physically mature adults emerge.

In general, the adolescent growth spurt begins at age 10 or 11 for females and at age 12 or 13 for males. It lasts about 2½ years. Before **puberty**, male and female body compositions differ only slightly, but during the adolescent spurt, differences between the genders become apparent in the skeletal system, lean body mass, and fat stores. In females, fat assumes a larger percentage of total body weight, and in males, the lean body mass—principally muscle and bone—increases much more than in females. On average, males grow 8 inches taller, and females, 6 inches taller. Males gain approximately 45 pounds, and females, about 35 pounds.

Energy and Nutrient Needs

The energy needs of adolescents vary greatly, depending on the current rate of growth, gender, body composition, and physical activity.[133] Boys' energy needs may be especially high; they typically grow faster than girls and, as mentioned, develop a greater proportion of lean body mass. An exceptionally active boy of 15 may need 3500 kcalories or more a day just to maintain his weight. Girls start growing earlier than boys and attain shorter heights and lower weights, so their energy needs peak sooner and decline earlier than those of their male peers. An inactive girl of 15 whose growth is nearly at a standstill may need fewer than 1800 kcalories a day if she is to avoid excessive weight gain. Thus, teenage girls need to pay special attention to being physically active and selecting foods of high nutrient density so that they will meet their nutrient needs without exceeding their energy needs.

Obesity The insidious problem of obesity becomes ever more apparent in adolescence and often continues into adulthood. Without intervention, overweight teens will face numerous physical and socioeconomic consequences for years to come. The consequences of obesity are so dramatic and our society's attitude toward obese people is so negative that even healthy-weight or underweight teens may perceive a need to lose weight. When taken to extremes, restrictive diets bring dramatic physical consequences of their own, as Nutrition in Practice 6 explains.

Vitamin D Recommendations for most vitamins increase during the teen years (see the tables on the inside front cover). Several of the vitamin recommendations for adolescents are similar to those for adults, including the recently revised recommendations for vitamin D.[134] Vitamin D is essential for bone growth and development. Recent studies of vitamin D status in adolescents show that many are vitamin D deficient; blacks, females, and overweight adolescents are most at risk.[135] Adolescents who do not receive enough vitamin D from fortified foods such as milk and cereals, or from sun exposure each day, may need a supplement.[136]

Iron The need for iron increases during adolescence for both females and males but for different reasons. Iron needs increase for females as they start to menstruate and for males as their lean body mass develops. Hence, the RDA increases at age 14 for both males and females. Because menstruation continues throughout a woman's childbearing years, the RDA for iron remains high for women into late adulthood. For males, the RDA returns to preadolescent values in early adulthood.

In addition, iron needs increase when the adolescent growth spurt begins, whether that occurs before or after age 14. Therefore, boys in a growth spurt need an additional 2.9 milligrams of iron per day above the RDA for their age; girls need an additional 1.1 milligrams per day. Furthermore, iron recommendations for girls before age 14 do not reflect the iron losses of menstruation, even though the average age of menarche (first menstruation) in the United States is 12.5 years. Therefore, for girls younger than age 14 who have started to menstruate, an additional 2.5 milligrams of iron per day is recommended. Thus, the RDA for iron depends not only on age and

puberty: the period in life in which a person becomes physically capable of reproduction.

© 2016 Cengage Learning®

TABLE 12-20 Iron Recommendations during Adolescence

Iron RDA for males:

- 9–13 yr: 8 mg/day
- 9–13 yr in growth spurt: 10.9 mg/day
- 14–18 yr: 11 mg/day
- 14–18 yr in growth spurt: 13.9 mg/day

Iron RDA for females:

- 9–13 yr: 8 mg/day
- 9–13 yr in menarche: 10.5 mg/day
- 9–13 yr in menarche and growth spurt: 11.6 mg/day
- 14–18 yr: 15 mg/day
- 14–18 yr in growth spurt: 16.1 mg/day

gender but also on whether the individual is in a growth spurt or has begun to menstruate, as listed in Table 12-20.

Iron intakes often fail to keep pace with increasing needs, especially for females, who typically consume fewer iron-rich foods such as meat and fewer total kcalories than males. Not surprisingly, iron deficiency is most prevalent among adolescent girls. Iron-deficient children and teens score lower on standardized tests than those who are not iron deficient.

Calcium Adolescence is a crucial time for bone development, and the requirement for calcium reaches its peak during these years.[137] Unfortunately, many adolescents, especially females, have calcium intakes below recommendations.[138] Low calcium intakes during times of active growth, especially if paired with physical inactivity, can compromise the development of peak bone mass, which is considered the best protection against adolescent fractures and adult osteoporosis. Increasing milk products in the diet to meet calcium recommendations greatly increases bone density.[139] Once again, however, teenage girls are most vulnerable, for their milk—and therefore their calcium—intakes begin to decline at the time when their calcium needs are greatest.[140] Furthermore, women have much greater bone losses than men in later life. In addition to dietary calcium, physical activity makes bones grow stronger. However, because some high schools do not require students to attend physical activity classes, many adolescents must make a point to be physically active during leisure time.

Food Choices and Health Habits

Teenagers like the freedom to come and go as they choose. They eat what they want if it is convenient and if they have the time. With a multitude of afterschool, social, and job activities, they almost inevitably fall into irregular eating habits. At any given time on any given day, a teenager may be skipping a meal, eating a snack, preparing a meal, or consuming food prepared by a parent or restaurant.[141] Adolescents who frequently eat meals with their families, however, eat more fruits, vegetables, grains, and calcium-rich foods and drink fewer soft drinks than those who seldom eat with their families.[142] Many adolescents begin to skip breakfast on a regular basis, missing out on important nutrients that are not made up at later meals during the day. Compared with those who skip breakfast, teenagers who do eat breakfast have higher intakes of vitamin A, vitamin C, and riboflavin, as well as calcium, iron, and zinc.[143] Teenagers who eat breakfast are therefore more likely to meet their nutrient recommendations.

Breakfast skipping may also lead to weight gain in adolescents. Eating breakfast each day, especially a breakfast rich in fiber and protein, improves satiety and reduces hunger and the desire to eat throughout the day.[144] As adolescents make the transition to adulthood, not only do they skip breakfast more often, but they also eat fast food more often. Both skipping breakfast and eating fast foods lead to weight gain.[145]

Ideally, in light of adolescents' busy schedules and desire for freedom, the adult becomes a **gatekeeper**, controlling the type and availability of food in the teenager's environment. Teenage sons and daughters and their friends should find plenty of nutritious, easy-to-grab food in the refrigerator (meats for sandwiches; low-fat cheeses; fresh, raw vegetables and fruits; fruit juices; and milk) and more in the cabinets (whole-grain breads, peanut butter, nuts, popcorn, and cereal). In many households today, all the adults work outside the home, and teenagers perform some of the gatekeeper's roles, such as shopping for groceries or choosing fast or prepared foods.

Snacks On average, about a fourth of an adolescent's total daily energy intake comes from snacks, which, if chosen carefully, can contribute some of the needed nutrients (see Table 12-16 on p. 345). A survey of more than 5000 adolescents found that those who ate snacks more often were less likely to be overweight or obese and had lower rates of abdominal obesity compared with those who ate snacks less often.[146]

gatekeeper: with respect to nutrition, a key person who controls other people's access to foods and thereby exerts a profound impact on their nutrition. Examples are the spouse who buys and cooks the food, the parent who feeds the children, and the caregiver in a day care center.

Beverages Most frequently, adolescents drink soft drinks instead of fruit juice or milk with lunch, supper, and snacks. About the only time they select fruit juices is at breakfast. When teens drink milk, they are more likely to consume it with a meal (especially breakfast) than as a snack. Because of their greater food intakes, boys are more likely than girls to drink enough milk to meet their calcium needs.[147]

Soft drinks, when chosen as the primary beverage, may affect bone density, partly because they displace milk from the diet. Over the past 3 decades, teens (especially girls) have been drinking more soft drinks and less milk. Adolescents who drink soft drinks regularly have a higher energy intake and a lower calcium intake than those who do not.[148]

Soft drinks and energy drinks containing caffeine present a different problem if caffeine intake becomes excessive.[149] Many adolescents consume energy drinks on a regular basis and these beverages contain much more caffeine than soft drinks.[150]* Caffeine seems to be relatively harmless, however, when used in moderate doses (less than 100 milligrams per day, roughly equivalent to fewer than three 12-ounce cola beverages a day). In greater amounts, it can cause the symptoms associated with anxiety—sweating, tenseness, and inability to concentrate.

Eating Away from Home Adolescents eat about one-third of their meals away from home, and their nutritional welfare is enhanced or hindered by the choices they make.[151] A lunch consisting of a hamburger, a chocolate shake, and french fries supplies substantial quantities of many nutrients at a kcalorie cost of about 800, an energy intake some adolescents can afford. When they eat this sort of lunch, teens can adjust their breakfast and dinner choices to include fruits and vegetables for vitamin A, vitamin C, folate, and fiber, and lean meats and legumes for iron and zinc. (See Appendix A for the nutrient contents of fast foods.) Fortunately, many fast-food restaurants are offering more nutritious choices than the standard hamburger meal.

Peer Influence Physical maturity and growing independence present adolescents with new choices whose consequences influence their health and nutrition status both today and throughout life. Many of the food and health choices adolescents make reflect the opinions and actions of their peers. When others perceive milk as "babyish," a teen may choose soft drinks instead; when others skip lunch and hang out in the parking lot, a teen may join in for the camaraderie, regardless of hunger. Some teenagers begin using drugs, alcohol, and tobacco; others wisely refrain. Adults can set up the environment so that nutritious foods are available and can stand by with reliable information and advice about health and nutrition, but the rest is up to the adolescents. Ultimately, they make the choices.

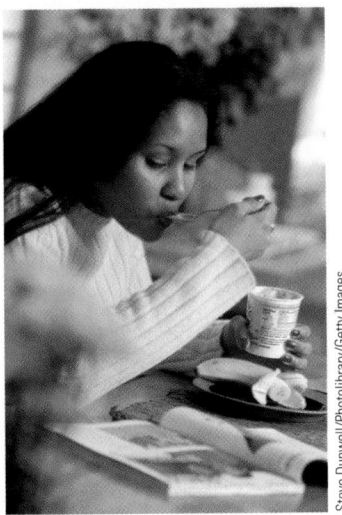

Nutritious snacks contribute valuable nutrients to an active teen's diet.

IN SUMMARY

▌ Nutrient needs rise dramatically as children enter the rapid growth phase of the teen years.

▌ The busy lifestyles of teenagers add to the challenge of meeting their nutrient needs, especially for iron and calcium.

Assessment of nutrition status in healthy infants, children and adolescents can confirm that development is normal or can catch potential problems early. (Chapter 14 offers details about nutrition assessment.) The Nutrition Assessment Checklist (on p. 352) highlights problems to look for when working with infants, children and adolescents.

*Caffeine-containing soft drinks typically deliver about 30 milligrams of caffeine per 12-ounce can; energy drinks typically deliver about 100 milligrams of caffeine for equivalent amounts. A pharmacologically active dose of caffeine is defined as 200 milligrams. Appendix A starts with a table listing the caffeine contents of selected foods, beverages, and drugs.

Nutrition Assessment Checklist FOR INFANTS, CHILDREN, AND ADOLESCENTS

Medical History

Check the medical record for:

- Alcohol, tobacco, or illicit drug abuse
- Attention deficit/hyperactivity disorder (ADHD)
- Diabetes or other chronic disorders
- Eating disorders
- Food allergies
- Lactose intolerance
- Obesity
- Pregnancy

Medications

For children or adolescents being treated with drug therapy for medical conditions, note:

- Side effects that might reduce food intake or change nutrient needs
- Proper administration of medication with respect to food intake

Dietary Intake

For infants, note:

- Method of feeding (breastfeeding, formula, or both)
- Frequency and duration of breastfeeding
- Amount of infant formula
- Practice of putting infant to bed with bottle
- Solid foods the infant is fed, if any
- Amount of food the infant is fed

For all children and adolescents, especially those considered at risk nutritionally, assess the diet for:

- Total energy
- Protein
- Calcium and iron
- Vitamin A, vitamin C, and folate
- Fiber

Note the following:

- Number of days each week a nutritious breakfast is eaten
- Number of hours the child or teen sleeps each day
- Number of soft drinks the child or teen drinks each day
- Number of fast-food meals eaten each day
- Number and type of snacks eaten each day
- Type and amount of physical activity
- Amount of caffeine consumed

Anthropometric Data

Measure baseline height and weight.

- Note infant birth weight.
- Reassess height, weight, and growth patterns at each medical checkup.
- Note weight, length, and head circumference of infants.
- Note significant obesity or underweight and any intervention strategies employed.

Laboratory Tests

Monitor the following laboratory tests for infants:

- Blood glucose of infants born to mothers with gestational diabetes
- Results of tests for inborn errors of metabolism (see Nutrition in Practice 16)

Monitor the following laboratory tests for children and adolescents:

- Hemoglobin, hematocrit, or other tests of iron status
- Blood glucose for children or adolescents with diabetes
- Blood lead concentrations

Physical Signs

Look for physical signs of:

- Protein-energy malnutrition
- Iron deficiency
- Vitamin A deficiency
- Vitamin C deficiency
- Folate deficiency

Clinical Applications

1. At 2½ years old, Travis is healthy, though slightly underweight, and headstrong. Travis's mother hovers over him at every meal and insists that he take several bites of every food on his plate, even if he dislikes the food or is not familiar with it. Even though Travis is hungry when he sits down to a meal, his mother's constant urging to get him to eat quickly quells any interest he had in eating. Travis simply folds his arms across his chest, closes his mouth tightly, and refuses to eat any more food. After more begging, pleading, and nagging, Travis's mother becomes angry and sends him away from the table. Travis is not allowed to snack between meals because his mother is concerned that snacks will ruin his appetite.

   ▌ What factors might be contributing to Travis's refusal to eat?

   ▌ Travis's mother is concerned about her son's underweight. What strategies would you suggest to help Travis gain weight?

Self Check

1. Breast milk is recommended for the first 12 months of life because it offers complete nutrition and ___ to the infant.
   a. fluoride
   b. fructose
   c. immunological protection
   d. pica

2. Which of the following is a characteristic of iron deficiency in children?
   a. It rarely develops in those with high intakes of milk.
   b. It affects brain function before anemia sets in.
   c. It is a primary factor in hyperactivity.
   d. Mild deficiency enhances mental performance by lowering physical activity level, thereby leading to increased attention span.

3. Three symptoms of lead toxicity are:
   a. diarrhea, irritability, and fatigue.
   b. low blood sugar, hair loss, and skin rash.
   c. increased heart rate, hyperactivity, and dry skin.
   d. bleeding gums, brittle fingernails, and swollen glands.

4. Allergic reactions to foods are most often caused by:
   a. corn, rice, or meats.
   b. eggs, peanuts, or milk.
   c. red meats, milk, or MSG.
   d. seafood, dark greens, or lactose.

5. When introducing new foods to children:
   a. reward children as they try new foods.
   b. offer many choices to encourage variety.
   c. offer one new food at the end of the meal.
   d. offer one new food at the beginning of the meal.

6. Which of the following is *not* true? Children who watch a lot of television are likely to:
   a. become obese.
   b. spend less time being physically active.
   c. learn healthy eating tips from programs.
   d. eat the foods most often advertised on television.

7. Which of the following strategies is *not* effective?
   a. Play first, eat later.
   b. Provide small portions.
   c. Encourage children to help prepare meals.
   d. Use dessert as a reward for eating vegetables.

8. During the growth spurt of adolescence:
   a. females gain more weight than males.
   b. males gain more fat, proportionately, than females.
   c. differences in body composition between males and females become apparent.
   d. similarities in body composition between males and females become apparent.

9. Two nutrients that are usually lacking in adolescents' diets are:
   a. zinc and fat.
   b. iron and calcium.
   c. protein and thiamin.
   d. vitamin A and riboflavin.

10. To help teenagers consume a balanced diet, parents can:
    a. monitor the teens' food intake.
    b. give up—parents can't influence teenagers.
    c. keep the cabinets and refrigerator well stocked.
    d. forbid snacking and insist on regular, well-balanced meals.

Answers to these questions can be found in Appendix H.

Notes

1. Formula feeding of term infants, in American Academy of Pediatrics, *Pediatric Nutrition*, 7th ed., ed. R. E. Kleinman (Elk Grove Village, IL.: American Academy of Pediatrics, 2014), pp. 61–81.

2. American Academy of Pediatrics, Policy statement: Breastfeeding and the use of human milk, Pediatrics 129 (2012): e827–e841, available at www.pediatrics.org/content/129/3/e827.full.

3. American Academy of Pediatrics, *New Mother's Guide to Breastfeeding*, 2nd ed., ed. J. Y. Meek (New York, Bantam Books, 2011), pp. 55–83.

4. P. V. Jeurink and coauthors, Mechanisms underlying immune effects of dietary oligosaccharides, *American Journal of Clinical Nutrition* 98 (2013): 572S–577S.

5. R. S. Kuipers and coauthors, Fetal intrauterine whole body linoleic, arachidonic and docosahexaenoic acid contents and accretion rates, *Prostaglandins, Leukotrienes, and Essential Fatty Acids*, 86 (2012): 13–20.

6. P. Willatts and coauthors, Effects of long-chain PUFA supplementation in infant formula on cognitive function in later childhood, *American Journal of Clinical Nutrition* 98 (2013): 536S–542S; S. J. Meldrum and coauthors, Achieving definitive results in long-chain polyunsaturated fatty acid supplementation trials of term infants: Factors for consideration, *Nutrition Reviews* 69 (2011): 205–214; E. E. Birch and coauthors, The DIAMOND (DHA Intake and Measurement of Neural Development) Study: A double-masked, randomized controlled clinical trial of the maturation of infant visual acuity as a function the dietary level of docosahexaenoic acid, *American Journal of Clinical Nutrition* 91 (2010): 848–859.

7. Meldrum and coauthors, 2011.

8. Willatts and coauthors, 2013.

9. S. A. Abrams, What are the risks and benefits to increasing dietary bone minerals and vitamin D intake in infants and small children? *Annual Review of Nutrition* 31 (2011): 285–297.

10. S. Gallo and coauthors, Effect of different dosages of oral vitamin D supplementation on vitamin D status in healthy, breastfed infants, *Journal of the American Medical Association* 309 (2013): 1785–1792; American Academy of Pediatrics, 2012.

11. C. G. Perrine and coauthors, Adherence to vitamin D recommendations among US infants, *Pediatrics* 125 (2010): 627–632.

12. D. E. W. Chatterton and coauthors Anti-inflammatory mechanisms of bioactive milk proteins in the intestine of newborns, *International Journal of Biochemistry and Cell Biology* 45 (2013): 1730–1747; B. Lonnerdal, Bioactive proteins in breast milk, *Journal of Paediatrics and Child Health* (Supplement S1) 49 (2013): 1–7;

American Academy of Pediatrics, 2012; Position of the American Dietetic Association, Promoting and supporting breastfeeding, 2009.

13. American Academy of Pediatrics, 2012; A. Walker, Breast milk as the gold standard for protective nutrients, *Journal of Pediatrics* 156 (2010): 53–57.

14. American Academy of Pediatrics, Breastfeeding, in *Pediatric* Nutrition, 7th ed., ed., RE Kleinman (Elk Grove Village, IL: American Academy of Pediatrics, 2014): pp. 41–59; American Academy of Pediatrics, 2012; Position of the American Dietetic Association, 2009.

15. American Academy of Pediatrics, 2012.

16. F. R. Hauck and coauthors, Breastfeeding and reduced risk of sudden infant death syndrome: A meta-analysis, *Pediatrics* 128 (2011): 103–110.

17. I. Labayen and coauthors, Association of exclusive breastfeeding duration and fibrinogen levels in childhood and adolescence: The European Youth Heart Study, *Archives of Pediatric and Adolescent Medicine* 166 (2012): 56–61; C. G. Owen, P. H. Whincup, and D. G. Cook, Breast-feeding and cardiovascular risk factors and outcomes in later life: Evidence from epidemiological studies, *Proceedings of the Nutrition Society* 70 (2011): 478–484; M. S. Fewtrell, Breast-feeding and later risk of CVD and obesity: Evidence from randomized trials, *Proceedings of the Nutrition Society* 70 (2011): 472–477.

18. K. Casazza, J. R. Fernandez, and D. B. Allison, Modest protective effects of breast-feeding on obesity, *Nutrition Today* 47 (2012): 33–38; L. Shields and coauthors, Breastfeeding and obesity at 21 years: A cohort study, *Journal of Clinical Nursing* 19 (2010): 1612–1617; L. Schack-Nielsen and coauthors, Late introduction of complementary feeding, rather than duration breastfeeding, may protect against adult overweight, *American Journal of Clinical Nutrition* 91 (2010): 619–627; L. Twells and L. A. Newhook, Can exclusive breastfeeding reduce the likelihood of childhood obesity in some regions of Canada? *Canadian Journal of Public Health* 101 (2010): 36–39; P. Chivers and coauthors, Body mass index, adiposity rebound and early feeding in a longitudinal cohort (Raine Study), *International Journal of Obesity* 34 (2010): 1169–1176.

19. Chivers and coauthors, 2010; Shields and coauthors, 2010.

20. Casazza, Fernandez, and Allison, 2012; K. L. Whitaker and coauthors, Comparing maternal and paternal intergenerational transmission of obesity risk in a large population-based sample, *American Journal of Clinical Nutrition* 91 (2010): 1560–1567; R. Li, S. B. Fein, and L. M. Grummer-Strawn, Do infants fed from bottles lack self-regulation of milk intake compared with directly breastfed infants? *Pediatrics* 125 (2010): e1386–e1393.

21. W. Jedrychowski and coauthors, Effect of exclusive breastfeeding on the development of children's cognitive function in the Krakow prospective birth cohort study, *European Journal of Pediatrics* 171 (2012): 151–158; M. A. Quigley and coauthors, Breastfeeding is associated with improved child cognitive development: A population-based cohort study, *Journal of Pediatrics* 160 (2012): 25–32; C. McCrory and R. Layte, The effect of breastfeeding on children's educational test scores at 9 years of age: Results of an Irish

cohort study, *Social Science and Medicine* 72 (2011); 1515–1521.

22. M. Guxens and coauthors, Breastfeeding, long-chain polyunsaturated fatty acids in colostrum, and infant mental development, *Pediatrics* 128 (2011): e880–e889.

23. American Academy of Pediatrics, Formula feeding of term infants, 2014.

24. U. S. Food and Drug Administration, FDA sets standards for infant formula, www.fda.gov/food/newsevents/constituentupdates/ucm384911.htm, updated June 6, 2014.

25. American Academy of Pediatrics, Formula feeding of term infants, 2014.

26. American Academy of Pediatrics, Formula feeding of term infants, 2014.

27. E. E. Ziegler, Consumption of cow's milk as a cause of iron deficiency in infants and toddlers, *Nutrition Reviews* 69 (2011): S37–S42.

28. Expert Panel on Integrated Guidelines for Cardiovascular Health and Risk Reduction in children and Adolescents, Summary report, *Pediatrics* 128 (2011): S213–S256.

29. Complementary feeding, in American Academy of Pediatrics, *Pediatric Nutrition Handbook*, 7th ed., ed. R. E. Kleinman (Elk Grove Village, IL.: American Academy of Pediatrics, 2014), pp. 123–139.

30. H. Przyrembel, Timing of introduction of complementary food: Short-and long-term health consequences, *Annals of Nutrition and Metabolism* 60 (2012): 8–20.

31. American Academy of Pediatrics, Complementary feeding, 2014.

32. American Academy of Pediatrics, Complementary feeding, 2014.

33. Feeding the child, in American Academy of Pediatrics, *Pediatric Nutrition*, 7th ed., ed. R. E. Kleinman (Elk Grove Village, IL.: American Academy of Pediatrics, 2014), pp. 143–173.

34. American Academy of Pediatrics, Feeding the child, 2014.

35. American Academy of Pediatrics, Complementary feeding, 2014.

36. American Academy of Pediatrics, Feeding the child, 2014; American Academy of Pediatrics, Policy statement—Prevention of choking among children, *Pediatrics* 125 (2010): 601–607.

37. R. P. Heaney, Diet, osteoporosis, and fracture prevention: The totality of the evidence, in A. Bendichand and R. J. Deckelbaum, eds., *Preventive Nutrition: The Comprehensive Guide for Health Professionals*, 4th ed. (New York: Human Press, 2010), pp. 443–469.

38. S. A. Ramsay and coauthors, "Are you done?" child care providers' verbal communication at mealtimes that reinforce or hinder children's internal cues of hunger and satiation, *Journal of Nutrition Education and Behavior* 42 (2010): 265–270.

39. Position of the Academy of Nutrition and Dietetics: Nutrition guidance for healthy children ages 2 to 11 years, *Journal of the Academy of Nutrition and Dietetics* 114 (2014): 1257–1276. American Academy of Pediatrics, Policy Statement—Children, adolescents, obesity, and the

media, *Pediatrics* 128 (2011): 201–208; V. C. Strasburger, A.B. Jordan, and E. Donnerstein, Health effects of media on children and adolescents, *Pediatrics* 125 (2010): 756–767.

40. J. L. Foltz and coauthors, Population-level intervention strategies and examples for obesity prevention in children, *Annual Review of Nutrition* 32 (2012): 391–415; Position of the American Dietetic Association: Benchmarks for nutrition in child care, *Journal of the American Dietetic Association* 111 (2011): 607–615; N. Larson and coauthors, What role can child-care settings play in obesity prevention? A review of the evidence and call for research efforts, *Journal of the American Dietetic Association* 111 (2011): 1343–1362.

41. Nutritional aspects of vegetarian diets, in R. E. Kleinman, ed., *Pediatric Nutrition*, 7th ed. (Elk Grove Village, IL: American Academy of Pediatrics, 2014), pp. 241–264.

42. Committee on the Scientific Evaluation of Dietary Reference Intakes, Food and Nutrition Board, Institute of Medicine, *Dietary Reference Intakes for Energy, Carbohydrate, Fiber, Fat, Fatty Acids, Cholesterol, Protein, and Amino Acids* (Washington, DC: National Academies Press, 2005), pp. 265–338.

43. Committee on the Scientific Evaluation of Dietary Reference Intakes, 2005, pp. 339–421.

44. Committee on the Scientific Evaluation of Dietary Reference Intakes, 2005, pp. 769–879.

45. Committee on the Scientific Evaluation of Dietary Reference Intakes, 2005, pp. 422–541.

46. R. D. Baker, F. R. Greer, and the Committee on Nutrition, Clinical Report: Diagnosis and prevention of iron deficiency and iron-deficiency anemia in infants and young children (0–3 years of age), *Pediatrics* 126 (2010): 1040–1050.

47. Expert Panel on Integrated Guidelines for Cardiovascular Health and Risk Reduction in Children and Adolescents, 2011.

48. Committee on Dietary Reference Intakes, *Dietary Reference Intakes for Calcium and Vitamin D* (Washington, DC: National Academies Press, 2011), pp. 345–402.

49. C. L. Wagner and F. R. Greer, and the Section on Breastfeeding and Committee on Nutrition, Prevention of rickets and vitamin D deficiency in infants, children, and adolescents, *Pediatrics* 122 (2008): 1142–1152.

50. American Academy of Pediatrics, Feeding the child, 2014; R. L. Bailey and coauthors, Do dietary supplements improve micronutrient sufficiency in children and adolescents? *Journal of Pediatrics* 161 (2012): 837–842.

51. Bailey and coauthors, 2012.

52. Position of the Academy of Nutrition and Dietetics, 2014.

53. R. R. Briefel and coauthors, The Feeding Infants and Toddlers Study 2008: Study design and methods, *Journal of the American Dietetic Association* 110 (2010): S16–S26; N. F. Butte and coauthors, Nutrient intakes of US infants, toddlers, and preschoolers meet or exceed dietary reference intakes, *Journal of the American Dietetic Association* 110 (2010): S27–S37.

54. M. K. Fox and coauthors, Food consumption patterns of young preschoolers: Are they starting

off on the right path? *Journal of the American Dietetic Association* 110 (2010): S52–S59.

55. Butte and coauthors, 2010;.

56. H. Skouteris and coauthors, Parental influence and obesity prevention in pre-schoolers: A systematic review of interventions, *Obesity Reviews* 12 (2011): 315–328.

57. R. B. Ervin and coauthors, Consumption of added sugar among U.S. children and adolescents, 2005–2008, *NCHS Data Brief* 87 (2012), available at www.cdc.gov/nchs/data/databriefs/db87.htm.

58. Bread for the World, Hunger facts: Domestic, available at www.bread.org/learn/hunger-basics/hunger-facts-domestic.html, June 24, 2014.

59. Position of the American Dietetic Association: Child and adolescent nutrition assistance programs, *Journal of the American Dietetic Association* 110 (2010): 791–799.

60. T. Coppinger and coauthors, Body mass, frequency of eating and breakfast consumption in 9–13-year-olds, *Journal of Human Nutrition and Dietetics* 25 (2012): 43–49; T. V. E. Kral and coauthors, Effects of eating breakfast compared with skipping breakfast on ratings of appetite and intake at subsequent meals in 8– to 10–y-old children, *American Journal of Clinical Nutrition* 93 (2011): 284–291; K. J. Smith and coauthors, Skipping breakfast: Longitudinal associations with cardiometabolic risk factors in the Childhood Determinants of Adult Health Study, *American Journal of Clinical Nutrition* 92 (2010): 1316–1325.

61. C. E. Basch, Breakfast and the achievement gap among urban minority youth, *Journal of School Health* 81 (2011): 635–640; S. B. Cooper, S. Bandelow, and M. E. Nevill, Breakfast consumption and cognitive function in adolescent schoolchildren, *Physiology & Behavior* 103 (2011): 431–439; S. P. P. Tin and coauthors, Breakfast skipping and change in body mass index in young children, *International Journal of Obesity* 35 (2011): 899–906; P. R. Deshmukh-Taskar and coauthors, The relationship of breakfast skipping and type of breakfast consumption with nutrient intake and weight status in children and adolescents: The National Health and Nutrition Examination Survey 1999–2006, *Journal of the American Dietetic Association* 110 (2010): 869–878.

62. K. Kordas, Iron, lead, and children's behavior and cognition, *Annual Review of Nutrition* 30 (2010): 123–148.

63. M. M. Black and coauthors, Iron deficiency and iron-deficiency anemia in the first 2 years of life: Strategies to prevent loss of developmental potential, *Nutrition Reviews* 69 (2011): S64–S70; M. K. Georgieff, Long-term brain and behavioral consequences of early iron deficiency, *Nutrition Reviews* 69 (2011): S43–S48; C. S. Wang and coauthors, Iron-deficiency anemia in infancy and social emotional development in preschool-aged Chinese children, *Pediatrics* 127 (2011): e927–e933; F. Corapci and coauthors, Longitudinal evaluation of externalizing and internalizing behavior problems following iron deficiency in infancy, *Journal of Pediatric Psychology* 35 (2010): 296–305.

64. Kordas, 2010.

65. Centers for Disease Control and Prevention, Lead, available at www.cdc.gov/nceh/lead/, updated June 19, 2014.

66. Centers for Disease Control and Prevention, Prevention tips, available at www.cdc.gov/nceh/lead/tips.htm, updated June 25, 2012.

67. R. S. Gupta and coauthors, The prevalence, severity, and distribution of childhood food allergy in the United States, *Pediatrics* 128 (2011): e9–e17; U. S. Food and Drug Administration, Food allergies: Reducing the risks, www.fda.gov/consumer/updates/foodallergies01229.htm, updated December 7, 2013.

68. U.S. Food and Drug Administration, 2013.

69. J. A. Boyce and coauthors, Guidelines for the diagnosis and management of food allergy in the United States: Summary of the NIAID-Sponsored Expert Panel Report, *Journal of the American Dietetic Association* 111 (2011): 17–27.

70. H. N. Cho and coauthors, Nutritional status according to sensitized food allergens in children with atopic dermatitis, *Allergy, Asthma, and Immunology Research* 3 (2010): 53–57.

71. Boyce and coauthors, 2011.

72. Gupta and coauthors, 2011.

73. S. Waserman and W. Watson, Food allergy, *Allergy, Asthma, and Clinical Immunology* 7 (2011): S7.

74. M. Pansare and D. Kamat, Peanut allergy, *Current Opinions in Pediatrics* 22 (2010): 642–646.

75. S. H. Sicherer, T. Mahr, and The Section on Allergy and Immunology, Clinical report—Management of food allergy in the school setting, *Pediatrics* 126 (2010): 1232–1239.

76. U.S. Food and Drug Administration, *Food Facts*, Food allergies: What you need to know, available at www.fda.gov/Food/ingredientspackaginglabeling/foodallergens/ucmo79311.htm, updated May 15, 2014.

77. Centers for Disease Control and Prevention, Attention-Deficit/Hyperactivity Disorder (ADHD), Data and statistics, www.cdc.gov/ncbddd/adhd/data/html, updated November 13, 2013.

78. Subcommittee on Attention-Deficit/Hyperactivity Disorder, Steering Committee on Quality Improvement and Management, ADHD: Clinical practice guideline for the diagnosis, evaluation, and treatment of attention-deficit/hyperactivity disorder in children and adolescents, *Pediatrics* 128 (2011): 1007–1022.

79. J. G. Millichap and M. M. Yee, The diet factor in attention-deficit/hyperactivity disorder, *Pediatrics* 129 (2012): 330–337.

80. L.J. Stevens and coauthors, Mechanisms of behavioral, atopic, and other reactions to artificial food colors in children, *Nutrition Reviews* 71 (2013): 268–281; R. B. Kanarek, Artificial food dyes and attention deficit hyperactivity disorder, *Nutrition Reviews* 69 (2011): 385–391; R. E. Kleinman and coauthors, A research model for investigating the effects of artificial food colorings on children with ADHD, *Pediatrics* 127 (2011): e1575–1584; T. E. Froehlich and coauthors, Update on environmental risk factors for attention-deficit/hyperactivity disorder, *Current Psychiatry Reports* 13 (2011): 333–344; A. Connolly and coauthors, Pattern of intake of food additives associated with hyperactivity in Irish children and teenagers, *Food Additives and Contaminants: Part A, Chemistry, Analysis, Control, Exposure and Risk Assessment* 27 (2010): 447–456; J. Stevenson and coauthors, The role of histamine degradation gene polymorphisms in moderating the effects of food additives on children's ADHD symptoms, *American Journal of Psychiatry* 167 (2010): 1108–1115.

81. Kanarek, 2011.

82. Food and Drug Administration, Overview of food ingredients, additives, and colors, available at www.fda.gov, revised April 2010, updated March 3, 2013.

83. C. L. Ogden and coauthors, Prevalence of childhood and adult obesity in the United States, 2011–2012, *Journal of the American Medical Association* 311 (2014): 806–814; S. A. Cunningham, M. R. Kramer, and K. M. Venkat Narayan, Incidence of childhood obesity in the United States, *New England Journal of Medicine* 370 (2014): 403–411.

84. Expert Panel on Integrated Guidelines for Cardiovascular Health and Risk Reduction in Children and Adolescents, 2011; J. J. Reilly, Assessment of obesity in children and adolescents: Synthesis of recent systematic reviews and clinical guidelines, *Journal of Human Nutrition and Dietetics* 23 (2010): 205–211.

85. A. C. Skinner and J. A. Skelton, Prevalence and trends in obesity and severe obesity among children in the United States, 1999–2012, *JAMA Pediatrics* 168 (2014): 581–586; G. Flores and H. Lin, Factors predicting severe childhood obesity in kindergarteners, *International Journal of Obesity* 37 (2013): 31–39.

86. Skinner and Skelton, 2014; Expert Panel on Integrated Guidelines for Cardiovascular Health and Risk Reduction in Children and Adolescents, 2011; N. S. The and coauthors, Association of adolescent obesity with risk of severe obesity in adulthood, *Journal of the American Medical Association* 304 (2010): 2042–2057; F. M. Biro and M. Wien, Childhood obesity and adult morbidities, *American Journal of Clinical Nutrition* 91 (2010): 1499S–1505S.

87. A. L. Thompson, Intergenerational impact of maternal obesity and postnatal feeding practices on pediatric obesity, *Nutrition Reviews* 71 (2013): S55–S61; A. Jaaskelainen and coauthors, Intergenerational transmission of overweight among Finnish adolescents and their parents: A 16–year follow-up study, *International Journal of Obesity* 35 (2011): 1289–1294; R. Cooper and coauthors, Associations between parental and offspring adiposity up to midlife: The contribution of adult lifestyle factors in the 1958 British Birth Cohort Study, *American Journal of Clinical Nutrition* 92 (2010): 946–953; Whitaker and coauthors, 2010.

88. Expert Panel, 2011; Biro and Wien, 2010.

89. Centers for Disease Control and Prevention, Overweight and obesity: A growing problem, www.cdc.gov/obesity/childhood/problem.html, updated April 27, 2012; Foltz and coauthors, 2012.

90. L. McGowan and coauthors, Healthy feeding habits: Efficacy results from a cluster-randomized, controlled exploratory trial of a novel, habit-based intervention with parents, *American Journal of Clinical Nutrition* 98 (2013): 769–777; S. J. Salvy and coauthors, Influence of parents and friends on children's and adolescents' food intake and food selection, *American Journal of*

Clinical Nutrition 93 (2011): 87–92; L. Hall and coauthors, Children's intake of fruit and selected energy-dense nutrient-poor foods is associated with fathers' intake, *Journal of the American Dietetic Association* 111 (2011): 1039–1044; H. A. Raynor and coauthors, The relationship between child and parent food hedonics and parent and child food group intake in children with overweight/obesity, *Journal of the American Dietetic Association* 111 (2011): 425–430; C. Sweetman and coauthors, Characteristics of family mealtimes affecting children's vegetable consumption and liking, *Journal of the American Dietetic Association* 111 (2011): 269–273; S. L. Anzman and coauthors, Parental influence on children's early eating environments and obesity risk: Implications for prevention, *International Journal of Obesity* 34 (2010): 1116–1124.

91. Hall and coauthors, 2011; L. R. Jones and coauthors, Influences on child fruit and vegetable intake: Sociodemographic, parental, and child factors in a longitudinal cohort study, *Public Health Nutrition* 13 (2010): 1122–1130.

92. J. Reedy and S. M. Krebs-Smith, Dietary sources of energy, solid fats, and added sugars among children and adolescents in the United States, *Journal of the American Dietetic Association* 110 (2010): 1477–1484.

93. E. C. Kosova, P. Auinger, and A. A. Bremer, The relationships between sugar-sweetened beverage intake and cardiometabolic markers in young children, *Journal of the Academy of Nutrition and Dietetics* 113 (2013): 219–227; Ervin and coauthors, 2012; J. A. Welsh and coauthors, Consumption of added sugars is decreasing in the United States, *American Journal of Clinical Nutrition* 94 (2011): 726–734.

94. M. D. BeBoer, R. J. Scharf, and R. T. Demmer, Sugar-sweetened beverages and weight gain in 2- to 5-year old children, *Pediatrics* 132 (2013): 413–420; G. L. Ambrosini and coauthors, Prospective associations between sugar-sweetened beverage intakes and cardiometabolic risk factors in adolescents, *American Journal of Clinical Nutrition* 98 (2013): 327–334; V. S. Malik and coauthors, Sugar-sweetened beverages and weight gain in children and adults: A systematic review and meta-analysis, *American Journal of Clinical Nutrition* 98 (2013): 1084–1092; D. F. Tate and coauthors, Replacing caloric beverages with water or diet beverages for weight loss in adults: Main results of the Choose Healthy Options Consciously Everyday (CHOICE) randomized clinical trial, *American Journal of Clinical Nutrition* 95 (2012): 555–563; V. S. Malik and coauthors, Sugar-sweetened beverages, obesity, type 2 diabetes mellitus, and cardiovascular disease risk, *Circulation* 121 (2010): 1356–1364; F. B. Hu and V. S. Malik, Sugar-sweetened beverages and risk of obesity and type 2 diabetes: epidemiologic evidence, *Physiology and Behavior* 100 (2010): 47–54; O. L. Bermudez and X. Gao, Greater consumption of sweetened beverages and added sugars is associated with obesity among US young adults, *Annals of Nutrition and Metabolism* 57 (2010): 211–218.

95. U. Ekelund and coauthors, Moderate to vigorous physical activity and sedentary time and caridometabolic risk factors in children and adolescents, *Journal of the American Medical Association* 307 (2012): 704–712.

96. Centers for Disease Control and Prevention, 2012.

97. A. E. Staiano and coauthors, Television, adiposity, and cardiometabolic risk in children and adolescents, *American Journal of Preventive Medicine* 44 (2013): 40–47; American Academy of Pediatrics, Council on Communications and Media, 2011; S. B. Sisson and coauthors, TVs in the bedrooms of children: Does it impact health and behavior? *Preventive Medicine* 52 (2011): 104–108.

98. American Academy of Pediatrics, Council on Communications and Media, Policy statement—Children, adolescents, obesity, and the media, *Pediatrics* 128 (2012): 201–208; S. B. Sisson and coauthors, Television-viewing time and dietary quality among U.S. children and adults, *American Journal of Preventive Medicine* 43 (2012): 196–200.

99. N. Pearson and S. J. Biddle, Sedentary behavior and dietary intake in children, adolescents, and adults: A systematic review, *American Journal of Preventive Medicine* 41 (2011): 178–188.

100. L. M. Powell, G. Szczypka, and F. J. Chaloupka, Trends in exposure to television food advertisements among children and adolescents in the United States, *Archives of Pediatric and Adolescent Medicine* 164 (2010): 794–802.

101. F. Folkvord and coauthors, The effect of playing advergames that promote energy-dense snacks or fruit on actual food intake among children, *American Journal of Clinical Nutrition* 97 (2013): 239–245.

102. J. L. Harris, and S. K. Graff, Protecting children from harmful food marketing: Options for local government to make a difference, Centers for Disease Control and Prevention, *Preventing Chronic Disease* 8 (September 2011), www.cdc.gov/ped/issues/2011/sep/10_0272.htm.

103. E. D. Kolish, Food advertising to children, *Nutrition Today* 49 (2014): 68–76.

104. J. P. Chaput and coauthors, Video game playing increases food intake in adolescents: A randomized crossover study, *American Journal of Clinical Nutrition* 93 (2011): 1196–1203; American Academy of Pediatrics, Council on Communications and Media, 2011.

105. K. White, G. Schofield, and A. E. Kilding, Energy expended by boys playing active video games, *Journal of Science and Medicine in Sport* 14 (2011): 130–134.

106. American Academy of Pediatrics, Council on Communications and Media, 2011.

107. W. Tu and coauthors, Intensified effect of adiposity on blood pressure in overweight and obese children, *Hypertension* 58 (2011): 818–824.

108. A. L. May, E. V. Kuklina, and P. W. Yoon, Prevalence of cardiovascular disease risk factors among US adolescents, 1999–2008, *Pediatrics* 129 (2012): 1035–1041; J. Ohman and coauthors, Early childhood overweight and asthma and allergic sensitization at 8 years of age, *Pediatrics* 129 (2012): 70–76; A. Tirosh and coauthors, Adolescent BMI trajectory and risk of diabetes versus coronary disease, *New England Journal of Medicine* 364 (2011): 1315–1325; J. C. Han, D. A. Lawlor, and S. Y. S. Kimm, Childhood obesity, *Lancet* 375 (2010): 1737–1748; Biro and Wien, 2010; P. W. Franks and coauthors, Childhood obesity, other cardiovascular risk factors, and premature death, *New England Journal of Medicine* 362 (2010): 458–493.

109. S. A. Taylor and coauthors, A qualitative study of the day-to-day lives of obese Mexican-American adolescent females, *Pediatrics* 131 (2013): 1132–1138.

110. D. M. Hoelscher and coauthors, Position of the Academy of Nutrition and Dietetics: Interventions for the prevention and treatment of pediatric overweight and obesity, *Journal of the Academy of Nutrition and Dietetics* 113 (2013): 1375–1394.

111. Hoelscher and coauthors, 2013.

112. American Heart Association, Overweight in children, 2012, available at http://www.heart.org/HEARTORG/GettingHealthy?Overweight-in-Children_UCM_304054_Article.jsp.

113. Hoelscher and coauthors, 2013.

114. P. J. Colllings and coauthors, Physical activity intensity, sedentary time, and body composition in preschoolers, *American Journal of Clinical Nutrition* 97 (2013): 1020–1028; C. L. Davis and coauthors, Exercise dose and diabetes risk in overweight and obese children, *Journal of American Medical Association* 308 (2012): 1103–1112.

115. Hoelscher and coauthors, 2013; A. L. Rogovik and R. D. Goldman, Pharmacologic treatment of pediatric obesity, *Canadian Family Physician* 57 (2011): 195–197.

116. S. Bondada, H.C. Jen, and D. A. Deugarte, Outcomes of bariatric surgery in adolescents, *Current Opinion in Pediatrics* 23 (2011): 552–556; P. E. O'Brien and coauthors, Laparoscopic adjustable gastric banding in severely obese adolescents, *Journal of the American Medical Association* 303 (2010): 519–526.

117. A. R. Ibele and S. G. Mattar, Adolescent bariatric surgery, *Surgical Clinics of North America* 91 (2011): 1339–1351.

118. K. W. Bauer, J. M. Berge, and D. Neumark-Sztainer, The importance of families to adolescents' physical activity and dietary intake, *Adolescent Medicine: State of the Art Reviews* 22 (2011): 601–613; Anzman and coauthors, 2010.

119. M. L. O'Connell and coauthors, Repeated exposure in a natural setting: A preschool intervention to increase vegetable consumption, *Journal of the Academy of Nutrition and Dietetics* 112 (2012): 230–234.

120. Position of the Academy of Nutrition and Dietetics, 2014.

121. B. Wansink, M. Shimizu, and A. Brumberg, Association of nutrient-dense snack combinations with calories and vegetable intake, *Pediatrics* 131 (2013): 22–29.

122. Position of the American Dietetic Association, 2011; Position of the American Dietetic Association, School Nutrition Association, and Society for Nutrition Education: Comprehensive school nutrition services, *Journal of the American Dietetic Association* 110 (2010): 1738–1749.

123. Position of the American Dietetic Association: Benchmarks for nutrition in child care, 2011.

124. The School Breakfast Program, www.fns.usda.gov/sbp/school-breakfast-program-sbp.htm, updated September 2013; Position of the American Dietetic Association: Local support for nutrition integrity in schools, *Journal of the American Dietetic Association* 110 (2010): 1244–1254.

125. Position of the American Dietetic Association: Local support for nutrition integrity in schools, 2010.

126. Centers for Disease Control and Prevention, School health guidelines to promote health eating and physical activity, *Morbidity and Mortality Weekly Report* 60 (Supplement), September 16, 2011, pp. 1–76.

127. National School Lunch Program, www.fns.usda .gov/nslp/national-school-lunch-program-nslp, updated September, 2013; Position of the American Dietetic Association: Local support for nutrition integrity in schools, 2010.

128. Food and Nutrition Services (FNS) USDA, Nutrition standards in the National School Lunch and School Breakfast Programs. Final rule, *Federal Register* 77 (2012): 4088–4167.

129. Position of the American Dietetic Association: Local support for nutrition integrity in schools, 2010.

130. Position of the American Dietetic Association: Local support for nutrition integrity in schools, 2010.

131. M. Kakarala, D. R. Keast, and S. Hoerr, Schoolchildren's consumption of competitive foods and beverages, excluding á la carte, *Journal of School Health* 80 (2010): 429–435; Position of the American Dietetic Association: Local support for nutrition integrity in schools, 2010.

132. United States Department of Agriculture, Smart snacks in school—USDA's "All Foods Sold in Schools" Standards, www.fns.usda.gov /school-meals/smart-snacks-school, updated June 20, 2014.

133. L. B. Shomaker and coauthors, Puberty and observed energy intake: Boy, can they eat! *American Journal of Clinical Nutrition* 92 (2010): 123–129; Committee on the Scientific Evaluation of Dietary Reference Intakes, 2005, pp. 177–182.

134. Committee on Dietary Reference Intakes, 2011, pp. 362– 402.

135. The Society for Adolescent Health and Medicine, Recommended vitamin D intake and management of low vitamin D status in adolescents: A position statement of the Society for Adolescent Health and Medicine, *Journal of Adolescent Health* 52 (2013): 801–803; L. E. Au and coauthors, Associations of vitamin D intake with 25-hydroxyvitamin D in overweight and racially/ ethnically diverse US children, *Journal of the Academy of Nutrition and Dietetics* 113 (2013): 1511–1516.

136. The Society for Adolescent Health and Medicine, 2013.

137. Committee on Dietary Reference Intakes, 2011, pp. 35–74.

138. D. K. Dror and L. H. Allen, Dairy product intake in children and adolescents in developed countries: Trends, nutritional contribution, and a review of association with health outcomes, *Nutrition Reviews* 72 (2014): 68–81; M. Mesias, I. Seiquer, and M. P. Navarro, Calcium nutrition in adolescence, *Critical Reviews in Food Science and Nutrition* 51 (2011): 195–209; Committee on Dietary Reference Intakes, 2011, pp.458–460; R. L. Bailey and coauthors, Estimation of total usual calcium and vitamin D intakes in the United States, *The Journal of Nutrition* 140 (2010): 817–822.

139. Dror and Allen, 2014; Mesias, Seiquer, and Navarro, 2011.

140. Dror and Allen, 2014; L. M. Fiorito and coauthors, Girls' early sweetened carbonated beverage intake predicts different patterns of beverage and nutrient intake across childhood and adolescence, *Journal of the American Dietetic Association* 110 (2010): 543–550.

141. A. Moag-Stahlberg, *Family Nutrition and Physical Activity Survey*, January 2011, available at www.eatright.org; G. J. Cutler and coauthors, Multiple sociodemographic and socioenvironmental characteristics are correlated with major patterns of dietary intake in adolescents, *Journal of the American Dietetic Association* 111 (2011): 230–240.

142. J. M. Berge and coauthors, Structural and interpersonal characteristics of family meals: Associations with adolescent body mass index and dietary patterns, *Journal of the Academy of Nutrition and Dietetics* 113 (2013): 816–822; A. J. Hammons and B. H. Fiese, Is frequency of shared family meals related to the nutritional health of children and adolescents? *Pediatrics* 127 (2011): e1565–e1574; D. Neumark-Sztainer and coauthors, Family meals and adolescents: What have we learned from Project EAT (Eating Among Teens)? *Public Health Nutrition* 13 (2010): 1113–1121.

143. Deshmukh-Taskar and coauthors, 2010; Smith and coauthors, 2010.

144. H. J. Leidy and coauthors, Beneficial effects of a higher-protein breakfast on the appetitive, hormonal, and neural signals controlling energy intake regulation in overweight/obese, "breakfast-skipping" late-adolescent girls, *American Journal of Clinical Nutrition* 97 (2013): 677–688; L. W. Jackson, The most important meal of the day: Why children skip breakfast and what can be done about it, *Pediatric Annals* 42 (2013): 184–187.

145. J. M. Poti, K. J. Duffey, and B. M. Popkin, The association of fast food consumption with poor dietary outcomes and obesity among children: Is it the fast food or the remainder of the diet? *American Journal of Clinical Nutrition* 99 (2014): 162–171; Smith and coauthors, 2010.

146. D. R. Keast, T. A. Nicklas, and C. E. O'Neil, Snacking is associated with reduced risk of overweight and reduced abdominal obesity in adolescents: National Health and Nutrition Examination survey (NHANES) 1999–2004, *American Journal of Clinical Nutrition* 92 (2010): 428–435.

147. Dror and Allen, 2014; N. D. Brener and coauthors, Beverage consumption among high school students—United States, 2010, *Morbidity and Mortality Weekly Report* 60 (2011): 778–780.

148. E. Han and L. M. Powell, Consumption patterns of sugar-sweetened beverages in the United States, *Journal of the Academy of Nutrition and Dietetics* 113 (2013): 43–53; D. T. Levy, K. B. Friend, and Y. C. Wang, A review of the literature on policies directed at the youth consumption of sugar sweetened beverages, *Advances in Nutrition* 2 (2011): 182S-200S.

149. S. M. Seifert and coauthors, Health effects of energy drinks on children, adolescents, and young adults, *Pediatrics* 127 (2011): 511–528.

150. Seifert and coauthors, 2011.

151. Poti, Duffey, and Popkin, 2014.

LO 12.4 Describe the lifestyle factors that can help prevent childhood obesity and the development of type 2 diabetes and heart disease.

When people think about the health problems of children and adolescents, they typically think of ear infections, colds, and acne—not heart disease, diabetes, or hypertension. Today, however, unprecedented numbers of U.S. children are being diagnosed with obesity and the serious "adult diseases," such as type 2 diabetes, that accompany overweight.[1] When type 2 diabetes develops before the age of 20, the incidence of diabetic kidney disease and death in middle age increases dramatically, largely because of the long duration of the disease. For children born in the United States in the year 2000, the risk of developing type 2 diabetes sometime in their lives is estimated to be 30 percent for boys and 40 percent for girls. U.S. children are not alone—rapidly rising rates of obesity threaten the health of an alarming number of children around the globe.[2] Without immediate intervention, millions of children are destined to develop type 2 diabetes and hypertension in childhood followed by **cardiovascular disease (CVD)** in early adulthood.[3]

Over the past three decades, researchers have been observing how changes in body weight, blood lipids, blood pressure, and individual behaviors correlate with the development of CVD over time—from infancy to childhood through adolescence and into young adulthood. Some major findings have emerged from this research:

▎ Changes inside the arteries—changes predictive of CVD—are evident in childhood.

▎ Obesity in children affects these changes.

▎ Behaviors that influence the development of obesity and of CVD are learned and begin early in life. These behaviors include overeating, physical inactivity, and cigarette smoking.

This Nutrition in Practice focuses on efforts to prevent childhood obesity, type 2 diabetes, and CVD (see Box NP12-1 for definitions of the relevant terms), but the benefits extend to other obesity-related diseases as well. The years of childhood (ages 2 to 18) are emphasized here, for the earlier in life health-promoting habits become established, the better they will stick.

What about genetics? Do some people inherit the tendency to become obese or develop diabetes or CVD regardless of the lifestyle habits they adopt?

For obesity, as well as for CVD, hypertension, and type 2 diabetes, genetics does not appear to play a *determining* role; that is, a person is not simply destined at birth to develop them. Instead, genetics appears to play a *permissive* role—the potential is inherited and will then develop, if given a push by factors in the

> **BOX NP12-1 GLOSSARY**
>
> **atherosclerosis (ATH-er-oh-scler-OH-sis):** a type of artery disease characterized by plaques (accumulations of lipid-containing material) on the inner walls of the arteries (see Chapter 22).
>
> ▎ *athero* = porridge or soft
>
> ▎ *scleros* = hard
>
> ▎ *osis* = condition
>
> **cardiovascular disease (CVD):** a general term for all diseases of the heart and blood vessels. Atherosclerosis is the main cause of CVD. When the arteries that carry blood to the heart muscle become blocked, the heart suffers damage, known as coronary heart disease (CHD).
>
> ▎ *cardio* = heart
>
> ▎ *vascular* = blood vessels
>
> **fatty streaks:** accumulation of cholesterol and other lipids along the walls of the arteries.
>
> **plaque (PLACK):** an accumulation of fatty deposits, smooth muscle cells, and fibrous connective tissue that develops in the artery walls. Plaque associated with atherosclerosis is known as **atheromatous** (ATH-er-OH-ma-tus) **plaque.**

environment such as poor diet, sedentary lifestyle, and cigarette smoking.[4] Researchers note that the relationship between genes and the environment is a synergistic one—their combined effects are greater than the sum of their individual effects.

Many experts agree that preventing or treating obesity in childhood will reduce the rate of chronic diseases in adulthood. Without intervention, most overweight children become overweight adolescents who become overweight adults, and being overweight exacerbates every chronic disease that adults face.[5] Fatty liver, a condition that correlates directly with BMI, was not even recognized in pediatric research until recently. Today, fatty liver disease affects about one in three obese children.[6]

What about events that take place during fetal development—malnutrition, for example? Can they affect a person's tendency to develop diseases later in life?

A theory called *fetal programming,* or *developmental origins of health and disease,* states that maternal malnutrition or other harmful conditions at a critical period of fetal development may have lifelong effects on an individual's pattern of genetic expression and therefore on the tendency to develop obesity and certain diseases.[7] Poor maternal diet or health during pregnancy may alter the infant's bodily functions that influence disease development, such as blood pressure, cholesterol metabolism, glucose metabolism, and immune functions.[8] For example, malnutrition during fetal development may encourage metabolic programming that promotes nutrient storage and thus provides a survival advantage in an environment of poor postnatal nutrition. In a postnatal environment of adequate nutrition or overnutrition, however, such adaptations can lead to the development of glucose intolerance, type 2 diabetes, cardiovascular disease, and hypertension.[9]

Why has type 2 diabetes become so prevalent?

In recent years, type 2 diabetes, a chronic disease closely linked with obesity, has been on the rise among children and adolescents as the prevalence of obesity in U.S. youth has increased.[10] Type 2 diabetes is most likely to occur in those who are obese and sedentary and have a family history of diabetes. Obesity is the most important risk factor—most of the children diagnosed with type 2 diabetes are obese. Most are diagnosed during puberty, but as children become more obese and less active, the disease is appearing in younger and younger children.

How does type 2 diabetes develop?

In type 2 diabetes, the body's cells become insulin resistant—that is, the cells become less sensitive to insulin, reducing the amount of glucose entering the cells from the blood. The combination of obesity and insulin resistance produces a cluster of symptoms, including high blood pressure and high blood lipids, which in turn promotes the development of atherosclerosis and the early development of CVD.[11] Other common problems evident by early adulthood include kidney disease, blindness, and miscarriages. The complications of diabetes, especially when encountered at a young age, can shorten life expectancy. Chapter 21 offers a detailed discussion of diabetes.

Prevention and treatment of type 2 diabetes depend on weight management, which can be particularly difficult in a young person's world of food advertising, video games, and pocket money for candy bars. The activity and dietary suggestions to help defend against heart disease later in this discussion apply to type 2 diabetes as well.

How does CVD develop, and when does its development begin?

Most CVD involves **atherosclerosis**—the accumulation of cholesterol and other blood lipids along the walls of the arteries. Frequently, atherosclerosis and its complications interfere with the flow of blood to the heart and can lead to coronary heart disease (CHD), which, in turn, raises the likelihood of a heart attack. When atherosclerosis interferes with blood flow to the brain, a stroke can result. Infants are born with healthy, smooth, clear arteries, but within the first decade of life, **fatty streaks** may begin to appear. During adolescence, these fatty streaks may begin to turn into **plaques** (Figure 22-2 in Chapter 22 shows the formation of plaques in atherosclerosis). By early adulthood, the fibrous plaques may begin to calcify and become raised lesions, especially in boys and young men. As the lesions grow more numerous and thicken, the heart disease rate begins to rise, and the rise becomes dramatic at about age 45 in men and 55 in women. From this point on, arterial damage and blockage progress rapidly, and heart attacks and strokes threaten life. In short, the consequences of atherosclerosis, which become apparent only in adulthood, have their beginnings in the first decades of life.[12]

Children with the highest risks of developing heart disease are sedentary and obese; they may also have diabetes, high blood pressure, and high blood cholesterol.[13] In contrast, children with

TABLE NP12-1 Cholesterol Values for Children and Adolescents

Disease Risk	Total Cholesterol (mg/dL)	LDL Cholesterol (mg/dL)
Acceptable	<170	<110
Borderline	170–199	110–129
High	≥200	≥130

Note: Adult values appear in Table 22-2 on p. 000.

© Cengage Learning®

the lowest risks of heart disease are physically active and of normal weight, with low blood pressure and favorable lipid profiles.

Parents do not need to worry about their children's blood cholesterol, do they?

Atherosclerotic lesion formation reflects blood cholesterol: as blood cholesterol rises, lesion coverage increases. Cholesterol values at birth are similar in all populations; differences emerge in early childhood. Standard values for cholesterol screening in children and adolescents are listed in Table NP12-1. Cholesterol concentrations change with age in children and adolescents, however, and are especially variable during puberty.[14] Thus, using a single cut point for all pediatric age groups has limitations.

In general, blood cholesterol tends to rise as dietary saturated fat intakes increase. Blood cholesterol also correlates with childhood obesity, especially abdominal obesity.[15] LDL cholesterol rises with obesity, and HDL declines. These relationships are apparent throughout childhood, and their magnitude increases with age.

Children who are both overweight and have high blood cholesterol are likely to have parents who develop heart disease early. For this reason, selective screening is recommended for children and adolescents of any age who are overweight or obese; those whose parents (or grandparents) have premature (≤55 years of age for men and ≤65 years of age for women) heart disease; those whose parents have elevated blood cholesterol; those who have other risk factors for heart disease such as hypertension, cigarette smoking, or diabetes; and those whose family history is unavailable. Because blood cholesterol in children is a good predictor of adult values, some experts recommend universal screening for all children aged 9 to 11.[16]

Early—but not advanced—atherosclerotic lesions are reversible, making screening and education a high priority. Both those with family histories of heart disease and those with multiple risk factors need intervention.

Is hypertension a concern for children and adolescents?

Pediatricians routinely monitor blood pressure in children and adolescents. High blood pressure may signal an underlying disease or the early onset of hypertension. Childhood hypertension, left untreated, can accelerate the development of atherosclerosis.[17] Diagnosing hypertension in children and adolescents requires consideration of age, gender, and height, and blood pressure cannot be assessed using the simple tables applied to adults.

Like atherosclerosis and high blood cholesterol, hypertension may develop in the first decades of life, especially among obese children, and worsen with time. Children can control their hypertension by participating in regular aerobic activity and by losing weight or maintaining their weight as they grow taller. Restricting dietary sodium also causes an immediate drop in most children's and adolescents' blood pressure.[18]

Regular physical activity lowers risks for heart disease and hypertension in adults; does it do so in children as well?

Yes. Research has confirmed an association between blood lipids and physical activity in children, similar to that seen in adults. Physically active children have a better lipid profile and lower blood pressure than physically inactive children, and these positive findings often persist into adulthood.[19] Table 12-12 on p. 341 offers examples of aerobic, muscle-strengthening, and bone-strengthening physical activities for children and adolescents.

Just as blood cholesterol and obesity track over the years, so does a child's level of physical activity.[20] Those who are inactive now are likely to still be inactive years later. Similarly, those who are physically active now tend to remain so. Compared with inactive teens, those who are physically active weigh less, smoke less, eat a diet lower in saturated fats, and have better blood lipid profiles. Both obesity and blood cholesterol correlate with the inactive pastime of watching television. The message is clear: physical activity offers numerous health benefits, and children who are active today are most likely to be active for years to come.

Are adult dietary recommendations appropriate for children?

Regardless of family history, all children older than age two should eat a variety of foods and maintain a desirable weight (see Table NP12-2). For heart health, children (2 to 18 years of age) should receive at least 25 percent and no more than 30 percent of total energy from fat, less than 10 percent from saturated fat, and less than 300 milligrams of cholesterol per day.[21]

Healthy children older than age two can begin the transition to these recommendations by eating fewer foods high in saturated fat and selecting more fruits and vegetables. Healthy meals can occasionally include moderate amounts of a child's favorite food, such as ice cream, even if it is high in saturated fat. A steady diet from the children's menus in some restaurants—which feature chicken nuggets, hot dogs, and french fries—easily exceeds a prudent intake of saturated fat, *trans* fat, and kcalories, however, and invites both nutrient shortages and weight gains.[22] Fortunately, most restaurant chains are changing children's menus to include steamed vegetables, fruit cups, and broiled or grilled chicken—additions welcomed by busy parents who often dine out or purchase take-out foods.

Other fatty foods, such as nuts, vegetable oils, and some varieties of fish such as tuna or salmon, contribute essential fatty acids. Low-fat milk and milk products also deserve special attention in a child's diet for the needed calcium and other nutrients they supply.

Parents and caregivers play a key role in helping children establish healthy eating habits. Balanced meals need to provide lean meat, poultry, fish, and legumes; fruits and vegetables; whole

TABLE NP12-2 American Heart Association Dietary Guidelines and Strategies for Children[a]

- Balance dietary kcalories with physical activity to maintain normal growth.
- Every day, engage in 60 minutes of moderate to vigorous play or physical activity.
- Eat vegetables and fruits daily. Use fresh, frozen, and canned vegetables and fruits and serve at every meal; limit those with added fats, salt, and sugar.
- Limit juice intake to 4 ounces per day.
- Use vegetable oils (canola, soybean, olive, safflower, or other unsaturated oils) and soft margarines low in saturated fat and *trans* fatty acids instead of butter or most other animal fats in the diet.
- Choose whole-grain breads and cereals rather than refined products; read labels and make sure that "whole grain" is the first ingredient.
- Limit or avoid the intake of sugar-sweetened beverages; encourage water.
- Consume low-fat and nonfat milk and milk products daily.
- Include two servings of fish per week, especially fatty fish such as broiled or baked salmon.
- Choose legumes and tofu in place of meat for some meals.
- Choose only lean cuts of meat and reduced-fat meat products; remove the skin from poultry.
- Use less salt, including salt from processed foods. Breads, breakfast cereals, and soups may be high in salt and/or sugar so read food labels and choose high-fiber, low-salt, low-sugar alternatives.
- Limit the intake of high-kcalorie add-ons such as gravy, Alfredo sauce, cream sauce, cheese sauce, and hollandaise sauce.
- Serve age-appropriate portion sizes on/in appropriately sized plates and bowls.

[a]These guidelines are for children 2 years of age and older.

Source: Adapted from Expert Panel on Integrated Guidelines for Cardiovascular Health and Risk Reduction in Children and Adolescents, Summary report, *Pediatrics* 128 (2011): S213–S256; American Heart Association, S. S. Gidding and coauthors, Dietary recommendations for children and adolescents: A guide for practitioners, *Pediatrics* 117 (2006): 544–559.

© Cengage Learning®

grains; and low-fat milk products. Such meals can provide enough energy and nutrients to support growth and maintain blood cholesterol within a healthy range.

Pediatricians warn parents to avoid extremes. Although intentions may be good, excessive food restriction may create nutrient deficiencies and impair growth. Furthermore, parental control over eating may instigate battles and foster attitudes about foods that can lead to inappropriate eating behaviors.

Do pediatricians ever prescribe drugs to lower blood cholesterol in children?

Experts agree that children with high blood cholesterol should first be treated with diet. If high blood cholesterol persists despite dietary intervention in children 10 years of age and older, then drugs may be necessary to lower blood cholesterol. Drugs can effectively lower blood cholesterol without interfering with adolescent growth or development.

Can parents or caregivers do anything else to help children reduce their risks of CVD?

Even though the focus of this text is nutrition, another risk factor for heart disease that starts in childhood and carries over into adulthood—cigarette smoking—must also be addressed. Each day more than 3000 young people between the ages of 12 and 17 light up for the first time, and an estimated 2000 become daily cigarette smokers.[23] One in seven high school students smokes regularly.[24] Approximately 90 percent of all adult smokers began smoking before the age of 18.

Of those teenagers who continue smoking, half will eventually die of smoking-related causes. Efforts to teach children about the dangers of smoking need to be aggressive. Children are not likely to consider the long-term health consequences of tobacco use. They are more likely to be struck by the immediate health consequences, such as shortness of breath when playing sports, or social consequences, such as having bad breath. Whatever the context, the message to all children and teens should be clear: Don't start smoking. If you've already started, quit.

In conclusion, *adult* heart disease is a major *pediatric* problem. Without intervention, some 60 million children are destined to suffer its consequences within the next 30 years. Optimal prevention efforts focus on children, especially on those who are overweight. Just as young children receive vaccinations against infectious diseases, they need screening for, and education about, chronic diseases. Many health education programs have been implemented in schools around the country. These programs are most effective when they include education in the classroom, heart-healthy meals in the lunchroom, fitness activities on the playground, and parental involvement at home.

Notes

1. C. L. Ogden and coauthors, Prevalence of childhood and adult obesity in the United States, 2011–2012, *Journal of the American Medical Association* 311 (2014): 806–814; D. Dabelea and coauthors, Prevalence of type 1 and type 2 diabetes among children and adolescents from 2001 to 2009, *Journal of the American Medical Association* 311 (2014): 1778–1776; Position of the American Academy of Nutrition and Dietetics: The role of nutrition in health promotion and chronic disease prevention, *Journal of the Academy of Nutrition and Dietetics* 113 (2013): 972–979; S. Saydah and coauthors, Cardiometabolic risk factors among US adolescents and young adults and risk of early mortality, *Pediatrics* 131 (2013): e679–e686; J. P. Reis and coauthors, Association between duration of overall and abdominal obesity beginning in young adulthood and coronary artery calcification in middle age, *Journal of the American Medical Association* 310 (2013): 280–288; A. Tirosh and coauthors, Adolescent BMI trajectory and risk of diabetes versus coronary disease, *New England Journal of Medicine* 364 (2011): 1315–1325; J. C. Han, D. A. Lawlor, and S. Y. S. Kimm, Childhood obesity, *Lancet* 375 (2010): 1737–1748; F. M. Biro and M. Wien,

Childhood obesity and adult morbidities, *American Journal of Clinical Nutrition* 91 (2010): 1499S–1505S; P. W. Franks and coauthors, Childhood obesity, other cardiovascular risk factors, and premature death, *New England Journal of Medicine* 362 (2010): 458–493.

2. M. de Onis and coauthors, Global prevalence and trends of overweight and obesity among preschool children, *American Journal of Clinical Nutrition* 92 (2010): 1257–1264; B. M. Popkin, Recent dynamics suggest selected countries catching up to US obesity, *American Journal of Clinical Nutrition* 91 (2010): 284S–288S.

3. A. L. May, E. V. Kuklina, and P. W. Yoon, Prevalence of cardiovascular disease risk factors among US adolescents, 1999–2008, *Pediatrics* 129 (2012): 1035–1041; C. Friedemann and coauthors, Cardiovascular disease risk in healthy children and its association with body mass index: Systematic review and meta-analysis, *British Medical Journal* 345 (2012): e4759; Expert Panel on Integrated Guidelines for Cardiovascular Health and Risk Reduction in Children and Adolescents, Summary report, *Pediatrics* 128 (2011): S212–S256; M. Juonola and coauthors, Childhood adiposity, adult adiposity, and cardiovascular risk factors, *New England Journal of Medicine* 365 (2011): 1876–1885.

4. R. N. H. Touwslager and coauthors, Genetic and environmental factors in associations between infant growth and adult cardiometabolic risk profile in twins, *American Journal of Clinical Nutrition* 98 (2013): 994–1001; L. Brazionis and coauthors, Diet spanning infancy and toddlerhood is associated with child blood pressure at age 7.5 y, *American Journal of Clinical Nutrition* 97 (2013): 1375–1386; D. K. Arnett and S. A. Claas, Preventing and controlling hypertension in the era of genomic innovation and environmental transformation, *Journal of the American Medical Association* 308 (2012): 1745–1746; M. Manco and B. Dallapiccola, Genetics of pediatric obesity, *Pediatrics* 130 (2012): 123–133; C. H. Llewellyn and coauthors, Inherited behavioral susceptibility to adiposity in infancy: A multivariate genetic analysis of appetite and weight in the Gemini birth cohort, *American Journal of Clinical Nutrition* 95 (2012): 633–639.

5. Juonaloa and coauthors, 2011; Franks and coauthors, 2010: 485–493.

6. B. G. Koot and coauthors, Lifestyle intervention for non-alcoholic fatty liver disease: Prospective cohort study of its efficacy and factors related to improvement, *Archives of Disease in Childhood* 96 (2011): 669–674.

7. M. L. Gusmão Correia and coauthors, Developmental origins of health and disease: Experimental and human evidence of fetal programming for metabolic syndrome, *Journal of Human Hypertension* 26 (2012): 405–419; J. L. Tarry-Adkins and S. E. Ozanne, Mechanisms of early life programming: Current knowledge and future directions, *American Journal of Clinical Nutrition* 94 (2011): 1765S–1771S; G. C. Burdge and K. A. Lillycrop, Nutrition, epigenetics, and developmental plasticity: Implications for understanding human disease, *Annual Review of Nutrition* 30 (2010): 315–339.

8. J. G. Eriksson, Early growth and coronary heart disease and type 2 diabetes: Findings from the Helsinki Birth Cohort Study (HBCS), *American Journal of Clinical Nutrition* 94 (2011): 1799S–1802S; B. Reusens and coauthors, Maternal malnutrition programs the endocrine pancreas in progeny, *American Journal of Clinical Nutrition* 94 (2011): 1824S–1829S; Tarry-Adkins and Ozanne, 2011; Burdge and Lillycrop, 2010.

9. Tarry-Adkins and Ozanne, 2011.

10. Dabelea and coauthors, 2014; Juonala and coauthors, 2011; Biro and Wien, 2010.

11. Biro and Wien, 2010.

12. Friedmann and coauthors, 2012; Expert Panel on Integrated Guidelines for Cardiovascular Health and Risk Reduction in Children and Adolescents, 2011.

13. Centers for Disease Control and Prevention, Prevalence of abnormal lipid levels among youths—United States, 1999–2006, *Morbidity and Mortality Weekly Report* 59 (2010): 29–33.

14. Expert Panel on Integrated Guidelines for Cardiovascular Health and Risk Reduction in Children and Adolescents, 2011.

15. Friedemann and coauthors, 2012; May, Kuklina, and Yoon, 2012.

16. Expert Panel on Integrated Guidelines for Cardiovascular Health and Risk Reduction in Children and Adolescents, 2011.

17. M. Barton, Childhood obesity: A lifelong health risk, *Acta Pharmacologica Sinica* 2 (2012): 189–193; J. Le and coauthors, "Vascular Age" is advanced in children with atherosclerosis-promoting risk factors, *Circulation Cardiovascular Imaging* 3 (2010): 8–14.

18. Q. Yang and coauthors, Sodium intake and blood pressure among US children and adolescents, *Pediatrics* 130 (2012): 611–619S. Stabouli and coauthors, The role of obesity, salt and exercise on blood pressure in children and adolescents, *Expert Review of Cardiovascular Therapy* 9 (2011): 753–761; J. Feber and M. Ahmed, Hypertension in children: New trends and challenges, *Clinical Science* 119 (2010): 151–161.

19. U. Ekelund and coauthors, Moderate to vigorous physical activity and sedentary time and cardiometabolic risk factors in children and adolescents, *Journal of the American Medical Association* 15 (2012): 704–712.

20. R. Telama and coauthors, Tracking of physical activity from early childhood through youth into adulthood, *Medicine and Science in Sports and Exercise* 46 (2014): 955–962.

21. Expert Panel on Integrated Guidelines for Cardiovascular Health and Risk Reduction in Children and Adolescents, 2011.

22. K. N. Boutelle and coauthors, Nutritional quality of lunch meal purchased for children at a fast-food restaurant, *Childhood Obesity* 7 (2011): 316–322.

23. Centers for Disease Control and Prevention, Youth and tobacco use, available at www.cdc.gov/tobacco/data_statistics/fact_sheets/youth_data/tobacco_use/index.htm, updated February 14, 2014.

24. R. A. Arrazola, S. R. Dube, and B. A. King, Tobacco product use among middle and high school students—United States, 2011 and 2012, *Morbidity and Mortality Weekly Report* 62 (2013): 893–897.

13

Nutrition through the Life Span: Later Adulthood

BananaStock/Alamy

FIGURE 13-1 The Aging of the U.S. Population

In 1940, 6.8 percent of the population was 65 or older. In 1990, 12.7 percent of us had reached age 65; by 2040, 21.7 percent will have reached age 65; and by 2090, nearly one out of four Americans will be 65 or older.

The last two chapters were devoted to stages of the life cycle that require special nutrition attention: pregnancy, lactation, infancy, childhood, and adolescence. Much of the text before that focused on nutrition to support wellness during adulthood. This chapter describes the special nutrition needs of the later adult years.

The most urgent nutrition need of older people, however, is to have made good food choices in the past! All of life's nutrition choices incur health consequences for the better or for the worse. A single day's intakes of nutrients may exert only a minute effect on body organs and their functions, but, over years and decades, the repeated effects accumulate to have major impacts. This being the case, it is of great importance for everyone, of every age, to pay close attention today to nutrition.

The "graying" of America is a continuing trend.[1] The majority of citizens are now middle aged, and the ratio of old people to young is increasing, as Figure 13-1 shows. Our society uses the arbitrary age of 65 to define the transition point between middle age and old age, but growing "old" happens day by day, with changes occurring gradually over time. Commonly used age groups include young old (65–74 years), old (75–84 years), and oldest old (≥85 years).

Since 1950 the population older than age 65 has almost tripled. Remarkably, the fastest-growing age group has been people older than age 85; since 1950 their numbers have increased sevenfold. The U.S. Bureau of the Census projects that by the year 2040 more than a million Americans will be 100 years old or older.

Life expectancy in the United States is 79 years, up from about 47 years in 1900.[2] Advances in medical science—antibiotics and other treatments—are largely responsible for almost doubling the life expectancy in the 20th century. Improved nutrition and an abundant food supply have also contributed to lengthening life expectancy. Ironically, this abundant food supply has also jeopardized the chances of further lengthening life expectancy as obesity rates increase.[3]

The human **life span,** currently estimated at 130 years, is the upper limit of human **longevity,** even given optimal nutrition. With work progressing in medical and genetic technologies, however, the human life span may be extended significantly.

Research in the field of aging is active—and difficult. Researchers are challenged by the diversity of older adults. When older adults experience health problems, it is hard to know whether to attribute these problems to genetics, aging, or other environmental factors such as nutrition. The idea that nutrition can influence the way the human body ages is particularly appealing because diet is a factor that people can control and change.

13.1 Nutrition and Longevity

LO 13.1 Describe the roles nutrition, physical activity, and other lifestyle choices play in longevity.

What has been learned so far about the effects of nutrition and environment on longevity provides incentive for researchers to keep asking questions about how and why human beings age. Among their questions are:

- To what extent is aging inevitable, and can it be slowed through changes in lifestyle and environment?

- What role does nutrition play in the aging process, and what role can it play in slowing aging?

life expectancy: the average number of years lived by people in a given society.

life span: the maximum number of years of life attainable by a member of a species.

longevity: long duration of life.

With respect to the first question, it seems that aging is an inevitable, natural process, programmed into the genes at conception. People can, however, slow the process within the natural limits set by heredity by adopting healthy lifestyle habits such as eating nutritious food and engaging in physical activity. In fact, a person's life expectancy depends on both individual health-related behaviors and genes.[4]

With respect to the second question, good nutrition helps to maintain a healthy body and can therefore ease the aging process in many significant ways.[5] Clearly, nutrition can improve the **quality of life** in the later years.[6]

Slowing the Aging Process

One approach researchers use to search out the secret of long life is to study older people. Some people are young for their ages, whereas others are old for their ages. What makes the difference?

Healthy Habits Some lifestyle habits seem to have a profound influence on people's health and therefore on their **physiological age**:[7]

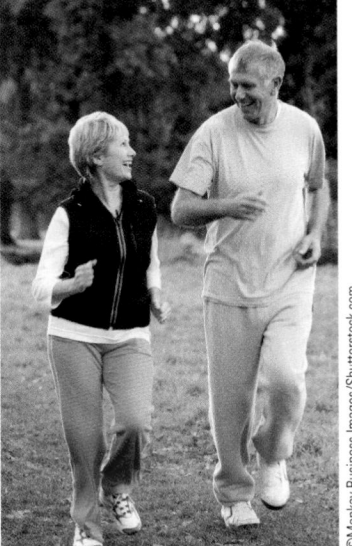

- Following a healthy, plant-based eating pattern such as the Mediterranean diet (rich in fruits, vegetables, whole grains, poultry, fish, and low-fat milk products)[8]

- Maintaining a healthy body weight

- Engaging in regular physical activity daily

- Not smoking

- Not using alcohol, or using it in moderation

- Sleeping regularly and adequately

- Having a sense of purpose

- Relieving stress (through meditation, prayer, naps, or other calming activity)

- Belonging to a community of loving family and friends (home, church, or other social network)

Over the years, the effects of these lifestyle choices accumulate—that is, those who follow all of these practices live longer and have fewer disabilities as they age. They are in better health, even if older in **chronological age**, than people who do not adopt these behaviors. Even though people cannot alter their birth dates, they may be able to add years to, and enhance the quality of, their lives. Physical activity seems to be most influential in preventing or slowing the many changes that many people seem to accept as an inevitable consequence of old age. In other words, physical activity and long life seem to go together.[9]

Regular physical activity promotes a healthy, independent lifestyle.

Physical Activity The many and remarkable benefits of regular physical activity are not limited to the young. Compared with those who are inactive, older adults who are active weigh less; have greater flexibility, more endurance, better balance, and better health; and live longer.[10] They reap additional benefits from various types of activities as well: aerobic activities improve cardiorespiratory endurance, blood pressure, and blood lipid concentrations; moderate endurance activities improve the quality of sleep; and resistance training significantly improves posture and mobility. In fact, regular physical activity is a powerful predictor of a person's mobility in the later years. Mobility, in turn, is closely associated with longevity.[11] Physical activity also increases blood flow to the brain, thereby preserving mental ability, alleviating depression, and supporting independence.[12]

Muscle mass and muscle strength tend to decline with aging, making older people vulnerable to falls and immobility. Falls are a major cause of fear, injury, disability, dependence, and even death among older adults. Regular physical activity tones,

quality of life: a person's perceived physical and mental well-being.

physiological age: a person's age as estimated from her or his body's health and probable life expectancy.

chronological age: a person's age in years from his or her date of birth.

firms, and strengthens muscles, helping to improve confidence, reduce the risk of falling, and minimize the risk of injury should a fall occur.

Even without a fall, older adults may become so weak that they can no longer perform life's daily tasks, such as climbing stairs, carrying packages, and opening jars. Resistance training helps older adults to maintain independence by strengthening the muscles needed to perform these tasks.[13] Even in frail, elderly people older than 85 years of age, resistance training has been shown not only to improve balance, muscle strength, and mobility but also to increase energy expenditure and energy intake. This finding highlights another reason to be physically active: a person spending energy on physical activity can afford to eat more food and, with it, more nutrients. People who are committed to an ongoing fitness program can benefit from higher energy and nutrient intakes and still maintain healthy body weights.

Ideally, physical activity should be part of each day's schedule and should be intense enough to prevent muscle atrophy and to speed up the heartbeat and respiration rate. Although aging affects both speed and endurance to some degree, older adults can still train and achieve exceptional performances. Healthy older adults who have not been active can ease into a suitable routine. They can start by walking short distances until they are walking at least 10 minutes continuously and then gradually increase the distance to a 30- to 60-minute walk at least 5 days a week. With persistence, people can achieve great improvements at any age. Table 13-1 provides exercise goals

TABLE 13-1 Exercise Guidelines for Older Adults

	Aerobic	Strength	Balance	Flexibility
Examples	Geoff Manasse/PhotoDisc/PictureQuest/Getty Images	IT Stock Free/PictureQuest/Getty Images	IT Stock Free/PictureQuest/Getty Images	Ron Chapple/Thinkstock/PictureQuest/Getty Images
Start easy and progress gradually	Be active five minutes on most or all days	Using 0- to 2-pound weights, do one set of 8–12 repetitions twice a week	Hold onto table or chair with one hand, then with one finger	Hold stretch for 10 seconds; do each stretch three times
Frequency	At least five days per week of moderate activity or at least four days per week of vigorous activity	At least two (nonconsecutive) days per week	Two to three days each week	At least two days per week, preferably on all days that aerobic or strength activities are performed
Intensity[a]	Moderate, vigorous, or combination	Moderate to high; 10 to 15 repetitions per exercise	—	Moderate
Duration	At least 30 minutes of moderate activity in bouts of at least 10 minutes each or at least 20 minutes of continuous vigorous activity	8 to 10 exercises involving the major muscle groups	—	Stretch major muscle groups for 10–30 seconds, repeating each stretch three to four times
Cautions and comments	Stop if you are breathing so hard you can't talk or if you feel dizziness or chest pain	Breathe out as you contract and in as you relax (do not hold your breath); use smooth, steady movements	Incorporate balance techniques with strength exercises as you progress	Stretch after strength and endurance exercises for 20 minutes, three times a week; use slow, steady movements; bend joints slightly

[a]On a 10-point scale, where sitting = 0 and maximum effort = 10, moderate intensity = 5 to 6 and vigorous intensity = 7 to 8.

Note: Activity recommendations are in addition to routine activities of daily living (such as getting dressed, cooking, and grocery shopping) and moderate activities lasting less than 10 minutes.

Source: C. E. Garber and coauthors, Quantity and quality of exercise for developing and maintaining cardiorespiratory, muscoskeletal, and neuromotor fitness in apparently healthy adults: Guidance for prescribing exercise, *Medicine and Science in Sports and Exercise* 43 (2011): 1334–1359; W. J. Chodzko-Zajko and coauthors, Position Stand of the American College of Sports Medicine: Exercise and physical activity for older adults, *Medicine and Science in Sports and Exercise* 41 (2009):1510–1530.

© 2016 Cengage Learning®

and guidelines for older adults. Relatively few older adults meet these goals. People with medical conditions should check with a physician before beginning an exercise routine, as should sedentary men older than 40 and sedentary women older than 50 who want to participate in a vigorous program.

Restriction of kCalories In their efforts to understand longevity, researchers have not only observed people but have also manipulated influencing factors, such as diet, in animals. This research has produced some interesting and suggestive findings. For example, animals live longer and have fewer age-related diseases when their energy intakes are restricted.[14] These life-prolonging benefits become evident when the diet provides enough food to prevent malnutrition and an energy intake of about 70 percent of normal; benefits decline as the age at which energy restriction begins is delayed.

Exactly how energy restriction prolongs life remains unexplained, although gene activity appears to play a key role. Energy restriction in animals prevents alterations in gene expression that are associated with aging. Food restriction may also extend the life span by preventing damaging lipid oxidation, thereby delaying the onset of age-related diseases such as cancer and atherosclerosis.[15] Other research suggests that energy restriction beneficially alters several aspects of fat cell metabolism, which may play a role in reducing chronic disease risk and extending life. Experiments with food restriction and longevity in animals have *not* suggested any direct applications to human nutrition.

Moderate energy restriction (80 to 90 percent of usual intake) in human beings may be valuable. When people restrict energy intake moderately, body weight, body fat, and blood pressure drop, and blood lipids and insulin response improve—favorable changes for preventing chronic diseases.[16] The reduction in oxidative damage that occurs with energy restriction in animals also occurs in people whose diets include antioxidant nutrients and phytochemicals. Diets such as the Mediterranean diet that include an abundance of fruits, vegetables, olive oil, whole grains, and legumes—with their array of antioxidants and phytochemicals—support good health and long life.[17]

Nutrition and Disease Prevention

Nutrition alone, even if ideal, cannot ensure a long and robust life. Nevertheless, nutrition clearly affects aging and longevity in human beings by way of its role in disease prevention. Among the better-known relationships between nutrition and disease are the following:

- Appropriate energy intake helps prevent *obesity, diabetes*, and related *cardiovascular diseases* such as atherosclerosis and hypertension (Chapters 7, 21, and 22) and may influence the development of some forms of *cancer* (Chapter 25).

- Adequate intakes of essential nutrients prevent *deficiency diseases* such as scurvy, goiter, and anemia (Chapters 8 and 9).

- Variety in food intake, as well as ample intakes of certain fruits and vegetables, may be protective against certain types of *cancer* (Chapter 25).

- Moderation in sugar intake helps prevent *dental caries* (Nutrition in Practice 17).

- Appropriate fiber intakes may help prevent disorders of the digestive tract such as *constipation, diverticulosis,* and possibly *colon cancer* (Chapters 2, 18, and 25).

- Moderate sodium intake and adequate intakes of potassium, calcium, and other minerals help prevent *hypertension* (Chapters 9 and 22).

- An adequate calcium intake throughout life helps protect against *osteoporosis* (Chapter 9).

Other, less well-established links between nutrition and disease are being discovered each day. Research that focuses on how life factors affect aging and disease processes is vital to ensuring that more and more people can look forward to long, healthy lives.

IN SUMMARY

▪ Life expectancy in the United States increased dramatically in the 20th century.

▪ Factors that enhance longevity include limited or no alcohol use, a plant-based eating pattern, weight control, adequate sleep, abstinence from smoking, and regular physical activity.

▪ Nutrition alone, even if ideal, cannot guarantee a long and robust life. At the very least, however, nutrition—especially when combined with regular physical activity—can influence aging and longevity in human beings by supporting good health and preventing disease.

13.2 Nutrition-Related Concerns during Late Adulthood

LO 13.2 Identify how nutrition might contribute to, or prevent, the development of age-related problems associated with vision, arthritis, and the brain.

Nutrition through the prime years may play a greater role than has been realized in preventing many changes once thought to be inevitable consequences of growing older. The following discussions of cataracts and macular degeneration, arthritis, and the aging brain show that nutrition may provide at least some protection against some of the conditions commonly associated with aging.

Cataracts and Macular Degeneration

Cataracts are age-related thickenings in the lenses of the eye that impair vision. If not surgically removed, they ultimately lead to blindness. Oxidative stress appears to play a significant role in the development of cataracts but supplements of the antioxidant nutrients (vitamin C, vitamin E, and carotenoids) do not seem to prevent or slow the progression.[18] By comparison, a healthy diet that includes plenty of fruits and vegetables rich in these antioxidants does seem to slow the progression or reduce the risk of developing cataracts.[19] Also, people who follow the *Dietary Guidelines for Americans* are reported to have fewer cataracts, though cataracts can occur even in well-nourished individuals due to exposure to ultraviolet light, oxidative damage, viral infections, toxic substances, genetic disorders, injury, or other trauma.[20] Most cataracts are vaguely called "senile" cataracts, meaning "caused by aging." In the United States, more than half of all adults age 65 and older have a cataract.

One other diet-related factor may play a role in cataract development: obesity.[21] How obesity may influence the development of cataracts is not known. Risk factors that typically accompany overweight, such as inactivity, diabetes, or hypertension, do not explain the association.

The leading cause of visual loss among older people is **macular degeneration**, a deterioration of the macular region of the eye. As with cataracts, risk factors for age-related macular degeneration include oxidative stress from sunlight. Preventive factors for macular degeneration may include supplements of the omega-3 fatty acid DHA, some B vitamins (folate, vitamin B_6, and vitamin B_{12}), and the carotenoids lutein and zeaxanthin.[22]

cataracts: clouding of the eye lenses that impairs vision and can lead to blindness.

macular (MACK-you-lar) **degeneration:** deterioration of the macular area of the eye that can lead to loss of central vision and eventual blindness. The **macula** is a small, oval, yellowish region in the center of the retina that provides the sharp, straight-ahead vision so critical to reading and driving.

Arthritis

More than 50 million people in the United States have some form of **arthritis.**[23] As the population ages, it is expected that the prevalence will increase to 70 million by 2030. The most common type of arthritis that disables older people is **osteoarthritis,** a painful swelling of the joints. During movement, the ends of bones are normally protected from wear by cartilage and by small sacs of fluid that lubricate the joint. With age, the cartilage sometimes disintegrates, and the joints become malformed and painful to move.

Obesity is common among adults with arthritis.[24] Weight loss can help overweight people with osteoarthritis, partly because the joints affected are often weight-bearing joints that are stressed and irritated by having to carry excess poundage. Interestingly, though, weight loss often relieves the worst pain of osteoarthritis in the hands as well, even though they are not weight-bearing joints. Jogging and other weight-bearing activities do not worsen osteoarthritis. In fact, both aerobic activity and weight training offer modest improvements in physical performance and pain relief, especially when accompanied by even modest weight loss.[25]

Nutrition quackery to treat arthritis is abundant, but no one universally effective diet for arthritis relief is known. Table 13-2 presents some of the many ineffective dietary treatments for osteoarthritis. Traditional medical intervention for arthritis includes medication and surgery. Two popular supplements for treating osteoarthritis—glucosamine and chondroitin—may alleviate pain and improve mobility, but mixed reports from studies emphasize the need for additional research.[26] Drugs and supplements used to relieve arthritis can impose nutrition risks; some affect appetite and alter the body's use of nutrients, as Chapter 15 explains.

Another type of arthritis, known as **rheumatoid arthritis,** has a possible link to diet through the immune system. In rheumatoid arthritis, the immune system mistakenly attacks the bone coverings as if they were made of foreign tissue. In some individuals, certain foods, notably a Mediterranean-type diet of fish, vegetables, and olive oil, may moderate the inflammatory responses and provide some relief.[27]

The omega-3 fatty acids commonly found in fish oil reduce joint tenderness and improve mobility in some people with rheumatoid arthritis. The same diet recommended for heart health—one low in saturated fat from meats and milk products and high in omega-3 fats from fish—helps prevent or reduce the inflammation in the joints that makes arthritis so painful.

The Aging Brain

Dementia affects an estimated 15 percent of adults older than 70 years of age in the United States and represents a financial burden of between $157 billion and $215 billion.[28] The brain, like all of the body's organs, ages in response to both genetic and environmental factors—such as physical activities, intellectual challenges, social interactions, and nutritious diets—that can enhance or diminish its amazing capacities. One of the challenges researchers face when studying the aging of the human brain is to distinguish among changes caused by normal, age-related, physiological processes; changes caused by diseases; and changes caused by cumulative, extrinsic factors such as diet.

The brain normally changes in some characteristic ways as it ages. For one thing, its blood supply decreases. For another, the number of **neurons,** the brain cells that specialize in transmitting information, diminishes as people age. Losses of neurons affect different functions depending on their location in the brain. For example, declines in the number of nerve cells in one part of the **cerebral cortex** affect hearing and speech, while losses in other parts of the cortex can impair memory and cognitive function. When the number of neurons in the hindbrain diminishes, balance and posture are affected.

TABLE 13-2 Ineffective Dietary Strategies for Arthritis

- Alfalfa tea
- Aloe vera liquid
- Amino acid supplements
- Blackstrap molasses
- Burdock root
- Calcium
- Celery juice
- Cod liver oil
- Copper supplements
- Dimethyl sulfoxide (DMSO)
- Fasting
- Fresh fruit
- Garlic
- Honey
- Inositol
- Kelp
- Lecithin
- Para-amino benzoic acid (PABA)
- Raw liver
- Superoxide dismutase (SOD)
- Vitamin D
- Vitamin megadoses
- Watercress
- Yeast

© Cengage Learning®

arthritis: inflammation of a joint, usually accompanied by pain, swelling, and structural changes.

osteoarthritis: a painful, chronic disease of the joints that occurs when the cushioning cartilage in a joint breaks down; joint structure is usually altered, with loss of function; also called *degenerative arthritis.*

rheumatoid arthritis: a disease of the immune system involving painful inflammation of the joints and related structures.

neurons: nerve cells; the structural and functional units of the nervous system. Neurons initiate and conduct nerve transmissions.

cerebral cortex: the outer surface of the cerebrum, which is the largest part of the brain.

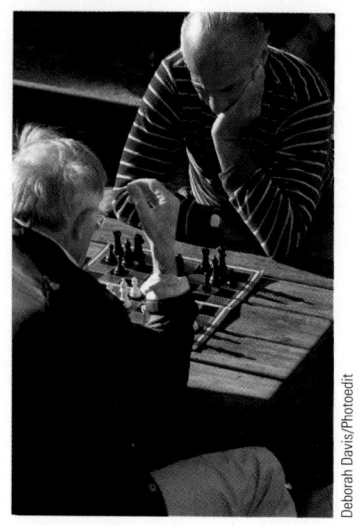

Both foods and mental challenges nourish the brain.

Nutrient Deficiencies and Brain Function Clinicians now recognize that much of the cognitive loss and forgetfulness generally attributed to aging is due in part to extrinsic, and therefore controllable, factors such as nutrient deficiencies. The ability of neurons to synthesize specific neurotransmitters depends in part on the availability of precursor nutrients that are obtained from the diet. The neurotransmitter serotonin, for example, derives from the amino acid tryptophan. In addition, the enzymes involved in neurotransmitter synthesis require vitamins and minerals to function properly. The B vitamins folate, vitamin B_6, and vitamin B_{12} slow brain atrophy and improve cognition and memory.[29] The fatty acid DHA counteracts the cognitive decline commonly seen in elderly adults.[30] Thus, nutrient deficiencies may contribute to the loss of memory and cognition that some older adults experience.[31] Such losses may be preventable or at least diminished or delayed through diet and exercise.

In some instances, the degree of cognitive loss is extensive. Such **senile dementia** may be attributable to a specific disorder such as a brain tumor or Alzheimer's disease.

Alzheimer's Disease In **Alzheimer's disease,** the most prevalent form of dementia, brain cell death occurs in the areas of the brain that coordinate memory and cognition. Alzheimer's disease afflicts more than 5 million people in the United States, and that number is expected to triple by the year 2050.[32] Diagnosis of Alzheimer's depends on its characteristic symptoms: the victim gradually loses memory, reasoning ability, the ability to communicate, physical capabilities, and, eventually, life itself. Table 13-3 compares the signs of Alzheimer's disease with typical age-related changes.

TABLE 13-3 **Signs of Alzheimer's and Typical Age-Related Changes Compared**

Signs of Alzheimer's	Typical Age-Related Changes
Memory loss that disrupts daily life such as asking for the same information repeatedly or asking others to handle tasks of daily living	Forgetting a name or missing an appointment
Challenges in planning or solving problems such as following a recipe or paying monthly bills	Missing a monthly payment or making an error when balancing the checkbook
Difficulty completing familiar tasks at home such as using the microwave, at work such as preparing a report, or at leisure such as playing a game	Needing help recording a television program
Confusion with time or place including current season and location	Not knowing today's date
Trouble understanding visual images and spatial relationships such as judging distances and recognizing self in a mirror	Experiencing visual changes due to cataracts
New problems with words in speaking or writing such as not knowing the name of a common object	Being unable to find the right word to use
Misplacing things and losing the ability to retrace steps such as putting the milk in the closet and having no idea when or where the milk was last seen	Misplacing a pair of glasses or the car keys
Decreased or poor judgment such as giving large sums of money to strangers	Making a bad decision on occasion
Withdrawal from work projects or social activities	Feeling too tired to participate in work, family, or social activities
Changes in mood and personality such as confusion, suspicion, depression, and anxiety, especially when in unfamiliar places or with unfamiliar people	Becoming irritable when routines are disrupted

Source: Adapted from Alzheimer's Association, www.alz.org/alzheimers_disease_10_signs_of_alzheimers.asp.

The primary risk factor for Alzheimer's disease is age, but the exact cause remains unknown.[33] Clearly, genetic factors are involved. Free radicals and oxidative stress also seem to be involved. Nerve cells in the brains of people with Alzheimer's disease show evidence of free-radical attack—damage to DNA, cell membranes, and proteins—and of the minerals that trigger these attacks—iron, copper, zinc, and aluminum.[34] Some research suggests that the antioxidant nutrients can limit free-radical damage and delay or prevent Alzheimer's disease, but more research is needed to confirm this possibility.[35]

Increasing evidence also suggests that overweight and obesity in middle age are associated with dementia in general, and with Alzheimer's disease in particular.[36] The possible relationship between obesity and Alzheimer's disease is disturbing given the current obesity epidemic. Efforts to prevent and treat obesity, however, may also help prevent Alzheimer's disease.

In Alzheimer's disease, the brain develops **senile plaques** and **neurofibrillary tangles.** Senile plaques are clumps of a protein fragment called beta-amyloid, whereas neurofibrillary tangles are snarls of the fibers that extend from the nerve cells. Both seem to occur in response to oxidative stress. The accumulation of beta-amyloid seems to be a consequence of both excessive production and impaired clearance.[37] Treatment research focuses on lowering beta-amyloid levels.

Research suggests that cardiovascular disease risk factors such as high blood pressure, diabetes, obesity, smoking, physical inactivity, and elevated levels of homocysteine may be related to the development of Alzheimer's disease.[38] Diets designed to support a healthy heart, which include the omega-3 fatty acids of oily fish, may benefit brain health as well.[39] Similarly, physical activity supports heart health and slows the cognitive decline of Alzheimer's disease.[40]

Treatment for Alzheimer's disease involves providing care to clients and support to their families. Drugs are used to improve or at least to slow the loss of short-term memory and cognition, but they do not cure the disease. Other drugs may be used to control depression, anxiety, and behavior problems.

Maintaining appropriate body weight may be the most important nutrition concern for the person with Alzheimer's disease. Depression and forgetfulness can lead to changes in eating behaviors and poor food intake. Furthermore, changes in the body's weight-regulation system may contribute to weight loss. Perhaps the best that a caregiver can do nutritionally for a person with Alzheimer's disease is to supervise food planning and mealtimes. Providing well-liked and well-balanced meals and snacks in a cheerful atmosphere encourages food consumption. To minimize confusion, offer a few ready-to-eat foods, in bite-size pieces, with seasonings and sauces. To avoid mealtime disruptions, control distractions such as music, television, children, and the telephone.

IN SUMMARY

■ Cataracts, age-related macular degeneration, and arthritis afflict millions of older adults, while others face senile dementia and other losses of brain function.

■ Oxidative stress plays a significant role in the development of cataracts, and the antioxidant nutrients and phytochemicals in fruits and vegetables may help minimize the damage.

■ Weight loss can help overweight people with osteoarthritis. For some people with rheumatoid arthritis, a Mediterranean-type diet of fish, vegetables, and olive oil may moderate the inflammatory responses and provide some relief.

■ Nutrient deficiencies may contribute to the loss of memory and cognition that some older adults experience. Such losses may be preventable or at least diminished or delayed through diet.

■ The primary risk factor for Alzheimer's disease is age, but the exact cause remains unknown.

senile dementia: the loss of brain function beyond the normal loss of physical adeptness and memory that occurs with aging.

Alzheimer's disease: a progressive, degenerative disease that attacks the brain and impairs thinking, behavior, and memory.

senile plaques: clumps of the protein fragment beta-amyloid on the nerve cells, commonly found in the brains of people with Alzheimer's dementia.

neurofibrillary tangles: snarls of the threadlike strands that extend from the nerve cells, commonly found in the brains of people with Alzheimer's dementia.

13.3 Energy and Nutrient Needs during Late Adulthood

LO 13.3 Explain why the needs for some nutrients increase or decrease as people age and describe healthful eating patterns for older adults.

Knowledge about the nutrient needs and nutrition status of older adults has grown considerably in recent years. The Dietary Reference Intakes (DRI) cluster people older than 50 into two age categories—51 to 70 years old and 71 years and older. Research is showing that the nutrition needs of people 50 to 70 years old may be very different from those of people older than 70—a pattern that makes sense considering the wide age span involved.

Setting standards for older people is difficult, though, because individual differences become more pronounced as people grow older. People start out with different genetic predispositions and ways of handling nutrients, and the effects of these differences become magnified with years of unique dietary habits. For example, one person may tend to omit fruits and vegetables from his diet, and by the time he is old, he may have a set of nutrition problems associated with a lack of fiber and antioxidants. Another person who omitted milk and milk products all her life may have nutrition problems related to a lack of calcium. Also, as people age, they may suffer different chronic diseases and take different medications—both have impacts on nutrient needs. Table 13-4 lists some changes of aging that can affect nutrition. For all these reasons, researchers have difficulty even defining "healthy aging," a prerequisite to developing recommendations that are designed to meet the "needs of practically all healthy persons." Still, some generalizations are valid. The next sections give special attention to a few nutrients of concern.

Energy and Energy Nutrients

Energy needs decline with advancing age. As a general rule, adult energy needs decline an estimated 5 percent per decade. One reason is that people usually reduce their physical activity as they age, although they need not do so. Another reason is that basal metabolic rate declines 1 to 2 percent per decade, in part because lean body mass and thyroid hormones diminish. Loss of muscle mass, known as **sarcopenia,** can be significant in the later years (its prevalence is more than 50 percent among those older than 75), and its consequences, dramatic (see Figure 13-2).[41] As skeletal muscle mass diminishes, people lose their ability to move and to maintain balance, making falls likely. The limitations

TABLE 13-4 **Examples of Physical Changes of Aging That Affect Nutrition**

Mouth	Tooth loss, gum disease, and reduced salivary output impede chewing and swallowing. Swallowing disorders and choking may become likely. Discomfort and pain associated with eating may reduce food intake.
Digestive tract	Intestines lose muscle strength, resulting in sluggish motility that leads to constipation (see Chapter 18). Stomach inflammation, abnormal bacterial growth, and greatly reduced acid output impair digestion and absorption. Pain may cause food avoidance or reduced intake.
Hormones	For example, the pancreas secretes less insulin and cells become less responsive, causing abnormal glucose metabolism.
Sensory organs	Diminished senses of smell and taste can reduce appetite; diminished sight can make food shopping and preparation difficult.
Body composition	Weight loss and decline in lean body mass lead to lowered energy requirements. May be preventable or reversible through physical activity.
Urinary tract	Increased frequency of urination may limit fluid intake.

© Cengage Learning®

sarcopenia (SAR-koh-PEE-nee-ah): age-related loss of skeletal muscle mass, muscle strength, and muscle function.

Courtesy of Dr. William Evans

that accompany the loss of muscle mass and strength play a key role in the diminishing health that often accompanies aging. To some extent, however, declines in lean body mass and energy needs may not be entirely inevitable. Optimal nutrition with sufficient protein and regular physical activity, especially resistance training, can help maintain muscle mass and strength and minimize the changes in body composition associated with aging.[42] Physical activity not only increases energy expenditure but also, along with sound nutrition, enhances bone density and supports many body functions as well.

The lower energy expenditures of many older adults require that they eat less food to maintain their weights. Accordingly, the estimated energy requirements for adults decrease steadily after age 19. Energy intakes typically decline in parallel with needs. Still, many older adults are overweight, indicating that their food intakes do not decline enough to compensate for their reduced energy expenditures. Chapter 6 presents the many health problems that accompany obesity and the BMI guidelines for a healthy body weight (18.5–24.9). These guidelines apply to all adults, regardless of age, but they may be too restrictive for older adults. The importance of body weight in defending against chronic diseases differs for older adults.[43] Being *moderately overweight* may not be harmful. Older adults who are *obese*, however, face serious medical complications and can improve their quality of life with weight loss.[44]

On limited energy allowances, people must select mostly nutrient-dense foods. There is little leeway for added sugars, solid fats, or alcohol. Older adults can follow the USDA Food Patterns (see pp. 16-17, making sure to choose the recommended daily amounts of food from each food group that are appropriate to their energy needs (see Table 1-5 on p. 18).

Protein The protein needs of older adults appear to be about the same as those of younger people. With advancing age, however, people take in fewer total kcalories from food and so may need a greater percentage of kcalories from protein at each meal in order to support a healthy immune system and prevent losing muscle tissue, bone tissue, and other lean body mass.[45]

As energy needs decrease, lower-kcalorie protein sources such as lean tender meats, poultry, fish, boiled eggs, fat-free milk products, and legumes can help hold weight to a healthy level. Underweight or malnourished older adults need the opposite—energy-dense protein sources such as eggs scrambled with margarine, tuna salad with mayonnaise, peanut butter on wheat toast, hearty soups, and milkshakes. Nutrient-fortified supplements in liquid, pudding, cookie, or other forms between meals can also boost energy and nutrient intakes.

Carbohydrate and Fiber As always, abundant carbohydrate is needed to protect protein from being used as an energy source. The recommendation to obtain ample amounts of mostly whole-grain breads, cereals, rice, and pasta holds true for older people. As for younger people, a steady supply of carbohydrate is essential for optimal brain functioning. With age, fiber takes on extra importance for its role in alleviating constipation, a common complaint among older adults and among residents of **health care communities** in particular.[46]

health care communities: living environments for people with chronic conditions, functional limitations, or need for supervision or assistance. Health care communities include assisted living facilities, group homes, short-term rehabilitation facilities, skilled nursing facilities, and hospice facilities.

Fruits and vegetables supply soluble fibers and phytochemicals to help ward off chronic diseases, but factors such as transportation problems, limited cooking facilities, and chewing problems limit some elderly people's intakes of fresh fruits and vegetables.[47] Even without such problems, most older adults fail to obtain the recommended daily 25 or more grams of fiber (14 grams per 1000 kcalories).[48] When low fiber intakes are combined with low fluid intakes, inadequate physical activity, and constipating medications, constipation becomes inevitable.

Fat As is true for people of all ages, dietary fat intake needs to be moderate for most older adults—enough to enhance flavors and provide valuable essential fatty acids and other nutrients, but not so much as to raise risks of cancer, atherosclerosis, and other degenerative diseases. The recommendation should not be taken too far; limiting fat too severely may lead to nutrient deficiencies and weight loss—two problems that carry greater health risks in the elderly than overweight.

Water

Dehydration is a risk for older adults, who may not notice or pay attention to their thirst or who find it difficult and bothersome to get a drink or to get to a bathroom.[49] Older adults who have lost bladder control may be afraid to drink too much water. Despite real fluid needs, older people do not seem to feel as thirsty or notice mouth dryness as readily as younger people. Many employees of health care communities such as assisted living facilities say it is hard to persuade their elderly clients to drink enough water and fruit juices.

Total body water decreases as people age, so even mild stresses such as fever or hot weather can precipitate rapid dehydration in older adults. Dehydrated older adults seem to be more susceptible to urinary tract infections, pneumonia, pressure ulcers, confusion, and disorientation.[50] An intake of 9 cups a day of total beverages, including water, is recommended for women; for men, the recommendation is 13 cups a day of total beverages, including water.[51]

Vitamins and Minerals

As research reveals more about how specific vitamins and minerals influence disease prevention and how age-related physiological changes affect nutrient metabolism, optimal intakes of vitamins and minerals for different groups of older adults are being defined. This section highlights the vitamins and minerals of greatest concern to older adults.

Vitamin D Older adults face a greater risk of vitamin D deficiency than younger people do. Vitamin D–fortified milk is the most reliable source of vitamin D, but many older adults drink little or no milk. Further compromising the vitamin D status of many older people, especially those in assisted living facilities or group homes, is their limited exposure to sunlight. Finally, aging reduces the skin's capacity to make vitamin D and the kidneys' ability to convert it to its active form. Not only are older adults not getting enough vitamin D, but they may actually need more to improve both muscle and bone strength. To prevent bone loss and to maintain vitamin D status, especially in those who engage in minimal outdoor activity, adults 51 to 70 years old need 15 micrograms daily and those 71 and older need 20 micrograms.[52] Supplements may be needed to achieve adequate levels of vitamin D.

Vitamin B$_{12}$ The DRI committee recommends that adults aged 51 years and older obtain 2.4 micrograms of vitamin B$_{12}$ daily *and* that vitamin B$_{12}$–fortified foods (such as fortified cereals) or supplements be used to meet much of the DRI recommended intake.[53] The committee's recommendation reflects the finding that many older adults lose the ability to produce enough stomach acid to make the protein-bound form of vitamin B_{12} available for absorption. Synthetic vitamin B_{12} is reliably absorbed, however. Given the poor cognition, anemia, and other devastating neurological effects associated with a vitamin B_{12} deficiency, an adequate intake is imperative.

One cause of the malabsorption of protein-bound vitamin B_{12} is a condition known as **atrophic gastritis.** An estimated 10 to 30 percent of adults older than 50 have atrophic gastritis.

Folate As is true of vitamin B_{12}, folate intakes of older adults typically fall short of recommendations. The elderly are also more likely to have medical conditions or to take medications that can compromise folate status.

Iron Among the minerals, iron deserves first mention. Iron-deficiency anemia is less common in older adults than in younger people, but it still occurs in some, especially in those with low food energy intakes. Aside from diet, other factors in many older people's lives make iron deficiency likely: chronic blood loss from disease conditions and medicines, and poor iron absorption due to reduced secretion of stomach acid and antacid use. Anyone concerned with older people's nutrition should keep these possibilities in mind.

Zinc Zinc intake is commonly low in older people. Zinc deficiency can depress the appetite and blunt the sense of taste, thereby leading to low food intakes and worsening of zinc status. Zinc deficiency may also increase the likelihood of infectious diseases such as pneumonia.[54] Many medications that older adults commonly use can impair zinc absorption or enhance its excretion and thus lead to deficiency.

Calcium The importance of abundant dietary calcium throughout life to protect against osteoporosis has been emphasized throughout this book. The calcium intakes of many people, especially women, in the United States are well below the recommendations. If milk causes stomach discomfort, as many older adults report, then lactose-modified milk or other calcium-rich foods should take its place.

Nutrient Supplements for Older Adults

People judge for themselves how to manage their nutrition, and many older adults turn to dietary supplements. Advertisers target older people with appeals to take supplements and eat "health" foods, claiming that these products prevent disease and promote longevity. Quite often those who take supplements are not deficient in the nutrients being supplemented.

Elderly people often benefit from a balanced low-dose vitamin and mineral supplement, however.[55] Such supplements supply many of the needed minerals along with the vitamins often lacking in older people's diets without providing too much of any one nutrient.

Nonetheless, food is still the best source of nutrients for everybody. Supplements are just that—supplements to foods, not substitutes for them. For anyone who is motivated to obtain the best possible health, it is never too late to learn to eat well, become physically active, and adopt other lifestyle changes such as quitting smoking and moderating alcohol use. Table 13-5 (on p. 376) summarizes the nutrient concerns of aging. Table 13-6 (on p. 376) offers strategies for growing old healthfully.

The Effects of Drugs on Nutrients

As people grow older, the use of medicines—from over-the-counter drugs such as aspirin and laxatives to prescription medications of all kinds—becomes commonplace. Most drugs interact with one or more nutrients in several ways, usually resulting in greater-than-normal needs for these nutrients. Chapter 15 offers a discussion of diet-drug interactions and describes the many reasons why elderly people are vulnerable to such interactions.

atrophic gastritis (a-TRO-fik gas-TRI-tis): a condition characterized by chronic inflammation of the stomach accompanied by a diminished size and functioning of the mucosa and glands.

TABLE 13-5 Summary of Nutrient Concerns of Aging

Nutrient	Effect of Aging	Comments
Water	Lack of thirst and decreased total body water make dehydration likely.	Mild dehydration is a common cause of confusion. Difficulty obtaining water or getting to the bathroom may compound the problem.
Energy	Need decreases as muscle mass decreases (sarcopenia).	Physical activity moderates the decline.
Fiber	Likelihood of constipation increases with low intakes and changes in the GI tract.	Inadequate water intakes and lack of physical activity, along with some medications, compound the problem.
Protein	Needs may stay the same or increase slightly.	Low-fat milk and other high-quality protein foods are appropriate. Low-fat, high-fiber legumes and grains meet both protein and other nutrient needs.
Vitamin B_{12}	Atrophic gastritis is common.	Deficiency causes neurological damage; supplements may be needed.
Vitamin D	Increased likelihood of inadequate intake; skin synthesis declines.	Daily sunlight exposure in moderation or supplements may be beneficial.
Calcium	Intakes may be low; osteoporosis is common.	Stomach discomfort commonly limits milk intake; calcium substitutes or supplements may be needed.
Iron	In women, status improves after menopause; deficiencies are linked to chronic blood losses and low stomach acid output.	Adequate stomach acid is required for absorption; antacid or other medicine use may aggravate iron deficiency; vitamin C and meat increase absorption.
Zinc	Intakes are often inadequate and absorption may be poor, but needs may also increase.	Medications interfere with absorption; deficiency may depress appetite and sense of taste.

© 2016 Cengage Learning®

TABLE 13-6 Strategies for Growing Old Healthfully

- Choose nutrient-dense foods.

- Be physically active. Walk, run, dance, swim, bike, or row for aerobic activity. Lift weights, do calisthenics, or pursue some other activity to tone, firm, and strengthen muscles. Practice balancing on one foot or doing simple movements with your eyes closed. Modify activities to suit changing abilities and preferences.

- Maintain appropriate body weight.

- Reduce stress—cultivate self-esteem, maintain a positive attitude, manage time wisely, know your limits, practice assertiveness, release tension, and take action.

- For women, discuss with a physician the risks and benefits of estrogen replacement therapy.

- For people who smoke, discuss with a physician strategies and programs to help you quit.

- Expect to enjoy sex, and learn new ways of enhancing it.

- Use alcohol only moderately, if at all; use drugs only as prescribed.

- Take care to prevent accidents.

- Expect good vision and hearing throughout life; obtain glasses and hearing aids if necessary.

- Take care of your teeth; obtain dentures if necessary.

- Be alert to confusion as a disease symptom, and seek diagnosis.

- Take medications as prescribed; see a physician before self-prescribing medicines or herbal remedies and a registered dietitian nutritionist before self-prescribing supplements.

- Control depression through activities and friendships; seek professional help if necessary.

- Drink six to eight glasses of water every day.

- Practice mental skills. Keep solving math problems and crossword puzzles, playing cards or other games, reading, writing, imagining, and creating.

- Make financial plans early to ensure security.

- Accept change. Work at recovering from losses; make new friends.

- Cultivate spiritual health. Cherish personal values. Make life meaningful.

- Go outside for sunshine and fresh air as often as possible.

- Be socially active—play bridge, join an exercise or dance group, take a class, teach a class, eat with friends, or volunteer time to help others.

- Stay interested in life—pursue a hobby, spend time with grandchildren, take a trip, read, grow a garden, or go to the movies.

- Enjoy life.

© 2016 Cengage Learning®

The most common drug that can affect nutrition in older people is alcohol. The effects of alcohol on people of all ages are explained in Nutrition in Practice 20.

IN SUMMARY

▌ Aging significantly affects nutrient needs and intakes, as summarized in Table 13-5.

▌ Elderly people often benefit from a balanced low-dose vitamin and mineral supplement. Food is still the best source of nutrients, however.

13.4 Food Choices and Eating Habits of Older Adults

LO 13.4 Discuss factors that influence adults' food choices and instruct an adult on how to seek food assistance if needed, shop for groceries, and prepare healthy meals for one person on a limited budget.

To provide any benefit, strategies and interventions to improve a person's nutrition status must be based on knowledge of food preferences and eating patterns. Menus and feeding programs for older adults must take into consideration not only the food likes and dislikes but also the living conditions, economic status, and medical conditions of this diverse group of people. If nutrition intervention is to be successful, it is essential to know what foods people will eat, in what settings they like to eat these foods, and whether they can buy and prepare meals.

Older people are, for the most part, independent, socially sophisticated, mentally lucid, fully participating members of society who report themselves to be happy and healthy. In fact, chronic disabilities among the elderly have declined dramatically in recent years. Older people spend more money per person on foods to eat at home than other age groups and less money on foods eaten away from home. Manufacturers would be wise to cater to the preferences of older adults by providing good-tasting, nutritious foods in easy-to-open, single-serving packages with labels that are easy to read. Such products enable older adults to maintain their independence; most of them want to take care of themselves and need to feel a sense of control and involvement in their own lives. As discussed earlier, another way older adults can take care of themselves is by remaining or becoming physically active. Physical activity helps preserve one's ability to perform daily tasks and so promotes independence.

Individual Preferences

Familiarity, taste, and health beliefs are most influential on older people's food choices. Eating foods that are familiar, especially ethnic foods that recall family meals and pleasant times, can be comforting. Older adults are choosing poultry and fish, low-fat milk and milk products, and high-fiber breads and grains, indicating that they recognize the importance of diet in supporting good health. Few older adults, however, consume the recommended amounts of milk products.

Meal Setting

The food choices and eating habits of older adults are also affected by the changes in lifestyle that often accompany aging in this society. Whether people live alone, with others, or in institutions affects the way they eat. For example, men living alone are most likely to be poorly nourished. Older adults who live alone do not make poorer food choices than those who live with companions; rather, they consume too little food: loneliness is directly related to inadequacies, especially of energy intakes.

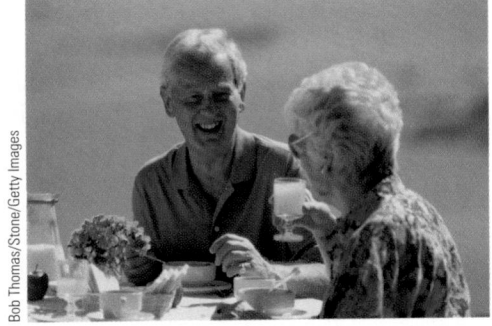

Shared meals can brighten the day and enhance the appetite.

Case Study BOX 13-1 ELDERLY MAN WITH A POOR DIET

Mr. Brezenoff is 75 years old and lives alone. He has slowly been losing weight since his wife died a year ago. At 5 feet 8 inches tall, he currently weighs 124 pounds. His previous weight was 150 pounds. In talking with Mr. Brezenoff, you realize that he doesn't even like to talk about food, let alone eat it. "My wife always did the cooking before, and I ate well. Now I just don't feel like eating." You manage to find out that he skips breakfast, has soup and bread for lunch, and sometimes eats a cold-cut sandwich or a frozen dinner for supper. He seldom sees friends or relatives. Mr. Brezenoff has also lost several teeth and doesn't eat any raw fruits or vegetables because he finds them hard to chew. He lives on a meager but adequate income.

1. Consult the BMI table (inside back cover), and judge whether Mr. Brezenoff is at a healthy weight. What other assessments might you use to back up your judgment? Is his weight loss significant?

2. What factors are contributing to Mr. Brezenoff's poor food intake? What nutrients are probably deficient in his diet?

3. Look at Mr. Brezenoff as an individual and suggest ways he can improve his diet and his lifestyle.

4. What other aspects of Mr. Brezenoff's physical and mental health should you consider in helping him improve his food intake?

TABLE 13-7 Risk Factors for Malnutrition in Older Adults

These questions help *determine* the risk of malnutrition in older adults:

- Disease: Do you have an illness or condition that changes the types or amounts of foods you eat?
- Eating poorly: Do you eat fewer than two meals a day? Do you eat fruits, vegetables, and milk products daily?
- Tooth loss or mouth pain: Is it difficult or painful to eat?
- Economic hardship: Do you have enough money to buy the food you need?
- Reduced social contact: Do you eat alone most of the time?
- Multiple medications: Do you take three or more different prescribed or over-the-counter medications daily?
- Involuntary weight loss or gain: Have you lost or gained 10 pounds or more in the last 6 months?
- Needs assistance: Are you physically able to shop, cook, and feed yourself?
- Elderly person: Are you older than 80?

Depression

Another factor affecting food intake and appetite in older people is depression. Loss of appetite and motivation to cook or even to eat frequently accompanies depression. An overwhelming feeling of grief and sadness at the death of a spouse, friend, or family member may leave many people, particularly elderly people, with a feeling of powerlessness to overcome the depression. The support and companionship of family and friends, especially at mealtimes, can help overcome depression and enhance appetite. The case study in Box 13-1 presents a man who has several of these problems. Use the suggestions here, and in the last section of this chapter, to help develop solutions. The Nutrition Assessment Checklist for Older Adults at the end of this chapter helps to pinpoint nutrition-related factors to look for when working with older adults. To *determine* the risk of malnutrition in older clients, health care providers can keep in mind the characteristics listed in Table 13-7.

Food Assistance Programs

Federally funded programs can provide food and nutrition services for older adults.[56] The Older Americans Act (OAA) provides many different support services to help older adults remain healthy and independent. An integral component of the OAA is the OAA Nutrition Program. Table 13-8 summarizes this and other food assistance programs available to the elderly.

Meals for Singles

Many older adults live alone, and singles of all ages face challenges in purchasing, storing, and preparing food. Large packages of meat and vegetables are often intended for families of four or more, and even a head of lettuce can spoil before one person can use it all. Many singles live in small dwellings and have little storage space for foods. A limited income presents additional obstacles. This section offers suggestions that can help to solve some of the problems singles face.

Avoid Foodborne Illness The risk of foodborne illness is greater for older adults than for other adults. The consequences of an upset stomach, diarrhea, fever, vomiting, abdominal cramps, and dehydration are oftentimes more severe, sometimes leading to paralysis, meningitis, or even death. For these reasons, older adults need to carefully follow the food safety suggestions presented in Nutrition in Practice 5.

TABLE 13-8 Food Assistance Programs for Older Adults

OAA Nutrition Program
Services: Provides congregate and home-delivered meals to improve older people's nutrition status. Includes transportation to congregate meal sites; shopping assistance; information and referral; and, to some extent, nutrition counseling and education.
Impact: Improves the nutrient content of high-risk older adults' diets and offers socialization and recreation. Many of the nutrition programs around the country go above and beyond federal requirements of congregate and home meals by offering lunch clubs, ethnic meals, and meals for older homeless people.

Supplemental Nutrition Assistance Program (SNAP)
Services: Supplements income for low-income households by means of a card similar to a debit card that can be used to purchase food.
Impact: Serves more as an income supplement for some elderly participants than as a device to improve nutrition status. For other elderly participants, nutrient intakes are higher than those of nonparticipants with similar incomes.

Meals on Wheels
Services: Delivers meals directly to the homebound elderly; integrated into the meal delivery services provided by the OAA Program.
Impact: Focuses on filling the need for weekend and holiday meals for the homebound elderly people, a service that is limited in the OAA Nutrition Program.

Senior Farmers Market Nutrition Program
Services: Provides low-income older adults with coupons that can be exchanged for fresh fruits, vegetables, and herbs at community-supported farmers' markets and roadside stands; administered by the USDA. State agencies may limit sales to specific foods that are locally grown to encourage recipients to support farmers in their own states.
Impact: Increases fresh fruit and vegetable consumption, provides nutrition information, and even reaches the homebound elderly, a group of people who normally do not have access to farmers' markets.

Spend Wisely People who have the means to shop and cook for themselves can cut their food bills just by being wise shoppers. Large supermarkets are usually less expensive than convenience stores. A grocery list helps reduce impulse buying, and specials and coupons can save money when the items featured are those that the shopper needs and uses.

Buying the right amount so as not to waste any food is a challenge for people eating alone. Fresh milk should be purchased in the size best suited for personal needs. Pint-size and even cup-size boxes of milk that can be stored unopened on a shelf for up to 3 months without refrigeration are available.*

Many foods that offer a variety of nutrients for practically pennies have a long shelf life; staples such as rice, pastas, dry powdered milk, and dried legumes can be purchased in bulk and stored for months at room temperature. Other foods that are usually a good buy include whole pieces of cheese rather than sliced or shredded cheese, fresh produce in season, variety meats such as chicken livers, and cereals that require cooking instead of ready-to-serve cereals.

A person who has ample freezing space can buy large packages of meat, such as pork chops, ground beef, or chicken, when they are on sale. Then the meat can be immediately wrapped in individual servings for the freezer. All the individual servings can be put in a bag marked appropriately with the contents and the date. Alternatively, grocers will break open a package of wrapped meat and rewrap the portion needed. Similarly, eggs can be purchased by the half-dozen. Eggs do keep for long periods, though, if stored properly in the refrigerator.

Frozen vegetables are more economical in large bags than in small boxes. The amount needed can be taken out, and the bag closed tightly with a twist tie or rubber band. If the package is returned quickly to the freezer each time, the vegetables will stay fresh for a long time. Fresh fruits and vegetables can be purchased individually. A person can buy fresh fruit at various stages of ripeness: a ripe one to eat right away, a semiripe one to eat soon after, and a green one to ripen on the windowsill.

*Boxes of milk that can be stored at room temperature have been exposed to temperatures above those of pasteurization just long enough to sterilize the milk—a process called *ultrahigh temperature (UHT)*.

If vegetables are packaged in large quantities, the grocer can break open the package so that a smaller amount can be purchased. Small cans of fruits and vegetables, even though they are more expensive per unit, are a reasonable alternative, considering that it is expensive to buy a regular-size can and let the unused portion spoil.

Finally, breads and cereals usually must be purchased in larger quantities. Again the amount needed for a few days can be taken out and the rest stored in the freezer.

Be Creative Creative chefs think of various ways to use foods when only large amounts are available. For example, a head of cauliflower can be divided into thirds. Then one-third is cooked and eaten hot, another third is put into a vinegar and oil marinade for use in a salad, and the last third can be used in a casserole or stew.

A variety of vegetables and meats can be enjoyed stir-fried; inexpensive vegetables such as cabbage, celery, and onion are delicious when crisp cooked in a little oil with herbs or lemon added. Interesting frozen vegetable mixtures are available in larger grocery stores. Cooked, leftover vegetables can be dropped in at the last minute. A bonus of a stir-fried meal is that there is only one pan to wash. Similarly, a microwave oven allows a home chef to use fewer pots and pans. Meals and leftovers can also be frozen or refrigerated in microwavable containers to re-heat as needed.

Many frozen dinners or grocery store take-out foods offer nutritious options. Adding a fresh salad, a whole-wheat roll, and a glass of milk can make a nutritionally balanced meal. Box 13-2 offers time-saving tips to turn convenience foods into nutritious meals.

Also, single people shouldn't hesitate to invite someone to share meals with them whenever there is enough food. It's likely that the person will return the invitation, and both parties will get to enjoy companionship and a meal prepared by others.

How To   BOX 13-2 TURN CONVENIENCE FOODS INTO NUTRITIOUS MEALS

These time-saving tips can turn convenience foods into nutritious meals:

- Add extra nutrients and a fresh flavor to canned stews and soups by tossing in some frozen ready-to-use mixed vegetables. Choose vegetables frozen without salty, fatty sauces—prepared foods generally contain enough salt to season the whole dish, including added vegetables.

- Buy frozen vegetables in a bag, toss in a variety of herbs, and use as needed.

- When grilling burgers or chicken, wrap a mixture of frozen broccoli, onion, and carrots in a foil packet with a tablespoon of Italian dressing and grill alongside the meat for seasoned grilled vegetables.

- Use fruits canned in their own juices as desserts. Toss in some frozen berries or peach slices and top with flavored yogurt for an instant fruit salad.

- Prepared rice or noodle dishes are convenient, but those claiming to contain broccoli, spinach, or other vegetables seldom contain enough to qualify as a serving of vegetables. Pump up the nutrient value by adding a half-cup of frozen vegetables per serving of pasta or rice just before cooking.

- Purchase frozen onion, mushroom, and pepper mixtures to embellish jarred spaghetti sauce or small frozen pizzas. Top with parmesan cheese.

- Use frozen shredded potatoes, sold for hash browns, in soups or stews or mix with a handful of shredded reduced-fat cheese or a can of fat-free "cream of anything" soup and bake for a quick and hearty casserole.

- Purchase a bag of triple-washed, ready-to-eat salad and add any or all of the following to make a hearty, healthy salad: a small can of garbanzo beans or a package of frozen edamame (immature soy beans); a handful of shredded reduced-fat cheese; a hard-boiled egg; a handful of toasted almonds or other nuts.

- Open a can of pinto beans or black beans, heat a tablespoon of olive oil, and sauté a little bit of frozen onion and pepper mixture. Add the beans and mash them in the oil and vegetables. Serve the bean mixture in a soft taco shell with shredded reduced-fat cheese, lettuce, and salsa for a tasty, nutritious bean taco.

- Food choices of older adults are affected by health status and changed life circumstances.

- Older people can benefit from both the nutrients provided and the social interaction available at congregate meals. Other government programs deliver meals to those who are homebound.

- With creativity and careful shopping, those living alone can prepare nutritious, inexpensive meals.

Nutrition Assessment Checklist FOR OLDER ADULTS

Medical History

Check the medical record for:

- Alcohol abuse
- Alzheimer's disease or other dementia or confusion
- Arthritis
- Cataracts
- Chronic diseases (cancer, heart disease, hypertension, diabetes)
- Cigarette, cigar, or pipe smoking; use of other tobacco products
- Constipation
- Dehydration
- Dental disease or tooth loss
- Depression
- Inflammation of the stomach (gastritis)
- Swallowing disorders

Medications

For older adults being treated with drug therapy for medical conditions, note:

- Use of multiple medications—prescription and/or over-the-counter medications, such as laxatives and pain relievers
- Side effects that might reduce food intake or change nutrient needs
- Proper administration of medication with respect to food intake
- Malnutrition—is the person's nutrition status questionable even before considering side effects of medications that worsen nutrition status?
- Diminished mental capacity that might interfere with taking correct medications and doses
- Dehydration (can alter effects of medications)

Dietary Intake

For all older adults, especially those at risk nutritionally, assess the diet for:

- Total energy
- Protein
- Calcium, iron, and zinc
- Vitamin B_6, vitamin B_{12}, folate, and vitamin D

Note the following:

- Number of meals eaten each day
- Number and ages of people in household
- Amount of milk consumed each day
- Type and frequency of outdoor activity
- Type and frequency of physical activity
- Financial resources
- Transportation resources
- Physical disabilities
- Mental alertness

Anthropometric Data

Measure baseline height and weight.

- Reassess height and weight at each medical checkup.
- Note significant overweight or underweight, which warrants intervention.
- Use skinfold measures to reveal altered body composition that may indicate malnutrition and loss of lean tissue.

Laboratory Tests

- Hemoglobin, hematocrit, or other tests of iron status
- Serum albumin or other measures of protein status
- Serum folate
- Serum B_{12}

Physical Signs

Look for physical signs of:

- Protein-energy malnutrition
- Iron and zinc deficiency
- Folate deficiency

Clinical Applications

1. Ms. Hamilton, an 80-year-old woman in excellent health, lives alone, eats a well-balanced diet, enjoys an active social life, and walks every day. Consider the way Ms. Hamilton's health and nutrition status might be affected by the following situations:

   ▮ Many of Ms. Hamilton's friends pass away or move into extended care facilities.

   ▮ Ms. Hamilton falls and breaks her hip.

   ▮ Ms. Hamilton begins to feel isolated and depressed.

   Describe interventions the health care professional can take to help Ms. Hamilton deal with each situation to prevent her from falling into a downward spiral.

Self Check

1. The fastest-growing age group in the United States is:
   a. under 21 years of age.
   b. 30 to 45 years of age.
   c. 50 to 70 years of age.
   d. over 85 years of age.

2. Which of the following lifestyle habits can enhance the length and quality of people's lives?
   a. Moderate smoking
   b. Six hours of sleep daily
   c. Regular physical activity
   d. Skipping breakfast

3. Which of the following is among the better-known relationships between nutrition and disease prevention?
   a. Appropriate fiber intake helps prevent goiter.
   b. Moderate sodium intake helps prevent obesity.
   c. Moderate sugar intake helps prevent hypertension.
   d. Appropriate energy intake helps prevent diabetes and cardiovascular disease.

4. A disease of the immune system that involves painful inflammation of the joints is:
   a. sarcopenia.
   b. osteoarthritis.
   c. senile dementia.
   d. rheumatoid arthritis.

5. Examples of low-kcalorie, high-quality protein foods include:
   a. cottage cheese, sour cream, and eggs.
   b. green and yellow vegetables and citrus fruits.
   c. potatoes, rice, pasta, and whole-grain breads.
   d. lean meats, poultry, fish, legumes, fat-free milk, and eggs.

6. For malnourished and underweight people, protein- and energy-dense snacks include:
   a. fresh fruits and vegetables.
   b. yogurt and cottage cheese.
   c. whole grains and high-fiber legumes.
   d. scrambled eggs and peanut butter on wheat toast.

7. Which of the following does *not* contribute to dehydration risk in older adults?
   a. They do not seem to feel thirsty.
   b. Total body water increases with age.
   c. They may find it difficult to get a drink.
   d. They may have difficulty swallowing liquids.

8. Inadequate milk intake and limited exposure to sunlight contribute to older adults' risk of:
   a. vitamin A deficiency.
   b. vitamin D deficiency.
   c. riboflavin deficiency.
   d. vitamin B_{12} deficiency.

9. Two risk factors for malnutrition in older adults are:
   a. loneliness and multiple medication use.
   b. increased energy needs and lack of fiber.
   c. decreased mineral absorption and antioxidant intake.
   d. high carbohydrate intake and lack of physical activity.

10. Strategies to improve nutrition status when growing old include:
    a. increasing vitamin A intake and exercising 30 minutes daily.
    b. choosing nutrient-dense foods and maintaining appropriate weight.
    c. avoiding high-fiber foods and taking a daily vitamin-mineral supplement.
    d. eating at least one big meal per day and drinking at least 10 glasses of water daily.

Answers to these questions appear in Appendix H.

Notes

1. Position of the Academy of Nutrition and Dietetics, Food and nutrition for older adults: Promoting health and wellness, *Journal of the Academy of Nutrition and Dietetics* 112 (2012): 1255–1277.

2. D. L. Hoyert and J. Xu, Deaths: Preliminary data for 2011, *National Vital Statistics Reports* 61 (2012): 1-51.

3. A. Fardet and Y. Boirie, Associations between diet-related diseases and impaired physiological mechanisms: A holistic approach based on meta-analysis to identify targets for preventive nutrition, *Nutrition Reviews* 71 (2013): 643–656; E. A. Finkelstein and coauthors, Individual and aggregate years-of-life-lost associated with overweight and obesity, *Obesity* 18 (2010): 333–339.

4. N. R. Eaton and coauthors, Genes, environments, personality, and successful aging: Toward a comprehensive developmental model in later life, *Journal of Gerontology* 67 (2012): 480–488.

5. Position of the Academy of Nutrition and Dietetics, 2012.

6. T. Ahmed and N. Haboubi, Assessment and management of nutrition in older people and its importance to health, *Clinical Interventions in Aging* 5 (2010): 207–216.

7. D. B. Panogiotakos and coauthors, Sociodemographic and lifestyle statistics of oldest old people (> 80 years) living in Ikaria island: The Ikaria Study, *Cardiology Research*, February 24, 2011, p. 679187; S. Sabia and coauthors, Influence of individual and combined healthy behaviours on successful aging, *Canadian Medical Association Journal* 184 (2012): 1985–1992; E. S. Ford and coauthors, Low-risk lifestyle behaviors and all-cause mortality: Findings from the National Health and Nutrition Examination Survey III Mortality Study, *American Journal of Public Health* 101 (2011): 1922–1929; A. L. Anderson and coauthors, Dietary patterns and survival of older adults, *Journal of the American Dietetic Association* 111 (2011): 84–91.

8. S. A. McNaughton, C. J. Bates, and G. D. Mishra, Diet quality is associated with all-cause mortality in adults aged 65 and older, *Journal of Nutrition* 142 (2012): 320–325; Anderson and coauthors, 2011.

9. L. Soares-Miranda and coauthors, Physical activity and heart rate variability in older adults: The cardiovascular health study, *Circulation* 129 (2014): 2100–2110; C. P. Wen and coauthors, Minimum amount of physical activity for reduced mortality and extended life expectancy: A prospective cohort study, *Lancet* 378 (2011): 1244–1253; S. W. Farrell and coauthors, Cardiorespiratory fitness, adiposity, and all-cause mortality in women, *Medicine and Science in Sports and Exercise* 42 (2010): 2006–2012; S. Q. Townsend and coauthors, Physical activity at midlife in relation to successful survival in women at age 70 years or older, *Archives of Internal Medicine* 170 (2010): 194–201.

10. W. J. Chodzko and coauthors, American College of Sports Medicine, Position stand: Exercise and physical activity for older adults, *Medicine and Science in Sports and Exercise* 41 (2009): 1510–1530.

11. S. Studenski and coauthors, Gait speed and survival in older adults, *Journal of the American Medical Association* 305 (2011): 50–58.

12. M. O. Melancon, D. Lorrain, and I. J. Dionne, Exercise increases tryptophan availability to the brain in older men age 57–70 years, *Medicine and Science in Sports and Exercise* 44 (2012): 881–887; J. C. Sieverdes and coauthors, Association between leisure time physical activity and depressive symptoms in men, *Medicine and Science in Sports and Exercise* 44 (2012): 260–265; G. F. Bertheussen and coauthors, Associations between physical activity and physical and mental health—A HUNT 3 Study, *Medicine and Science in Sports and Exercise* 43 (2011): 1220–1228; L. D. Baker and coauthors, Effects of aerobic exercise on mild cognitive impairment, *Archives of Neurology* 67 (2010): 71–79.

13. L. Krist, F. Dimeo, and T. Keil, Can progressive resistance training twice a week improve mobility, muscle strength, and quality of life in very elderly nursing-home residents with impaired mobility? A pilot study, *Clinical Interventions in Aging* 8 (2013): 443–448.

14. H. W. Park, Longevity, aging, and caloric restriction: Clive Main McCay and the construction of a multidisciplinary research program, *Historical Studies in the Natural Sciences* 40 (2010): 79–124.

15. R. Pallavi, M. Giogio, and P. G. Pelicci, Insights into the beneficial effect of caloric/dietary restriction for healthy and prolonged life, *Frontiers in Physiology* 3 (2012): 318.

16. L. M. Redman and E. Ravussin, Caloric restriction in humans: Impact on physiological, psychological, and behavioral outcomes, *Antioxidants and Redox Signaling* 14 (2011): 275–287.

17. C. Samieri and coauthors, The association between dietary patterns at midlife and health in aging: An observational study, *Annals of Internal Medicine* 159 (2013): 584–591; F. Sofi and coauthors, Accruing evidence on benefits of adherence to the Mediterranean diet on health: An updated systematic review and meta-analysis, *American Journal of Clinical Nutrition* 92 (2010): 1189–1196.

18. M. C. Mathew and coauthors, Antioxidant vitamin supplementation for preventing and slowing the progression of age-related cataract, *Cochrane Database of Systematic Reviews* 6 (2012): CD004567.

19. K. A. Weikel and coauthors, Nutritional modulation of cataract, *Nutrition Reviews* 72 (2014): 30–47; Y. Chi, C. Jing, and H. Pan, Association of blood antioxidants and vitamins with risk of age-related cataract: A meta-analysis of observational studies, *American Journal of Clinical Nutrition* 98 (2013): 778–786.

20. J. A. Mares and coauthors, Healthy diets and the subsequent prevalence of nuclear cataract in women, *Archives of Ophthalmology* 128 (2010): 738–749.

21. C. W. Pan and Y. Lin, Overweight, obesity, and age-related cataract: A meta-analysis, *Optometry and Vison Science* 91 (2014): 478–483; J. Ye and coauthors, Body mass index and risk of age-related cataract: A meta-analysis of prospective cohort studies, *PLoS One* 9 (2014): e89923.

22. B. Gopinath and coauthors, Homocysteine, folate, vitamin B-12, and 10–y incidence of age-related macular degeneration, *American Journal of Clinical Nutrition* 98 (2013): 129–135; The Age-Related Eye Disease Study 2 (AREDS2) Research Group, Lutein + zeaxanthin and omega-3 fatty acids for age-related macular degeneration, *Journal of the American Medical Association* 309 (2013): 2005–2015; L. Ma and coauthors, Lutein and zeaxanthin intake and the risk of age-related macular degeneration: A systematic review and meta-analysis, *British Journal of Nutrition* 107 (2012): 350–359; J. R. Evans and J. G. Lawrenson, Antioxidant vitamin and mineral supplements for preventing age-related macular degeneration, *Cochrane Database of Systematic Reviews* 6 (2012): CD000253; J. P. SanGiovanni and M. Neuringer, The putative role of lutein and zeaxanthin as protective agents against age-related macular degeneration: Promise of molecular genetics for guiding mechanistic and translational research in the field, *American Journal of Clinical Nutrition* 96 (2012): 1223S-1233S; E. J. Johnson, Age-related macular degeneration and antioxidant vitamins: Recent findings, Current Opinion in *Clinical Nutrition and Metabolic Care* 13 (2010): 28–33.

23. K. E. Barbour and coauthors, Prevalence of doctor-diagnosed arthritis and arthritis-attributable activity limitation: United States, 2010–2012, *Morbidity and Mortality Weekly Report* 62 (2013): 869–873.

24. Prevalence of obesity among adults with arthritis—United States, 2003–2009, *Morbidity and Mortality Weekly Report* 60 (2011): 509–513.

25. E. M. Ross and C. B. Juhl, Osteoarthritis 2012 year in review: Rehabilitation and outcomes, *Osteoarthritis Cartilage* 20 (2012): 1477–1483; K. R. Vincent and H. K. Vincent, Resistance exercise for knee osteoarthritis, *PM & R* 4 (2012): S45–S52; K. L. Bennell and R. S. Hinman, A review of the clinical evidence for exercise in osteoarthritis of the hip and knee, *Journal of Science and Medicine in Sport* 14 (2011): 4–9.

26. M. Fransen and coauthors, Glucosamine and chondroitin for knee osteoarthritis: A double-blind randomized placebo-controlled clinical trial evaluating single and combination regimens, *Annals of the Rheumatic Diseases*, January 6, 2014, doi: 10.1136/annrheumdis-2013-203954, epub ahead of print; R. L. Ragle and A. D. Sawitzke, Nutraceuticals in the management of osteoarthritis: A critical review, *Drugs and Aging* 29 (2012): 17–31; N. Burdett and J. D. McNeil, Difficulties with assessing the benefit of glucosamine sulphate as treatment for osteoarthritis, *International Journal of Evidence Based Healthcare*, 10 (2012): 222–226.

27. G. Smedslund and coauthors, Effectiveness and safety of dietary interventions for rheumatoid arthritis: A systematic review of randomized controlled trials, *Journal of the American Dietetic Association* 110 (2010): 727–735.

28. M. D. Hurd and coauthors, Monetary costs of dementia in the United States, *New England Journal of Medicine* 368 (2013): 1326–1334.

29. J. G. Walker and coauthors, Oral folic acid and vitamin B-12 supplementation to prevent cognitive decline in community-dwelling older adults with depressive symptoms—the Beyond Ageing Project: A randomized controlled trial, *American Journal of Clinical Nutrition* 95 (2012): 194–203; D. Smith and coauthors, Homocysteine-lowering by B vitamins slows the rate of accelerated brain atrophy in mild cognitive impairment: A randomized controlled trial, *PLoS One* 5 (2010): e12244; J. Selhub, A. Troen, and I. H. Rosenberg, B vitamins and the aging brain, *Nutrition Reviews* 68 (2010): S60–S64.

30. N. G. Bazan, M. F. Molina, and W. C. Gordon, Docosahexaenoic acid signalolipidomics in nutrition: Significance in aging, neuroinflammation, macular degeneration, Alzheimer's and other neurodegenerative diseases, *Annual Review of Nutrition* 31 (2011): 321–351.

31. Walker and coauthors, 2012; Bazan, Molina, and Gordon, 2011.

32. Centers for Disease Control and Prevention, Alzheimer's disease, www.cdc.gov/aging/aginginfo /alzheimers.htm, updated February 23, 2011.

33. H. W. Querfurth and F. M. LaFeria, Mechanisms of disease: Alzheimer's disease, *New England Journal of Medicine* 362 (2010): 329–344.

34. Querfurth and LaFeria, 2010.

35. F. E. Harrison, A critical review of vitamin C for the prevention of age-related decline and Alzheimer's disease, *Journal of Alzheimer's Disease* 29 (2012): 11–26; J. Viña and coauthors, Antioxidant pathways in Alzheimer's disease: Possibilities of intervention, *Current Pharmaceutical Design* 17 (2011): 3861–3864.

36. B. Misiak, J. Leszek, and A. Kiejna, Metabolic syndrome, mild cognitive impairment and Alzheimer's disease—The emerging role of systemic low-grade inflammation and adiposity, *Brain Research Bulletin* 89 (2012): 144–149.

37. V. J. DePaula and coauthors, Alzheimer's disease, *Sub-cellular Biochemistry* 65 (2012): 329–352.

38. P. K. Crane and coauthors, Glucose levels and risk of dementia, *New England Journal of Medicine* 369 (2013): 540–548; D. E. Barnes and K. Yaffe, The projected effect of risk factor reduction on Alzheimer's disease prevalence, *Lancet Neurology* 10 (2011): 819–828; S. M. De La Monte,

Metabolic derangements mediate cognitive impairment and Alzheimer's disease: Role of peripheral insulin-resistance diseases, *Panminerva Medica* 54 (2012): 171–178; Misiak, Leszek, and Kiejan, 2012; J. D. Doecke and coauthors, Blood-based protein biomarkers for diagnosis of Alzheimer Disease, *Archives of Neurology* 69 (2012): 1318–1325.

39. I. Lourida and coauthors, Mediterranean diet, cognitive function, and dementia: A systematic review *Epidemiology* 24 (2013): 479–489; G. M. Cole and S. A. Frautschy, DHA may prevent age-related dementia, *Journal of Nutrition* 140 (2010): 869–874; Y. Gu and coauthors, Food combination and Alzheimer disease risk: A protective diet, *Archives of Neurology* 67 (2010): 699–706.

40. L. E. Middleton and coauthors, Activity energy expenditure and incident cognitive impairment in older adults, *Archives of Internal Medicine* 171 (2011): 1251–1257.

41. Position of the Academy of Nutrition and Dietetics, 2012.

42. L. A. Burton and D. Sumukadas, Optimal management of sarcopenia, *Clinical Interventions in Aging* 5 (2010): 217–228.

43. Position of the Academy of Nutrition and Dietetics, 2012; J. Cohen-Mansfield and R. Perach, Is there a reversal in the effect of obesity on mortality in old age? *Journal of Aging Research* 2011 (2011): 765071; D. K. Childers and D. B. Allison, The "obesity paradox": A parsimonious explanation for relations among obesity, mortality rate and aging? *International Journal of Obesity* 34 (2010): 1231–1238.

44. N. Napoli and coauthors, Effect of weight loss, exercise, or both on cognition and quality of life in obese older adults, *American Journal of Clinical Nutrition* 100 (2014): 189–198; Position of the Academy of Nutrition and Dietetics, 2012; L. M. Donini and coauthors, A systematic review of the literature concerning the relationship between obesity and mortality in the elderly, *Journal of Nutrition, Health & Aging* 16 (2012): 89–98.

45. J. E. Morley and coauthors, Nutritional recommendations for the management of sarcopenia, *Journal of the American Medical Directors Association* 11 (2010): 391–396; A. K. Surdykowski and coauthors, Optimizing bone

health in older adults: The importance of dietary protein, *Aging Health* 6 (2010): 345–357.

46. J. Slavin, Fiber and prebiotics: Mechanisms and health benefits, *Nutrients* 5 (2013): 1417–1435.

47. Position of the Academy of Nutrition and Dietetics, 2012.

48. D. E. King, A. G. Mainous III, and C. A. Lambourne, Trends in dietary fiber intake in the United states, 1999–2008, *Journal of the Academy of Nutrition and Dietetics* 112 (2012): 642–648.

49. Position of the Academy of Nutrition and Dietetics, 2012.

50. Position of the Academy of Nutrition and Dietetics, 2012; Standing Committee on the Scientific Evaluation of Dietary Reference Intakes, Food and Nutrition Board, Institute of Medicine, *Dietary Reference Intakes for Water, Potassium, Sodium, Chloride, and Sulfate* (Washington, DC: National Academies Press, 2005), pp. 118–127.

51. Standing Committee on the Scientific Evaluation of Dietary Reference Intakes, *Dietary Reference Intakes for Water, Potassium, Sodium, Chloride, and Sulfate,* 2005, pp. 149–150.

52. Committee on Dietary Reference Intakes, *Dietary Reference Intakes for Calcium and Vitamin D* (Washington, DC: National Academies Press, 2011), pp. 345–402.

53. Committee on Dietary Reference Intakes, *Dietary Reference Intakes for Thiamin, Riboflavin, Niacin, Vitamin B6, Folate, Vitamin B12, Pantothenic Acid, Biotin, and Choline* (Washington, DC: National Academies Press, 2000), p. 338.

54. J. B. Barnett, D. H. Hamer, and S. N. Meydani, Low zinc status: A new risk factor for pneumonia in the elderly? *Nutrition Reviews* 68 (2010): 30–37.

55. Position of the Academy of Nutrition and Dietetics, 2012.

56. Position of the Academy of Nutrition and Dietetics, 2012; Position of the American Dietetic Association, American Society for Nutrition, and Society for Nutrition Education: Food and nutrition programs for community-residing older adults, *Journal of the American Dietetic Association* 110 (2010): 463–472

LO 13.5 Identify some reasons why hunger is present in a country as wealthy as the United States and describe the resources available to those in need.

Worldwide, one person in every eight experiences persistent hunger—not the healthy appetite triggered by anticipation of a hearty meal but the painful sensation caused by a lack of food.[1] Hunger deprives a person of the physical and mental energy needed to enjoy a full life and often leads to severe malnutrition and death. In 2011, more than 2 million children younger than the age of 5 died as a result of hunger and malnutrition.[2]

In the United States, where most people enjoy a life of relative abundance, 6.8 million households live with **very low food security**—one or more members of these households, many of them children, repeatedly had little or nothing to eat because of a lack of money.[3] Another 11 million households experience **low food security** or **marginal food security,** somewhat less dire conditions. Given the agricultural bounty and enormous wealth in this country, do these numbers surprise you? The limited or uncertain availability of nutritionally adequate and safe foods is known as **food insecurity** and is a major social problem in our nation

today.[4] Table NP13-1 presents questions used in national surveys to identify food insecurity in the United States, and Figure NP13-1 (on p. 386) presents the most recent findings. Surveys like these provide crude, but necessary, data to estimate the degree of hunger in this country. Box NP13-1 (on p. 386) defines related terms.

Why is hunger a problem in developed countries such as the United States where food is abundant?

Hunger has many causes, but in developed countries, the primary cause is **food poverty**. People are hungry not because there is no food available nearby, but because they lack sufficient money with which to buy nutritious food and pay for other necessities, such as housing, clothing, medicines, and utilities. An estimated 15 percent of the population of the United States lives in poverty.[5] Even those above the poverty line may not have **food security.** Physical and mental illnesses and disabilities, sudden job losses, and high living expenses threaten their financial stability. Further contributing to food poverty are other problems such as abuse of alcohol and other drugs; lack of awareness of food assistance programs; and the reluctance of people, particularly the elderly, to accept what they perceive as "welfare" or "charity." Lack of financial resources remains

---

TABLE NP13-1 Questions to Identify Food Insecurity in a U.S. Household

To determine the extent of food insecurity in a household, surveys ask questions about behaviors and conditions known to characterize households having difficulty meeting basic food needs during the past 12 months. Most often, adults tend to protect their children from hunger. In the most severe cases, children also suffer from hunger and eat less.

1. Did you worry whether food would run out before you got money to buy more?
2. Did you find that the food you bought just didn't last and you didn't have money to buy more?
3. Were you unable to afford to eat balanced meals?
4. Did you or other adults in your household ever cut the size of your meals or skip meals because there wasn't enough food?
5. Did this happen in 3 or more months during the previous year?
6. Did you ever eat less than you should because there wasn't enough money for food?

7. Were you ever hungry but didn't eat because you couldn't afford enough food?
8. Did you lose weight because you didn't have enough money to buy food?
9. Did you or other adults in your household ever not eat for a whole day because you were running out of money to buy food?
10. Did this happen in 3 or more months during the previous year?
11. Did you rely on only a few kinds of low-cost food to feed your children because you were running out of money to buy food?
12. Were you unable to feed your children a balanced meal because you couldn't afford it?
13. Were your children not eating enough because you just couldn't afford enough food?
14. Did you ever cut the size of your children's meals because there wasn't enough money for food?
15. Were your children ever hungry but you just couldn't afford more food?

16. Did your children ever skip a meal because there wasn't enough money for food?
17. Did this happen in 3 or more months during the previous year?
18. Did your children ever not eat for a whole day because there wasn't enough money for food?

The more positive responses, the greater the food insecurity. Households with children answer all of the questions and are categorized as follows:

- ≤2 positive responses = food secure
- 3–7 positive responses = low food security
- ≥8 positive responses = very low food security

Households without children answer the first 10 questions and are categorized as follows:

- ≤2 positive responses = food secure
- 3–5 positive responses = low food security
- ≥6 positive responses = very low food security

Figure NP13-1 shows the results of the 2012 surveys.

Source: U.S. Department of Agriculture, *Food Security in the U.S.,* www.ars.gov, updated August 19, 2013.

FIGURE NP13-1 **Prevalence of Food Security of U.S. Households**

Source: A. Coleman-Jensen, M. Nord, and A. Singh, *Household Food Security in the United States in 2012*, Economic Research Service, U.S. Department of Agriculture, www.ers.usda.gov, September 2013.

Very low food security (5.7%)

Low food security (8.8%)

Food secure (85.5%)

U.S. Department of Agriculture

BOX NP13-1 GLOSSARY

emergency kitchens: programs that provide meals to be eaten on-site; often called *soup kitchens*.

food banks: facilities that collect and distribute food donations to authorized organizations feeding the hungry.

food deserts: urban and rural low-income areas with limited access to affordable and nutritious foods (also defined in Chapter 7).

food insecurity: limited or uncertain access to foods of sufficient quality or quantity to sustain a healthy and active life. Food insecurity categories include:

▌ *low food security:* reduced dietary quality, variety, or desirability but with little or no indication of reduced food intake; formerly known as *food insecurity without hunger.*

▌ *very low food security:* multiple indications of disrupted eating patterns and reduced food intake; formerly known as *food insecurity with hunger.*

food pantries: community food collection programs that provide groceries to be prepared and eaten at home.

food poverty: hunger occurring when enough food exists in an area but some of the people cannot obtain it because they lack money, are being deprived for political reasons, live in a country at war, or suffer from other problems such as lack of transportation.

food recovery: the collection of wholesome food for distribution to low-income people who are hungry. Four common methods of food recovery are:

▌ *Field gleaning:* collecting crops from fields that either have already been harvested or are not profitable to harvest.

▌ *Perishable food rescue or salvage:* collection of perishable produce from wholesalers and markets.

▌ *Prepared food rescue:* collection of prepared foods from commercial kitchens.

▌ *Nonperishable food collection:* collection of processed foods from wholesalers and markets.

food security: access to enough food to sustain a healthy and active life. Food security categories include:

▌ *high food security:* no indications of food-access problems or limitations.

▌ *marginal food security:* one or two indications of food-access problems but with little or no change in food intake.

---

the major cause of food poverty in developed countries, and solving this problem would do a lot to relieve hunger.

In the United States, poverty and hunger reach across various segments of society, touching some more than others—notably, single parents living in households with their children, Hispanics, African Americans, and those living in the inner cities. People living in poverty are simply unable to buy sufficient amounts of nourishing foods, even if they are skilled in food shopping. Consequently, their diets tend to be inadequate. For many of the children in these families, school lunch (and breakfast, where available) may be the only nourishment for the day. Otherwise, they go hungry, waiting for an adult to find money for food. Not surprisingly, these children are more likely to have health problems and iron-deficiency anemia than those who eat regularly. They also tend to perform poorly in school and in social situations. For adults, the risk of developing chronic diseases increases.[6] For pregnant women, the risk of developing gestational diabetes more than doubles.[7]

Is it true that hunger and obesity often exist side by side—sometimes within the same household or even the same person?

Ironically, it is true—food insufficiency and obesity often exist side by side.[8] Food insecurity and obesity may logically seem to be mutually exclusive, but research studies consistently show that the highest rates of obesity occur among those living in the greatest poverty and food insecurity.[9]

Low-income urban and rural communities that offer little or no access to affordable nutritious foods—**food deserts** (first mentioned in Chapter 7)—lack markets that sell fresh produce.[10] Not surprisingly, people living in food deserts often lack fruits and vegetables in their diets and often fail to meet intake recommendations of the *Dietary Guidelines*.[11] High-fat, high-sugar, refined, energy-dense foods that are readily available in food deserts infamously lack other needed nutrients. Doughnuts, packaged sweet cakes, sugary punches, hamburgers, and french fries fill the stomach, are affordable, are easily obtained at any hour, are easily carried, require no preparation, and taste good. It is not surprising, then, that these high-kcalorie foods edge nutrient-dense staple foods out of the diet.

Economic uncertainty and stress greatly influence the prevalence of obesity.[12] People who are unsure about their next meal may overeat when food or money become available. Interestingly, food insecure people who do *not* participate in food assistance programs have a greater risk of obesity than those who do—it seems that providing a reliable supply of nutritious food may help to prevent obesity among those living with food insecurity.[13]

What U.S. food programs are directed at relieving hunger in the United States?

The Academy of Nutrition and Dietetics calls for aggressive action to bring an end to domestic hunger and to achieve food and nutrition security for all residents of the United States.[14] Many federal and local programs aim to prevent or relieve malnutrition and hunger.

An extensive network of federal assistance programs provides life-giving food daily to millions of U.S. citizens. An estimated one out of every seven Americans receives food assistance of some kind, at a total cost of almost $95 billion per year.[15] Even so, the programs are not fully successful in preventing hunger, though they do seem to improve the nutrient intakes of those who participate. Programs described in the life cycle chapters include the WIC program for low-income pregnant women, breastfeeding mothers, and their young children (Chapter 11); the school lunch and breakfast programs for children (Chapter 12); and the food assistance programs for older adults such as congregate meals and Meals on Wheels (Chapter 13).

The centerpiece of food programs for low-income people in the United States is the Supplemental Nutrition Assistance Program (SNAP), administered by the U.S. Department of Agriculture (USDA). The USDA issues debit cards through state agencies to households—people who buy and prepare food together. The amount a household receives depends on its size, resources, and income. Recipients may use the cards to purchase food and food-bearing plants and seeds but not to buy tobacco, cleaning items, alcohol, or other nonfood items. Box NP13-2 offers tips for both saving money and preventing food waste.

SNAP is the largest of the federal food assistance programs, both in amount of money spent and in number of people participating. It provides assistance to more than 46 million people at a cost of $75 billion per year; about half of the recipients are children.

Why do health care professionals need to know about food assistance programs?

Health care professionals who work in public health are generally well acquainted with food assistance programs, and often many of their clients receive such assistance. Regardless of the setting in which health care professionals see clients, however, it is important to encourage those who may be having financial problems to talk with a social worker who can assess their eligibility for food assistance programs. The subject of food assistance must be approached in a nonjudgmental and tactful manner—the client may feel uncomfortable about seeking assistance.

Are there other programs aimed at reducing hunger in the United States?

Efforts to resolve the problem of hunger in the United States do not depend solely on federal assistance programs. National **food recovery** programs such as Feeding America coordinate the efforts of **food banks, food pantries, emergency kitchens,** and homeless shelters that provide food to tens of millions of people a year. Table NP13-2 (on p. 388) lists websites for Feeding America and other hunger relief organizations.

Each year, a tremendous amount of our food supply is wasted in fields, commercial kitchens, grocery stores, and

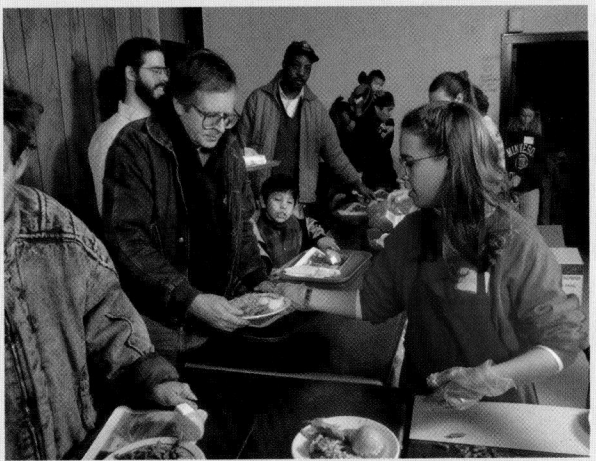

Skjold/The Image Works

Feeding the hungry in the United States.

BOX NP13-2 HOW TO STRETCH FOOD DOLLARS AND REDUCE WASTE

Eating well on a budget can pose a challenge, but these tips ease the task. For daily menus and recipes for healthy, thrifty meals, visit the USDA Center for Nutrition Policy and Promotion: *www.cnpp.usda.gov.*

Plan Ahead

▌ Plan your menus, write grocery lists, and shop only for foods on your list to avoid expensive "impulse" buying.

▌ Center meals on whole grains, legumes, and vegetables; use smaller quantities of meat, poultry, fish, or eggs.

▌ Use cooked cereals such as oatmeal instead of ready-to-eat breakfast cereals.

▌ Cook large quantities when time and money allow; freeze portions for convenient later meals.

▌ Check for sales and use coupons for products you need; plan meals to take advantage of sale items.

Shop Smart

▌ Do not shop when hungry.

▌ Select whole foods instead of convenience foods (raw whole potatoes instead of refrigerated prepared mashed potatoes, for example).

▌ Try store brands.

▌ Buy fresh produce in season; buy canned or frozen items at other times.

▌ Buy large bags of frozen items or dry goods; use as needed and store the remainder.

▌ Buy fat-free dry milk; mix and refrigerate quantities needed for a day or two. Buy fresh milk by the gallon or half-gallon only if you can use it up before it spoils.

▌ Buy less expensive cuts of meat, such as beef chuck and pork shoulder roasts; cook with liquid long enough to make the meat tender.

▌ Buy whole chickens instead of pieces; ask a butcher to show you how to cut them up.

▌ Frequent discount stores instead of grocery stores for nonfood items such as toilet paper and detergent.

Reduce Waste

▌ Change your thinking from "what do I want to eat" to "what do I have available to eat." You paid for the food you have on hand—so use it up.

▌ Buy only the amount of fresh foods that you will eat before it spoils.

▌ Peel away the tough outer layers from stems of asparagus and broccoli; slice and cook the tender stems or add raw to salads.

▌ Scrub, but don't peel, potatoes before cooking—the skins add color, texture, and nutrients to the dish.

▌ Before buying food in bulk, plan how to store it properly. If it spoils before use, you'll throw away your savings.

▌ If your "bargain" bulk food is more than you can use but is still fresh, donate it to your local food bank or homeless shelter. (It won't save you money, but it will provide a wealth of satisfaction.)

▌ If space permits, compost fruit and vegetable scraps to feed shrubs and other outdoor plants.

TABLE NP13-2 **Hunger Relief Organizations**

Organization	Mission Statement
Bread for the World *www.bread.org*	Nonpartisan, Christian citizens' movement seeking to influence reform in policies, programs, and conditions that allow hunger and poverty to persist globally.
Catholic Relief Services *www.crs.org*	Humanitarian service agency assisting the impoverished and disadvantaged through community-based, sustainable development initiatives.
Congressional Hunger Center *www.hungercenter.org*	Bipartisan organization training and inspiring leaders with the intent to end hunger and advocating public policies to create a food-secure world.
Feeding America www.feedingamerica.org	Domestic charity organization providing food assistance through a nationwide network of member food banks and facilitating education to end hunger nationally.
Food and Agriculture Organization (FAO) of the United Nations *www.fao.org*	International organization leading efforts to achieve food security for all by helping to develop and modernize countries' agriculture, forestry, and fishery practices.
Idealist *www.idealist.org*	International organization seeking to connect people, organizations, and resources to help build a world where all people can live free and dignified lives.
Institute for Food and Development Policy *www.foodfirst.org*	North American organization working to catalyze food systems that are healthy, sustainable, just, and democratic by building community voice and capacity for change.
Oxfam America *www.oxfamamerica.org*	International relief and development organization aiming to create lasting solutions to poverty, hunger, and injustice.
Pan American Health Organization *www.paho.org*	International public health agency aiming to strengthen national and local health systems with the purpose of improving the quality of, and lengthening, the lives of the peoples in the Americas.
Society of St. Andrew *www.endhunger.org*	Ecumenical Christian ministry salvaging and redirecting large amounts of fresh produce to hunger agencies for distribution to the poor.
The Hunger Project *www.thp.org*	International relief organization attempting to end hunger and poverty by pioneering sustainable, grassroots, women-centered strategies and advocating for their widespread adoption in countries throughout the world.
United Nations Children's Fund (UNICEF) *www.unicef.org*	International organization advocating for the protection of children's rights, to help meet their basic needs and to expand their opportunities to reach their full potentials.
WhyHunger *www.whyhunger.org*	Domestic organization supporting and funding community-based organizations intent on empowering individuals and building self-reliance to provide long-term solutions to end hunger and poverty.
World Food Programme *www.wfp.org*	Food aid branch of the United Nations aiming to prepare for, protect during, and provide assistance after emergencies, as well as reduce hunger and undernutrition.
World Health Organization (WHO) *www.who.int*	United Nations agency acting as the authority on international public health by influencing policy, setting research agendas, establishing standards, and providing technical support to monitor and assess health trends.

restaurants—enough food to feed millions of people. Food recovery programs collect and distribute good food that would otherwise go to waste. Volunteers might pick corn left in an already harvested field, a grocer might deliver ripe bananas to a local food bank, and a caterer might take leftover chicken salad to a community shelter, for example. All of these efforts help to feed the hungry in the United States.

What about local efforts and community nutrition programs?

Food recovery programs depend on volunteers. Concerned citizens work through local agencies and churches to feed the hungry. Community-based food pantries provide groceries, and soup kitchens serve prepared meals. Meals often deliver adequate nourishment, but most homeless people receive fewer than one and a half

Community-based efforts to feed citizens include food pantries that provide groceries.

meals a day, so many are still inadequately nourished. Health care professionals can serve as valuable members of community groups seeking to provide food assistance.

Notes

1. *The State of Food Insecurity in the World, 2012, Executive Summary,* retrieved from Food and Agriculture Organization, www.fao.org.

2. World Health Organization, *Children: Reducing mortality,* Fact sheet, September 2012, retrieved from www.who.int/mediacentre/factsheets/fs178/en/index.html.

3. A. Coleman-Jensen and coauthors, *Economic Research Service Report Summary,* September 2012, Household food security in the United States, 2011, retrieved from www.ers.usda.gov/publications/err-economic-research-report/err141.aspx.

4. Position of the American Dietetic Association, Food insecurity in the United States, *Journal of the American Dietetic Association* 110 (2010): 1368–1377.

5. US Census Bureau, *Social, Economic, and Housing Statistics Division: Poverty* (Washington, DC: U.S. Government Printing Office, 2011).

6. H. K. Seligman and D. Schillinger, Hunger and socioeconomic disparities in chronic disease, *New England Journal of Medicine* 363 (2010): 6–9.

7. C. M. Olson, Food insecurity and maternal health during pregnancy, *Journal of the American Dietetic Association* 110 (2010): 690–691.

8. L. Pan and coauthors, Food insecurity is associated with obesity among US adults in 12 states, *Journal of the Academy of Nutrition and Dietetics* 112 (2012): 1403–1409; J. C. Eisenmann and coauthors, Is food insecurity related to overweight and obesity in children and adolescents? A summary of studies, 1995–2009, *Obesity Reviews* 12 (2011): e73–e83.

9. D. S. Ludwig, S. J. Blumenthal, and W. C. Willett, Opportunities to reduce childhood hunger and obesity: Restructuring the Supplemental Nutrition Assistance Program (the Food stamp Program), *Journal of the American Medical Association* 308 (2012): 2567-2568; J. Levine, Poverty and obesity in the U.S., *Diabetes* 60 (2011): 2667–2668; B. M. Popkin, L. S. Adair, and S. W. Ng, Global nutrition transition and the pandemic of obesity in developing countries, *Nutrition Reviews* 70 (2011): 3–21.

10. A. M. Fretts and coauthors, Associations of processed meat and unprocessed red meat intake with incident diabetes: The Strong Heart Family Study, *American Journal of Clinical Nutrition* 95 (2012): 752–758; H. J. Song and coauthors, Understanding a key feature of urban food stores to develop nutrition intervention, *Journal of Hunger & Environmental Nutrition* 7 (2012): 77–90.

11. B. T. Izumi and coauthors, Associations between neighborhood availability and individual consumption of dark-green and orange vegetables among ethnically diverse adults in Detroit, *Journal of the American Dietetic Association* 111 (2011): 274–279.

12. Ludwig, Blumenthal, and Willett, 2012; A. Offer, R. Pechey, and S. Ulijaszek, Obesity under affluence varies by welfare regimes: The effect of fast food, insecurity, and inequality, *Economics and Human Biology* 8 (2010): 297–308.

13. A. Karnik and coauthors, Food insecurity and obesity in New York City primary care clinics, *Medical Care* 49 (2011): 658–661; N. I. Larson and M. T. Story, Food insecurity and weight status among U.S. children and families: A review of the literature, *American Journal of Preventative Medicine* 40 (2011): 166–173.

14. Position of the American Dietetic Association, 2010.

15. USDA Economic Research Service, Economic Bulletin 6–8, The food assistance landscape: 2010 annual report, retrieved from www.ers.usda.gov/media/129642/eib6-8.pdf.

14

Illness and Nutrition Care

14.1 Nutrition in Health Care

LO 14.1 Describe the interrelationships between illness and malnutrition and explain how health professionals identify and treat patients at risk for nutrition problems.

14.2 Nutrition Assessment

LO 14.2 Discuss the various types of data used for evaluating an individual's nutrition and health status and describe how energy requirements can be estimated in the hospital setting.

14.3 Implementing Nutrition Care

LO 14.3 Discuss the different types of dietary modifications available to patients with medical problems and explain how each of these is used during patient care.

14.4 Nutrition in Practice: Nutritional Genomics

LO 14.4 Explain how nutritional genomics research may improve our understanding of the relationship between illness and nutrition care.

Previous chapters of this book introduced the nutrients and described how the appropriate dietary choices can support good health. Turning now to clinical nutrition, this chapter introduces the process used for providing nutrition care and the implementation of nutrition care in clinical practice. Ensuring that nutrient needs are met is a key part of this process, so the chapter also describes methods used for estimating energy requirements and common nutrition modifications.

14.1 Nutrition in Health Care

LO 14.1 Describe the interrelationships between illness and malnutrition and explain how health professionals identify and treat patients at risk for nutrition problems.

Malnutrition is frequently reported in patients hospitalized with acute illness, and acutely ill individuals without nutrition problems on admission often exhibit a subsequent decline in nutrition status. Depending on the patient population, estimates of malnutrition in hospital patients range from 15 to 60 percent.[1] Poor nutrition status weakens immune function and compromises a person's healing ability, influencing both the course of disease and the body's response to treatment. Thus, preventing and correcting nutrition problems may improve the outcome of medical treatments and help to prevent complications. In addition, patients are often concerned about the impact their diet has on their medical condition.

Effects of Illness on Nutrition Status

Illnesses and their treatments may lead to malnutrition by reducing food intake, interfering with digestion and absorption, or altering nutrient metabolism and excretion (see Figure 14-1). For example, the nausea caused by some illnesses or treatments can diminish appetite and reduce food intake; similarly, inflammation in the mouth or esophagus can cause discomfort when an individual consumes food. Some medications may cause **anorexia** (loss of appetite) or gastrointestinal (GI)

anorexia: loss of appetite.

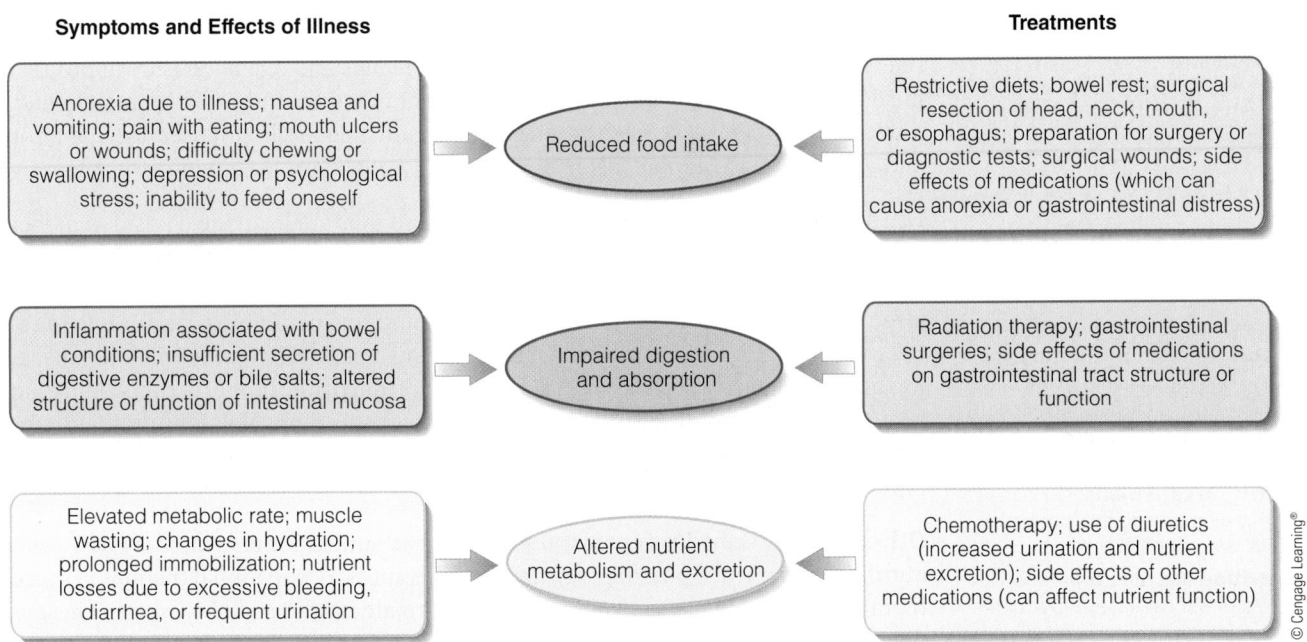

Symptoms and Effects of Illness

Treatments

Anorexia due to illness; nausea and vomiting; pain with eating; mouth ulcers or wounds; difficulty chewing or swallowing; depression or psychological stress; inability to feed oneself → Reduced food intake ← Restrictive diets; bowel rest; surgical resection of head, neck, mouth, or esophagus; preparation for surgery or diagnostic tests; surgical wounds; side effects of medications (which can cause anorexia or gastrointestinal distress)

Inflammation associated with bowel conditions; insufficient secretion of digestive enzymes or bile salts; altered structure or function of intestinal mucosa → Impaired digestion and absorption ← Radiation therapy; gastrointestinal surgeries; side effects of medications on gastrointestinal tract structure or function

Elevated metabolic rate; muscle wasting; changes in hydration; prolonged immobilization; nutrient losses due to excessive bleeding, diarrhea, or frequent urination → Altered nutrient metabolism and excretion ← Chemotherapy; use of diuretics (increased urination and nutrient excretion); side effects of other medications (can affect nutrient function)

© Cengage Learning®

FIGURE 14-1 Ways in Which Illness Can Affect Nutrition Status

discomfort or interfere with nutrient function and metabolism. Prolonged bed rest often results in **pressure sores,** which increase metabolic stress and raise protein and energy needs.

The dietary changes required during an acute illness are usually temporary and can be tailored to accommodate an individual's preferences and lifestyle. However, chronic illnesses (those lasting 3 months or longer) may require long-term modifications. For example, diabetes treatment requires lifelong changes in diet and lifestyle that some people may find difficult to adhere to. The challenge for health professionals is to help their patients understand the potential benefits of nutrition treatments and accept the dietary adjustments that can improve their health.

Responsibility for Nutrition Care

Members of the health care team work together to ensure that the nutritional needs of patients are met during illness. The roles of health professionals may vary among different institutions, however, and their responsibilities can sometimes overlap. In some cases, the patient's nutrition care is incorporated into the medical care plan developed by the entire health care team. Such plans, called **clinical pathways,** outline coordinated plans of care for specific medical diagnoses, procedures, or treatments.

Physicians Physicians are responsible for meeting all of a patient's medical needs, including nutrition. They prescribe **diet orders** (also called *nutrition prescriptions*) and other instructions related to nutrition care, including referrals for nutrition assessment and dietary counseling. Physicians rely on nurses, registered dietitians, and other health professionals to alert them to nutrition problems, suggest strategies for handling nutrition care, and provide nutrition services.

Registered Dietitians A **registered dietitian** is a food and nutrition expert who is qualified to provide **medical nutrition therapy.** Registered dietitians conduct nutrition and dietary assessments; diagnose nutrition problems; develop, implement, and evaluate **nutrition care plans** (described later); plan and approve menus; and provide dietary counseling and nutrition education services. Registered dietitians may also manage food and cafeteria services in health care institutions.

Registered Dietetic Technicians Registered dietetic technicians often work in partnership with registered dietitians and assist in the implementation and monitoring of nutrition services. Depending on their background and experience, they may screen patients for nutrition problems, develop menus and recipes, ensure appropriate meal delivery, monitor patients' food choices and intakes, and provide patient education and counseling. Dietetic technicians sometimes supervise foodservice operations and may have roles in purchasing, inventory, quality control, sanitation, or safety.

Nurses Nurses interact closely with patients and thus are in an ideal position to identify people who would benefit from nutrition services. Nurses often screen patients for nutrition problems and may participate in nutrition and dietary assessments. Nurses also provide direct nutrition care, such as encouraging patients to eat, finding practical solutions to food-related problems, recording a patient's food intake, and answering questions about special diets. As members of **nutrition support teams,** nurses are responsible for administering tube and intravenous feedings. In facilities that do not employ registered dietitians, nurses often assume responsibility for much of the nutrition care.

Other Health Care Professionals Other heath practitioners who may assist with nutrition care include pharmacists, physical therapists, occupational therapists, speech therapists, nursing assistants, home health care aides, and social workers. These individuals can be instrumental in alerting dietitians or nurses to nutrition problems or may share relevant information about a patient's health status or personal needs.

pressure sores: regions of skin and tissue that are damaged due to prolonged pressure on the affected area by an external object, such as a bed, wheelchair, or cast; vulnerable areas of the body include buttocks, hips, and heels. Also called *decubitus* (deh-KYU-bih-tus) *ulcers.*

clinical pathways: coordinated programs of treatment that merge the care plans of different health practitioners; also called *care pathways, care maps,* or *critical pathways.*

diet orders: specific instructions regarding dietary management; also called *nutrition prescriptions.*

registered dietitian: a food and nutrition expert who has completed the education and training specified by the Academy of Nutrition and Dietetics (or Dietitians of Canada), including a bachelor's degree in nutrition or dietetics, a supervised internship, and a national registration examination.

medical nutrition therapy: nutrition care provided by a registered dietitian; includes assessing nutrition status, diagnosing nutrition problems, and providing nutrition care.

nutrition care plans: strategies for meeting an individual's nutritional needs.

nutrition support teams: health care professionals responsible for the provision of nutrients by tube feeding or intravenous infusion.

TABLE 14-1 Criteria for Identifying Malnutrition Risk

Category	Specific Examples
Admission data	Age, medical diagnosis, severity of illness or injury
Anthropometric data	Height and weight, body mass index (BMI), unintentional weight changes, loss of muscle or subcutaneous fat
Functional assessment data	Low hand grip strength, general weakness, impaired mobility
Historical information	History of diabetes, renal disease, or other chronic illness; use of medications that can impair nutrition status; extensive dietary restrictions; food allergies or intolerances; requirement for nutrition support; depression, social isolation, or dementia
Laboratory test results	Blood test results that suggest the presence of inflammation (such as low serum protein levels) or anemia
Signs and symptoms	Reduced appetite or food intake, problems that interfere with food intake (such as chewing or swallowing difficulties or nausea and vomiting), localized or general edema, presence of pressure sores

© 2016 Cengage Learning®

Nutrition Screening

A referral for nutrition care may result from a **nutrition screening,** an assessment procedure that helps to identify patients who are malnourished or at risk of malnutrition. The screening should be sensitive enough to identify patients who require nutrition care but simple enough to be completed within 10 to 15 minutes. The information collected in a nutrition screening may include the admitting diagnosis, physical measurements and test results obtained during the admission process, relevant signs and symptoms, and information about nutrition and health status provided by the patient or caregiver (see Table 14-1 for examples). The **Joint Commission,** a nonprofit organization that confers accreditation to health care institutions, recommends that a nutrition screening be conducted within 24 hours of a patient's admission to a hospital or other extended-care facility. Nutrition screening is also frequently included in outpatient services and community health programs.

A number of nutrition screening tools have become popular in recent years; one example is the Subjective Global Assessment, which ranks nutrition-related elements of the medical history and physical examination to assess malnutrition risk (see Table 14-2, p. 394). Briefer screening methods may use just two or three variables; for example, several tools screen for malnutrition risk by evaluating health status, unintentional weight changes, and reduced appetite or food intake.[2]

FIGURE 14-2 The Nutrition Care Process

© Cengage Learning®

The Nutrition Care Process

Registered dietitians use a systematic approach to medical nutrition therapy called the **nutrition care process.**[3] Figure 14-2 presents the four distinct, yet interrelated, steps of the nutrition care process:

1. Nutrition assessment
2. Nutrition diagnosis
3. Nutrition intervention
4. Nutrition monitoring and evaluation

Although the nutrition care process is easiest to visualize as a series of steps, the steps are frequently revisited to reassess and revise diagnoses and intervention strategies.

nutrition screening: a brief assessment of health-related variables to identify patients who are malnourished or at risk for malnutrition.

Joint Commission: a nonprofit organization that sets standards for health care performance and safety and confers accreditation to health care organizations and programs that meet those standards.

nutrition care process: a systematic approach used by dietetics professionals to evaluate and treat nutrition-related problems.

TABLE 14-2 Subjective Global Assessment

The Subjective Global Assessment evaluates a person's risk of malnutrition by ranking key variables of the medical history and physical examination. These variables are each given an A, B, or C rating: A for well nourished, B for potential or mild malnutrition, and C for severe malnutrition. Patients are classified according to the final numbers of A, B, and C ratings.

Medical History

▪ Body weight changes: percentage weight loss in past 6 months; weight change in past 2 weeks

▪ Dietary changes: suboptimal, low kcalorie, liquid diet, or starvation

▪ GI symptoms: nausea, diarrhea, vomiting, or anorexia for more than 2 weeks

▪ Functional ability: full capacity versus suboptimal, walking versus bedridden

▪ Degree of disease-related metabolic stress: low, medium, or high

Physical Examination

▪ Subcutaneous fat loss (triceps or chest)

▪ Muscle loss (quadriceps or deltoids)

▪ Ankle edema

▪ Sacral (lower spine) edema

▪ Ascites (abdominal edema)

Classification:

A: Well nourished: if no significant loss of weight, fat, or muscle tissue and no dietary difficulties, functional impairments, or GI symptoms; also applies to patients with recent weight gain and improved appetite, functioning, or medical prognosis

B: Moderate malnutrition: if 5 to 10 percent weight loss, mild loss of muscle or fat tissue, decreased food intake, and digestive or functional difficulties that impair food intake; the B classification usually applies to patients with an even mix of A, B, and C ratings

C: Severe malnutrition: if more than 10 percent weight loss, severe loss of muscle or fat tissue, edema, multiple GI symptoms, and functional impairments

Sources: P. Charney and M. Marian, Nutrition screening and nutrition assessment, in P. Charney and A. M. Malone, eds., *ADA Pocket Guide to Nutrition Assessment* (Chicago: American Dietetic Association, 2009), pp. 1–19; A. S. Detsky and coauthors, What is subjective global assessment of nutritional status? *Journal of Parenteral and Enteral Nutrition* 11 (1987): 8–13.

Each step of the nutrition care process must be documented in the medical record, providing a record for future reference and facilitating communication among members of the health care team.

Nutrition Assessment A nutrition assessment involves the collection and analysis of health-related information in order to identify specific nutrition problems and their underlying causes. The information may be obtained from the medical record, physical examination, laboratory analyses, medical procedures, an interview with the patient or caregiver, and consultation with other health professionals. The assessment data are used to develop a plan of action to prevent or correct nutrient imbalances or to determine whether a care plan is working. The next section of this chapter describes the components of nutrition assessment in more detail.

Nutrition Diagnosis Each nutrition problem receives a separate diagnosis, which is formatted as a **PES statement,** a statement that includes the specific problem (P), etiology or cause (E), and signs and symptoms that provide evidence of the problem (S).[4] For example, a potential nutrition diagnosis might be, "Unintentional weight gain (*the problem*) related to long-term use of corticosteroids (*the etiology or cause*) as evidenced by an involuntary weight gain of 10 percent of body weight over the past 6 months (*the sign or symptom*)." A nutrition diagnosis often changes during the course of an illness.

Nutrition Intervention After nutrition problems are identified, the appropriate nutrition care can be planned and implemented. A nutrition intervention may include counseling or education about appropriate dietary and lifestyle practices, a change in medication or other treatment, or adjustments in the meals or services provided to a hospital patient. To be successful, the intervention must consider the individual's food habits, lifestyle, and other personal factors. Goals are stated in terms of measurable outcomes; for example, the goals for an overweight person with diabetes might

PES statement: a statement that describes a nutrition problem in a format that includes the problem (P), the etiology or cause (E), and the signs and symptoms (S).

include improvements in blood glucose levels and body weight. Other goals may be positive changes in dietary behaviors and lifestyle; for example, a diabetes patient may learn how to control carbohydrate intake or portion sizes or begin a regular exercise program.

Nutrition Monitoring and Evaluation The effectiveness of the nutrition care plan must be evaluated periodically: the patient's progress should be monitored closely, and updated assessment data or diagnoses may require adjustments in goals or outcome measures. Sometimes a new situation alters nutritional needs; for example, a change in the medical treatment or a new medication may alter a person's tolerance to certain foods. The nutrition care plan must be flexible enough to adapt to the new situation.

If progress is slow or a patient is unable or unwilling to make the suggested changes, the care plan should be redesigned and take into account the reasons why the earlier plan was not successful. This new plan may need to include motivational techniques or additional patient education. If the patient remains unwilling to modify behaviors despite the expected benefits, the health care provider can try again at a later time when the patient may be more receptive.

IN SUMMARY

▌ Illnesses and their treatments can alter food intake and nutrient needs, leading to malnutrition. In turn, poor nutrition status can influence the course of illness and reduce the effectiveness of medical treatments.

▌ The combined efforts of each member of the health care team ensure that patients receive optimal nutrition care.

▌ Nutrition screening identifies individuals who can benefit from nutrition assessment and follow-up nutrition care. The nutrition care process includes four interrelated steps: nutrition assessment, nutrition diagnosis, nutrition intervention, and nutrition monitoring and evaluation.

14.2 Nutrition Assessment

LO 14.2 Discuss the various types of data used for evaluating an individual's nutrition and health status and describe how energy requirements can be estimated in the hospital setting.

As described earlier, a nutrition assessment provides the information needed for diagnosing nutrition problems and designing a nutrition care plan; follow-up assessments can determine whether the care plan has been effective. Ideally, the assessment should be sensitive enough to detect subtle nutrition problems and specific enough to identify problem nutrients. For most nutrient imbalances, a variety of tests are necessary to identify nutrition problems.

Historical Information

Historical information provides valuable clues about the patient's nutrition status and nutrient requirements; it also reveals personal preferences that need consideration when developing a nutrition care plan. Table 14-3 (p. 396) summarizes the various types of historical data that contribute to a nutrition assessment. This information can be obtained from the medical record or by interviewing the patient or caregiver.

Medical History The medical history helps the practitioner identify health problems or medical treatments that may interfere with food intake or require dietary

TABLE 14-3 Historical Information Used in Nutrition Assessment[a]

Medical History	Medication and Supplement History	Personal and Social History	Food and Nutrition History
Age	Prescription drugs	Cognitive abilities	Food intake
Current complaint(s)	Over-the-counter drugs	Cultural/ethnic identity	Food availability
Past medical problems	Dietary and herbal supplements	Educational level	Recent weight changes
Ongoing medical treatments		Employment status	Dietary restrictions
Surgical history		Home/family situation	Food allergies or intolerances
Family medical history		Religious beliefs	Nutrition and health knowledge
Chronic disease risk		Socioeconomic status	Physical activity level and exercise habits
Mental/emotional health status		Use of tobacco, alcohol, or illegal drugs	

© 2016 Cengage Learning®

[a]Historical information is classified in different ways among medical institutions.

TABLE 14-4 Medical Problems Often Associated with Malnutrition

▪ Acquired immune deficiency syndrome (AIDS)
▪ Alcoholism
▪ Anorexia nervosa or bulimia
▪ Burns (extensive or severe)
▪ Cancer and cancer treatments
▪ Cardiovascular diseases
▪ Celiac disease
▪ Chewing or swallowing difficulties
▪ Chronic kidney disease
▪ Dementia or other mental illness
▪ Diabetes mellitus
▪ Feeding disabilities
▪ Infections
▪ Inflammatory bowel diseases
▪ Liver disease
▪ Malabsorption
▪ Pressure sores
▪ Surgery (major)
▪ Vomiting (prolonged or severe)

© 2016 Cengage Learning®

changes; Table 14-4 lists examples. Many other conditions can lead to malnutrition, especially if nutrition problems are not recognized and corrected before they become serious.

Medication and Supplement History Many medications can have detrimental effects on nutrition status, and various components of foods and dietary supplements can alter the absorption and metabolism of drugs. Chapter 15 provides examples of diet-drug interactions that may need consideration when planning nutrition care.

Personal and Social History Personal and social factors influence both food choices and the ability to manage health and nutrition problems. For example, cultural background or religious beliefs can affect food preferences, whereas financial concerns may restrict access to health care and nutritious foods. Some individuals may depend on others to prepare or procure food. A person who lives alone or is depressed may eat poorly or be unable to follow complex dietary instructions.

Food and Nutrition History A food and nutrition history (often called a *diet history*) is a detailed account of a person's dietary practices. It includes information about food intake, lifestyle habits, and other factors that affect food choices. The procedure often includes an interview about recent food intake (for example, a *24-hour dietary recall*) and a survey about usual food choices (such as a *food frequency questionnaire*). The following section describes the most common methods of gathering food intake information.

Food Intake Data

Obtaining accurate food intake data is challenging, as the results may vary depending on an individual's memory and honesty and the assessor's skill and training. Each method has its own strengths and weaknesses, so the best results are obtained using a combination of approaches. Table 14-5 summarizes the methods commonly used as well as each method's advantages and disadvantages.

The 24-Hour Dietary Recall The **24-hour dietary recall** is a guided interview in which an individual recounts all of the foods and beverages consumed in the past 24 hours or during the previous day. The interview includes questions about the times when meals or snacks were eaten, amounts consumed, and ways in which foods were prepared (see Figure 14-3).

24-hour dietary recall: a record of foods consumed during the previous day or in the past 24 hours; sometimes modified to include foods consumed in a typical day.

TABLE 14-5 Methods for Obtaining Food Intake Data

Method	Description	Advantages	Disadvantages
24-hour dietary recall	Guided interview in which the foods and beverages consumed in a 24-hour period are described in detail.	▪ Results are not dependent on literacy or educational level of respondent. ▪ Interview occurs after food is consumed, so method does not influence dietary choices. ▪ Results are obtained quickly; method is relatively easy to conduct. ▪ Method does not require reading or writing ability.	▪ Process relies on memory. ▪ Underestimation and overestimation of food intakes are common. ▪ Food items that cause embarrassment (alcohol, desserts) may be omitted. ▪ Data from a single day cannot accurately represent the respondent's usual intake. ▪ Seasonal variations may not be addressed. ▪ Skill of interviewer affects outcome.
Food frequency questionnaire	Written survey of food consumption during a specific period of time, often a 1-year period.	▪ Process examines long-term food intake, so day-to-day and seasonal variability should not affect results. ▪ Questionnaire is completed after food is consumed, so method does not influence food choices. ▪ Method is inexpensive to administer.	▪ Process relies on memory. ▪ Food lists often include common foods only. ▪ Serving sizes are often difficult for respondents to evaluate without assistance. ▪ Calculated nutrient intakes may not be accurate. ▪ Food lists for the general population are of limited value in special populations. ▪ Method is not effective for monitoring short-term changes in food intake.
Food record	Written account of food consumed during a specified period, usually several consecutive days. Accuracy is improved by including weights or measures of foods.	▪ Process does not rely on memory. ▪ Recording foods as they are consumed may improve accuracy of food intake data. ▪ Process is useful for controlling intake because keeping records increases awareness of food choices.	▪ Recording process itself influences food intake. ▪ Underreporting and portion size errors are common. ▪ Process is time-consuming and burdensome for respondent; requires high degree of motivation. ▪ Method requires literacy and the physical ability to write. ▪ Seasonal changes in diet are not taken into account.
Direct observation	Observation of meal trays or shelf inventories before and after eating; possible only in residential facilities.	▪ Process does not rely on memory. ▪ Method does not influence food intake. ▪ Method can be used to evaluate the acceptability of a prescribed diet.	▪ Process is possible only in residential situations. ▪ Method is labor intensive.

© 2016 Cengage Learning®

The *multiple-pass method* is considered the most effective approach for conducting a 24-hour dietary recall.[5] In this procedure, the interview includes four or five separate passes through the 24-hour period of interest. In the first pass, the respondent provides a "quick list" of foods consumed without prompts by the interviewer. The second pass is conducted to help the respondent remember foods that are often forgotten, such as beverages, bread, additions to foods (such as butter on toast), savory snacks, and sweets. The third and fourth passes elicit additional details about the foods consumed, such as the amounts eaten, preparation methods, and places where foods were obtained or consumed. A final pass is conducted to provide a final opportunity to recall foods and to probe for additional details. The entire multiple-pass interview can be conducted in about 30 to 45 minutes.

Recall interviews may be conducted on several nonconsecutive days to get a better representation of a person's usual diet. A disadvantage of the 24-hour dietary recall is that it does not take into account fluctuations in food intake

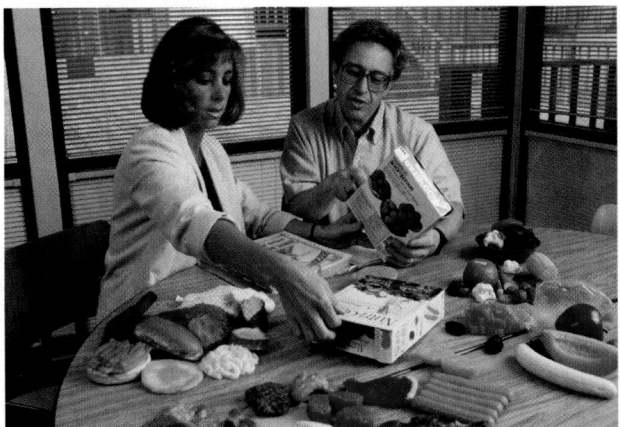

Nathan Benn/CORBIS

FIGURE 14-3 Collecting Food Intake Data
The use of food models and measuring utensils can help an individual visualize portion sizes, improving the accuracy of food intake data.

FRUIT	HOW OFTEN								HOW MUCH			
	Never or less than once per month	1 per mon.	2–3 per mon.	1 per week	2 per week	3–4 per week	5–6 per week	Every day	MEDIUM SERVING	YOUR SERVING SIZE		
										S	M	L
EXAMPLE: Bananas	○	○	○	●	○	○	○	○	1 medium	○ 1/2	● 1	○ 2
Bananas	○	○	○	○	○	○	○	○	1 medium	○ 1/2	○ 1	○ 2
Apples, applesauce	○	○	○	○	○	○	○	○	1 medium or 1/2 cup	○ 1/2	○ 1	○ 2
Oranges (not including juice)	○	○	○	○	○	○	○	○	1 medium	○ 1/2	○ 1	○ 2
Grapefruit (not including juice)	○	○	○	○	○	○	○	○	1/2 medium	○ 1/4	○ 1/2	○ 1
Cantaloupe	○	○	○	○	○	○	○	○	1/4 medium	○ 1/8	○ 1/4	○ 1/2
Peaches, apricots (fresh, in season)	○	○	○	○	○	○	○	○	1 medium	○ 1/2	○ 1	○ 2
Peaches, apricots (canned or dried)	○	○	○	○	○	○	○	○	1 medium or 1/2 cup	○ 1/2	○ 1	○ 2
Prunes, or prune juice	○	○	○	○	○	○	○	○	1/2 cup	○ 1/4	○ 1/2	○ 1
Watermelon (in season)	○	○	○	○	○	○	○	○	1 slice	○ 1/2	○ 1	○ 2
Strawberries, other berries (in season)	○	○	○	○	○	○	○	○	1/2 cup	○ 1/4	○ 1/2	○ 1
Any other fruit, including kiwi, fruit cocktail, grapes, raisins, mangoes	○	○	○	○	○	○	○	○	1/2 cup	○ 1/4	○ 1/2	○ 1

© Cengage Learning®

FIGURE 14-4 Sample Section of a Food Frequency Questionnaire

or seasonal variations. Moreover, food intakes are often underestimated because the process relies on an individual's memory and reporting accuracy.

Food Frequency Questionnaire A **food frequency questionnaire** surveys the foods and beverages regularly consumed during a specific time period. Some questionnaires are qualitative only: food lists contain common foods, organized by food group, with check boxes to indicate frequency of consumption. Other types of questionnaires can collect semiquantitative information by including portion sizes as well. Figure 14-4 shows a sample section of a semiquantitative questionnaire that surveys fruit intake over the previous year. Because the respondent is often asked to estimate food intakes over a 1-year period, the results should not be affected by seasonal changes in diet. Conversely, a disadvantage of this method is its inability to determine recent changes in food intake.

Some shortened versions of food frequency questionnaires focus on food categories relevant to a person's medical condition. For example, a questionnaire designed to evaluate calcium intake may include only milk products, fortified foods, certain fruits and vegetables, and dietary supplements that contain calcium. A computer analysis can then quickly estimate the individual's calcium intake and compare it to recommendations.

Food Record A **food record** is a written account of foods and beverages consumed during a specified time period, usually several consecutive days. Foods are recorded as they are consumed in order to obtain the most complete and accurate record possible; thus, the process does not rely on memory. A detailed food record includes the types and amounts of foods and beverages consumed, times of consumption, and methods of preparation. It provides valuable information about food intake as well as a person's response to and compliance with nutrition therapy. Unfortunately, food records require a great deal of time to complete, and people need to be highly motivated to keep accurate records. Another drawback is that the recording process itself may influence food intake. Furthermore, it is difficult to obtain accurate estimates of nutrient intakes in just a few days or even a week due to day-to-day and seasonal variations in food intake.

food frequency questionnaire: a survey of foods routinely consumed. Some questionnaires ask about the types of food eaten and yield only qualitative information; others include questions about portions consumed and yield semiquantitative data as well.

food record: a detailed log of food eaten during a specified time period, usually several days; also called a *food diary*. A food record may also include information regarding medications, disease symptoms, and physical activity.

Direct Observation In facilities that serve meals, food intakes can be directly observed and analyzed. This method can also reveal a person's food preferences, changes in appetite, and any problems with a prescribed diet. Health practitioners use direct observation to conduct patients' **kcalorie counts,** which are estimates of the food energy (and often, protein) consumed by patients during a single day or several consecutive days. To perform a kcalorie count, the clinician records the dietary items that a patient is given at meals and subtracts the amounts remaining after meals are completed; this procedure allows an estimate of the kcaloric content of foods and beverages actually consumed. Although a useful means of discerning patients' intakes, direct observation requires regular and careful documentation and can be labor intensive and costly.

Anthropometric Data

Measures of body size, known as **anthropometric** measurements, can reveal problems related to both **protein-energy malnutrition (PEM)** and overnutrition. Height (or **length**) and weight are the most common anthropometric measurements and are used to evaluate growth in children and nutrition status in adults. Other helpful values include the results of body composition tests (see Appendix E) and circumferences of the head, waist, and limbs.

Height (or Length) Poor growth in children can be a sign of malnutrition. In adults, height measurements alone do not reflect current nutrition status but can be used for estimating a person's energy needs or appropriate body weight. Length is measured in infants and children younger than 24 months of age, and height is usually measured in older children and adults. Length can also be measured in adults and children who cannot stand unassisted due to physical or medical reasons. Box 14-1 describes some standard techniques for measuring length and height.

In adults who are bedridden or unable to stand, height can be estimated from equations that include either the knee height or the full arm span, both of which correlate

kcalorie counts: estimates of food energy (and often, protein) consumed by patients for one or more days.

anthropometric (AN-throw-poe-MEH-trik)**:** related to physical measurements of the human body, such as height, weight, body circumferences, and percentage of body fat.

protein-energy malnutrition (PEM): a state of malnutrition characterized by depletion of tissue proteins and energy stores, usually accompanied by micronutrient deficiencies.

length: the distance from the top of the head to the soles of the feet while a person is recumbent (lying down). In contrast, *height* is measured while a person is standing upright.

How To BOX 14-1 MEASURE LENGTH AND HEIGHT

To improve the accuracy of length and height measurements, keep the following in mind:

▌ Always measure—never ask. Self-reported heights are less accurate than measured heights. If height is not measured, document that the height is self-reported.

▌ Measure the length of infants and young children by using a measuring board with a fixed headboard and a movable footboard. It generally takes two people to measure length: one person gently holds the infant's head against the headboard; the other straightens the infant's legs and moves the footboard to the bottom of the infant's feet.

▌ Measure height next to a wall on which a nonstretchable measuring tape or board has been fixed. Ask the

person to stand erect without shoes and with heels together. The person's eyes and head should be facing forward, with heels, buttocks, and shoulder blades touching the wall. Place a ruler or other flat, stiff object on the top of the head at a right angle to the wall and carefully note the height measurement. Immediately record length and height measurements to the nearest ⅛ inch or 0.1 centimeter.

▌ For evaluating the growth rate of young children, use the appropriate growth chart (Appendix E) when plotting results. If length is measured, use the growth chart for children between 0 and 36 months; if height is measured, use the chart for individuals between 2 and 20 years.

▌ Higher values are obtained from supine measurements than from vertical height measurements due to gravity.

It generally takes two people to measure the length of an infant.

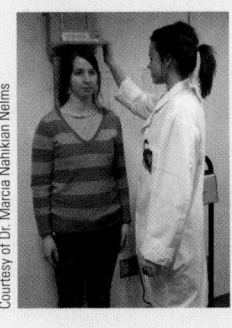

Standing erect allows for an accurate height measurement.

Tips for measuring weight include:

- Always measure—never ask. Self-reported weights are often inaccurate. If weight is not measured, document that the weight is self-reported.

- Valid weight measurements require scales that have been carefully maintained, calibrated, and checked for accuracy at regular intervals. Beam balance and electronic scales are the most accurate. Bathroom scales are inaccurate and inappropriate for clinical use.

- Measure an infant's weight with a scale that allows the infant to sit or lie down. The tray should be large enough to support an infant or young child up to 40 pounds, and weight graduations should be in ½-ounce or 10-gram increments. For accurate results, weigh

infants without clothes or diapers. Excessive movement by the infant can reduce accuracy.

- Children who can stand are weighed in the same way as adults, using beam balance or electronic scales with platforms large enough for standing comfortably.

- If repeated weight measurements are needed, each weighing should take place at the same time of day (preferably before breakfast), in the same amount of clothing, after the person has voided, and using the same scale. Record weights to the nearest ¼ pound or 0.1 kilogram.

- Special scales and hospital beds with built-in scales are available for weighing people who are bedridden.

G. DeGrazia/Custom Medical Stock

Infants are weighed on scales that allow them to sit or lie down.

Image Source/Jupiter Images

Beam balance scales allow accurate weight measurements for older children and adults.

well with height.[6] Knee height, which extends from the heel to the top of the knee when the leg is bent at a 90-degree angle, can be measured in either a sitting or supine position with a knee-height caliper; specific formulas are available for different age, gender, and ethnic groups. The full arm span is the distance from the tip of one middle finger to the other while the arms are extended horizontally. In children with disabilities that affect stature, alternative measures of linear growth include the full arm span, lower-leg lengths (knee to heel, similar to the knee-height measure), and upper-arm lengths (shoulder to elbow), all of which can be compared with reference percentiles.

Body Weight During clinical care, health care providers monitor body weights closely: weight changes may reflect changes in body water due to illness, and an involuntary loss of weight can be a sign of PEM. Body weights can be compared with healthy ranges on height-weight tables and growth charts or used to calculate the **body mass index (BMI).** A healthy body weight typically falls within a BMI range of 18.5 to 25; thus, an appropriate body weight can usually be estimated by using a BMI table or graph (see the inside back cover of this book). Box 14-2 includes suggestions for improving the accuracy of weight measurements.

Head Circumference A measurement of head circumference helps to assess brain growth and malnutrition in children up to 3 years of age, although the measure is not necessarily reduced in a malnourished child. Head circumference values can also track brain development in premature and small-for-gestational-age infants. To measure head circumference, the assessor encircles the largest circumference measure of a child's head with a nonstretchable measuring tape: the tape is placed just above the eyebrows and ears and around the occipital prominence at the back of the head (see Figure 14-5). The measurement is read to the nearest ⅛th inch or 0.1 centimeter.

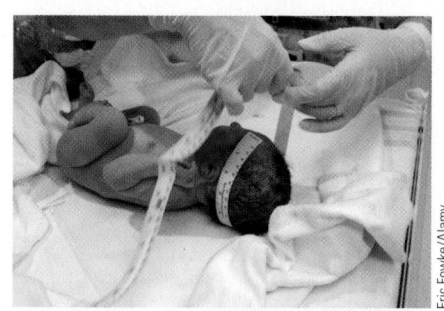

Eric Fowke/Alamy

FIGURE 14-5 Head circumference measurements can help to assess brain growth.

body mass index (BMI): a person's weight in relation to height; determined by dividing one's weight (in kilograms) by the square of the height (in meters).

Circumferences of Waist and Limbs Circumferences of the waist and limbs are useful for evaluating body fat and muscle mass, respectively. The waist circumference correlates with intra-abdominal fat and can help in assessing overnutrition. Circumferences of the mid-upper arm, mid-thigh, and mid-calf regions can help in evaluating the effects of illness, aging, and PEM on skeletal muscle tissue. For improved accuracy, circumference measurements are often used together with skinfold measurements to correct for the subcutaneous fat in limbs.

Anthropometric Assessment in Infants and Children To evaluate growth patterns, anthropometric data can be plotted on growth charts, such as those provided in Appendix E. The most commonly used growth charts compare height (or length) to age, weight to age, head circumference to age, weight to length, and BMI to age. Although individual growth patterns vary, a child's growth will generally stay at about the same percentile throughout childhood; a sharp drop in a previously steady growth pattern suggests malnutrition. Growth patterns that fall below the 5th percentile may also be cause for concern, although genetic influences must be considered when interpreting low values. Growth charts with BMI-for-age percentiles can be used to assess risk of underweight and overweight in children over 2 years of age: the 5th and 85th percentiles are used as cutoffs to identify children who may be malnourished or overweight, respectively.[7]

Anthropometric Assessment in Adults To evaluate the nutritional risks associated with illness, clinicians monitor both the total reduction in weight and the rate of weight loss over time. An unintended weight loss of more than 5 percent within 1 month or more than 10 percent within 6 months suggests PEM.[8] Weight changes must be evaluated carefully, however: although unintentional weight loss can indicate malnutrition, weight gain may result from fluid retention rather than recovery of muscle tissue or overnutrition. Fluid retention often accompanies worsening disease in patients with heart failure, liver cirrhosis, and kidney failure and it can mask the weight loss associated with PEM. Some medications can also contribute to weight changes.

Weight data are often expressed as a percentage of usual body weight (%UBW) or ideal body weight (%IBW). The %UBW is more effective than %IBW for interpreting weight changes that occur in underweight, overweight, or obese individuals. In overweight persons, the %IBW may fail to identify significant weight loss. Conversely, in underweight individuals, the %IBW can overstate the degree of weight loss due to illness. Box 14-3 (p. 402) describes how to estimate and evaluate changes in body weight, and Table 14-6 shows how to interpret the %UBW and %IBW.

Some illnesses discussed in later chapters are associated with losses in muscle tissue that resist nutrition intervention. In older adults, losses in both muscle tissue and height are common even though body weights may remain stable. Including measures such as skinfold thicknesses and limb circumferences in a nutrition assessment may help the clinician identify changes in body composition that need to be addressed in the treatment plan.

TABLE 14-6 Body Weight and Nutritional Risk

%UBW	%IBW	Nutritional Risk
85–95	80–90	Risk of mild malnutrition
75–84	70–79	Risk of moderate malnutrition
<75	<70	Risk of severe malnutrition

© Cengage Learning®

Biochemical Analyses

Biochemical data are based on analyses of blood and urine samples, which contain nutrients, proteins, and metabolites that reflect nutrition and health status. Repeated measures are more helpful than single values, as serial data can indicate whether a condition is improving or worsening. Table 14-7 (pp. 402–403) lists and describes common blood tests that may have nutritional implications. Laboratory tests relevant to specific diseases will be discussed in the chapters that follow.

Interpreting laboratory values can be challenging because a number of factors influence test results. For example, fluid imbalances can alter test values: fluid retention

% Weight Loss: The percentage weight loss is calculated by dividing the amount of weight lost by the weight that the person generally maintains:

$$\% \text{ weight loss} = \frac{\text{weight loss}}{\text{usual weight}} \times 100$$

For example, a woman who loses 10 pounds from a usual body weight of 120 pounds will have lost about 8% of her usual weight (10 lb ÷ 120 lb = 0.083 = 8.3%).

%UBW: To estimate %UBW, compare an individual's current weight with the usual body weight:

$$\%\text{UBW} = \frac{\text{current weight}}{\text{usual weight}} \times 100$$

For example, if a man loses 32 pounds during illness and his usual weight is 180 pounds, his current weight would be 148 pounds. These values can be incorporated into the previous equation:

$$\%\text{UBW} = \frac{148}{180} \times 100 = 82.2\%$$

The man in this example weighs 82.2 percent of his usual weight. A look at Table 14-6 shows that a person who is at 82 percent of UBW may be moderately malnourished.

%IBW: To estimate %IBW, compare an individual's current weight with a reasonable (ideal) weight from a BMI table or other appropriate reference:

$$\%\text{IBW} = \frac{\text{current weight}}{\text{ideal weight}} \times 100$$

For example, suppose you wish to calculate the %IBW for a woman who is 5 feet 8 inches tall and weighs 116 pounds. The midpoint of the healthy BMI range is approximately 22, so using a BMI table (as shown on the inside back cover of this book), you estimate that a reasonable weight for this woman would be about 144 pounds:

$$\%\text{IBW} = \frac{116}{144} \times 100 = 80.6\%$$

The woman in this example weighs about 80.6 percent of her ideal body weight. A look at Table 14-6 suggests that, at 80.6 percent of IBW, she may be mildly malnourished. Keep in mind that the calculation of "ideal body weight" is somewhat arbitrary because the BMI table and various other references provide a range of weights for individuals of a given height.

TABLE 14-7   Routine Laboratory Tests with Nutritional Implications

This table lists some commonly performed blood tests that have implications for nutritional problems. Unless whole blood is used, results are generally reported in terms of either *plasma* or *serum* levels. *Plasma* is the yellow fluid that remains after cells are removed and still contains clotting factors. *Serum* is the fluid remaining after both cells and clotting factors are removed.

Laboratory Test	Acceptable Range	Description
Hematology (whole blood samples)		
Red blood cell (RBC) count	Male: 4.3–5.7 million/μL Female: 3.8–5.1 million/μL	RBC number; helps with anemia diagnosis.
Hemoglobin (Hb)	Male: 13.5–17.5 g/dL Female: 12.0–16.0 g/dL	RBC hemoglobin content; helps with anemia diagnosis.
Hematocrit (Hct)	Male: 39–49% Female: 35–45%	Percent RBC volume in blood; helps with anemia diagnosis.
Mean corpuscular volume (MCV)	80–100 fL	RBC size; helps to distinguish microcytic and macrocytic anemia.
Mean corpuscular hemoglobin concentration (MCHC)	31–37% Hb/cell	RBC Hb concentration; helps with diagnosis of iron-deficiency anemia.
White blood cell (WBC) count	4500–11,000 cells/μL	WBC number; may indicate immune status, infection, or inflammation.
Serum Proteins		
Total protein	6.4–8.3 g/dL	Levels are not highly sensitive or specific to disease; may reflect body protein content, illness, infection, inflammation, changes in hydration or metabolism, pregnancy, or use of certain medications.
Albumin	3.4–4.8 g/dL	Levels may reflect illness or PEM; slow to respond to improvement or worsening of disease.

(continued)

TABLE 14-7 (continued)

Laboratory Test	Acceptable Range	Description
Transferrin	200–400 mg/dL >60 yr: 180–380 mg/dL	Levels may reflect illness, PEM, or iron deficiency; slightly more sensitive to changes in health status than albumin.
Transthyretin (prealbumin)	10–40 mg/dL	Levels may reflect illness or PEM; more responsive to changes in health status than albumin or transferrin.
C-reactive protein	68–8200 ng/mL	Elevated levels may indicate inflammation or infection.
Serum Enzymes		
Creatine kinase (CK)	Male: 38–174 U/L Female: 26–140 U/L	Different forms are found in the muscle, brain, and heart. Elevated blood levels may indicate a heart attack, brain tissue damage, or skeletal muscle injury.
Lactate dehydrogenase (LDH)	208–378 U/L	Found in many tissues; specific types may be elevated after a heart attack, lung damage, or liver disease.
Alkaline phosphatase	>20 yr: 25–100 U/L	Found in many tissues; often measured to evaluate liver function.
Aspartate aminotransferase (AST; formerly SGOT)	10–30 U/L	Elevated levels may indicate liver disease or liver damage; somewhat increased after muscle injury.
Alanine aminotransferase (ALT; formerly SGPT)	Male: 10–40 U/L Female: 7–35 U/L	Elevated levels may indicate liver disease or liver damage; somewhat increased after muscle injury.
Serum Electrolytes		
Sodium	136–146 mEq/L	Helps with assessment of hydration status or neuromuscular, kidney, and adrenal functions.
Potassium	3.5–5.1 mEq/L	Helps with assessment of acid–base balance or kidney function; can also detect potassium imbalances.
Chloride	98–106 mEq/L	Helps with assessment of hydration status or detection of acid–base and electrolyte imbalances.
Other		
Glucose (fasting),[a] serum	Adult: 74–106 mg/dL >60 yr: 80–115 mg/dL	Helps with diagnosis of glucose intolerance, diabetes mellitus, and hypoglycemia; also used for monitoring diabetes treatment.
Glycated hemoglobin (HbA_{1c}), whole blood	4.0–6.0% of total Hb	Used for monitoring long-term blood glucose control (approximately 1 to 3 months prior).
Blood urea nitrogen (BUN), serum or plasma	6–20 mg/dL	Primarily used for monitoring kidney function; value altered by liver failure, dehydration, or shock.
Uric acid, serum	Male: 3.5–7.2 mg/dL Female: 2.6–6.0 mg/dL	Used for detection of gout or changes in kidney function; levels affected by age and diet and vary among different ethnic groups.
Creatinine, serum or plasma	Male: 0.7–1.3 mg/dL Female: 0.6–1.1 mg/dL	Used for monitoring renal function.

[a]Fasting glucose levels that repeatedly exceed 100 mg/dL suggest prediabetes.

Note: μL = microliter; dL = deciliter; fL = femtoliter; ng = nanogram; U/L = units per liter; mEq = milliequivalents.

Source: L. Goldman and A. I. Schafer, eds., *Goldman's Cecil Medicine* (Philadelphia: Saunders, 2012).

can cause lab results to be deceptively low, whereas dehydration may cause the values to be deceptively high. Serum protein levels may be influenced by fluid status, infections, inflammation, pregnancy, and other factors. Similarly, serum levels of vitamins and minerals are often poor indicators of nutrient deficiency due to the effects of other physiological factors. Taken together with other assessment data, however, laboratory test results help to present a clearer picture than is possible to obtain otherwise.

Serum Proteins Serum protein levels can aid in the assessment of protein-energy status, but as mentioned earlier, the levels may fluctuate for other reasons as well.[9] Because serum proteins are synthesized in the liver, blood levels of these proteins can reflect liver function. Metabolic stress alters serum proteins because the liver responds to stress by increasing its synthesis of some proteins and reducing the synthesis of others. Values may also be influenced by hydration status, pregnancy, kidney function, zinc status, blood loss, and some medications. Because serum proteins are affected by so many factors, their values must be considered along with other data in order to evaluate nutrition status.

Albumin Albumin is the most abundant protein in blood plasma, and its levels are routinely monitored in hospital patients to help gauge the severity of illness. Although many medical conditions influence albumin, it is slow to reflect changes in nutrition status because of its large body pool and slow rate of degradation. (Box 14-4 lists the **half-life** for albumin and other proteins discussed in this section.) In people with chronic PEM, albumin levels remain normal for a long period despite significant protein depletion, and levels fall only after prolonged malnutrition. Likewise, albumin levels increase slowly when malnutrition is treated, so albumin is not a sensitive indicator of effective treatment.

Transferrin Transferrin is an iron-transport protein, and its blood concentrations respond to iron status, PEM, and various illnesses. Transferrin levels rise as iron status worsens and fall as iron status improves, so using transferrin values to evaluate protein-energy status is difficult if an iron deficiency is also present. Transferrin degrades more rapidly than albumin but its levels change relatively slowly in response to nutrition therapy.

Transthyretin and Retinol-Binding Protein Blood concentrations of transthyretin (also called *prealbumin*) and retinol-binding protein decrease rapidly during PEM and respond quickly to improved protein intakes. Thus, these proteins are more sensitive than albumin to short-term changes in protein status. Although sometimes used to evaluate malnutrition risk or improvement in nutrition status, they are more expensive to measure than albumin so they are not routinely included during nutrition assessment. Like other serum proteins, their usefulness is somewhat limited because they are affected by a number of different factors, including metabolic stress, zinc deficiency, and various medical conditions.

C-Reactive Protein C-reactive protein (CRP) levels rise rapidly in response to inflammation or infection and are often elevated in individuals with critical illness, heart disease, and certain cancers. Elevated CRP values may help to identify individuals at risk for malnutrition, as well as aid in the interpretation of other serum protein tests.[10]

Physical Examinations

As with other assessment methods, interpreting physical signs of malnutrition requires skill and clinical judgment. Most physical signs are nonspecific; they can reflect any of several nutrient deficiencies, as well as conditions unrelated to nutrition. For example, cracked lips may be caused by several B vitamin deficiencies but may also result from sunburn, windburn, or dehydration. Dietary and biochemical data are usually needed as additional evidence to confirm suspected nutrient deficiencies.

Clinical Signs of Malnutrition Signs of malnutrition tend to appear most often in parts of the body where cell replacement occurs at a rapid rate, such as the hair, skin, and digestive tract (including the mouth and tongue). Table 14-8 lists some clinical signs of nutrient deficiencies, and Figure 14-6 illustrates some signs of malnutrition in a child with kwashiorkor. Note that many signs of nutrient deficiency appear only in the advanced stages. Chapters 8 and 9 provide additional examples of the clinical signs of nutrient imbalances.

Hydration Status As mentioned, fluid imbalances may accompany some illnesses and can also result from the use of certain medications. Recognizing the signs of fluid retention or dehydration is necessary for the correct interpretation of blood test results and the body weight measurement.

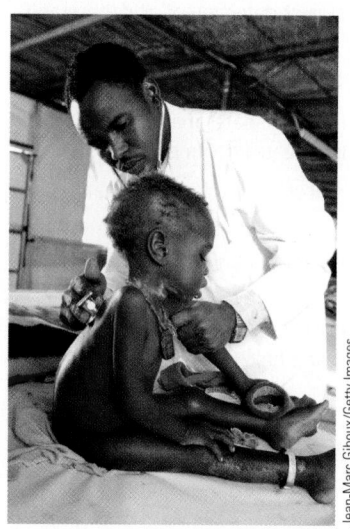

Jean-Marc Giboux/Getty Images

FIGURE 14-6 Physical Examination

In a child with kwashiorkor, physical signs of malnutrition may include sparse, brittle hair; loss of hair color; a swollen abdomen; and dermatitis.

half-life: in blood tests, refers to the time it takes for the concentration of a substance to be reduced by half. Albumin has a half-life of 14 to 20 days, meaning that half of the amount circulating in plasma is degraded in this time period.

TABLE 14-8 Clinical Signs of Nutrient Deficiencies

Body System	Acceptable Appearance	Signs of Malnutrition	Other Causes of Abnormalities
Hair	Shiny, firm in scalp	Dull, brittle, dry, loose; falls out (PEM); corkscrew hair (vitamin C)	Excessive hair bleaching; hair loss from aging, chemotherapy, or radiation therapy
Eyes	Bright; clear; shiny; pink, moist membranes; adjust easily to light	Pale membranes (iron); spots, dryness, night blindness (vitamin A); redness at corners of eyes (B vitamins)	Anemia that is unrelated to nutrition, eye disorders, allergies, aging
Lips	Smooth	Dry, cracked, or with sores in the corners of the lips (B vitamins)	Sunburn, windburn, excessive salivation from ill-fitting dentures or various disorders
Mouth and gums	Oral tissues without lesions, swelling, or bleeding; red tongue; normal sense of taste; teeth without caries; ability to chew and swallow	Bleeding gums (vitamin C); smooth or magenta tongue (B vitamins); poor taste sensation (zinc)	Medications, periodontal disease (poor oral hygiene)
Skin	Smooth, firm, good color	Poor wound healing (PEM, vitamin C, zinc); dry, rough, lack of fat under skin (essential fatty acids, PEM, vitamin A, B vitamins); bruising or bleeding under skin (vitamins C and K); pale (iron)	Poor skin care, diabetes mellitus, aging, medications
Nails	Smooth, firm, uniform, pink	Ridged (PEM); spoon shaped, pale (iron)	—
Other	—	Dementia, peripheral neuropathy (B vitamins); swollen glands at front of neck (PEM, iodine); bowed legs (vitamin D)	Disorders of aging (dementia), diabetes mellitus (peripheral neuropathy)

© 2016 Cengage Learning®

Fluid retention (also called *edema*) may be caused by malnutrition, infection, injury, and some medications. It can also result from impaired blood circulation or disorders of the kidneys, liver, and lungs. Physical signs of fluid retention include weight gain, facial puffiness, swelling of limbs, abdominal distention, and tight-fitting shoes.

Dehydration may be caused by vomiting, diarrhea, sweating, fever, excessive urination, blood loss, and burns (due to fluid loss through skin lesions). Risk of dehydration is especially high in older adults, who have a reduced thirst response and various other impairments in fluid regulation. Signs or symptoms include thirst, weight loss, dry skin or mouth, reduced skin tension, dark yellow or amber urine, and low urine volume.

Functional Assessment Nutrient deficiencies sometimes impair physiological functions, so clinicians may conduct tests or procedures to evaluate some aspects of malnutrition. For example, both PEM and zinc deficiency can depress immunity, which can be evaluated by testing the skin response to antigens that cause redness and swelling when immune function is adequate. Muscle weakness due to **wasting** (loss of muscle tissue) may be assessed by testing hand grip strength. Exercise tolerance, which is reduced in heart and lung disorders, may be evaluated using a treadmill or cycle ergometer.

Determining Energy Requirements

To estimate the energy needs of hospital patients, clinicians often measure or calculate the resting metabolic rate (RMR) and then adjust the RMR value with a "stress factor" that accounts for the medical problem.[11] In ambulatory patients, a factor for activity level may also be applied. Table 14-9 (p. 406) lists examples of RMR equations in common use, and Box 14-5 (p. 406) presents an example of this method. Note that in overweight and obese individuals who not critically ill, the Mifflin–St. Jeor equation has been found to yield the most accurate results.[12]

wasting: the gradual atrophy (loss) of body tissues; associated with protein-energy malnutrition or chronic illness.

TABLE 14-9 Selected Equations for Estimating Resting Metabolic Rate (RMR)

Harris–Benedict[a]

Women: RMR = 655.1 + [9.563 × weight (kg)] + [1.85 × height (cm)] − [4.676 × age (years)]
Men: RMR = 66.5 + [13.75 × weight (kg)] + [5.003 × height (cm)] − [6.755 × age (years)]

Mifflin–St. Jeor

Women: RMR = [9.99 × weight (kg)] + [6.25 × height (cm)] − [4.92 × age (years)] − 161
Men: RMR = [9.99 × weight (kg)] + [6.25 × height (cm)] − [4.92 × age (years)] + 5

[a]Although these equations are sometimes used for estimating basal metabolic rate (BMR), they were derived from data measured during resting conditions in most cases.

RMR Calculations (handwritten)

© Cengage Learning®

How To BOX 14-5 ESTIMATE APPROPRIATE ENERGY INTAKES FOR HOSPITAL PATIENTS

To determine the appropriate energy intake for a hospital patient, the health practitioner may measure or calculate the patient's resting metabolic rate (RMR) and then apply a "stress factor" to accommodate the additional energy needs imposed by illness. The stress factor 1.25 has been shown to be reasonably accurate for many hospitalized patients; other examples are listed in Box 24-2 on p. 633.

The following example uses the Mifflin–St. Jeor equation (shown in Table 14-9) and the stress factor 1.25 to determine the energy needs of a 57-year-old female patient who is 5 feet 3 inches tall, weighs 115 pounds, and is confined to bed.

Step 1: The patient's weight and height are converted to the units used in the equation:

Weight in kilograms = 115 lb ÷ 2.2 lb/kg = 52.3 kg
Height in centimeters = 63 in × 2.54 cm/in = 160 cm

Step 2: Using the Mifflin–St. Jeor equation for estimating RMR in women:

RMR = [9.99 × weight (kg)] + [6.25 × height (cm)] −
[4.92 × age (years)] − 161
= (9.99 × 52.3) + (6.25 × 160) − (4.92 × 57) − 161
= 522 + 1000 − 280 − 161 = 1081 kcal

Step 3: The RMR value is multiplied by the appropriate stress factor:

RMR × stress factor = 1081 × 1.25 = 1351 kcal

Thus, an appropriate energy intake for this patient would be approximately 1351 kcal. Her weight should be monitored to determine if her actual needs are higher or lower.

For a patient who is not confined to bed, an additional activity factor can be applied to accommodate the extra energy needs. For example, if the patient in the example begins limited activity while in the hospital, an activity factor of 1.2 can be multiplied by the results obtained in Step 3:

1351 × activity factor = 1351 × 1.2 = 1621 kcal

The activity factor for a hospitalized patient often falls between 1.1 and 1.4, and it is likely to change as the patient's condition improves.

In patients who are critically ill, energy needs may be higher than normal due to fever, mechanical ventilation, restlessness, or the presence of open wounds. Patients who are critically ill are usually bedridden and inactive, however, so the energy needed for physical activity is minimal. Energy requirements for critical-care patients are described in Chapter 24.

IN SUMMARY

▌ Nutrition assessments include historical information, anthropometric data, biochemical analyses, and physical examinations. Health care providers assess food intake using 24-hour dietary recall interviews, food frequency questionnaires, food records, and direct observation.

▌ Anthropometric measurements, such as height, weight, and body circumferences, help clinicians evaluate growth patterns, overnutrition and undernutrition, and body composition.

Lisa Sawrey is an 80-year-old retired businesswoman who has been a widow for 10 years. She uses a walker and has poorly fitting dentures. She was recently admitted to the hospital with pneumonia and also has congestive heart failure and diabetes. She routinely takes several medications to control her blood glucose levels, hypertension, and heart function. In addition to these medications, the physician has recently ordered antibiotics to treat the pneumonia. During an initial nutrition screening, Mrs. Sawrey stated that she had been eating very poorly over the past 2 weeks. She said that she usually weighs about 125 pounds—a fact that was documented in her medical chart from a previous visit. Although she felt she was losing weight, she didn't know how much weight she may have lost or when she started losing weight. Upon admission to the hospital, Mrs. Sawrey weighed 110 pounds and was 5 feet 3 inches tall. Her serum albumin level was 3.0 grams per deciliter. A physical exam revealed edema, and several other laboratory tests confirmed that she was retaining fluid. As a result of the nutrition screening, Mrs. Sawrey was referred to a registered dietitian for a nutrition assessment.

1. From the brief description provided, which items in Mrs. Sawrey's medical history, personal and social history, and food and nutrition history might alert the dietitian that this patient is at risk of malnutrition?

2. Identify a healthy body weight for Mrs. Sawrey, and calculate her %UBW and %IBW. What do the results reveal? How does the presence of edema influence your evaluation of Mrs. Sawrey's weight loss?

3. How might fluid retention alter Mrs. Sawrey's serum protein levels? What physical symptoms may have indicated that she was retaining excess fluid?

4. What tools can be used to estimate Mrs. Sawrey's usual food intake? What medical, physical, and personal factors are likely to influence her diet?

5. Describe other types of assessment information the dietitian may need before developing a nutrition care plan.

■ Biochemical analyses may indicate nutrient imbalances but are also influenced by various other medical problems.

■ Physical examinations can reveal signs of nutrient deficiencies, fluid imbalances, and functional impairments related to nutritional problems.

■ The energy needs of hospital patients can be estimated by multiplying a person's resting metabolic rate (RMR) by factors that account for the medical condition and activity level.

The case study in Box 14-6 can help you review the different components of a nutrition assessment.

14.3 Implementing Nutrition Care

LO 14.3 Discuss the different types of dietary modifications available to patients with medical problems and explain how each of these is used during patient care.

Once the health care professional has collected assessment information, the next steps of the nutrition care process can be carried out. A nutrition care plan often includes both dietary adjustments and nutrition education. Note that some aspects of nutrition care fall within the scope of dietetics practice, whereas others require the assistance of other health professionals.

Dietary Modifications

During illness, many patients can meet energy and nutrient needs by following a **regular diet.** Other patients may require a **modified diet,** which is altered by changing food consistency or texture, nutrient content, or the foods included in the diet.

regular diet: a diet that includes all foods and meets the nutrient needs of healthy people; may also be called a *standard diet* or *house diet.*

modified diet: a diet that contains foods altered in texture, consistency, or nutrient content or that includes or omits specific foods; may also be called a *therapeutic diet.*

TABLE 14-10 Examples of Modified Diets

Type of Diet[a]	Description of Diet	Appropriate Uses
Modified Texture and Consistency		
Mechanically altered diets	Contain foods that are modified in texture. Pureed food diets include only pureed foods; mechanically altered and soft food diets may include solid foods that are mashed, minced, ground, or soft.	Pureed food diets are used for people with swallowing difficulty, poor lip and tongue control, or oral hypersensitivity. Mechanically altered and soft food diets are appropriate for people with limited chewing ability or certain swallowing impairments.
Blenderized liquid diet	Contains fluids and foods that are blenderized to liquid form.	For people who cannot chew, swallow easily, or tolerate solid foods.
Clear liquid diet	Contains clear fluids or foods that are liquid at room temperature and leave minimal residue in the colon.	For preparation for bowel surgery or colonoscopy, for acute GI disturbances (such as after GI surgeries), or as a transition diet after intravenous feeding. For short-term use only.
Modified Nutrient or Food Content		
Fat-restricted diet	Limits dietary fat to low (<50 g/day) or very low (<25 g/day) intakes.	For people who have certain malabsorptive disorders or symptoms of diarrhea, flatulence, or steatorrhea (fecal fat) resulting from dietary fat intolerance.
Low-fiber diet	Limits dietary fiber; degree of restriction depends on the patient's condition and reason for restriction.	For acute phases of intestinal disorders or to reduce fecal output before surgery. Not recommended for long-term use.
Low-sodium diet	Limits dietary sodium; degree of restriction depends on symptoms and disease severity.	To help lower blood pressure or prevent fluid retention; used in hypertension, congestive heart failure, renal disease, and liver disease.
High-kcalorie, high-protein diet	Contains foods that are kcalorie and protein dense.	Used for patients with high kcalorie and protein requirements (due to cancer, AIDS, burns, trauma, and other conditions); also used to reverse malnutrition, improve nutritional status, or promote weight gain.

[a]Registered dietitians may use the term *nutrition therapy* in place of *diet* when they provide nutrition care; for example, the *low-fiber diet* may be called *low-fiber nutrition therapy*.

Source: Academy of Nutrition and Dietetics, *Nutrition Care Manual* (Chicago: Academy of Nutrition and Dietetics, 2014).

Table 14-10 lists examples of modified diets that are often prescribed during illness.[13] Diets that contain foods with altered texture and consistency may be recommended for individuals with chewing or swallowing impairments. Other dietary modifications may relieve disease symptoms or prevent certain types of complications; for example, restricting dietary fat or fiber may be helpful for people with certain kinds of intestinal disorders, and controlling sodium intake may help to prevent fluid accumulation. A high-kcalorie, high-protein diet may be prescribed to prevent or reverse malnutrition. Note that a person may have several medical problems and a number of modifications may be needed.

Modified diets should be adjusted to satisfy individual preferences and tolerances and may need to be altered as a patient's condition changes. Later chapters include more specific information about modified diets and additional dietary strategies for treating nutritional problems.

Diet Progression A change in diet as a patient's food tolerance improves is called **diet progression.** For example, the diet order may read, "progress diet from clear liquids to a regular diet as tolerated." In practice, this means that the patient would be given clear beverages initially, and then gradually be provided with other beverages or solid foods that are unlikely to cause discomfort. As another example, the diet may progress from small, frequent feedings to larger meals as tolerance improves. Symptoms such as nausea, vomiting, diarrhea, and gastrointestinal pain suggest intolerance.

diet progression: a change in diet as a patient's tolerances permit.

Diet Manual When designing menus for modified diets, the dietary and foodservice personnel refer to a **diet manual,** which details the exact foods or preparation methods to include in or exclude from a modified diet. The diet manual may also outline the rationale and indications for use of the diets and include sample menus. The manual may be compiled by the dietetics staff or adopted from another health care facility or a dietetics organization.

Alternative Feeding Routes In most cases, patients can meet their nutrient needs by consuming regular foods. If their nutrient needs are high or their appetites poor, oral supplements can be added to their diets to improve their intakes. Sometimes, however, a person's medical condition makes it difficult to meet nutrient needs orally. Two options remain: **tube feedings** or **parenteral nutrition,** described more fully in Chapter 16.

- *Tube feedings.* Nutritionally complete formulas can be delivered through a tube placed directly into the stomach or intestine. Tube feedings are preferred to parenteral nutrition if the GI tract is functioning normally.

- *Parenteral nutrition.* A person's medical condition sometimes prohibits the use of the GI tract to deliver nutrients. If the person is malnourished and the GI tract cannot be used for a significant period of time, parenteral nutrition, in which nutrients are supplied intravenously, can meet nutritional needs.

Nothing by Mouth (NPO) An order to not give a patient anything at all—food, beverages, or medications—is indicated by NPO, an abbreviation for *non per os,* meaning "nothing by mouth." For example, an order may read "NPO for 24 hours" or "NPO until after X-ray." The NPO order is commonly used during certain acute illnesses or diagnostic tests involving the GI tract.

Approaches to Nutrition Care

A nutrition care plan often involves significant dietary modifications. To ensure better compliance, the plan must be compatible with the desires and abilities of the person it is designed to help. The challenge is greater if dietary changes are required for extended periods.

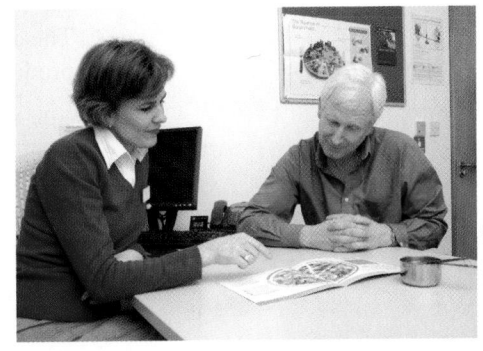

FIGURE 14-7 Nutrition Counseling
Nutrition counseling requires sensitivity to cultural orientation, educational background, and motivation for change.

Long-Term Dietary Intervention When long-term changes are necessary, a care plan must take into account a person's current food practices, lifestyle, and degree of motivation (see Figure 14-7). Behavior change is a process that occurs in stages; therefore, more than one consultation is usually necessary. The following approaches may be helpful in implementing long-term dietary changes:[14]

- *Determine the individual's readiness for change.* Some people have little desire to change their food practices, and even those who are willing may not be fully prepared to take the necessary steps. The health practitioner needs to consider a patient's readiness to adopt new dietary behaviors before attempting to implement an ambitious care plan.

- *Emphasize what to eat, rather than what not to eat.* Emphasizing foods to include in the diet, rather than those to restrict, can make dietary changes more appealing. For example, encouraging additional fruits and vegetables is a more attractive message than telling the patient to restrict butter, cream sauces, and ice cream.

- *Suggest only one or two changes at a time.* People are more likely to adopt a nutrition care plan that does not deviate too much from their usual diet. If they succeed in adopting one or two changes, they are more likely to stick to the plan and be open to additional suggestions. Stricter plans may yield quicker results but are useful only for highly motivated people.

diet manual: a resource that specifies the foods or preparation methods to include in or exclude from modified diets and provides sample menus.

tube feedings: liquid formulas delivered through a tube placed in the stomach or intestine.

parenteral nutrition: the provision of nutrients by vein, bypassing the intestine.

Nutrition Education Nutrition education allows patients to learn about the dietary factors that affect their particular medical condition. Ideally, this knowledge can motivate them to change their diet and lifestyle in order to improve their health status.

A nutrition education program should be tailored to a person's age, level of literacy, and cultural background. Learning style must also be considered: some people learn best by discussion supplemented with written materials, whereas others prefer a demonstration with visual examples, such as food models and measuring devices.[15] Information can be provided in one-on-one sessions or group discussions. The meeting should include an assessment of the person's understanding of the material and commitment to making changes. Follow-up sessions can reveal whether the person has successfully adopted a dietary plan. For example, a dietitian who counsels a woman who is lactose intolerant and hesitant to use milk products might proceed as follows:

- The dietitian provides sample menus of a nutritionally adequate diet that limits milk and milk products. Together, the dietitian and the woman design menus that consider her food preferences.

- The dietitian describes the types and amounts of milk products that would likely be tolerated without causing symptoms and explains how to gradually incorporate these foods into the diet.

- Using diet analysis software, the dietitian demonstrates how altering intakes of calcium- and vitamin D–containing foods changes a meal's nutrient content.

- The dietitian explains how to use the Daily Values on food labels to estimate the calcium content of packaged foods.

- The dietitian provides information about the advantages and disadvantages of different calcium and vitamin D supplements.

- The dietitian assesses the woman's understanding by having her identify nonmilk products that are high in calcium or vitamin D.

Ideally, the dietitian would be able to monitor the woman's progress in a subsequent counseling session.

Documenting Nutrition Care

Each step of the nutrition care process must be documented in the patient's medical record. The entries should be as succinct as possible so that they can be quickly read and easily understood by other members of the health care team. In addition, electronic (computerized) medical records, which have been widely adopted in the past decade, have standardized templates that require concise language. Before making entries in medical records, health care professionals need to learn the particular charting methods preferred by their medical facility. Although a variety of charting styles are in use, the content is more relevant than the particular format used.

ADIME Format The ADIME format closely reflects the steps of the nutrition care process. The letters represent the different steps: *A*ssessment, *D*iagnosis, *I*ntervention, and *M*onitoring and *E*valuation. Using this format, the nutrition care plan is recorded as follows:

- *Assessment.* The assessment section summarizes relevant assessment results, such as the medical problem, historical information, height, weight, BMI, laboratory test results, and relevant symptoms.

- *Diagnosis.* The diagnosis section lists and prioritizes the nutrition diagnoses.

- *Intervention.* The intervention section describes treatment goals and expected outcomes, specific interventions, and the patient's responses to nutrition care.

Monitoring and Evaluation. The monitoring and evaluation section records the patient's progress, changes in the patient's condition, and adjustments in the care plan.

SOAP Format. The SOAP format is the oldest method used for documenting nutrition care and is still in popular use. The letters represent the types of information included in each section: *S*ubjective, *O*bjective, *A*ssessment, and the *P*lan for care.

- *Subjective* information is obtained in an interview with the patient or caregiver and includes the chief medical problem and relevant symptoms.

- *Objective* information includes nutrition screening or assessment data, such as the results of anthropometric and laboratory tests and the physical examination.

- The *Assessment* section contains a brief evaluation of the subjective and objective data and provides concise diagnoses of the nutrition problems.

- The *Plan* includes recommendations that can help solve the problem, including the nutrition prescription, plan for nutrition education and counseling, and referrals to other professionals or agencies.

Figure 14-8 shows an example of a SOAP note, although many variations are possible.

Improving Food Intake

People in hospitals and other medical facilities often lose their appetites as a result of their medical condition, treatment, or emotional distress. Moreover, some medications and other treatments can dramatically alter taste perceptions. Patients may receive meals at specified times, whether they are hungry or not, and often must eat in bed without companionship. Under these types of conditions, eating can become

SOAP NOTE

Patient Name: James Steiner   **ID:** 009821   **Date/Time:** 09/15/2015, 11:15 a.m.

Age: 58   **Gender:** Male   **Medical diagnosis:** Hypercholesterolemia

Subjective
Patient reports excessive snacking at work, little exercise, recent weight gain of 10 lb in past year; willing to attempt 5% weight loss and dietary/lifestyle changes to reduce LDL-C before trying statin medication

Objective
Height: 6'1"; Weight: 268 lb
Total cholesterol: 288 mg/dL
LDL-C: 214 mg/dL; HDL-C: 48 mg/dL
Triglycerides: 132 mg/dL

BMI: 35.4, obesity II
Waist circumference: 45"
EER: 2725 kcal
Diet order: Weight reduction; heart-healthy diet

Assessment
Abdominal obesity; dietary recall indicates ~3700 kcal intake per day and diet high in fat, saturated fat, *trans* fat
Nutrition Diagnoses: 1. Obesity related to excess energy intake of ~1000 kcal/day and physical inactivity as evidenced by elevated BMI; 2. Less than optimal fat intake related to poor food choices as evidenced by elevated LDL cholesterol and body weight

Plan
Goal: 15 lb weight loss over next 6 months; patient to walk 45-min/day
Nutrition prescription: 2700 kcal/day weight reduction with ~30% kcal from fat, 7% of kcal from saturated fat, minimal *trans* fat

Initial education: discussed food portions, low-kcal foods, sources of saturated and *trans* fats, pre-planning meals and snacks
Referral: Heart-healthy workshop on 9/22; patient to attend with wife
Follow-up visit: 10/15 (1 month); patient to bring 3-day food record and identify appropriate portions, saturated/*trans* fat sources

Signature: Genevieve Johnson, M.S., R.D.   **Position:** Dietitian, Nutrition Services

© Cengage Learning®

FIGURE 14-8 Example of a SOAP Note

1. Empathize with the patient. Show that you understand how difficult eating may be when a person feels too sick to move or too tired to sit up. Help to motivate the patient by explaining how important good nutrition is to recovery.

2. Help patients select the foods they like and mark menus appropriately. When appropriate and permissible, let family members or friends bring favorite foods from outside the hospital.

3. For patients who are weak, suggest foods that require little effort to eat. Eating a roast beef sandwich, for example, requires less effort than cutting and eating a steak. Drinking soup from a cup may be easier than eating it with a spoon.

4. During mealtimes, make sure the patient's room is quiet and has sufficient lighting for viewing the food. See that the room is free of odors that may interfere with the appetite.

5. Help patients prepare for meals. Help them wash their hands and get comfortable, either in bed or in a chair. Adjust the extension table to a comfortable distance and height and make sure it is clean. Take these steps before the food tray arrives so that the meal can be served promptly and at the right temperature.

6. When the food cart arrives, check the patient's tray. Confirm that the patient is receiving the right diet, the foods on the tray are those selected from the menu, and the foods look appealing. Order a new tray if the foods are not appropriate.

7. Help with eating, if necessary. Help patients open containers or cut foods, and assist with feeding if patients cannot feed themselves. Encourage patients with little appetite to eat the most nutritious foods first and to drink liquids between meals.

8. Take a positive attitude toward the hospital's food. Never say something like "I couldn't eat this either." Instead, say, "The foodservice department really tries to make foods appetizing. I'm sure we can find a solution."

more of a chore than a pleasurable experience. Meals may also be unwelcome if the person is in pain or has been sedated.

To improve food intakes, health professionals should ensure that the patient's room remains calm and quiet during mealtime. Excessive activity, like room maintenance or ward rounds, can distract patients and reduce appetite. If the patient's appetite or sense of taste is affected by illness, the patient can be asked to identify foods that are the most enjoyable. Box 14-7 lists additional suggestions that may help to improve food intake at mealtimes. The case study in Box 14-8 provides an opportunity for you to review the implementation of nutrition care.

IN SUMMARY

▪ Dietary modifications prescribed during illness include changes in food texture or consistency, modified energy or nutrient content, or the inclusion or exclusion of certain foods. Some medical conditions may require the use of tube feedings or parenteral nutrition.

Case Study   BOX 14-8 IMPLEMENTING NUTRITION CARE

Max is a 14-year-old boy who was admitted to the hospital after he passed out while playing with friends. Tests confirm a diagnosis of type 1 diabetes mellitus. Max remains in the hospital for several days until his blood glucose and ketone levels are under control. During this time, he and his family learn about diabetes, the diet Max needs to follow, the use of insulin, the monitoring of blood glucose levels, and the required coordination of diet, insulin, and physical activity. The details of diabetes mellitus are reserved for Chapter 21, but for now you can consider the steps that are necessary for implementing Max's nutrition care.

1. Given the chronic nature of Max's illness and his age, what approaches should the health care provider use when discussing the required meal plan and insulin treatment with Max and his family?

2. What factors need consideration when designing a nutrition education program for Max and his parents?

3. Max will need additional care to learn more about diabetes and to make the adjustments that will allow him to cope with his condition. Why is it important to address follow-up care before Max leaves the hospital?

- A nutrition care plan should take into account a person's food practices, lifestyle, and degree of motivation. Nutrition education should be individualized to accommodate a patient's needs and learning style.

- Nutrition care must be clearly documented in the medical record; the ADIME and SOAP formats are popular styles of documentation.

- Hospital patients may need assistance at mealtime and encouragement to consume adequate amounts of food.

Clinical Applications

1. Describe the potential nutritional implications of these findings from a patient's medical, personal, and social histories: age 78, lives alone, recently lost spouse, uses a walker, has no natural teeth or dentures, has a history of hypertension and diabetes, uses medications that cause frequent urination, sleeps poorly, often feels depressed.

2. Calculate the %UBW and %IBW for a man who is 5 feet 11 inches tall with a current weight of 150 pounds and a usual body weight of 180 pounds. What additional information do you need to interpret the implications of his weight loss?

3. Jacob is a 29-year-old male who is 6 feet 2 inches tall and has a usual body weight of 180 pounds. He was admitted to the hospital following an automobile accident and was treated for minor injuries. Using the method described in Box 14-5 on p. 408, estimate an appropriate energy intake for Jacob using the Mifflin–St. Jeor equation. Use the stress factor 1.25, with no additional activity factor.

4. A healthy 70-year-old woman, admitted to the hospital for a hip replacement surgery, develops an infection after the surgery and recovery is slower than expected. You notice that she seems uninterested in meals and has eaten only small amounts of food for several days. What steps can be taken to uncover and address problems that the woman might be having with food?

Self Check

1. Mr. Hom experiences loss of appetite, difficulty swallowing, and mouth pain as a consequence of illness. Mr. Hom is at risk of malnutrition due to:
   a. altered metabolism.
   b. reduced food intake.
   c. altered excretion of nutrients.
   d. altered digestion and absorption.

2. Of the following data collected during a nutrition screening, which item does *not* place the person at risk for malnutrition?
   a. Having a health problem that is frequently associated with PEM
   b. Using prescription medications that affect nutrient needs
   c. Residing with a spouse in a middle-income neighborhood
   d. Significantly reducing food intake over the past five or more days

3. The nutrition care process is a systematic approach for:
   a. identifying the nutrient content of foods.
   b. ordering special diets.
   c. conducting a nutrition screening.
   d. meeting the nutritional needs of patients.

4. Which dietary assessment method does a health practitioner use to conduct a kcalorie count?
   a. Direct observation
   b. 24-hour recall interview
   c. Food frequency questionnaire
   d. Food record

5. The %UBW of a person who weighs 135 pounds and has a usual body weight of 150 pounds is:
   a. 111 percent.
   b. 90 percent.
   c. 86 percent.
   d. 74 percent.

6. A malnourished, acutely ill patient has just begun to eat after days without significant amounts of food. Which of the following blood test results would change most quickly as the patient's nutrition and health status improves?
   a. Albumin
   b. Transferrin
   c. Serum electrolytes
   d. Retinol-binding protein

7. Fluid retention may cause all of the following effects *except:*
   a. swelling of limbs.
   b. facial puffiness.
   c. weight loss.
   d. tight-fitting shoes.

8. A nurse notices a food on a patient's tray and is not sure if the food is allowed on the patient's diet. An appropriate action for the nurse to take would be to check the:
   a. diet manual.
   b. diet order.
   c. nutrition care plan.
   d. medical record.

9. A successful nutrition intervention would include a long list of:
   a. dietary changes that the patient should consider making.
   b. foods that the patient should avoid.
   c. appetizing meals and foods that the patient can include in the diet.
   d. reasons why the patient should make dietary changes.

10. The most important factor(s) that affect(s) how nutrition education is presented is (are):
   a. the person's nutrient needs and nutrition status.
   b. the person's abilities and motivation.
   c. the person's medical history.
   d. the entries in the medical record.

Answers to these questions can be found in Appendix H.

Notes

1. J. V. White and coauthors, Consensus statement of the Academy of Nutrition and Dietetics/ American Society for Parenteral and Enteral Nutrition: Characteristics recommended for the identification and documentation of adult malnutrition (undernutrition), *Journal of the Academy of Nutrition and Dietetics* 112 (2012): 730–738.

2. E. Saltzman and K. M. Mogensen, Physical and clinical assessment of nutrition status, in A. M. Coulston, C. J. Boushey, and M. G. Ferruzzi, eds., *Nutrition in the Prevention and Treatment of Disease* (London: Academic Press/Elsevier, 2013), pp. 65–79.

3. The Academy Quality Management Committee and Scope of Practice Subcommittee of the Quality Management Committee, Academy of Nutrition and Dietetics: Revised 2012 standards of practice in nutrition care and standards of professional performance for registered dietitians, *Journal of the Academy of Nutrition and Dietetics* 113 (2013): S29–S45.

4. The Academy Quality Management Committee and Scope of Practice Subcommittee of the Quality Management Committee, 2013.

5. F. E. Thompson and A. F. Subar, Dietary assessment methodology, in A. M. Coulston, C. J.

Boushey, and M. G. Ferruzzi, eds., *Nutrition in the Prevention and Treatment of Disease* (London: Academic Press/Elsevier, 2013), pp. 5–46; K. S Stote and coauthors, The number of 24 h dietary recalls using the U.S. Department of Agriculture's automated multiple-pass method required to estimate nutrient intake in overweight and obese adults, *Public Health Nutrition* 14 (2011): 1736–1742.

6. E. Saltzman and K. M. Mogensen, Physical and clinical assessment of nutrition status, in A. M. Coulston, C. J. Boushey, and M. G. Ferruzzi, eds., *Nutrition in the Prevention and Treatment of Disease* (London: Academic Press/Elsevier, 2013), pp. 65–79.

7. S. Going, M. Hingle, and J Farr, Body composition, in A. C. Ross and coeditors, eds., *Modern Nutrition in Health and Disease* (Baltimore: Lippincott Williams & Wilkins, 2014), pp. 635–648.

8. A. Malone and C. Hamilton, Academy of Nutrition and Dietetics/American Society for Parenteral and Enteral Nutrition consensus malnutrition characteristics: Application in practice, *Nutrition in Clinical Practice* 28 (2013): 639–650.

9. C. W. Thompson, Laboratory assessment, in P. Charney and A. M. Malone, eds., *ADA Pocket*

Guide to Nutrition Assessment (Chicago: American Dietetic Association, 2009), pp. 62–153.

10. Malone and Hamilton, 2013.

11. E. Leistra and coauthors, Predictors for achieving protein and energy requirements in undernourished hospital patients, *Clinical Nutrition* 30 (2011): 484–489.

12. D. C. Frankenfield, Bias and accuracy of resting metabolic rate equations in non-obese and obese adults, *Clinical Nutrition* 32 (2013): 976–982.

13. Academy of Nutrition and Dietetics, *Nutrition Care Manual* (Chicago: Academy of Nutrition and Dietetics, 2014).

14. L. E. Burke and coauthors, Current theoretical bases for nutrition intervention and their uses, in A. M. Coulston, C. J. Boushey, and M. G. Ferruzzi, eds., *Nutrition in the Prevention and Treatment of Disease* (London: Academic Press/Elsevier, 2013), pp. 141–155.

15. L. M. Delahanty and J. M. Heins, Tools and techniques to facilitate nutrition intervention, in A. M. Coulston, C. J. Boushey, and M. G. Ferruzzi, eds., *Nutrition in the Prevention and Treatment of Disease* (London: Academic Press/Elsevier, 2013), pp. 169–189.

LO 14.4 Explain how nutritional genomics research may improve our understanding of the relationship between illness and nutrition care.

Consider this situation: A physician scrapes your cheek to collect a sample of cells and submits the sample to a **genomics** lab. In a short time, you receive a report that reveals your disease susceptibilities and suggests dietary and lifestyle changes that can improve your health. You may even be given a prescription for food choices or a dietary supplement that will best meet your personal nutrient requirements. Unlikely? Perhaps, but these possibilities are being explored by scientists working in the field of **nutritional genomics,** the study of dietary effects on **gene expression.** Recent research suggests that some dietary factors may be more helpful (or more harmful) in people who have particular genetic variations. The promise of nutritional genomics is a custom-designed dietary prescription that fits each person's specific needs. The accompanying glossary (see Box NP14-1, p. 416) defines genomics and related terms.

What is a genome?

Genetic information is encoded in DNA molecules within the nuclei of almost all of the cells in our bodies. Figure NP14-1 shows how the genetic material is organized within the **genome,** the complete set of genetic information within our cells. The DNA molecules are tightly packed along with associated proteins within the 46 **chromosomes.** Segments of a DNA strand that can eventually be translated into proteins are called **genes.** The sequence of **nucleotides** within each gene encodes the amino acid sequence of a particular protein. Scientists estimate that there are between 20,000 and 25,000 genes in the human genome.[1] However, only a small percentage (about 2 percent) of the genome codes for proteins; most DNA consists of **noncoding sequences,** which may help to regulate gene expression or have other functions.

When proteins are made, the information in the DNA sequence is first transcribed (copied) to messenger RNA molecules, which carry the genetic information from the nucleus to the cytoplasm. Gene expression can be measured by determining the amounts of messenger RNA in a tissue sample. The expression of thousands of genes can be measured simultaneously using **microarray technology** (see Figure NP14-2 on p. 416).

FIGURE NP14-1 **The Human Genome**

1 The human genome is a complete set of genetic material organized into 46 chromosomes, located within the nucleus of a cell.

2 A chromosome is made of DNA and associated proteins.

3 The double helical structure of a DNA molecule is made up of two long chains of nucleotides. Each nucleotide is composed of a phosphate group, a 5-carbon sugar, and a base.

4 The sequence of nucleotide bases (C, G, A, T) determines the amino acid sequence of proteins. These bases are connected by hydrogen bonding to form base pairs: adenine (A) with thymine (T) and guanine (G) with cytosine (C).

5 A gene is a segment of DNA that includes the information needed to synthesize one or more proteins.

© Cengage Learning®

A DNA microarray allows researchers to monitor the expression of thousands of genes simultaneously.

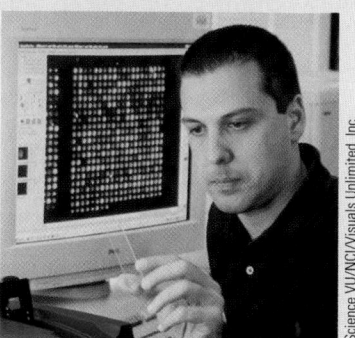

Science VU/NCI/Visuals Unlimited, Inc.

How do nutrients alter gene expression?

Various nutrients can switch gene expression on or off.[2] The **promoter** region of a gene (a DNA sequence involved with gene activation) acts as the master switch. A large variety of proteins known as **transcription factors** can bind to areas on the promoter and either enhance or inhibit gene expression. A combination of dietary factors and hormones influences the types of transcription factors that reach the nucleus and their tendency to bind to DNA. Specific examples of how nutrients can influence transcription factors include:

- The transcription factor that enhances the gene expression of enzymes required for cholesterol synthesis enters the nucleus only when the cellular cholesterol content is low.

- The transcription factor that inhibits the expression of ferritin, an iron-storage protein, changes its affinity for DNA based on the iron content of the cell.

Gene expression is also influenced by modifications in the structure of DNA and its packaging in chromosomes. For example, **methylation** of DNA molecules (the addition of methyl groups) alters the expression of numerous genes and depends on both inherited factors and the availability of certain nutrients. In individuals who are susceptible to a disease that is influenced by DNA methylation, an altered diet or nutrient supplementation can potentially reduce the risk of disease.[3] The field of **epigenetics** investigates processes that cause heritable changes in gene expression that are separate from the underlying DNA nucleotide sequence.

How much genetic variation is there among people?

Except for identical twins, no two individuals are genetically identical. However, the variation in the genomes of any two persons is only about 1 to 3 percent,[4] a difference of approximately one base in every few hundred. Genetic differences, known as **polymorphisms,** are variations in the DNA sequence of a particular gene. The most common type of polymorphism is a *single-nucleotide polymorphism,* characterized by a nucleotide

insertion, deletion, or substitution in the DNA molecule. Genetic variations are significant only if they affect a protein's amino acid sequence in a way that alters the protein's function, or if the change in the DNA molecule changes how a particular gene is regulated.

Genetic variation gives rise to the diversity among human beings—it explains most of the differences in our physical appearances and metabolic characteristics. Along with environmental factors, it also determines our susceptibilities to disease. Diseases affected by a single gene tend to be relatively rare and usually exert their effects early in life. In contrast, common diseases such as heart disease and cancer are influenced by many genes and typically develop over several decades or even longer. In these more complex **multigene,** or **polygenic,** disorders, many genes

---

BOX NP14-1 GLOSSARY

chromosomes: structures within the nucleus of a cell that contain the cell's DNA and associated proteins.

epigenetics: processes that cause heritable changes in gene expression that are separate from the DNA nucleotide sequence.

gene expression: the process by which a cell converts the genetic code into RNA and protein.

genes: segments of DNA that contain the information needed to make proteins.

genome (JEE-nome)**:** the full complement of genetic material in the chromosomes of a cell.

genomics (jee-NO-miks)**:** the study of genomes.

methylation: the addition of methyl ($-CH_3$) groups.

microarray technology: research technology that monitors the expression of thousands of genes simultaneously.

multigene or **polygenic:** involving a number of genes, rather than a single gene.

noncoding sequences: regions of DNA that do not code for proteins. Some noncoding sequences may have regulatory or structural properties, but most have no known function.

nucleotides: the subunits of DNA and RNA molecules. These compounds—cytosine (C), thymine (T), uracil (U), guanine (G), and adenine (A)—are each composed of a phosphate group, a 5-carbon sugar (ribose), and a nitrogen-containing base. A DNA molecule is made up of two long chains of nucleotides held together by hydrogen bonding between nucleotide bases on opposing strands; each hydrogen-bonded nucleotide couple is called a *base pair.*

nutritional genomics: the study of dietary effects on genetic expression; also known as *nutrigenomics.*

polymorphisms: variations in DNA sequences of a particular gene. A *single-nucleotide polymorphism,* the most common type of polymorphism, involves the insertion, deletion, or substitution of a single nucleotide in the DNA strand.

- *poly* = many
- *morph* = form
- *ism* = condition

promoter: a region of DNA involved with gene activation.

transcription factors: proteins that bind DNA at specific sequences to regulate gene expression.

can contribute to disease risk, but no single gene may be sufficient to cause the disease on its own. In addition, the specific genes that influence a person's susceptibility to disease may vary substantially among different individuals.

What are some examples of single-gene disorders?

Examples of single-gene disorders include phenylketonuria (discussed in Nutrition in Practice 16), sickle-cell anemia, and the iron-overload disease hemochromatosis. Single-gene disorders may seriously disrupt metabolism and often require significant dietary or medical intervention. However, not all single-gene disorders have life-threatening ramifications. For example, lactose intolerance is related to an alteration in the promoter of the lactase gene; the condition may cause gastrointestinal discomfort but is readily managed by simple dietary changes.

How are multigene disorders different from single-gene disorders?

Multigene disorders are usually sensitive to a number of environmental influences, including diet and lifestyle; these environmental factors can directly influence the expression of the genes involved. Multigene disorders tend to develop over many years, so determining genetic susceptibility may allow a person to modify diet and lifestyle appropriately and reduce their disease risk before signs and symptoms appear.

Heart disease is an example of a disease with multiple gene influences.[5] Its many risk factors represent the involvement of an assortment of genes, which affect disparate aspects of physiology and metabolism. Consider that the major risk factors for heart disease include elevated blood cholesterol levels, hypertension, type 2 diabetes, and obesity. The underlying cause of any of these risk factors is rarely known; currently, clinicians screen for the presence of risk factors but not for the reasons why they occur. Should genomic research prove successful, a future assessment might be to identify specific genetic variations that can lead to the development of individual risk factors. For example, tests may determine whether a person's high blood cholesterol levels are due to excessive cholesterol absorption, excessive cholesterol production in the liver, or reduced cholesterol degradation. This information could then guide health care providers to the most appropriate intervention, allowing a better match between treatment recommendations and a person's genetic profile.

Can genomic research be used to explore the differences in nutrient needs among people?

Even though most people apparently can meet their nutrient needs by consuming nutrients at recommended levels, it would be useful to learn more about genetic variations within healthy populations. The techniques that have emerged from genomic research may provide a means for fine-tuning nutrient recommendations for different individuals. Moreover, ideal indicators of nutrient status are still lacking for several of the minerals, such as zinc, magnesium, and chromium. Scientists hope to eventually produce genomic maps that will indicate how various nutrient deficiencies and combinations of deficiencies affect gene expression. These maps may eventually provide data that can help diagnose nutrient deficiencies.

Will knowledge about the human genome substantially change the manner in which health care is provided?

The enthusiasm surrounding genomic research should be put into perspective in terms of both the status of clinical medicine at present and people's willingness to make difficult lifestyle choices. Critics have questioned whether genetic markers for disease are more useful than simple and inexpensive clinical measurements, which reflect both genetic and environmental influences.[6] In other words, knowing that a person is genetically predisposed toward high cholesterol levels is not necessarily more useful than knowing the person's actual blood cholesterol level. Furthermore, a person's family history is already a simple genomic tool that indicates a higher genetic risk for certain illnesses. Understanding the family's medical history allows the clinician to use risk-reduction strategies that are appropriate to the culture and literacy of the patient, rather than focusing on genetic risk alone.[7]

Obtaining additional knowledge about disease risk is not necessarily useful unless people are motivated to make serious lifestyle changes. For example, despite the present abundance of disease prevention recommendations, many people seem unwilling or unable to make the changes known to improve health.[8] Researchers have estimated that heart disease and type 2 diabetes are 80 percent and 90 percent preventable, respectively, by changing one's lifestyle to include an appropriate diet, a healthy body weight, and regular exercise, among other factors.[9] Given the difficulty that people have with current recommendations, it is unlikely that they will enthusiastically adopt an even more detailed list of dietary and lifestyle modifications.

What ethical concerns are raised by having extensive knowledge about an individual's genome?

A primary concern with our newfound ability to obtain detailed genetic information is confidentiality: should information about a person's susceptibility to disease be released to others (including other family members at risk) without that person's consent? Concern about privacy issues has led to federal and state legislation that prevents discrimination by group health plans, health insurers, and employers on the basis of an individual's genetic predisposition to disease.[10]

Another consideration is whether genetic testing is always in the best interest of children. Although early knowledge of a child's predisposition to illnesses may be useful for parents who want to provide optimal care, the release of this information could threaten the child's privacy and increase the potential for genetic discrimination in the future. In addition, children at high risk of developing a serious illness may grow up believing that their future choices are limited and may alter their life course to accommodate a disease that may never develop.[11]

Although genomic research has the potential to improve our ability to diagnose and treat disease, it is still unclear how knowledge of the genome will be translated into useful medical treatments. Health care professionals will need to keep informed of the ethical, legal, and social implications of nutritional and medical genomics as this remarkable research continues.

Notes

1. P. Stankiewicz and J. R. Lupski, Gene, genomic, and chromosomal disorders, in L. Goldman and A. I. Schafer, eds., *Goldman's Cecil Medicine* (Philadelphia: Saunders, 2012), pp. 187–195.

2. R. J. Cousins and L. A. Lichten, Nutritional regulation of gene expression and nutritional genomics, in A. C. Ross and coeditors, eds., *Modern Nutrition in Health and Disease* (Baltimore: Lippincott Williams & Wilkins, 2014), pp. 515–522.

3. S.-W. Choi and S. Friso, Epigenetics: A new bridge between nutrition and health, *Advances in Nutrition* 1 (2010): 8–16; G. C. Burdge and K. A. Lillycrop, Nutrition, epigenetics, and developmental plasticity: Implications for understanding human disease, *Annual Review of Nutrition* 30 (2010): 315–339.

4. P. J. Stover and Z. Gu, Genetic variation: Effect on nutrient utilization and metabolism, in A. C. Ross and coeditors, eds., *Modern Nutrition in Health and Disease* (Baltimore: Lippincott Williams & Wilkins, 2014), pp. 523–533.

5. C. J. O'Donnell and E. G. Nabel, Genomics of cardiovascular disease, *New England Journal of Medicine* 365 (2011): 2098–2109.

6. R. San-Cristobal, F. I. Milagro, and J. A. Martinez, Future challenges and present ethical considerations in the use of personalized nutrition based on genetic advice, *Journal of the Academy of Nutrition and Dietetics* 113 (2013): 1447–1454; W. C. Willett, Balancing life-style and genomics research for disease prevention, *Science* 296 (2002): 695–698.

7. M. J. Khoury and coauthors, Do we need genomic research for the prevention of common diseases with environmental causes? *American Journal of Epidemiology* 161 (2005): 799–805.

8. R. W. Grant and coauthors, Personalized genetic risk counseling to motivate diabetes prevention, *Diabetes Care* 36 (2013): 13–19; J. P. Evans and coauthors, Deflating the genomic bubble, *Science* 331 (2011): 861–862.

9. Khoury and coauthors, 2005.

10. P. R. Reilly and R. M. DeBusk, Ethical and legal issues in nutritional genomics, *Journal of the American Dietetic Association* 108 (2008): 36–40.

11. B. R. Korf, Principles of genetics, in L. Goldman and A. I. Schafer, eds., *Goldman's Cecil Medicine* (Philadelphia: Saunders, 2012), pp. 184–187.

15

Medications, Diet-Drug Interactions, and Herbal Supplements

15.1 Medications in Disease Treatment

LO 15.1 Explain how medications are used in patient care and discuss the potential risks associated with their use.

15.2 Diet-Drug Interactions

LO 15.2 Identify the different types of diet-drug interactions and give examples of each.

15.3 Herbal Supplements

LO 15.3 Give examples of some popular herbal products and explain why they are not considered reliable treatments during illness.

15.4 Nutrition in Practice: Complementary and Alternative Therapies

LO 15.4 Explain how complementary and alternative therapies differ from those used in conventional medicine and describe the various types of alternative therapies currently available.

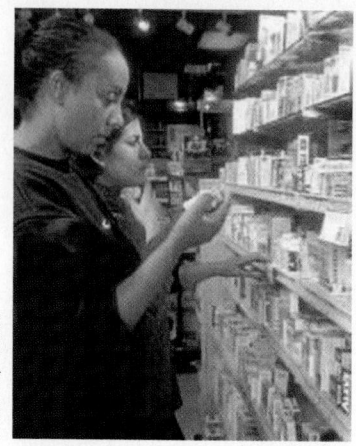

FIGURE 15-1 Consumers Shopping for OTC Drugs
OTC drugs are considered safe enough for self-medication but can cause adverse effects when used inappropriately.

Although many people rely on medications to treat or prevent medical problems, some may not realize that the drugs may have dangerous effects when taken incorrectly. Certain medications can alter body processes and cause serious side effects; others may disrupt nutrient metabolism or cause toxicity due to interactions with dietary substances. This chapter introduces the use of medications in clinical care, describes potential diet-drug interactions, and discusses herbal supplements, which many individuals use in hope of improving their health in some way. Nutrition in Practice 15 describes the various categories and uses of complementary and alternative therapies.

15.1 Medications in Disease Treatment

LO 15.1 Explain how medications are used in patient care and discuss the potential risks associated with their use.

Drugs must be proved to be safe and effective before they can be marketed in the United States. The Food and Drug Administration (FDA) is responsible for approving sales of new drugs and inspecting facilities where drugs are manufactured. By law, drugs are divided into two categories:[1]

▎ *Prescription drugs* are usually given to treat serious conditions and may cause severe side effects. For these reasons, they are sold by prescription only, which ensures that a physician has evaluated the patient's medical condition and determined that the benefits of using the medication outweigh the risks of incurring side effects.

▎ *Over-the-counter (OTC) drugs* are those that individuals can use safely and effectively without medical supervision (see Figure 15-1). People use them to treat less serious illnesses that are easily self-diagnosed. Examples include aspirin to treat headaches or pain and antacids to combat acid reflux. The FDA regulates labels on OTC drugs to make sure they provide accurate information about the drugs' appropriate uses and dosages and potential adverse effects. Prescription drugs considered safe enough for self-medication are often given OTC status, sometimes in smaller doses than are available by prescription.

Brand-name drugs are usually given patent protection for 20 years after the patent is submitted. After the patent expires, a less-expensive **generic drug** may be sold. To gain FDA approval, the generic version of a drug must have similar biological effects as compared with the original drug: it must contain the same active ingredients; be identical in strength, dosage form, and route of administration; and meet the same requirements for purity and quality. In some cases, the bioavailability (amount absorbed) of a brand-name drug and generic drug may differ due to differences in the drugs' solubility or the types of inactive ingredients present; thus, greater benefit may be obtained by using the brand-name drug.[2] Most often, however, consumers can be confident that generic drugs are as safe and effective as the brand-name products they replace.

Risks from Medications

The risk of an adverse reaction always accompanies the use of a medicine. Thus, a medication should be used only when the benefits of using it outweigh the potential risks. The risks become greater when a drug is incorrectly prescribed or administered. This section discusses the types of risks associated with medications and suggests some steps for managing risk.

Side Effects By the time a drug reaches the marketplace, large-scale clinical trials have revealed the majority of side effects associated with its use. However, rare side effects are sometimes detected only after a drug has been more widely used. In some

generic drug: a drug that lacks patent protection. Examples include the sedative *diazepam*, which is equivalent to the brand-name drug *Valium,* and the diuretic *furosemide,* equivalent to the brand-name drug *Lasix.*

instances, these effects occur because the drugs are used for longer periods or in different circumstances than originally anticipated.

The FDA monitors adverse events after drugs are marketed. Manufacturers are required to submit periodic reports, and individuals using the drugs are encouraged to report unexpected effects directly to the FDA. The FDA's MedWatch program encourages health professionals and consumers to report medication problems by mail, fax, telephone, or the Internet (see details at *www.fda.gov/Safety/MedWatch/default .htm*). The FDA may decide to change labeling information or even withdraw drugs from the marketplace if the drugs are believed to cause unacceptable risks to health.

Because OTC drugs are available without a prescription, patients may not realize that adverse effects can occur if the drugs are used inappropriately. Under certain circumstances, the active ingredients in these drugs may worsen a medical condition, produce complications, or interact with other medications. Furthermore, people who use products with several active ingredients may inadvertently take toxic amounts of a substance when using several drugs simultaneously. For example, a person with a cold may take one medication to treat a cough and another medication for a headache without realizing that both contain an **analgesic** (pain medication).

Drug-Drug Interactions When a person uses multiple drugs, one drug may alter the effects of another drug, and the risk of side effects increases. These problems are common in older adults, who often use several medications daily over long periods. Although primary care physicians typically supervise medication use, some individuals use drugs prescribed by a number of different physicians. Others may use OTC medications and dietary supplements in addition to prescription drugs without being aware of the risks associated with certain combinations of substances.

Diet-Drug Interactions Substances in the diet may alter the effectiveness of drugs, and drugs may affect food intake or the digestion, absorption, metabolism, or excretion of nutrients. Later sections of this chapter describe these interactions in detail.

Medication Errors A medication error is any preventable event that causes inappropriate drug use or patient harm due to mistakes made by the health professional, patient, or caregiver. Many medication errors involve the use of incorrect drugs or improper dosages.[3] The wrong drug is sometimes administered when two different drugs have similar packaging or have names that look or sound alike (for example, *hydralazine* is used to treat hypertension, whereas *hydroxyzine* treats anxiety). In other cases, the physician's prescription may be misread or misinterpreted; for example, a 1.0 milligram dose could be misread as a 10 milligram dose, or an order for 10 milligrams of an injectable drug could be misinterpreted as a 10 milliliter dose.

Several policy changes and programs are helping to reduce medication errors. The bar codes currently used on medications and patient identification bracelets allow health practitioners to verify that the correct medication and dosage are administered: error messages alert personnel if the drug, dose, or timing of administration is inappropriate. In addition, a national education campaign is attempting to eliminate one of the most common but preventable sources of medication errors—the use of ambiguous medical abbreviations (see examples in Table 15-1, p. 422). Because terms such as these are easily misread or misinterpreted, they should no longer be used in clinical documentation related to patient care.

Patients at High Risk of Adverse Effects

Health care professionals should be aware that some patients are more vulnerable than others to adverse effects from drugs. This category includes the populations that rarely participate in clinical trials that determine product safety: pregnant and lactating women, children, and people with medical conditions that are not the main focus of the study. In these groups, side effects may be discovered only after a drug has

analgesic: a drug that relieves pain.

TABLE 15-1 Terms Prohibited on Prescriptions or Medication Records

Prohibited Terms	Intended Meaning	Potential Problem	Correct Term for Documentation
U	Unit	Can be misread as the number 0 or 4; may cause 10-fold overdose or higher.	Write out "unit."
IU	International unit	Can be misread as IV (intravenous) or 10.	Write out "international unit."
Trailing zero (1.0 mg) or lack of leading zero (.1 mg)	1 mg; 0.1 mg	Decimal point can be missed, leading to 10-fold error in dosages.	On medication orders, never use zero by itself after a decimal. Always use zero before a decimal point.
μg	Microgram	Can be misread as mg (milligram).	Write out "microgram."
Q.D. (q.d.), Q.O.D. (q.o.d.)	*Q.D.* means "every day"; *Q.O.D.* means "every other day."	Can be mistaken for one another or misread as "q.i.d." (four times daily).	Write out "daily" or "every other day."

been marketed. Children may react in different ways to drugs than adults do, and the appropriate dosage for their age and size is often unknown. Also, limited data are available on drug safety in older adults. Elderly people with chronic diseases that require multiple medications are especially susceptible to adverse effects (see Figure 15-2). They are also more likely to have impaired function of the liver or kidneys—the two organs critical to metabolizing and eliminating drugs from the body.

To reduce the likelihood of adverse effects, health professionals should discuss with patients the potential benefits and risks of using medications before prescribing them. These suggestions may help:

- Advise the patient that drugs should not be taken unless absolutely necessary. Discuss dietary or lifestyle practices that have benefits similar to those of drugs. For example, laxatives may not be necessary if an individual increases consumption of foods high in fiber and begins exercising regularly.

- Request a complete list of prescription medications, OTC drugs, and dietary supplements that the patient is taking. Ensure that at least one physician is coordinating the patient's drug use. Encourage the patient to purchase all medications at the same pharmacy so that the pharmacist can alert physicians and patients to potential problems.

- Verify that the patient understands how to take medications properly. Alert the patient to potential drug-drug and diet-drug interactions.

- Encourage the patient to keep track of side effects. Inform the patient that new or unusual symptoms may be due to a new medication rather than the medical condition. In some cases, another medication that treats the condition may have fewer side effects.

IN SUMMARY

- Both prescription and OTC drugs must be shown to be safe and effective before they are sold. The benefits of using a medication should be greater than the risks associated with its use. Potential risks include side effects, drug-drug and diet-drug interactions, and medication errors.

- Common medication errors include the use of incorrect drugs or improper dosages. Bar coding is required on medications sold to health institutions, and confusing terms are being eliminated from documents related to patient care.

- Patients at highest risk of experiencing adverse effects from medications include pregnant and nursing women, children, and the elderly.

- Health professionals should discuss the risks and benefits of medications with patients and alert them to potential dangers and possible solutions.

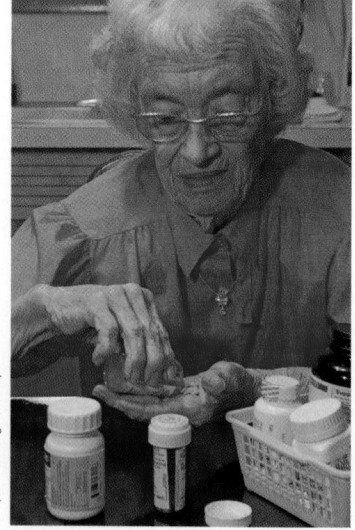

Terry Smith Images/Alamy

FIGURE 15-2
Elderly people using multiple medications are especially susceptible to adverse effects from drugs.

15.2 Diet-Drug Interactions

LO 15.2 Identify the different types of diet-drug interactions and give examples of each.

When working with patients, medical personnel should be alert to possible interactions between drugs and dietary substances. These interactions can raise health care costs and result in serious, and sometimes fatal, complications. Accordingly, health professionals must learn to take steps to prevent or lessen their adverse consequences. Diet-drug interactions (also called *food-drug interactions* or *drug-nutrient interactions*) generally fall into the following categories:

- Drugs may alter food intake by reducing the appetite or by causing complications that make food consumption difficult or unpleasant. Other drugs may increase the appetite and cause weight gain.

- Drugs may alter the absorption, metabolism, or excretion of nutrients. Conversely, nutrients and other food components may alter the absorption, metabolism, and excretion of drugs.

- Some interactions between dietary components and drugs can cause drug toxicity.

Examples of these types of diet-drug interactions are shown in Table 15-2 (p. 424).[4]

Drug Effects on Food Intake

Some drugs can make food intake difficult or unpleasant: they may suppress the appetite, cause mouth dryness, alter the sense of taste, lead to inflammation or lesions in the mouth or gastrointestinal (GI) tract, or induce nausea or vomiting. Certain side effects of drugs, including abdominal discomfort, constipation, and diarrhea, may be worsened by food consumption. Medications that cause drowsiness, such as sedatives and some painkillers, can make a person too tired to eat.

Drug complications that reduce food intake are significant only when they continue for a long period. Although many drugs can cause nausea in certain individuals, the nausea often subsides after the first few doses of the drug and therefore has little effect on nutrition status. If side effects persist, other medications may be prescribed to treat them; for example, antinauseants and **antiemetics** may help to reduce nausea and vomiting and thereby improve food intake.

Some medications stimulate the appetite and encourage weight gain. Unintentional weight gain may result from the use of some antidepressants, antipsychotics, antidiabetic drugs, and corticosteroids (such as prednisone).[5] For some conditions, however, weight gain is desirable. Patients with diseases that cause wasting, such as cancer or AIDS, are sometimes prescribed appetite enhancers such as megestrol acetate (Megace), a progesterone analog, or dronabinol (Marinol), which is derived from the active ingredient in marijuana.

Drug Effects on Nutrient Absorption

The medications that most often cause nutrient malabsorption are those that either upset GI function or damage the intestinal mucosa. **Antineoplastic drugs** and **antiretroviral drugs** are especially detrimental, whereas nonsteroidal anti-inflammatory drugs (NSAIDs) and some antibiotics can have similar, though milder, effects. This section describes additional ways in which medications may alter nutrient absorption.

Drug-Nutrient Binding Some medications bind to nutrients in the GI tract, preventing their absorption. For example, bile acid binders (such as cholestyramine,

antiemetics: drugs that prevent vomiting.

antineoplastic drugs: drugs that control or kill cancer cells.

antiretroviral drugs: drugs that treat retrovirus infections, such as infection with human immunodeficiency virus (HIV).

TABLE 15-2 Examples of Diet-Drug Interactions

Drugs may alter food intake by:

▪ Altering the appetite (amphetamines suppress appetite; corticosteroids increase appetite).

▪ Interfering with taste or smell (amphetamines change taste perceptions).

▪ Inducing nausea or vomiting (digitalis may do both).

▪ Interfering with oral function (some antidepressants may cause dry mouth).

▪ Causing sores or inflammation in the mouth (methotrexate may cause painful mouth ulcers).

Drugs may alter nutrient absorption by:

▪ Changing the acidity of the digestive tract (antacids may interfere with iron and folate absorption).

▪ Damaging mucosal cells (cancer chemotherapy may damage mucosal cells).

▪ Binding to nutrients (bile acid binders bind to fat-soluble vitamins).

Foods and nutrients may alter drug absorption by:

▪ Stimulating the secretion of gastric acid (the antifungal agent ketoconazole is absorbed better with meals due to increased acid secretion).

▪ Altering the rate of gastric emptying (drug absorption may be delayed when the drug is taken with food).

▪ Binding to drugs (calcium binds to tetracycline, reducing the absorption of both substances).

▪ Competing for absorption sites in the small intestine (dietary amino acids interfere with levodopa absorption).

Drugs and nutrients may interact and alter metabolism by:

▪ Acting as structural analogs (as do warfarin and vitamin K).

▪ Using similar enzyme systems (phenobarbital induces liver enzymes that increase the metabolism of folate, vitamin D, and vitamin K).

▪ Competing for transport on plasma proteins (fatty acids and drugs may compete for the same sites on the plasma protein albumin).

Drugs may alter nutrient excretion by:

▪ Altering nutrient reabsorption in the kidneys[a] (some diuretics increase the excretion of sodium and potassium).

▪ Causing diarrhea or vomiting (diarrhea and vomiting may cause electrolyte losses).

Food substances may alter drug excretion by:

▪ Inducing the activities of liver enzymes that metabolize drugs, increasing drug excretion (components of charcoal-broiled meats increase the metabolism of warfarin, theophylline, and acetaminophen).

Food substances and drugs may interact and cause toxicity by:

▪ Increasing side effects of the drug (the caffeine in beverages can increase the adverse effects of stimulants).

▪ Increasing drug action to excessive levels (grapefruit components inhibit the enzymes that degrade certain drugs, increasing drug concentrations in the body).

[a]When the kidneys reabsorb a substance, they retain it in the blood. Substances that are not reabsorbed are excreted in the urine.

or Questran), which are used to reduce cholesterol levels, may bind to fat-soluble vitamins. Some antibiotics, notably tetracycline and ciprofloxacin (Cipro), bind to the calcium in foods and supplements, reducing the absorption of both the calcium and the antibiotic. Other minerals that may bind to these antibiotics include iron, magnesium, and zinc. Consumers are advised to use dairy products and all mineral supplements at least two hours apart from these medications.

Altered Stomach Acidity Medications that reduce stomach acidity can impair the absorption of vitamin B_{12}, folate, and iron. Examples include antacids, which neutralize stomach acid by acting as weak bases, and antiulcer drugs (such as proton pump inhibitors and H2 blockers), which interfere with acid secretion.

Direct Inhibition Several drugs impede nutrient absorption by interfering with their transport into mucosal cells. For example, the antibiotics trimethoprim (Proloprim) and pyrimethamine (Daraprim) compete with folate for absorption into intestinal cells. The anti-inflammatory medication colchicine, a treatment for gout, inhibits vitamin B_{12} absorption.

CHAPTER FIFTEEN

Dietary Effects on Drug Absorption

Major influences on drug absorption include the stomach-emptying rate, the level of acidity in the stomach, and direct interactions with dietary components. The drug's formulation may also influence its absorption. The instructions included with medications typically advise whether food should be included or avoided with use.

Stomach-Emptying Rate Drugs reach the small intestine more quickly when the stomach is empty. Therefore, taking a medication with meals may delay its absorption, although the total amount absorbed may not be lower. As an example, aspirin works faster when taken on an empty stomach, although taking it with food is often encouraged to reduce stomach irritation.

Slow stomach emptying can sometimes enhance drug absorption because the drug's absorption sites in the small intestine are less likely to become saturated. However, a slow drug absorption rate (due to slow stomach emptying) can be a problem if high drug concentrations are needed for effectiveness, as when a hypnotic is taken to induce sleep.

Stomach Acidity Some drugs are better absorbed in an acidic environment, whereas others are absorbed better under alkaline conditions. For example, reduced stomach acidity (due to secretory disorders or antacid medications) may reduce the absorption of ketoconazole (Nizoral, an antifungal medication) and atazanavir (an antiretroviral medication), but increase the absorption of digoxin (Lanoxin, which treats heart failure) and alendronate (Fosamax, which treats osteoporosis).[6] Some drugs can be damaged by acid and are available in coated forms that resist the stomach's acidity.

Interactions Between Drugs and Dietary Components Various dietary substances can bind to drugs and inhibit their absorption. As mentioned earlier, minerals can bind to some antibiotics, reducing absorption of both the minerals and the drugs. High-fiber meals can decrease the absorption of some tricyclic antidepressants due to binding between the fiber and the drugs. Conversely, the absorption of many lipophilic drugs (those with fat-soluble structures) is improved when the drugs are taken with a fat-containing meal.[7]

Drug Effects on Nutrient Metabolism

Drugs and nutrients share similar enzyme systems in the small intestine and liver. Consequently, some drugs may enhance or inhibit the activities of enzymes needed for nutrient metabolism. For example, the **anticonvulsants** phenobarbital and phenytoin increase levels of the liver enzymes that metabolize folate, vitamin D, and vitamin K; therefore, persons using these drugs may require supplements of these vitamins.

The drug methotrexate, which treats cancer (and some inflammatory conditions), acts by interfering with folate metabolism and thus depriving rapidly dividing cancer cells of the folate they need to multiply. Methotrexate resembles folate in structure (see Figure 15-3, p. 426) and competes with folate for the enzyme that converts folate to its active form. The adverse effects of using methotrexate therefore include symptoms of folate deficiency. These adverse effects can be reduced by using a preactivated form of folate (called leucovorin), which is often prescribed along with methotrexate to ensure that the body's rapidly dividing cells (skin cells, cells of the digestive tract, and red blood cells) receive adequate folate.

Isoniazid is an antibacterial agent that is used to treat and prevent tuberculosis. The drug inhibits the conversion of vitamin B_6 to its coenzyme form (pyridoxal phosphate), which is involved with neurotransmitter synthesis. Some patients using isoniazid therapy may develop peripheral neuropathy unless they take supplemental vitamin B_6 during the course of treatment.[8]

anticonvulsants: drugs that treat epileptic seizures.

FIGURE 15-3 **Folate and Methotrexate**

By competing for the enzyme that activates folate, methotrexate prevents cancer cells from obtaining the folate they need to multiply. In the process, normal cells are also deprived of the folate they need.

Folate

Methotrexate

Dietary Effects on Drug Metabolism

Some food components alter the activities of enzymes that metabolize drugs or may counteract drug effects in other ways. Compounds in grapefruit juice (or whole grapefruit) have been found to inhibit or inactivate enzymes that metabolize a number of different drugs. As a result of the reduced enzyme action, blood concentrations of the drugs increase, leading to stronger physiological effects. The effect of the grapefruit juice can last for a substantial period, possibly as long as several days after the juice is consumed;[9] thus, the interaction cannot be avoided by separating grapefruit juice consumption from drug administration. Table 15-3 provides examples of drugs that interact with grapefruit juice, as well as some drugs that are unaffected.

A number of dietary substances can alter the activity of the anticoagulant drug warfarin (Coumadin). One important interaction is with vitamin K, which is structurally similar to warfarin. Warfarin acts by blocking the enzyme that activates vitamin K, thereby preventing the synthesis of blood-clotting factors (vitamin K is required for the synthesis of prothrombin and various other blood-clotting proteins). The amount of warfarin prescribed is dependent, in part, on how much vitamin K is in the diet. If vitamin K consumption from foods or supplements changes substantially, it can alter the effect of the drug. Individuals using warfarin are advised to consume similar

TABLE 15-3 **Examples of Grapefruit Juice–Drug Interactions**

Drug Category	Drugs Affected by Grapefruit Juice	Drugs Unaffected by Grapefruit Juice
Anticoagulants	—	Acenocoumarol Warfarin
Anti-diabetic drugs	Repaglinide Saxagliptin	Glyburide Metformin
Anti-infective drugs	Erythromycin Saquinavir	Clarithromycin Indinivir
Cardiovascular drugs	Amiodarone Felodipine Nicardipine	Amlodipine Digoxin Diltiazem
Central nervous system drugs	Buspirone Carbamazepine Diazepam	Haloperidol Lorazepam Risperidone
Cholesterol-lowering drugs	Atorvastatin Lovastatin Simvastatin	Fluvastatin Pravastatin Rosuvastatin
Immunosuppressants	Cyclosporine Tacrolimus	Prednisone

amounts of vitamin K daily to keep warfarin activity stable. The dietary sources highest in vitamin K are green leafy vegetables.

Several popular herbs contain natural compounds that affect blood coagulation or warfarin metabolism and therefore should be avoided during warfarin treatment. These herbs include St. John's wort, garlic, ginseng, dong quai, danshen, and others.[10]

Drug Effects on Nutrient Excretion

Drugs that increase urine production may reduce nutrient reabsorption in the kidneys, resulting in greater urinary losses of the nutrients. For example, some **diuretics** can increase losses of calcium, potassium, magnesium, and thiamin; thus, dietary supplements may be necessary to avoid deficiency. Risk of nutrient depletion is higher if multiple drugs with the same effect are used, if kidney function is impaired, or if the medications are used for long periods. Note that some diuretics can cause certain minerals to be retained, rather than excreted.

Corticosteroids, which are used as anti-inflammatory agents and immunosuppressants, promote sodium and water retention and increase urinary potassium excretion.[11] Long-term use of corticosteroids can have multiple adverse effects, which include muscle wasting, bone loss, weight gain, and hyperglycemia, with eventual development of osteoporosis and diabetes.

Dietary Effects on Drug Excretion

Inadequate excretion of medications can cause toxicity, whereas excessive losses may reduce the amount available for therapeutic effect. Some food components influence drug excretion by altering the amount reabsorbed in the kidneys. For example, the amount of lithium (a mood stabilizer) reabsorbed in the kidneys is similar to the amount of sodium that is reabsorbed. Consequently, both dehydration and sodium depletion, which promote sodium reabsorption, can result in lithium retention. Similarly, a person with a high sodium intake will excrete more sodium in the urine and, therefore, more lithium. Individuals using lithium are advised to maintain a consistent sodium intake from day to day to maintain stable blood concentrations of lithium.

Urine acidity can affect drug excretion due to the effects of pH on a compound's ionic (chemical) form. The medication quinidine, used to treat arrhythmias, is excreted more readily in acidic urine. Foods or drugs that cause urine to become more alkaline may reduce quinidine excretion and raise blood levels of the medication.

Diet-Drug Interactions and Toxicity

Interactions between food components and drugs can cause toxicity or exacerbate a drug's side effects. The combination of tyramine, a food component, and monoamine oxidase (MAO) inhibitors, which treat depression and Parkinson's disease, can be fatal. MAO inhibitors block an enzyme that normally inactivates tyramine, as well as the hormones epinephrine and norepinephrine. When people who take MAO inhibitors consume excessive tyramine, the increased tyramine in the blood can induce a sudden release of stored norepinephrine. This surge in norepinephrine results in severe headaches, rapid heartbeat, and a dangerous rise in blood pressure. For this reason, people taking MAO inhibitors are advised to restrict their intakes of foods rich in tyramine.

Foods that often contain significant amounts of tyramine are listed in Table 15-4. Note that the tyramine content of foods depends on storage conditions and processing; thus the amounts in similar products can vary substantially.

TABLE 15-4 Examples of Foods with a High Tyramine Content[a]

- Aged cheeses (Cheddar, Gruyère)
- Aged or cured meats (sausage, salami)
- Beer
- Fermented vegetables (sauerkraut, kim chee)
- Fish or shrimp sauce
- Prepared soy foods (miso, tempeh, tofu)
- Soy sauce
- Yeast extract (Marmite, Vegemite)

[a]Although tyramine occurs naturally in foods, it is also formed when bacteria degrade food proteins; thus, the tyramine content increases when a food ages or spoils. Individuals at risk of tyramine toxicity are advised to buy mainly fresh foods and consume them promptly.

© 2016 Cengage Learning®

diuretics: drugs that promote urine production.

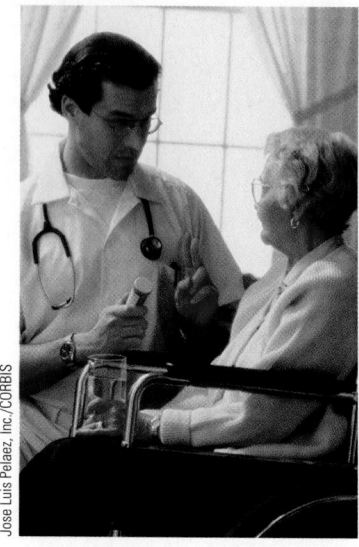
Jose Luis Pelaez, Inc./CORBIS

FIGURE 15-4 Medication Management
To help prevent diet-drug interactions, ask about *all* of the drugs and supplements the patient takes, including prescription and over-the-counter medications, herbal products, and other dietary supplements.

Considering the many ways in which drugs and dietary substances can interact, health professionals should attempt to understand the mechanisms underlying diet-drug interactions, identify them when they occur, and prevent them whenever possible. Figure 15-4 and Box 15-1 offer some practical advice about preventing diet-drug interactions.

IN SUMMARY

■ Medications can alter food intake and affect the absorption, metabolism, or excretion of nutrients. Components of foods can similarly affect drug activity.

■ Drugs can alter food intake by increasing or decreasing the appetite, altering the sense of taste, causing GI discomfort, or damaging the lining of the GI tract.

■ Drugs can affect nutrient absorption by binding to nutrients, altering stomach acidity, or interfering with nutrient transport into intestinal cells. Dietary substances can influence drug absorption by altering the stomach emptying rate, altering stomach acidity, or directly binding to the drug.

■ Drugs and nutrients may interfere with each other's metabolism because they use similar enzymes in the small intestine and liver.

■ Diet-drug interactions may lead to nutrient losses in urine and alter the urinary excretion of drugs. Some interactions between food components and drugs may result in toxicity.

How To BOX 15-1 PREVENT DIET-DRUG INTERACTIONS

The Joint Commission, an accreditation agency for health care organizations, has recommended that all patients be educated about potential diet-drug interactions. Health professionals can help by informing patients of precautions related to medications and watching for signs of problems that may arise.

To prevent diet-drug interactions, first list the types and amounts of over-the-counter drugs, prescription drugs, and dietary supplements that the patient uses on a regular basis. Look up each of these substances in a drug reference and make a note of:

■ The appropriate method of administration (twice daily or at bedtime, for example).

■ How the drug should be administered with respect to foods, beverages, and specific nutrients (for example, take on an empty stomach, take with food, do not take with milk, or do not drink alcoholic beverages while using the medication).

■ How the drug should be used with respect to other medications.

■ The side effects that may influence food intake (nausea and vomiting, diarrhea, constipation, or sedation, for example) or nutrient needs (interference with nutrient absorption or metabolism, for example).

A similar process can be used to review the dietary supplements that a person is taking. A reliable reference may list their

appropriate uses, possible side effects, and potential interactions with food and medications.

Patients who take multiple medications may need to time their intakes carefully to avoid drug-drug or diet-drug interactions. The health professional can use information from a patient's food and nutrition history (see Chapter 14) to help the patient coordinate meals and drugs so as to avoid interactions.

Some medications have well-known effects on nutritional status. The health professional should remain alert for signs of problems, especially when:

■ Nutritional problems are a frequent result of using the medication.

■ A patient requires multiple medications.

■ The patient is in a high-risk group; for example, a child, a pregnant or lactating woman, an older adult, or a person who is malnourished, abuses alcohol, or has impaired liver or kidney function.

■ The patient needs to use the medications for an extended period.

Check with the pharmacist for additional information about drugs and their potential adverse effects.

15.3 Herbal Supplements

LO 15.3 Give examples of some popular herbal products and explain why they are not considered reliable treatments during illness.

The use of herbal supplements has grown rapidly in the past decade. About 20 percent of adults in the United States report using herbal supplements.[12] Consumers use these products in the hope of improving their general health and preventing or treating specific diseases. Top-selling herbal supplements include echinacea (see Figure 15-5), garlic, ginkgo, ginseng, and St. John's wort.[13] Table 15-5 (p. 430) lists these and other popular herbal products along with their common uses and potential risks associated with their use.

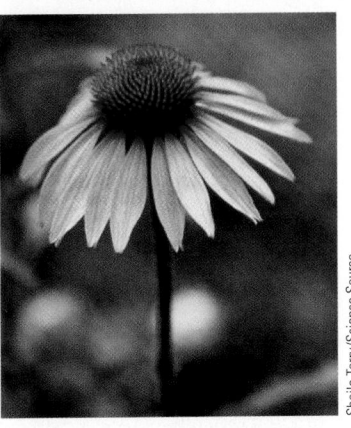

FIGURE 15-5 Echinacea Flower
Despite the popularity of echinacea, its benefits for treating the common cold have not been supported by some well-designed clinical studies.

Effectiveness and Safety of Herbal Products

Despite the popularity of herbal products in the United States, the benefits of their use are uncertain. Although many medicinal herbs contain naturally occurring compounds that exert physiological effects, few herbal products have been rigorously tested, many make unfounded claims, and some may contain contaminants or produce toxic effects.[14]

Efficacy Herbs have been used for centuries to treat medical conditions, and many have acquired reputations for being beneficial for individuals with specific diseases. Unfortunately, only a limited number of clinical studies support the traditional uses,* and the results of studies that suggest little or no benefit are rarely publicized by the supplement industry. The National Center for Complementary and Alternative Medicine (a division of the National Institutes of Health) is currently funding large, controlled trials of several popular herbal treatments in an effort to obtain reliable efficacy and safety data.

Although labels on herbal products cannot make claims about preventing or treating specific diseases, suggestive statements are common. For example, a label may claim that a product "promotes restful sleep" but cannot state that it treats insomnia. Stores often shelve herbal products by health condition; for example, posted signs may indicate the products suggested for "liver health" or "digestive health." Publicity materials with misleading information are often positioned near the products. In addition, salespersons often give inappropriate advice about the use of herbal supplements for improving one's health.[15]

Consistency of Herbal Ingredients Herbs contain numerous compounds, and it is often unclear which of these ingredients, if any, might produce the implied beneficial effects. Because the compounds in herbs vary among species and are affected by a plant's growing conditions, different samples of an herb can have different chemical compositions. The preparation method may also cause variations in the composition of an herbal product. Some manufacturers attempt to standardize the herbal extracts they sell so that the compound believed to be beneficial is more likely to be obtained from each dose.

Even when certain substances in an herb have been shown to be effective, the product purchased by the consumer might not provide the ingredients required for benefit. For example, a consumer group (ConsumerLab.com) that regularly analyzes dietary and herbal supplements often reports finding lower amounts of herbal ingredients than are listed on product labels.[16] In a university study that evaluated the authenticity of 44 single-herb supplements, 32 percent of the products were found to contain a completely different plant species than was listed on the label.[17]

Safety Issues Consumers often assume that because plants are "natural," herbal products must be harmless. Many herbal remedies have toxic effects, however.[18] The most common adverse effects of herbs include diarrhea, nausea, and vomiting.

*For example, some studies suggest that St. John's wort may be effective for treating mild depression, ginger may help to prevent motion sickness, and garlic supplements may improve blood pressure in people with hypertension.

TABLE 15-5 Popular Herbal Products, Their Common Uses, and Adverse Effects

Herb[a]	Scientific Name	Common Uses	Potential Adverse Effects
Black cohosh	*Cimicifuga racemosa*	Relief of menopausal symptoms	Rare; occasional stomach upset, headache, weight gain
Chaparral	*Larrea tridentata*	General tonic; treatment of infection, cancer, and arthritis	Hepatitis, liver failure
Comfrey	*Symphytum officinale*	Wound healing (topical use), treatment of lung and GI disorders	Liver damage
Echinacea	*Echinacea augustifolia, E. pallida, E. purpurea*	Prevention and treatment of upper respiratory infections	Rare; allergic reactions
Feverfew	*Tanacetum parthenium*	Prevention of migraine headache	Mouth and tongue sores, swelling of lips and mouth, stomach upset
Garlic	*Allium sativum*	Reduction of blood clotting, atherosclerosis, blood pressure, and blood cholesterol	Breath and body odor, nausea, hypotension, allergy, excessive bleeding
Ginger	*Zingiber officinale*	Prevention and treatment of nausea and motion sickness	Rare; occasional heartburn
Ginkgo	*Ginkgo biloba*	Treatment of dementia, memory defects, and circulatory impairment	Rare; nausea, stomach upset, diarrhea, allergy, anxiety, insomnia, excessive bleeding
Ginseng	*Panax ginseng, P. quinquefolius*	General tonic, reduction of blood glucose levels	Rare
Kava	*Piper methysticum*	Treatment of anxiety, stress, and insomnia	Rare; stomach upset, restlessness, drowsiness, tremor, headache, allergic skin reactions, occasional hepatitis and liver failure
St. John's wort	*Hypericum perforatum*	Treatment of mild to moderate depression	Skin photosensitivity
Saw palmetto	*Serenoa repens*	Reduction of symptoms associated with enlarged prostate	Rare; abdominal pain, nausea, diarrhea, fatigue, headache, decreased libido
Valerian	*Valeriana officinalis*	Sedation, treatment of insomnia	Rare
Yohimbe	*Pausinystalia yohimbe*	Treatment of erectile dysfunction	Anxiety, dizziness, headache, nausea, rapid heartbeat, hypertension, increased urinary frequency

© 2016 Cengage Learning®

[a]An *herb* is a non-woody, seed-producing plant; *herbal products* include other types of plant products, such as garlic and ginkgo.

The popular herbs chaparral, germander, kava, and pennyroyal have caused liver damage.[19] The use of yohimbe (promoted for bodybuilding and erectile dysfunction) has been linked to heart arrhythmias, high blood pressure, anxiety, and seizures. Note that such adverse effects are rarely listed on supplement labels.

Contamination of herbal products is another safety concern. Many products have been found to contain lead and other toxic metals in excessive amounts.[20] Other contaminants frequently found in herbal supplements include molds, bacteria, and pesticides that have been banned for use on food crops.[21] Adulteration of herbal supplements is a serious concern: chemical analyses have frequently identified synthetic drugs that were not declared on the label.[22] There are sometimes reports of illnesses and fatalities occurring from the intentional or accidental substitutions of one plant species for another.[23] Although not mentioned on the label, fillers made from rice, soybean, and wheat have been found in herbal supplements and may be a health risk for persons with allergies to these substances.[24]

Unlike drugs, herbal products do not need FDA approval before they are marketed. According to the Dietary Supplement Health and Education Act (DSHEA) of 1994, the companies that produce or distribute dietary (including herbal) supplements are responsible for determining their safety, yet these companies are not required to provide any evidence or conduct safety studies. If a company receives reports of illness or injury related to the use of its products, it is not required to submit this information to the FDA. In addition, the FDA must show that a supplement is unsafe before it can take action to remove the product from the marketplace.

Herb-Drug Interactions Like drugs, herbs may either intensify or interfere with the effects of other herbs and drugs or they may raise the risk of toxicity.[25] For example, garlic, ginger, and goldenseal contain compounds that lower blood pressure and they may therefore strengthen the effects of antihypertensive drugs. Garlic, ginkgo, and ginseng may increase the risk of bleeding when used with anticoagulant drugs. St. John's wort has been found to diminish the actions of oral contraceptives, anticoagulants, and other drugs. Unfortunately, information about herb-drug interactions is limited, and much of what is known has been obtained from case studies rather than controlled clinical trials. Table 15-6 provides some examples of herb-drug interactions.

Use of Herbal Products in Illness

When people self-medicate or ask the advice of store clerks instead of seeking effective medical treatment, the consequences are sometimes serious and irreversible. Purchasing an herbal remedy may be less stressful than a visit to the doctor, but it may delay getting an appropriate treatment and allow an illness to progress. Although retailers are not legally permitted to provide medical advice, sellers of herbal products routinely make improper claims that the products are able to treat, prevent, or cure specific illnesses.[26]

Patients are often unaware that herbal products may be unsafe or can interact with medications. Elderly individuals (65 years old and older) are at highest risk of herb-drug interactions because most individuals in this age group take three or more prescription drugs over the course of a year.[27] Some pharmacology textbooks and handbooks now contain information about herbal supplements and potential herb-drug interactions, and various consumer websites and periodicals provide information about the safety of brand-name herbal products. Health professionals should turn to these resources to help patients who plan to use herbal supplements.

TABLE 15-6 Examples of Herb-Drug Interactions

Herb	Drugs	Interaction
Chamomile	Anticoagulants, sedatives	May intensify or prolong drug effects
Echinacea	Immunosuppressant drugs	May suppress drug effects
Feverfew	Anticoagulants, antiplatelet drugs, aspirin	May increase risk of bleeding
Garlic, ginger, ginkgo, ginseng	Anticoagulants, antiplatelet drugs	May increase risk of bleeding
Goldenseal	Anticoagulants, antihypertensives	May oppose anticoagulant effects, increasing risk of clot formation (anticoagulants); may strengthen effect of antihypertensives
Licorice	Antiarrhythmics, antihypertensives, diuretics	May cause toxicity (antiarrhythmics), oppose drug effects (antihypertensives), cause excessive potassium losses (diuretics)
St. John's wort	Various	May suppress drug effects
Valerian	Sedatives	May intensify or prolong sedative effects

Source: R. S. Porter and J. L. Kaplan, eds., *Merck Manual of Diagnosis and Therapy* (Whitehouse Station, NJ: Merck Sharp and Dohme Corp., 2011): 3421–3432; P. A. Cohen and E. Ernst, Safety of herbal supplements: A guide for cardiologists, *Cardiovascular Therapeutics* 28 (2010): 246–253.

© 2016 Cengage Learning®

- Herbal products are not reliable treatments for medical conditions; there is little evidence demonstrating their effectiveness and safety, and the concentrations of active ingredients in herbal products can vary greatly. Safety concerns include adverse effects, contamination, and herb-drug interactions.

- Manufacturers and distributors of herbal supplements are responsible for determining product safety but are not required to conduct safety studies. The FDA must prove that a supplement is unsafe before removing it from the market.

- Consumers using herbs may delay getting an appropriate treatment for their condition and may receive questionable advice from supplement retailers.

Clinical Applications

1. An elderly woman in a residential home has been losing weight since her arrival there. She has been taking several medications to treat both a heart problem and a mild case of bronchitis. You notice that she eats only a few bites at mealtimes and seems uninterested in food. Describe several steps you can take to learn whether the medications are interfering with her food intake in some way.

2. A patient mentions that he regularly takes six to seven dietary and herbal supplements and that he has not told the physician that he uses them. His prescription medications include an antihypertensive agent (to reduce blood pressure) and warfarin. What approach might you take to learn the details about his supplement use and his reasons for taking them? If you discover that some of the supplements may pose a risk for diet-drug or herb-drug interactions with his prescription medications, what steps should you take?

Self Check

1. Over-the-counter drugs:
   a. rarely cause adverse effects.
   b. are unlikely to interact with dietary components.
   c. are usually taken for longer periods than prescription medications.
   d. are used to treat illnesses that are typically self-diagnosed and self-treated.

2. Recommendations for reducing the incidence of medication errors include:
   a. avoiding the use of confusing terms on clinical documents.
   b. advising patients to take only one medication at a time.
   c. requiring that prescriptions be handwritten instead of typed.
   d. physician supervision whenever drugs are administered.

3. Adverse drug effects are most likely when:
   a. multiple medications are used.
   b. generic drugs are substituted for brand-name drugs.
   c. patients begin using a new medication.
   d. medications are taken for just one or two days.

4. Examples of medication-related symptoms that can significantly limit food intake include:
   a. ringing in the ears.
   b. persistent nausea and vomiting.
   c. insomnia.
   d. skin rash.

5. Medications that reduce stomach acidity can impair the absorption of:
   a. fat-soluble vitamins.
   b. thiamin and riboflavin.
   c. sodium and potassium.
   d. vitamin B_{12}, folate, and iron.

6. Compounds in grapefruit juice:
   a. bind to antibiotics, reducing their absorption.
   b. cause excessive drug excretion.
   c. strengthen the effects of certain drugs.
   d. alter acidity in the stomach, impairing drug absorption.

7. Vitamin K consumption should be consistent in patients using:
   a. tetracycline.
   b. warfarin.
   c. lithium.
   d. isoniazid.

8. People who use MAO inhibitors must limit consumption of:
   a. whole milk and yogurt.
   b. aged cheeses.
   c. dark green leafy vegetables.
   d. grapefruit juice.

9. An important step that health practitioners can take to limit the risk of medication-related side effects is to:
   a. recommend use of over-the-counter drugs instead of prescription medications.
   b. encourage use of herbal supplements rather than prescription medications.
   c. advise patients to take medications separately from meals.
   d. ask patients to fully describe the types and amounts of medications and dietary supplements they are using.

10. An important difference between medications and herbal products that reach the marketplace is that:
    a. medications that cause adverse effects cannot be sold.
    b. medications are subject to contamination with toxic metals, molds, and bacteria.
    c. herbal products are not required to prove safety and effectiveness.
    d. herbal products must provide standard amounts of active ingredients.

Answers to these questions appear in Appendix H.

Notes

1. R. L. Corelli, Therapeutic and toxic potential of over-the-counter agents, in B. G. Katzung, ed., *Basic and Clinical Pharmacology* (New York: Lange Medical Books/McGraw-Hill, 2012), pp. 1115–1124.

2. P. W. Lofholm and B. G. Katzung, Rational prescribing and prescription writing, in B. G. Katzung, ed., *Basic and Clinical Pharmacology* (New York: Lange Medical Books/McGraw-Hill, 2012), pp. 1139–1148.

3. Lofholm and Katzung, 2012.

4. L.-N. Chan, Drug-nutrient interactions, in A. C. Ross and coeditors, eds., *Modern Nutrition in Health and Disease* (Baltimore: Lippincott Williams & Wilkins, 2014), pp. 1440–1452; J. I. Boullata and L. M. Hudson, Drug-nutrient interactions: A broad view with implications for practice, *Journal of the Academy of Nutrition and Dietetics* 112 (2012): 506–517.

5. J. M. Gervasio, Drug-induced changes to nutritional status, in J. I. Boullata and V. T. Armenti, eds., *Handbook of Drug-Nutrient Interactions* (New York: Humana Press, 2010), pp. 427–445.

6. E. Lahner and coauthors, Systematic review: Impaired drug absorption related to the co-administration of antisecretory therapy, *Alimentary Pharmacology and Therapeutics* 29 (2009): 1219–1229.

7. D. Fleisher and coauthors, Drug absorption with food, in J. I. Boullata and V. T. Armenti, eds., *Handbook of Drug-Nutrient Interactions* (New York: Humana Press, 2010), pp. 209–241.

8. I. F. Btaiche, B. V. Sweet, and M. D. Kraft, Positive drug-nutrient interactions, in J. I. Boullata and V. T. Armenti, eds., *Handbook of Drug-Nutrient Interactions* (New York: Humana Press, 2010), pp. 303–339.

9. Chan, 2014; D. G. Bailey, Grapefruit and other fruit juices interactions with medications, in J. I. Boullata and V. T. Armenti, eds., *Handbook of Drug-Nutrient Interactions* (New York: Humana Press, 2010), pp. 267–302.

10. C. E. Dennehy and C. Tsourounis, Dietary supplements and herbal medications, in B. G. Katzung, ed., *Basic and Clinical Pharmacology* (New York: McGraw-Hill, 2012), pp. 1125–1137; L.-N. Chan, Interaction of natural products with medication and nutrients, in J. I. Boullata and V. T. Armenti, eds., *Handbook of Drug-Nutrient Interactions* (New York: Humana Press, 2010), pp. 341–366.

11. G. W. Cannon, Immunosuppressing drugs including corticosteroids, in L. Goldman and A. I. Schafer, eds., *Goldman's Cecil Medicine* (Philadelphia: Saunders, 2012), pp. 159–165.

12. R. L. Bailey and coauthors, Dietary supplement use in the United States, 2003–2006, *Journal of Nutrition* 141 (2011): 261–266.

13. U.S. Government Accountability Office (GAO), Herbal dietary supplements: Examples of deceptive or questionable marketing practices and potentially dangerous advice, GAO-10-662T (Washington, DC: May 26, 2010).

14. M. E. Gershwin and coauthors, Public safety and dietary supplementation, *Annals of the New York Academy of Sciences* 1190 (2010): 104–117; U.S. Government Accountability Office (GAO), 2010.

15. U.S. Government Accountability Office (GAO), 2010.

16. ConsumerLab.com, Product Reviews (various reports), available at www.consumerlab.com, site visited January 3, 2014.

17. S. G. Newmaster and coauthors, DNA barcoding detects contamination and substitution in North American herbal products, *BMC Medicine* 11 (2013): 222–233.

18. Dennehy and Tsourounis, 2012.

19. C. Bunchorntavakul and K. R. Reddy, Review article: Herbal and dietary supplement hepatotoxicity, *Alimentary Pharmacology and Therapeutics* 37 (2013): 3–17.

20. U.S. Government Accountability Office (GAO), 2010.

21. U.S. Government Accountability Office (GAO), 2010; V. H. Tournas, E. Katsoudas, and E. J. Miracco, Moulds, yeasts, and aerobic plate counts in ginseng supplements, *International Journal of Food Microbiology* 108 (2006): 178–181.

22. P. A. Cohen and E. Ernst, Safety of herbal supplements: A guide for cardiologists, *Cardiovascular Therapeutics* 28 (2010): 246–253; Gershwin and coauthors, 2010.

23. M. L. Coghlan and coauthors, Deep sequencing of plant and animal DNA contained within traditional Chinese medicines reveals legality issues and health safety concerns, *PLoS Genetics* 8 (2012): e1002657, doi:10.1371/journal.pgen.1002657; R. B. van Breemen, H. H. S. Fong, and N. R. Farnsworth, Ensuring the safety of botanical dietary supplements, *American Journal of Clinical Nutrition* 87 (2008): 509S–513S.

24. Bunchorntavakul and Reddy, 2013.

25. Dennehy and Tsourounis, 2012; Cohen and Ernst, 2010.

26. U.S. Government Accountability Office (GAO), 2010.

27. U.S. Government Accountability Office (GAO), 2010.

LO 15.4 Explain how complementary and alternative therapies differ from those used in conventional medicine and describe the various types of alternative therapies currently available.

The medical treatments described in the clinical chapters are based upon current scientific understanding of human physiology and biochemistry and are generally supported by well-conducted clinical research. This Nutrition in Practice examines therapies that have *not* been scientifically validated and are therefore not currently promoted by conventional health professionals; these therapies fall into a category called *complementary and alternative medicine (CAM)*. When the therapies are used together with conventional medicine, they are called *complementary*; when used in place of conventional medicine, they are called *alternative*.[1] Note that the term "alternative" may be misleading in that it inappropriately implies that unproven methods of treatment are valid alternatives to conventional treatments.

How popular is CAM in the United States?

Nearly 40 percent of adults in the United States use some form of CAM (excluding the use of prayer).[2] CAM is especially prevalent among persons with chronic pain or debilitating illness; for example, 80 percent of cancer patients reportedly use CAM.[3] Many patients use CAM as an adjunct to conventional medicine—often for symptoms or illnesses that are not sufficiently helped by conventional treatments. CAM therapies remain popular despite the dearth of evidence demonstrating their effectiveness. Reasons for their popularity include consumers' growing interest in self-help measures, the noninvasive nature of many CAM therapies, and the positive interactions consumers have with CAM practitioners.[4]

In response to the enormous popularity of CAM in the United States, in 1998 Congress established the National Center for Complementary and Alternative Medicine (NCCAM), which is now one of the 27 institutes that make up the National Institutes of Health (NIH). NCCAM's missions are to investigate complementary and alternative therapies by funding well-designed scientific studies and to provide authoritative information for consumers and health professionals. If enough evidence is found to support the use of a complementary or alternative therapy, it will likely become incorporated into mainstream medical practice.[5]

Why should mainstream health professionals learn more about CAM?

Due to the significant consumer interest in trying novel treatments, health professionals need to be familiar with CAM therapies so that they can better communicate with patients regarding their medical care and advise them when an alternative approach conflicts with standard therapy or presents a danger to health. To provide medical students with objective information about CAM, many medical schools in the United States now offer elective courses about alternative forms of treatment. Physicians who practice *integrative medicine* may refer patients for complementary therapies while continuing to provide standard treatments.

What kinds of practices are considered CAM therapies?

CAM encompasses any and all therapies that are not normally part of conventional medicine. Consequently, the list of CAM approaches includes hundreds of advertised therapies purchased and used by consumers. Unfortunately, CAM has become a marketing buzzword and is used by unscrupulous sellers of worthless treatments. NCCAM categorizes CAM therapies as shown in Table NP15-1 and defined in Box NP15-1 on p. 435. Several popular examples are described in this Nutrition in Practice; other examples are discussed on the NCCAM website (*http://nccam.nih.gov/health*).

TABLE NP15-1 Examples of Complementary and Alternative Medicine

Alternative Medical Systems
- Ayurveda
- Homeopathic medicine
- Naturopathic medicine
- Traditional Chinese medicine

Biologically Based Therapies
- Aromatherapy
- Dietary supplements
- Foods and special diets
- Herbal products
- Hormones

Energy Therapies
- Bioelectrical therapies (including electrical and magnetic fields)
- Biofield therapies (including acupuncture, qi gong, and therapeutic touch)

Manipulative and Body-Based Methods
- Chiropractic
- Massage therapy
- Osteopathic manipulation
- Reflexology

Mind-Body Interventions
- Biofeedback
- Faith healing (prayer)
- Meditation
- Mental healing (including hypnotherapy)
- Music, art, and dance therapy

acupuncture (AK-you-PUNK-chur)**:** a therapy that involves inserting thin needles into the skin at specific anatomical points, allegedly to correct disruptions in the flow of energy within the body.

bioelectrical or **bioelectromagnetic therapies:** therapies that involve the unconventional use of electric or magnetic fields to cure illness.

biofeedback training: instruction in techniques that allow individuals to gain voluntary control of certain physiological processes, such as skin temperature or brain wave activity, to help reduce stress and anxiety.

biofield therapies: healing methods based on the belief that illnesses can be healed by manipulating energy fields that purportedly surround and penetrate the body. Examples include *acupuncture, qi gong,* and *therapeutic touch.*

chiropractic (KYE-roh-PRAK-tic)**:** a method of treatment based on the unproven theory that spinal manipulation can restore health.

▌ A *subluxation* is a misaligned vertebra or other spinal alteration that may cause illness.
▌ *Adjustment* is the manipulative therapy practiced by chiropractors.

faith healing: the use of prayer or belief in divine intervention to promote healing.

homeopathic (HO-mee-oh-PATH-ic) **medicine:** a practice based on the theory that "like cures like"; that is, substances believed to cause certain symptoms are prescribed at extremely low concentrations for curing diseases with similar symptoms.

▌ *homeo* = like
▌ *pathos* = suffering

imagery: the use of mental images of things or events to aid relaxation or promote self-healing.

massage therapy: manual manipulation of muscles to reduce tension, increase blood circulation, improve joint mobility, and promote healing of injuries.

meditation: a self-directed technique of calming the mind and relaxing the body.

naturopathic (NAY-chur-oh-PATH-ic) **medicine:** an approach to health care using practices alleged to enhance the body's natural healing abilities. Treatments may include a variety of alternative therapies including dietary supplements, herbal remedies, exercise, and homeopathy.

qi gong (chee-GUNG)**:** a traditional Chinese system that combines movement, meditation, and breathing techniques and allegedly cures illness by enhancing the flow of qi (energy) within the body.

therapeutic touch: a technique of passing hands over a patient to purportedly identify energy imbalances and transfer healing power from therapist to patient; also called *laying on of hands.*

traditional Chinese medicine (TCM): an approach to health care based on the concept that illness can be cured by enhancing the flow of qi (energy) within a person's body. Treatments may include herbal therapies, physical exercises, meditation, acupuncture, and remedial massage.

How do alternative medical systems differ from conventional medicine?

Alternative medical systems are based on beliefs that lack the scientific basis of the theories underlying conventional medicine. Virtually all of these alternative systems were developed well over a hundred years ago, before our bodies' biochemical and physiological processes were well understood. The alternative treatments may appeal to consumers because the interventions are nontechnical and seem nonthreatening. In general, however, the alternative theories and practices remain rooted in the past and have not been updated to include current knowledge. Examples of alternative medical systems include the following:

▌ **Naturopathic medicine** proposes that a person's natural "life force" can foster self-healing. This life force is allegedly stimulated by certain health-promoting factors and suppressed by excesses and deficiencies. Naturopathic therapies aim to enhance the natural healing powers of the body and may include special diets or fasting, herbal remedies and other dietary supplements, **acupuncture,** homeopathy, massage, and various other interventions.

▌ **Homeopathic medicine** is based on the dubious theory that "like cures like." Homeopaths believe that a substance that causes a particular set of symptoms can be used to cure a disease that has similar symptoms. Homeopathic medicines are usually natural substances that are substantially diluted in the belief that dilution increases potency, and most remedies are so extremely diluted that the original substance is no longer present. Homeopaths theorize that even though their remedies no longer contain a diluted substance, they still have powerful healing effects because the water structure is somehow altered during the dilution process used to prepare homeopathic medicines. This theory, however, conflicts with scientific understanding of water structure and properties.

▌ **Traditional Chinese medicine (TCM)** includes a large number of folk practices that originated in China. TCM is based on the theory that the body has pathways (called *meridians*) that conduct energy (called *qi*; pronounced "chee"). The interrupted flow of qi is believed to cause illness. TCM practices allegedly improve the flow of qi and include acupuncture, **qi gong,** herbal remedies, dietary practices, and massage. Ironically, the Western approach to managing illness is now the primary system of health care used in China.[6]

What is the theory underlying mind-body interventions?

Mind-body interventions attempt to improve a person's sense of well-being despite the presence of illness. The treatments are also used in the hope of reducing stress, dealing with pain, or lowering blood pressure. Some of these therapies have been incorporated into mainstream medicine for stress reduction or relaxation. For example, **biofeedback training,** in which individuals learn to monitor skin temperature, muscle tension, or brain wave activity while practicing relaxation techniques, is frequently taught by behavioral medicine specialists to help patients reduce stress or anxiety (see Figure NP15-1 on p. 436). Other techniques to reduce stress and promote relaxation include **meditation,** art and music therapy, and prayer.

The clinical applications of other mind-body therapies are far more questionable. One example is guided **imagery,** in which a person tries to reverse the disease process (for example, shrink a tumor) by using mental pictures. Another example is the use of **faith healing** in place of proven conventional treatments to cure disease.

© Cindy Charles/PhotoEdit

Which alternative practices involve physical manipulation, and how do they work?

Manipulative interventions include physical touch, forceful movement of different parts of the body, and the application of pressure. Some practitioners maintain that special energy fields are manipulated during the physical treatment and that proper energy flow induces healing. Popular practices include the following:

- **Chiropractic** theory proposes that keeping the nervous system free from obstruction allows the body to heal itself, allegedly because the healing process stems from the brain and is conducted via the spinal cord and nerves to all parts of the body. Chiropractors claim to diagnose illnesses by detecting subluxations in the spine, which are variously described as misaligned vertebrae or pinched nerves that allegedly cause subtle interferences within the nervous system. The main treatment is the *adjustment,* a manual manipulation that is said to correct a subluxation and restore the body's natural healing ability. Although spinal manipulation has mainly been found to be helpful for improving back pain, many chiropractors still assert that chiropractic can cure disease rather than simply relieve symptoms. For example, many chiropractors promote spinal manipulation to treat infectious diseases and prevent cancer, even though the nervous system and spinal alignment do not play roles in the pathology of these conditions.

- **Massage therapy** is the manipulation of muscle and connective tissue to improve muscle function, reduce pain, or promote relaxation. Massage therapists may also apply heat or cold and give advice about exercises that may improve muscle tone and range of motion. Massage is often integrated into conventional physical therapy, although some massage therapists may incorrectly suggest that massage is a valid treatment for a wide range of medical conditions.

What are the alleged effects of "energy" therapies?

Two categories of therapies involve the alleged curative power of "energy":

- **Biofield therapies** are said to influence the energy that surrounds or pervades the human body, and their proponents claim that an energy therapy can strengthen or restore a person's "energy flow" and induce healing. Acupuncture, qi gong, and **therapeutic touch** are among the therapies that subscribe to these theories. Note that CAM adherents often use the term "energy" unscientifically and that there is no objective evidence of this sort of energy flow.

- **Bioelectrical** or **bioelectromagnetic therapies** use electric or magnetic fields to allegedly promote healing; for example, magnets have been marketed with claims that they can improve circulation, reduce inflammation, and speed recovery from injuries.

Acupuncture is probably the best-known therapy involving "energy flow." The practice involves the shallow insertion of stainless steel needles into the skin at designated points on the body, sometimes accompanied by a low-frequency current to produce greater stimulation. Practitioners believe that the treatment restores health by improving the flow of energy in the body.

Do conventional health practitioners consider CAM treatments to be safe and effective?

CAM treatments are generally excluded from mainstream medical practice because there is no evidence proving that they are effective for treating the diseases and medical conditions for which they are used. Many consumers think otherwise and seem satisfied that these treatments "work." How is this dichotomy to be explained?

Surveys suggest that consumers perceive their visits to CAM therapists as far more pleasant than their visits to conventional health practitioners. As explained earlier, CAM therapists often spend more time with patients, are more attentive, and use less invasive interventions. Self-help measures are encouraged, so the consumer has more control over the treatment. The therapies appear to be more "natural" and to have fewer side effects. Possible explanations for "cures" include the following:

- A person may seem cured because of misdiagnosis; that is, the condition diagnosed by the CAM practitioner may not have actually existed.

- The condition may have been self-limiting, or it may have gone into temporary remission after the treatment.

- Undue credit may be inappropriately assigned to the CAM therapy when the improvement was actually due to a previous or concurrent conventional treatment.

- The placebo effect may have had an influence on the course of disease.

The central question remains: Do the CAM therapies merely make people *feel* better, or do they really *get* better? This question can be answered only by well-controlled research studies.

Are any potential dangers associated with the use of CAM?

One of the attractions of alternative therapies is the assumption that they are safe. Recall, however, the concerns associated with the use of herbal products discussed in Chapter 15, which include the potential toxicity of herbal ingredients, product contamination or adulteration, and interactions with conventional medications. Another concern is that use of CAM therapies may delay the use of reliable treatments that have demonstrable benefits.[7] Various reports have described people with treatable medical conditions who suffered permanent disability or death when they were misdiagnosed or improperly treated by CAM practitioners. For example, a rare but well-known risk of spinal cord injury or stroke is associated with a type of cervical manipulation performed by chiropractors.[8] Unfortunately, because most CAM therapies are not regulated or monitored, there are no accurate estimates of their adverse effects.

What should health practitioners do if they think their patients are using CAM?

Health practitioners should routinely inquire about the use of CAM therapies and educate patients about the hazards of postponing or stopping conventional treatment. Patients should also be told about potential interactions between conventional treatments and CAM therapies. Some patients may want to learn about differences between evidence-based medical practices and untested CAM theories and may be interested in the integrative medicine options available.

All alternative therapies have one characteristic in common: their effectiveness is, for the most part, unproven. Because patients often choose CAM therapies because of positive interactions with alternative practitioners, health care practitioners should realize that empathizing with patients may go a long way toward winning their trust and improving their compliance with therapy. Furthermore, health practitioners should stay informed about

unconventional practices by obtaining reliable, objective resources so that they can knowledgeably discuss these options with patients.

Notes

1. S. Rosenzweig, Complementary and alternative medicine, in R. S. Porter and J. L. Kaplan, eds., *Merck Manual of Diagnosis and Therapy* (Whitehouse Station, NJ: Merck Sharp and Dohme Corp., 2011), pp. 3411–3420.

2. Rosenzweig, 2011.

3. M. Charlson, Complementary and alternative medicine, in L. Goldman and A. I. Schafer, *Goldman's Cecil Medicine* (Philadelphia: Saunders, 2012), pp. 177–181.

4. Charlson, 2012; A. M. McCaffrey, G. F. Pugh, and B. B. O'Connor, Understanding patient preference for integrative medical care: Results from patient focus groups, *Journal of General Internal Medicine* 22 (2007): 1500–1505.

5. S. E. Straus, Complementary and alternative medicine, in L. Goldman and D. Ausiello, eds., *Cecil Medicine* (Philadelphia: Saunders, 2008), pp. 206–209.

6. D. R. Haley and coauthors, Five myths of the Chinese health care system, *Health Care Manager* 27 (2008): 147–158.

7. Rosenzweig, 2011.

8. F. C. Albuquerque and coauthors, Craniocervical arterial dissections as sequelae of chiropractic manipulation: Patterns of injury and management, *Journal of Neurosurgery* 115 (2011): 1197–1205.

Specialized Nutrition Support: Enteral and Parenteral Nutrition

16.1 Enteral Nutrition

LO 16.1 Identify patients who may benefit from enteral nutrition and describe the feeding routes, enteral formulas, and administration considerations for tube feedings.

16.2 Parenteral Nutrition

LO 16.2 Identify patients who may benefit from parenteral nutrition and describe the components of parenteral solutions and administration techniques.

16.3 Nutrition Support at Home

LO 16.3 Give examples of individuals who may be candidates for home nutrition support and discuss the considerations involved in using enteral or parenteral nutrition in the home.

16.4 Nutrition in Practice: Inborn Errors of Metabolism

LO 16.4 Describe the possible metabolic effects of inborn errors of metabolism and discuss the complications and treatments of phenylketonuria and galactosemia.

David Gee 2/Alamy

Patients are often too sick to consume a regular diet. Moreover, some illnesses may interfere with eating, digestion, or absorption to such a degree that oral intakes alone cannot supply the necessary nutrients. In such cases, **nutrition support**—the delivery of nutrients using a feeding tube or intravenous infusions—can meet a patient's nutritional needs. **Enteral nutrition,** the provision of nutrients using the gastrointestinal (GI) tract, usually refers to the use of tube feedings, which deliver nutrient-dense formulas directly to the stomach or small intestine via a thin, flexible tube. **Parenteral nutrition** provides nutrients intravenously to patients who do not have sufficient GI function to handle enteral feedings. If the GI tract remains functional, enteral nutrition is preferred over parenteral nutrition because it is associated with fewer infectious complications and is significantly less expensive.[1] Figure 16-1 summarizes the decision-making process for selecting the most appropriate feeding method.

16.1 Enteral Nutrition

LO 16.1 Identify patients who may benefit from enteral nutrition and describe the feeding routes, enteral formulas, and administration considerations for tube feedings.

If GI function is normal and a poor appetite is the primary nutrition problem, patients may be able to improve their diets by using oral supplements. If patients are unable to meet their nutrient needs by oral intakes alone, tube feedings can be used to deliver the required nutrients.

Oral Supplements

Patients who are weak or debilitated may find it easier to consume oral supplements than to consume meals (see Figure 16-2, p. 440). Moreover, a patient who can improve nutrition

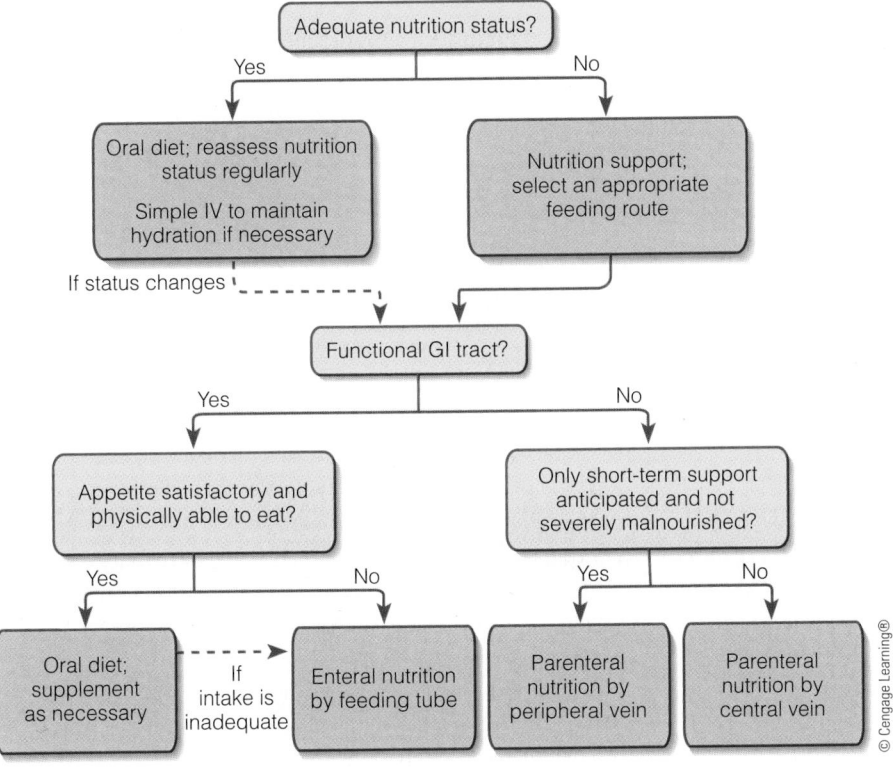

FIGURE 16-1 **Selecting a Feeding Route**

nutrition support: the delivery of nutrients using a feeding tube or intravenous infusions.

enteral (EN-ter-al) **nutrition:** the provision of nutrients using the GI tract; usually refers to the use of tube feedings.

parenteral (par-EN-ter-al) **nutrition:** the intravenous provision of nutrients that bypasses the GI tract.

- *par* = beside
- *entero* = intestine

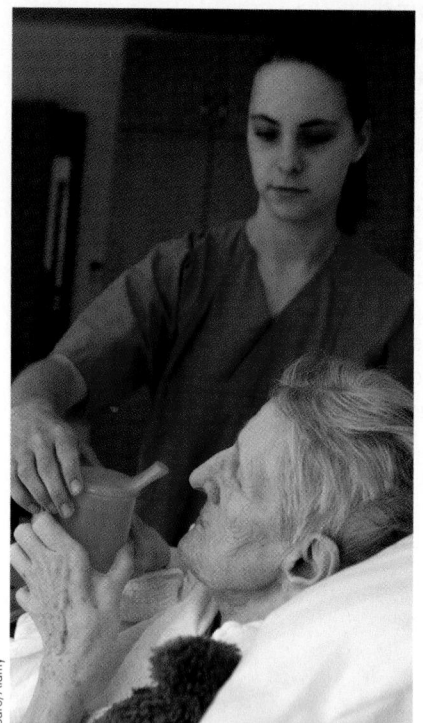

Caro/Alamy

FIGURE 16-2 Use of Oral Supplements
Patients can drink nutrient-dense formulas when they are unable to consume enough food from a regular diet.

fistulas (FIST-you-luz)**:** abnormal passages between organs or tissues (or between an internal organ and the body's surface) that permit the passage of fluids or secretions.

intractable: not easily managed or controlled.

status with supplements may be able to avoid the stress, complications, and expense associated with tube feedings. Hospitals usually stock a variety of nutrient-dense formulas, milkshakes, fruit drinks, and snack bars to provide to patients at risk of becoming malnourished. Note that similar products are sold in pharmacies and grocery stores for home use; examples of popular liquid supplements include Ensure, Boost, and Carnation Breakfast Essentials. These types of products can add energy and protein to the diets of patients and be a reliable source of nutrients.

When a patient uses an oral supplement, taste becomes an important consideration. Allowing patients to sample different products and select the ones they prefer helps to promote acceptance. Box 16-1 offers additional suggestions for helping patients improve their intakes using oral supplements.

Candidates for Tube Feedings

Tube feedings are typically recommended for patients at risk of developing protein-energy malnutrition who are unable to consume adequate food and/or oral supplements to maintain their health. The following medical conditions or treatments may indicate the need for tube feedings:

- Severe swallowing disorders
- Impaired motility in the upper GI tract
- GI obstructions and **fistulas** that can be bypassed with a feeding tube
- Certain types of intestinal surgeries
- Little or no appetite for extended periods, especially if the patient is malnourished
- Extremely high nutrient requirements
- Mechanical ventilation
- Mental incapacitation due to confusion, neurological disorders, or coma

Contraindications for tube feedings include severe GI bleeding, high-output fistulas, **intractable** vomiting or diarrhea, and severe malabsorption. The procedure may also be contraindicated if the expected need for nutrition support is less than 5 to 7 days in a malnourished patient or less than 7 to 9 days in an adequately nourished patient.[2]

How To BOX 16-1 HELP PATIENTS IMPROVE INTAKES WITH ORAL SUPPLEMENTS

Patients in hospitals are often quite ill and have poor appetites. Even when a person enjoys an oral supplement, the taste may become monotonous in time. Health practitioners may be able to motivate patients to improve intakes by trying these suggestions:

- Let the patient sample different products that are appropriate for his or her needs, and provide only those that the patient enjoys.

- Serve supplements attractively. For example, a liquid formula offered in a glass on an attractive plate may be more appealing than a formula served from a can with an unfamiliar name.

- Try keeping a liquid supplement in an ice bath so that it is cool and refreshing when the patient drinks it. Check with the patient to make sure the colder temperature is suitable.

- If a patient finds the smell of a formula unappealing, it may help to cover the top of the glass with plastic wrap or a lid, leaving just enough room for a straw.

- For patients with little appetite, offer the drink or snack food in small amounts that are easy to tolerate, and serve it more frequently during the day.

- Provide easy access. Keep the supplement close to the patient's bed where it can be reached with little effort and within sight so that the patient is reminded to consume it.

- If the patient stops enjoying a particular product, suggest an alternative. Maintain an updated list of oral supplements that are available at your institution so that you can advise patients about the possible options.

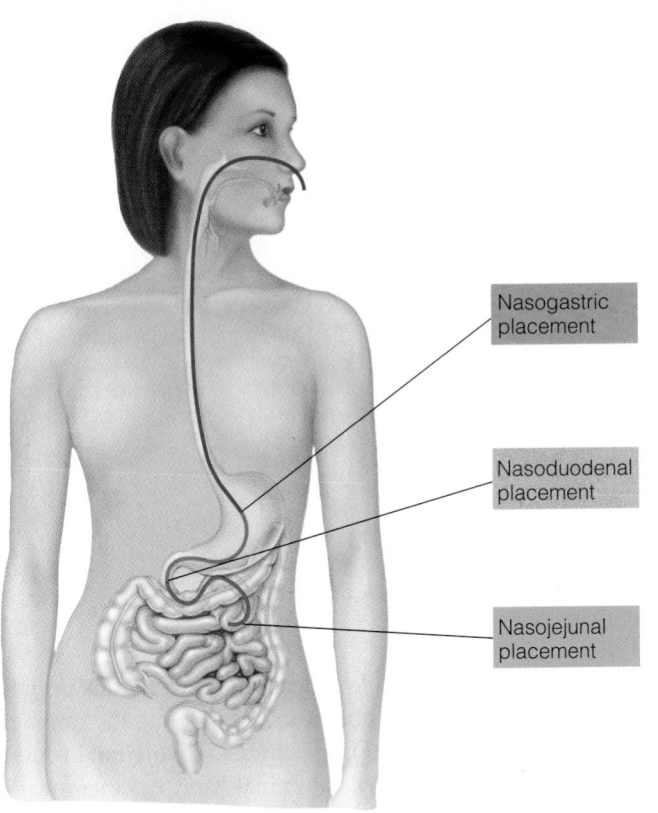

Nasogastric placement

Nasoduodenal placement

Nasojejunal placement

Gastrostomy

Jejunostomy

© Cengage Learning®

Transnasal feeding tube placements

Enterostomies

FIGURE 16-3 Tube Feeding Routes

LTH NHS Trust/Science Source

A transnasal feeding tube accesses the GI tract via the nose. The patient in this photo is being fed through a nasogastric tube; he is also attached to a respirator to help him breathe.

Dr. P. Marazzi/Science Source

In a gastrostomy, the feeding tube accesses the GI tract through the abdominal wall.

FIGURE 16-4 Examples of Tube Feeding Routes

Tube Feeding Routes

The feeding route chosen depends on the patient's medical condition, the expected duration of tube feeding, and the potential complications of a particular route. Figures 16-3 and 16-4 illustrate the main feeding routes, and Box 16-2 (p. 442) describes each route.

Gastrointestinal Access When a patient is expected to be tube fed for less than four weeks, the feeding tube is generally routed into the GI tract via the nose (**nasogastric** or **nasoenteric** routes). The patient is frequently awake during **transnasal**

BOX 16-2 GLOSSARY OF TUBE FEEDING ROUTES

For each type of tube placement, the terms are listed in order from the upper to lower organs of the digestive system.

transnasal: a *transnasal feeding tube* is one that is inserted through the nose.

- **nasogastric (NG):** tube is placed into the stomach via the nose.
- **nasoenteric:** tube is placed into the GI tract via the nose; most often refers to *nasoduodenal* and *nasojejunal* feeding routes (also known as *nasointestinal* feeding routes).
- **nasoduodenal (ND):** tube is placed into the duodenum via the nose.
- **nasojejunal (NJ):** tube is placed into the jejunum via the nose.

orogastric: tube is inserted into the stomach through the mouth. This method is often used to feed infants because a nasogastric tube may hinder the infant's breathing.

enterostomy (EN-ter-AH-stoe-mee): an opening into the GI tract through the abdominal wall.

- **gastrostomy** (gah-STRAH-stoe-mee): an opening into the stomach through which a feeding tube can be passed. A nonsurgical technique for creating a gastrostomy under local anesthesia is called *percutaneous endoscopic gastrostomy (PEG)*.
- **jejunostomy** (JEH-ju-NAH-stoe-mee): an opening into the jejunum through which a feeding tube can be passed. A nonsurgical technique for creating a jejunostomy is called *percutaneous endoscopic jejunostomy (PEJ)*. The tube can either be guided into the jejunum via a gastrostomy or passed directly into the jejunum *(direct PEJ)*.

Corpak MedSystems

FIGURE 16-5 The feeding tube shown here has centimeter marks to help with insertion and to check migration. The Y-port at the upper end of the tube allows the administration of water or medications during feedings.

aspiration: drawing in by suction or inhalation; a common complication of enteral feedings in which substances from the GI tract are drawn into the lungs. Aspiration risk is high in patients with esophageal disorders, neuromuscular diseases, and conditions that reduce consciousness or cause dementia.

French units: units of measure for a feeding tube's outer diameter; 1 French equals 1/3 millimeter.

gastric decompression: the removal of stomach contents (such as GI secretions, air, or blood) in patients with motility problems or obstructions that prevent stomach emptying; the procedure may be used to reduce discomfort, vomiting, or various complications during critical illness or after certain surgeries.

(through-the-nose) placement of a feeding tube. While the patient is in a slightly upright position with head tilted, the tube is inserted into a nostril and passed into the stomach (nasogastric route), duodenum (**nasoduodenal** route), or jejunum (**nasojejunal** route). The final position of the feeding tube tip is verified by abdominal X-ray or other means. In infants, **orogastric** placement, in which the feeding tube is passed into the stomach via the mouth, is sometimes preferred over transnasal routes; this placement allows the infant to breathe more normally during feedings.

When a patient will be tube fed for longer than four weeks, or if the nasoenteric route is inaccessible due to an obstruction or other medical reasons, a direct route to the stomach or intestine may be created by passing the tube through an **enterostomy,** an opening in the abdominal wall that leads to the stomach (**gastrostomy**) or jejunum (**jejunostomy**). An enterostomy can be made by either surgical incision or needle puncture.

Selecting a Feeding Route Gastric feedings (nasogastric and gastrostomy routes) are preferred whenever possible. These feedings are more easily tolerated and less complicated to deliver than intestinal feedings because the stomach controls the rate at which nutrients enter the intestine. Gastric feedings are not possible, however, if patients have gastric obstructions or motility disorders that interfere with the stomach's ability to empty. Gastric feedings are also avoided in patients at high risk of **aspiration,** a common complication in which substances from the GI tract (either GI secretions or refluxed stomach contents) are drawn into the lungs, potentially leading to pneumonia (note that studies have not consistently shown that gastric feedings are associated with a higher pneumonia risk[3]). Table 16-1 summarizes the advantages and disadvantages of the various tube feeding routes.

Feeding Tubes Feeding tubes are made from soft, flexible materials (such as silicone or polyurethane) and come in a variety of lengths and diameters (see Figure 16-5). The tube selected largely depends on the patient's age and size, the feeding route, and the formula viscosity.

The outer diameter of a feeding tube is measured in **French units,** in which each unit equals 1/3 millimeter; thus, a "12 French" feeding tube has a 4-millimeter diameter ($12 \times 1/3$ mm = 4 mm). The inner diameter depends on the thickness of the tubing material. Double-lumen tubes are also available; these allow a single tube to be used for both intestinal feedings and **gastric decompression,** a procedure in which the stomach contents of patients with motility problems or obstructions are removed by suction.

TABLE 16-1 Comparison of Tube Feeding Routes[a]

Insertion Method or Feeding Site	Advantages	Disadvantages
Transnasal	Does not require surgery or incisions for placement; tubes can be placed by a nurse or trained dietitian.	Easy to remove by disoriented patients; long-term use may irritate the nasal passages, throat, and esophagus.
▪ Nasogastric	Easiest to insert and confirm placement; least expensive method; feedings can often be given intermittently and without an infusion pump.	Highest risk of aspiration in compromised patients;[b] risk of tube migration to the small intestine.
▪ Nasoduodenal and nasojejunal	Lower risk of aspiration in compromised patients;[b] allows for earlier tube feedings than gastric feedings during acute stress; may allow enteral feedings even when obstructions, fistulas, or other medical conditions prevent gastric feedings.	More difficult to insert and confirm placement; risk of tube migration to the stomach; feedings require an infusion pump for administration.
Tube enterostomies	Allow the lower esophageal sphincter to remain closed, reducing the risk of aspiration;[b] more comfortable than transnasal insertion for long-term use; site is not visible under clothing.	Tubes must be placed by a physician or surgeon; general anesthesia may be required for surgically placed tubes; risk of complications from the insertion procedure; risk of infection at the insertion site.
▪ Gastrostomy	Feedings can often be given intermittently and without a pump; easier insertion procedure than a jejunostomy.	Moderate risk of aspiration in high-risk patients;[b] feedings often withheld for 12 to 24 hours before and 48 to 72 hours after the insertion procedure.
▪ Jejunostomy	Lowest risk of aspiration;[b] allows for earlier tube feedings than gastrostomy during critical illness; may allow enteral feedings even when obstructions, fistulas, or medical conditions prevent gastric feedings.	Most difficult insertion procedure; most costly method; feedings require an infusion pump for administration.

© 2016 Cengage Learning®

[a]Relative to other tube feeding routes. The actual advantages and disadvantages of different insertion procedures depend on the person's medical condition.
[b]The risk of aspiration associated with the different feeding routes is controversial and still under investigation.

Enteral Formulas

Most enteral formulas can supply all of an individual's nutrient requirements when consumed in sufficient volume, a necessity for the patient who is using a tube feeding for more than a few days. The formulas can be used alone or provided along with other foods.

Types of Enteral Formulas More than 75 enteral formulas are currently marketed;[4] Appendix G lists examples. The main types of formulas include the following:

▪ **Standard formulas,** also called *polymeric formulas*, are provided to individuals who can digest and absorb nutrients without difficulty. They contain intact proteins extracted from milk or soybeans (called **protein isolates**) or a combination of such proteins. The carbohydrate sources include hydrolyzed cornstarch, glucose polymers (such as maltodextrin and corn syrup solids), and sugars. A few formulas, called **blenderized formulas,** are produced from whole foods such as chicken, vegetables, fruits, and oil, along with some added vitamins and minerals.

▪ **Elemental formulas,** also called *hydrolyzed, chemically defined, or monomeric formulas,* are prescribed for patients who have compromised digestive or absorptive functions. Elemental formulas contain proteins and carbohydrates that have been partially or fully broken down to fragments that require little (if any) digestion. The formulas are often low in fat and may provide fat from **medium-chain triglycerides (MCT)** to ease digestion and absorption.

▪ **Specialized formulas,** also called *disease-specific* or *specialty formulas,* are intended to meet the nutrient needs of patients with particular illnesses. Products have been

standard formulas: enteral formulas that contain mostly intact proteins and polysaccharides; also called *polymeric formulas.*

protein isolates: proteins that have been isolated from foods.

blenderized formulas: enteral formulas that are prepared by using a food blender to mix and puree whole foods.

elemental formulas: enteral formulas that contain proteins and carbohydrates that are partially or fully hydrolyzed; also called *hydrolyzed, chemically defined,* or *monomeric formulas.*

medium-chain triglycerides (MCT): triglycerides that contain fatty acids that are 8 to 10 carbons in length. MCT do not require digestion and can be absorbed in the absence of lipase or bile.

specialized formulas: enteral formulas for patients with specific illnesses; also called *disease-specific formulas* or *specialty formulas.*

developed for individuals with liver, kidney, and lung diseases; glucose intolerance; severe wounds; and metabolic stress (later chapters provide details). Specialized formulas are generally expensive, and their effectiveness is controversial.

▌ **Modular formulas,** created from individual macronutrient preparations called *modules,* are sometimes prepared for patients who require specific nutrient combinations. Vitamin and mineral preparations are also included in the formulas so that they can meet all of a person's nutrient needs. In some cases, one or more modules are added to other enteral formulas to adjust their nutrient composition.

Macronutrient Composition The amounts of protein, carbohydrate, and fat in enteral formulas vary substantially. The protein content of most standard formulas ranges from 12 to 20 percent of total kcalories;[5] note that protein needs are high in patients with severe metabolic stress, whereas protein restrictions are necessary for patients with chronic kidney disease. Carbohydrate and fat provide most of the energy in enteral formulas; standard formulas generally provide 30 to 60 percent of kcalories from carbohydrate and 15 to 30 percent of kcalories from fat.

Energy Density The energy density of most enteral formulas ranges from 1.0 to 2.0 kcalories per milliliter of fluid. The formulas that have higher energy densities can meet energy and nutrient needs in a smaller volume of fluid and therefore benefit patients who have high nutrient needs or fluid restrictions.

Fiber Content Fiber-containing formulas may be helpful for improving fecal bulk and colonic function, treating diarrhea or constipation, and maintaining blood glucose control. Conversely, fiber-containing formulas are avoided in patients with acute intestinal conditions or pancreatitis and before or after some intestinal examinations and surgeries.

Osmolality Osmolality refers to the moles of osmotically active solutes (or *osmoles*) per kilogram of solvent. An enteral formula with an osmolality similar to that of blood serum (about 300 milliosmoles per kilogram) is an **isotonic formula,** whereas a **hypertonic formula** has an osmolality greater than that of blood serum.

Most enteral formulas have osmolalities between 300 and 700 milliosmoles per kilogram; generally, elemental formulas and nutrient-dense formulas have higher osmolalities than standard formulas. Most people are able to tolerate both isotonic and hypertonic feedings without difficulty.[6] When medications are infused along with enteral feedings, however, the osmotic load increases substantially and may contribute to the diarrhea experienced by many tube-fed patients.

Formula Selection Some of the factors considered when choosing a formula are shown in Figure 16-6. Generally, the formula chosen should meet the patient's medical and nutrient needs with the lowest risk of complications and the lowest cost. The main factors that influence formula selection include:

▌ *GI function.* Although the vast majority of patients can use standard formulas, a person with a functional but impaired GI tract may require an elemental formula.

▌ *Nutrient and energy needs.* As with patients consuming regular diets, the tube-fed patient may require adjustments in nutrient and energy intakes. If fluids are restricted, the formula should have adequate nutrient and energy densities to provide the required nutrients in the volume prescribed.

▌ *Fiber modifications.* The choice of formulas is narrower if fiber intake needs to be low or high.

▌ *Individual tolerances (food allergies and sensitivities).* Nearly all formulas are lactose free and gluten free and can accommodate the needs of patients with lactose intolerance or gluten sensitivity. For patients with food allergies, ingredient lists should be checked before providing a formula.

modular formulas: enteral formulas prepared in the hospital from modules that contain single macronutrients; used for people with unique nutrient needs.

osmolality (OZ-moe-LAL-ih-tee): the concentration of osmotically active solutes in a solution, expressed as milliosmoles (mOsm) per kilogram of solvent. Osmotically active solutes affect *osmosis,* the movement of water across semipermeable membranes.

isotonic formula: a formula with an osmolality similar to that of blood serum (about 300 milliosmoles per kilogram).

▌ *iso* = equal
▌ *tono* = pressure

hypertonic formula: a formula with an osmolality greater than that of blood serum.

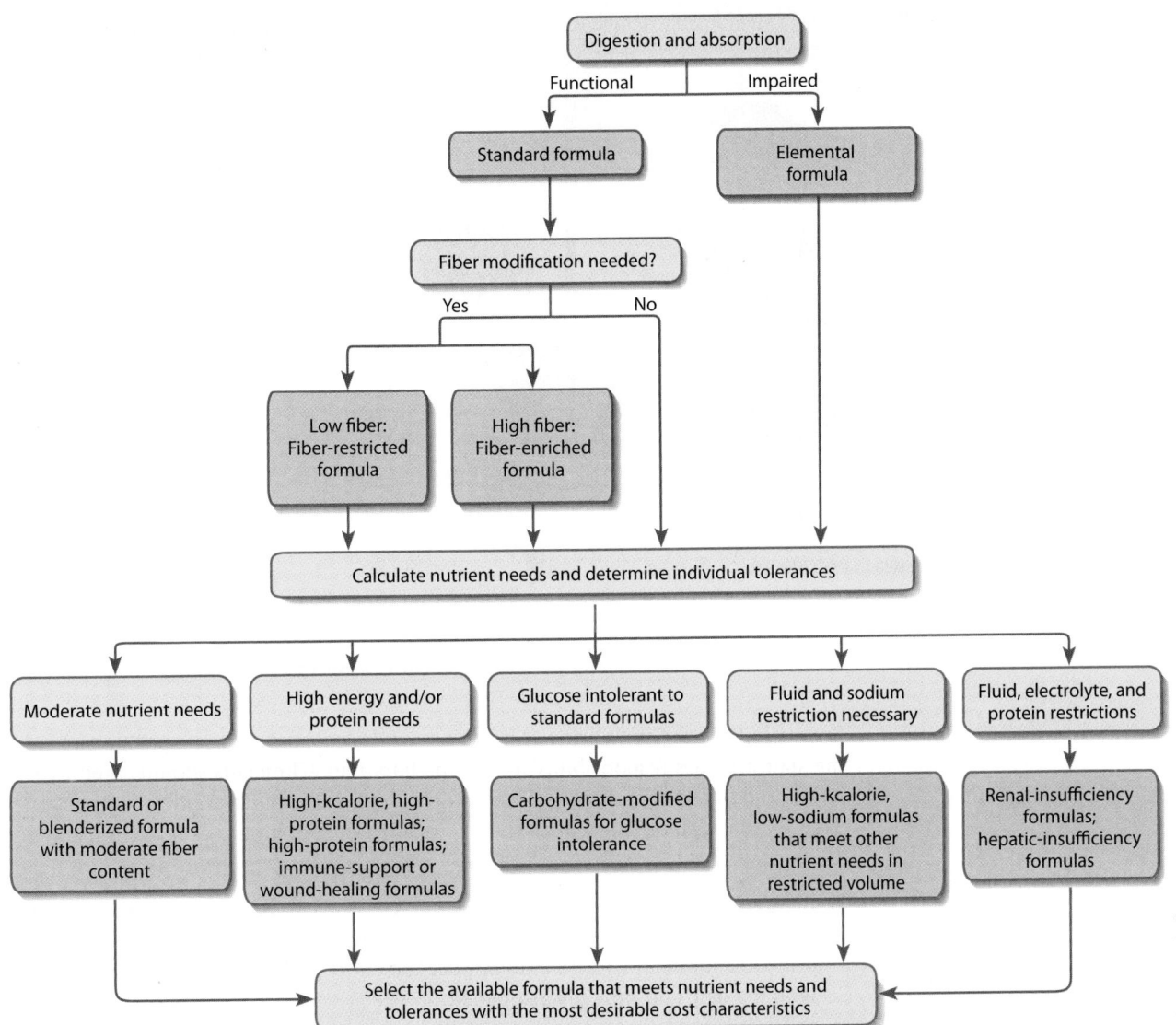

FIGURE 16-6 **Selecting a Formula**

Health care facilities stock a limited number of formulas, so formula selection is influenced by availability. The medical staff may initially choose a formula based on the criteria previously mentioned and then reevaluate the decision according to the patient's response to the formula.

Safe Handling Individuals who are ill or malnourished often have suppressed immune systems, making them vulnerable to infection from foodborne illness. Thus, the personnel involved with preparing or delivering formula should be aware of the specific protocols at their facility that prevent formula contamination (such as the **Hazard Analysis and Critical Control Points [HACCP] system**).

Formulas may be delivered using an **open feeding system** or a **closed feeding system** (see Figure 16-7, p. 446). With an open system, the formula needs to be transferred from its original packaging to a feeding container. Examples include formulas that are packaged in cans or bottles, concentrates that need to be diluted, and powders that require reconstitution. In a closed system, the sterile formula is prepackaged in a container that can be connected directly to a feeding tube. Closed systems are less likely to become contaminated, require less nursing time, and can hang for longer periods of time than open systems. Although closed systems cost more initially, they may be less expensive in the long run because they prevent bacterial contamination and thus avoid the costs of treating infections.

Hazard Analysis and Critical Control Points (HACCP) system: a management system to identify and correct potential microbial hazards in the preparation, storage, handling, and administration of food products; commonly referred to as *HASS-ip*.

open feeding system: a formula delivery system that requires the transfer of the formula from its original packaging to a feeding container.

closed feeding system: a formula delivery system in which the sterile formula comes prepackaged in a container that can be attached directly to the feeding tube for administration.

In an open feeding system, the formula is transferred from its original packaging to a feeding container.

In a closed feeding system, the formula is prepackaged in a container that can be attached directly to a feeding tube, such as the bottle shown on the left. The formula in the can at right can be used in an open feeding system.

FIGURE 16-7 **Comparison of Open and Closed Feeding Systems**

Formula Safety Guidelines After the formula reaches the nursing station, the nursing staff assumes responsibility for its safe handling. Clinicians should carefully wash hands and put on disposable gloves before handling formulas and feeding containers. The following steps can reduce the risk of formula contamination when using open feeding systems:[7]

- Before opening a can of formula, clean the lid with a disposable alcohol wipe and wash the can opener (if needed) with detergent and hot water. (Check HACCP protocols for details.) If you do not use the entire can at one feeding, label the can with the date and time it was opened.

- Store opened cans or mixed formulas in clean, closed containers. Refrigerate the unused portion of formula promptly. Discard unlabeled or improperly labeled containers and all open containers of formula that are not used within 24 to 48 hours.

- Hang no more than an 8-hour supply of formula (or a 4-hour supply for newborn infants) when using liquid formula from a can. Formulas prepared from powders or modules should hang no longer than 4 hours. Discard any formula that remains, rinse the feeding bag and tubing, and add fresh formula to the feeding bag. A new feeding container and tubing (except for the feeding tube itself) is necessary every 24 hours.

For closed systems, the hang time should be no longer than 24 to 48 hours. Contamination is more likely with the longer time periods.

Administration of Tube Feedings

The methods of tube feeding administration vary somewhat from one health care facility to the next. The procedures presented in the following sections are suggested guidelines.

Preparing for Tube Feedings Before starting a tube feeding, health practitioners can ease fears by fully discussing the procedure with the patient and family members, who may feel anxious about the use of a feeding tube. The discussion should address the reasons why tube feeding is appropriate as well as the benefits and risks of the procedure. Box 16-3 offers suggestions that may help ease the concerns of patients who may benefit from tube feeding.

Although many patients are initially apprehensive about receiving tube feedings, they may be less resistant once they understand the insertion method, the expected duration of the tube feeding, and the strategic role that nutrition plays in recovery from illness. The pointers that follow can help health practitioners prepare patients for transnasal tube feedings:

▌ Allow the patient to see and touch the feeding tube. Understanding that the tube is soft and narrow (only about half the diameter of a pencil) often alleviates anxiety.

▌ Show the patient how the feeding equipment is attached to the feeding tube, and explain how the feeding will work. For young children, use dolls or stuffed toys to demonstrate tube insertion and feeding procedures.

▌ Explain that the patient remains fully alert during the procedure and helps to pass the tube by swallowing. A numbing solution sprayed on the back of the throat minimizes discomfort and prevents gagging during the procedure.

▌ Inform the patient that after the tube has been inserted, most people become accustomed to its presence within a few hours. In most cases, the patient can continue to swallow foods and beverages with the tube in place.

Tube feedings may cause some patients to feel that they have lost control over an important aspect of their lives. They may also feel self-conscious about how the feeding tube looks or feel awkward when moving around with the equipment. A few measures can help:

▌ Assure the patient that the tube feeding is temporary, if such assurance is appropriate.

▌ Involve patients in the decision-making and care process whenever possible. Patients can help to arrange their daily feeding schedules and can perform some of the feeding procedures themselves.

▌ Show patients how to manipulate the feeding equipment so that they can get out of bed and move around.

Serious complications can develop if a transnasal tube is accidentally inserted into the respiratory tract or if formula or GI secretions are aspirated into the lungs. To minimize the risk of incorrect tube placement, clinicians use X-rays to verify the position of the feeding tube before a feeding is initiated. After the tube's placement has been confirmed, the nurse secures the tube to the patient's nose and cheek with tape and monitors the position of the tubing throughout the day. Tube placement can also be monitored by testing the pH of a sample of body fluid drawn into the feeding tube, as the pH in the stomach (5 or lower) is lower than the pH in the small intestine or respiratory tract (6 or higher).

To reduce the risk of aspiration, the patient's upper body is elevated to a 30- to 45-degree angle during the feeding and for 30 to 60 minutes after the feeding whenever possible.[8] The addition of blue food coloring to formula was formerly suggested as a means of identifying aspirated formula in lung secretions; however, the practice was discontinued after it was found to be associated with various complications and even deaths.[9]

Formula Delivery Methods Nutrient needs may be met by delivering relatively large amounts of formula several times per day (**intermittent feedings**) or smaller amounts continuously (**continuous feedings**). A patient may also start with continuous feedings and gradually transition to intermittent feedings. Each method has specific uses, advantages, and disadvantages.

Intermittent feedings are best tolerated when they are delivered into the stomach (not the intestine). Generally, a total of about 250 to 400 milliliters of formula is delivered over 30 to 45 minutes using a gravity drip method or an infusion pump (see Figure 16-8, p. 448). The exact amount is determined by dividing the required volume of formula into several daily feedings, as shown in Box 16-4 (p. 448). Due to the relatively high volume of formula delivered at one time, intermittent feedings may be difficult for some patients to tolerate, and the risk of aspiration may be higher than with continuous feedings. An advantage of intermittent feedings is that they are similar to the usual pattern of eating and allow the patient freedom of movement between meals.

Rapid delivery of a large volume of formula into the stomach (250 to 500 milliliters over 5 to 15 minutes) is called a **bolus feeding.** This type of feeding may be given every 3 to 4 hours using a syringe. Bolus feedings are convenient for patients and staff because they are rapidly administered, do not require an infusion pump, and allow

intermittent feedings: delivery of about 250 to 400 milliliters of formula over 30 to 45 minutes.

continuous feedings: slow delivery of formula at a constant rate over an 8- to 24-hour period.

bolus (BOH-lus) **feeding:** delivery of about 250 to 500 milliliters of formula over a 5- to 15-minute period.

FIGURE 16-8 The delivery of intermittent and continuous feedings can be controlled with an infusion pump.

greater independence for patients. However, bolus feedings can cause abdominal discomfort, nausea, and cramping in some patients, and the risk of aspiration is greater than with other methods of feeding. For these reasons, bolus feedings are used only in patients who are not critically ill.

Continuous feedings are delivered slowly and at a constant rate over a period of 8 to 24 hours, and are most often used for intestinal feedings. The slower delivery rate is easier to tolerate, so continuous feedings are generally recommended for critically ill patients or patients who cannot tolerate intermittent feedings. An infusion pump is usually used to ensure accurate and steady flow rates; consequently, the feedings can limit the patient's freedom of movement and are also more costly. Continuous feedings conducted for shorter periods (8 to 16 hours; called **cyclic feedings**) allow greater patient mobility and GI rest and may be used to help patients transition to intermittent feedings or an oral diet.

Initiating and Advancing Tube Feedings Formula administration techniques vary widely among institutions, so protocols should be reviewed carefully before working with patients. In addition, patient tolerance must be considered when adjusting formula delivery rates. Some general guidelines include the following:[10]

Formulas are typically provided full-strength; diluting them is not recommended because this reduces the nutrients provided and increases contamination risk.

cyclic feedings: continuous feedings conducted for 8 to 16 hours daily, allowing patient mobility and bowel rest during the remaining hours of the day.

How To   BOX 16-4 PLAN A TUBE FEEDING SCHEDULE

After selecting a suitable formula, the clinician must determine the volume of formula that meets the patient's nutritional needs. Consider a patient who needs 2000 kcalories daily and is receiving a standard formula that provides 1.0 kcalorie per milliliter. The total volume of formula required would be 2000 milliliters per day:

$$x \text{ mL} \times 1.0 \text{ kcal/mL} = 2000 \text{ kcal}$$
$$x \text{ mL} = \frac{2000 \text{ kcal}}{1.0 \text{ kcal/mL}} = 2000 \text{ mL}$$

If the patient is to receive intermittent feedings six times a day, he will need about 333 milliliters of formula at each feeding:

$$2000 \text{ mL} \div 6 \text{ feedings} = 333 \text{ mL/feeding}$$

Alternatively, if he is to receive intermittent feedings eight times a day, he will need 250 milliliters (or about one can of ready-to-feed formula) at each feeding:

$$2000 \text{ mL} \div 8 \text{ feedings} = 250 \text{ mL/feeding}$$

If the patient is to receive the formula continuously over 24 hours, he will need about 83 milliliters of formula each hour:

$$2000 \text{ mL} \div 24 \text{ hours} = 83 \text{ mL/hr}$$

Intermittent feedings can start with 60 to 120 milliliters at the initial feeding and be increased by 60 to 120 milliliters every 8 to 12 hours until the goal volume is reached. Continuous feedings may start at rates of about 10 to 40 milliliters per hour and be increased by 10 to 20 milliliters per hour every 8 to 12 hours until the goal rate is reached. If the patient cannot tolerate an increased rate of delivery, the feeding rate is slowed until the person adapts.

Goal rates can usually be achieved over 24 to 48 hours, although in some patients, formula delivery can be started at the goal rate immediately.[11] Slower rates of delivery may be better tolerated by critically ill patients, when concentrated formulas are used, or in patients who have undergone an extended period of bowel rest due to surgery, intestinal disease, or the use of parenteral nutrition.

Checking the Gastric Residual Volume To ensure that the stomach is emptying properly, the nurse may measure the **gastric residual volume,** the volume of formula and GI secretions remaining in the stomach after feeding. In this procedure, the gastric contents are gently withdrawn through the feeding tube using a syringe, usually before intermittent feedings and every 4 to 8 hours during continuous feedings in critically ill patients. Although the practice is controversial,[12] some experts recommend that feedings be withheld and an evaluation be conducted if the gastric residual volume exceeds 500 milliliters.[13] If the tendency to accumulate fluids persists, the physician may recommend intestinal feedings or begin drug therapy to stimulate gastric emptying.

Meeting Water Needs Although water needs vary, many patients require about 30 to 40 milliliters of water per kilogram body weight daily.[14] Additional water is required in patients with severe vomiting, diarrhea, fever, excessive sweating, high urine output, high-output ostomies, blood loss, or open wounds. Fluids may be restricted in persons with kidney, liver, or heart disease.

The water in formulas meets a substantial portion of water needs: most enteral formulas contain about 70 to 85 percent water, or about 700 to 850 milliliters of water per liter of formula. In addition to the water in formulas, water can be provided by flushing water separately through the feeding tube. Water flushes are also conducted to prevent feeding tubes from clogging; the water used for flushes (20 to 30 milliliters before and after intermittent feedings and about every 4 hours during continuous feeding) should be included when estimating fluid intakes.

Medication Delivery during Tube Feedings

Patients receiving tube feedings sometimes require one or more medications that need to be delivered through feeding tubes. Because medications can interact with the components of enteral formulas in the same ways that they interact with substances in foods, potential diet-drug interactions must be considered. Medications can also cause feeding tubes to clog. Box 16-5 (p. 450) provides some guidelines that may help to prevent complications.

Medications and Continuous Feeding Continuous feedings are ordinarily stopped before and after medication administration to prevent interactions that may clog the feeding tube or interfere with the medication's absorption. Some medications may require a prolonged formula-free interval; for example, feedings need to be stopped for at least one hour before and after administering phenytoin, a medication that controls seizures.[15] In such cases, the formula's delivery rate needs to be increased so that the correct amount of formula can be delivered.

Diarrhea Medications are a major cause of the diarrhea that frequently accompanies tube feedings. Diarrhea is especially associated with the administration of sorbitol-containing medications, laxatives, and some types of antibiotics.[16] The high osmolality of many liquid medications can also cause diarrhea, so dilution of hypertonic medications may be helpful.

gastric residual volume: the volume of formula and GI secretions remaining in the stomach after a previous feeding.

The pharmacist is your best resource for learning how and when medications can be administered via feeding tubes, especially when you are dealing with an unfamiliar drug. Check with the pharmacist to learn the following:

▪ Whether a particular medication is known to be incompatible with formulas.

▪ The proper timing of medication administration to avoid diet-drug interactions.

▪ For patients using intestinal feedings, whether a medication can be absorbed without exposure to stomach acid.

▪ Whether a liquid form of a medication is available and, if so, the appropriate dosage of the liquid form.

▪ If only tablets are available, whether the tablets can be crushed and mixed with water. Enteric-coated and sustained-release medications should not be crushed due to the potential for adverse effects.

In general, it is best to give medications by mouth instead of by tube whenever possible. In some cases, the injectable form of a medication may be the best option. For medications that must be given by feeding tube:

▪ Do not mix medications with enteral formulas. Do not mix medications together.

▪ Before administering medications, ensure that the feeding tube is placed correctly, that it is not clogged, and that the gastric residual volume is not excessive.

▪ Position the patient in a semi-upright position (30 degrees or higher) to prevent aspiration.

▪ Flush the feeding tube with 15 to 30 milliliters of warm water before and after administering a medication. When more than one medication is administered, flush the feeding tube with water between medications.

▪ Use liquid forms of medications whenever possible. Dilute viscous or hypertonic liquid medications with at least 30 milliliters of water before administering them through the feeding tube.

▪ If tablets are used, crush tablets to a fine powder and mix with about 30 milliliters of warm water before administering.

Tube Feeding Complications

Complications of tube feedings include gastrointestinal problems, such as constipation and diarrhea; mechanical problems related to the tube feeding process; and metabolic problems, such as nutrient deficiencies and changes in the body's biochemistry. Examples of the most common complications, along with some preventive and corrective measures, are summarized in Table 16-2.

Transition to Table Foods

After the patient's condition improves, the volume of formula can be tapered off as the patient gradually shifts to an oral diet. Individuals receiving continuous feedings are often switched to intermittent feedings initially. Patients using elemental formulas may begin the transition by using a standard formula, either orally or via tube feeding. Oral intake should supply about two-thirds of estimated nutrient needs before the tube feeding is discontinued completely.[17] The Case Study in Box 16-6 (p. 452) allows you to review the many factors involved in tube feedings.

IN SUMMARY

▪ Transnasal feeding routes are preferred for short-term tube feedings, whereas enterostomies are used for longer-term feedings. Gastric feedings are preferred but may be avoided in patients at risk of aspiration.

▪ Patients may receive standard, elemental, specialized, or modular formulas; the formulas can be delivered intermittently, in bolus feedings, or continuously.

▪ Formulas can meet a substantial portion of the patient's water requirements. Medications should be given separately and accompanied by water flushes to prevent tube clogging.

▪ Complications of tube feedings can be gastrointestinal, mechanical, or metabolic in nature.

TABLE 16-2 Causes and Management of Tube Feeding Complications

Complications	Possible Causes	Preventive/Corrective Measures
Aspiration of formula	Inappropriate tube placement	Ensure correct placement of feeding tube.
	Delayed gastric emptying	Elevate head of bed during and after feeding; decrease formula delivery rate if gastric residual volume is excessive; consider using intestinal feedings in high-risk patients.
	Excessive sedation	Minimize use of medications that cause sedation.
Clogged feeding tube	Excessive formula viscosity	Ensure that tube size is appropriate; flush tubing with water before and after giving formula. Remedies to unclog feeding tubes include flushes with warm water or solutions that contain pancreatic enzymes and sodium bicarbonate; consult pharmacist for more options.
	Improper administration of medications	Use oral, liquid, or injectable medications whenever possible; flush tubing with water before and after a medication is given; avoid mixing medications with formula; dilute thick or sticky liquid medications before administering; crush tablets to a fine powder and mix with water (except enteric-coated or sustained-release medications).
Constipation	Inadequate dietary fiber	Use a formula with appropriate fiber content.
	Dehydration	Provide additional fluids.
	Lack of exercise	Encourage walking and other activities, if appropriate.
	Medication side effect	Consult physician about minimizing or replacing medications that cause constipation.
Diarrhea	Medication intolerance	Dilute hypertonic medications before administering; avoid using poorly tolerated medications.
	Infection in GI tract	Consult physician about specific diagnosis and appropriate treatment.
	Formula contamination	Review safety guidelines for formula preparation and delivery.
	Excessively rapid formula administration	Decrease formula delivery rate or use continuous feedings.
	Lactose or gluten intolerance	Use lactose-free or gluten-free formulas and supplements in patients with intolerances.
Fluid and electrolyte imbalances	Diarrhea	See items under *Diarrhea.*
	Inappropriate fluid intake or excessive losses	Monitor daily weights, intake and output, serum electrolyte levels, and clinical signs that indicate dehydration or overhydration; ensure that water intake and formula delivery rates are appropriate.
	Inappropriate insulin, diuretic, or other therapy	Ensure that medication doses are appropriate.
	Inappropriate nutrient intake	Use a formula with appropriate nutrient content; ensure that malnourished patients do not receive excessive nutrients.[a]
Nausea and vomiting, cramps	Delayed stomach emptying	Decrease formula delivery rate or use continuous feedings; halt feeding if gastric residual volume is excessive (>500 mL); evaluate for obstruction; consider use of medications to improve emptying rate.
	Formula intolerance	Ensure that formula is at room temperature, delivery rate is appropriate, and formula odor is not objectionable; consider using formula that is low in fat, low in fiber, or elemental.
	Medication intolerance	Consult physician about replacing medications that are poorly tolerated.
	Response to disease or disease treatment	Consider use of medications that control nausea and vomiting.

© Cengage Learning®

[a]An excessive nutrient intake in malnourished patients may cause *refeeding syndrome,* a disorder that can lead to fluid and electrolyte imbalances; see p. 458 for details.

Sharyn Bartell is a 24-year-old student who suffered multiple fractures when she fell from a cliff while hiking. She has been in the hospital for 2 weeks and has no appetite. Due to her injuries, she is in traction and is immobile, although the head of her bed can be elevated 45 degrees. Sharyn weighed 140 pounds upon her arrival in the hospital, but she has lost 8 pounds over the course of her hospitalization. The health care team agrees that nasoduodenal tube feeding should be instituted before her nutrition status deteriorates further. A standard formula is selected for the feeding, and Sharyn's nutrient requirements can be met with 2200 milliliters of the formula per day.

1. What steps can be taken to prepare Sharyn for tube feeding? What are some general reasons why nasoduodenal placement of the feeding tube might be preferred over nasogastric placement?

2. The physician's orders specify that the feeding should be given continuously over 18 hours. Using the method shown in Box 16-4, determine an appropriate tube feeding schedule.

3. Describe precautions that should be taken if Sharyn is to receive medications through the feeding tube.

4. After 3 days of feeding, Sharyn develops diarrhea. Check Table 16-2 to determine the possible causes. What measures can be taken to correct the diarrhea?

16.2 Parenteral Nutrition

LO 16.2 Identify patients who may benefit from parenteral nutrition and describe the components of parenteral solutions and administration techniques.

The first half of this chapter described how oral supplements and enteral formulas can improve or replace a regular diet. Such products cannot be used when intestinal function is inadequate, however, and therefore the ability to meet nutrient needs intravenously is a lifesaving option for critically ill persons. The procedure is costly, however, and is associated with a number of potentially dangerous complications. As previous sections suggested, enteral nutrition support is preferred if the GI tract is functional.

Candidates for Parenteral Nutrition

Parenteral nutrition is typically recommended for patients who are unable to digest or absorb nutrients and who are either malnourished or likely to become so (review Figure 16-1). The following conditions may require use of parenteral nutrition:

▍ Intractable vomiting or diarrhea

▍ Severe GI bleeding

▍ Intestinal obstructions or fistulas

▍ Paralytic ileus (intestinal paralysis)

▍ Short bowel syndrome (a substantial portion of the small intestine has been removed)

▍ Bone marrow transplants

▍ Severe malnutrition and intolerance to enteral nutrition

Venous Access

The access sites for parenteral nutrition fall into two main categories: the **peripheral veins** located in the hand or forearm, and the large-diameter **central veins** located near the heart.

Peripheral Parenteral Nutrition In **peripheral parenteral nutrition (PPN),** nutrients are delivered using only the peripheral veins (see Figure 16-9). Peripheral veins can be damaged by overly concentrated solutions, however—**phlebitis** may develop,

peripheral veins: the small-diameter veins that carry blood from the limbs.

central veins: the large-diameter veins located close to the heart.

peripheral parenteral nutrition (PPN): the infusion of nutrient solutions into peripheral veins, usually a vein in the arm or back of the hand.

phlebitis (fleh-BYE-tiss)**:** inflammation of a vein.

characterized by redness, swelling, and tenderness at the infusion site. To prevent phlebitis, the **osmolarity** of parenteral solutions used for PPN is generally kept below 900 milliosmoles per liter,[18] a concentration that limits the amounts of energy and protein the solution can provide. PPN is used most often in patients who require short-term nutrition support (less than 2 weeks) and who do not have high nutrient needs or fluid restrictions. The use of PPN is not possible if the peripheral veins are too weak to tolerate the procedure. In many cases, clinicians must rotate venous access sites to avoid damaging veins.

Total Parenteral Nutrition Most patients meet their nutrient needs using the larger central veins, where blood volume is greater and nutrient concentrations do not need to be limited. This method can reliably provide all of a person's nutrient requirements and therefore is called **total parenteral nutrition (TPN).** Because the central veins carry a large volume of blood, the parenteral solutions are rapidly diluted; thus, patients with high nutrient needs or fluid restrictions can receive the nutrient-dense solutions they require. TPN is also preferred for patients who require long-term parenteral nutrition.

To access central veins, the tip of a central venous **catheter** can either be placed directly into a large-diameter central vein or threaded into a central vein through a peripheral vein (see Figure 16-10). Peripheral insertion of central catheters is less invasive and lower in cost than direct insertion into central veins.

Parenteral Solutions

The pharmacies located within health care institutions are often responsible for preparing parenteral solutions; this arrangement is convenient because the pharmacist can customize the solutions to meet patients' nutrient needs and because the solutions have a limited shelf life. The physician typically submits an order form such as the one shown in Figure 16-11 (p. 454) to the pharmacy. Prescriptions for parenteral solutions are highly individualized and may need to be recalculated daily until the patient's condition is stable. Because the nutrients are provided intravenously, they must be given in forms that are safe to inject directly into the bloodstream.

© Ed Eckstein/PhotoTake

FIGURE 16-9 Peripheral Parenteral Nutrition
The peripheral veins can provide access to the blood for delivery of parenteral solutions.

osmolarity: the concentration of osmotically active solutes in a solution, expressed as milliosmoles per liter of solution (mOsm/L). *Osmolality* (mOsm/kg) is an alternative measure used to describe a solution's osmotic properties.

total parenteral nutrition (TPN): the infusion of nutrient solutions into a central vein.

catheter: a thin tube placed within a narrow lumen (such as a blood vessel) or body cavity; can be used to infuse or withdraw fluids or keep a passage open.

FIGURE 16-10 Accessing Central Veins for Total Parenteral Nutrition

Physician Orders
PARENTERAL NUTRITION (PN) – ADULT

Primary Diagnosis: _____ Ht: _____ cm **Dosing Wt:** _____ kg

PN Indication: _____ Allergies _____

Instructions: This form must be completed for a new order or continuation of PN and faxed to the Pharmacy by [Insert Time] to receive same day preparation. PN administration begins at [Insert Time]. Contact the Nutrition Support Service at (XXX) XXX-XXXX for additional information.

Administration Route: CVC or PICC   *Note: Proper tip placement of the CVC or PICC must be confirmed prior to PN infusion*

Peripheral IV (PIV) *(Final PN Osmolarity ≤ _____ mOsm/L)*

Monitoring: Daily weights, Strict input & output, Bedside glucose monitoring every _____ hours

Na, K, Cl, CO_2, Glucose, BUN, Scr, Mg, PO_4 every _____

T, Bili, Alk Phos, AST, ALT, Albumin, Triglycerides, Calcium every _____

Base Solution: *Parenteral nutrition MUST be administered through a dedicated infusion port and filtered with a 1.2-micron in-line*
Select one *filter at all times. Discard any unused volume after 24 hours.*

PERIPHERAL 2-in-1	**CENTRAL 2-in-1**	**CENTRAL 3-in-1**
Dextrose _____ g	Dextrose _____ g	Dextrose _____ g
Amino Acids (*Brand _____*) _____ g	Amino Acids (*Brand _____*) _____ g	Amino Acids (*Brand _____*) _____ g
For patients with PIV and established glucose tolerance; Provides _____ kcal; Maximum Rate not to exceed _____ mL/hour	*For patients with CVC or PICC and established glucose tolerance; Provides _____ kcal; Maximum Rate not to exceed _____ mL/hour*	Fat Emulsion (*Brand _____*) _____ g
		For patients with CVC or PICC and established glucose/fat emulsion tolerance; Provides _____ kcal; Maximum Rate not to exceed _____ mL/hour

RATE & VOLUME: _____ mL/hour for _____ hours = _____ mL/day
Must specify

Use of additional fat emulsion not required with 3-in-1 base solution

or CYCLIC INFUSION: _____ mL/hour for _____ hours, then _____ mL/hour for _____ hours = _____ mL/day

---

Fat Emulsion (*Brand _____*) – via PIV or CVC with 2-in-1 base solutions   (Select caloric density & volume)

10%	250 mL	Infuse at _____ mL/hour over _____ hours	Frequency _____
20%	500 mL	*(Note: infusions < 4 or > 12 hours not recommended)*	*Discard any unused volume after 12 hours.*

Additives: *(per day)* | ***Normal Dosages***

Sodium Chloride	_____ mEq	*1-2 mEq Sodium/kg/day*
as Acetate	_____ mEq	*pH or CO_2 dependent*
as Phosphate	_____ mmol of PO_4	*Consider if hyperkalemic*
Potassium Chloride	_____ mEq	*1-2 mEq Potassium/kg/day*
as Acetate	_____ mEq	*pH or CO_2 dependent*
as Phosphate	_____ mmol of PO_4	*20-40 mmol/day (1 mmol Phos = 1.5 mEq K)*
Calcium **Gluconate**	_____ mEq	*5-15 mEq/day*
Magnesium **Sulfate**	_____ mEq	*8-24 mEq/day*
Adult **Multivitamins**	_____ mL/day	*Contains Vitamin K 150 mcg*
Adult **Trace Elements**	_____ mL/day	*Zn ___ mg, Cu ___ mg, Mn ___ mg, Cr ___ mcg, Se ___ mcg (with normal hepatic function)*
H_2 **Antagonist** _____	_____ mg	*_____ mg/day with normal renal function*
Other:		

Additives: *(per day)*
Regular Insulin _____ units
Recommend if hyperglycemic, start with 1 unit for every 10 g of dextrose

Pharmacy Use Only: Ca/PO_4
Limit Checked _____
(Note: Some brands of amino acids contain phosphate)

Physician's Signature: _____   **Pager Number:** _____   Date/time: _____

Orders transcribed by: _____   Date/time: _____   Orders verified by: _____   Date/time: _____

SEND COMPLETED ORDERS TO PHARMACY

© Cengage Learning®

FIGURE 16-11 Sample Parenteral Nutrition Order Form

Amino Acids Parenteral solutions contain all of the essential amino acids and various combinations of the nonessential amino acids. The amino acid concentrations in commercial solutions range from 3 to 20 percent (see Box 16-7); the more concentrated solutions are used only for TPN. Just as in regular foods, the amino acids provide 4 kcalories per gram. Disease-specific products are available for patients with liver disease, kidney disease, and metabolic stress, but they are rarely used in practice due to lack of evidence of their benefit.[19]

Carbohydrate Glucose is the main source of energy in parenteral solutions. It is provided in the form dextrose monohydrate, in which each glucose molecule is associated with a single water molecule. Dextrose monohydrate provides 3.4 kcalories per gram, slightly less than pure glucose, which provides 4 kcalories per gram. Commercial dextrose solutions are available in concentrations between 2.5 and 70 percent; concentrations greater than 10 percent are usually used only in TPN solutions.[20]

Lipids Lipid emulsions supply essential fatty acids and are a significant source of energy. The emulsions available in the United States contain triglycerides from either soybean oil or a mixture of olive oil and soybean oil, egg phospholipids to serve as emulsifying agents, and glycerol to make the solutions isotonic.[21] Lipid emulsions are available in 10, 20, and 30 percent solutions, containing 1.1, 2.0, and 3.0 kcalories per milliliter, respectively. Therefore, a 500-milliliter container of 10 percent lipid emulsion would provide 550 kcalories; the same volume of a 20 percent lipid emulsion would provide 1000 kcalories (see Box 16-8). In the United States, the 30 percent lipid emulsion can be used for preparing mixed parenteral solutions but is not approved for direct infusion into patients (see Figure 16-12).[22]

Lipid emulsions are often provided daily and may supply 20 to 30 percent of total kcalories. Including lipids as an energy source reduces the need for energy from dextrose and thereby lowers the risk of hyperglycemia in glucose-intolerant patients. Lipid infusions must be restricted in patients with hypertriglyceridemia, however. There is also some concern that lipid emulsions that contain excessive amounts of linoleic acid may suppress some aspects of the immune response.[23]

Fluids and Electrolytes Daily fluid needs range from 30 to 40 milliliters per kilogram body weight in stable patients. The amount of fluid provided is adjusted according to daily fluid losses and the results of hydration assessment.

The electrolytes added to parenteral solutions include sodium, potassium, chloride, calcium, magnesium, and phosphate. The amounts infused differ from DRI values because they are not influenced by absorption, as they are when consumed orally. In the parenteral nutrition order, most electrolyte concentrations are expressed in *milliequivalents (mEq),* which are units that indicate the number of ionic charges provided by the electrolyte (see Box 16-9). The body's fluids and parenteral solutions are neutral solutions that contain equal numbers of positive and negative charges.

Because electrolyte imbalances can be lethal, electrolyte management by experienced professionals is necessary whenever intravenous therapies are used. Blood tests are administered daily to monitor electrolyte levels until patients have stabilized.

Vitamins and Trace Minerals All vitamins are usually included in parenteral solutions, although a preparation without vitamin K is available for patients using warfarin therapy (see Chapter 15, pp. 426–427). The trace minerals typically added to parenteral solutions include chromium, copper, manganese, selenium, and zinc. Iron is often excluded because it can destabilize parenteral solutions that contain lipid emulsions; therefore, special forms of iron may need to be injected separately.

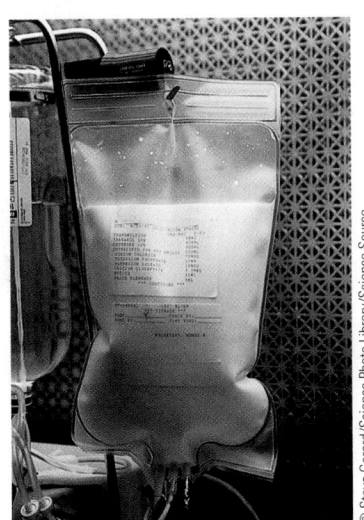

FIGURE 16-12 A lipid emulsion gives the parenteral solution a milky white color.

© Steve Gerard/Science Photo Library/Science Source

BOX 16-7

To convert nutrient concentrations to grams per milliliter:

- 10% amino acid solution = 10 g amino acids/100 mL
- 10% dextrose solution = 10 g dextrose monohydrate/100 mL

BOX 16-8

To determine the kcalories in lipid emulsions:

- 500 mL of a 10% lipid emulsion: 500 mL × 1.1 kcal/mL = 550 kcal
- 500 mL of a 20% lipid emulsion: 500 mL × 2 kcal/mL = 1000 kcal

BOX 16-9

Milliequivalents are determined by dividing an ion's molecular weight (MW) by its number of charges. For example:

- For calcium, MW = 40, and the ion has 2 positive charges: 40 ÷ 2 = 20. Thus, 1 mEq of Ca^{++} is equivalent to 20 mg of calcium.
- For sodium, MW = 23, and the ion has 1 positive charge: 23 ÷ 1 = 23. Thus, 1 mEq of Na^+ is equivalent to 23 mg of sodium.
- *1 mEq of Ca^{++} has the same number of charges as 1 mEq of Na^+.*

Medications To avoid the need for a separate infusion site, medications are occasionally added directly to parenteral solutions or infused through a separate port in the catheter.

Parenteral Formulations When a parenteral solution contains dextrose, amino acids, and lipids, it is called a **total nutrient admixture (TNA),** a **3-in-1 solution,** or an **all-in-one solution.** A **2-in-1 solution** excludes lipids, and the lipid emulsion is administered separately, often using a second port in the catheter. Although the administration of TNA solutions is simpler because only one infusion pump is required, the addition of lipid emulsion to solutions may reduce their stability, a major concern when TNA solutions are compounded. Thus, lipids are often administered separately when they are not a major energy source and are used only to provide essential fatty acids. Box 16-10 describes a method for calculating the macronutrient and energy content of a parenteral solution.

Osmolarity Recall that the osmolarity of PPN solutions is limited to 900 milliosmoles per liter because peripheral veins are sensitive to high nutrient concentrations, whereas TPN solutions may be as nutrient dense as necessary. Amino acids, dextrose, and electrolytes contribute the most to a solution's osmolarity. Because lipids contribute little to osmolarity, lipid emulsions can be used to increase the energy provided in PPN solutions.

Administering Parenteral Nutrition

Parenteral nutrition is a complex treatment that requires skills from a variety of disciplines. Many hospitals organize nutrition support teams, consisting of physicians, nurses, dietitians, and pharmacists, that specialize in the provision of both enteral and parenteral nutrition. The nurse, who performs direct patient care, plays a central role in administering and monitoring parenteral infusions.

Care of Intravenous Catheters Catheter-related problems frequently cause complications (see Table 16-3). Catheters may be improperly positioned or may dislodge after placement. Air can leak into catheters and escape into the bloodstream, obstructing blood flow. Catheters in peripheral veins may cause phlebitis, necessitating

total nutrient admixture (TNA): a parenteral solution that contains dextrose, amino acids, and lipids; also called a **3-in-1 solution** or an **all-in-one solution.**

2-in-1 solution: a parenteral solution that contains dextrose and amino acids, but excludes lipids.

How To BOX 16-10 CALCULATE THE MACRONUTRIENT AND ENERGY CONTENT OF A PARENTERAL SOLUTION

Suppose a patient is receiving 1.25 liters (1250 milliliters) of a parenteral solution that contains 5 percent amino acids and 30 percent dextrose, supplemented with 250 milliliters of a 20 percent lipid emulsion daily. How many grams of protein and carbohydrate is the person receiving, and what is the total energy intake for the day?

Amino acids:

$$5\% \text{ amino acids} = \frac{5 \text{ g amino acids}}{100 \text{ mL}}$$

$$\frac{5 \text{ g amino acids}}{100 \text{ mL}} \times 1250 \text{ mL} = 62.5 \text{ g of amino acids}$$

62.5 g amino acids × 4.0 kcal/g = 250 kcal

Carbohydrate:

$$30\% \text{ dextrose} = \frac{30 \text{ g dextrose}}{100 \text{ mL}}$$

$$\frac{30 \text{ g dextrose}}{100 \text{ mL}} \times 1250 \text{ mL} = 375 \text{ g of dextrose}$$

375 g dextrose × 3.4 kcal/g = 1275 kcal

Lipids:

Recall that a 20 percent lipid emulsion provides 2.0 kcalories per milliliter. If the patient is given 250 milliliters of the emulsion:

250 mL × 2.0 kcal/mL = 500 kcal

Total energy intake:

250 kcal + 1275 kcal + 500 kcal = 2025 kcal

reinsertion at an alternate site. A catheter may become clogged from blood clotting or from a buildup of scar tissue around the catheter tip. Catheters are also a leading cause of infection: contamination may be introduced during insertion or may develop at the placement site.

To reduce the risk of complications, nurses use aseptic techniques when inserting catheters, changing tubing, or changing a dressing that covers the catheter site. Unusual bleeding or a wet dressing suggests a problem with catheter placement. A change in infusion rate may indicate a clogged catheter. Infection may be indicated by redness or swelling around the catheter site or by an unexplained fever. Routine inspections of equipment and frequent monitoring of patients' symptoms help to minimize the problems associated with catheter use.

Administration of Parenteral Solutions Infusion protocols vary among institutions. One approach is to start the infusion at a slow rate (with a solution that is either full strength or nutrient dilute) and increase the rate gradually over a 2- to 3-day period. For example, 40 milliliters per hour can be infused during the first 24 hours of administration (supplying 960 milliliters), and the volume increased to the goal rate on the second day. Another method is to give the full volume of a nutrient-dilute solution on the first day and advance nutrient concentrations as tolerated. Solutions can often be started at full volume and full strength, unless there is a risk of fluid overload, hyperglycemia, or other complications.[24]

Parenteral solutions are usually infused continuously over 24 hours (**continuous parenteral nutrition**) in acutely ill patients.[25] Patients who require long-term parenteral nutrition often receive infusions for 10- to 14-hour periods only (**cyclic parenteral nutrition**), allowing more freedom of movement during the day. For this method, patients must be able to start and stop daily infusions without complication and tolerate the nutrient-dense solutions that allow them to meet their nutritional needs in shorter time periods. Some patients may begin with continuous infusions and transition to cyclic infusions as their condition improves.

Regular monitoring can help to prevent complications. The parenteral solution and tubing are checked frequently for signs of contamination. Routine testing of glucose, lipid, and electrolyte levels helps to determine tolerance to solutions. Frequent reassessment of nutrition status may be necessary until a patient has stabilized.

Discontinuing Parenteral Nutrition The patient must have adequate GI function before parenteral nutrition can be tapered off and enteral feedings begun. During the transition to oral feedings, a combination of methods is often necessary. Parenteral infusions are usually tapered off at the same time that tube feedings or oral feedings are begun, such that the two methods can together supply the needed nutrients. Once about two-thirds to three-fourths of nutrient needs can be provided by other means, the parenteral infusions may be discontinued. Transitioning to an oral diet is sometimes difficult because a person's appetite remains suppressed for several weeks after parenteral nutrition is terminated.

Managing Metabolic Complications

As discussed previously, the catheters used for intravenous infusions may cause a number of serious complications. This section discusses some metabolic complications that may result from parenteral nutrition (review Table 16-3) and some suggestions for managing them.[26]

Hyperglycemia Hyperglycemia (blood glucose levels that exceed about 180 mg/dL during parenteral infusions) most often occurs in patients who are glucose intolerant, receiving excessive energy or dextrose, undergoing severe metabolic stress, or receiving corticosteroid medications. It can be prevented by providing insulin along

TABLE 16-3 **Potential Complications of Parenteral Nutrition**

Catheter-Related
- Air embolism
- Blood clotting at catheter tip
- Clogging of catheter
- Dislodgment of catheter
- Improper placement
- Infection, sepsis
- Phlebitis
- Tissue injury

Metabolic
- Electrolyte imbalances
- Gallbladder disease
- Hyperglycemia, hypoglycemia
- Hypertriglyceridemia
- Liver disease
- Metabolic bone disease
- Nutrient deficiencies
- Refeeding syndrome

© 2016 Cengage Learning®

continuous parenteral nutrition: continuous administration of parenteral solutions over a 24-hour period.

cyclic parenteral nutrition: administration of parenteral solutions over a 10- to 14-hour period each day.

with parenteral solutions, avoiding overfeeding or overly rapid infusion rates, and restricting the amount of dextrose in the solution. Dextrose infusions are generally limited to less than 5 milligrams per kilogram of body weight per minute in critically ill adult patients so that the carbohydrate intake does not exceed the maximum glucose oxidation rate.

Hypoglycemia Although uncommon, hypoglycemia sometimes occurs when parenteral nutrition is interrupted or discontinued or if excessive insulin is given. In patients at risk, such as young infants, infusions may be tapered off over several hours before discontinuation. Another option is to infuse a dextrose solution at the same time that parenteral nutrition is interrupted or stopped.

Hypertriglyceridemia Hypertriglyceridemia may result from dextrose overfeeding or overly rapid infusions of lipid emulsion. If blood triglyceride levels exceed 400 milligrams per deciliter, lipid infusions should be reduced or stopped.

Refeeding Syndrome Severely malnourished patients who are aggressively fed (parenterally or otherwise) may develop **refeeding syndrome,** characterized by electrolyte and fluid imbalances and hyperglycemia. These effects occur because dextrose infusions raise levels of circulating insulin, which promotes anabolic processes that quickly remove potassium, phosphate, and magnesium from the blood. The altered electrolyte levels can lead to fluid retention and life-threatening changes in various organ systems. To prevent refeeding syndrome, health practitioners start parenteral infusions slowly and carefully monitor electrolyte and glucose levels when malnourished patients begin receiving nutrition support.

Liver Disease Fatty liver often results from parenteral nutrition, but it is usually corrected after the parenteral infusions are discontinued. Long-term parenteral nutrition, however, can result in progressive liver disease. To minimize the risk, clinicians avoid giving the patient excess energy, dextrose, or lipids (which promote fat deposition in the liver) and monitor liver enzyme levels weekly. Cyclic infusions may be less problematic than continuous infusions.

Gallbladder Disease When parenteral nutrition continues for more than a few weeks, sludge (thickened bile) may build up in the gallbladder and eventually lead to gallstone formation. Patients requiring long-term parenteral nutrition may be given medications to stimulate gallbladder contractions or improve bile flow or may have their gallbladders removed surgically.

Metabolic Bone Disease Long-term parenteral nutrition is associated with lower bone mineralization and bone density, which may be related to altered intakes or metabolism of calcium, phosphorus, magnesium, and vitamin D. Interventions may include adjustments in parenteral nutrients, medications, and weight-bearing physical activity.

IN SUMMARY

▌ Peripheral parenteral nutrition is provided to patients who need short-term parenteral support and do not have high nutrient needs or fluid restrictions. Total parenteral nutrition supplies nutrient-dense solutions for long-term parenteral support.

▌ Parenteral solutions include amino acids, dextrose, electrolytes, vitamins, and minerals. Lipid emulsions may be included in the mixture or may be administered separately.

refeeding syndrome: a condition that sometimes develops when a severely malnourished person is aggressively fed; characterized by electrolyte and fluid imbalances and hyperglycemia.

Michael Reyes, a 27-year-old man with an inflammatory intestinal disease, underwent a surgical procedure in which a substantial portion of his small intestine was removed. He had received TPN prior to surgery and continued to receive it afterwards. After 10 days, tube feeding was begun and initially delivered very small feedings.

1. List some reasons that the nutrition support team initially chose TPN as a means of nutrition support for this patient. How would you explain the need for parenteral nutrition to Michael?

2. Describe the components of a typical TPN solution. Calculate the energy content of 1 liter of a solution that provides 140 grams of dextrose monohydrate, 45 grams of amino acids, and 90 milliliters of 20 percent lipid emulsion. If Michael's energy requirement is 2100 kcalories per day, how many liters of solution will he need each day?

3. Why is it important that Michael begin enteral feedings as soon as possible? Assuming that Michael eventually tolerates a tube feeding, in what ways can the health care team help him make the transition from parenteral nutrition to tube feedings? Consider some of the physiological problems that Michael might face when he begins a regular diet.

4. If Michael is unable to meet his nutrient needs orally, he may need to continue tube feeding or TPN at home. As you read through the section on nutrition support at home, consider the factors that would make Michael a good candidate for a home nutrition support program. Consider both the benefits of a proposed program and the problems he could encounter.

▌ Parenteral solutions may be initiated gradually or provided at full volume and full strength in selected patients. Critically ill patients may require continuous infusions, whereas long-term users may prefer cyclic infusions.

▌ Complications involving catheters include improper placement or dislodgment, infection, clotting, embolism, and phlebitis. Metabolic complications include hyperglycemia, hypoglycemia, hypertriglyceridemia, refeeding syndrome, and diseases of the liver, gallbladder, and bone.

The Case Study in Box 16-11 checks your understanding of the concepts introduced in this section.

16.3 Nutrition Support at Home

LO 16.3 Give examples of individuals who may be candidates for home nutrition support and discuss the considerations involved in using enteral or parenteral nutrition in the home.

Some individuals may require nutrition support—either tube feedings or parenteral nutrition—after a medical condition has stabilized and they no longer require hospital services. For such a person, home nutrition support may be a suitable option. Current medical technology allows for the safe administration of nutrition support in the home, and insurance coverage often pays a substantial portion of the costs.

Candidates for Home Nutrition Support

Individuals referred for home nutrition support usually need long-term nutrition care for chronic medical conditions. Users of home nutrition services (or their caregivers) must be capable of learning the required procedures and managing any complications that arise. Candidates for home nutrition support include the following:

▌ For home enteral nutrition, people who have disorders that prevent food from reaching the intestines or interfere with nutrient absorption. Examples include

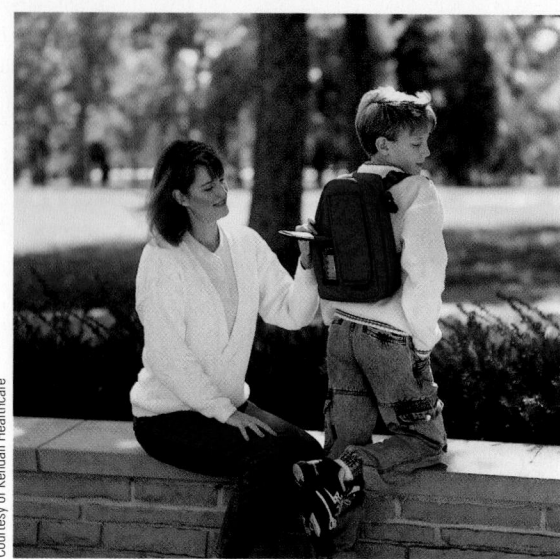

FIGURE 16-13 Home Nutrition Support
Portable pumps and convenient carrying cases allow freedom of movement for individuals using home nutrition support.

people with severe dysphagia, gastroparesis, gastric outlet or duodenal obstructions, and pancreatic or intestinal conditions that cause malabsorption.[27]

▮ For home parenteral nutrition, people who have disorders that severely impede nutrient absorption or interfere with intestinal motility. Examples include patients with short bowel syndrome, certain types of motility disorders, and radiation enteropathy.[28]

Planning Home Nutrition Care

As with the nutrition support provided in health care facilities, home nutrition care involves decisions about access sites, formulas, and nutrient delivery methods. Users of these services should be involved in the decision making to ensure long-term compliance and satisfaction.

Home Enteral Nutrition Access to the GI tract is possible using either nasal tubes or enterostomies. Although people can learn to place nasogastric tubes themselves, active individuals often prefer low-profile gastrostomy or jejunostomy tubes, which allow a more normal lifestyle. For gastric feedings, bolus infusions are most easily delivered. If intermittent feedings require slow or reliable delivery rates, infusion pumps may be needed. Portable pumps can free individuals from the need to infuse formula at home (see Figure 16-13).

Insurance reimbursements do not always include the cost of enteral formulas, which are considered food products. For this reason, some people choose to prepare simple formulas at home. Blenderizing regular foods is possible, but the resulting mixture needs to be strained to remove particles or clumps that may obstruct the tube. Closed (ready-to-hang) feeding systems are useful for avoiding contamination risk but are not appropriate for intermittent feedings that require smaller amounts of formula.

Home Parenteral Nutrition Although both peripheral parenteral nutrition and total parenteral nutrition (TPN) can be provided at home, long-term therapy requires access to the larger central veins appropriate for TPN. The catheter's exit site is generally placed in a region accessible to the patient. Most people prefer cyclic infusions over continuous infusions and transition to cyclic infusions before discharge from the hospital. Because infusion pumps are required for home TPN, sufficient battery backup is necessary in case electrical service is interrupted. Portable pumps are useful for individuals who prefer to infuse during the day or have active lifestyles.

Parenteral solutions need to be sterile and aseptically prepared, and individuals who mix their own solutions must be carefully trained. Ready-made parenteral solutions require refrigeration and are stable for limited periods; for example, 3-in-1 solutions may be stable for only one week when refrigerated.

Quality-of-Life Issues

Individuals who depend on home nutrition support face unique challenges that can affect quality of life. Activities and work schedules must be planned around feedings. People receiving nocturnal feedings often cite disturbed sleep as a major problem. Among social issues, the inability to share meals with family and friends is often a great concern.[29] The Oley Foundation (*www.oley.org*) is a good source of current information and emotional support for people who require home nutrition services.

- Candidates for home enteral nutrition have disorders that interfere with swallowing ability, GI motility, or nutrient absorption. Candidates for home parenteral nutrition have disorders that severely impair nutrient absorption or intestinal motility.

- Patients and caregivers can participate in decisions about access sites, formulas, and nutrient delivery methods. Enteral formulas and parenteral solutions can be purchased or prepared in the home.

- The use of portable pumps helps individuals lead a normal lifestyle; nevertheless, lifestyle adjustments to nutrition support may be difficult and stressful.

Nutrition Assessment Checklist FOR PEOPLE RECEIVING ENTERAL NUTRITION SUPPORT

Medical History

Check the medical record for medical conditions that:

- Alter nutrient needs and influence formula selection
- Influence the selection of tube placement sites and feeding routes
- Suggest the length of time that the tube feeding will be needed

Monitor the medical record for complications or risks that may influence the formula selection or delivery technique, including:

- Aspiration
- Constipation
- Fluid and electrolyte imbalances
- Diarrhea
- Hyperglycemia
- Nausea and vomiting
- Skin irritation

Medications

Check medications for those that can cause side effects similar to the complications of tube feeding, such as:

- Nausea and vomiting
- Diarrhea
- Constipation
- GI discomfort

For medications delivered through the feeding tube, check:

- Form of medication and possible alternatives
- Viscosity of liquid medications
- Potential for diet-drug interactions

Dietary Intake

To assess nutritional adequacy, check to see whether:

- The formula is appropriate for the patient's needs
- Supplemental water is provided to meet needs
- The formula is administered as prescribed

Anthropometric Data

Measure baseline height and weight, and monitor body weight regularly. If weight is not appropriate:

- Determine whether energy needs have been correctly assessed
- Check to see if the formula is being delivered as prescribed
- Check for signs of dehydration or overhydration

Laboratory Tests

Check serum and urine tests for signs of:

- Fluid and electrolyte imbalances
- Hyperglycemia
- Improvement or deterioration of the medical condition

Physical Signs

Look for physical signs of:

- Dehydration or overhydration
- Delayed gastric emptying
- Malnutrition

Nutrition Assessment Checklist FOR PEOPLE RECEIVING PARENTERAL NUTRITION SUPPORT

Medical History

Check the medical record for medical conditions that:

- Prevent the use of enteral nutrition
- Indicate the appropriate infusion route (peripheral versus central)
- Suggest the length of time that parenteral nutrition will be required

Monitor the medical record for complications or risks that may influence the parenteral solution formulation or delivery technique, including:

- Acid-base imbalances
- Fluid and electrolyte imbalances
- Hyperglycemia or hypoglycemia
- Hypertriglyceridemia
- Preexisting liver disease
- Refeeding syndrome

Medications

For medications added to the parenteral solution, determine the:

- Medication's compatibility with the parenteral solution
- Length of time that the medication can remain stable in solution

For medications infused separately, determine:

- Length of time that the infusion may need to be stopped
- Necessary adjustments in parenteral infusions to compensate for medication delivery

Dietary Intake

To assess nutritional adequacy, check to see whether:

- Patient's nutrient needs were correctly determined
- Solution is administered as prescribed
- Infusion pump is operating correctly

Anthropometric Data

Measure baseline height and weight, and monitor daily weights. If weight is not appropriate:

- Determine whether energy needs have been correctly assessed
- Check to see if the parenteral solution is being delivered as prescribed
- Check for signs of dehydration or overhydration

Laboratory Tests

Check serum and urine tests for signs of:

- Fluid, electrolyte, and acid-base imbalances
- Hyperglycemia or hypoglycemia
- Hypertriglyceridemia
- Abnormal liver function
- Improvement or deterioration of the medical condition

Physical Signs

Routinely monitor the following:

- Catheter insertion site for signs of infection or inflammation
- Blood pressure, temperature, pulse, and respiration for signs of fluid, electrolyte, and acid-base imbalances

Look for physical signs of:

- Dehydration or overhydration
- Malnutrition

Clinical Applications

1. Appendix G provides examples of enteral formulas on the market and lists their energy and macronutrient contents. Select one standard formula and one elemental formula from Tables G-1 and G-2, respectively. For the two formulas you selected, calculate the volume of formula that would meet the energy needs of a patient who requires about 1750 kcalories daily. Use these results in answering the following questions:

   a. What is the amount of protein, carbohydrate, and fat that the patient would obtain in a typical day? Determine the percentages of kcalories that come from carbohydrate and fat. Do these percentages fall within the Acceptable Macronutrient Distribution Ranges described in Chapter 1 (p. 10)?

   b. Tables G-1 and G-2 show the formula volumes that would meet the Reference Daily Intakes (RDI). Would the volumes you obtained meet typical vitamin and mineral needs?

2. A liter of a TPN solution contains 500 milliliters of 50 percent dextrose solution and 500 milliliters of 5 percent amino acid solution. Determine the daily energy and protein intakes of a person who receives 2 liters per day of such a solution.

Calculate the average daily energy intake if the person also receives 500 milliliters of a 20 percent fat emulsion three times a week.

3. Consider the clinical, financial, psychological, and social ramifications of using home parenteral nutrition, with no foods allowed by mouth, in answering the following questions:
   a. What would be the advantages of living at home instead of in a hospital or other residential facility? Can you think of some disadvantages?
   b. Think about how you, as the patient, might manage daily infusions: consider the time, cost, and commitment required to maintain the therapy.
   c. If not allowed to consume foods, what possible difficulties might you encounter? How would you handle holidays and special occasions that center around food?

Self Check

1. For a patient who is at high risk of aspiration and is not expected to be able to eat table foods for several months, an appropriate placement of a feeding tube might be:
   a. nasogastric.
   b. nasoenteric.
   c. gastrostomy.
   d. jejunostomy.

2. In selecting an appropriate enteral formula for a patient, the primary consideration is:
   a. formula osmolality.
   b. the patient's nutrient needs.
   c. availability of infusion pumps.
   d. formula cost.

3. An important measure that may prevent bacterial contamination in tube feeding formulas is:
   a. nonstop feeding of formula.
   b. using the same feeding bag and tubing each day.
   c. discarding opened containers of formula not used within 24 hours.
   d. adding formula to the feeding container before it empties completely.

4. A difference between continuous and intermittent feedings is that continuous feedings:
   a. require an infusion pump.
   b. allow greater freedom of movement.
   c. are more similar to normal patterns of eating.
   d. are associated with more GI side effects.

5. A patient needs 1800 milliliters of formula a day. If the patient is to receive formula intermittently every four hours, how many milliliters of formula will she need at each feeding?
   a. 225
   b. 300
   c. 400
   d. 425

6. The nurse using a feeding tube to deliver medications recognizes that:
   a. medications given by feeding tube generally do not cause GI complaints.
   b. medications can usually be added directly to the feeding container.
   c. enteral formulas do not interact with medications in the same way that foods do.
   d. thick or sticky liquid medications and crushed tablets can clog feeding tubes.

7. For a patient receiving central TPN who also receives intravenous lipid emulsions two or three times a week, the lipid emulsions serve primarily as a source of:
   a. essential fatty acids.
   b. cholesterol.
   c. fat-soluble vitamins.
   d. concentrated energy.

8. Iron is typically excluded from parenteral solutions, in part, because:
   a. requirements for iron vary substantially from person to person.
   b. iron can destabilize solutions that include lipid emulsions.
   c. iron restriction is necessary in persons using warfarin therapy.
   d. iron promotes fat deposition in the liver.

9. Refeeding syndrome is associated with dangerous fluctuations in:
   a. serum electrolytes.
   b. serum liver enzyme levels.
   c. blood triglyceride levels.
   d. ketone bodies.

10. Patients using home parenteral nutrition:
    a. usually prefer continuous rather than cyclic infusions.
    b. are unable to travel or work away from home.
    c. require infusion pumps for use at home.
    d. can only obtain 2-in-1 solutions and so must infuse lipids separately.

Answers to these questions can be found in Appendix H.

Notes

1. K. L. Coughlin, S. I. Austhof, and C. Hamilton, Nutrition support: Indication and efficacy, in A. Skipper, ed., *Dietitian's Handbook of Enteral and Parenteral Nutrition* (Sudbury, MA: Jones and Bartlett Learning, 2012), pp. 22–45.

2. B. Brown, Patient selection and indications for enteral feedings, in P. Charney and A. Malone, eds., *Pocket Guide to Enteral Nutrition* (Chicago: Academy of Nutrition and Dietetics, 2013), pp. 14–51.

3. A. Skipper, Enteral nutrition, in A. Skipper, ed., *Dietitian's Handbook of Enteral and Parenteral Nutrition* (Sudbury, MA: Jones and Bartlett Learning, 2012), pp. 259–280; R. Bankhead and coauthors, A.S.P.E.N. enteral nutrition practice recommendations, *Journal of Parenteral and Enteral Nutrition* 33 (2009): 122–167.

4. A. M. Malone, Enteral formula selection, in P. Charney and A. Malone, eds., *Pocket Guide to Enteral Nutrition* (Chicago: Academy of Nutrition and Dietetics, 2013), pp. 120–152.

5. L. E. Matarese and M. M. Gottschlich, Enteral feeding, in A. C. Ross and coeditors, eds., *Modern Nutrition in Health and Disease* (Baltimore: Lippincott Williams & Wilkins, 2014), pp. 1126–1135.

6. Skipper, Enteral nutrition, 2012.

7. M. Shelton, Monitoring and evaluation of enteral feedings, in P. Charney and A. Malone, eds., *Pocket Guide to Enteral Nutrition* (Chicago: Academy of Nutrition and Dietetics, 2013), pp. 153–169; Bankhead and coauthors, 2009.

8. Skipper, Enteral nutrition, 2012.

9. M. K. Russell, Complications of enteral feedings, in P. Charney and A. Malone, eds., *Pocket Guide to Enteral Nutrition* (Chicago: Academy of Nutrition and Dietetics, 2013), pp. 170–197.

10. C. Thompson and M. Romano, Initiation, advancement, and transition of enteral feedings, in P. Charney and A. Malone, eds., *Pocket Guide to Enteral Nutrition* (Chicago: Academy of Nutrition and Dietetics, 2013), pp. 88–119; Bankhead and coauthors, 2009.

11. V. M. Zhao and T. R. Ziegler, Specialized nutrition support, in J. W. Erdman, I. A. Macdonald, and S. H. Zeisel, eds., *Present Knowledge in Nutrition* (Ames, IA: Wiley-Blackwell, 2012), pp. 982–999.

12. T. W. Rice, Gastric residual volume: End of an era, *Journal of the American Medical Association* 309 (2013): 283–284.

13. Russell, 2013.

14. P. Ayers and coeditors, *A.S.P.E.N. Parenteral Nutrition Handbook* (Silver Spring, MD: American Society for Pareneral and Enteral Nutrition, 2014); E. Schiavo and A. Skipper, Water and micronutrients, in A. Skipper, ed., *Dietitian's Handbook of Enteral and Parenteral Nutrition* (Sudbury, MA: Jones and Bartlett Learning, 2012), pp. 82–101.

15. P. D. Wohlt and coauthors, Recommendations for the use of medications with continuous enteral nutrition, *American Journal of Health-Systems Pharmacy* 66 (2009): 1458–1467.

16. Russell, 2013.

17. Thompson and Romano, 2013.

18. A. Skipper, Parenteral nutrition, in A. Skipper, ed., *Dietitian's Handbook of Enteral and Parenteral Nutrition* (Sudbury, MA: Jones and Bartlett Learning, 2012), pp. 281–300.

19. Skipper, Parenteral nutrition, 2012.

20. P. Ayers and coeditors, 2014.

21. P. Ayers and coeditors, 2014.

22. P. Ayers and coeditors, 2014.

23. V. W. Vanek and coauthors, A.S.P.E.N. position paper: Clinical role for alternative intravenous fat emulsions, *Nutrition in Clinical Practice* 27 (2012): 150–192.

24. S. Roberts, Initiation, advancement, and acute complications, in P. Charney and A. Malone, eds., *ADA Pocket Guide to Parenteral Nutrition* (Chicago: American Dietetic Association, 2007), pp. 76–102.

25. P. Ayers and coauthors, A.S.P.E.N. parenteral nutrition safety consensus recommendations, *Journal of Parenteral and Enteral Nutrition* 38 (2014): 296–333.

26. P. Ayers and coeditors, 2014; R. O. Brown, G. Minard, and T. R. Ziegler, Parenteral nutrition, in A. C. Ross and coeditors, eds., *Modern Nutrition in Health and Disease* (Baltimore: Lippincott Williams & Wilkins, 2014), pp. 1136–1161.

27. A. Pattinson and L. Epp, Home enteral nutrition, in P. Charney and A. Malone, eds., *Pocket Guide to Enteral Nutrition* (Chicago: Academy of Nutrition and Dietetics, 2013), pp. 198–229.

28. V. J. Kumpf and E. M. Tillman, Home parenteral nutrition: Safe transition form hospital to home, *Nutrition in Clinical Practice* 27 (2012): 749–757.

29. M. F. Winkler, Living with enteral and parenteral nutrition: How food and eating contribute to quality of life, *Journal of the American Dietetic Association* 110 (2010): 169–177.

LO 16.4 Describe the possible metabolic effects of inborn errors of metabolism and discuss the complications and treatments of phenylketonuria and galactosemia.

An **inborn error of metabolism** is an inherited trait, caused by a genetic **mutation,** that results in the absence, deficiency, or dysfunction of a protein that has a critical metabolic role.[1] The severity of the inborn error's effects is ultimately related to the degree of impairment caused by the missing or altered protein. This Nutrition in Practice describes some inborn errors of metabolism and discusses the role of diet in two of these disorders: phenylketonuria and galactosemia. Box NP16-1 defines terms related to inborn errors of metabolism.

What problems can result from inborn errors of metabolism?

The protein affected by an inborn error may function as an enzyme, receptor, transport protein, or structural protein. When the body fails to make a protein, the functions that depend on that protein are impaired. For example, when an enzyme is missing or malfunctioning in a metabolic pathway that typically converts compound A to compound

B, compound A will accumulate and compound B will not be made. The excess of compound A and the lack of compound B may have harmful effects. Furthermore, the imbalances in one pathway may affect other pathways and ultimately cause a number of metabolic and physiologic disturbances. Table NP16-1 (p. 466) lists some examples of inborn errors related to defects in nutrient metabolism.

What role can diet play in treating inborn errors of metabolism?

Nutrition therapy is the primary treatment for many inborn errors that involve nutrient metabolism. Once the biochemical pathway affected by an inborn error is identified, the individual may be able to alter the diet to compensate for deficiencies and excesses. The typical dietary intervention involves restricting substances that cannot be properly metabolized and including substances that cannot be produced. Thus, dietary changes may be able to improve outcomes of some inborn errors by:

- Preventing the accumulation of toxic **metabolites** (metabolic products)

- Replacing nutrients that are deficient as a result of a defective metabolic pathway

- Providing a diet that supports normal growth and development and maintains health

Successful treatment of an inborn error of metabolism depends on the ability to screen newborns and diagnose metabolic diseases before irreversible damage can occur. After a genetic defect is identified, family members may undergo **genetic counseling** to evaluate the likelihood that they may pass on the disorder to future offspring. During counseling, couples may learn about reproductive options such as artificial insemination, *in vitro* fertilization, or prenatal monitoring after conception.

Are there treatments for inborn errors that don't involve dietary changes?

Nondietary therapies can treat some inborn errors of metabolism, although the options are somewhat limited. In some cases, the missing protein is infused; this is the primary means of treating **hemophilia,** caused by deficiency of one of the plasma proteins needed for clotting blood. Drug therapy is the main treatment for some inborn errors, including **cystic fibrosis** (discussed in Chapter 19), which is characterized by a defect that prevents normal chloride transport across cell membranes. Future approaches may include **gene therapy,** a treatment that introduces DNA sequences into the chromosomes of affected cells, prompting the cells to express the protein needed to correct the abnormality.

What is an example of an inborn error that benefits from dietary treatment?

A classic example is **phenylketonuria (PKU),** a metabolic disorder that affects amino acid metabolism. PKU occurs in approximately 1

BOX NP16-1 GLOSSARY

cystic fibrosis: an inherited disorder that affects the transport of chloride across epithelial cell membranes; primarily affects the gastrointestinal and respiratory systems.

galactosemia (ga-LAK-toe-SEE-me-ah)**:** an inherited disorder that impairs galactose metabolism; may cause damage to the brain, liver, kidneys, and lens in untreated patients.

gene therapy: treatment for inherited disorders in which DNA sequences are introduced into the chromosomes of affected cells, prompting the cells to express the protein needed to correct the disease.

genetic counseling: support for families at risk of genetic disorders; involves diagnosis of disease, identification of inheritance patterns within the family, and review of reproductive options.

hemophilia (HE-moh-FEEL-ee-ah)**:** an inherited bleeding disorder characterized by deficiency or malfunction of a plasma protein needed for clotting blood.

inborn error of metabolism: an inherited trait (one that is present at birth) that causes the absence, deficiency, or malfunction of a protein that has a critical metabolic role.

metabolites: products of metabolism; compounds produced by a biochemical pathway.

mutation: an heritable change in the DNA sequence of a gene.

phenylketonuria (FEN-il-KEY-toe-NU-ree-ah) or **PKU:** an inherited disorder characterized by a defect in the enzyme phenylalanine hydroxylase, which normally converts the essential amino acid phenylalanine to the amino acid tyrosine. The condition is named after the phenylalanine metabolites—called *phenylketones*—that are excreted in the urine of individuals who have the disorder.

Disorder	Affected Nutrient(s) or Substance	Metabolic Defect	Nutritional Treatment
Amino acid metabolism			
Maple syrup urine disease	Branched-chain amino acids (isoleucine, leucine, and valine)	Impaired metabolism of branched-chain amino acids	Restriction of branched-chain amino acids; thiamin supplementation
Phenylketonuria	Phenylalanine	Impaired conversion of phenylalanine to tyrosine	Phenylalanine-restricted diet; tyrosine supplementation
Carbohydrate metabolism			
Galactosemia	Galactose	Impaired conversion of galactose to glucose	Galactose-restricted diet
Glycogen storage disease	Glycogen	Impaired metabolism or transport of glycogen, resulting in glycogen accumulation in tissues	Varies; may require frequent feedings, cornstarch supplementation, high-protein diet
Lipid metabolism			
Carnitine transporter deficiency	Fatty acids	Impaired transport of fatty acids into the mitochondria for oxidation	Carnitine supplementation; avoidance of fasting and strenuous exercise
X-adrenoleukodystrophy[a]	Very long-chain fatty acids	Impaired breakdown of very long-chain fatty acids in peroxisomes	Under investigation; limited benefit from a low-fat diet with restriction of very long-chain fatty acids, supplementation with various fatty acid mixtures,[a] and avoidance of fasting
Mineral metabolism			
Hemochromatosis	Iron	Excessive iron absorption (causes iron accumulation)	Avoidance of iron and vitamin C supplements and alcoholic beverages (routine blood draws remove excess iron from the body)
Wilson's disease	Copper	Impaired copper excretion (causes copper accumulation)	Avoidance of copper-rich foods; zinc therapy (reduces copper absorption)

© 2016 Cengage Learning®

[a]The disease X-adrenoleukodystrophy was featured in the 1992 film *Lorenzo's Oil.*

out of every 15,000 births in the United States each year.[2] In PKU, the missing or defective protein is the liver enzyme *phenylalanine hydroxylase,* which converts the essential amino acid phenylalanine to the amino acid tyrosine. This chemical reaction is also the first step in the breakdown of excess phenylalanine. Without the enzyme, phenylalanine and its by-products accumulate in the blood and tissues, resulting in severe damage to the developing brain. The impairment in the metabolic pathway also prevents the liver synthesis of tyrosine and tyrosine-derived compounds (such as the neurotransmitter epinephrine, the skin pigment melanin, and the hormone thyroxin). Under these conditions, tyrosine becomes essential: the body cannot produce tyrosine, and therefore the diet must supply it.

Although PKU's most debilitating effect is on brain development, other signs may manifest if the condition is untreated. Infants with PKU may have poor appetites and grow slowly. They may be irritable or have tremors or seizures. Their bodies and urine may have a musty odor. Their skin may be unusually pale, and they may develop skin rashes. In older children and adults who discontinue treatment, neurological and psychological problems are common. Individuals with elevated phenylalanine levels may exhibit impaired reasoning, a reduced attention span, and poor memory, among other deficits.[3]

How is PKU diagnosed?

PKU must be diagnosed soon after birth so that early treatment can prevent its devastating effects. For this reason, newborns are screened for PKU in all 50 states. A standard blood test for phenylalanine is typically conducted by heel puncture after the infant has consumed several meals containing protein (see Figure NP16-1). Abnormal results require further testing.

The screening of newborns for PKU is one of the most common genetic tests in the United States and many other countries. Before widespread newborn screening, infants with PKU demonstrated

FIGURE NP16-1 A simple blood test screens newborns for PKU—a common inborn error of metabolism.

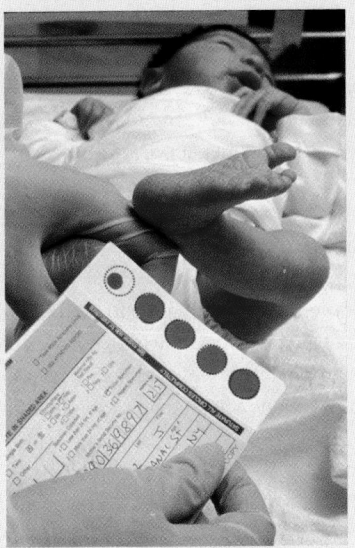

Ted Horowitz/Corbis

FIGURE NP16-2 Phenylalanine-free formulas help patients with PKU maintain safe blood levels of the amino acid phenylalanine.

Mead Johnson Nutrition

developmental delays (for example, inability to crawl) by 6 to 9 months of age. By the time parents recognized the problem, the damage was irreversible. Most of the damaging consequences of this disorder are now prevented due to the early detection and treatment of PKU.

What is the treatment for PKU?

The treatment for PKU is a diet that restricts phenylalanine and supplies tyrosine so that the blood levels of these amino acids are maintained within safe ranges. Because phenylalanine is an essential amino acid, the diet cannot exclude it completely. Children with PKU need phenylalanine to grow, but they cannot handle excesses without detrimental effects. Therefore, their diets must provide enough phenylalanine to support growth and health but not so much as to cause harm. The diets must also provide tyrosine, which is an essential nutrient for individuals with PKU. To ensure that blood concentrations of phenylalanine and tyrosine are close to normal, blood tests are performed periodically, and diets are adjusted when necessary. If the dietary treatment is conscientiously followed, it can prevent the effects described earlier. Older children and adults with PKU must continue to follow the PKU diet to prevent deterioration in brain function.

What are the main features of the PKU diet?

Central to the PKU diet is the use of an enteral formula that is phenylalanine-free yet supplies energy, amino acids, vitamins, and minerals (see Figure NP16-2). For infants, the phenylalanine-free formula can be supplemented with measured amounts of breast milk or regular infant formula to provide the phenylalanine needed for growth. Low-phenylalanine formulas are available for infants who must meet all of their nutrient needs with formula. Formula requirements need to be recalculated periodically to accommodate the growing infant's shifting needs for protein, phenylalanine, tyrosine, and energy.

Once food consumption begins, a phenylalanine-free formula supplies the needed amino acids, and foods that contain

phenylalanine are carefully monitored. All protein foods contain some phenylalanine; therefore, high-protein foods such as meat, fish, poultry, milk, cheese, legumes, and nuts (including peanut butter) are omitted. Fruit, vegetables, and cereals also contain phenylalanine, so only limited amounts are allowed. Low-protein flours and mixes are available for making low-phenylalanine bread, pasta, cake, and cookies. Foods that do not contain phenylalanine, such as jam, jelly, and most sweeteners, can be used freely. Growth rates and nutrition status are monitored to ensure that the diet is adequate. Older children, teens, and adults with PKU should continue to use the phenylalanine-free formulas to help them meet their protein and energy needs.

Individuals with PKU should be encouraged to develop creative ways to make their diet enjoyable. The formula can be flavored or combined with fruit or juice to make smoothies or frozen juice bars. Sandwiches can be made with low-phenylalanine bread and fillings such as mashed bananas or avocados, shredded carrots and olives, or tomato slices with mayonnaise. Food variety can be expanded by using products made from the protein *glycomacropeptide*, which is a phenylalanine-free protein derived from whey; available products include milk substitutes, shakes, and protein bars.

How long should a person with PKU continue the dietary treatment?

Lifelong adherence to a phenylalanine-restricted diet is currently recommended for all individuals with PKU, as elevated phenylalanine levels can adversely affect cognitive function at any age. It is especially important that women with PKU maintain safe phenylalanine concentrations during pregnancy. Elevated phenylalanine levels, especially during the first trimester, have been associated with mental disability, birth defects, and growth retardation in the offspring of PKU mothers who have discontinued dietary treatment.[4]

Although consuming a low-phenylalanine diet is the main treatment for patients with PKU, a number of other therapies have been investigated. The medication sapropterin dihydrochloride (Kuvan) improves phenylalanine hydroxylase function in some patients with PKU, thereby allowing an increased intake of regular

467

protein foods.[5] Supplementation with large neutral amino acids (such as tyrosine and threonine), which compete with phenylalanine for transport across cell membranes, may improve both blood phenylalanine levels and neurologic function; different amino acid mixtures are being studied as potential therapies for PKU patients who are unable to remain on the PKU diet long term.[6]

What is another example of an inborn error that requires dietary changes?

Galactosemia is an example of an inborn error of carbohydrate metabolism. Individuals with galactosemia are deficient in one of the enzymes needed to metabolize galactose, a sugar that is primarily found in milk products (recall that lactose molecules contain galactose). An accumulation of galactose metabolites can cause damage in multiple tissues. Infants with galactosemia who are given milk react with severe vomiting and liver jaundice within days of the initial feeding. Serious liver damage can develop and progress to symptomatic cirrhosis. Other complications may include kidney failure, cataracts, and brain damage. Treatment in the first weeks of life can prevent the most detrimental effects of galactosemia, but if treatment is delayed, the damage to the brain is irreversible.[7]

What is the dietary treatment for galactosemia?

Patients with galactosemia must consume a galactose-restricted diet. The diet is much simpler than the diet for PKU because galactose is not an essential nutrient and is not in a metabolic pathway that produces a required substance. In addition, dietary galactose is primarily obtained from lactose (the milk sugar), so the main focus of dietary treatment is the exclusion of milk and milk products. Other foods that contain galactose in substantial amounts, such as organ meats and some legumes, fruits, and vegetables, must also be avoided or restricted. Prepared foods and medications that include lactose as an additive must be avoided as well. Galactosemia patients or their caregivers are generally given food lists that identify common sources of galactose.

Infants diagnosed with galactosemia are given lactose-free formulas to meet their nutrient needs. Once a child can consume adequate amounts of regular foods, special formulas are unnecessary; however, care must be taken to ensure that the diet supplies adequate calcium. Individuals with galactosemia must remain on the galactose-restricted diet throughout their lives to avoid potential damage to the brain, liver, kidney, and lens.[8]

How effective is the dietary treatment for galactosemia?

Although the early introduction of a galactose-restricted diet can eliminate the acute toxic effects of galactosemia, complications of the disease may develop despite an individual's compliance with diet therapy. For example, many patients experience difficulties with language, abstract thinking, and visual perception. Ovarian failure and cataracts are common. The reasons for these long-term complications are not fully understood.

For many inborn errors of metabolism, effective management requires early diagnosis and treatment, as well as control of the environmental factors that may cause toxicity. In some cases, dietary changes are central to treatment and can prevent serious complications. Other inborn errors, however, may not be as easily treated. Future developments in biotechnology may allow gene therapy to assist in the medical treatment of some of these disorders.

Notes

1. J. Elsas II, Approach to inborn errors of metabolism, in L. Goldman and A. I. Schafer, eds., *Goldman's Cecil Medicine* (Philadelphia: Saunders, 2012), pp. 1340–1346.

2. N. Blau, F. J. van Spronsen, and H. L. Levy, Phenylketonuria, *Lancet* 376 (2010): 1417–1427.

3. Blau, van Spronsen, and Levy, 2010.

4. Blau, van Spronsen, and Levy, 2010.

5. M. Giovannini and coauthors, Phenylketonuria: Nutritional advances and challenges, *Nutrition and Metabolism* 9 (2012): 7, doi: 10.1186/1743-7075-9-7.

6. Giovannini and coauthors, 2012; F. J. van Spronsen and coauthors, Large neutral amino acids in the treatment of PKU: From theory to practice, *Journal of Inherited Metabolic Disease* 33 (2010): 671–676.

7. L. J. Elsas II and P. B. Acosta, Inherited metabolic disease: Amino acids, organic acids, and galactose, in A. C. Ross and coeditors, eds., *Modern Nutrition in Health and Disease* (Baltimore: Lippincott Williams & Wilkins, 2014), pp. 906–969.

8. Elsas II and Acosta, 2014.

17

Foods and Food Consistency for Upper GI Disorders

17.1 Modifications in Food Texture and Consistency

LO 17.1 Describe the different types of mechanically altered diets and the clear liquid diet and explain how these diets are used during patient care.

17.2 Conditions Affecting the Mouth and Esophagus

LO 17.2 Describe the causes, consequences, and nutrition management of dry mouth, dysphagia, and gastroesophageal reflux disease.

17.3 Conditions Affecting the Stomach

LO 17.3 Identify some common stomach disorders and summarize the medical treatments and dietary

strategies that may promote healing or improve symptoms.

17.4 Gastric Surgery

LO 17.4 Describe the different types of gastric surgery and the nutrition care required after these procedures.

17.5 Nutrition in Practice: Nutrition and Oral Health

LO 17.5 Describe the causes, effects, and treatments of dental caries and periodontal disease and discuss the relationships between these conditions and chronic illness.

Photodisc/Getty Images

469

Gastrointestinal (GI) illnesses account for a significant fraction of hospital admissions and visits to health practitioners each year. Diagnosis is not always straightforward, however, because many patients with GI complaints exhibit no physical abnormalities. Evaluation therefore requires a detailed review of a patient's symptoms and responses to dietary adjustments. Because GI complications frequently accompany other illnesses, the medical history can sometimes uncover the underlying source of distress.

17.1 Modifications in Food Texture and Consistency

LO 17.1 Describe the different types of mechanically altered diets and the clear liquid diet and explain how these diets are used during patient care.

Mechanically altered diets, which contain foods that are modified in texture or consistency, are frequently recommended for individuals with chewing or swallowing difficulties. The foods in these diets are typically liquid, pureed, ground, chopped, minced, or soft in texture. A **clear liquid diet** may be prescribed before or after certain types of medical procedures.

Mechanically Altered Diets

Table 17-1 and Figure 17-1 provide examples of foods that are usually included in mechanically altered diets. Although the names for these diets vary, a more restrictive diet may contain mostly pureed foods (*pureed diet*), whereas a less restrictive diet may include ground or minced foods (*ground/minced diet* or *mechanically altered diet*) or moist, soft-textured foods that easily form a bolus (*soft diet*). Because chewing and swallowing problems vary in severity and may fluctuate over time, individual tolerances ultimately determine whether foods are included or excluded. A later section provides details about the specific diets used for treating swallowing difficulties (see *Dysphagia*, pp. 472–475).

A *blenderized diet* is most often recommended following oral or facial surgeries (for example, jaw wiring). Foods that can be blenderized (often with added liquid) are available from all food groups: they include breads and cereals; boiled rice and pasta; cooked vegetables; fresh or cooked fruit without skins or seeds; and cooked, tender

mechanically altered diets: diets that contain foods that have been mechanically altered to modify texture or consistency; foods may be liquid, pureed, ground, chopped, minced, or tenderized.

clear liquid diet: a diet that consists of foods that are liquid at room temperature, require minimal digestion, and leave little residue (undigested material) in the colon.

TABLE 17-1 Foods Included in Mechanically Altered Diets

Depending on the feeding problem, a pureed, mechanically altered, or soft diet may include foods that are pureed, mashed, ground, minced, or soft textured. Foods used in the different diets may overlap. Individual tolerances ultimately determine whether foods are included or excluded.

Pureed Diets	Mechanically Altered or Soft Diets
Milk products: Milk, smooth yogurt, pudding, custard	**Milk products:** Milk, yogurt with soft fruit, pudding, cottage cheese
Fruit: Pureed fruit and fruit juice without pulp, seeds, skin, or chunks; well-mashed fresh bananas; applesauce	**Fruit:** Canned or cooked fruit without seeds or skin, fruit juice with small amounts of pulp, ripe bananas
Vegetables: Pureed cooked vegetables without seeds, skin, or chunks; mashed potatoes; pureed potatoes with gravy	**Vegetables:** Soft, well-cooked vegetables that are not rubbery or fibrous; well-cooked, moist potatoes
Meat and meat substitutes: Pureed meat; smooth, homogenous souffles; hummus or other pureed legume spreads	**Meat and meat substitutes:** Ground, minced, or tender meat, poultry, or fish with gravy or sauce; tofu; well-cooked, moist legumes; scrambled or soft-cooked eggs
Breads and cereals: Smooth cooked cereals such as Cream of Wheat, slurried bread or pancakes,[a] pureed rice and pasta	**Breads and cereals:** Cooked cereals or moistened dry cereals with minimal texture, soft bread or pancakes, well-cooked noodles or dumplings in sauce or gravy

© Cengage Learning®

[a] Slurried foods are foods that have been mixed with liquid to achieve an appropriate consistency; they may be gelled and shaped to improve their appearance.

A meal of pureed foods can include meats, beans, breads, cereals, fruits, and vegetables that are pureed to a pudding-like consistency. Foods should be homogeneous and cohesive. Sticky foods, such as melted cheese or peanut butter, are generally not included.

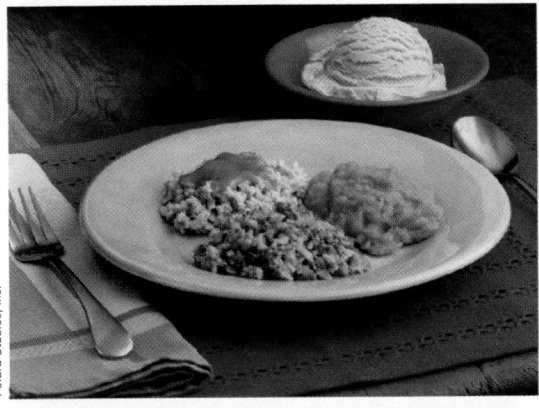

Most foods can be ground or minced so that chewing is not required. The diet can include ground meats; soft, moist casseroles; scrambled eggs and egg salad; bite-sized pasta; smooth cooked cereals; and mashed or minced fruits and vegetables.

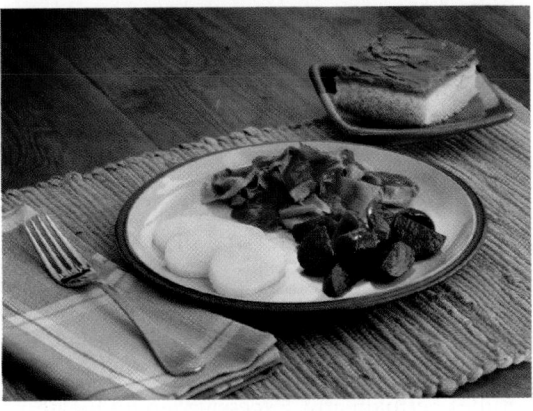

A diet with soft-textured, easy-to-swallow foods may include moist, shaved, tender meats; baked fish; cooked or cold cereals with milk; well-cooked vegetables; thinly sliced cucumber without skin or seeds; soft breads and cookies without nuts or seeds; and fruits without seeds or tough skins.

FIGURE 17-1 Diets for People with Chewing or Swallowing Problems

meats and fish. Foods that do not blend well should be excluded; examples include hard or rubbery foods such as nuts and seeds, coconut, dried fruit, hard cheese, sausages and frankfurters, and some raw vegetables.

Clear Liquid Diet

Clear liquids, which require minimal digestion and are easily tolerated by the GI tract, are often the foods recommended before some GI procedures (such as GI examinations, X-rays, or surgeries), after GI surgery, or after fasting or intravenous feeding. The *clear liquid diet* consists of clear fluids and foods that are liquid at room temperature and leave little undigested material (called **residue**) in the colon. Permitted foods include clear or pulp-free fruit juices, carbonated beverages, clear meat and vegetable broths (such as consommé and bouillon), fruit-flavored gelatin, fruit ices made from clear juices, frozen juice bars, and plain hard candy. Although the clear liquid diet

residue: material left in the intestine after digestion; includes mostly dietary fiber and undigested starches and proteins.

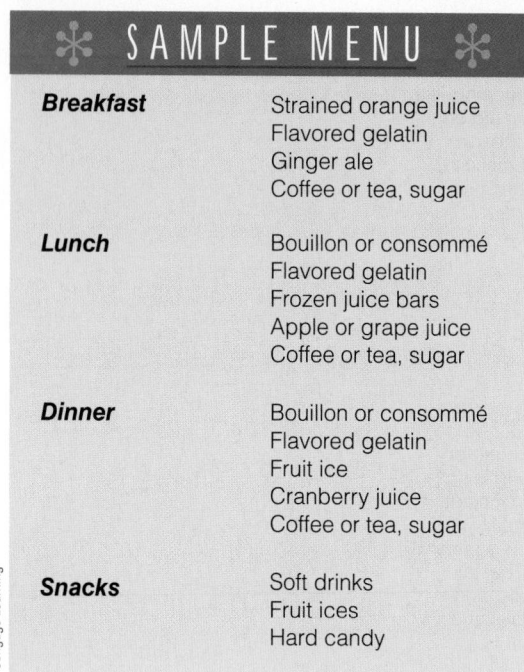

SAMPLE MENU

Breakfast	Strained orange juice Flavored gelatin Ginger ale Coffee or tea, sugar
Lunch	Bouillon or consommé Flavored gelatin Frozen juice bars Apple or grape juice Coffee or tea, sugar
Dinner	Bouillon or consommé Flavored gelatin Fruit ice Cranberry juice Coffee or tea, sugar
Snacks	Soft drinks Fruit ices Hard candy

FIGURE 17-2 Menu—Clear Liquid Diet

provides fluid and electrolytes, its nutrient and energy contents are extremely limited. If used for longer than a day or two, this diet should be supplemented with commercially prepared low-residue formulas that provide required nutrients. Figure 17-2 gives an example of a one-day clear liquid menu.

A liquid diet that includes milk and other opaque liquids (such as fruit nectars, yogurt, and oral supplements) is called a **full liquid diet.** Although rarely necessary, it is sometimes used as a transitional diet between the clear liquid diet and diets that contain solid foods.

IN SUMMARY

- Mechanically altered diets are often prescribed for people with swallowing and chewing difficulties.

- Clear liquid diets may be used briefly before some GI procedures, after GI surgery, or after fasting or intravenous feeding.

17.2 Conditions Affecting the Mouth and Esophagus

LO 17.2 Describe the causes, consequences, and nutrition management of dry mouth, dysphagia, and gastroesophageal reflux disease.

This section describes how to relieve the discomfort of dry mouth and examines the causes and treatments of the two most common disorders affecting the esophagus: dysphagia (difficulty swallowing) and gastroesophageal reflux disease.

Dry Mouth

Dry mouth (**xerostomia**), caused by reduced salivary flow, is a side effect of many medications and is associated with a number of diseases and disease treatments.[1] Antidepressants, antihistamines, antihypertensives, antineoplastics, bronchodilators, and other medications can cause dry mouth. Poorly controlled diabetes is often associated with dry mouth, as are conditions that directly affect salivary gland function, such as **Sjögren's syndrome.** Radiation therapy that treats head and neck cancers often damages salivary glands, sometimes permanently. Excessive mouth breathing is also a common cause of dry mouth.

Dry mouth can impair health in a variety of ways.[2] It can interfere with speaking and swallowing. Mouth infections, bad breath, and dental diseases are more common. Dentures may be uncomfortable to wear, and ulcerations may develop where they contact the mouth. Taste sensation is often diminished, and salty or spicy foods may cause pain. Dry mouth may cause a person to reduce food intake and may thereby increase malnutrition risk. Table 17-2 offers suggestions that may help to manage dry mouth.

Dysphagia

Dysphagia is generally caused by either a problem affecting the muscles involved with swallowing or a physical obstruction between the mouth and stomach. Table 17-3 lists some potential causes of dysphagia, which are categorized according to the location of the swallowing difficulty.[3]

Oropharyngeal Dysphagia A person with **oropharyngeal dysphagia** has difficulty transferring food from the mouth and pharynx to the esophagus. The condition

full liquid diet: a liquid diet that includes clear liquids, milk, yogurt, ice cream, and liquid nutritional supplements (such as Ensure).

xerostomia (ZEE-roh-STOE-me-ah): dry mouth caused by reduced salivary flow.

- *xero* = dry
- *stoma* = mouth

Sjögren's (SHOW-grenz) **syndrome:** an autoimmune disease characterized by the destruction of secretory glands, resulting in dry mouth and dry eyes.

dysphagia (dis-FAY-jah)**:** difficulty swallowing.

oropharyngeal dysphagia (OR-oh-fah-ren-JEE-al diss-FAY-jah)**:** an inability to transfer food from the mouth and pharynx to the esophagus; usually caused by a neurological or muscular disorder.

TABLE 17-2 Suggestions for Managing Dry Mouth

Food and Beverage Tips

- Take frequent sips of water or another sugarless beverage.
- Suck on ice cubes or frozen fruit juice bars (unless their coldness causes discomfort).
- Consume foods that have a high fluid content, such as soups, stews, sauces and gravies, yogurt, and pureed fruit.
- Avoid dry foods like toast, chips, and crackers.
- Avoid citrus juices and spicy or salty foods if they cause mouth irritation.

Lifestyle Practices

- Chew sugarless gum to help stimulate salivary flow.
- Avoid caffeine, alcohol, and smoking, which may dry the mouth.
- Use a humidifier during the night.

Saliva Substitutes

- Use over-the-counter saliva substitutes (available as gels, sprays, and tablets), especially just before meals and at bedtime.
- Try rinsing the mouth with a teaspoonful of vegetable oil or softened margarine.

Dental Care

- Pay strict attention to oral hygiene, brushing teeth and flossing at least twice daily. Try to brush immediately after each meal.
- Avoid alcohol- and detergent-containing mouthwashes that may dry and irritate the mouth.
- Ask your dentist about fluoride treatments that help to prevent tooth decay.

Medications

- If dry mouth is caused by a medication, ask your physician about possible alternatives.
- Ask your physician if using a medication to stimulate saliva secretion may be of benefit; examples include cevimeline (Evoxac) and pilocarpine (Salagen).

© Cengage Learning®

TABLE 17-3 Selected Causes of Dysphagia

Oropharyngeal Dysphagia

- Alzheimer's disease (advanced stages)
- Amyotrophic lateral sclerosis (Lou Gehrig's disease)
- Brain injury
- Cerebral palsy
- Multiple sclerosis
- Muscular dystrophy
- Myasthenia gravis
- Parkinson's disease
- Poliomyelitis
- Stroke

Esophageal Dysphagia

- Achalasia
- Esophageal cancer
- Esophageal spasm
- External compression (from a tumor, enlarged thyroid gland, or enlarged left atrium)
- Scleroderma
- Strictures (from inflammation, scarring, or a congenital abnormality)

© Cengage Learning®

is typically due to a neuromuscular disorder that inhibits the swallowing reflex or impairs the strength or coordination of the muscles involved with swallowing. Symptoms include an inability to initiate swallowing, coughing during or after swallowing (due to aspiration), and nasal regurgitation. Other signs include a gurgling noise after swallowing, a hoarse or "wet" voice, or a speech disorder. Oropharyngeal dysphagia is common in elderly persons and frequently follows a stroke.

Esophageal Dysphagia A person with **esophageal dysphagia** has difficulty passing materials through the esophageal lumen and into the stomach, usually due to an obstruction in the esophagus or a motility disorder. The main symptom is the sensation of food "sticking" in the esophagus after it is swallowed. An obstruction can be caused by a **stricture** (abnormal narrowing), tumor, or compression of the esophagus by surrounding tissues. Whereas an obstruction can prevent the passage of solid foods but may not affect liquids, a motility disorder hinders the passage of both solids and liquids. **Achalasia,** the most common motility disorder, is a degenerative nerve condition affecting the esophagus; it is characterized by impaired peristalsis and incomplete relaxation of the lower esophageal sphincter when swallowing.

Complications of Dysphagia If dysphagia restricts food consumption, malnutrition and weight loss may occur. Individuals who cannot swallow liquids are at increased risk of dehydration. If aspiration occurs, it may cause choking, airway obstruction, or respiratory infections, including pneumonia.

Nutrition Intervention for Dysphagia The National Dysphagia Diet, developed in 2002 by a panel of dietitians, speech and language therapists, and a food scientist, has helped to standardize the nutrition care of dysphagia patients.[4] Table 17-4 (p. 474)

esophageal dysphagia: an inability to move food through the esophagus; usually caused by an obstruction or a motility disorder.

stricture: abnormal narrowing of a passageway; often due to inflammation, scarring, or a congenital abnormality.

achalasia (ack-ah-LAY-zhah): an esophageal disorder characterized by weakened peristalsis and impaired relaxation of the lower esophageal sphincter.

- *a* = without
- *chalasia* = relaxation

presents brief descriptions of the different levels of the diet and some sample meals. After the appropriate dietary level is selected, the diet must be adjusted to suit the person's swallowing abilities and tolerances. In many cases, the most appropriate foods may be determined only by trial and error. A consultation with a swallowing expert, such as a speech and language therapist, is often necessary. Because a person's swallowing ability can fluctuate over time, the dietary plan may need frequent reassessment.

TABLE 17-4 **National Dysphagia Diet**

Level 1: Dysphagia Pureed

Foods should be pureed or well mashed, homogeneous, and cohesive. This diet is for patients with moderate to severe dysphagia and poor oral or chewing ability.

Sample menus:

▪ *Breakfast:* Cream of Wheat, slurried muffins or pancakes,[a] pureed scrambled eggs, plain or vanilla yogurt, well-mashed bananas, fruit juice without pulp (thickened as needed), coffee or tea (if thin liquids are acceptable).

▪ *Lunch or dinner:* Pureed tomato soup, slurried crackers, pureed meat or poultry, zucchini soufflé, mashed potatoes with gravy, pureed carrots or green beans, smooth applesauce, pureed peaches, chocolate pudding.

Foods to avoid: Dry breads and cereals, oatmeal, rice, fruit yogurt, cheese (including cottage cheese), peanut butter, nuts and seeds, raw fruits and vegetables, chunky applesauce, fruit preserves with chunks or seeds, tomato sauce with seeds, beverages with pulp, coarsely ground pepper, herbs.

Level 2: Dysphagia Mechanically Altered

Foods should be moist, cohesive, and soft textured and should easily form a bolus. This diet is for patients with mild to moderate dysphagia; some chewing ability is required.

Sample menus:

▪ *Breakfast:* Moist oatmeal, cornflakes or puffed rice cereal with milk (thickened as needed), moist pancakes or muffins (with butter, margarine, or jam; without nuts or seeds), soft scrambled eggs, cottage cheese, ripe bananas or cooked fruit without skin or seeds, fruit juice (thickened as needed), coffee or tea (if thin liquids are allowed).

▪ *Lunch or dinner:* Soup with easy-to-chew meat and vegetables; slurried bread or crackers; minced, tender-cooked meat; well-cooked pasta with moist meatballs and tomato sauce; baked potato with gravy; soft, tender-cooked vegetables (not fibrous or rubbery); canned peach slices; soft fruit pie (with bottom crust only); soft, smooth chocolate bar.

Foods to avoid: Dry or coarse foods; breads and cereals with nuts, seeds, or dried fruit; frankfurters and sausages; hard-cooked eggs; corn and clam chowders; sandwiches; pizza; sliced cheese; rice; French fries; potato skin; raw vegetables; fibrous, rubbery, or non-tender cooked vegetables such as asparagus, broccoli, brussels sprouts, cabbage, celery, corn, and peas; peanut butter; coconut; nuts and seeds; raw fruit (except banana); cooked fruit with skin or seeds; pineapple; mango; uncooked dried fruit; popcorn; chewy candies (such as caramel or licorice).

Level 3: Dysphagia Advanced

Foods should be moist and in bite-sized pieces when swallowed; foods with mixed textures are included. This diet is for patients with mild dysphagia and adequate chewing ability.

Sample menus:

▪ *Breakfast:* Cereal with milk, moist pancakes or muffins (with butter, margarine, or jam; without nuts or seeds), poached or scrambled eggs, fruit yogurt, soft fresh fruit (peeled) or berries, coffee or tea (if thin liquids are tolerated).

▪ *Lunch or dinner:* Chicken noodle soup; moistened crackers or moist bread; thin-sliced tender meat; cheese; moist, soft-cooked potatoes or rice; tender-cooked vegetables; shredded lettuce with dressing; fresh, peeled peach or melon; canned fruit salad; moist chocolate chip cookie (without nuts).

Foods to avoid: Dry or coarse foods; breads and cereals with nuts, seeds, or dried fruit; corn and clam chowders; potato skin; raw vegetables (except shredded lettuce); corn; chunky peanut butter; coconut; nuts and seeds; hard fruit (such as apples or pears); fruit with skin, seeds, or a stringy texture (such as mango or pineapple); uncooked dried fruit; fruit leather; popcorn; chewy candies (such as caramel or licorice).

Liquid Consistencies (only those tolerated are allowed in the diet)

▪ *Thin:* Watery fluids; may include milk, coffee, tea, juices, carbonated beverages.

▪ *Nectarlike:* Fluids thicker than water that can be sipped through a straw; may include buttermilk, eggnog, tomato juice, cream soups.

▪ *Honeylike:* Fluids that can be eaten with a spoon but do not hold their shape; may include honey, some yogurt products, tomato sauce.

▪ *Spoon-thick:* Thick fluids that must be eaten with a spoon and can hold their shape; may include milk pudding, thickened applesauce.

[a] Slurried foods are foods that have been mixed with liquid to achieve an appropriate consistency; they may be gelled and shaped to improve their appearance.

Take a moment to think about a meal of pureed or ground foods. A typical dinner of baked chicken, potatoes, carrots, and green beans can look like mounds of differently colored mush. The foods may taste great, but a person may have little appetite before trying a first bite. To improve appetite, be creative when preparing and serving meals:

■ Help to stimulate the appetite by preparing favorite foods and foods with pleasant smells. Enliven food flavors with aromatic spices and seasonings.

■ Substitute brightly colored vegetables for white vegetables; for example, replace mashed potatoes with mashed sweet potatoes. If serving more than one vegetable, place contrasting colors (such as spinach and carrots) side by side or swirl the two together.

■ Shape pureed and ground foods so they resemble traditional dishes; for example, meats can be flattened to form a patty or rounded to resemble meatballs. Use food molds to restore slurried breads and pureed meats to their traditional shapes.

■ Try layering ingredients so that the food looks like a fancy casserole or popular hors d'oeuvre. For example, food items can resemble lasagna, moussaka, tamales, or sushi.

■ Use attractive plates and silverware to improve the visual appeal of a meal. Colorful garnishes can add interest and eye appeal.

Efforts to improve the appearance of foods can go a long way toward helping people eat nourishing meals and maintain a healthy weight.

Food Properties and Preparation Foods included in dysphagia diets should have easy-to-manage textures and consistencies. Soft, cohesive foods are easier to swallow than hard or crumbly foods. Moist foods are better tolerated than dry foods. Some foods within a category may be acceptable and others may not; for example, some cookies are soft and tender, whereas others are hard and brittle. Sticky or gummy foods, such as peanut butter and cream cheese, may be difficult to clear from the mouth and throat.

The textures of foods are typically altered to make them easier to swallow. Solid foods are often pureed, mashed, ground, or minced (review Table 17-1 on p. 470). Foods that have more than one texture, such as vegetable soup or cereal with milk, are difficult to manage, so ingredients may be blended to a single consistency with items such as nuts and seeds omitted. Semi-liquid foods such as sauces and gravies may be thickened with food starches (such as cornstarch or potato flakes) during cooking or mixed with commercial food thickeners after cooking until the desired consistency is reached. A variety of pre-thickened food products, including pureed meats, eggs, vegetables, and pasta, are commercially available.

Consuming foods that have a similar consistency can quickly become monotonous. Including a variety of flavors and colors can make a meal more appealing. Box 17-1 and Figure 17-3 present suggestions for improving the acceptance of pureed and other mechanically altered foods.

Properties of Liquids Thickened liquids are easier to swallow than thin liquids such as water or juice. Table 17-4 describes the four levels of liquid consistencies prescribed for dysphagia patients, referred to as thin, nectarlike, honeylike, and spoon-thick. To increase viscosity, commercial thickeners can be stirred into beverages and other liquid foods, such as soup broths. Some beverages may lose their appeal when thickened; for example, individuals may find thickened coffee and tea unacceptable.

Alternative Feeding Strategies for Dysphagia Some patients may be able to learn alternative feeding techniques to help them compensate for their swallowing problem. For example, changing the position of the head and neck while eating and drinking can minimize some swallowing difficulties. (As an example, cups designed for dysphagia patients allow drinking without tilting the head back.) Individuals with oropharyngeal dysphagia can be taught exercises that strengthen the jaws, tongue, or larynx, or they can learn new methods of swallowing that allow them to consume a normal diet. Speech and language therapists are often responsible for teaching patients these techniques.

Diamond Crystal Specialty Foods, Inc.

FIGURE 17-3 Meal of Pureed Foods
Pureed foods can be formed into attractive shapes using commercial thickeners and food molds.

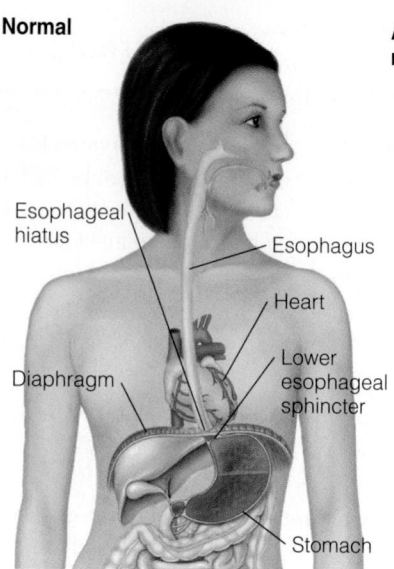

Normal

Esophageal hiatus

Esophagus

Heart

Lower esophageal sphincter

Diaphragm

Stomach

The stomach normally lies below the diaphragm, and the esophagus passes through the esophageal hiatus. The lower esophageal sphincter prevents reflux of stomach contents.

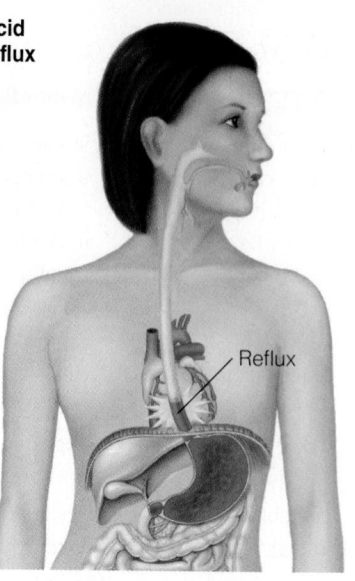

Acid reflux

Reflux

Whenever the pressure in the stomach exceeds the pressure in the esophagus, as can occur with overeating and overdrinking, the chance of reflux increases. The resulting "heartburn" is so-named because it is felt in the area of the heart.

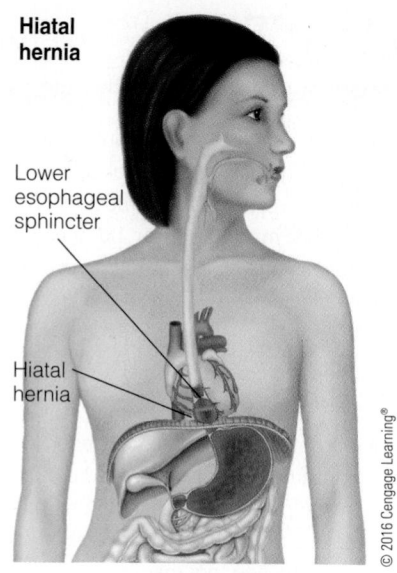

Hiatal hernia

Lower esophageal sphincter

Hiatal hernia

Risk of acid reflux may increase as a consequence of a hiatal hernia. A "sliding" hiatal hernia occurs when part of the stomach, along with the lower esophageal sphincter, rises into the area above the diaphragm.

© 2016 Cengage Learning®

FIGURE 17-4 The Upper GI Tract, Acid Reflux, and Hiatal Hernia

Gastroesophageal Reflux Disease

Gastroesophageal reflux disease (GERD) is characterized by frequent reflux (backward flow) of the stomach's acidic contents into the esophagus, leading to pain, inflammation, and, possibly, tissue damage. People who suffer from GERD often refer to these symptoms as *heartburn* or *acid indigestion*. The reflux itself does not necessarily cause symptoms or injury—it occurs occasionally in healthy people and is a problem only if it creates complications and requires lifestyle changes or medical treatment.

Causes of GERD The lower esophageal sphincter is the main barrier to gastric reflux, so GERD can result if the sphincter muscle is weak or relaxes inappropriately. Other factors that predispose a person to GERD include high stomach pressures and inadequate acid clearance from the esophagus. Conditions associated with high rates of GERD include obesity, pregnancy, and **hiatal hernia,** in which a portion of the stomach protrudes above the diaphragm (see Figure 17-4). During pregnancy, nearly two-thirds of women report heartburn, which typically worsens during the third trimester.[5] Many medications can increase the risk of reflux, as does the use of nasogastric tubes in tube feedings. Various other conditions or substances can exacerbate GERD by increasing stomach pressures or weakening the lower esophageal sphincter; Table 17-5 lists examples.

Consequences of GERD If gastric acid remains in the esophagus long enough to damage the esophageal lining, the resulting inflammation is called **reflux esophagitis.** Severe and chronic inflammation may lead to esophageal ulcers, with consequent bleeding. After healing begins, the scar tissue may narrow the inner diameter of the esophagus, causing esophageal stricture. A slowly progressive dysphagia for solid foods sometimes results, and swallowing occasionally becomes painful. Pulmonary disease may develop if gastric contents are aspirated into the lungs. Chronic reflux is also associated with **Barrett's esophagus,** a condition in which damaged esophageal cells are gradually replaced by cells that resemble those in gastric or intestinal tissue; such cellular changes increase the risk of developing esophageal cancer. GERD can also damage tissues in the mouth, pharynx, and larynx, resulting in eroded tooth enamel, sore throat, and laryngitis.[6]

gastroesophageal reflux disease (GERD): condition characterized by frequent reflux (backward flow) of the stomach's acidic contents into the esophagus.

hiatal hernia: a condition in which the upper portion of the stomach protrudes above the diaphragm; most cases are asymptomatic.

reflux esophagitis: inflammation in the esophagus resulting from the reflux of acidic stomach contents.

Barrett's esophagus: a condition in which esophageal cells damaged by chronic exposure to stomach acid are replaced by cells that resemble those in the stomach or small intestine, sometimes becoming cancerous.

Treatment of GERD Treatment objectives are to alleviate symptoms and facilitate the healing of damaged tissue. Severe ulcerative disease may require immediate acid-suppressing medication, whereas a mild case may be managed with dietary and life-style changes. Box 17-2 (p. 478) lists lifestyle modifications that may help to prevent the recurrence of gastrointestinal reflux.

Medications that suppress gastric acid secretion help the healing process by reducing the damaging effects of acid on esophageal tissue. **Proton-pump inhibitors** are the most effective of the antisecretory agents and are used both for rapid healing of esophagitis and as a maintenance treatment. Other antisecretory drugs include **histamine-2 receptor blockers** (often referred to as *H2 blockers*) and antacids, which neutralize gastric acid. Antacids are frequently used to relieve occasional heartburn, but they are not necessarily appropriate for GERD because they have only short-term effects and are ineffective for healing esophagitis. The Case Study in Box 17-3 (p. 478) will help you review the treatments available for a patient with GERD.

IN SUMMARY

▪ Dry mouth can diminish taste sensation, lead to reduced food intake, and increase the risk of developing oral infections. It can be managed with oral hygiene, dietary changes, and saliva substitutes.

▪ Dysphagia may interfere with food intake and increase the risk of aspiration. Treatment may include dietary adjustments, strengthening exercises, and using different swallowing techniques.

▪ Gastroesophageal reflux disease (GERD) may lead to inflammation, esophageal ulcers, bleeding, and stricture. Treatment includes lifestyle changes and use of acid-suppressing drugs.

17.3 Conditions Affecting the Stomach

LO 17.3 Identify some common stomach disorders and summarize the medical treatments and dietary strategies that may promote healing or improve symptoms.

Stomach disorders range from occasional bouts of discomfort to severe conditions that require surgery. This section begins with a discussion of *dyspepsia* (often called "indigestion"), the sensation of pain or discomfort in the upper abdomen that occurs after food consumption. More serious stomach conditions that may benefit from dietary adjustments include *gastritis* and *peptic ulcers*, which most often result from bacterial infection or the use of medications that damage the stomach lining.

Dyspepsia

Dyspepsia refers to general symptoms of pain or discomfort in the upper abdominal region, which may include stomach pain or burning, after-meal fullness, early satiation, nausea, and bloating. These symptoms sometimes indicate the presence of more serious illnesses, such as GERD or peptic ulcer disease. Although about 25 percent of the population experiences dyspepsia, only about half of those affected seek medical attention.[7]

Causes of Dyspepsia Abdominal symptoms don't always lead to a clear diagnosis. Various medical conditions can cause abdominal discomfort, including foodborne illness, GERD, peptic ulcers, gastric motility disorders, gallbladder and pancreatic diseases, and tumors in the upper GI tract. Chronic diseases such as diabetes mellitus, heart disease, and hypothyroidism are sometimes accompanied by gastric symptoms. Some medications and dietary supplements can cause gastrointestinal problems.

TABLE 17-5 Conditions and Substances Associated with Esophageal Reflux

Conditions/Substances That Increase Pressure within the Stomach

▪ Ascites (abdominal fluid accumulation)
▪ Carbonated beverages
▪ Delayed gastric emptying
▪ Eating large meals
▪ Lying down after eating
▪ Obesity
▪ Pregnancy
▪ Wearing tight clothing around the waist or abdomen

Conditions/Substances That Weaken the Lower Esophageal Sphincter

▪ Alcohol
▪ Anticholinergic drugs
▪ Antihistamines
▪ Caffeinated beverages
▪ Calcium channel blockers
▪ Chocolate
▪ Cigarette smoking
▪ Diazepam
▪ Estrogen, progesterone
▪ Fatty foods
▪ Peppermint and spearmint
▪ Theophylline
▪ Tricyclic antidepressants

© Cengage Learning®

proton-pump inhibitors: a class of drugs that inhibit the enzyme that pumps hydrogen ions (protons) into the stomach. Examples include omeprazole (Prilosec) and lansoprazole (Prevacid).

histamine-2 receptor blockers: a class of drugs that suppress acid secretion by inhibiting receptors on acid-producing cells; commonly called *H2 blockers*. Examples include cimetidine (Tagamet), ranitidine (Zantac), and famotidine (Pepcid).

dyspepsia: symptoms of pain or discomfort in the upper abdominal area, often called "indigestion"; a symptom of illness rather than a disease itself.

▪ *dys* = bad; impaired
▪ *pepsis* = digestion

How To   BOX 17-2 MANAGE GASTROESOPHAGEAL REFLUX DISEASE

Management of GERD may require modifications in diet and life-style to reduce the recurrence of acid reflux or minimize discomfort. Recommendations typically include the following:

- Consume only small meals and drink liquids between meals so that the stomach does not become overly distended, which can exert pressure on the lower esophageal sphincter.

- Limit foods or substances that increase gastric acid secretion (such as alcohol and coffee) or weaken the pressure of the lower esophageal sphincter (such as alcohol, chocolate, fried or fatty foods, peppermint, and spearmint).

- During periods of esophagitis, avoid foods and beverages that may irritate the esophagus, such as citrus fruits and juices, tomato products, garlic, onions, pepper, spicy foods, carbonated beverages, and very hot or very cold foods (depending on individual tolerances).

- Avoid eating bedtime snacks or lying down after meals. Meals should be consumed at least three hours before bedtime.

- Reduce nighttime reflux by elevating the head of the bed on 6-inch blocks, inserting a foam wedge under the mattress, or propping pillows under the head and upper torso.

- Avoid bending over and wearing tight-fitting garments; both can cause pressure in the stomach to increase, heightening the risk of reflux.

- Avoid cigarette smoking, which relaxes the lower esophageal sphincter.

- Avoid using nonsteroidal anti-inflammatory drugs (NSAIDs) such as aspirin, naproxen, and ibuprofen, which can damage the esophageal mucosa.

Food tolerances among people with GERD can vary markedly. Health practitioners can help patients pinpoint food intolerances by advising them to keep a record of the foods and beverages they consume, as well as any resulting symptoms.

Case Study   BOX 17-3 WOMAN WITH GERD

Joanne Rinaldi is a 39-year-old accountant who is 5 feet 4 inches tall and weighs 165 pounds. During a recent physical examination, she mentioned to her physician that she had been feeling fairly well until she began experiencing heartburn, which has progressively become more frequent and painful. The heartburn often occurs after she eats a large meal and is particularly bad after she goes to bed at night. By directly examining the esophageal lumen using an endoscope (a thin, flexible tube equipped with an optical device), the physician found evidence of reflux esophagitis and a slight narrowing throughout the length of the esophagus.

Ms. Rinaldi's medical history does not indicate any significant health problems. During her last physical exam, her physician advised her to stop smoking cigarettes and to lose 20 pounds, but she has not attempted to do either. The nutrition assessment reveals that Ms. Rinaldi is feeling stressed because it is the middle of the tax season. She usually has little time for breakfast, eats a lunch of fast foods while continuing to work at her desk, and eats a large dinner at around 8 P.M.

She generally has wine with dinner and another alcoholic beverage later in the evening.

1. Explain to Ms. Rinaldi the meaning of the medical diagnoses *reflux esophagitis* and *esophageal stricture*.

2. Based on the brief history provided, list the factors and behaviors that increase Ms. Rinaldi's risks of experiencing reflux. What recommendations can you make to help her change these behaviors?

3. What medications might the physician prescribe, and why?

Intestinal conditions such as irritable bowel syndrome or lactose intolerance may mimic dyspepsia. Although pinpointing the cause of gastric symptoms can be difficult, a complete examination is in order if the individual experiences unintentional weight loss, dysphagia, persistent vomiting, GI bleeding, or anemia, which suggest the presence of serious illness.[8]

Potential Food Intolerances Although many people believe their symptoms are caused by consuming certain types of meals, foods, or spices, research studies have yielded mixed results.[9] Fatty foods and high-fat meals, which slow gastric emptying, may exacerbate symptoms in some individuals. Other substances reported to cause symptoms include alcohol, chocolate, coffee, peppers, spices and spicy foods, and citrus fruits.[10] To minimize symptoms, people with dyspepsia may be advised to consume small, frequent meals; avoid fatty or highly spiced foods; and avoid the specific foods believed to trigger symptoms.

Bloating and Stomach Gas The feeling of bloating may be caused by excessive gas in the stomach, which accumulates when air is swallowed. Air swallowing often accompanies gum chewing, smoking, rapid eating, drinking carbonated beverages, and using a straw. Omitting these practices generally helps to correct the problem.

Nausea and Vomiting

Nausea and vomiting accompany many illnesses and are common side effects of medications. Although occasional vomiting is not dangerous, prolonged vomiting can cause fluid and electrolyte imbalances and may require medical care. Chronic vomiting can reduce food intake and lead to malnutrition and nutrient deficiencies.

The symptoms that accompany vomiting may give clues about its cause.[11] If abdominal pain is present, a GI disorder or obstruction is usually the cause. If abdominal pain is not present, possible causes of vomiting include medications, foodborne illness, pregnancy, motion sickness, neurological disease, inner ear disorders, hepatitis, and various chronic illnesses.

Treatment of Nausea and Vomiting Most cases are short lived and require no treatment. When treatment is necessary, the main goal is to find and correct the underlying disorder. Restoring hydration may also be necessary in some individuals. If a medication is the cause, taking it with food may help. If the cause is unknown or the underlying disorder cannot be corrected, medications that suppress nausea and vomiting can be prescribed. People with **intractable vomiting**—severe vomiting that is not easily controlled—may require intravenous nutrition support.

Dietary Interventions Sometimes nausea can be prevented or improved with dietary measures. To minimize stomach distention, patients should consume small meals and drink beverages between meals rather than during a meal. Dry, starchy foods such as toast, crackers, and pretzels may help to reduce nausea, whereas fatty or spicy foods and foods with strong odors may worsen symptoms. Foods that are cold or at room temperature may be better tolerated than hot foods. Individuals often have strong food aversions when nauseated, and tolerances vary greatly.

Gastritis

Gastritis is a general term that refers to inflammation of the gastric mucosa. Acute cases of gastritis typically result from irritating substances or treatments that damage stomach tissue, resulting in tissue erosions, ulcers, or hemorrhaging (severe bleeding). Chronic gastritis may be caused by long-term infection or autoimmune disease; it can progress to widespread inflammation and tissue atrophy and is also a risk factor for gastric cancer. In most cases, gastritis results from *Helicobacter pylori* infection or the use of nonsteroidal anti-inflammatory drugs (NSAIDs), which are both primary causes of peptic ulcer disease as well. Table 17-6 lists some potential causes of gastritis.

Complications of Gastritis The extensive tissue damage that sometimes develops in chronic gastritis can disrupt gastric secretory functions. If hydrochloric acid secretions become abnormally low (**hypochlorhydria**) or absent (**achlorhydria**), absorption of nonheme iron and vitamin B_{12} can be impaired, increasing the risk of deficiency. Pernicious anemia, characterized by autoimmune destruction of the gastric cells that produce hydrochloric acid and intrinsic factor, is a form of **atrophic gastritis** that is usually associated with the macrocytic anemia of vitamin B_{12} deficiency (see p. 209).[12]

Dietary Interventions for Gastritis Dietary recommendations depend on an individual's symptoms. In asymptomatic cases, no dietary adjustments are needed. If

TABLE 17-6 Potential Causes of Gastritis

Infection
- Bacterial: *Helicobacter pylori*
- Fungal: *Candida albicans*
- Parasitic: *Anisakis* (nematode infection)
- Viral: *Cytomegalovirus*

Chemical Substances
- Alcohol
- Cancer chemotherapy
- Drugs (especially aspirin and other NSAIDs)
- Ingestion of toxins or corrosive materials

Internal (Bodily) Causes
- Autoimmune disease
- Bile reflux
- Severe stress or sepsis

Miscellaneous
- Foreign bodies
- High salt intake
- Radiation therapy

© Cengage Learning®

intractable vomiting: vomiting that is not easily managed or controlled.

gastritis: inflammation of stomach tissue. (The suffix *-itis* refers to the presence of inflammation in an organ or tissue.)

Helicobacter pylori (H. pylori): a species of bacterium that colonizes the GI mucosa; a primary cause of gastritis and peptic ulcer disease.

hypochlorhydria (HIGH-poe-clor-HIGH-dree-ah): abnormally low gastric acid secretions.

achlorhydria (AY-clor-HIGH-dree-ah): absence of gastric acid secretions.

atrophic gastritis: a form of gastritis characterized by destruction of gastric mucosal tissue due to chronic inflammation; eventually the gastric epithelium may be replaced with another type of tissue.

FIGURE 17-5 Peptic Ulcer Disease

A peptic ulcer, such as the gastric ulcer shown here, damages mucosal tissue and may cause pain and bleeding. Duodenal ulcers are more common than gastric ulcers in the United States and other Western countries.

pain or discomfort is present, the patient should avoid irritating foods and beverages; these often include alcohol, coffee (including decaffeinated), cola beverages, spicy foods, and fried or fatty foods. If food consumption increases pain or causes nausea and vomiting, food intake should be avoided for 24 to 48 hours to rest the stomach. If hypochlorhydria or achlorhydria is present, supplementation of iron and vitamin B_{12} may be warranted.

Peptic Ulcer Disease

A **peptic ulcer** is an open sore that develops in the GI mucosa when gastric acid and pepsin overwhelm mucosal defenses and destroy mucosal tissue (see Figure 17-5). A primary factor in peptic ulcer development is *H. pylori* infection, which is present in approximately 30 to 60 percent of patients with gastric ulcers and 70 to 90 percent of those with duodenal ulcers.[13] Another major factor is the use of NSAIDs, which have both topical and systemic effects that can damage the GI lining. In rare cases, ulcers may develop from disorders that cause excessive acid secretion. Ulcer risk can also be increased by cigarette smoking and psychological stress. Note that the specific reasons why ulcers develop are unknown; only 10 to 15 percent of people with chronic *H. pylori* infection actually develop a peptic ulcer.[14]

Effects of Emotional Stress Although most ulcers are associated with *H. pylori* infection or NSAID use, about 5 to 20 percent of ulcers develop for other reasons.[15] Psychological stress by itself is not believed to cause ulcers, but it has effects on physiological processes and behaviors that may increase a person's vulnerability. The physiological effects of stress vary among individuals but may include hormonal changes that impair immune responses and wound healing, increased secretions of hydrochloric acid and pepsin, and rapid stomach emptying (which increases the acid load in the duodenum). Stress may also lead to behavioral changes, including the increased use of cigarettes, alcohol, and NSAIDs—all potential risk factors for ulcers. Thus, stress may contribute to ulcer development although its precise effects are not fully understood.

Symptoms of Peptic Ulcers Peptic ulcer symptoms vary. Some people are asymptomatic or experience only mild discomfort. In others, ulcer pain may be experienced as a hunger pain, a sensation of gnawing, or a burning pain in the stomach region. The pain or discomfort of ulcers may be relieved by food and recur several hours after a meal, especially if the ulcer is duodenal. Gastric ulcers may be aggravated by food and can cause loss of appetite and eventual weight loss. Ulcer symptoms tend to go into remission regularly and recur every few weeks or months.[16]

Complications of Peptic Ulcers Peptic ulcers are a major cause of GI bleeding, which occurs in up to 15 percent of ulcer cases.[17] Bleeding is a potential cause of death and, if severe, may indicate the need for surgical intervention. Severe bleeding is evidenced by black, tarry stool samples or, occasionally, vomit that resembles coffee grounds. Other serious complications of ulcers include perforations of the stomach or duodenum and **gastric outlet obstruction** due to scarring or inflammation.

Drug Therapy for Peptic Ulcers The goals of ulcer treatment are to relieve pain, promote healing, and prevent recurrence. In most cases, treatment requires using a combination of antibiotics to eradicate *H. pylori* infection and/or discontinuing the use of aspirin and other NSAIDs, which can irritate the gastric mucosa and delay healing. The antibiotics used to treat *H. pylori* infection most often include amoxicillin, clarithromycin, metronidazole, and tetracycline. Antisecretory drugs are prescribed to relieve pain and allow healing; these include proton-pump inhibitors, H2 blockers, and antacids (as used in GERD; see p. 477). Bismuth preparations (such as Pepto-Bismol) and the medication sucralfate may also help to heal ulcers by coating ulcerated tissue and preventing further erosion. Box 17-4 provides examples of the nutrition-related effects of some of these medications.

peptic ulcer: an open sore in the gastrointestinal mucosa; may develop in the esophagus, stomach, or duodenum.

peptic = related to digestion

gastric outlet obstruction: an obstruction that prevents the normal emptying of stomach contents into the duodenum.

BOX 17-4 DIET-DRUG INTERACTIONS

Check this table for notable nutrition-related effects of the medications discussed in this chapter.

Antacids (aluminum hydroxide, magnesium hydroxide, calcium carbonate)	**Gastrointestinal effects:** Constipation (aluminum- or calcium-containing antacids), diarrhea (magnesium-containing antacids) **Dietary interactions:** May decrease iron, calcium, folate, and vitamin B_{12} absorption **Metabolic effects:** Electrolyte imbalances
Antibiotics (for *H. pylori* infection; include amoxicillin, metronidazole, tetracycline)	**Gastrointestinal effects:** Diarrhea, nausea and vomiting (tetracycline, metronidazole), altered taste sensation (metronidazole) **Dietary interactions:** Avoid alcohol with metronidazole; tetracycline can bind to calcium, iron, magnesium, and zinc, reducing absorption of both the tetracycline and the minerals
Antisecretory drugs (proton-pump inhibitors, H2 blockers)	**Gastrointestinal effects:** Diarrhea, constipation, nausea and vomiting, abdominal pain (proton-pump inhibitors) **Dietary interactions:** May decrease iron, calcium, folate, and vitamin B_{12} absorption
Octreotide	**Gastrointestinal effects:** Abdominal cramps, diarrhea, nausea and vomiting, flatulence **Dietary interactions:** May decrease absorption of fat, fat-soluble vitamins, and vitamin B_{12} **Metabolic effects:** Hyperglycemia, hypothyroidism

Nutrition Care for Peptic Ulcers The goals of nutrition care are to correct nutrient deficiencies, if necessary, and encourage dietary and lifestyle practices that minimize symptoms.[18] Patients should avoid dietary items that increase acid secretion or irritate the GI lining; examples include alcohol, coffee and other caffeine-containing beverages, chocolate, and pepper, although individual tolerances vary. Small meals may be better tolerated than large ones. Patients should avoid food consumption for at least two hours before bedtime. There is no evidence that dietary adjustments alter the rate of healing or prevent recurrence.[19]

IN SUMMARY

▌ *Dyspepsia* refers to general symptoms of pain or discomfort in the upper abdominal region; dietary measures may include avoiding large meals, fatty or spicy foods, and foods that trigger symptoms.

▌ Gastritis and peptic ulcer disease are most often associated with *H. pylori* infection, which can be eradicated by antibiotic therapy. NSAID use may promote gastritis and peptic ulcer disease by damaging the mucosal lining.

▌ Nutrition care for gastritis and peptic ulcer disease includes correcting any nutritional deficiencies that develop and eliminating dietary substances that cause pain or discomfort.

17.4 Gastric Surgery

LO 17.4 Describe the different types of gastric surgery and the nutrition care required after these procedures.

Gastric surgery is sometimes necessary for treating stomach cancer, some ulcer complications, and ulcers that are resistant to drug therapy. In recent years, gastric surgeries have also become popular treatments for severe obesity. This section describes **gastrectomy,** the surgery that removes diseased areas of the stomach, and **bariatric surgery,** the type of surgery that treats obesity (bariatric surgery was introduced in Chapter 7).

gastrectomy (gah-STREK-ta-mie): the surgical removal of part of the stomach (partial gastrectomy) or the entire stomach (total gastrectomy).

bariatric (BAH-ree-AH-trik) **surgery:** surgery that treats severe obesity.

▌ *baros* = weight

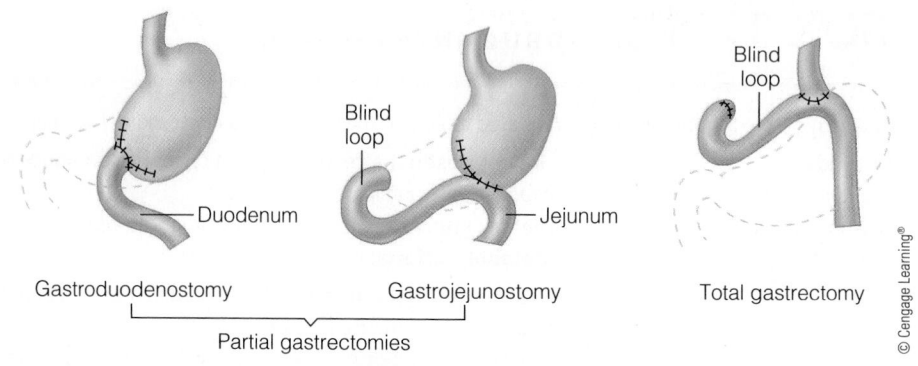

Duodenum

Gastroduodenostomy

Blind loop

Jejunum

Gastrojejunostomy

Partial gastrectomies

Blind loop

Total gastrectomy

© Cengage Learning®

FIGURE 17-6 Gastrectomy Procedures
In a gastrectomy, part or all of the stomach is surgically removed. The dashed lines show the removed section.

Gastrectomy

Figure 17-6 illustrates some typical gastrectomy procedures. In a partial gastrectomy, only part of the stomach is removed, and the remaining portion is connected to the duodenum or jejunum. In a total gastrectomy, the surgeon removes the entire stomach and connects the esophagus directly to the small intestine.

Nutrition Care after Gastrectomy Following a gastrectomy, the oral ingestion of fluids and foods is suspended until some healing has occurred, and fluids are supplied intravenously. Oral intakes begin with small sips of water, ice chips (melted in the mouth), and broth. Once fluids are tolerated, patients may be offered liquid meals (with no sugars) at first; after solid foods are started, meals may contain only one or two food items at a time so that tolerance can be evaluated. Tube feedings may be necessary if complications prevent a normal progression to solid foods.[20]

Dietary measures after a gastrectomy are determined by the size of the remaining stomach, which influences meal size, and the stomach emptying rate, which affects food tolerances. Depending on the amount of food tolerated, the patient may require as many as five to eight small meals and snacks per day. A protein food (fish, lean meats, eggs, or cheese) should be included in each meal so that adequate protein is obtained. Patients should avoid sweets and sugars because they increase osmolarity in the small intestine and potentiate the **dumping syndrome** (discussed below). Some patients may need to avoid milk products due to lactose intolerance. Soluble fibers may be added to meals to slow stomach emptying and to reduce the risk of diarrhea. Liquids are restricted during meals (and for up to 30 to 60 minutes after meals) due to limited stomach capacity and because liquids can increase the stomach emptying rate. Table 17-7 lists foods that are often permitted or limited in postgastrectomy diets.

Dumping Syndrome The dumping syndrome, a common complication of gastrectomy, is characterized by a group of symptoms resulting from rapid gastric emptying. Ordinarily, the pyloric sphincter controls the rate of flow from the stomach into the duodenum. After some types of stomach surgery, stomach emptying is no longer regulated, and the stomach's hyperosmolar contents rush into the small intestine more quickly after meals, causing a number of unpleasant effects. Early symptoms can occur within 30 minutes after eating and may include nausea, vomiting, abdominal cramping, diarrhea, lightheadedness, rapid heartbeat, and others (see Table 17-8). These symptoms are due to a shift of fluid from the bloodstream to the intestinal lumen that increases intestinal distention and lowers blood volume; in addition, the accelerated release of GI hormones may alter both intestinal motility and blood flow. Several hours later, symptoms of hypoglycemia

dumping syndrome: a cluster of symptoms that result from the rapid emptying of an osmotic load from the stomach into the small intestine.

bacterial overgrowth: excessive bacterial colonization of the stomach and small intestine; may be due to reduced gastric acid secretions, altered motility of intestinal contents, or changes in intestinal anatomy due to surgical reconstruction. (Chapter 19 describes bacterial overgrowth in detail.)

TABLE 17-7 Postgastrectomy Diet

Food Category	Foods Recommended (as tolerated)	Foods to Limit (unless tolerated)
Meat and meat alternates	Lean tender meat, fish, poultry, and shellfish; eggs; smooth nut butters	Fried, tough, or chewy meat, fish, poultry, and shellfish; frankfurters and sausages; bacon; luncheon meat; dried peas and beans; nuts; chunky nut butters
Milk and milk products	Milk, plain yogurt, cheese	Milk shakes, chocolate milk, sweetened yogurt
Breads and cereals	Bread, crackers, bagels, pasta, and breakfast cereals made from enriched white flour (cereals should contain no added sugars)	Breads and cereals with more than 2 grams of fiber per serving; baked goods with dried fruit, nuts, or seeds; granola; frosted cereals; pastry; doughnuts
Vegetables	Tender-cooked vegetables without peels, skin, or seeds; raw lettuce	Raw vegetables (except lettuce), beets, broccoli, brussels sprouts, cabbage, cauliflower, collard and mustard greens, corn, potato skin
Fruit	Canned fruit without added sugar, bananas, melon	Canned fruit in syrup, raw fruit (except bananas and melons), dried fruit, fruit juice
Beverages	Decaffeinated coffee and tea, beverages sweetened with artificial sweeteners	Caffeinated beverages; alcoholic beverages; beverages sweetened with sugar, corn syrup, or honey

© Cengage Learning®

may occur because the unusually large spike in blood glucose following the meal (due to rapid nutrient influx and absorption) can result in an excessive insulin response.

Dietary adjustments can greatly minimize or prevent dumping syndrome. The goals are to slow the rate of gastric emptying, limit the amount of food material that reaches the intestine, and reduce foods that increase osmolarity. Therefore, fluids are restricted during meals, meal size is limited, and sugars (including milk sugar) are restricted. In some cases, a medication that inhibits GI motility may be prescribed to lessen symptoms. Box 17-5 (p. 484) lists practical suggestions for reducing the occurrence of dumping syndrome. The Case Study in Box 17-6 (p. 484) provides the opportunity to design a menu for a postgastrectomy patient who is at risk of dumping syndrome.

Postsurgical Complications and Nutrition Status After a gastrectomy, it may take time for the patient to learn the amount of food that can be consumed without discomfort. The symptoms associated with meals may lead to food avoidance, substantial weight loss, and eventually, malnutrition. Other nutrition problems that may occur after a gastrectomy include the following:

▪ *Fat malabsorption.* Fat digestion and absorption may become impaired for a number of reasons after a gastrectomy. The accelerated transit of food material may prevent the normal mixing of fat with lipase and bile. If the duodenum has been removed or bypassed, less lipase is available for fat digestion. **Bacterial overgrowth,** a common consequence of gastric surgeries, can lead to changes in bile acids that upset bile function. The fat malabsorption that results from these changes can eventually cause deficiencies of fat-soluble vitamins and some minerals. Supplemental pancreatic enzymes are sometimes provided to improve fat digestion.

▪ *Bone disease.* Fat malabsorption can lead to malabsorption of both vitamin D and calcium;* furthermore, patients at risk of dumping syndrome may need to avoid milk products, which are among the best sources of these nutrients. Bone density should be monitored during the years following surgery, and supplementation of calcium and vitamin D is often recommended.

TABLE 17-8 Symptoms of Dumping Syndrome

Early Dumping Syndrome

Symptoms may begin within 30 minutes after eating.[a]

▪ Abdominal cramps, bloating

▪ Diarrhea

▪ Flushing, sweating

▪ Lightheadedness

▪ Nausea and vomiting

▪ Rapid heartbeat

▪ Weakness, feeling faint

Late Dumping Syndrome

Symptoms may begin 1 to 3 hours after eating.[b]

▪ Anxiety

▪ Confusion

▪ Headache, dizziness

▪ Hunger

▪ Palpitations

▪ Sweating

▪ Weakness, feeling faint

[a] Symptoms are due to rapid gastric emptying, which leads to a fluid shift from the bloodstream to the intestinal lumen, intestinal distention, and decreased blood volume.

[b] Symptoms are due to rapid glucose absorption and the excessive release of insulin, resulting in hypoglycemia.

© Cengage Learning®

*Fat malabsorption reduces calcium absorption because the negatively charged fatty acids combine with calcium (which is positively charged) and prevent its absorption.

Dietary adjustments can greatly minimize or prevent symptoms of dumping syndrome. The following suggestions may help:

- Eat smaller meals that suit the reduced capacity of the stomach. Increase the number of meals consumed daily so that energy intake is adequate.

- Eat in a relaxed setting. Eat slowly, and chew food thoroughly.

- Include fiber-rich foods in each meal. Adding soluble fibers like pectin or guar gum to meals may help to control symptoms.

- If symptoms of hypoglycemia continue, try including a protein-rich food in each meal.

- Limit the amount of fluid included in meals. Avoid drinking beverages within 30 to 60 minutes before and after meals, but be sure to consume adequate fluid to avoid dehydration.

- Avoid juices, sweetened beverages, and foods that contain high amounts of sugar. Use artificial sweeteners to sweeten beverages and desserts.

- Avoid milk and most milk products, which are high in lactose. Avoid enzyme-treated milk as well, because the breakdown products of lactose (glucose and galactose) can also cause dumping symptoms. Cheese may be better tolerated than milk because its lactose content is low. Make an effort to consume nonmilk calcium sources such as green leafy vegetables, fish with bones, and tofu.

- Avoid carbonated beverages if they cause bloating.

- Avoid foods and beverages that are very hot or very cold, unless tolerated.

- Lie down for 20 to 30 minutes (or longer) after eating to help slow the transit of food to the small intestine. While eating a meal, sit upright.

Case Study BOX 17-6 NUTRITION CARE AFTER GASTRIC SURGERY

Ed Hanson, a 58-year-old biology teacher, was admitted to the hospital for gastric surgery after numerous medical treatments failed to manage severe complications related to his peptic ulcer disease. A gastrojejunostomy was performed, and after about 24 hours, Mr. Hanson was able to take small sips of warm water. The health care team anticipates multiple nutrition-related problems and is taking measures to prevent them.

1. Review Figure 17-6 to better understand Mr. Hanson's surgical procedure. Consider the possibilities that he might experience the following symptoms: early satiety, nausea and vomiting, weight loss, dumping syndrome, fat malabsorption, anemia, and bone disease. Explain why each of these conditions may occur.

2. What type of diet will the physician prescribe for Mr. Hanson after he begins eating solid foods? Create a day's worth of menus, using foods from Table 17-7.

3. What advice can you give Mr. Hanson that will help to prevent dumping syndrome? List several foods from each major food group that may cause symptoms of dumping syndrome.

- *Anemia.* After a gastrectomy, the reduced secretion of gastric acid and intrinsic factor impairs the absorption of both iron and vitamin B_{12}, often leading to anemia. If the duodenum has been removed or is bypassed, the risk of iron deficiency increases because the duodenum is a major site of iron absorption. Supplementation of both iron and vitamin B_{12} is often warranted after surgery.

Bariatric Surgery

Bariatric surgery is currently considered the most effective and durable treatment for morbid obesity.[21] Candidates for bariatric surgery are obese individuals who have a body mass index (BMI) greater than 40, or a BMI between 35 and 40 accompanied by severe weight-related problems such as diabetes, hypertension, or debilitating osteoarthritis (a healthy BMI usually falls between 20 and 25). In addition, the patient should have attempted a variety of nonsurgical weight-loss measures prior to seeking surgery. Bariatric surgery patients should have realistic expectations about the amount of weight they are likely to lose, the diet they will

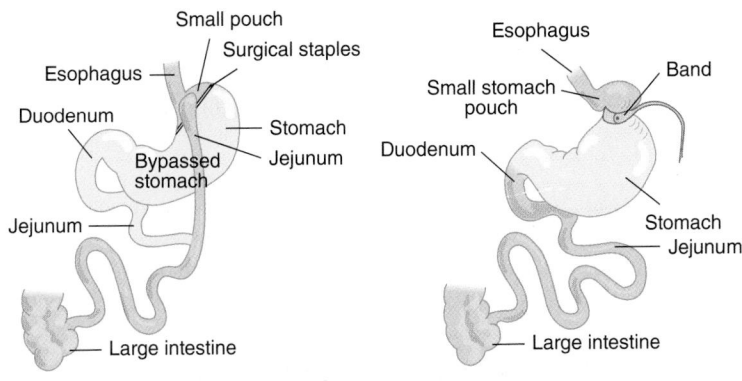

In the gastric bypass operation, the surgeon constructs a small gastric pouch and connects it directly to the jejunum so that the flow of food bypasses a substantial portion of the small intestine. The dark pink area highlights the altered flow of food through the GI tract. The pale pink area indicates the bypassed sections.

In the gastric banding procedure, the surgeon creates a small gastric pouch using an inflatable band placed near the top of the stomach. The band is tightened or loosened by adding or removing fluid via an access port placed under the skin.

In the sleeve gastrectomy procedure, the surgeon removes 70 to 85 percent of stomach tissue and staples the remaining portions together to create a vertical, tube-shaped stomach with limited capacity. The sleeve gastrectomy is often a stand-alone procedure but may also be performed as the first stage of a more complex surgery if greater weight loss is desired.

FIGURE 17-7 Surgical Procedures for Severe Obesity

need to follow, and the complications that may ensue. Some types of bariatric surgery can dramatically affect health and nutrition status, and many patients require lifelong management.

Bariatric Surgical Procedures Figure 17-7 illustrates the most popular surgical options for weight reduction. The *gastric bypass* operation, which accounts for about 60 to 70 percent of bariatric surgeries,[22] constructs a small gastric pouch that reduces stomach capacity and thereby restricts meal size. In addition, the gastric pouch is connected directly to the jejunum, resulting in significant nutrient malabsorption because the flow of food bypasses a significant portion of the small intestine. In the *gastric banding* procedure, a fluid-filled inflatable band is placed around the uppermost portion of the stomach; adjusting the band's fluid level can tighten or loosen the band and alter the size of the opening to the rest of the stomach. A smaller opening slows the rate at which the upper region is emptied and prolongs the sense of fullness after a meal. The *sleeve gastrectomy* procedure removes a large portion of the stomach, leaving a narrow gastric tube (or "sleeve") that holds only about 3 to 5 ounces (about ½ cup) of food. This operation may be converted to a gastric bypass or other type of malabsorptive surgery if weight loss is inadequate. Whereas the gastric bypass and sleeve gastrectomy operations are permanent, the gastric banding procedure is fully reversible.

Clinical studies indicate that the gastric bypass and sleeve gastrectomy surgeries usually result in greater weight loss than the gastric banding procedure. Although study results vary, gastric bypass patients typically lose 60 to 70 percent of their excess body weight, patients with a sleeve gastrectomy lose about 57 percent of their excess weight, and individuals who undergo gastric banding lose about 50 percent of their excess weight.[23]

Nutrition Care after Bariatric Surgery After bariatric surgery, patients initially consume only sugar-free, noncarbonated clear liquids and low-fat broths; afterward, they progress to a liquid diet (high in protein, low in sugars and fat), followed by pureed foods and then solid foods; the diet is advanced as tolerated. Once the diet progresses to solid foods, patients consume between three and six small meals per day. Only small portions of food can be consumed at each meal because overeating may stretch the gastric region or result in vomiting or regurgitation. Similarly, fluids must be consumed separately from meals to avoid excessive distention. Although precise

Patients need to learn new dietary habits after bariatric surgery. The following recommendations may help:

- Consume only small portions of food and chew food thoroughly. Use a small spoon, and take small bites. Relax and enjoy the meal, taking at least 15 to 20 minutes to eat.

- Understand that, at first, the appropriate amount of each food served at mealtime may be only a few spoonfuls. Learn to recognize the sensations that occur when the gastric pouch is full. Signs of fullness may include pressure in the stomach region, a slight feeling of nausea, or pain in the upper chest or shoulder.

- To control vomiting, try eating smaller volumes of food, eating more slowly, and avoiding foods known to cause difficulty. Continued vomiting may be a sign that some food choices or amounts are inappropriate.

- Consume food only during designated mealtimes (usually 3 to 6 small meals per day), and avoid consuming foods at other times of the day. Snacking throughout the day can become a bad habit that causes weight to be regained.

- Learn to recognize foods that cause problems. Foods that are dry, sticky, or fibrous may be difficult to tolerate during the weeks after surgery.

- Avoid consuming liquids within 30 minutes of mealtime. Avoid high-kcalorie drinks like sweetened soda, milk shakes, and alcoholic beverages. Avoid drinking carbonated beverages or using a straw, as these practices can increase stomach gas and cause bloating.

- Sip water and other beverages throughout the day to obtain sufficient fluids. Aim to consume between 6 and 8 cups of water and other noncaloric beverages daily. Remember that most people meet a significant fraction of their fluid needs by eating food, but a person who has undergone bariatric surgery must limit food intake.

- Engage in regular physical activity. Activity is a valuable aid to weight maintenance and can help to maintain lean tissue while weight is being lost.

dietary guidelines vary depending on the type of procedure performed, other recommendations usually include the following:[24]

- *Protein intake.* Recommendations range from about 1.0 to 1.5 grams of protein per kilogram of ideal body weight per day; however, intakes are often lower than recommended. Patients are generally instructed to consume liquid protein supplements regularly and to eat high-protein foods before consuming other foods in a meal.

- *Vitamin and mineral supplementation.* Daily multivitamin/mineral supplements help to prevent nutrient deficiencies. Due to nutrient malabsorption, patients who have had the gastric bypass surgery usually require additional supplementation of vitamin B_{12}, vitamin D, calcium, and iron.

- *Foods to avoid.* Some foods may obstruct the gastric outlet; these include doughy or sticky breads and pasta products; melted cheese; raw vegetables; fibrous vegetables such as asparagus and celery; foods with seeds, hulls, peels, or skins; nuts; popcorn; and tough, chewy meats.

- *Dumping syndrome.* To avoid symptoms of dumping syndrome, gastric bypass patients must carefully control food portions, avoid foods high in sugars, and consume liquids between meals.

After bariatric surgery, patient education and counseling are critical for weight loss and weight management, and patients also need to learn the elements of a healthy diet. Box 17-7 includes additional dietary suggestions for patients who have undergone bariatric surgery.

Postsurgical Concerns Common complaints after bariatric surgery include nausea, vomiting, and constipation.[25] Although the cause of these problems varies among patients, dietary noncompliance and inadequate fluid intake are often contributing factors, and improved dietary intakes can help in resolving these conditions. Rapid weight loss increases a person's risk of developing gallbladder disease; patients at especially high risk sometimes have their gallbladders removed while undergoing bariatric surgery. After gastric bypass surgery, long-term complications may include fat malabsorption, bone disease, and anemia.

IN SUMMARY

▌ Gastric surgeries, used to treat cancer, peptic ulcer complications, and obesity, require dietary adjustments after surgery and are associated with complications that may affect nutrition status. Common postsurgical complications include fat malabsorption, bone disease, anemia, and dumping syndrome.

▌ After gastric surgery, patients must learn to consume appropriate food portions, meet fluid needs, use dietary supplements to prevent nutrient deficiencies, and choose foods that are unlikely to cause abdominal discomfort, vomiting, or dumping syndrome.

Nutrition Assessment Checklist FOR PEOPLE WITH DISORDERS OF THE UPPER GI TRACT

Medical History

Check the medical history to uncover conditions or treatments that may:

- Interfere with chewing or swallowing
- Lead to dry mouth
- Lead to dyspepsia, nausea, or vomiting

Check for a medical diagnosis of:

- Gastritis or peptic ulcer
- GERD
- Hiatal hernia
- Pernicious anemia

For a patient who has undergone gastric surgery, check for the following complications:

- Anemia
- Bone disease
- Dumping syndrome
- Fat malabsorption

Medications

Record all medications and note:

- Aspirin or NSAID use in patients with gastritis or peptic ulcer disease
- Medications that may cause dry mouth
- Medications that may cause nausea and vomiting

To help alleviate nausea, suggest that medications be taken with food, when possible.

Dietary Intake

To devise an acceptable meal plan, obtain:

- An accurate and thorough record of food intake
- A thorough record of dietary supplement intake, including both vitamin/mineral supplements and herbal products

- A record of food allergies and intolerances, as well as food preferences
- A record of foods that provoke symptoms of GERD, dyspepsia, gastritis, peptic ulcers, or dumping syndrome

For patients on long-term dysphagia diets, monitor appetite, food tolerances, and the variety of foods consumed.

Anthropometric Data

Measure baseline height and weight. Address weight loss early to prevent malnutrition in patients with:

- Difficulty chewing or swallowing
- Dumping syndrome
- Dyspepsia
- Frequent nausea and vomiting
- Malabsorption

Laboratory Tests

Check laboratory tests for signs of dehydration for patients with:

- Constipation
- Dumping syndrome
- Persistent vomiting

Check laboratory tests for nutrition-related anemia in patients with:

- Gastritis
- Long-term use of antisecretory drugs
- Previous gastric surgeries

Physical Signs

Look for physical signs of:

- Dehydration—in patients with constipation, dumping syndrome, or persistent vomiting
- Iron and vitamin B_{12} deficiencies—in patients with hypochlorhydria or achlorhydria

Clinical Applications

1. Although some individuals require a mechanically altered diet for just a few weeks, others have medical problems that require long-term use of such diets. Consider the difference between working with a person who has had a swallowing problem for years and a person who recently had mouth surgery and is just beginning to eat again.

   ▪ Explain how the needs of these individuals may differ. What nutrition-related problems may develop if a person has been following a restrictive dysphagia diet for several years?

   ▪ Using Table 17-1, Table 17-4, and Box 17-1, create a day's worth of menus for a person who requires long-term use of a pureed dysphagia diet and tolerates only liquids that have a honeylike or spoon-thick consistency.

2. Jillian, a 35-year-old woman who is 5 feet 4 inches tall and weighs 227 pounds, has had severe hip and knee osteoarthritis for several years and was recently diagnosed with type 2 diabetes. After trying numerous weight-loss programs without success, she finally visits a bariatric surgeon to learn about the surgical options for treating her obesity.

   ▪ Calculate Jillian's BMI, and explain why Jillian would or would not be a good candidate for bariatric surgery.

   ▪ Should Jillian decide to undergo gastric bypass surgery, she will need to permanently change her dietary habits. Describe the dietary recommendations and nutrition concerns following bariatric surgery. Summarize the measures necessary for preventing vomiting, distention of the gastric pouch, gastric outlet obstruction, and dumping syndrome.

   ▪ Explain why dehydration is a frequent complication following bariatric surgery. What tips can you give Jillian to help her avoid this problem?

Self Check

1. Foods permitted on the clear liquid diet include all of the following *except:*
   a. milk.
   b. fruit ices.
   c. flavored gelatin.
   d. consommé.

2. If a patient with dysphagia has difficulty swallowing solids but can easily swallow liquids:
   a. the problem is most likely a motility disorder.
   b. the patient may have achalasia.
   c. the problem is probably an esophageal obstruction.
   d. the patient most likely has oropharyngeal dysphagia.

3. The clinican working with a patient with dysphagia should recognize that:
   a. the patient should eat only pureed foods to minimize the risk of aspiration.
   b. the foods allowed are those that can be comfortably and safely chewed and swallowed.
   c. highly seasoned foods are often restricted.
   d. regular diets do not meet nutrient needs, so supplements are required.

4. Possible consequences of GERD include all of the following *except:*
   a. reflux esophagitis.   c. Barrett's esophagus.
   b. dysphagia.   d. gastric ulcer.

5. Treating GERD with proton-pump inhibitors is effective because they:
   a. reduce gastric acid secretion.
   b. reduce pressure within the stomach.
   c. strengthen the lower esophageal sphincter.
   d. provide a protective barrier between gastric acid and the esophageal mucosa.

6. Chronic gastritis may increase risk of:
   a. dumping syndrome.
   b. bone disease.
   c. iron and vitamin B_{12} deficiencies.
   d. gallbladder disease.

7. The primary cause of most peptic ulcers is:
   a. consumption of spicy foods.
   b. psychological stress.
   c. smoking cigarettes.
   d. *Helicobacter pylori* infection.

8. The main dietary recommendation for patients with gastritis or peptic ulcers is to consume foods that:
   a. neutralize stomach acidity.
   b. are well tolerated and do not cause discomfort.
   c. coat the stomach lining.
   d. promote healing of mucosal tissue.

9. Following a gastrectomy, patients can greatly minimize the risk of dumping syndrome by:
   a. increasing intake of carbohydrates and avoiding fatty foods.
   b. consuming liquids between meals and avoiding foods that supply sugars.
   c. consuming a high-fiber diet and minimizing meat and cheese intake.
   d. including milk products with each meal to provide protein.

10. After a gastric bypass operation, the patient should be monitored for all of the following conditions *except:*
    a. anemia.
    b. bone disease.
    c. hiatal hernia.
    d. fat-soluble vitamin deficiencies.

Answers to these questions appear in Appendix H.

Notes

1. T. E. Daniels, Diseases of the mouth and salivary glands, in L. Goldman and A. I. Schafer, eds., *Goldman's Cecil Medicine* (Philadelphia: Saunders, 2012), pp. 2449–2454; R. B. Cohen, Approach to dental and oral symptoms, in R. S. Porter and J. L. Kaplan, eds., *Merck Manual of Diagnosis and Therapy* (Whitehouse Station, NJ: Merck Sharp and Dohme Corp., 2011), pp. 494–516.

2. S. Naguwa and M. E. Gershwin, Sjögren's syndrome, in L. Goldman and A. I. Schafer, eds., *Goldman's Cecil Medicine* (Philadelphia: Saunders, 2012), pp. 1713–1716.

3. A. Chaudhury and H. Mashimo, Oropharyngeal and esophageal motility disorders, in N. J. Greenberger, ed., *Current Diagnosis and Treatment: Gastroenterology, Hepatology, and Endoscopy* (New York: McGraw-Hill Companies, 2012), pp. 164–182.

4. Academy of Nutrition and Dietetics, *Nutrition Care Manual* (Chicago: Academy of Nutrition and Dietetics, 2014).

5. S. Friedman and J. R. Agrawal, Gastrointestinal and biliary complications of pregnancy, in N. J. Greenberger, ed., *Current Diagnosis and Treatment: Gastroenterology, Hepatology, and Endoscopy* (New York: McGraw-Hill Companies, 2012), pp. 79–104.

6. G. W. Falk and D. A. Katzka, Diseases of the esophagus, in L. Goldman and A. I. Schafer, eds., *Goldman's Cecil Medicine* (Philadelphia: Saunders, 2012), pp. 874–886.

7. W. W. Chan and R. Burakoff, Functional (nonulcer) dyspepsia, in N. J. Greenberger, ed., *Current Diagnosis and Treatment: Gastroenterology, Hepatology, and Endoscopy* (New York: McGraw-Hill Companies, 2012), pp. 203–213.

8. Chan and Burakoff, 2012.

9. B. E. Lacy and coauthors, Review article: Current treatment options and management of functional dyspepsia, *Alimentary Pharmacology and Therapeutics* 36 (2012): 3–15.

10. Chan and Burakoff, 2012.

11. K. McQuaid, Approach to the patient with gastrointestinal disease, in L. Goldman and A. I. Schafer, eds., *Goldman's Cecil Medicine* (Philadelphia: Saunders, 2012), pp. 828–844.

12. E. Andres and K. Serraj, Optimal management of pernicious anemia, *Journal of Blood Medicine* 3 (2012): 97–103; A. C. Antony, Megaloblastic anemias, in L. Goldman and A. I. Schafer, eds., *Goldman's Cecil Medicine* (Philadelphia: Saunders, 2012), pp. 1075–1083.

13. E. Lew, Peptic ulcer disease, in N. J. Greenberger, ed., *Current Diagnosis and Treatment: Gastroenterology, Hepatology, and Endoscopy* (New York: McGraw-Hill Companies, 2012), pp. 187–197.

14. Lew, 2012.

15. E. J. Kuipers and M. J. Blaser, Acid peptic disease, in L. Goldman and A. I. Schafer, eds., *Goldman's Cecil Medicine* (Philadelphia: Saunders, 2012), pp. 886–895.

16. Kuipers and Blaser, 2012.

17. Lew, 2012.

18. Academy of Nutrition and Dietetics, 2014.

19. S. Cohen, Gastritis and peptic ulcer disease, in R. S. Porter and J. L. Kaplan, eds., *Merck Manual of Diagnosis and Therapy* (Whitehouse Station, NJ: Merck Sharp and Dohme Corp., 2011), pp. 128–138.

20. Academy of Nutrition and Dietetics, 2014.

21. M. K. Robinson and N. J. Greenberger, Treatment of obesity: The impact of bariatric surgery, in N. J. Greenberger, ed., *Current Diagnosis and Treatment: Gastroenterology, Hepatology, and Endoscopy* (New York: McGraw-Hill Companies, 2012), pp. 224–236.

22. K. Tymitz, T. Magnuson, and M. Schweitzer, Bariatric surgery, in A. C. Ross and coeditors, eds., *Modern Nutrition in Health and Disease* (Baltimore: Lippincott Williams & Wilkins, 2014), pp. 800–807.

23. P. Sieber and coauthors, Five-year results of laparoscopic sleeve gastrectomy, *Surgery for Obesity and Related Diseases* (2013): doi: 10.1016/j.soard.2013.06.024; Weight Management Dietetic Practice Group, *ADA Pocket Guide to Bariatric Surgery* (Chicago: American Dietetic Association, 2009), pp. 1–16.

24. Tymitz, Magnuson, and Schweitzer, 2014; J. I. Mechanick and coauthors, Clinical practice guidelines for the perioperative nutritional, metabolic, and nonsurgical support of the bariatric surgery patient—2013 update, *Endocrine Practice* 19 (2013): 337–372.

25. Robinson and Greenberger, 2012.

LO 17.5 Describe the causes, effects, and treatments of dental caries and periodontal disease and discuss the relationships between these conditions and chronic illness.

Various aspects of nutrition and oral health have been discussed in this book. Chapters 2 and 9 describe the effects of carbohydrates and fluoride, respectively, on the development of dental caries. Chapter 12 discusses the development of tooth decay in babies who are given bottles for prolonged periods. This Nutrition in Practice provides additional information about dental caries and introduces other problems related to oral health. The glossary in Box NP17-1 defines related terms.

What is dental caries, and what factors influence its development?

Dental caries is an oral infectious disease that affects the structures and integrity of the teeth. Caries develops when the bacteria that reside in **dental plaque** metabolize dietary carbohydrates and produce acids that attack tooth enamel. If allowed to progress, the decay can penetrate the dentin and destroy other structures that support and maintain the tooth (see Figure NP17-1). The development of dental caries is influenced by the type of carbohydrate consumed, the frequency of carbohydrate intake, the stickiness of the foods that contain carbohydrate, and the availability of saliva to rinse the teeth and neutralize acid. Other factors include oral hygiene, fluoride intake, and the composition of tooth enamel,

---

FIGURE NP17-1 Development of Dental Caries

Dental caries begins when acid dissolves the enamel that covers the tooth. If not repaired, the decay may penetrate the dentin and spread into the pulp of the tooth, causing inflammation, abscess, and possible loss of the tooth.

© Cengage Learning®

---

which together influence a person's susceptibility to caries. Poor nutrition during pregnancy, infancy, or early childhood can impair the development of healthy teeth and increase vulnerability to dental caries. Table NP17-1 lists examples of nutrient deficiencies that influence the development of dental caries.[1]

Which foods promote caries development?

The most **cariogenic** foods are carbohydrate-containing foods that remain in contact with the teeth for prolonged periods, are difficult to clear from the mouth, or are consumed frequently or over an

---

BOX NP17-1 GLOSSARY

cariogenic (KAH-ree-oh-JEN-ic): conducive to development of dental caries.

dental calculus: mineralized dental plaque, often associated with inflammation and bleeding.

dental caries (KAH-reez): infectious disease of the teeth that causes the gradual decay and disintegration of tooth structures.

dental plaque (PLACK): a film of bacteria and bacterial by-products that accumulates on the tooth surface.

gingiva (jin-JYE-va, JIN-jeh-va): the gums.

gingivitis (jin-jeh-VYE-tus): inflammation of the gums, characterized by redness, swelling, and bleeding.

periodontal disease: disease that involves the connective tissue that supports the teeth.

periodontitis: inflammation or degeneration of the tissues that support the teeth.

periodontium: the tissues that support the teeth, including the gums, cementum (bonelike material covering the dentin layer of the tooth), periodontal ligament, and underlying bone.

▎ *peri* = around, surrounding

▎ *odont* = tooth

TABLE NP17-1 Nutrient Deficiencies Affecting Development of Dental Caries

Nutrient Deficiency	Effect on Dental Tissues
Protein	Delayed tooth development, decreased tooth size, increased solubility of tooth enamel, degradation of salivary glands
Vitamin A	Impaired formation of tooth enamel, degradation of salivary glands
Vitamin D, calcium, and phosphorus	Impaired formation of tooth enamel, reduced enamel mineralization, decreased resistance to dental caries
Fluoride	Increased susceptibility to enamel demineralization, reduced protection against decay-causing bacteria

© Cengage Learning®

extended period. Examples include hard candies or lozenges that dissolve slowly in the mouth; sticky or chewy foods such as dried fruit or chewy bread; starchy snack foods such as pretzels or chips, and sweetened beverages that are repeatedly sipped. These foods can be eaten without provoking tooth decay if they are consumed quickly and removed from tooth surfaces promptly.

Acidic foods and beverages, such as cola drinks, citrus fruits and juices, pickles, and some herbal teas, also contribute to the erosion of tooth enamel. Acidic food items are more cariogenic when consumed after or between meals because they are less likely to be rinsed away by saliva or neutralized by alkaline foods that may be consumed during the meal.[2]

Do any foods help to prevent caries?

Yes, foods that stimulate saliva flow, neutralize mouth acidity, or induce the clearance of food particles from the teeth can help to prevent caries formation. Examples include cheese, which increases salivary secretions and contains nutrients that neutralize acid; milk, which reduces mouth acidity due to its nearly neutral pH; and raw vegetables, which require vigorous chewing and therefore stimulate saliva flow. Some foods contain substances that reduce enamel solubility, such as the fluoride in tea and an unidentified compound in cocoa. The sequence in which foods are eaten influences caries development; for example, eating cheese after consuming an acidic fruit dessert can raise plaque pH and reduce caries risk, whereas drinking sugared coffee at the end of the meal can prolong plaque acidity. Chewing sugarless gum after or between meals can help to prevent caries by stimulating salivary flow, pushing saliva into hard-to-reach crevices in and around teeth, and removing food particles from the teeth.[3]

How does saliva protect against caries formation?

In addition to rinsing away the sugars and food particles that remain on the teeth, saliva contains substances (such as proteins, bicarbonate, and phosphates) that dilute and neutralize mouth acidity. Furthermore, saliva contains antimicrobial proteins (immunoglobulins and lysozyme) that defend against bacteria and fungi. Finally, the calcium, phosphate, and fluoride ions in saliva help to prevent dissolution of enamel and promote remineralization. If salivary secretions are low or absent, the risk of developing dental caries and other dental diseases greatly increases.

Does dental plaque contribute to other dental diseases?

Yes, the deposits of plaque can thicken and lead to other dental problems. As plaque accumulates on the tooth surface, it fills with calcium and phosphate, eventually forming **dental calculus.**[4] Calculus develops either at the gum surface or in the crevice between the gum and a tooth; its presence may lead to additional plaque retention. The buildup of plaque and calculus increases the likelihood of infection and subsequent inflammation.

Periodontal disease is the name given to inflammatory conditions that involve the **periodontium,** the structures that support the tooth in its bony socket (see Figure NP17-2). The periodontium includes the gums (called **gingiva**), other connective tissues surrounding the tooth, and the bone underneath. Inflammation of

FIGURE NP17-2 Periodontal disease destroys the tissues and bones that hold teeth in place.

CNRI/Science Source

the gums, called **gingivitis,** is characterized by redness, bleeding, and swelling of gum tissue. **Periodontitis** is an inflammation of the other tissues surrounding the tooth. As plaque invades the space below the gum line, the combination of toxic bacterial by-products and the body's immune responses can damage the tissues holding a tooth in place. Left untreated, the tissues and bone of the peridontium may ultimately be destroyed, leading to permanent tooth loss.

What are the risk factors for periodontal disease, and how is it treated?

Dental plaque is the primary risk factor associated with periodontal disease, and the severity of disease is related to the amount of plaque present. Tobacco smoking is another factor, possibly due to its destructive effects on cellular immune responses.[5] The likelihood of developing periodontal disease is increased if a person has a chronic illness that impairs immune status, such as diabetes mellitus or HIV infection. Other risk factors include stress, pregnancy, use of certain medications (including oral contraceptives, antiepileptic drugs, and anticancer drugs), and dental conditions that increase plaque accumulation, such as poorly aligned teeth or ill-fitting bridges. Strategies for reducing risk focus on improving oral hygiene (proper brushing and flossing) and encouraging smoking cessation. Table NP17-2 (p. 492) provides suggestions that may help to decrease the risk of developing oral diseases.

Treatment of periodontal disease depends on the extent of damage. In mild cases, deep cleaning (removal of plaque and calculus deposits) and proper oral hygiene may reverse the condition. Antimicrobial mouth rinses and topical antibiotics may be prescribed to control infection. Surgical approaches may be used to eliminate gum pockets by reshaping tooth and bone surfaces or to replace tissues that have been destroyed.

How do chronic illnesses influence a person's risk for dental and oral diseases?

Some chronic illnesses can alter the structure and function of dental tissues, impair immune responses, or cause reduced salivary flow. Furthermore, certain medications can reduce salivary secretions, along with the immune protection that saliva provides. Examples of conditions that may upset oral health and increase the risks of developing dental problems include the following:

▎ *Diabetes mellitus.* Periodontal disease is more prevalent among people with diabetes mellitus, especially those whose diabetes

TABLE NP17-2 Suggestions for Preventing Oral Diseases

Personal hygiene

- Brush your teeth twice daily for at least 2 minutes with a fluoride toothpaste. Replace your toothbrush every 3 or 4 months or whenever the bristles become frayed.

- Floss between your teeth at least once a day.

- Avoid smoking. If you smoke, look into tobacco cessation programs in your area.

- Avoid consuming excessive amounts of alcohol.

Dietary practices

- Reduce your consumption of sugary foods. Avoid consuming sugary and starchy snacks between meals.

- After consuming carbohydrate-containing foods, sugary beverages, or acidic soft drinks or teas, rinse your mouth or clean your teeth.

- If you chew gum, use a sugarless gum.

- Avoid putting an infant or child to bed with a nursing bottle containing anything except plain water.

- In communities that do not provide fluoridated water, provide children at high risk of dental caries with a fluoride supplement.

Professional dental care

- Visit a dentist at least once a year to have your teeth and mouth examined and teeth cleaned. Visit the dentist more often if necessary.

- Ask the dentist if you are a candidate for topical fluoride treatments or tooth sealants, which protect susceptible tooth surfaces.

© 2016 Cengage Learning®

is poorly controlled.[6] People with diabetes often have impaired immune responses and a greater susceptibility to infection. Diabetes also favors the growth of bacteria that infect periodontal tissues. Compared with healthy individuals, people with diabetes tend to have increased plaque accumulations and reduced salivary flow.

- *Human immunodeficiency virus (HIV)/AIDS.* HIV infection is characterized by compromised immunity, and the risk of developing periodontal disease is closely linked to the degree of immunosuppression present. Those at greatest risk include smokers and individuals with poor oral hygiene.[7] In untreated persons, fungal and viral infections are common and may cause burning in the mouth and painful ulcerations. Many HIV-infected individuals develop dry mouth as a result of medications or salivary gland dysfunction.

- *Oral cancers.* The radiation treatment required for oral cancers often causes serious oral and dental complications.[8] Inflammation and tissue damage can be so severe that the radiation treatment may need to be halted or the intensity significantly reduced. Other complications include dry mouth, changes in taste sensation, fungal and viral infections, and tissue and muscle scarring (which often reduces chewing ability).

To minimize complications, dental care is often initiated before radiation therapy begins.

Can dental diseases have adverse effects on health beyond their effects on the teeth?

Yes, the bacteria that reside on dental tissues can enter the bloodstream and travel to other tissues; therefore, they may be able to trigger immune responses or cause infections elsewhere in the body.[9] Evidence supports a link between dental bacteria and other medical conditions, including the following:

- *Atherosclerosis and heart disease.* The inflammatory process induced by periodontal pathogens may increase levels of cytokines and other mediators that accelerate the progression of atherosclerosis. In addition, periodontal bacteria may enter into the bloodstream and contribute to the processes of plaque formation or blood clotting.[10]

- *Diabetes mellitus.* The chronic inflammation caused by periodontal disease can exacerbate insulin resistance and provoke events leading to type 2 diabetes. Severe periodontal disease has also been linked to poor glycemic control in persons with diabetes.[11]

- *Respiratory illnesses.* Clinical studies suggest a link between pneumonia and poor oral health. In addition, dental treatment and improvements in oral health have been associated with significant reductions in respiratory diseases in institutionalized elderly adults.[12]

Research studies are in progress to confirm cause-and-effect relationships between oral bacteria and the medical conditions described above, as well as the specific mechanisms involved.

Developing sound eating habits and maintaining good dental hygiene are practices that can promote dental health and possibly reduce the risk of developing other medical problems. Additional studies will help to clarify the complex interactions between dental disease and chronic illnesses.

Notes

1. R. Touger-Decker, D. R. Radler, and D. P. DePaola, Nutrition and dental medicine, in A. C. Ross and coeditors, eds., *Modern Nutrition in Health and Disease* (Baltimore: Lippincott Williams & Wilkins, 2014), pp. 1016–1040.

2. Touger-Decker, Radler, and DePaola, 2014.

3. Touger-Decker, Radler, and DePaola, 2014; S. K. Stookey, The effect of saliva on dental caries, *Journal of the American Dental Association* 139 (2008): 11S–17S.

4. J. T. Ubertalli, Common dental disorders, in R. S. Porter and J. L. Kaplan, eds., *Merck Manual of Diagnosis and Therapy* (Whitehouse Station, NJ: Merck Sharp and Dohme Corp., 2011), pp. 516–523.

5. J. B. C. Neto and coauthors, Smoking and periodontal tissues: A review, *Brazilian Oral Research* 26 (2012): 25–31.

6. Touger-Decker, Radler, and DePaola, 2014.

7. C. N. John, L. X. Stephen, and C. W. J. Africa, Is human immunodeficiency virus (HIV) stage an independent risk factor for altering the periodontal status of HIV-positive patients? A South African study, *BMC Oral Health* 13 (2013): 69, doi: 10.1186/1472-6831-13-69.

8. Touger-Decker, Radler, and DePaola, 2014; Academy of Nutrition and Dietetics, Position of the Academy of Nutrition and Dietetics: Oral health and nutrition, *Journal of the Academy of Nutrition and Dietetics* (2013): 693–701.

9. R. V. Oppermann, P. Weidlich, and M. L. Musskopf, Periodontal disease and systemic complications, *Brazilian Oral Research* 26 (2012): 39–47.

10. P. B. Lockhart and coauthors, Periodontal disease and atherosclerotic vascular disease: Does the evidence support an independent association? *Circulation* 125 (2012): 2520–2544.

11. P. M. Preshaw and coauthors, Periodontitis and diabetes: A two-way relationship, *Diabetologia* 55 (2012): 21–31.

12. A. Azarpazhooh and H. C. Tenenbaum, Separating fact from fiction: Use of high-level evidence from research syntheses to identify diseases and disorders associated with periodontal disease, *Journal of the Canadian Dental Association* 78 (2012): c25.

18

Fiber-Modified Diets for Lower Gastrointestinal Tract Disorders

18.1 Modifying Dietary Fiber Intake

LO 18.1 Identify medical problems that may be treated with a modified fiber intake and describe the use of high-fiber diets in nutrition practice.

18.2 Disorders of Bowel Function

LO 18.2 Summarize the medical treatments and dietary strategies that may be helpful for individuals with constipation, diarrhea, and irritable bowel syndrome.

18.3 Inflammatory Bowel Diseases

LO 18.3 Describe the effects of the inflammatory bowel diseases on health and nutrition status and discuss their medical and nutrition treatments.

18.4 Diverticular Disease of the Colon

LO 18.4 Identify potential risk factors for diverticular disease of the colon and describe its treatment.

18.5 Colostomies and Ileostomies

LO 18.5 Discuss the various dietary concerns of people with colostomies and ileostomies.

18.6 Nutrition in Practice: Probiotics and Intestinal Health

LO 18.6 Describe the potential benefits of consuming probiotics and prebiotics and identify some common dietary sources.

The lower gastrointestinal (GI) tract, which includes the small intestine and large intestine, continues the digestion of food that arrives from the stomach and facilitates nutrient absorption. This chapter discusses the potential benefits of adjusting dietary fiber intake when treating some lower GI disorders.

18.1 Modifying Dietary Fiber Intake

LO 18.1 Identify medical problems that may be treated with a modified fiber intake and describe the use of high-fiber diets in nutrition practice.

Diets can be modified by either increasing or decreasing dietary fiber. As discussed in Chapter 2, *insoluble fibers* increase stool weight and speed the passage of wastes through the large intestine. *Soluble, viscous fibers* slow the passage of food through the GI tract, which increases satiety and delays glucose absorption in the small intestine. Table 18-1 lists some medical problems that may be treated with modifications in dietary fiber intake.

People can increase their intake of fiber-rich foods by emphasizing the consumption of whole grains, legumes, nuts and seeds, and fruits and vegetables. Individuals who must restrict dietary fiber can limit their consumption of these foods. Chapter 2 and Appendix A provide detailed information about the fiber content of foods. Figure 18-1 (p. 496) shows a one-day menu that includes about 38 grams of fiber, which is the DRI for men who are 19 to 50 years of age (the fiber DRI for women in this age range is 25 grams per day).

Increased intestinal gas (**flatulence**) may be an unpleasant side effect of consuming a high-fiber diet. Because dietary fibers are not digested, they pass into the colon and are fermented by bacteria, which produce gas as a by-product (soluble fibers are more readily fermented than the insoluble fibers). Therefore, health practitioners advise that fiber-containing foods be added gradually at first and portions increased as tolerance improves. Intestinal gas also develops when people consume other incompletely digested or poorly absorbed carbohydrates; these include fructose, sugar alcohols (sorbitol, xylitol, mannitol), the indigestible carbohydrates in beans (raffinose and stachyose), and some forms of resistant starch, found in grain products and potatoes. Table 18-2 lists examples of foods commonly associated with excessive gas production, although individual responses vary. Malabsorption disorders (discussed in Chapter 19) can cause considerable flatulence because the undigested nutrients can be metabolized by colonic bacteria. Swallowed air that is not expelled by belching may travel to the intestines and be a source of intestinal gas as well. Note that many people attribute abdominal bloating and pain to excessive gas, but these symptoms do not correlate well with an increase in intestinal gas.[1]

IN SUMMARY

▍ Insoluble dietary fibers increase stool volume and reduce transit time in the large intestine. Soluble fibers slow the passage of food in the GI tract, which increases satiety and delays glucose absorption in the small intestine.

▍ Because fiber-containing foods can increase intestinal gas, they should be added gradually and portions increased as tolerance improves.

18.2 Disorders of Bowel Function

LO 18.2 Summarize the medical treatments and dietary strategies that may be helpful for individuals with constipation, diarrhea, and irritable bowel syndrome.

Many different factors alter the fluid content of stools or transit time and lead to constipation or diarrhea. Consequently, these conditions accompany a wide variety of

TABLE 18-1 Indications for Modifying Fiber Intake

Increasing Fiber Intake
▪ Constipation
▪ Diabetes mellitus
▪ Diverticulosis (prevention)
▪ Heart disease
▪ Irritable bowel syndrome
▪ Prediabetes or diabetes
▪ Weight management

Reducing Fiber Intake
▪ Inflammatory bowel diseases (active episodes)
▪ Post-surgical diet (depending on tolerance)
▪ Ostomy surgery

© 2016 Cengage Learning®

TABLE 18-2 Foods That May Increase Intestinal Gas

▪ Apples
▪ Artichokes
▪ Asparagus
▪ Beans and peas
▪ Beer
▪ Broccoli
▪ Brussels sprouts
▪ Cabbage
▪ Carbonated beverages
▪ Carrots
▪ Cauliflower
▪ Corn
▪ Fructose-sweetened products
▪ Fruit juices
▪ Green beans
▪ Leeks
▪ Milk products (if lactose intolerant)
▪ Onions
▪ Peanuts
▪ Pears
▪ Turnips
▪ Wheat

© 2016 Cengage Learning®

flatulence: the condition of having excessive intestinal gas, which causes abdominal discomfort.

High-Fiber Diet

Breakfast

1 c multigrain cereal
½ c strawberries
1 c fat-free milk
2 slices whole wheat toast
2 tbs peanut butter
1 c coffee

Lunch

1 c black bean soup
3 oz broiled chicken
½ c steamed broccoli
½ c baked sweet potatoes
1 fresh pear
1 whole wheat dinner roll
1 tsp margarine

Dinner

3 oz baked fish
½ c brown rice
½ c peas
1 whole wheat dinner roll
2 tsp margarine
1 piece carrot cake
1 c fat-free milk

Snack

3 c popcorn
1 c tomato juice

FIGURE 18-1 Sample One-Day Menu Containing 38 g Fiber

FIGURE 18-2 High-fiber foods promote regular bowel movements.

health problems. Because dietary fiber affects GI transit time as well as stool volume and composition, modifying the fiber intake can often improve bowel function.

Constipation

A diagnosis of constipation is based, in part, on a defecation frequency of fewer than three bowel movements per week. Other symptoms may include the passage of hard stools and excessive straining during defecation. In some cases, a person's perception of constipation may be due to a mistaken notion of what constitutes "normal" bowel habits, so the person's expectations about bowel function may need to be addressed. Constipation is particularly prevalent among women and all adults over 70 years of age.[2]

Causes of Constipation The risk of constipation is increased in individuals with a low-fiber diet, low food intake, inadequate fluid intake, or low level of physical activity. All of these factors can extend transit time, leading to increased water reabsorption within the colon and dry, hard stools that are difficult to pass. Medical conditions often associated with constipation include diabetes mellitus and hypothyroidism. Neurological conditions such as Parkinson's disease, spinal cord lesions, and multiple sclerosis may cause motor problems that lead to constipation. During pregnancy, women often experience constipation because the enlarged uterus presses against the rectum and colon. Constipation is also a common side effect of several classes of medications and some dietary supplements, including opiate-containing analgesics, tricyclic antidepressants, diuretics, calcium channel blockers, beta-blockers, and iron and calcium supplements.

Treatment of Constipation In individuals with a low fiber intake, the primary treatment for constipation is a gradual increase in fiber intake to at least 25 grams per day.[3] High-fiber diets increase stool weight and fecal water content and promote a more rapid transit of materials through the colon. Foods that increase stool weight the most include wheat bran, fruits, and vegetables (see Figure 18-2). Bran intake can be increased by adding bran cereals and whole-wheat bread to the diet or by mixing bran powder with beverages or foods. The transition to a high-fiber diet may be difficult for some people because it can increase intestinal gas, so high-fiber foods should be added gradually, as tolerated. Fiber supplements like methylcellulose (Citrucel), psyllium (Metamucil, Fiberall), and polycarbophil (Fiber-Lax) are also effective (see Table 18-3); these supplements can be mixed with beverages and taken several times daily. Unlike other fibers, methylcellulose and polycarbophil do not increase intestinal gas.

Several other dietary measures may also help to relieve constipation. Consuming adequate fluid (usually 1.5 to 2 liters daily) can help to increase stool frequency in people who are already consuming a high-fiber diet. An appropriate fluid intake prevents excessive reabsorption of water from the colon, resulting in wetter stools. Adding prunes or prune juice to the diet is often recommended because prunes contain compounds that have a mild laxative effect.

Laxatives Laxatives may relieve constipation by increasing stool weight, increasing the water content of stool, or stimulating peristaltic contractions. Table 18-3 includes examples of common laxatives and describes their modes of action. Enemas and suppositories (chemicals introduced into the rectum) are also used to promote defecation; they work by distending and stimulating the rectum or by lubricating the stool.

Medical Interventions For patients with severe constipation who do not respond to dietary or laxative treatments, physicians may

TABLE 18-3 Laxatives and Bulk-Forming Agents

Laxative Type	Active Ingredients	Product Examples	Method of Action	Cautions
Fiber (bulk-forming agents)	Malt soup extract, methylcellulose, polycarbophil, psyllium	Citrucel, Fiberall, Fiber-Lax, Metamucil	Increase stool weight and aid in the formation of soft, bulky stools. Similar effects are achieved by adding bran to the diet. For mild constipation. Safe for long-term use.	Some fiber supplements may increase flatulence. Psyllium may cause an allergic reaction.
Osmotic laxatives: nonabsorbable salts	Magnesium citrate, magnesium hydroxide	Epsom salts, milk of magnesia, Citromag	Attract water and increase liquidity of stools, which stimulates contractions.	May cause bloating and watery stools or diarrhea. Should be used with caution. Avoid using in renal patients and children.
Osmotic laxatives: nonabsorbable sugars	Lactulose, polyethylene glycol, sorbitol	Cephulac, Chronulac, CoLyte	Attract water and increase liquidity of stools, which stimulates contractions. Must be used for several days to take effect. Safe for long-term use.	May cause flatulence and cramps. Can lose effectiveness over time.
Stimulant or irritant laxatives	Aloe, bisacodyl, cascara, castor oil, senna	Correctol, Dulcolax, Ex-Lax	Act as local irritants to colonic tissue; stimulate peristalsis and mucosal secretions. For moderate to severe constipation. Long-term use is discouraged.	Usually given only after milder treatments fail. May alter fluid and electrolyte balances. May lead to laxative dependency.
Stool surfactant agents (stool softeners)	Docusate sodium	Colace, Surfak	Promotes the mixing of water with stools; prevents formation of dry, hard stools.	Do not increase stool weight. Limited effectiveness.

prescribe medications that stimulate colonic contractions. Biofeedback techniques are sometimes successful in training patients to relax their pelvic muscles more effectively.

Diarrhea

Diarrhea is characterized by the passage of frequent, watery stools. In most cases, it lasts for only a day or two and subsides without complication. Severe or persistent diarrhea, however, can cause dehydration and electrolyte imbalances. Diarrhea may be accompanied by other symptoms, such as fever, abdominal cramps, dyspepsia, or bleeding, which help in diagnosing the cause.

Causes of Diarrhea Diarrhea is a complication of multiple GI disorders and may also be caused by infections, medications, or dietary substances.[4] It results from inadequate fluid reabsorption in the intestines, sometimes in conjunction with an increase in intestinal secretions. In *osmotic diarrhea,* unabsorbed nutrients or other substances attract water to the colon and increase fecal water content; common causes include high intakes of poorly absorbed sugars (such as sorbitol, mannitol, or fructose) and lactase deficiency (which causes lactose malabsorption). In *secretory diarrhea,* the fluid secreted by the intestines exceeds the amount that can be reabsorbed by intestinal cells. Secretory diarrhea is often due to foodborne illness but can also be caused by intestinal inflammation and various chemical substances (such as medications or unabsorbed bile acids). *Motility disorders* may also result in diarrhea because they accelerate the transit of colonic residue, reducing the contact time available for fluid reabsorption.

Medical Treatment of Diarrhea Correcting the underlying medical problem is the first step in treating diarrhea. For example, antibiotics are prescribed to treat intestinal infections. If a medication is the cause of diarrhea, a different drug may be prescribed. If certain foods are responsible, they can be omitted from the diet. Bulk-forming agents such as psyllium (Metamucil) or methylcellulose (Citrucel) can help to reduce the liquidity of the stool. If chronic diarrhea does not respond to treatment,

BOX 18-1

An oral rehydration solution
can be mixed from the
following ingredients:

- ½ tsp sodium chloride
  (table salt)

- ⅓ tsp potassium chloride
  (salt substitute)

- ¾ tsp sodium bicarbonate
  (baking soda)

- 1⅓ tbs sugar

- 1 qt water

antidiarrheal drugs may be prescribed to slow GI motility or reduce intestinal secretions. Probiotics (live bacteria provided in foods or dietary supplements) may be beneficial for treating certain types of diarrhea (especially infectious diarrhea), but standard treatment protocols have not been developed.[5]

Oral Rehydration Therapy Severe diarrhea requires the replacement of lost fluid and electrolytes. Oral rehydration solutions can be purchased or easily mixed using water, salts, and glucose or sucrose (see Box 18-1 for a recipe that includes ingredients found in the home). The addition of carbohydrate to the solution facilitates sodium and water absorption. Commercial sports drinks are not ideal fluids for rehydration because their sodium content is too low, but they can be used if accompanied by salty snack foods. When diarrhea results in extreme dehydration, intravenous solutions are used to quickly replenish fluid and electrolytes.

Nutrition Therapy for Diarrhea Nutrition care depends on the cause of diarrhea and its severity and duration. The dietary treatment often recommended is a low-fiber, low-fat, lactose-free diet,[6] which limits foods that contribute to stool volume, such as those with significant amounts of fiber, resistant starch, fructose, sugar alcohols, and lactose (in lactose-intolerant individuals). Avoidance of fatty foods may be advised if they aggravate diarrhea. Gas-producing foods (those with poorly digested or absorbed carbohydrates) can increase intestinal distention and cause additional discomfort. Although fluid intakes must usually be increased to replace fluid losses, patients should avoid caffeinated coffee and tea because caffeine stimulates GI motility and can thereby reduce water reabsorption. In the treatment of formula-fed infants, apple pectin or banana flakes are sometimes added to formulas to help thicken stool consistency. Table 18-4 lists foods that may worsen diarrhea, although individual tolerances vary.

Irritable Bowel Syndrome

People with **irritable bowel syndrome** experience chronic and recurring intestinal symptoms that cannot be explained by specific physical abnormalities. The symptoms usually include disturbed defecation (diarrhea and/or constipation), flatulence, and abdominal discomfort or pain; the pain is often aggravated by eating and relieved by defecation. In some patients, symptoms are mild; in others, the disturbances in colonic function can interfere with work and social activities enough to dramatically alter the person's lifestyle and sense of well-being.[7]

TABLE 18-4 Foods That May Worsen Diarrhea

Foods to Avoid	Rationale	Selected Examples[a]
High-fiber foods	They increase colonic residue.	Breads and cereals with more than 2 g fiber per serving, fruits and vegetables with peels or skins
Foods with indigestible carbohydrates	They contribute to osmotic diarrhea.	Artichokes, asparagus, brussels sprouts, cabbage, dried beans and peas, fruit, garlic, green beans, leeks, onions, wheat, zucchini
Foods that contain fructose or sugar alcohols	They contribute to osmotic diarrhea.	Dried fruit, fresh fruit (except bananas), fruit juices, fructose-sweetened soft drinks, sugar-free gums and candies
Milk products, if person is lactose intolerant	They contribute to osmotic diarrhea.	Milk and milk products
Gas-producing foods	They increase abdominal discomfort.	Foods with poorly digested or absorbed carbohydrates (including foods listed in the three rows directly above)
Caffeine-containing beverages	They increase intestinal motility.	Coffee, tea, colas, energy drinks

[a]Individual tolerances vary; the foods to avoid are best determined by trial and error.

irritable bowel syndrome: an intestinal disorder of unknown cause that disturbs the functioning of the large intestine; symptoms include abdominal pain, flatulence, diarrhea, and constipation.

© 2016 Cengage Learning®

Although the causes of irritable bowel syndrome remain elusive, people with the disorder tend to have excessive colonic responses to meals, GI hormones, and psychological stress. Many individuals exhibit hypersensitivity to a normal degree of intestinal distention and feel discomfort when experiencing normal meal transit or typical amounts of intestinal gas. Intestinal motility after meals may be excessive, leading to diarrhea, or be reduced, causing constipation. Some patients show signs of low-grade intestinal inflammation; others may have had a bacterial infection that initiated their GI problems. Symptoms may worsen during periods of psychological stress. Diagnosing irritable bowel syndrome is difficult because its symptoms are typical of other GI disorders and laboratory tests for the condition are nonexistent.

Treatment of Irritable Bowel Syndrome Medical treatment of irritable bowel syndrome often includes dietary adjustments, stress management, and behavioral therapies. Medications may be prescribed to manage symptoms but they are not always helpful. The drugs prescribed may include laxatives, antidiarrheal agents, antidepressants, antispasmotics (which reduce pain by relaxing GI muscles), and antibiotics (which alter bacterial populations in the colon).

Nutrition Therapy for Irritable Bowel Syndrome Although dietary adjustments may reduce symptoms, responses among patients vary considerably. The most common recommendation is to gradually increase fiber intake from food or supplements to relieve constipation and improve stool bulk. However, clinical studies suggest that additional fiber has little or no effectiveness in improving symptoms and may worsen flatulence.[8] Psyllium supplementation may be helpful for individuals with constipation. Some individuals have fewer symptoms when they consume small, frequent meals instead of larger ones. Foods that aggravate symptoms may include fried or fatty foods, gas-producing foods, milk products (not necessarily due to lactose intolerance), wheat products, and coffee (with or without caffeine); however, individual tolerances are best determined by trial and error. A careful evaluation of the dietary patterns that exacerbate symptoms may uncover the foods and habits most closely associated with intestinal discomfort.

Treatments under investigation for irritable bowel syndrome include peppermint oil, which relaxes smooth muscle within the GI tract, and various types of probiotics.[9] The Case Study in Box 18-2 can help you apply your knowledge about irritable bowel syndrome to a clinical situation.

Case Study BOX 18-2 YOUNG ADULT WITH IRRITABLE BOWEL SYNDROME

Dara Calloway is a 22-year-old recent college graduate who began her first professional job in a bank 1 month ago. As a college student, she occasionally experienced abdominal pain and cramping after eating. She also had frequent bouts of diarrhea and felt somewhat better after bowel movements. Once Dara began her new job, her symptoms occurred more frequently. At first, she attributed her symptoms to job stress, but when the symptoms continued for several months, she decided to see her physician. After taking a careful history and conducting tests to rule out other bowel disorders, the physician diagnosed irritable bowel

syndrome. The physician prescribed bulk-forming fibers and advised Dara to keep a record of her food intake and symptoms for 1 week. Dara was then referred to a dietitian for a review of her dietary record. The dietitian noticed that Dara routinely drank several cups of coffee in the morning and had large meals for lunch and dinner. Dara often ate out in Mexican restaurants and favored spicy foods, refried beans, and fatty desserts. Between meals, she snacked on low-carbohydrate foods sweetened with sugar alcohols and drank several cans of soda daily. Her dietary fiber intake, however, totaled only about 13 grams daily.

1. Describe the characteristics of irritable bowel syndrome to Dara, and indicate the role that stress might play in her illness.

2. Explain how the record of food intake and symptoms might be helpful in devising an appropriate dietary plan for Dara. Could any of the foods that are currently in Dara's diet be aggravating her symptoms?

3. What dietary measures might benefit individuals with irritable bowel syndrome? What problems might some of the dietary changes cause?

■ Constipation accompanies many different health problems; a high-fiber diet or fiber supplements are often beneficial.

■ Diarrhea can result from malabsorption, intestinal infections, motility disorders, or medications; a low-fiber, low-fat, lactose-free diet may be recommended.

■ Irritable bowel syndrome is characterized by chronic, recurring intestinal symptoms such as diarrhea and/or constipation, abdominal pain, and flatulence; dietary measures may include increasing fiber intake, consuming small meals, and omitting certain foods from the diet.

18.3 Inflammatory Bowel Diseases

LO 18.3 Describe the effects of the inflammatory bowel diseases on health and nutrition status and discuss their medical and nutrition treatments.

Inflammatory bowel diseases are chronic inflammatory illnesses characterized by abnormal immune responses to microbes that inhabit the GI tract.[10] Although both genetic and environmental factors contribute to the development of these diseases, the exact triggers are unknown. Table 18-5 compares the two major forms of inflammatory bowel disease, **Crohn's disease** and **ulcerative colitis.** Crohn's disease usually involves the small intestine and may lead to nutrient malabsorption, whereas ulcerative colitis affects the large intestine, where little nutrient absorption occurs. Both diseases are characterized by periods of active disease interspersed with periods of remission. Nutrient losses can result from tissue damage, bleeding, and diarrhea.

Complications of Crohn's Disease Crohn's disease may occur in any region of the GI tract, but most cases involve the ileum and/or large intestine (see Figure 18-3). Lesions may develop in different areas in the intestine, with normal tissue separating affected regions (called "skip" lesions). During exacerbations, the inflammation may extend deeply into intestinal tissue and be accompanied by ulcerations, fissures, and **fistulas.** The resultant scar tissue can eventually thicken, narrowing the lumen and possibly causing strictures or obstructions. About 40 percent of patients require surgery within 10 years of diagnosis.[11] Patients with Crohn's disease are also at increased risk of developing intestinal cancers.

Crohn's disease: an inflammatory bowel disease that usually occurs in the lower portion of the small intestine and the colon; the inflammation may pervade the entire intestinal wall.

ulcerative colitis (ko-LYE-tis)**:** an inflammatory bowel disease that involves the rectum and colon; the inflammation affects the mucosa and submucosa of the intestinal wall.

fistulas (FIST-you-luz)**:** abnormal passages between organs or tissues that allow the passage of fluids or secretions.

TABLE 18-5 Comparison of Crohn's Disease and Ulcerative Colitis

	Crohn's Disease	Ulcerative Colitis
Location of inflammation	Approximately 35% of cases involve the ileum and colon, 28% are in the small intestine only, and 32% are confined to the colon	Confined to the rectum and colon; always involves the rectum but often extends into the colon
Pattern of inflammation	Discrete areas separated by normal tissue ("skip" lesions)	Continuous inflammation throughout the affected region
Depth of damage	Damage throughout all layers of tissue; causes deep fissures that give intestinal tissue a "cobblestone" appearance	Damage primarily in the mucosa and submucosa (the layers of intestinal tissue closest to the lumen)
Fistulas	Common	Usually do not occur
Cancer risk	Increased	Greatly increased

The healthy colon has a smooth surface with a visible pattern of fine blood vessels.

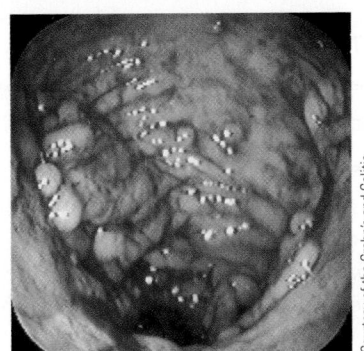

In Crohn's disease, the mucosa has a "cobblestone" appearance due to deep fissuring in the inflamed mucosal tissue.

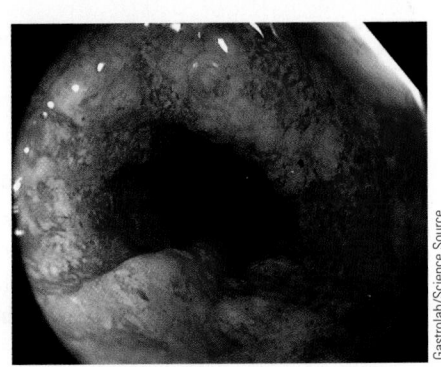

In ulcerative colitis, the colon appears inflamed and reddened, and ulcers are visible.

FIGURE 18-3 Comparison of Crohn's Disease and Ulcerative Colitis

Malnutrition may result from poor food intake, malabsorption, diarrhea, bleeding, nutrient losses (especially of protein) from inflamed tissues, increased needs due to inflammation, and surgical resections that shorten the small intestine. If the ileum is affected, bile acids may become depleted,* causing malabsorption of fat, fat-soluble vitamins, calcium, magnesium, and zinc (the minerals bind to the unabsorbed fatty acids). Because the ileum is the site of vitamin B_{12} absorption, deficiency can develop unless the patient is given vitamin B_{12} injections. Anemia may result from bleeding, inadequate absorption of the nutrients (iron, folate, and vitamin B_{12}) involved in blood cell formation, or the metabolic effects of chronic illness (see Nutrition in Practice 19).

Complications of Ulcerative Colitis Ulcerative colitis always involves the rectum and usually extends into the colon (see Figure 18-3). Tissue inflammation is continuous along the length of intestine affected, ending abruptly at the area where healthy tissue begins. The erosion or ulceration affects the mucosa and submucosa only (the tissue layers closest to the lumen). During active episodes, patients may have frequent, urgent bowel movements that are small in volume and contain blood and mucus. Symptoms may include diarrhea, constipation, rectal bleeding, and abdominal pain.

Although mild disease may cause few complications, weight loss, fever, and weakness are common when much of the colon is involved. Severe disease is often associated with anemia (due to blood loss), dehydration, and electrolyte imbalances. Protein losses from the inflamed tissue can be substantial. A **colectomy** (removal of the colon) is performed in 25 to 40 percent of patients and prevents future recurrence.[12] Colon cancer risk is substantially increased in ulcerative colitis patients.

Drug Treatment of Inflammatory Bowel Diseases Medications help to control symptoms, reduce inflammation, and minimize complications. The drugs prescribed include antidiarrheal agents, immunosuppressants, anti-inflammatory drugs (usually corticosteroids and salicylates), and antibiotics. The Diet-Drug Interactions feature in Box 18-3 (p. 502) lists some nutrition-related effects of these medications.

Nutrition Therapy for Inflammatory Bowel Diseases Crohn's disease often requires aggressive dietary management because it can lead to protein-energy malnutrition, nutrient deficiencies, and growth failure in children. Specific dietary measures depend on the symptoms and complications that develop. High-kcalorie, high-protein diets may be prescribed to prevent or treat malnutrition or promote

colectomy: removal of a portion or all of the colon.

*Most of the bile used during digestion is eventually reabsorbed in the ileum and returned to the liver.

BOX 18-3 DIET-DRUG INTERACTIONS

Check this table for notable nutrition-related effects of the medications discussed in this chapter.

Antidiarrheal drugs	**Gastrointestinal effect:** Constipation
Anti-inflammatory drugs (sulfasalazine, corticosteroids)	**Gastrointestinal effects:** Nausea, vomiting (sulfasalazine) **Dietary interactions:** Sulfasalazine may decrease folate absorption; supplementation is recommended **Metabolic effects:** Anemia (sulfasalazine); fluid retention, hyperglycemia, hypocalcemia, hypokalemia, hypophosphatemia, increased appetite, protein catabolism (corticosteroids)
Laxatives	**Gastrointestinal effects:** Diarrhea, flatulence, abdominal discomfort **Metabolic effects:** Dehydration, electrolyte imbalances, laxative dependency

healing. Oral supplements may help to increase energy intake and improve weight gain. Vitamin and mineral supplements are usually necessary, especially if nutrient malabsorption is present. During disease exacerbations, a low-fiber, low-fat diet provided in small, frequent feedings can minimize stool output and reduce symptoms of malabsorption. In some instances, tube feedings are used to supplement the diet or may be the sole means of providing nutrients. Table 18-6 includes some other adjustments that may be beneficial.

In most cases, the diet for ulcerative colitis requires few adjustments. As in Crohn's disease, the symptoms and complications that arise are managed with appropriate dietary measures. During disease exacerbations, emphasis is given to restoring fluid

TABLE 18-6 Management of Symptoms and Complications in Crohn's Disease

Symptom or Complication	Possible Dietary Measures
Growth failure, weight loss, or muscle wasting	▪ High-kcalorie, high-protein diet ▪ Oral supplements ▪ Tube feedings
Anorexia or pain with eating	▪ Small, frequent meals ▪ Oral supplements, as tolerated ▪ Tube feedings if long-term (>5–7 days)
Malabsorption	▪ High-kcalorie diet ▪ Nutrient supplementation
Steatorrhea (fat malabsorption)	▪ Low-fat diet ▪ Medium-chain triglycerides ▪ Nutrient supplementation
Diarrhea	▪ Fluid and electrolyte replacement ▪ Nutrient supplementation
Lactose intolerance	▪ Avoidance of lactose-containing foods
Nutrient deficiencies	▪ Nutrient-dense diet ▪ Nutrient supplementation
Strictures, partial obstruction, or fistulas	▪ Low-fiber diet ▪ Liquid supplements
Severe bowel obstruction, high-output fistulas, or severe exacerbations of disease	▪ Total parenteral nutrition

© 2016 Cengage Learning®

and electrolyte balances and correcting deficiencies that result from protein and blood losses. A low-fiber diet may reduce irritation by minimizing fecal volume. If colon function becomes severely impaired, food and fluids may be withheld and fluids and electrolytes supplied intravenously until colon function returns.

IN SUMMARY

▌ Crohn's disease can severely damage small intestinal tissue and lead to nutrient malabsorption. The damage from ulcerative colitis is confined to the large intestine, where little nutrient absorption occurs.

▌ Dietary measures for inflammatory bowel diseases aim to reduce symptoms, manage complications, and correct deficiencies. A low-fiber diet can reduce irritation during active episodes of illness.

18.4 Diverticular Disease of the Colon

LO 18.4 Identify potential risk factors for diverticular disease of the colon and describe its treatment.

Diverticulosis refers to the presence of pebble-sized herniations (outpockets) in the intestinal mucosa, known as diverticula (see Figure 18-4). Most people with diverticulosis are symptom free and remain unaware of the condition until a complication develops. The prevalence of diverticulosis increases with age, occurring in 50 to 65 percent of 80-year-old individuals.[13]

Although the cause of diverticulosis is unclear, changes in connective tissue proteins that occur with aging may contribute to its development.[14] Epidemiological studies and controlled studies in rats have suggested that low-fiber diets may increase risk due to fiber's influence on transit time, stool volume, and intraluminal pressures;[15] however, some recent clinical studies were unable to find an association between low-fiber intakes and the incidence of diverticulosis.[16]

diverticulosis (dye-ver-tic-you-LOH-sis)**:** an intestinal condition characterized by the presence of small herniations (called diverticula) in the intestinal wall.

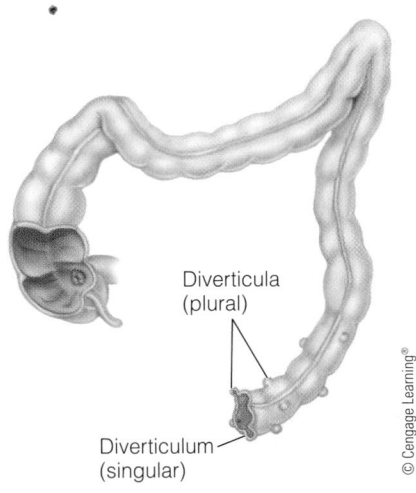

Diverticula (plural)

Diverticulum (singular)

© Cengage Learning®

Diverticula are small pouches that develop in weakened areas of the intestinal wall. The condition of having diverticula is known as *diverticulosis*.

David M. Martin, M.D./Science Source

Diverticula are frequently seen during a colonoscopy, a procedure that uses a flexible, lighted tube to examine the inside of the colon.

FIGURE 18-4 Diverticula in the Colon

FIBER-MODIFIED DIETS FOR LOWER GASTROINTESTINAL TRACT DISORDERS

Diverticulitis Inflammation or infection sometimes develops in the area around a diverticulum. This condition, called **diverticulitis,** is the most common complication of diverticulosis, affecting 10 to 25 percent of individuals with the condition.[17] It is thought to result from erosion of the diverticular wall due to high intraluminal pressure or particulate matter, leading to inflammation and eventually a microperforation that causes subsequent infection. If the infection spreads to adjacent organs, fistulas may develop. Symptoms of diverticulitis may include persistent abdominal pain, tenderness in the affected area, fever, constipation, and diarrhea.

Treatment for Diverticular Disease Medical treatment for diverticulosis is necessary only if symptoms develop. Patients are often advised to increase fiber intake to relieve constipation and other symptoms, although high-fiber diets have not been shown to reverse diverticulosis or prevent disease progression.[18] Fiber should be increased gradually to ensure tolerance; emphasis should be on insoluble fiber sources such as wheat bran, whole grains, fruits, and vegetables. Bulk-forming agents, such as psyllium, can help to increase fiber intake if food sources are insufficient. Avoiding nuts, seeds, and popcorn is sometimes suggested to prevent complications, but no evidence is available to justify the recommendation.[19]

Patients with diverticulitis may need antibiotics to treat infections and, possibly, pain-control medications. In mild cases, a clear liquid diet may be advised initially, with progression to solid foods as tolerated. In severe cases, oral fluids and food are withheld and fluids are given intravenously. After pain and diarrhea have resolved, an oral diet is reintroduced, beginning with clear liquids and progressing to a low-fiber diet.[20] Once the inflammation has subsided, a high-fiber diet is recommended to help prevent symptom recurrence.

IN SUMMARY

▌ Diverticulosis, the presence of small herniations in the intestinal wall, is often asymptomatic unless complications develop; its prevalence increases with advancing age.

▌ Diverticulitis, which involves inflammation or infection of the diverticula, may require medical treatment and temporary bowel rest.

18.5 Colostomies and Ileostomies

LO 18.5 Discuss the various dietary concerns of people with colostomies and ileostomies.

An *ostomy* is a surgically created opening (called a **stoma**) in the abdominal wall through which dietary wastes can be eliminated. Whereas a permanent ostomy is necessary after a partial or total colectomy, a temporary ostomy is sometimes constructed to bypass the colon after injury or extensive surgery. To create the stoma, the cut end of the remaining segment of functional intestine is routed through an opening in the abdominal wall and stitched in place so that it empties to the exterior. The stoma can be formed from a section of the colon (**colostomy**) or ileum (**ileostomy**), as shown in Figure 18-5. Conditions that may require these procedures include inflammatory bowel diseases, diverticulitis, and colorectal cancers.

To collect wastes, a disposable bag is affixed to the skin around the stoma and emptied during the day as needed. In some cases, an internal pouch is constructed from ileal tissue and attached to the anus so that the anal sphincter can control output. Stool consistency varies according to the length of colon that is functional. If a small portion of the colon is absent or bypassed, the stools may continue to be semi-solid.

diverticulitis (dye-ver-tic-you-LYE-tis)**:** an inflammation or infection involving diverticula.

stoma (STOE-ma)**:** a surgically created opening in a body tissue or organ.

colostomy (co-LAH-stoe-me)**:** a surgical passage through the abdominal wall into the colon.

ileostomy (ill-ee-AH-stoe-me)**:** a surgical passage through the abdominal wall into the ileum.

Colostomy

In a colostomy, a portion of the colon is removed or bypassed, and the stoma is formed from the remaining section of functional colon.

Ileostomy

In an ileostomy, the entire colon is removed or bypassed, and the stoma is formed from the ileum.

© Cengage Learning®

FIGURE 18-5 Colostomy and Ileostomy

If the entire colon has been removed or is bypassed, the ability to absorb fluid and electrolytes is substantially reduced, and the output is liquid.

Nutrition Care for Patients with Ostomies Dietary adjustments are individualized according to the surgical procedure and symptoms that develop afterward. Following surgery, the diet may progress from clear liquids (low in sugars) to regular foods, as tolerated. To reduce stool output, a low-fiber diet may be recommended. Small, frequent meals may be more acceptable than larger ones. To determine food tolerances, patients should try small amounts of questionable foods and assess their effects; a food that causes problems can be tried again later. Appropriate fluid and electrolyte intakes should be encouraged when a large portion of the colon has been removed.

People with ileostomies need to chew thoroughly to ensure that foods are adequately digested and to prevent obstructions, a common complication due to the small diameter of the ileal lumen. Foods high in insoluble fibers are sometimes discouraged because they reduce transit time, may cause obstructions, and increase stool output. To replace electrolyte losses, patients are encouraged to use salt liberally and to ingest beverages with added electrolytes (such as sports drinks and rehydration beverages), if necessary. If a large portion of the ileum has been removed, fat malabsorption may occur due to bile acid depletion, and vitamin B_{12} injections may be required.

Dietary concerns after colostomies depend on the length of colon remaining. Most patients have no dietary restrictions and can return to a regular diet. Patient concerns may include stool odors, excessive gas production, and diarrhea. If a large portion of colon was removed, recommendations may be similar to those given to ileostomy patients.

Obstructions As mentioned, foods that are incompletely digested can cause obstructions, a primary concern of ileostomy patients. Although these patients can consume almost any food that is cut in small pieces and carefully chewed, the following foods may cause difficulty: celery, coconut, coleslaw, mushrooms, peas, salad greens, dried fruit, unpeeled fresh fruits, pineapple, nuts, seeds, popcorn, frankfurters, sausages, and tough, chewy meats.[21]

Reducing Gas and Odors Persons with ostomies are often concerned about foods that may increase gas production or cause strong odors. Foods that may cause excessive gas were discussed earlier (p. 495). Foods that sometimes produce unpleasant odors include asparagus, beer, broccoli, brussels sprouts, cabbage, cauliflower, dried beans and peas, eggs, fish, garlic, and onions. Foods that may help to reduce odors include buttermilk, cranberry juice, parsley, and yogurt.[22]

Diarrhea Examples of foods that aggravate diarrhea are listed in Table 18-4 (p. 498). Foods that may thicken stool include applesauce, banana, cheese, pasta, potatoes, smooth peanut butter, tapioca, and white rice.[23] What works may differ for each individual, however, and is best determined by trial and error.

IN SUMMARY

■ Colostomies and ileostomies are surgically created openings in the abdominal wall using the cut end of the colon or ileum. Fluid and electrolyte requirements are greater after an ostomy if colon function is reduced or absent.

■ Poorly digested foods may cause obstructions in people with ostomies, although thorough chewing can reduce risk. Other concerns include excessive gas production, food odors, and diarrhea.

Nutrition Assessment Checklist FOR PEOPLE WITH LOWER GI TRACT DISORDERS

Medical History

Check the medical record for diseases that:

■ Cause chronic GI symptoms, such as irritable bowel syndrome or an inflammatory bowel disease
■ Interfere with nutrient absorption, such as Crohn's disease

Check for surgical procedures involving the lower GI tract, such as:

■ Intestinal resections
■ Ileostomy or colostomy

Check for the following symptoms or complications:

■ Anemia
■ Constipation
■ Diarrhea, dehydration
■ Fistulas
■ Nutrient deficiencies
■ Strictures or obstructions
■ Poor growth, in children

Medications

Check for medications or dietary supplements that may:

■ Cause constipation or diarrhea
■ Alter appetite or nutrient needs

Dietary Intake

Note the following problems, and contact the dietitian if you suspect difficulties such as:

■ Poor appetite or food intake
■ Food intolerances

■ Inadequate fiber intake, in patients with constipation
■ Malabsorbed carbohydrates, in patients with diarrhea
■ Inadequate fluid intake

Anthropometric Data

Measure baseline height and weight. Address weight loss early to prevent malnutrition in patients with:

■ Severe or persistent diarrhea
■ Nutrient malabsorption

Laboratory Tests

Check laboratory tests for signs of dehydration, electrolyte imbalances, nutrient deficiencies, and anemia in patients with:

■ Severe or persistent diarrhea
■ Nutrient malabsorption
■ Intestinal resections

Physical Signs

Look for physical signs of:

■ Dehydration
■ Fat-soluble vitamin deficiencies
■ Vitamin B_{12} deficiency
■ Mineral deficiencies
■ Protein-energy malnutrition

Clinical Applications

1. A health practitioner working with a patient with a constipation problem provides him with detailed information about a high-fiber diet. At a follow-up appointment, the patient reports no change in symptoms. His food diary for that day shows that he consumed an omelet and toast for breakfast and a sandwich with juice for lunch.

   ▮ Considering these two meals only, what additional information would help the health practitioner evaluate the man's compliance with the diet he was given?

   ▮ Review the discussion about fiber in Chapter 2 and create a one-day menu that provides the DRI for fiber for an adult male, using the fiber values listed in Appendix A.

2. A number of symptoms and disorders of the GI tract, as described in this chapter and the previous one, are associated with aging. Review both chapters and list these symptoms and disorders. Referring back to Chapter 13, describe some effects of aging on the GI tract and explain how these changes might relate to the GI symptoms and disorders you listed.

3. The diets described in this chapter are highly individualized: a particular food may cause discomfort for one person and have no effect on another. Describe some practical ways to keep track of food intolerances.

Self Check

1. Foods that do *NOT* supply fiber include:
   a. cabbage and broccoli.
   b. beef and pork.
   c. oats and corn.
   d. beans and peas.

2. The health practitioner advising an elderly patient with constipation encourages the patient to:
   a. consume a low-fat diet low in sodium.
   b. consume a high-protein diet rich in calcium.
   c. gradually add high-fiber foods to the diet.
   d. eliminate gas-forming foods from the diet.

3. Laxatives help to promote bowel movements by:
   a. stimulating peristalsis.
   b. increasing stool weight.
   c. increasing the water content of stools.
   d. All of the above

4. Osmotic diarrhea often results from:
   a. excessive colonic contractions.
   b. excessive fluid secretion by the intestines.
   c. nutrient malabsorption.
   d. viral, bacterial, or protozoal infections.

5. An oral rehydration solution can be mixed at home using:
   a. water, vinegar, honey, and table salt.
   b. water, table salt, and salt substitute.
   c. water, milk, sugar, and table salt.
   d. water, table salt, baking soda, potassium chloride, and sugar.

6. Symptoms of irritable bowel syndrome most often include:
   a. constipation and/or diarrhea and flatulence.
   b. weight loss and malnutrition.
   c. strong odors and obstructions.
   d. nauea and vomiting.

7. A patient with Crohn's disease may develop all of the following nutrition problems, *except:*
   a. fat malabsorption.
   b. dumping syndrome.
   c. vitamin B_{12} deficiency.
   d. anemia.

8. Ulcerative colitis may afflict which region of the digestive tract?
   a. Ileum, rectum, and colon
   b. Rectum and colon
   c. Stomach and duodenum
   d. Most regions of the GI tract can be affected

9. Diverticulosis is most often associated with:
   a. aging.
   b. inadequate exercise.
   c. intestinal surgery.
   d. a high-fiber diet.

10. After an ileostomy, the most serious concern is that:
    a. the diet is too restrictive to meet nutrient needs.
    b. waste disposal causes frequent daily interruptions.
    c. incompletely digested foods may cause obstructions.
    d. fluid restrictions prevent patients from drinking beverages freely.

Answers to these questions appear in Appendix H.

Notes

1. A. E. Bharucha, Approach to the patient with lower GI complaints, in R. S. Porter and J. L. Kaplan, eds., *Merck Manual of Diagnosis and Therapy* (Whitehouse Station, NJ: Merck Sharp and Dohme, 2011), pp. 83–94; F. Azpiroz and M. D. Levitt, Intestinal gas, in M. Feldman, L. S. Friedman, and L. J. Brandt, eds., *Sleisenger and Fordtran's Gastrointestinal and Liver Disease* (Philadelphia: Saunders, 2010), pp. 233–240.

2. L. Leung and coauthors, Chronic constipation: An evidence-based review, *Journal of the American Board of Family Medicine* 24 (2011): 436–451.

3. Academy of Nutrition and Dietetics, *Nutrition Care Manual* (Chicago: Academy of Nutrition and Dietetics, 2014).

4. J. S. Trier, Acute diarrheal disorders, in N. J. Greenberger, ed., *Current Diagnosis and Treatment: Gastroenterology, Hepatology, and Endoscopy* (New York: McGraw-Hill Companies, 2012), pp. 47–67.

5. M. E. Sanders and coauthors, An update on the use and investigation of probiotics in health and disease, *Gut* 62 (2013): 787–796; D. Wolvers and coauthors, Guidance for substantiating the evidence for beneficial effects of probiotics: Prevention and management of infections by probiotics, *Journal of Nutrition* 140 (2010): 698S–712S.

6. Academy of Nutrition and Dietetics, 2014.

7. S. Friedman, Irritable bowel syndrome, in N. J. Greenberger, ed., *Current Diagnosis and Treatment: Gastroenterology, Hepatology, and Endoscopy* (New York: McGraw-Hill Companies, 2012), pp. 297–309.

8. L. Ruepert and coauthors, Bulking agents, antispasmodics and antidepressants for the treatment of irritable bowel syndrome, *Cochrane Database of Systematic Reviews* 8 (2011), article no. CD003460, doi: 10.1002/14651858.CD003460.pub3.

9. G. Clarke and coauthors, Review article: Probiotics for the treatment of irritable bowel syndrome—focus on lactic acid bacteria, *Alimentary Pharmacology and Therapeutics* 35 (2012): 403–413; P. Moayyedi and coauthors, The efficacy of probiotics in the treatment of irritable bowel syndrome: A systematic review, *Gut* 59 (2010): 325–332.

10. R. S. Blumberg and S. B. Snapper, Inflammatory bowel disease: Immunologic considerations and therapeutic implications, in N. J. Greenberger, ed., *Current Diagnosis and Treatment: Gastroenterology, Hepatology, and Endoscopy* (New York: McGraw-Hill Companies, 2012), pp. 12–22.

11. G. R. Lichtenstein, Inflammatory bowel disease, in L. Goldman and A I. Schafer, eds., *Goldman's Cecil Medicine* (Philadelphia: Saunders, 2012), pp. 913–921.

12. J. L. Irani, A. Ramsanahie, and R. Bleday, Inflammatory bowel disease: Surgical considerations, in N. J. Greenberger, ed., *Current Diagnosis and Treatment: Gastroenterology, Hepatology, and Endoscopy* (New York: McGraw-Hill Companies, 2012), pp. 36–46.

13. A. C. Travis and R. S. Blumberg, Diverticular disease of the colon, in N. J. Greenberger, ed., *Current Diagnosis and Treatment: Gastroenterology, Hepatology, and Endoscopy* (New York: McGraw-Hill Companies, 2012), pp. 259–272.

14. Travis and Blumberg, 2012; J. M. Fox and N. H. Stollman, Diverticular disease of the colon, in M. Feldman, L. S. Friedman, and L. J. Brandt, eds., *Sleisenger and Fordtran's Gastrointestinal and Liver Disease* (Philadelphia: Saunders, 2010), pp. 2073–2089.

15. Travis and Blumberg, 2012; Fox and Stollman, 2010.

16. A. F. Peery and coauthors, A high-fiber diet does not protect against asymptomatic diverticulosis, *Gastroenterology* 142 (2012): 266–272; L. L. Strate, Lifestyle factors and the course of diverticular disease, *Digestive Diseases* 30 (2012): 35–45.

17. Travis and Blumberg, 2012.

18. C. Ünlü and coauthors, A systematic review of high-fibre dietary therapy in diverticular disease, *International Journal of Colorectal Disease* 27 (2012): 419–427.

19. S. Tarleton and J. K. DiBaise, Low-residue diet in diverticular disease: Putting an end to a myth, *Nutrition in Clinical Practice* 26 (2011): 137–142.

20. Academy of Nutrition and Dietetics, 2014.

21. Academy of Nutrition and Dietetics, 2014.

22. Academy of Nutrition and Dietetics, 2014.

23. Academy of Nutrition and Dietetics, 2014.

LO 18.6 Describe the potential benefits of consuming probiotics and prebiotics and identify some common dietary sources.

Soon after birth, the warm, nutrient-rich environment within the gastrointestinal tract is colonized by a wide variety of bacterial species. In fact, the approximately 10 trillion bacterial cells inhabiting our bodies (**flora**) represent more than 90 percent of the cells in the body. Most bacterial cells reside in our colon, which harbors over 500 different species.[1] Although the exact composition of intestinal bacteria varies among individuals, the pattern within an individual tends to remain constant over time, fluctuating somewhat due to age, illness, antibiotic treatment, and, to some extent, dietary factors. Table NP18-1 lists the predominant types of bacteria that colonize the human intestines, and Table NP18-2 shows how the bacterial populations vary within different regions of the GI tract.

Over the past several decades, nutritional scientists and microbiologists have tried to determine whether **probiotics**—live, **nonpathogenic** microorganisms supplied in sufficient numbers to possibly benefit our health—can be useful for preventing or treating various medical conditions. Although the diseases of interest include gastrointestinal disorders, researchers have also been studying the effects of bacterial probiotics on cancer, immune system disorders, and other illnesses. This Nutrition in Practice discusses some of the research and explains some of the issues involved in selecting and consuming probiotics. The accompanying glossary in Box NP18-1 defines some relevant terms.

TABLE NP18-1 Intestinal Flora

Predominant Types	Subdominant Types
Bacteroides	Enterobacteria
Bifidobacteria	Enterococci
Clostridia	Escherichia
Eubacteria	Klebsiella
Peptococci	Lactobacilli
Peptostreptococci	Micrococci
Ruminococci	Staphylococci

© 2016 Cengage Learning®

TABLE NP18-2 Bacterial Populations in the Gastrointestinal Tract

Organ	Total Bacteria (per mL of contents)
Stomach, duodenum	10–1000
Jejunum, ileum	10^4–10^8
Colon	10^{10}–10^{12}

© 2016 Cengage Learning®

BOX NP18-1 GLOSSARY

bacterial translocation: movement of bacteria across the intestinal mucosa, allowing access to body tissues.

flora: the bacteria that normally reside in a person's body.

nonpathogenic: not capable of causing disease.

pathogenic: capable of causing disease.

prebiotics: indigestible substances in foods that stimulate the growth of nonpathogenic bacteria within the large intestine.

probiotics: live microorganisms provided in foods and dietary supplements for the purpose of preventing or treating disease.

How do our intestinal bacteria influence health?

Intestinal bacteria can benefit our health in a number of different ways. First, the bacteria degrade much of our undigested or unabsorbed dietary carbohydrate, including certain dietary fibers, starch that is resistant to digestion, and poorly absorbed sugars and sugar alcohols. In turn, the bacteria produce some vitamins, as well as short-chain fatty acids that our colonic epithelial cells and other body cells can use as an energy source. Intestinal bacteria also assist in the development and maintenance of mucosal tissue, protect intestinal tissue from **pathogenic** bacteria, and stimulate immune defenses in mucosal cells and other body tissues.[2]

Certain nondigestible substances in food, called **prebiotics,** can stimulate the growth or activity of the resident bacteria within the large intestine. Prebiotics include some of the carbohydrates found in artichokes, asparagus, bananas, chicory root, garlic, Jerusalem artichokes, leeks, onions, and other foods.[3] Because the intestinal bacteria that degrade these substances produce gas as a by-product, people who consume high amounts of these foods may experience more flatulence than usual.

Why are certain types of bacteria considered "probiotic"?

For microbes to be "probiotic"—that is, beneficial to health—they must be nonpathogenic when consumed. They must survive their transit through the digestive tract; therefore, they must be resistant to destruction by stomach acid, bile, and other digestive substances. They should be able to alter the intestinal environment in some way that is beneficial to the human host, such as by producing antimicrobial substances, altering immune defenses, metabolizing undigested foodstuffs, or protecting the intestinal walls.

Probiotic bacteria must be consumed in large amounts—between 100 million and 100 billion live bacteria per day—to survive in sufficient numbers to influence the bacterial populations in the large intestine; a serving of yogurt usually provides these amounts. Carefully controlled studies have not found that probiotic bacteria actually *colonize* the intestine, however, as they are no longer detected in fecal or intestinal samples once ingestion of the probiotic product stops. Note that only a few different types of bacteria are used in foods, and the relatively small amounts consumed cannot compete with the huge populations that normally reside in our digestive tract.

What types of medical problems are helped by probiotics?

Although the results of research studies vary, probiotics may help to prevent and treat some gastric and intestinal disorders (including inflammatory bowel diseases and irritable bowel syndrome), alter susceptibility to food allergens and alleviate some allergy symptoms, and improve the availability and digestibility of various nutrients. Other potential benefits include improved immune responses, reduced symptoms of lactose intolerance, and reduced cancer risk.[4]

Much of the research investigating probiotics and intestinal illness has focused on the prevention and treatment of infectious diarrhea. For example, controlled trials have suggested that certain strains of probiotic bacteria may shorten the duration of diarrhea caused by rotavirus infection in infants and children, decrease the incidence of traveler's diarrhea in tourists visiting high-risk areas, and prevent the recurrence of infectious diarrhea in hospitalized patients.[5] In studies of children and adults using antibiotics, some strains of probiotic bacteria have been shown to reduce the incidence and duration of antibiotic-associated diarrhea.[6] As another example, some studies have suggested that probiotic treatment may help to reduce the recurrence of *pouchitis,* an inflammation of the surgical pouch created in some patients who have had an ileostomy or colostomy.[7]

Despite promising research results thus far, there are no clear conclusions about the appropriate probiotic doses or durations of treatment for many of these conditions. Moreover, the beneficial effects of one bacterial strain cannot be extrapolated to other strains of the same species, as different strains can have contrasting effects.[8] Thus, individuals who decide to consume probiotic-containing foods and supplements to benefit their health cannot be certain that the substances they use will help their condition. At best, probiotics should be considered an adjunct therapy rather than a primary treatment for an illness.

What are the main dietary sources of probiotics?

Probiotics are provided mainly by fermented foods (see Figure NP18-1). In the United States, yogurt and acidophilus milk are produced using various species of lactobacilli and bifidobacteria, although the species are chosen for their ability to produce desirable food products rather than their potential health benefits. In Europe and Asia, food products containing probiotic bacteria include yogurt, milk, ice cream, oatmeal gruel, and soft drinks. Although lactobacilli are used to produce various other fermented food products, such as sauerkraut, pickles, brined olives, and sausages, these foods retain few, if any, live bacteria after they undergo typical food processing methods.

A number of companies market probiotic supplements, which are available in capsules, tablets, and powders.[9] Because probiotic products contain living organisms, storage conditions may affect viability—heat, moisture, and oxygen can reduce survival times—and therefore consumers should check the expiration date before purchasing a product. When a consumer group (ConsumerLab.com)

FIGURE NP18-1 Various species of *Lactobacillus* are used in the production of fermented food products, such as the foods shown in this photo.

Polara Studios, Inc

tested 19 probiotic supplements, they found that 5 of the products contained only 16 to 56 percent of the organisms claimed on the label.[10] Thus, there is no guarantee that a dietary supplement will contain the numbers of microbes expected.

Are there any potential problems associated with the use of probiotics?

Yes. One major concern is the possibility that probiotic bacteria may cause infection in immune-compromised individuals. Various species of probiotic bacteria, including *Lactobacillus* species, have been isolated from the infection sites of severely ill individuals who were consuming the probiotic.[11] Risk is increased by the use of antibiotic therapy (which reduces intestinal flora populations), illnesses or medications that suppress immunity, and illnesses that increase risk of **bacterial translocation** (including inflammatory bowel illnesses and intestinal infections). Care should be taken to inquire about probiotic use in these patients.

Other safety concerns are related to the lack of industry standards for probiotics in foods and supplements: the concentrations and strains of probiotic organisms in foods may vary substantially. Thus, a consumer who wishes to try probiotics would find it difficult to determine how much of a product to consume in order to achieve the desired effect.

The microbes that inhabit the GI tract have critical roles in maintaining the integrity of intestinal tissues and influence health in various other ways. Preliminary research suggests that altering our bacterial populations by consuming probiotics or prebiotics may help to improve our defenses against certain illnesses. Additional studies are needed to verify the beneficial effects of probiotics and prebiotics and to develop standard protocols that can be used for treating illness.

Notes

1. M. W. Ariefdjohan, O. N. Brown-Esters, and D. A. Savaiano, Intestinal microflora and diet in health, in A. M. Coulston, C. J. Boushey, and M. G. Ferruzzi, eds., *Nutrition in the Prevention and Treatment of Disease* (London: Academic Press/Elsevier, 2013), pp. 719–738.

2. Ariefdjohan, Brown-Esters, and Savaiano, 2013.

3. E. M. M. Quigley, Prebiotics and probiotics: Their role in the management of gastrointestinal disorders in adults, *Nutrition in Clinical Practice* 27 (2012): 195–200.

4. Ariefdjohan, Brown-Esters, and Savaiano, 2013; M. E. Sanders and coauthors, An update on the use and investigation of probiotics in health and disease, *Gut* 62 (2013): 787–796.

5. Ariefdjohan, Brown-Esters, and Savaiano, 2013.

6. S. Tejero and coauthors, Probiotics and prebiotics as modulators of the gut microbiota, in A. C. Ross and coeditors, eds., *Modern Nutrition in Health and Disease* (Baltimore: Lippincott Williams & Wilkins, 2014), pp. 506–512.

7. Tejero and coauthors, 2014.

8. Quigley, 2012.

9. L. E. Morrow, V. Gogineni, and M. A. Malesker, Probiotics in the intensive care unit, *Nutrition in Clinical Practice* 27 (2012): 235–241.

10. ConsumerLab.com, Product review: Probiotics for adults, children, and pets, available at www.consumerlab.com; site visited February 14, 2014.

11. K. Whelan and C. E. Myers, Safety of probiotics in patients receiving nutritional support: A systematic review of case reports, randomized controlled trials, and nonrandomized trials, *American Journal of Clinical Nutrition* 91 (2010): 687–703.

19

Carbohydrate- and Fat-Modified Diets for Malabsorption Disorders

19.1 Malabsorption Syndromes

LO 19.1 Describe some procedures that can help to identify a malabsorption problem and discuss the potential causes and consequences of fat malabsorption and bacterial overgrowth.

19.2 Lactose Intolerance

LO 19.2 Identify the causes of lactose intolerance and describe the current treatment approaches for this condition.

19.3 Disorders of the Pancreas

LO 19.3 Identify the effects of pancreatitis and cystic fibrosis on health and nutrition status and describe the nutrition therapies used in treatment.

19.4 Disorders of the Small Intestine

LO 19.4 Summarize the effects of celiac disease and short bowel syndrome on health and nutrition status and describe their nutrition care.

19.5 Nutrition in Practice: Anemia in Illness

LO 19.5 Describe the process of erythropoiesis and explain how nutrient deficiencies, diseases, or disease treatments may lead to anemia.

The gastrointestinal (GI) illnesses that are the most detrimental to nutrition status are those that cause nutrient malabsorption. Malabsorption can lead to nutrient deficiencies and weight loss and cause serious complications. This chapter describes disorders that require carbohydrate- and fat-modified diets to treat malabsorption.

19.1 Malabsorption Syndromes

LO 19.1 Describe some procedures that can help to identify a malabsorption problem and discuss the potential causes and consequences of fat malabsorption and bacterial overgrowth.

To digest and absorb nutrients, we depend on normal digestive secretions and healthy intestinal mucosa. Malabsorption can therefore be caused by pancreatic disorders that cause enzyme or bicarbonate deficiencies, disorders that result in bile deficiency, and inflammatory diseases or medical treatments that damage intestinal tissue. In some cases, the treatment of an intestinal disease requires surgical removal of a section (**resection**) of the small intestine, leaving minimal absorptive capacity in the portion that remains. In addition, various medications can damage the mucosa and impair the digestive and absorptive functions of the small intestine. Table 19-1 lists examples of diseases and treatments that are frequently associated with malabsorption.

Malabsorption rarely involves a single nutrient. When malabsorption is caused by pancreatic enzyme deficiencies, all macronutrients—protein, carbohydrate, and fat—may be affected. When fat is malabsorbed, fat-soluble nutrients and some minerals are usually malabsorbed as well. Malabsorption disorders and their treatments can tax nutritional status further by causing complications that alter food intake, raise nutrient needs, or promote additional nutrient losses.

Evaluating Malabsorption

A number of clinical procedures and laboratory tests are used to determine whether an individual has a malabsorption problem. Examples include the following:[1]

- *Endoscopy or biopsy.* Direct examination of the duodenal mucosa with an **endoscope** may reveal physical changes characteristic of intestinal diseases that cause malabsorption. A **biopsy** can be taken during the procedure for further analysis.

- *Stool fat analysis.* Fat malabsorption can be determined by placing the patient on a high-fat diet (80 to 100 grams per day), performing a 48- to 72-hour stool collection, and measuring the stool's fat content. Healthy individuals generally eliminate less than 7 grams of fat per day under these conditions. Excessive fat in the stools is known as **steatorrhea.**

- *Hydrogen breath test.* When carbohydrate is malabsorbed, colonic bacteria digest the carbohydrate and produce hydrogen gas, which is absorbed and later can be measured in the breath. The hydrogen breath test is often used to diagnose lactose intolerance, but it can diagnose malabsorption of other types of carbohydrate as well. This test is also used to determine the presence of excessive bacteria in the small intestine.

- *Xylose absorption.* Xylose, a sugar that is readily absorbed but is not well metabolized, can be used to test whether the small intestine is able to absorb nutrients normally. In the xylose absorption test, the patient is given an oral dose of xylose, and blood and urine tests determine whether appropriate amounts of xylose were absorbed.

TABLE 19-1 Potential Causes of Malabsorption

Genetic disorders
- Enzyme deficiencies

Intestinal disorders
- AIDS-related enteropathy
- Bacterial overgrowth
- Celiac disease
- Crohn's disease
- Radiation enteritis

Intestinal infections
- Giardiasis
- Nematode (roundworm) infections

Liver disease (bile insufficiency)

Pancreatic disorders
- Chronic pancreatitis
- Cystic fibrosis

Surgeries
- Gastric or intestinal bypass surgery
- Intestinal resection (short bowel syndrome)

© Cengage Learning®

resection: the surgical removal of part of an organ or body structure.

endoscope: a flexible fiber optic tube used for viewing internal cavities of the body.

biopsy: removal of a tissue sample to determine the cause of an illness.

steatorrhea (stee-AH-tor-REE-ah): excessive fat in the stool due to fat malabsorption; characterized by stools that are loose, frothy, and foul smelling due to a high fat content.
- steat = fat
- rheo = flow

Fat Malabsorption

Fat is the nutrient most frequently malabsorbed because both digestive enzymes and bile must be present for its digestion. Thus, fat malabsorption often develops when an illness reduces either pancreatic or bile secretions. For example, both pancreatitis and cystic fibrosis can decrease the secretion of pancreatic lipase, whereas severe liver disease can cause bile insufficiency. Motility disorders that accelerate gastric emptying or intestinal transit can cause fat malabsorption because they prevent the normal mixing of dietary fat with lipase and bile. Fat malabsorption can also be caused by conditions or treatments that damage the intestinal mucosa, such as inflammatory bowel diseases, AIDS, and radiation treatments for cancer.

Consequences of Fat Malabsorption Fat malabsorption is associated with losses of food energy, essential fatty acids, fat-soluble vitamins, and some minerals (see Figure 19-1). Weight loss may result if the individual does not consume alternative sources of energy. Deficiencies of fat-soluble vitamins and essential fatty acids are common in chronic conditions. Malabsorption of some minerals, including calcium, magnesium, and zinc, often occurs because the minerals form **soaps** with the unabsorbed fatty acids and bile acids. Calcium deficiency may lead to bone loss, which is further aggravated by the vitamin D deficiency that often develops due to fat malabsorption.

Another consequence of fat malabsorption is an increased risk of kidney stones, which are most often composed of calcium oxalate.* The oxalates in foods ordinarily bind to calcium in the small intestine and are eliminated in the stool. If calcium instead binds to fatty acids or bile acids, the oxalates are free to be absorbed into the blood and are ultimately excreted in the urine. The risk of developing oxalate stones increases when urinary oxalate levels are high. Kidney stones are discussed further in Chapter 23.

soaps: chemical compounds formed from fatty acids and positively charged minerals.

FIGURE 19-1 The Consequences of Fat Malabsorption

*Oxalates are plant compounds found in green leafy vegetables and some other foods. The oxalates can bind to minerals in the GI tract and form complexes that the body cannot absorb.

TABLE 19-2 Fat-Restricted Diet

A fat-restricted diet includes mostly low-fat and fat-free foods. For a fat intake of 50 grams per day, limit meats and meat substitutes to 6 ounces per day, and limit fats and oils to 8 teaspoons per day.[a] Foods from other food groups should provide less than 1 gram of fat per serving.

Food Category	Foods Recommended	Foods to Avoid
Meat and meat alternates	Lean meat, fish, or skinless poultry prepared by broiling, roasting, grilling, or boiling; low-fat luncheon meat such as sliced turkey breast; meat alternates such as dried beans or peas; low-fat egg substitutes; egg whites	Meat with visible fat, ground beef (unless extra lean), sausage, bacon, frankfurters, spareribs, duck, tuna packed in oil, whole eggs and egg yolks
Milk and milk products	Fat-free milk, fat-free yogurt, fat-free sour cream substitutes, fat-free half-and-half and cream substitutes, fat-free cheese; low-fat milk products can be used in moderation	Milk products that are not fat free or low fat
Breads, cereals, rice, and pasta	Whole-grain and enriched breads, cooked cereals and most cold breakfast cereals, plain tortillas, bagels, English muffins, fat-free muffins, saltine crackers, graham crackers, pretzels, plain rice, plain noodles and pasta	Biscuits, pancakes, waffles, granola, snack crackers made with fat, cornbread, doughnuts, corn chips, fried rice, buttered or butter-flavored popcorn
Vegetables	All vegetables prepared without added fat	Buttered, creamed, breaded, or fried vegetables; vegetables prepared au gratin style; french-fried potatoes; potato chips, olives
Fruit	All types of fruit except avocados	Avocado; fruit dishes prepared with fat, nuts, or coconut
Desserts	Sherbet; fruit ices; flavored gelatin; fat-free pudding; angel food cake; meringue; fat-free bakery products; fat-free ice cream or frozen yogurt; fat-free candy such as marshmallows, jelly beans, and hard candy	Cake, cookies, pie, and pastry made with fat; pudding made with whole milk or eggs; ice cream; candy made with fat, such as caramel or chocolate
Fats and oils	Vegetable oils, soft or liquid margarines and spreads, limited amounts of butter or stick margarine (1 tsp provides about 3½–4½ g fat) Each of these foods can replace 1 tsp fat in the amounts specified: 1 tbs salad dressing, 2 tbs low-fat salad dressing, ½ tbs peanut butter, 1 tbs chopped nuts, 2 tbs mashed avocado	Dietary fat that exceeds the amount specified in the nutrition prescription
Beverages	Fruit juices, soft drinks, fat-free milk, coffee, tea, coffee substitutes	Beverages made with milk (unless fat free) or added cream, chocolate milk, eggnog, milk shakes

Sample Menu (contains about 50 g fat):

Breakfast: 6 oz orange juice, 1 c oatmeal with nonfat milk and raisins, 1 slice whole-wheat toast with 1 tsp margarine, coffee with fat-free half-and-half

Lunch: Turkey breast sandwich (2 slices whole-wheat bread, 2 oz lean turkey breast, 2 tomato slices, lettuce leaf, and 2 tsp mayonnaise), 2 c salad greens with 1 tbs salad dressing, fruit cup (1 c peaches and ½ c berries) with ½ c orange sherbet

Snack: 6 oz nonfat fruit yogurt, 6 saltine crackers with 1 tbs peanut butter and ½ tbs honey

Dinner: 4 oz cod with sliced lemon, 1 slice French bread with 1 tsp butter, 1 c steamed rice with herbs and walnut oil (includes ½ tsp oil), 1 c steamed broccoli and carrots with ½ tsp margarine, 1 piece angel food cake with fat-free whipped cream

© 2016 Cengage Learning®

[a]To achieve a fat intake that is less than 50 grams, additional reductions may be necessary. For example, for a fat intake of 25 grams per day, limit meats and meat substitutes to 4 ounces per day, and limit fats and oils to 2 teaspoons per day.

Nutrition Therapy for Fat Malabsorption If steatorrhea does not improve, a fat-restricted diet may be recommended (see Table 19-2). The diet may help to relieve intestinal symptoms that are aggravated by fat intake (such as diarrhea and flatulence) and reduce vitamin and mineral losses. Because fat is a primary energy source, it should not be restricted more than necessary. **Medium-chain triglycerides (MCT),** which do not require lipase or bile for digestion and absorption, can be used as an alternative source of dietary fat, although MCT oil does not provide essential fatty acids. Box 19-1 (p. 516) offers suggestions for following a fat-restricted diet and for using MCT oil.

medium-chain triglycerides (MCT): triglycerides with fatty acids that are 8 to 10 carbons in length. MCT do not require digestion and can be absorbed in the absence of lipase or bile.

For some individuals, fat-restricted diets may be difficult to follow. Fats add flavors, aromas, and textures to foods—characteristics that make foods more enjoyable. Unlike some dietary changes that can be introduced gradually, fat restriction is often implemented immediately, allowing little time for adaptation. These suggestions may help:

▌ Fat is better tolerated if provided in small portions. Divide the day's allotment into several servings that can be consumed throughout the day.

▌ Use variety to enhance enjoyment of meals: vary flavors, textures, colors, and seasonings.

▌ Look for fat-free items when grocery shopping. Incorporate fat-free ingredients when preparing favorite recipes.

▌ Try fat-free and low-fat condiments to improve the diet's palatability. Experiment with herbs and spices. Instead of butter, use fruit butter on toast. Use butter-flavored granules on vegetables. Replace mayonnaise in sandwiches with a spicy mustard. Replace salad dressing with a flavored vinegar.

▌ Avoid products that contain the fat substitute olestra, which may aggravate GI symptoms.

If patients are interested in using medium-chain triglyceride (MCT) oil:

▌ Explain that MCT products are expensive but that the cost is sometimes covered by medical insurance.

▌ Advise patients to add MCT oil to the diet gradually. Diarrhea and abdominal cramps may result if too much is used at once. Tolerance to MCT oil may improve in time.

▌ Advise patients that MCT oil may have an unpleasant taste when used alone. Suggest using MCT oil in recipes as a substitute for regular oil. MCT oil can replace the oil in salad dressings, be incorporated into sauces, and be used in cooking or baking. It can also be added to fat-free milk products to make milk shakes.

▌ Point out that MCT oil should not be used to fry foods because it decomposes at lower temperatures than most cooking oils.

Bacterial Overgrowth

Ordinarily, the GI tract is protected from **bacterial overgrowth** by gastric acid, which destroys bacteria; peristalsis, which flushes bacteria through the small intestine before they multiply; and immunoglobulins secreted into the GI lumen.[2] When bacterial overgrowth does occur, it can lead to fat malabsorption because the bacteria dismantle the bile acids needed for fat emulsification. Deficiencies of the fat-soluble vitamins A, D, and E may eventually develop. The bacteria also produce enzymes and toxins that disturb the intestinal mucosa, destroying some mucosal enzymes (especially lactase) and possibly reducing the absorptive surface area. Some types of bacteria metabolize vitamin B_{12}, reducing its absorption and increasing the risk of deficiency. Although symptoms of bacterial overgrowth are often minor and nonspecific, severe cases may lead to chronic diarrhea, steatorrhea, flatulence, bloating, and weight loss.

Causes of Bacterial Overgrowth Conditions that impair intestinal motility and allow material to stagnate can greatly increase susceptibility to bacterial overgrowth. For example, in some types of gastric surgery, a portion of the small intestine is bypassed, preventing the flow of material in the bypassed region and allowing bacteria to flourish (see the "blind loop" shown in Figure 17-6 on p. 482). Intestinal motility can also be reduced by strictures, obstructions, and diverticula in the small intestine, as well as by some chronic illnesses, including diabetes mellitus and scleroderma.[3]

Reduced secretions of gastric acid can also lead to bacterial overgrowth. Possible causes include atrophic gastritis, acid-suppressing medications, and some gastrectomy procedures.

Treatment for Bacterial Overgrowth Treatment may include antibiotics to suppress bacterial growth and surgical correction of the anatomical defects that contribute to a motility disorder. Medications may be given to stimulate peristalsis, and acid-suppressing medications should be discontinued. A lactose-restricted diet may reduce flatulence and diarrhea in some individuals. Dietary supplements can correct nutrient deficiencies, especially deficiencies of fat-soluble vitamins, calcium (which combines with malabsorbed fatty acids), and vitamin B_{12}.

bacterial overgrowth: excessive bacterial colonization of the stomach and small intestine; may be due to low gastric acidity, altered GI motility, mucosal damage, or contamination.

▋ Nutrient malabsorption can result from an undersupply of digestive secretions, motility disorders, or damaged intestinal mucosa. Clinical procedures or laboratory tests may reveal the underlying conditions causing a malabsorption problem.

▋ Fat malabsorption can cause losses of food energy and deficiencies of essential fatty acids, fat-soluble vitamins, and some minerals. In severe cases, nutrition therapy may include a fat-restricted diet and use of MCT oil.

▋ Bacterial overgrowth may result from conditions that reduce gastric acidity or intestinal motility; it typically causes malabsorption of fat and some essential nutrients.

19.2 Lactose Intolerance

LO 19.2 Identify the causes of lactose intolerance and describe the current treatment approaches for this condition.

Approximately 75 percent of people worldwide have some degree of **lactose intolerance,** which is caused by the loss or reduction of lactase, the intestinal enzyme that digests the lactose in milk products.[4] Lactose intolerance is especially prevalent among individuals of certain ethnic groups, including Asians, African Americans, Native Americans, Ashkenazi Jews, and Latinos. It may also result from GI disorders, medications, or medical treatments that damage the small intestinal mucosa. The primary symptoms of lactose intolerance are diarrhea and increased intestinal gas.

Lactose intolerance is rarely serious and is easily managed by simple dietary adjustments. Although people with the condition are sometimes reluctant to consume milk products, clinical studies have found that individuals with lactose intolerance can tolerate up to 2 cups of milk daily without significant symptoms.[5] In addition, the regular consumption of milk products increases the amount of lactose metabolized by intestinal bacteria, which improves lactose tolerance.[6] People who avoid milk for fear of intestinal discomfort can be urged to gradually increase their consumption of lactose-containing foods. They may more readily tolerate milk when intake is divided throughout the day and the milk is taken with food (see Figure 19-2). Most aged cheeses are well tolerated because they contain little lactose. Yogurts that contain live bacterial cultures are often acceptable because the bacteria contain lactase, which may aid in lactose digestion. Other options are to add a lactase preparation to milk or to take enzyme tablets before consuming milk products. Lactose-free milk is also commercially available.

People who develop lactose intolerance as a result of intestinal illness are often advised to temporarily restrict milk and milk products. Foods that contain lactose can be reintroduced in small amounts once the condition improves. Individuals who restrict milk products should be encouraged to consume alternative food sources of calcium and vitamin D.

Courtesy of Trinh Tran

FIGURE 19-2 Milk and Lactose Intolerance
Most people with lactose intolerance can drink milk, especially if they drink it along with other foods and limit the amount they consume at any one time.

lactose intolerance: intolerance to lactose-containing foods due to the loss or reduction of intestinal lactase; symptoms may include flatulence, bloating, and diarrhea.

IN SUMMARY

▋ Lactose intolerance, caused by lactase deficiency, can be managed by adjusting the amount and timing of lactose consumption.

CARBOHYDRATE- AND FAT-MODIFIED DIETS FOR MALABSORPTION DISORDERS

■ Most people with lactose intolerance can consume up to 2 cups of milk daily without significant symptoms; tolerance may be improved by consuming small portions of milk at one time and consuming the milk with foods.

19.3 Disorders of the Pancreas

LO 19.3 Identify the effects of pancreatitis and cystic fibrosis on health and nutrition status and describe the nutrition therapies used in treatment.

As mentioned previously, pancreatic disorders can lead to maldigestion and malabsorption due to the impaired secretion of digestive enzymes. This section describes several diseases that disrupt pancreatic function and cause widespread malabsorption.

Pancreatitis

Pancreatitis is an inflammatory disease of the pancreas. Although mild cases may subside in a few days, other cases can persist for weeks or months. Chronic pancreatitis can lead to irreversible damage to pancreatic tissue and permanent loss of function.

Acute Pancreatitis In acute pancreatitis, the digestive enzymes within pancreatic cells become prematurely activated, causing destruction of pancreatic tissue and subsequent inflammation. About 70 to 80 percent of acute cases are caused by gallstones or alcohol abuse; less frequent causes include elevated blood triglyceride levels or exposure to various toxins.[7] Common symptoms include severe abdominal pain, nausea and vomiting, and abdominal distention. In most patients, the condition resolves within a week with no complications. More serious cases may lead to chronic pancreatitis, infection, the systemic inflammatory response syndrome (see p. 631), or multiple organ failure.

Nutrition Therapy for Acute Pancreatitis The initial treatment for acute pancreatitis is supportive and includes pain control and intravenous hydration. In cases of mild-to-moderate pancreatitis, oral fluids and food are withheld until the patient is pain free and experiences no nausea or vomiting.[8] Afterward, patients can usually consume a regular diet; a fat-restricted diet may be helpful for patients with symptoms of fat malabsorption (such as steatorrhea and abdominal pain). In severe pancreatitis, continuous tube feedings, started within the initial 48 hours of treatment, may lead to improved outcomes compared with withholding intakes; the use of elemental formulas (formulas that contain hydrolyzed nutrients) may improve patient tolerance.[9] Protein needs are generally high in pancreatitis patients (between 1.2 and 1.5 grams per kilogram body weight per day[10]) due to the catabolic effects of inflammation. Patients should be given multivitamin/mineral supplements until food intakes can meet their nutritional needs.

Chronic Pancreatitis Chronic pancreatitis is characterized by progressive, permanent damage to pancreatic tissue, resulting in the impaired secretion of digestive enzymes and bicarbonate. About 70 to 80 percent of cases are caused by excessive alcohol consumption.[11] Most patients with chronic pancreatitis experience persistent abdominal pain, which may worsen with eating and be accompanied by nausea and vomiting. Although all macronutrients are maldigested, the symptoms of fat malabsorption are typically the most severe. Long-term illness is associated with reduced secretion of insulin and glucagon, and diabetes eventually develops in 30 to 50 percent of patients.[12]

Nutrition Therapy for Chronic Pancreatitis The objectives of nutrition therapy are to reduce malabsorption and correct malnutrition. Pancreatic enzyme replacement is the main treatment for steatorrhea and other symptoms of malabsorption. Most enzyme preparations are **enteric coated** to resist the acidity of the stomach and do not dissolve until they reach the small intestine. If nonenteric-coated preparations

enteric coated: refers to medications or enzyme preparations that are coated to withstand gastric acidity and dissolve only at the higher pH of the small intestine.

BOX 19-2 DIET-DRUG INTERACTIONS

Check this table for notable nutrition-related effects of the medications discussed in this chapter.

Antisecretory drugs (proton-pump inhibitors, H2 blockers)	**Gastrointestinal effects:** Diarrhea, constipation, nausea and vomiting, abdominal pain (proton-pump inhibitors) **Dietary interactions:** May decrease iron, calcium, folate, and vitamin B_{12} absorption
Pancreatic enzyme replacements	**Gastrointestinal effects:** Constipation, nausea and vomiting, diarrhea, abdominal cramps, irritation of GI mucosa **Dietary interactions:** May decrease folate and iron absorption **Metabolic effects:** Elevated serum or urinary uric acid levels (with high doses), allergic reactions (rare)

are used, acid-suppressing drugs are also required (Box 19-2 lists nutrition-related side effects of these medications). Fecal fat concentrations can be monitored to determine if the enzyme treatment has been effective.

Patients with chronic pancreatitis who are hypermetabolic and underweight have high protein and energy requirements; protein needs may range between 1.0 and 1.5 grams per kilogram body weight per day and energy intakes should be about 35 kcalories per kilogram daily.[13] Dietary supplements are used to correct nutrient deficiencies, which may be due to malabsorption or to the alcohol abuse that caused the disease. Patients should avoid alcohol completely and quit smoking cigarettes, as these substances can exacerbate illness and interfere with healing.[14]

Cystic Fibrosis

Cystic fibrosis is the most common life-threatening genetic disorder among Caucasians, with an incidence of approximately 1 in 3000 to 5000 white births.[15] The condition is characterized by a mutation in the protein that regulates chloride transport across epithelial cell membranes. The abnormality alters the ion concentration and/or viscosity of **exocrine** secretions, causing a broad range of serious complications. Until a few decades ago, few infants born with cystic fibrosis survived to adulthood. Now, with early detection and advances in medical treatment, the median life span has reached 38 years of age, with many patients surviving into their 50s.[16]

Consequences of Cystic Fibrosis Cystic fibrosis is characterized by abnormal chloride and sodium levels in exocrine secretions. These altered secretions ultimately disrupt the functioning of multiple tissues and organs. Common complications of cystic fibrosis involve the lungs, pancreas, and sweat glands.

- *Lungs.* Changes in bronchial secretions lead to an impaired ability to clear airway mucus, resulting in chronic respiratory infections, progressive inflammation, and airway obstruction (see Figure 19-3, p. 520). The eventual lung damage causes breathing difficulties, chronic coughing, and lower exercise tolerance. Nutrition status may become impaired due to hypermetabolism, the greater energy cost of labored breathing, and anorexia (loss of appetite).

- *Pancreas.* Most patients produce thickened pancreatic secretions that obstruct the pancreatic ducts.[17] The trapped pancreatic enzymes eventually damage pancreatic tissue, leading to progressive atrophy and scarring. Few pancreatic enzymes reach the small intestine, resulting in severe malabsorption of protein, fat, and fat-soluble vitamins.

- *Sweat glands.* Salt losses in sweat are usually excessive, increasing the risk of dehydration.

Children with cystic fibrosis are chronically undernourished, grow poorly, and have difficulty maintaining normal body weight. Complications that may develop over time

cystic fibrosis: a genetic disorder characterized by abnormal chloride and sodium levels in exocrine secretions; often leads to respiratory illness and pancreatic insufficiency.

exocrine: pertains to external secretions, such as those of the mucous membranes or the skin. Opposite of *endocrine,* which pertains to hormonal secretions into the blood.

include pancreatitis, glucose intolerance or diabetes (due to destruction of insulin-producing cells), and gallbladder and liver diseases.

Nutrition Therapy for Cystic Fibrosis

Patients with cystic fibrosis have high energy requirements, which range from 120 to 150 percent of DRI values; however, intakes are often much lower than these levels.[18] To achieve normal growth and appropriate weight, patients are typically encouraged to eat a high-kcalorie, high-protein diet, consume high-fat foods freely, eat frequent meals and snacks, and supplement meals with milk shakes or oral supplements. Supplemental tube feedings can help to improve nutrition status if energy intakes are inadequate.

Pancreatic enzyme replacement therapy is a central feature of cystic fibrosis treatment. Supplemental enzymes must be included with every meal or snack. For young children, the contents of capsules are mixed in small amounts of liquid or a soft food (such as applesauce) and fed with a spoon. Enzyme dosages may need to be adjusted if malabsorption continues, as evidenced by poor growth or GI symptoms such as steatorrhea, intestinal gas, or abdominal pain.

The risk of nutrient deficiency depends on the degree of malabsorption; nutrients of greatest concern include the fat-soluble vitamins, essential fatty acids, calcium, iron, and zinc. Multivitamin/mineral supplements are routinely recommended. The liberal use of table salt and salty foods is encouraged to make up for sodium losses in sweat. The Case Study in Box 19-3 reviews the care of a patient with cystic fibrosis.

Mauro Fermariello/Science Source

FIGURE 19-3 Postural Drainage Therapy
Postural drainage, a type of physical therapy used in cystic fibrosis, helps to clear the thick, sticky secretions that block airways and increase infection risk. The therapy involves maintaining a position that helps fluid drain out of the lungs, sometimes helped by soft claps or vibration over the areas that require drainage.

IN SUMMARY

❚ Whereas acute pancreatitis is short lived and does not cause permanent damage, chronic pancreatitis can lead to digestive enzyme deficiencies and may require pancreatic enzyme replacement therapy.

❚ Cystic fibrosis can cause obstructive lung disease and pancreatic damage; the nutrition treatment includes a high-kcalorie, high-protein diet and pancreatic enzyme replacement therapy.

Case Study BOX 19-3 CHILD WITH CYSTIC FIBROSIS

Julie is a 7-year-old girl diagnosed with cystic fibrosis. Symptoms of steatorrhea and poor growth during infancy prompted the tests that led to the diagnosis. She is currently 45 inches tall and weighs 42 pounds. Her height for age and weight for age fall near the 10th percentile (see Appendix E). Julie eats regular foods during the day and receives additional nutrients by tube feedings delivered overnight.

1. What do the height and weight percentiles tell you about Julie's nutrition status? Why is growth failure common in children with cystic fibrosis?

2. Explain why Julie's energy needs are so much higher than normal. Describe the elements of the diet that Julie should follow to improve growth.

3. Explain to Julie's parents how to use enzyme replacement therapy effectively.

4. Julie's parents are hoping to discontinue the nightly tube feedings. Do you think the tube feedings are necessary? Why or why not?

19.4 Disorders of the Small Intestine

19.4 Summarize the effects of celiac disease and short bowel syndrome on health and nutrition status and describe their nutrition care.

Malabsorption is a frequent consequence when the intestinal mucosa is damaged due to inflammation, infection, or other causes. One intestinal illness characterized by severe inflammation—Crohn's disease—was described in Chapter 18. This section discusses *celiac disease,* an intolerance to wheat, barley, and rye that can damage the intestinal mucosa, and *short bowel syndrome,* the malabsorption disorder that results when a significant portion of the small intestine is surgically removed.

Celiac Disease

Celiac disease is an immune disorder characterized by an abnormal immune response to a protein fraction in **wheat gluten** and to related proteins in barley and rye. The reaction to gluten causes severe damage to the intestinal mucosa and subsequent malabsorption. Celiac disease affects approximately 1 percent of Caucasians, although it is less common in other ethnic groups.[19]

Consequences of Celiac Disease The immune reaction to gluten can cause striking changes in intestinal tissue (see Figure 19-4). In affected areas, the villi may be shortened or absent, resulting in a significant reduction in mucosal surface area (and, therefore, in the number of cells that digest and absorb nutrients). The damage may be restricted to the duodenum or may involve the full length of the small intestine. Individuals with severe disease may malabsorb all nutrients to some degree; in mild cases, the nutrients malabsorbed vary according to the extent of damage and portion of intestine affected.

Symptoms of celiac disease include GI disturbances such as diarrhea, steatorrhea, and flatulence. Because lactase deficiency can result from the mucosal damage, milk products may exacerbate GI symptoms. Due to nutrient malabsorption, children with celiac disease often exhibit poor growth, low body weight, muscle wasting, and anemia.

celiac (SEE-lee-ack) **disease:** an immune disorder characterized by an abnormal immune response to wheat gluten and related proteins; also called *gluten-sensitive enteropathy* or *celiac sprue.*

wheat gluten (GLU-ten)**:** a family of water-insoluble proteins in wheat; includes the gliadin (GLY-ah-din) fractions that are toxic to persons with celiac disease.

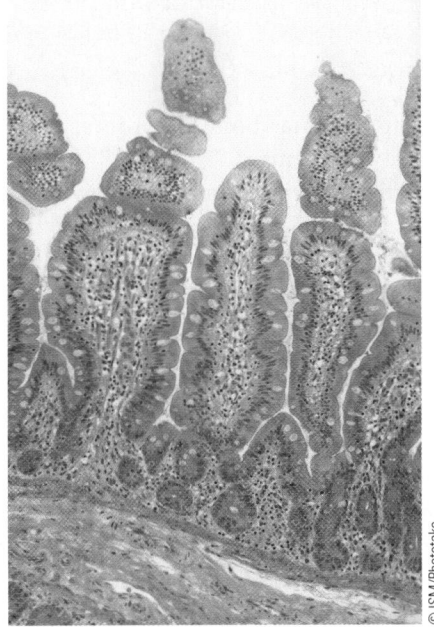

In the healthy intestine, the villi greatly increase the absorptive surface area.

In celiac disease, the villi may be shortened or absent, resulting in substantial reductions in nutrient absorption.

FIGURE 19-4 Effect of Celiac Disease on Intestinal Tissue

TABLE 19-3 Gluten-Free Diet

Food Category	Gluten-Free Choices	Potential Gluten Sources
Meat and meat alternates	Fresh meat, fish, or poultry; shellfish; dried peas and beans; tofu; nuts and seeds; eggs	Luncheon meats, sandwich spreads, meatloaf, meatballs, frankfurters, sausage, poultry injected with broth, imitation meat products, imitation seafood, meat extenders, miso, egg substitutes, dried egg products, dry roasted nuts, peanut butter. *Avoid*: products made with hydrolyzed vegetable protein (HVP), marinades, and soy sauce; breaded foods; foods prepared with cream sauces or gravies.
Milk and milk products	Milk, buttermilk, half-and-half, cream, plain yogurt, cheese, cottage cheese, cream cheese	Chocolate milk, milk shakes, frozen yogurt, flavored yogurt, cheese spreads, cheese sauces. *Avoid*: malted milk, malted milk powders.
Breads, cereals, rice, and pasta	Breads, bakery products, and cereals made with amaranth, arrowroot, buckwheat, corn, flax, hominy grits, millet, potato flour or potato starch, quinoa, rice, sorghum, soybean flour, tapioca, and teff; pasta and noodles made with the grains or starches listed above; corn tacos and corn tortillas	Oatmeal and oat bran (due to possible contamination), rice crackers, rice cakes, corn cakes. *Avoid*: breads, bakery products, cereals, tortillas, matzo, pasta, and pancake or baking mixes made with wheat, rye, barley, and triticale. *Wheat products* include bulghur, couscous, durum flour, einkorn, emmer, farina, graham flour, kamut, semolina, spelt, wheat bran, and wheat germ. *Barley products* include malt, malt flavoring, and malt extract.
Fruits and vegetables	Any fresh, frozen, or canned fruits or vegetables	French fries from fast-food restaurants, commercial salad dressings, fruit pie fillings, dried fruit (may be dusted with flour). *Avoid*: scalloped potatoes (usually made with wheat flour), creamed vegetables, vegetables dipped in batters.
Desserts	Bakery products made with gluten-free flours, most ice creams, sherbet, sorbet, Italian ices, popsicles, gelatin desserts, egg custards, most chocolate bars, chocolate chips, hard candies, marshmallows, whipped toppings	Some ice creams (especially if made with cookie dough, brownies, nuts, and other added ingredients), candies, and candy bars. *Avoid*: bakery products or doughnuts made with wheat, rye, or barley; pudding made with wheat flour; ice cream or sherbets that contain gluten stabilizers; ice cream cones; licorice.
Beverages	Coffee; tea; cocoa made with pure cocoa powder; soft drinks; wine; distilled alcoholic beverages such as rum, gin, whiskey, and vodka	Instant tea or coffee, coffee substitutes, chocolate drinks, hot cocoa mixes. *Avoid*: beer, ale, lager, malt beverages, cereal beverages, beverages that contain nondairy cream substitutes.

© 2016 Cengage Learning®

FIGURE 19-5 Gluten-Free Foods
Gluten-free products help people with celiac disease enjoy a wider variety of foods.

Polara Studios, Inc

dermatitis herpetiformis: a gluten-sensitive disorder characterized by a severe skin rash.

Adults may develop anemia, bone disorders, neurological symptoms, and fertility problems.

Some gluten-sensitive individuals may have few GI symptoms but react to gluten by developing a severe, itchy rash. This condition is called **dermatitis herpetiformis** and requires dietary adjustments similar to those for celiac disease.

Nutrition Therapy for Celiac Disease The treatment for celiac disease is lifelong adherence to a gluten-free diet. Improvement in symptoms often occurs within several weeks, although mucosal healing can sometimes take years. If lactase deficiency is suspected, patients should avoid lactose-containing foods until the intestine has recovered.

The gluten-free diet eliminates foods that contain wheat, barley, and rye (see Table 19-3 and Figure 19-5). Because many foods contain ingredients derived from these grains, foods that are problematic are not always obvious. Gluten sources that may be overlooked include beer, brewer's yeast, caramel coloring, coffee substitutes, communion wafers, imitation meats, malt syrup, medications, salad dressings, and soy sauce. Gluten-free products can be purchased to replace common food items such as bread, pasta, and cereals.

Patients should also be instructed in food preparation methods that prevent cross-contamination from utensils, cutting boards, and toasters. Figure 19-6 shows an example of a menu for a gluten-free diet.

Although most people with celiac disease can safely consume moderate amounts of oats, most oats grown in the United States are contaminated with wheat, barley, or rye. Oats are usually grown in rotation with other grains and may become contaminated during harvesting or processing. Some oat manufacturers now produce oats in dedicated facilities and test products to ensure that they are gluten free. Individuals who wish to include oats in their diet should purchase only uncontaminated oats and limit intakes to the amounts found to be safe (about ½ cup of dry rolled oats per day).

Short Bowel Syndrome

The treatment of Crohn's disease, intestinal cancers, and other conditions may include the surgical resection of a major portion of the small intestine. **Short bowel syndrome** is the malabsorption syndrome that results when the absorptive capacity of the remaining intestine is insufficient for meeting nutritional needs. Without appropriate dietary adjustments, short bowel syndrome can result in fluid and electrolyte imbalances and multiple nutrient deficiencies. Symptoms include diarrhea, steatorrhea, dehydration, weight loss, and growth impairment in children.

Figure 19-7 (p. 524) reviews nutrient absorption in the GI tract and describes how absorption is affected by surgical resections. Generally, up to 50 percent of the small intestine can be resected without serious nutritional consequences.[20] More extensive resections lead to generalized malabsorption, and patients may need lifelong parenteral nutrition to supplement oral intakes.

Intestinal Adaptation After an intestinal resection, the remaining intestine undergoes **intestinal adaptation**, which dramatically improves the intestine's absorptive capacity. Adaptation—which depends on the presence of nutrients and GI secretions in the lumen—begins soon after surgery and continues for several years. During this period, the remaining section of intestine develops taller villi and deeper crypts and also grows in length and diameter; these changes dramatically increase the absorptive surface area. The ileum has a greater capacity for adaptation than the jejunum; thus, removal of the ileum has more severe consequences than removal of the jejunum. Loss of the ileum permanently disrupts vitamin B_{12} and bile acid absorption, and depletion of bile acids exacerbates fat malabsorption. Adaptation is achieved more easily if the colon is present because the colon's resident bacteria can metabolize unabsorbed carbohydrates and produce some usable nutrients. An intact colon also helps to reduce losses of fluids and electrolytes.

Nutrition Therapy for Short Bowel Syndrome Total parenteral nutrition meets nutritional needs after surgery and is gradually replaced by tube feedings and/or oral feedings. To promote intestinal adaptation, the feedings may be started within a week after surgery, after diarrhea subsides somewhat and some bowel function is restored. Initial oral intake may consist of sips of clear, sugar-free liquids, progressing to larger amounts of liquid formulas and then to solid foods, as tolerated. Very small, frequent feedings can utilize the remaining intestine most effectively. To compensate for malabsorption and reduce the need for nutrition support, a high-kcalorie diet may be encouraged.[21]

The exact diet prescribed depends on the portion of intestine removed, the length of remaining intestine, and whether the colon is still intact. If a high-kcalorie diet is advised and fat is well tolerated, a high-fat, low-carbohydrate diet may help to increase energy intakes. Conversely, a high-complex-carbohydrate, low-fat diet may be suggested for patients who have an intact colon, because the colon bacteria can metabolize the unabsorbed carbohydrate and produce short-chain fatty acids (which are absorbed in the colon), and the fat restriction may improve steatorrhea. Patients should avoid

---

Gluten-Free Menu

Breakfast

- Orange juice
- Gluten-free pancake with maple syrup
- Plain yogurt with banana and strawberries
- Coffee with half-and-half

Lunch

- Grilled chicken breast with cranberry chutney
- Baked potato topped with grated cheddar cheese
- Sliced tomato with chopped basil
- Raspberry sherbet

Snack

- Tortilla chips and guacamole
- Hot cocoa (made with cocoa powder)

Dinner

- Sauteed catfish with sliced lemon and dill
- Wild rice pilaf
- Collard greens and garlic sauteed in olive oil
- Green salad with oil and vinegar dressing
- Vanilla egg custard

© Cengage Learning®

FIGURE 19-6 Sample Menu—Gluten-Free Diet

short bowel syndrome: the malabsorption syndrome that follows resection of the small intestine; characterized by inadequate absorptive capacity in the remaining intestine.

intestinal adaptation: physiological changes in the small intestine that increase its absorptive capacity after resection.

WHAT IS ABSORBED

Duodenum/jejunum
- Simple carbohydrates
- Fats
- Amino acids
- Vitamins[a]
- Minerals[a]
- Water

Ileum
- Bile salts
- Vitamin B_{12}
- Water
(Can adapt to assume absorptive functions of the duodenum and jejunum)

Colon
- Water
- Electrolytes
- Short-chain fatty acids

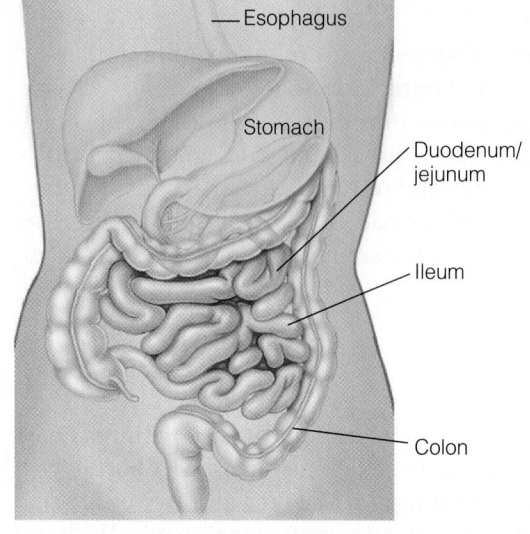

— Esophagus

Stomach

Duodenum/jejunum

Ileum

Colon

POSSIBLE CONSEQUENCES OF RESECTION

Duodenum/jejunum
- Minimal consequences if the ileum remains intact
- Calcium and iron malabsorption if duodenum resected

Ileum
- Fat malabsorption
- Protein malabsorption
- Malabsorption of fat-soluble vitamins and vitamin B_{12}
- Reduced calcium, magnesium, and zinc absorption
- Fluid losses
- Diarrhea/steatorrhea

Colon
- Fluid and electrolyte losses
- Diarrhea
(Losses are compounded if ileum is also resected)

© 2016 Cengage Learning®

[a]The absorption of vitamins and minerals begins in the duodenum and continues throughout the length of the small intestine.

FIGURE 19-7 Nutrient Absorption and Consequences of Intestinal Surgeries

concentrated sweets (which attract fluids) or milk products if they worsen diarrhea. Vitamin and mineral supplementation can help to prevent deficiencies. The Case Study in Box 19-4 can help you review the material on short bowel syndrome.

IN SUMMARY

▌ Celiac disease is characterized by an abnormal immune response to gluten, resulting in malabsorption; a gluten-free diet is the primary treatment.

▌ Short bowel syndrome may result from major intestinal resections. Although intestinal adaptation can improve absorptive capacity over time, individuals with extensive resections may require lifelong parenteral nutrition support.

Case Study BOX 19-4 PATIENT WITH SHORT BOWEL SYNDROME

Judi Morel is a 28-year-old economist with an eight-year history of Crohn's disease. Judi is 5 feet 7 inches tall. Three years ago, she underwent a small bowel resection and remained free of active disease for two years. During that time, her symptoms subsided; she was able to tolerate most foods without any problem and gained weight. Ten months ago, Judi experienced a severe flare-up of her Crohn's disease. Since that time, she has lost 15 pounds and currently weighs 118 pounds. She has experienced severe abdominal pain and fatigue that have persisted despite aggressive medical management that included

intravenous nutrition. Five days ago, Judi underwent another resection, which left her with 40 percent of healthy small intestine. Her colon is intact. She is experiencing extensive diarrhea.

1. Describe the manifestations of Crohn's disease, and explain why surgery is sometimes performed as part of the treatment (review Chapter 18). Describe the complications of disease that may affect nutrient needs.

2. Using the BMI table in the back of the book, check the ideal weight range for a person of Judi's height. What

nutrition-related concerns are suggested by Judi's recent weight loss? What other nutrition problems did Judi probably experience as a consequence of Crohn's disease?

3. Discuss the complications that may follow an extensive intestinal resection. What factors may affect a person's ability to meet nutrient needs with an oral diet?

4. Describe the dietary progression recommended after an extensive intestinal resection. After Judi is able to eat solid foods, what factors may affect the type of diet that is recommended for her?

Nutrition Assessment Checklist FOR PEOPLE WITH MALABSORPTION DISORDERS

Medical History

Check the medical record for medical diagnoses of:

- Celiac disease
- Crohn's disease
- Chronic pancreatitis
- Cystic fibrosis
- Lactose intolerance
- Short bowel syndrome

Check for surgical procedures involving the GI tract, such as:

- Gastrectomy
- Gastric bypass surgery
- Intestinal bypass surgery
- Intestinal resections

Check for the following symptoms or complications:

- Anemia
- Bacterial overgrowth
- Bone disease
- Diarrhea, dehydration
- Fistulas
- Kidney stones
- Lactose intolerance
- Obstructions
- Poor growth, in children
- Steatorrhea

Medications

Check for medications or dietary supplements that may:

- Interfere with appetite or food intake
- Irritate the mucosal lining
- Reduce gastric acid secretion

Dietary Intake

Note the following problems and contact the dietitian if you suspect difficulties such as:

- Food intolerances
- Inadequate fluid intake
- Poor appetite or food intake

Anthropometric Data

Measure baseline height and weight. Address weight loss early to prevent malnutrition in patients with:

- Gastric or intestinal bypass surgeries
- Gastric or intestinal resections
- Malabsorption
- Severe or persistent diarrhea
- Steatorrhea

Laboratory Tests

Check laboratory tests for signs of dehydration, electrolyte imbalances, and nutrient deficiencies in patients with:

- Intestinal resections
- Malabsorption
- Severe or persistent diarrhea
- Steatorrhea

Physical Signs

Look for physical signs of:

- Dehydration
- Essential fatty acid and fat-soluble vitamin deficiencies
- Folate and vitamin B_{12} deficiencies
- Mineral deficiencies
- Protein-energy malnutrition

Clinical Applications

1. Using Table 19-2 on p. 515 as a guide, plan a day's menus for a diet containing approximately 50 grams of fat. Take care to make the meals both palatable and nutritious. How can these menus be improved using the suggestions in Box 19-1?

2. As stated in this chapter, the treatment of celiac disease is deceptively simple—eliminate wheat, barley, and rye, and possibly oats. Remaining on a gluten-free diet is more challenging than it appears, however.

   ▌ Randomly select 10 of your favorite snack and convenience foods. Take a trip to the grocery store, and check the labels of the products you selected to see if they would be allowed on a gluten-free diet. Keep in mind that the labels may not list all offending ingredients.

   ▌ Find acceptable substitutes for the products that are not allowed, either by substituting other foods or by checking for gluten-free products in the grocery store. If you have access to the Internet, you may want to investigate websites that advertise gluten-free products to get an idea of what's available.

Self Check

1. Possible causes of malabsorption include all of the following *except:*
   a. inflammatory bowel disease.
   b. pancreatic dysfunction.
   c. liver disease.
   d. flatulence.

2. The hydrogen breath test can help to diagnose:
   a. B vitamin deficiencies.
   b. fat malabsorption.
   c. carbohydrate malabsorption.
   d. pancreatic disorders.

3. Nutrition problems that may result from fat malabsorption include all of the following *except:*
   a. weight loss.
   b. essential amino acid deficiencies.
   c. bone loss.
   d. oxalate kidney stones.

4. Common nutrition problems associated with bacterial overgrowth in the stomach and small intestine include:
   a. sensitivity to gluten.
   b. fat malabsorption and vitamin B_{12} deficiency.
   c. constipation.
   d. permanent loss of digestive enzymes.

5. Lactose intolerance is a direct consequence of:
   a. insufficient lactase.
   b. milk allergy.
   c. fluid imbalance.
   d. pancreatic dysfunction.

6. The majority of chronic pancreatitis cases can be attributed to:
   a. bacterial and viral infections.
   b. gallstones.
   c. alcohol abuse.
   d. elevated triglyceride levels.

7. The most appropriate diet for a person with cystic fibrosis is a:
   a. high-kcalorie diet.
   b. high-fiber diet.
   c. gluten-free diet.
   d. fat-controlled diet.

8. Chronic pancreatitis and cystic fibrosis are both treated with:
   a. intestinal resection.
   b. postural drainage.
   c. enzyme replacement therapy.
   d. stool softeners.

9. A person on a gluten-free diet must avoid products containing:
   a. wheat, barley, and rye.
   b. lactose.
   c. excessive fat.
   d. corn, rice, and millet.

10. Despite the intestine's capacity for adaptation, removal of which section of the intestine will likely result in fat malabsorption and multiple nutrient deficiencies?
    a. Duodenum
    b. Jejunum
    c. Colon
    d. Ileum

Answers to these questions appear in Appendix H.

Notes

1. C. E. Semrad, Approach to the patient with diarrhea and malabsorption, in L. Goldman and A. I. Schafer, eds., *Goldman's Cecil Medicine* (Philadelphia: Saunders, 2012), pp. 895–913; J. S. Trier, Intestinal malabsorption, in N. J. Greenberger, ed., *Current Diagnosis and Treatment: Gastroenterology, Hepatology, and Endoscopy* (New York: McGraw-Hill Companies, 2012), pp. 237–257.

2. Trier, 2012.

3. Semrad, 2012.

4. S. Hertzler and coauthors, Nutrient considerations in lactose intolerance, in A. M. Coulston, C. J. Boushey, and M. G. Ferruzzi, eds., *Nutrition in the Prevention and Treatment of Disease* (London: Academic Press/Elsevier, 2013), pp. 757–772.

5. Hertzler and coauthors, 2013.

6. A. Szilagyi and coauthors, Differential impact of lactose/lactase phenotype on colonic microflora, *Canadian Journal of Gastroenterology* 24 (2010): 373–379.

7. B. U. Wu, D. L. Conwell, and P. A. Banks, Acute pancreatitis, in N. J. Greenberger, ed., *Current Diagnosis and Treatment: Gastroenterology, Hepatology, and Endoscopy* (New York: McGraw-Hill Companies, 2012), pp. 311–318.

8. Academy of Nutrition and Dietetics, *Nutrition Care Manual* (Chicago: Academy of Nutrition and Dietetics, 2014); C. E. Forsmark, Pancreatitis, in L. Goldman and A. I. Schafer, eds., *Goldman's Cecil Medicine* (Philadelphia: Saunders, 2012), pp. 937–944.

9. J. M. Mirtallo, International consensus guidelines for nutrition therapy in pancreatitis, *Journal of Parenteral and Enteral Nutrition* 36 (2012): 284–291.

10. Mirtallo, 2012.

11. Forsmark, 2012.

12. S. N. Duggan and K. C. Conlon, A practical guide to the nutritional management of chronic pancreatitis, *Practical Gastroenterology* (June 2013): 24–32.

13. Duggan and Conlon, 2013.

14. Forsmark, 2012; D. L. Conwell, B. Wu, and P. A. Banks, Chronic pancreatitis, in N. J. Greenberger, ed., *Current Diagnosis and Treatment: Gastroenterology, Hepatology, and Endoscopy* (New York: McGraw-Hill Companies, 2012), pp. 319–327.

15. F. J. Accurso, Cystic fibrosis, in L. Goldman and A. I. Schafer, eds., *Goldman's Cecil Medicine* (Philadelphia: Saunders, 2012), pp. 544–548.

16. C. L. Rogers, Nutritional management of the adult with cystic fibrosis—part I, *Practical Gastroenterology* (January 2013): 10–24.

17. Accurso, 2012.

18. Rogers, 2013.

19. A. Rubio-Tapia and coauthors, Prevalence of celiac disease in the United States, *American Journal of Gastroenterology* 107 (2012): 1538–1544.

20. K. N. Jeejeebhoy, Short bowel syndrome, in A. C. Ross and coeditors, eds., *Modern Nutrition in Health and Disease* (Baltimore: Lippincott Williams & Wilkins, 2014), pp. 1069–1079.

21. Jeejeebhoy, 2014.

LO 19.5 Describe the process of erythropoiesis and explain how nutrient deficiencies, diseases, or disease treatments may lead to anemia.

Anemia is usually defined as a significant reduction in the blood's red blood cell mass or hemoglobin content, which lowers the blood's oxygen-carrying capacity. It is frequently the first sign of illness and may be the disorder that initially drives an individual to seek medical attention. Anemia is associated with a great number of diseases and is common among hospital patients. Earlier chapters in this textbook describe some of the relationships between nutrient deficiencies and anemia. This Nutrition in Practice explains how and why anemia develops during the course of illness. The Glossary in Box NP19-1 defines the relevant terms.

How does anemia develop?

Anemia develops when red blood cells (also called *erythrocytes*) are unable to be produced in sufficient numbers, are too quickly destroyed, or are lost due to bleeding.[1] Because red blood cells contain the hemoglobin that supplies oxygen to tissues, their absence can result in fatigue and reduced stamina. The deficiency of oxygen in tissues is the main stimulus for the production of additional red blood cells. Table NP19-1 provides an overview of some different categories of anemia and their underlying causes.

TABLE NP19-1 Types of Anemia

Type of Anemia	General Mechanism
Anemia of chronic disease	Reduced iron availability due to disease or inflammatory processes; results in reduced red blood cell (RBC) production and increased RBC degradation
Aplastic anemia	Failure of stem cells to develop into RBCs; may be due to immune disease, viruses, drugs and toxins, or genetic defects
Folate- or vitamin B_{12}-deficiency anemia	Reduced availability of folate or vitamin B_{12}, which are required for DNA synthesis and cell division; results in large, immature RBCs (megaloblastic anemia)
Hemolytic anemia	Premature destruction of red blood cells; results in shortened RBC life span and fewer RBCs
Hemorrhagic anemia	Blood loss; causes reduction in circulating RBCs
Iron-deficiency anemia	Reduced iron availability; interferes with hemoglobin production and results in small, hypochromic RBCs (microcytic anemia)
Sickle cell anemia	Genetic mutation that results in altered hemoglobin molecules; causes production of abnormal, sickle-shaped RBCs
Thalassemia	Genetic mutation that reduces hemoglobin synthesis; results in reduced RBC production

© 2016 Cengage Learning®

BOX NP19-1 GLOSSARY

anemia of chronic disease: anemia that develops in persons with chronic illness; may resemble iron-deficiency anemia even though iron stores are often adequate. Also called *anemia of chronic inflammation*.

aplastic anemia: anemia characterized by the inability of bone marrow to produce adequate numbers of blood cells. Causes include drug toxicity, viruses, and genetic defects.

erythropoiesis (eh-RIH-throh-poy-EE-sis)**:** production of red blood cells within the bone marrow.

erythropoietin (eh-RIH-throh-POY-eh-tin)**:** a hormone produced by kidney cells that stimulates red blood cell production.

hemolytic (hee-mo-LIH-tic) **anemia:** anemia characterized by the breakdown of red blood cells.

megaloblastic anemia: anemia characterized by large (macrocytic), immature red blood cells, as occurs in folate or vitamin B_{12} deficiency; also called *macrocytic anemia*.

microcytic anemia: anemia characterized by small, hypochromic (pale) red blood cells, as occurs in iron deficiency.

peripheral blood smear: a blood sample spread on a glass slide and stained for analysis under a microscope. *Peripheral* refers to the use of circulating blood rather than tissue blood.

reticulocytes: immature red blood cells released into blood by bone marrow.

How are red blood cells produced?

The production of red blood cells (**erythropoiesis**) takes place in the bone marrow, a soft tissue found in certain types of bone. The process begins when kidney cells sense the low oxygen content of blood and release the hormone **erythropoietin** (see Figure NP19-1, p. 528). Erythropoietin travels to the bone marrow, where it stimulates precursor cells (stem cells) to divide and differentiate into red blood cells. The cells that are released from the bone marrow are immature red blood cells called **reticulocytes.** Reticulocytes develop into mature red blood cells over a 24- to 48-hour period while they circulate in the bloodstream. Reticulocytes generally constitute 0.5 to 1.5 percent of the red blood cell population.[2]

Which nutrient deficiencies can interfere with red blood cell production?

The nutrient deficiencies that most often upset red blood cell production are those of iron, folate, and vitamin B_{12}. Iron is required for hemoglobin production, and deficiency results in **microcytic anemia,** characterized by small, hypochromic cells (see pp. 240–241). Vitamin B_{12} and folate participate in DNA synthesis, and deficiency of either nutrient leads to **megaloblastic anemia,** characterized by large (macrocytic), immature cells (see pp. 208–209). Other nutrient

FIGURE NP19-1 Erythropoiesis

Kidney

① When the kidneys detect reduced oxygen in the blood, they secrete the hormone erythropoietin.

Erythropoietin

Bone Marrow

② Erythropoietin stimulates erythropoiesis (red blood cell production) in the bone marrow.

③ Immature red blood cells (called reticulocytes) are released into the blood.

Reticulocytes (immature red blood cells)

④ Reticulocytes mature into red blood cells over a 24- to 48-hour period.

Erythrocytes (red blood cells)

© Cengage Learning®

deficiencies may cause anemia, although not as frequently. Vitamin E helps to maintain cell membrane integrity, and its deficiency is associated with **hemolytic anemia** (red blood cell breakdown). Vitamin B_6 plays a role in hemoglobin production, and a deficiency may occasionally cause microcytic anemia. Vitamin C supports blood vessel integrity; fragile and bleeding capillaries may result from its deficiency. Protein-energy malnutrition leads to anemia because red blood cell development depends on protein synthesis. Although nutrient deficiencies may result from dietary inadequacy, they can also arise during the course of illness due to the effects of disease on intestinal absorption, nutrient metabolism, and nutrient losses.

How can illnesses cause the nutrient deficiencies that lead to anemia?

There are numerous ways in which illnesses can lead to iron, folate, or vitamin B_{12} deficiencies, the main causes of the nutritional anemias. Blood loss, common to many illnesses, is a primary cause of iron deficiency. Some illnesses may result in a reduction in food intake, as discussed throughout the clinical chapters. The liver's stores of iron and vitamin B_{12} are often adequate to prevent deficiencies during transient illnesses, but reserves of folate are limited; thus, a folate deficiency can develop within a few months if dietary intakes are low. If several nutrient deficiencies occur simultaneously, it may be difficult to identify the cause of anemia using standard blood tests (see Appendix E) because both megaloblastic anemia and microcytic anemia may be present.

Which illnesses are associated with blood loss?

Gastrointestinal conditions are often associated with bleeding; examples include peptic ulcers, inflammatory bowel diseases, and gastrointestinal varices (enlarged veins) that develop in advanced

liver disease. Excessive bleeding can also accompany coagulation disorders, which are often due to liver disease, genetic defects, or vitamin K deficiency. Frequent blood draws or surgical procedures can contribute to blood loss and result in iron deficiency. Unfortunately, slow, chronic bleeding is sometimes difficult to identify before anemia develops.

How do malabsorption disorders contribute to the development of anemia?

Chapters 18 and 19 explain how disorders that damage the small intestine can lead to nutrient malabsorption. Diseases like Crohn's disease and celiac disease can destroy the intestinal mucosa and reduce the absorption of all nutrients. Iron is primarily absorbed in the duodenum and upper jejunum, and its absorption is impaired by conditions that reduce hydrochloric acid secretion or result in surgical resection (removal) of the upper intestine. Resection of the stomach or ileum can hasten the onset of vitamin B_{12} deficiency because both organs have roles in vitamin B_{12} absorption: recall from Chapter 8 that the stomach produces a protein called *intrinsic factor* that transports vitamin B_{12} through the small intestine, and that the ileum is the site of vitamin B_{12} absorption.

Why is anemia present during many chronic illnesses, even when the illnesses are not accompanied by nutrient deficiencies or bleeding disorders?

Chronic disease itself can cause anemia, and anemia is sometimes the initial sign that chronic disease is present. In fact, the **anemia of chronic disease** is the most common type of anemia affecting hospitalized patients and patients with chronic illnesses.[3] This type of anemia usually occurs in individuals who have inflammatory diseases, autoimmune diseases, acute and chronic infections, chronic kidney disease, or cancers. Although often a mild form of anemia, it can progress and become severe enough to require blood transfusions.

The anemia of chronic disease is characterized by alterations both in the distribution of iron among tissues and in the rates of red blood cell production and destruction.[4] During chronic illness, inflammatory mediators induce the production of the protein *hepcidin*, which blocks the release of iron from storage and thereby renders iron unavailable for red blood cell production. Furthermore, hepcidin inhibits iron's release from intestinal cells into the blood and therefore interferes with iron absorption. Finally, inflammatory processes cause red blood cells to be degraded more quickly than usual, and the reduced production of red blood cells cannot keep pace. Eventually, outright iron deficiency may be a consequence of the impaired iron absorption.

How is the anemia of chronic disease diagnosed?

Blood tests help to distinguish between the anemia of chronic disease and iron-deficiency anemia (see Table NP19-2). The combination of low serum iron and low total iron-binding capacity suggests the presence of the anemia of chronic disease rather than iron deficiency. In addition, serum ferritin levels may be normal or elevated during chronic illness, whereas they are typically low in iron deficiency. Diagnosis is more complicated if both types of anemia are present.

Can medications cause anemia?

Yes, anemia is among the adverse effects that may result from medication use. Various medications can disrupt nutrient metabolism, impair blood coagulation and erythropoiesis, or increase red blood cell destruction. Because the life span of red blood cells is about 120 days, the long-term use of such medications is more likely to result in anemia than short-term use.

How do medications alter nutrient metabolism?

There are numerous ways in which medications can alter nutrient metabolism; the most common are listed in Table 15-2 on p. 424. As an example, a number of medications are known to influence the absorption or metabolism of folate and lead to megaloblastic anemia. Sulfasalazine (used in ulcerative colitis) and pyrimethamine

(an antimalarial) inhibit folate absorption, and methotrexate (an immunosuppressant) and phenytoin (an anticonvulsant) interfere with folate metabolism.[5] If a medication is known to result in deficiency, nutrient supplementation is usually recommended as an adjunct therapy.

How do medications impair blood coagulation?

Anticoagulants, which are prescribed specifically to reduce blood clotting, sometimes lead to excessive bleeding. These medications work by interfering with one of the processes involved in blood clotting, such as platelet function, vitamin K function, or the synthesis of clotting proteins. Other than anticoagulants, a large number of other drugs can impair coagulation, including commonly used drugs such as aspirin and other nonsteroidal anti-inflammatory drugs. The anticoagulant effects may be augmented if several of these drugs are used simultaneously. The slow, chronic bleeding that sometimes develops may go unnoticed until excessive blood loss has occurred.

Which categories of drugs inhibit erythropoiesis?

The categories of drugs that can inhibit erythropoiesis include anticonvulsants, antibiotics, antidiabetic drugs, antihistamines, diuretics, antithyroid drugs, and anticancer agents.[6] The anemia that occurs when the bone marrow fails to produce adequate numbers of blood cells is called **aplastic anemia.** Aplastic anemia can also be caused by viral infections, exposure to toxins, and genetic defects.

How can medications cause blood cell destruction?

Some patients may develop hemolytic anemia as a result of drug interactions with red blood cells. For example, a drug may implant itself into the red blood cell membrane and elicit an antibody response that destroys the cell.[7] Drugs that may cause this response include cephalosporin (an antibiotic) and fludarabine (an anti-leukemia agent). Withdrawal of these drugs can eventually reverse the anemia, and sometimes medications are given to suppress the immune response.

With all the possible ways in which anemia can develop, how can its cause be determined?

Identifying the cause of anemia is often quite challenging. In some cases, anemia may be a well-known consequence of disease, as when renal failure impairs the synthesis of the hormone erythropoietin. When anemia develops rapidly, blood loss is often the cause, whereas a more gradual onset suggests malnutrition, chronic illness, or slow, chronic bleeding. As mentioned earlier, the results of laboratory tests provide valuable clues, although conditions such as dehydration and inflammation can influence the values. Laboratory results are especially difficult to analyze if several disturbances are present simultaneously. A **peripheral blood smear** (see Figure NP19-2, p. 530) is often used to study abnormalities in red blood cell shape and may also reveal an underlying cause.

Anemia is a disorder associated with many different diseases, and it may also be caused by disease treatment. When it occurs during illness, its causes must be investigated before it leads to

TABLE NP19-2 Laboratory Tests for Evaluating Iron Deficiency and Anemia of Chronic Disease

Laboratory Test	Effect of Iron Deficiency	Effect of Chronic Disease
Red blood cell (RBC) size and number	Microcytic; reduced RBC count	Normocytic or microcytic; reduced RBC count
Serum iron	Low	Low
Serum ferritin	Low	Normal or elevated
Serum transferrin	Elevated	Low
Total iron-binding capacity	High	Normal or low
Bone marrow iron	Low	Normal or elevated

complications that worsen the prognosis. The medical history, blood tests, and peripheral blood smears may all help to determine the reasons why anemia has developed.

FIGURE NP19-2 Peripheral Blood Smear

A peripheral blood smear provides information about the number and shape of blood cells. The blood smear shown here includes two white blood cells (a basophil and a neutrophil) among the group of healthy red blood cells.

Carolina Biological/Encyclopedia/Corbis

Notes

1. A. E. Lichtin, Approach to the patient with anemia, in R. S. Porter and J. L. Kaplan, eds., *Merck Manual of Diagnosis and Therapy* (Whitehouse Station, NJ: Merck Sharp and Dohme Corp., 2011), pp. 918–924.

2. Lichtin, 2011.

3. G. D. Ginder, Microcytic and hypochromic anemias, in L. Goldman and A. I. Schafer, eds., *Goldman's Cecil Medicine* (Philadelphia: Saunders, 2012), pp. 1039–1044.

4. Ginder, 2012.

5. A. C. Antony, Megaloblastic anemias, in L. Goldman and A. I. Schafer, eds., *Goldman's Cecil Medicine* (Philadelphia: Saunders, 2012), pp. 1075–1083.

6. G. C. Bagby, Aplastic anemia and related disorders, in L. Goldman and A. I. Schafer, eds., *Goldman's Cecil Medicine* (Philadelphia: Saunders, 2012), pp. 1083–1090.

7. R. S. Schwartz, Autoimmune and intravascular hemolytic anemias, in L. Goldman and A. I. Schafer, eds., *Goldman's Cecil Medicine* (Philadelphia: Saunders, 2012), pp. 1045–1052.

20

Nutrition Therapy for Liver and Gallbladder Diseases

20.1 Fatty Liver and Hepatitis

LO 20.1 Identify potential causes of fatty liver and hepatitis and describe the medical or nutrition care that may be helpful for these conditions.

20.2 Cirrhosis

LO 20.2 Discuss the potential causes and consequences of liver cirrhosis and describe its medical treatments and nutrition therapies.

20.3 Liver Transplantation

LO 20.3 Identify the potential health concerns of patients who undergo liver transplantation.

20.4 Gallstone Disease

LO 20.4 Explain why gallstones develop and discuss the major risk factors and treatment approaches for gallstone disease.

20.5 Nutrition in Practice: Alcohol in Health and Disease

LO 20.5 Describe how alcohol is metabolized in the body and discuss the potential risks and benefits associated with its use.

The liver is the most metabolically active organ in the body. It plays a central role in processing, storing, and redistributing the nutrients provided by the foods we eat. The liver also produces the bile that emulsifies fat during digestion; between meals, this bile is stored and concentrated in the gallbladder. The liver synthesizes most of the proteins that circulate in plasma, including albumin, blood clotting proteins, and transport proteins. In addition, the liver detoxifies drugs and alcohol and processes excess nitrogen so that it can be safely excreted as urea. If damage or disease hinders the liver's ability to perform its numerous functions, the effects on health and nutrition status can be profound.

Liver disease progresses slowly. Its primary symptom, fatigue, often goes unnoticed. Other symptoms may be so mild that complications develop before liver disease is diagnosed. Once liver disease is recognized, health practitioners emphasize the need to preserve the remaining liver function, as the liver can regenerate some healthy tissue, improving the prognosis. Preventing additional damage is the principal means of avoiding liver failure or transplantation.

20.1 Fatty Liver and Hepatitis

LO 20.1 Identify potential causes of fatty liver and hepatitis and describe the medical or nutrition care that may be helpful for these conditions.

Fatty liver and hepatitis are the two most common disorders affecting the liver. Although both conditions may be mild and are usually reversible, each may progress to more serious illness and eventually cause liver damage.

Fatty Liver

Fatty liver is an accumulation of fat in liver tissue. Ordinarily, the liver's excess triglycerides are packaged into very-low-density lipoproteins (VLDL) and exported to the bloodstream. Fatty liver represents an imbalance between the amount of fat produced in the liver or picked up from the blood and the amount the liver uses or exports to the blood via VLDL. Fatty liver is estimated to affect 20 percent or more of the adult population in the United States.[1]

Fatty liver is a clinical finding that is common to many conditions. It may be caused by defects in metabolism, excessive alcohol ingestion, or exposure to various drugs and toxins. In cases unrelated to alcohol, insulin resistance (reduced sensitivity to insulin in liver, muscle, and adipose cells) is the primary risk factor; thus, fatty liver frequently accompanies diabetes mellitus, metabolic syndrome, and obesity. Other causes of fatty liver include protein-energy malnutrition and long-term total parenteral nutrition.

Consequences of Fatty Liver In many individuals, fatty liver is asymptomatic and causes no harm. In other cases, it may be associated with inflammation (**steatohepatitis**), liver enlargement (**hepatomegaly**), and fatigue. If liver damage and scarring develop, fatty liver may progress to cirrhosis (discussed in a later section), liver failure, or liver cancer.[2]

Fatty liver is the most common cause of abnormal liver enzyme levels in the blood. Laboratory findings typically include elevated blood concentrations of the liver enzymes ALT and AST (see Table 20-3, p. 535), as well as increased levels of triglycerides, cholesterol, and glucose.

Treatment of Fatty Liver The usual treatment for fatty liver is to eliminate the factors that cause it. For example, if fatty liver is due to alcohol abuse or drug treatment, it may improve after the patient discontinues use of the substance. In patients with elevated blood lipids, fatty liver may improve after blood lipid levels are lowered. An appropriate treatment for obese or diabetic patients might be weight reduction,

fatty liver: an accumulation of fat in liver tissue; also called *hepatic steatosis* (STEE-ah-TOE-sis).

▪ *hepatic* = pertaining to the liver

▪ *steato* = fat

steatohepatitis (STEE-ah-to-HEP-ah-TYE-tis)**:** liver inflammation that is associated with fatty liver.

hepatomegaly (HEP-ah-toe-MEG-ah-lee)**:** enlargement of the liver.

TABLE 20-1 Features of Hepatitis Viruses

Hepatitis Virus	Major Mode of Transmission	New Cases (United States, 2011)	Chronic Disease Rate (% of cases)	Chronic Cases[a] (United States, 2011)	Vaccine
A	Fecal-oral	2,800	None	0	Available
B	Bloodborne, sexual transmission	18,800	Newborn infants: 90% Children (1 to 5 years): 30–50% Adults: 5%	0.7–1.4 million	Available
C	Bloodborne	16,500	75–85%	2.7–3.9 million	None

[a]Chronic cases of hepatitis are those that last 6 months or longer.

Note: There are fewer new cases of hepatitis C virus (HCV) infection than of hepatitis B virus (HBV) infection each year, but more HCV cases become chronic. Therefore, there are more HCV carriers than HBV carriers.

Source: Centers for Disease Control and Prevention, *Viral hepatitis surveillance: United States, 2011* (Atlanta: U.S. Department of Health and Human Services, 2013).

increased physical activity, or medications that improve insulin sensitivity. Rapid weight loss should be discouraged, however, because it may accelerate the progression of liver disease.[3] Note that lifestyle modifications are not always successful in reversing fatty liver, especially in patients who lack the usual risk factors.

Hepatitis

Hepatitis, a condition of liver inflammation, results from damage to liver tissue. Most often, the damage is caused by infection with specific viruses, designated by the letters *A*, *B*, *C*, *D*, and *E*. Other causes include excessive alcohol intake, fatty liver disease, autoimmune disease, and exposure to some drugs, herbal substances, and toxic chemicals. Long-term hepatitis can lead to cirrhosis (discussed in a later section) and liver cancer.

Viral Hepatitis Acute hepatitis is most often caused by infection with hepatitis viruses A, B, or C (see Table 20-1). Specific features of these viruses include the following:

▌ *Hepatitis A virus* (HAV) is primarily spread via fecal-oral transmission, which usually involves the ingestion of foods or beverages that have been contaminated with fecal material. Outbreaks of HAV infection are often associated with floods and other natural disasters, when inadequately treated sewage contaminates water supplies. Vaccinations against HAV are recommended for high-risk individuals, such as international travelers, food handlers, and newborn infants. HAV infection usually resolves within a few months and does not cause chronic illness or permanent liver damage.

▌ *Hepatitis B virus* (HBV) is transmitted by infected blood or needles, by sexual contact with an infected person, or from mother to infant during childbirth. A major global health concern, HBV has infected about one-third of the world population, although chronic illness develops in less than 10 percent of cases.[4] Vaccinations are currently recommended for newborn infants and children, health-care workers, dialysis patients, recipients of blood products, sex partners of infected persons, and users of injected drugs.

▌ *Hepatitis C virus* (HCV) is spread via infected blood or needles but is not readily spread by sexual contact or childbirth. Most HCV cases progress to chronic illness, and currently HCV is the leading cause of chronic liver disease in the United States.[5] No vaccine is available to protect against HCV infection. Preventive measures include blood donor screening, viral inactivation of blood products, infection control practices in health care settings, and risk reduction counseling to high-risk individuals.

Symptoms and Signs of Hepatitis The effects of hepatitis depend on the cause and severity of the condition. Individuals with mild or chronic cases are often asymptomatic. The onset of acute hepatitis may be accompanied by fatigue, malaise, nausea, anorexia, and pain in the liver area. The liver is often slightly enlarged and

hepatitis (hep-ah-TYE-tis)**:** inflammation of the liver.

FIGURE 20-1 Jaundice is a yellow discoloration of the tissues that is most easily seen in the sclera. Jaundice results when liver dysfunction impairs the metabolism of bilirubin, a breakdown product of hemoglobin that is normally excreted in bile and urine. Accumulation of bilirubin in the bloodstream leads to yellow discoloration of tissues.

jaundice (JAWN-dis)**:** yellow discoloration of the skin and eyes due to an accumulation of bilirubin, a breakdown product of hemoglobin that normally exits the body via bile secretions.

cirrhosis (sih-ROE-sis)**:** an advanced stage of liver disease in which extensive scarring replaces healthy liver tissue, causing impaired liver function and liver failure.

pruritis: itchy skin.

hepatic portal vein: the blood vessel that conducts nutrient-rich blood from the digestive tract to the liver.

tender. **Jaundice** (yellow discoloration of tissues) may develop, causing yellowing of the skin, urine, and sclera (see Figure 20-1). Other symptoms of hepatitis may include fever, muscle weakness, joint pain, and skin rashes. Serum levels of the liver enzymes ALT and AST are typically elevated. Chronic hepatitis can cause complications that are typical of liver cirrhosis and may lead to liver cancer.

Treatment of Hepatitis Hepatitis is treated with supportive care, such as bed rest (if necessary) and an appropriate diet. Hepatitis patients should avoid substances that irritate the liver, such as alcohol, drugs, and dietary supplements that cause liver damage. Hepatitis A infection usually resolves without the use of medications, whereas antiviral drugs may be used to treat HBV and HCV infections. Nonviral forms of hepatitis may be treated with anti-inflammatory and immunosuppressant drugs. Hospitalization is not required for hepatitis unless other medical conditions or complications hamper recovery.

Nutrition care varies according to a patient's symptoms and nutrition status. Most individuals require no dietary changes. Those with anorexia or abdominal discomfort may find small, frequent meals easier to tolerate. Patients with persistent vomiting may require fluid and electrolyte replacement. Malnourished individuals need to consume adequate protein and energy to replenish nutrient stores; the diet should include about 1.0 to 1.2 grams of protein per kilogram of body weight each day.[6] Oral supplements can be helpful for improving nutrient intakes.

IN SUMMARY

■ Fatty liver can result from metabolic defects, exposure to some drugs and toxins, or excessive alcohol intake. Insulin resistance is a primary risk factor for fatty liver; thus, the condition often accompanies diabetes mellitus, metabolic syndrome, and obesity. Hepatitis is frequently caused by viral infection but can also result from alcohol abuse, drug toxicity, and other causes.

■ Although fatty liver is often benign, hepatitis can become chronic and lead to cirrhosis and liver cancer. Hepatitis treatment involves supportive care, such as bed rest, elimination of liver toxins, and dietary measures that maintain or improve nutrition status.

20.2 Cirrhosis

LO 20.2 Discuss the potential causes and consequences of liver cirrhosis and describe its medical treatments and nutrition therapies.

Cirrhosis is a late stage of chronic liver disease. Long-term liver disease gradually destroys liver tissue, leading to scarring (fibrosis) in some regions and small areas of regenerated, healthy tissue in others (see Figure 20-2). As the disease progresses, the

Normal liver tissue is smooth and has a regular texture.

A cirrhotic liver has an irregular, nodular appearance. The nodules represent clusters of regenerating cells within the damaged liver tissue.

FIGURE 20-2 Cirrhosis of the Liver

scarring becomes more extensive, leaving fewer areas of healthy tissue. A cirrhotic liver is often shrunken in size and has an irregular, nodular appearance. Cirrhosis is characterized by impaired liver function and may eventually result in liver failure. Together, chronic liver disease and cirrhosis rank as the 12th leading cause of death in the United States.[7]

The chief causes of cirrhosis in the United States are chronic hepatitis C infection and alcoholic liver disease, followed by nonalcoholic fatty liver disease and chronic hepatitis B infection.[8] Additional causes include other types of chronic hepatitis, drug-induced liver injury, some inherited metabolic disorders, and bile duct blockages, which cause bile acids to accumulate to toxic levels in the liver (see Table 20-2).

Consequences of Cirrhosis

Many patients with liver disease remain asymptomatic for years. Because liver damage progresses slowly, the effects of chronic liver disease may be subtle at first. Initial symptoms are usually nonspecific and may include fatigue, malaise, anorexia, and weight loss. Later, the decline in liver function can lead to metabolic disturbances: patients may develop anemia, bruise easily, and be more susceptible to infections. If bile obstruction occurs, jaundice, fat malabsorption, and **pruritis** (itchy skin) are likely. The physical changes in liver tissue may interfere with blood flow, causing fluid to accumulate in blood vessels and body tissues. Advanced cirrhosis can disrupt kidney, lung, and brain function, and is usually associated with malnutrition. Figure 20-3 illustrates some common clinical effects of liver cirrhosis.

Table 20-3 lists laboratory tests that are used to monitor the extent of liver damage. Serum liver enzyme levels are elevated in liver disease because the injured liver tissue releases the enzymes into the bloodstream. Serum levels of bilirubin may be increased if the liver is too damaged to process it or if bile ducts are blocked and prevent its excretion. The impaired synthesis of plasma proteins by the liver reduces albumin levels and extends blood-clotting time. Liver damage also reduces the conversion of ammonia to urea, causing ammonia levels in the blood to rise.

Portal Hypertension A large volume of blood normally flows through the liver. The **hepatic portal vein** and hepatic artery together supply approximately 1500 milliliters (about 1.5 quarts) of blood each minute

TABLE 20-2 Causes of Cirrhosis

Alcoholic liver disease

Autoimmune hepatitis

Bile duct obstructions
- Biliary cirrhosis
- Cystic fibrosis

Drug-induced liver injury

Metabolic disorders
- Galactosemia
- Glycogen storage diseases
- Hemochromatosis (causes excessive liver iron)
- Wilson's disease (causes excessive liver copper)

Nonalcoholic fatty liver disease

Viral hepatitis
- Hepatitis B
- Hepatitis C

© 2016 Cengage Learning®

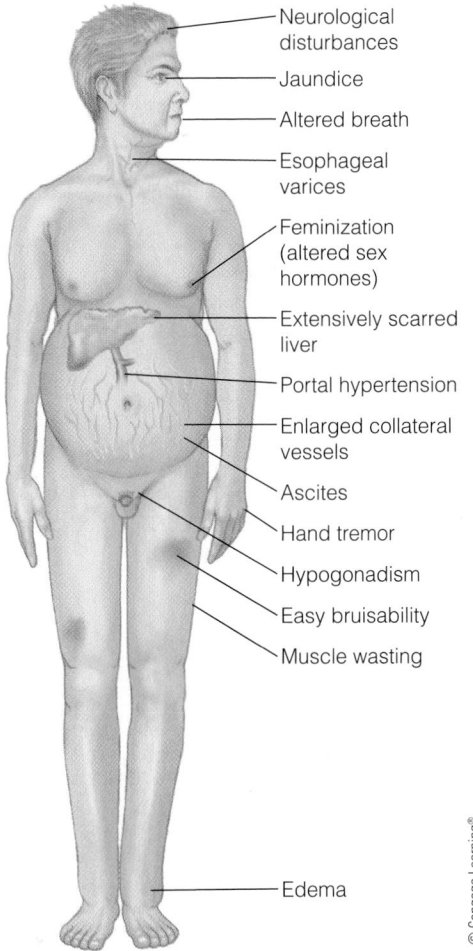

- Neurological disturbances
- Jaundice
- Altered breath
- Esophageal varices
- Feminization (altered sex hormones)
- Extensively scarred liver
- Portal hypertension
- Enlarged collateral vessels
- Ascites
- Hand tremor
- Hypogonadism
- Easy bruisability
- Muscle wasting
- Edema

© 2016 Cengage Learning®

FIGURE 20-3 Clinical Effects of Liver Cirrhosis

TABLE 20-3 Laboratory Tests for Evaluation of Liver Disease

Laboratory Test	Normal Ranges (serum)	Values in Liver Disease
Alanine aminotransferase (ALT)	Male: 10–40 U/L Female: 7–35 U/L	Increased
Albumin	3.4–4.8 g/dL	Decreased
Alkaline phosphatase	25–100 U/L	Normal or increased
Ammonia	15–45 µg N/dL	Increased
Aspartate aminotransferase (AST)	10–30 U/L	Increased
Bilirubin (total)	0.3–1.2 mg/dL	Increased
Blood urea nitrogen (BUN)	6–20 mg/dL	Normal or decreased
Gamma-glutamyl transpeptidase (GGT)	Male: 2–30 U/L Female: 1–24 U/L	Increased
Prothrombin time[a]	11–15 seconds	Prolonged

© 2016 Cengage Learning®

[a] The test for prothrombin time evaluates the clotting ability of blood.

Note: U/L = units per liter; dL = deciliter; µg = micrograms; N = nitrogen

FIGURE 20-4 Esophageal varices, such as those shown here, may protrude into the lumen and be vulnerable to rupture and bleeding.

FIGURE 20-5 Ascites can be caused by various illnesses, but cirrhosis is the underlying cause in most patients with the condition.

portal hypertension: elevated blood pressure in the hepatic portal vein due to obstructed blood flow through the liver and a greater inflow of portal blood.

collateral vessels: blood vessels that enlarge or newly form to allow an alternative pathway for diverted blood.

varices (VAH-rih-seez)**:** abnormally dilated blood vessels (singular: *varix*).

ascites (ah-SIGH-teez)**:** an abnormal accumulation of fluid in the abdominal cavity.

sinusoids: the small capillary-like passages that carry blood through liver tissue.

hepatic encephalopathy (en-sef-ah-LOP-ah-thie)**:** a neurological complication of advanced liver disease that is characterized by changes in personality, mood, behavior, mental ability, and motor functions.

▪ *encephalo* = brain

▪ *pathy* = disease

hepatic coma: loss of consciousness resulting from severe liver disease.

to the extensive network of vessels in the liver. The scarred tissue of a cirrhotic liver impedes the flow of blood, three-fourths of which is supplied by the hepatic portal vein. The restricted blood flow within the liver (and increased blood flow in nearby arteries*) results in a greater volume of portal blood, which causes a rise in blood pressure in the portal vein known as **portal hypertension.**

Collateral Vessels and Gastroesophageal Varices When portal blood flow is impeded, the blood is forced backward into nearby veins and then diverted to the systemic circulation via **collateral vessels,** which develop and expand throughout the gastrointestinal (GI) tract and in regions near the abdominal wall. As portal pressure builds, some of these collaterals can become enlarged and engorged with blood, forming abnormally dilated vessels called **varices** (see Figure 20-4). The varices that develop in the esophagus *(esophageal varices)* and stomach *(gastric varices)* are vulnerable to rupture because they have thin walls and often bulge into the lumen. If ruptured, they can cause massive bleeding that is sometimes fatal. The blood loss is exacerbated by the liver's reduced production of blood-clotting factors.

Ascites Within 10 years of disease onset, about 50 percent of cirrhosis patients develop **ascites,** an accumulation of fluid in the abdominal cavity (see Figure 20-5). The development of ascites indicates that liver damage has reached a critical stage, as half of patients with ascites die within 5 years.[9] Ascites is primarily a consequence of portal hypertension, sodium and water retention in the kidneys, and reduced albumin synthesis in the diseased liver. As a result of portal hypertension, the distorted blood flow elsewhere in the body alters kidney function, leading to sodium and water retention and an accumulation of body fluid. The elevated pressure within the liver's small blood vessels (**sinusoids**) causes fluid to leak into lymphatic vessels and, ultimately, the abdominal cavity. The movement of water into the abdomen is exacerbated by low levels of serum albumin, a protein that helps to retain fluid in blood vessels. Ascites can cause abdominal discomfort and early satiety, which contribute to malnutrition. Because ascites can raise the body's water weight considerably, weight changes may be difficult to interpret.

Hepatic Encephalopathy Advanced liver disease often leads to **hepatic encephalopathy,** a disorder characterized by abnormal neurological functioning. Signs of hepatic encephalopathy include adverse changes in personality, behavior, mood, mental ability, and motor functions (see Table 20-4). At worst, amnesia, unresponsiveness, and **hepatic coma** may develop. Although hepatic encephalopathy is fully reversible with medical treatment, the prognosis is poor when it progresses to the advanced stages.

The exact causes of hepatic encephalopathy remain elusive, although elevated blood ammonia levels are thought to play a key role in its development due to ammonia's

TABLE 20-4 Clinical Features of Hepatic Encephalopathy

Early Stages	Middle Stages	Later Stages
▪ Personality changes	▪ Mood and behavior changes	▪ Confusion, amnesia
▪ Short attention span	▪ Disorientation	▪ Somnolence to semi-stupor
▪ Depression, irritability	▪ Lethargy	▪ Involuntary eye movements
▪ Lack of coordination	▪ Slurred speech	▪ Muscular rigidity
▪ Tremor	▪ Pronounced tremor	▪ Abnormal reflexes
▪ Sleep disturbances	▪ Changes in sleep–wake cycle	▪ Coma

*Restricted blood flow within the liver stimulates the release of vasodilators—and therefore, increased blood flow—in nearby arteries.

TABLE 20-5 Possible Causes of Malnutrition in Liver Disease

Mechanism	Examples
Reduced nutrient intake	Abdominal discomfort, altered mental status, altered taste sensation, anorexia, early satiety (due to ascites), effects of medications (including GI disturbances and taste changes), fasting for medical procedures, fatigue, nausea and vomiting, dietary restrictions
Malabsorption or nutrient losses	Diarrhea, effects of medications (including malabsorption and nutrient losses from diuretic use), fat malabsorption (due to reduced bile flow), GI bleeding, vomiting
Altered metabolism or increased nutrient needs	Hypermetabolism, impaired protein synthesis, infections or inflammation, muscle catabolism, reduced nutrient storage and metabolism in the liver

neurotoxicity. Other substances that may accumulate in brain tissue and disturb brain function include sulfur compounds, naturally occurring benzodiazepines, short-chain fatty acids, and manganese.[10] Some research shows that severe liver damage may lead to reduced serum levels of the **branched-chain amino acids** and increased levels of the **aromatic amino acids,** which may alter the types of neurotransmitters produced in the brain.[11] Most likely, a combination of abnormalities contributes to the disruption in neurological functioning.

Elevated Ammonia Levels Much of the body's free ammonia is produced by bacterial action on unabsorbed dietary protein in the colon. Normally, the liver extracts this ammonia from portal blood and converts it to urea, which is then excreted by the kidneys. In advanced liver disease, the liver is unable to process the ammonia sufficiently. In addition, much of the ammonia-laden portal blood bypasses the liver by way of collateral vessels and reaches the general blood circulation, causing a substantial increase in the ammonia that reaches brain tissue. Although blood ammonia levels do not correlate well with the degree of neurological impairment in hepatic encephalopathy, ammonia-reducing medications can successfully reverse the neurological symptoms.[12]

Malnutrition and Wasting Most patients with advanced cirrhosis develop protein-energy malnutrition and experience some degree of wasting. Malnutrition is usually caused by a combination of factors (see Table 20-5). Patients may consume less food due to reduced appetite, GI symptoms, early satiety associated with ascites, or fatigue. If the diet is restricted in sodium (to treat ascites), foods may seem unpalatable. Fat malabsorption is common due to reduced bile availability, which may lead to steatorrhea and deficiencies of the fat-soluble vitamins and some minerals. Additional nutrient losses may result from diarrhea, vomiting, and GI bleeding. If cirrhosis is a consequence of alcohol abuse, multiple nutrient deficiencies may be present.

Treatment of Cirrhosis

Medical treatment for cirrhosis aims to correct the underlying cause of disease and prevent or treat complications. Supportive care, including an appropriate diet, abstinence from alcohol, and avoidance of liver toxins, promotes recovery and helps to prevent further damage. Antiviral medications may be prescribed to treat viral infections. Patients should be screened and treated for life-threatening complications, such as gastroesophageal varices and liver cancer. Liver transplantation may be necessary in advanced cirrhosis.

Medications can effectively treat many of the complications that accompany cirrhosis. Individuals with portal hypertension and varices may be given propranolol (Inderal) or octreotide (Sandostatin), which reduce portal blood pressure and bleeding risk. Diuretics can help to control portal hypertension and ascites; common examples

branched-chain amino acids: the essential amino acids leucine, isoleucine, and valine, which have side groups with a branched structure.

aromatic amino acids: the amino acids phenylalanine, tyrosine, and tryptophan, which have carbon rings in their side groups.

BOX 20-1 DIET-DRUG INTERACTIONS

Check this table for notable nutrition-related effects of the medications discussed in this chapter.

Appetite stimulants (megestrol acetate, dronabinol)	**Gastrointestinal effects:** Nausea, vomiting, diarrhea **Dietary interaction:** Dronabinol potentiates the effects of alcohol **Metabolic effect:** Hyperglycemia (megestrol acetate)
Diuretics (furosemide, spironolactone[a])	**Gastrointestinal effects:** Dry mouth, anorexia, decreased taste perception **Dietary interactions:** Furosemide's bioavailability is reduced when taken with food; licorice root may interfere with the effects of diuretics **Metabolic effects:** Fluid and electrolyte imbalances,[a] hyperglycemia, hyperlipidemias, thiamin deficiency (furosemide), elevated uric acid levels (furosemide)
Immunosuppressants (cyclosporine, tacrolimus)	**Gastrointestinal effects:** Nausea, vomiting, abdominal discomfort, diarrhea, constipation, anorexia **Dietary interactions:** Limit alcohol intake due to the potential for toxic effects; grapefruit juice can raise serum concentrations of these drugs to toxic levels; the bioavailability of tacrolimus is reduced when the drug is taken with food **Metabolic effects:** Electrolyte imbalances, hyperglycemia, hyperlipidemias, anemia
Lactulose	**Gastrointestinal effects:** Nausea, vomiting, diarrhea, flatulence **Dietary interactions:** Calcium and magnesium supplements may reduce the effectiveness of lactulose **Metabolic effects:** Fluid and electrolyte imbalances

[a] *Furosemide* is a "potassium-wasting" diuretic; patients should increase intakes of potassium-rich foods. *Spironolactone* is a "potassium-sparing" diuretic; patients should avoid supplemental potassium and potassium-containing salt substitutes.

include spironolactone (Aldactone) and furosemide (Lasix). Lactulose, a nonabsorbable disaccharide, treats hepatic encephalopathy by reducing ammonia production and absorption in the colon. The antibiotic rifaximin is an alternative treatment for elevated ammonia that works by altering bacterial populations. To stimulate the appetite and promote weight gain, megestrol acetate (Megace) or dronabinol (Marinol) may be prescribed. Box 20-1 lists potential nutritional problems associated with these medications.

Nutrition Therapy for Cirrhosis

Nutrition care for cirrhosis depends on the patient's general health, extent of liver damage, and accompanying complications. Common problems include protein-energy malnutrition and muscle wasting; thus, protein and energy intakes must be sufficient for maintaining nitrogen balance and body weight. Dietary substances that may cause additional liver injury should be avoided; examples include alcohol, some herbal supplements, and vitamin or mineral megadoses. If esophageal varices are present, a soft diet (which contains only moist, soft-textured foods; see Chapter 17) may be prescribed to reduce the risk of bleeding. Table 20-6 lists the general dietary guidelines for cirrhosis.

Energy Energy needs range from 25 to 40 kcalories per kilogram of dry body weight per day; recommendations for patients with stable cirrhosis usually fall in the lower part of this range, whereas patients with malnutrition or multiple complications usually require higher intakes.[13] Requirements may be further increased in patients with hypermetabolism, catabolism, infection, nutrient malabsorption, or recent unintentional weight loss. In patients with ascites, a value for dry weight can be obtained after diuretic therapy or after a medical procedure that directly removes excess abdominal fluid.

Many patients with cirrhosis have difficulty consuming enough food to achieve good nutrition status. Some individuals may find four to six small meals easier to tolerate than three large meals each day. Oral supplements, including liquid formulas and energy bars, can be used to improve energy intakes. Box 20-2 offers additional suggestions that can help a patient meet energy needs.

TABLE 20-6 Nutrition Therapy for Liver Cirrhosis

Energy	■ Energy needs range from 25 to 40 kcal/kg body weight per day; patients with stable cirrhosis usually require 25 to 35 kcal/kg per day, whereas those with multiple complications or malnutrition may require 30 to 40 kcal/kg per day. ■ Energy requirements may be higher in patients with hypermetabolism, catabolism, infection, malabsorption, or recent unintentional weight loss. Energy requi rements may be lower in patients who would benefit from weight loss. ■ In patients with ascites, a value for dry body weight should be used for calculating nutrition needs.
Meal frequency	■ To improve food intake, patients should consume small meals four to six times daily.
Protein	■ Patients should consume 1.0 to 1.5 g protein/kg dry body weight per day to maintain or improve nitrogen balance. ■ In patients with hepatic encephalopathy, the protein intake should be spread throughout the day; protein restriction is rarely recommended as it may worsen malnutrition.
Carbohydrate and fat	■ Carbohydrate and fat recommendations are similar to those for the general population. ■ Persons with insulin resistance or diabetes should monitor carbohydrate intakes and consume a diet that maintains blood glucose control. ■ If fat is malabsorbed, medium-chain triglycerides (MCT) can be used to increase kcalories.
Sodium	■ Patients should restrict sodium as necessary to control ascites; 2000 mg sodium per day is adequate restriction in most cases.
Vitamins and minerals	■ Patients may require dietary supplements to obtain adequate amounts of vitamins and minerals.

© 2016 Cengage Learning®

How To   BOX 20-2 HELP THE CIRRHOSIS PATIENT EAT ENOUGH FOOD

Individuals with cirrhosis often have difficulty consuming enough food to prevent malnutrition and its consequences. Ascites and GI symptoms such as nausea and vomiting may interfere with food intake. Fatigue may cause a lack of interest in food preparation. Sodium restrictions may make foods unpalatable. To improve food intake:

■ If nutrient restrictions are necessary, make sure the patient fully understands how to modify the diet so that food intake is not restricted unnecessarily. Provide lists of acceptable foods and menus. Explain how recipes can be altered so that favorite foods can still be incorporated into the diet.

■ Suggest between-meal snacks during the day and a snack at bedtime. A liquid supplement like Boost or Ensure can substitute for a snack and requires no preparation. Snacks should not be consumed within two hours of meals, or they may reduce appetite at mealtime.

■ If the patient has little appetite or is quickly satiated, suggest foods that are higher in food energy, such as whole milk instead of reduced-fat milk or canned fruit that is packed in heavy syrup instead of fruit juice. Suggest that beverages be consumed separately from meals.

■ Recommend energy boosters. Cream sauces and gravies can add kcalories to entrées. Fruit juices and fruit nectars can substitute for drinking water. The following additions can boost the energy content of meals:

  ■ Sour cream and butter—on vegetables and potatoes

  ■ Mayonnaise—in sandwiches and salads

■ Half-and-half and light cream—in soups and on cereal

■ Hard-cooked eggs—in casseroles and meat loaf

■ Cheese—in salads and casseroles and melted on steamed vegetables

■ Peanut butter, nut butters, and cream cheese—on crackers or celery and in milk shakes

■ Chopped nuts—in salads, cooked cereals, and bakery products

Sodium-restricted diets are recommended for treating ascites and other medical conditions, including kidney and heart disorders. Box 22-6 (p. 594) and Table 23-1 (p. 607) provide information about restricting dietary sodium. To improve the palatability of low-sodium meals:

■ Suggest that patients replace salt with strong-flavored herbs and spices such as chili powder, coriander, cumin, curry powder, garlic, ginger, lemon, mint, and parsley.

■ Advise patients to check food labels to learn the sodium content of packaged foods. Similar products may be available that are lower in sodium. (Persons using potassium-sparing diuretics should be cautioned to avoid salt substitutes that replace sodium with potassium.)

Offer support and encouragement to the patient with cirrhosis. Significant weight loss is less likely to occur if dietary advice is provided before problems progress.

Protein To maintain or improve nitrogen balance, the protein recommendation is 1.0 to 1.5 grams of protein per kilogram of body weight per day based on dry weight or an appropriate weight for height (the protein RDA for healthy adults is 0.8 g/kg).[14] In patients with hepatic encephalopathy, the protein intake should be spread throughout the day so that only modest amounts are consumed at each meal. Protein restriction is rarely recommended because an inadequate protein intake can worsen malnutrition and wasting.

Clinical studies have suggested that oral supplementation with branched-chain amino acids (BCAA) may improve neurological functioning in patients with hepatic encephalopathy.[15] BCAA supplementation may also improve insulin resistance and immune responses in patients with advanced cirrhosis.[16] The benefit of BCAA supplementation on survival rates of cirrhosis patients, however, is still in question.

Carbohydrate and Fat Carbohydrate and fat recommendations for cirrhosis patients are similar to those for the general population.[17] Many patients with cirrhosis are insulin resistant, however, and require medications or insulin to manage their hyperglycemia. These individuals should follow the dietary guidelines for diabetes: monitor carbohydrate intakes and consume a diet that maintains blood glucose levels within a normal range (see Chapter 21). In addition, carbohydrate intakes should be fairly consistent from day to day for improved blood glucose control. If fat is malabsorbed, medium-chain triglycerides (MCT) can be used to provide additional energy. Severe steatorrhea warrants supplementation of the fat-soluble vitamins, calcium, magnesium, and zinc (see Chapter 19).

Sodium Patients with ascites are generally advised to restrict sodium. Because ascites is partly caused by sodium and water retention in the kidneys, treatment usually includes both sodium restriction (to no more than 2000 milligrams of sodium per day) and diuretic therapy to promote fluid loss. Potassium intake should be monitored if a potassium-wasting diuretic (such as furosemide) is used.

Many patients find low-sodium diets unpalatable, so some health practitioners may allow a more liberal sodium intake and depend on diuretics to remove excess fluid. If patients do not respond to sodium restriction and diuretic therapy, excess fluid may be removed from the abdomen by surgical puncture (**paracentesis**). In another procedure, the portal pressure (which contributes to the development of ascites) is relieved by creating a passage between the portal vein and hepatic vein using a stent (**transjugular intrahepatic portosystemic shunt**). Note that fluid restrictions are occasionally implemented when ascites is accompanied by severe **hyponatremia** (serum sodium less than about 125 milliequivalents per liter) but other methods of reducing the body's water volume are preferable.[18]

Vitamins and Minerals Vitamin and mineral deficiencies are common in patients with cirrhosis due to the effects of illness, disease complications, or the alcohol abuse that may have induced liver disease. Therefore, nutrient supplementation is often necessary. If steatorrhea is present, fat-soluble nutrients can be provided in water-soluble forms. Patients with esophageal varices may find it easier to ingest supplements in liquid form.

Food Safety Because people with cirrhosis are susceptible to infections, they should avoid foods that may increase risk of foodborne illness, such as unpasteurized milk products; undercooked meat, fish, poultry, and eggs; unwashed fruits and vegetables; raw vegetable sprouts; and unpasteurized juices.[19] Nutrition in Practice 5 provides additional information about safe food practices (pp. 125–131).

Enteral and Parenteral Nutrition Support In hospitalized patients who are unable to consume enough food, tube feedings may be infused overnight as a supplement to oral intakes or may replace oral feedings entirely. Although standard formulas are often appropriate, an energy-dense formula (supplying at least 1.5 kcalories

paracentesis (pah-rah-sen-TEE-sis)**:** a surgical puncture of a body cavity with an aspirator to draw out excess fluid.

transjugular intrahepatic portosystemic shunt: a passage within the liver that connects a portion of the portal vein to the hepatic vein using a stent; access to the liver is gained via the jugular vein in the neck.

hyponatremia: abnormally low sodium levels in the blood; a possible result of fluid overload.

Lenny Levitt, a 49-year-old carpenter, has just been diagnosed with cirrhosis, which is a consequence of his alcohol abuse over the past 25 years. Although he understands that he has an alcohol problem and recently entered an alcohol rehabilitation program, he is still drinking. At 5 feet 8 inches tall, Mr. Levitt, who formerly weighed 160 pounds, now weighs 130 pounds. According to family members, he is showing signs of mental deterioration, such as forgetfulness and an inability to concentrate. He is jaundiced and appears thin, although his abdomen is distended with ascites. Laboratory findings indicate elevated serum concentrations of AST, ALT, and ammonia; reduced albumin levels; and hyperglycemia.

1. Do Mr. Levitt's laboratory values suggest liver disease? Compare the results of his laboratory tests with the values shown in Table 20-3.

2. From the limited information available, evaluate Mr. Levitt's nutrition status. What medical problem makes it difficult to interpret his present weight? Describe the development of that type of problem in liver disease, and explain how the diet is usually adjusted for such a patient.

3. Estimate Mr. Levitt's energy and protein needs. Describe the general diet you might recommend for him. What suggestions do you have for increasing his energy intake?

4. Explain the significance of Mr. Levitt's elevated blood ammonia levels. What signs may indicate that he is undergoing mental decline?

5. Describe each of the following complications of liver disease: portal hypertension, jaundice, and gastroesophageal varices. What complication may result if the esophageal varices are not treated?

per milliliter) should be provided for patients with ascites.[20] In patients with esophageal varices, the feeding tube should be as narrow and flexible as possible to prevent rupture and bleeding. Parenteral nutrition support should be considered for patients who are unable to tolerate enteral feedings due to intestinal obstruction, GI bleeding, or uncontrollable vomiting. To avoid excessive fluid delivery, patients with ascites typically require concentrated parenteral solutions, which are infused into central veins. The Case Study in Box 20-3 can help you apply your knowledge of cirrhosis to a clinical situation.

IN SUMMARY

▌ Liver cirrhosis is characterized by extensive fibrosis and progressive liver dysfunction. The primary causes of cirrhosis in the United States are hepatitis C infection and alcoholic liver disease.

▌ Symptoms of cirrhosis include fatigue, GI disturbances, anorexia, and weight loss; eventually, patients may bruise easily and be more susceptible to infections. Complications of cirrhosis include portal hypertension, gastroesophageal varices, ascites, hepatic encephalopathy, and malnutrition.

▌ Treatment of cirrhosis is highly individualized and depends on the accompanying symptoms and complications. Both drug therapies and dietary adjustments are usually necessary. Many patients with cirrhosis need to consume a high-kcalorie, high-protein diet to prevent weight loss and wasting. Patients with ascites may be advised to restrict sodium.

20.3 Liver Transplantation

LO 20.3 Identify the potential health concerns of patients who undergo liver transplantation.

Acute or chronic liver disease can lead to liver failure, in which case liver transplantation is the only remaining treatment option. The most common illnesses that precede liver transplantation are chronic hepatitis C infection and alcoholic liver disease, which account for about 50 percent of liver transplant cases.[21] The 5-year survival rate among transplant recipients ranges from 54 to 81 percent, depending on the cause of illness.[22] Complications such as ascites and hepatic encephalopathy worsen the prognosis.

Nutrition Status of Transplant Patients As mentioned earlier, advanced liver disease is usually associated with malnutrition, which can increase the risk of complications following a liver transplant. Evaluating nutrition status in transplant candidates can be difficult, however, because liver dysfunction and malnutrition often have similar metabolic effects. If fluid retention is present, it can mask weight loss and alter anthropometric and laboratory values. Correcting malnutrition prior to transplant surgery can help speed recovery after the surgery.

Posttransplantation Concerns The immediate concerns following a transplant are organ rejection and infection. Immunosuppressive drugs, including prednisone, cyclosporine, and tacrolimus, help to reduce the immune responses that cause rejection, but they also raise the risk of infection. Infections are a potential cause of death following a liver transplant; therefore, antibiotics and antiviral medications are prescribed to reduce infection risk.

Immunosuppressive drugs can affect nutrition status in numerous ways. Gastrointestinal side effects include nausea, vomiting, diarrhea, abdominal pain, and mouth sores. Some medications may alter appetite and taste perception. Some of the drugs may cause hyperglycemia or outright diabetes, which may need to be controlled with insulin. Electrolyte and fluid imbalances are common. Other possible effects include hypertension, hyperlipidemias, kidney toxicity, protein catabolism, and increased osteoporosis risk.[23]

Protein and energy requirements are increased after transplantation due to the stress of surgery. High-kcalorie, high-protein snacks and oral supplements can help the transplant patient meet postsurgical needs. Vitamin and mineral supplementation is also an integral part of nutrition care. To help transplant patients avoid developing foodborne illnesses, health practitioners should provide information about food safety measures, such as cooking meats adequately, washing fresh produce, and avoiding foods that may be contaminated. Nutrition in Practice 5 (pp. 125–131) provides additional information about food safety.

IN SUMMARY

▌ Liver transplantation has improved the long-term outlook for patients with advanced liver disease. Transplant patients are usually malnourished, however, and may have medical problems that affect transplant success.

▌ Due to the potential for organ rejection, immunosuppressive drugs are prescribed following an organ transplant. Use of these drugs increases the risk of infection, and the drugs have side effects that can impair nutrition status and general health.

20.4 Gallstone Disease

LO 20.4 Explain why gallstones develop and discuss the major risk factors and treatment approaches for gallstone disease.

The gallbladder concentrates and stores the bile produced by the liver until the bile is needed for fat digestion (see Figure 20-6). Disorders that obstruct the liver's release of bile can damage the liver. More commonly, disorders of the **biliary system**—the gallbladder and bile ducts—involve the formation of **gallstones.** Gallstone disease affects 10 to 15 percent of the adult population in the United States.[24]

biliary system: the gallbladder and ducts that deliver bile from the liver and gallbladder to the small intestine.

gallstones: stones that form in the gallbladder from crystalline deposits of cholesterol or bilirubin; also called *choleliths*.

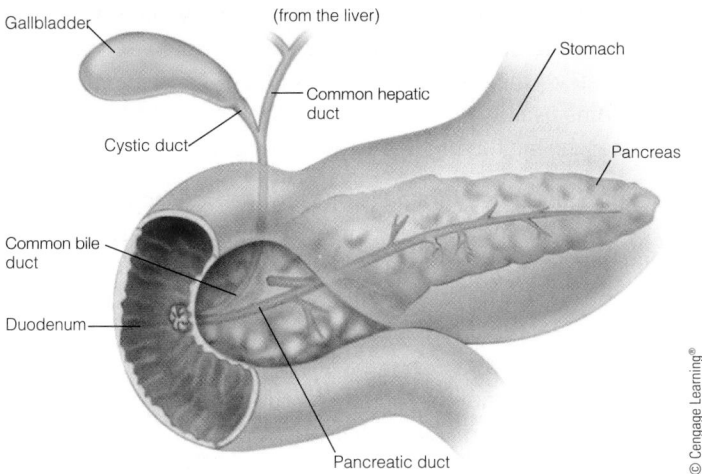

Gallbladder

(from the liver)

Stomach

Common hepatic
duct

Cystic duct

Pancreas

Common bile
duct

Duodenum

Pancreatic duct

© Cengage Learning®

FIGURE 20-6 The Gallbladder and Bile Ducts

Types of Gallstones

Gallstone formation, or **cholelithiasis,** results from the excessive concentration and crystallization of compounds in bile. Bile is composed of water, bile salts, cholesterol, phospholipids (primarily lecithin), proteins, and bile pigment (bilirubin). During storage in the gallbladder, bile's concentration increases approximately 10-fold as its water content is extracted. The formation of gallstones is favored by factors that increase bile's cholesterol concentration, promote crystal formation and development, or reduce gallbladder motility.

Cholesterol Gallstones In about 90 percent of cases, gallstones are composed primarily of cholesterol, although they also contain calcium salts and bilirubin.[25] The cholesterol in bile can precipitate out of solution and form small crystals, which eventually coalesce to form stones. The stones can be as small as a pea or as large as a golf ball (see Figure 20-7). Some people tend to form many small stones, while others may form only one or two large ones.

Cholesterol gallstones often develop after the bile concentrate thickens and forms a type of **sludge** that cannot be easily expelled by gallbladder contraction. Biliary sludge may develop after rapid weight loss or fasting, gastric bypass surgery, or long-term total parenteral nutrition, and it can also occur during pregnancy.

Pigment Gallstones Although pigment stones account for a minority of cases in the United States, they are the predominant type of gallstone in some Asian countries. Pigment stones are primarily made up of the calcium salt of bilirubin (calcium bilirubinate). They often develop as a result of bacterial infection, which alters the structure of bilirubin and causes it to precipitate out of bile and form stones. Other cases result from excessive red blood cell breakdown, leading to an abnormal accumulation of bilirubin. Conditions associated with pigment stone formation include biliary tract infections, pancreatitis, and red blood cell disorders, such as sickle-cell anemia. Pigment stones may form in either the gallbladder or a bile duct. Unlike the crystalline cholesterol stones, pigment stones are soft and easily crushed.

Consequences of Gallstones

About 85 percent of gallstones are asymptomatic and are discovered accidentally while testing for other conditions.[26] In other cases, patients may experience an aggressive course of illness with recurring symptoms.

Gallstone Symptoms Gallstone pain (often called *biliary colic*) usually arises when a gallstone temporarily blocks the cystic duct, which leads from the gallbladder to the

Courtesy of Dr. David King © Myrna Engler/Photo Researchers, Inc.

FIGURE 20-7 Gallstones
Most gallstones are made primarily of cholesterol; they can be as small as a pea or as large as a golf ball. Cholesterol stones are usually yellow-green in color, whereas pigment stones can be brown or black.

cholelithiasis (KOH-leh-lih-THIGH-ah-sis)**:** formation of gallstones.

▮ *chole* = bile
▮ *lithiasis* = formation of stones

sludge: literally, a semi-solid mass. Biliary sludge is made up of mucus, cholesterol crystals, and bilirubin granules.

common bile duct (review Figure 20-6). The pain is steady and severe and may last for several minutes or several hours. Although the pain is usually located in the upper abdomen, it may radiate to the chest, back, or shoulder. Nausea and vomiting may also be present. Symptoms usually develop after meals, especially after eating fatty foods. Pain may also occur during the night and awaken a person from sleep.

Complications of Gallstones If a gallstone remains lodged in the cystic duct, it can obstruct bile flow to the duodenum and cause **cholecystitis**—distention and inflammation of the gallbladder. Cholecystitis can lead to infection or to more severe complications, including perforation of the gallbladder, **peritonitis,** and fistulas. If gallstones obstruct the common bile duct, they can block bile flow from the liver and lead to jaundice or damage to liver tissue. An impacted stone within the bile ducts may lead to infection and the condition known as **bacterial cholangitis,** which causes severe pain, sepsis, and fever and is often a medical emergency. Gallstones can block the pancreatic duct as well—a primary cause of acute pancreatitis. Due to the potential danger of these complications, individuals should seek medical attention if gallstone pain does not resolve over time or if fever, jaundice, or persistent nausea and vomiting develop.

Risk Factors for Cholesterol Gallstones

The risk of developing cholesterol gallstones is influenced by a number of genetic and lifestyle factors. As described in the sections that follow, the risk factors may either cause an increase in bile's cholesterol concentration or a reduction in gallbladder motility, thereby promoting gallstone crystallization or subsequent stone growth.

Ethnicity Although the genetic factors involved are not well understood, ethnicity exerts a strong influence on gallstone formation. The Pima Indians are an exceptionally high-risk population, as gallstones develop in about 75 percent of adult women.[27] African Americans tend to have a lower prevalence of gallstones than white or Mexican-American populations.[28]

Aging Because gallstones do not dissolve spontaneously, gallstone prevalence increases with age. Moreover, bile composition tends to change with aging: the cholesterol concentration increases while bile salts decrease, leading to a greater likelihood of cholesterol crystallization.

Gender The prevalence of cholesterol gallstones is about twice as high in women as in men;[29] this is because estrogen alters cholesterol metabolism, causing an increased secretion of cholesterol into bile. Similarly, the use of estrogen replacement therapy after menopause increases gallstone risk.

Pregnancy Gallstone risk is increased in pregnancy due to hormonal changes: the higher estrogen levels raise bile's cholesterol concentration, and the increase in progesterone levels reduces gallbladder motility. The risk of gallstones worsens as the pregnancy progresses and is especially high during the third trimester.

Obesity and Weight Loss Obesity predisposes to gallstone formation because it is associated with increased cholesterol synthesis in the liver, which results in higher cholesterol concentrations in bile. Gallstones may also develop as a result of rapid weight loss, which both increases the secretion of cholesterol into bile and decreases gallbladder motility. Another effect of rapid weight loss is an increased production of the gallbladder's *mucin* proteins, which are a major component of biliary sludge and also serve as a matrix for cholesterol crystals during stone growth. The oral ingestion of bile salts has been shown to reduce the risk of gallstone formation during rapid weight loss.

Other Risk Factors Long-term total parenteral nutrition usually reduces gallbladder motility, which promotes the development of biliary sludge. Some medications (such as octreotide) may have similar effects. The medication clofibrate, used for heart

cholecystitis (KOH-leh-sih-STY-tis)**:** inflammation of the gallbladder, usually caused by obstruction of the cystic duct by gallstones.

peritonitis: inflammation of the peritoneal membrane, which lines the abdominal cavity.

bacterial cholangitis (KOH-lan-JYE-tis)**:** bacterial infection involving the bile ducts.

CHAPTER TWENTY

disease, increases the cholesterol concentration of bile, promoting gallstone crystallization. High triglyceride levels in blood are also associated with increased gallstone risk, as are spinal cord injuries and diseases affecting the ileum.

Treatment of Gallstones

Asymptomatic gallstones generally do not require treatment. Gallstones that cause symptoms or complications are usually treated with gallbladder surgery or nonsurgical procedures that dissolve or fragment the stones. To minimize symptoms before the gallbladder or gallstones are removed, a low-fat diet (with less than 30 percent of total kcalories from fat) may be prescribed; some individuals may tolerate small, frequent meals better than large meals.[30]

Surgery Gallbladder removal, or **cholecystectomy,** is the primary treatment for patients with recurring gallstones. The standard surgical approach is a **laparoscopic** method, which relies on narrow surgical telescopes (laparoscopes) to view and perform the necessary procedures via small incisions in the abdomen. The procedure takes only one or two hours, and many patients are discharged on the same day as the surgery. In patients with complications that make organ removal difficult, open cholecystectomy—which requires opening the abdominal cavity—may be necessary.

Once the gallbladder has been removed, the common bile duct collects bile between meals and releases it into the duodenum at mealtimes; thus, patients can usually tolerate a regular diet. Some individuals may experience diarrhea due to an increased amount of bile in the large intestine, which has a laxative effect. Abdominal pain is sometimes caused by the presence of residual stones within the common bile duct that were overlooked during surgery or that formed within the duct itself. Bile duct injuries occasionally result from the surgical procedure.

Nonsurgical Procedures Nonsurgical methods are used primarily in patients who have small cholesterol stones and transient conditions associated with gallstone formation. The gallstones can be treated by oral intake of ursodeoxycholic acid (ursodiol), a bile acid that reduces the bile's cholesterol content and eventually allows the cholesterol crystals in gallstones to dissolve. Ursodeoxycholic acid must be used for 6 to 18 months and is best suited for stones that are 5 to 10 millimeters (about ¼ to ½ inch) in diameter or smaller. Recurrence rates after dissolution are as high as 50 percent within 5 years after treatment.[31]

Cholesterol gallstones can be fragmented using **shock-wave lithotripsy,** a procedure that is also used to fragment kidney stones. This technique uses high-amplitude sound waves (called shock waves) to break gallstones into pieces that are small enough to either pass into the intestine without causing symptoms or be dissolved with ursodeoxycholic acid. Shock-wave lithotripsy can be performed only in patients with few gallstones. Due to high gallstone recurrence rates (up to 80 percent recurrence after 10 years), the procedure is used mainly to remove bile duct stones that are difficult to extract by other means.[32]

IN SUMMARY

▌ Gallstones are the most common disorder affecting the gallbladder. They are formed by the concentration of compounds in bile, especially cholesterol and the bile pigment bilirubin.

▌ Although most gallstones are asymptomatic, some gallstones can cause recurring pain and GI problems that appear after meals and may persist for several hours.

▌ The risk of gallstone disease is influenced by ethnicity, gender, pregnancy, obesity, rapid weight loss, and other factors.

▌ Treatments for gallstones include gallbladder removal and gallstone dissolution or fragmentation.

cholecystectomy (KOH-leh-sis-TEK-toe-mee)**:** surgical removal of the gallbladder.

laparoscopic: pertaining to procedures that use a laparoscope for internal examination or surgery. A laparoscope is a narrow surgical telescope that is inserted into the abdominal cavity through a small incision. A video camera is usually attached so that the procedure can be viewed on a television monitor.

shock-wave lithotripsy: a nonsurgical procedure that uses high-amplitude sound waves to fragment gallstones or kidney stones.

Nutrition Assessment Checklist FOR PEOPLE WITH DISORDERS OF THE LIVER AND GALLBLADDER

Medical History

Check the medical record to determine:

- Type of liver disorder
- Cause of the liver disorder
- If the patient has received a liver transplant
- If the patient has a history of gallstones

Review the medical record for complications that may alter nutritional needs, including:

- Abdominal pain
- Anemia
- Ascites
- Esophageal varices
- Hepatic encephalopathy
- Impaired kidney or lung function
- Infections
- Insulin resistance or diabetes mellitus
- Malabsorption
- Malnutrition
- Pancreatitis

Medications

In patients with liver dysfunction, the risk of diet-drug interactions is high because most drugs are metabolized in the liver. Risk of interactions is intensified for patients with:

- Ascites (medications may take a long time to reach the liver)
- Renal failure (medications often undergo further metabolism in the kidneys and are excreted in the urine)
- Malnutrition
- Multiple prescriptions
- Long-term medication use

Dietary Intake

For patients with fatty liver, pay special attention to:

- Energy intake, if the patient is overweight or malnourished, has diabetes, or is receiving total parenteral nutrition
- Carbohydrate intake, if the patient has diabetes or is receiving total parenteral nutrition
- Alcohol abuse

For patients with hepatitis, cirrhosis, or ascites:

- Check appetite.
- Ensure that energy and nutrient intakes are appropriate.

- Determine whether alcohol is being consumed.
- Determine whether sodium restriction is warranted.
- Base energy intakes on desirable weight or an estimated dry weight to avoid overfeeding.

Anthropometric Data

Take baseline height and weight measurements, and monitor weight regularly. For patients with ascites and edema:

- Monitor weight changes to evaluate the degree of fluid retention.
- Remember that the patient may be malnourished, and weight may be deceptively high.

Laboratory Tests

Note that albumin and serum proteins are often reduced in people with liver disease and are not appropriate indicators of nutrition status. Review the following laboratory test results to assess liver function:

- Albumin
- Alkaline phosphatase
- ALT and AST
- Ammonia
- Bilirubin
- Gamma-glutamyl transpeptidase
- Prothrombin time

Check laboratory test results for complications associated with liver failure, including:

- Anemia
- Decreased renal function
- Fluid retention
- Hyperglycemia

Physical Signs

Look for physical signs of:

- Fluid retention (ascites and edema)
- Protein-energy malnutrition (muscle wasting and unintentional weight loss)
- Nutrient deficiencies

Clinical Applications

1. Vijaya Reddy is a college student who visited relatives near her parents' birthplace in Anantapur, India, during summer vacation. Although her relatives provided boiled or purified water at their home, they occasionally took Vijaya to local restaurants, where she drank tap water. Several weeks after Vijaya returned home, she developed flu-like symptoms and started feeling extremely tired. She also experienced upper abdominal pain and felt nauseous after meals. After her roommate told her that her eyes and

skin appeared yellow, she knew something was definitely wrong. A physician at the student health center diagnosed hepatitis.

- Which type of hepatitis did Vijaya most likely have?
- What additional symptoms may develop? Is Vijaya's condition likely to become chronic?
- What medical treatment is suggested for Vijaya's condition? Describe the dietary modifications that may be necessary in some cases.

2. As discussed in the section on cirrhosis, many patients develop protein-energy malnutrition and wasting during the course of illness. Review Table 20-5 to find examples of problems that may lead to malnutrition. Select three nutrition or medical problems (from the "Examples" column), and discuss the complications of liver disease that may cause the problems you selected. What dietary or medical treatments can help in managing these problems?

Self Check

1. In cases of fatty liver that are unrelated to excessive alcohol intakes, the primary risk factor is:
   a. following a high-protein diet.
   b. use of illicit drugs.
   c. following a high-fat diet.
   d. insulin resistance.

2. Which of the following statements about hepatitis is true?
   a. Chronic hepatitis can progress to cirrhosis.
   b. Whatever the cause of hepatitis, symptoms are typically severe.
   c. Vaccines are available to protect against hepatitis A, B, and C viruses.
   d. HCV infection can be spread through contaminated foods and water.

3. Esophageal varices are a dangerous complication of liver disease primarily because they:
   a. interfere with food intake.
   b. can lead to massive bleeding.
   c. divert blood flow from the GI tract.
   d. contribute to hepatic encephalopathy.

4. A complication of cirrhosis that contributes to the development of ascites is:
   a. portal hypertension.
   b. elevated serum ammonia levels.
   c. bile obstruction.
   d. insulin resistance.

5. Lactulose, a nonabsorbable disaccharide, is generally prescribed to patients who develop which complication of cirrhosis?
   a. Portal hypertension
   b. Hepatic encephalopathy
   c. Bile insufficiency
   d. Ascites

6. With respect to protein intake, patients with hepatic encephalopathy should:
   a. consume a high-protein diet.
   b. restrict protein intake to avoid elevations in serum ammonia.
   c. spread protein intake evenly throughout the day.
   d. use formulas enriched with aromatic amino acids to meet their protein needs.

7. People with ascites must often restrict their dietary intake of:
   a. fat.
   b. protein.
   c. sugars.
   d. sodium.

8. Dietary concerns after a liver transplant include all of the following *except*:
   a. severe protein restrictions that are difficult to adhere to.
   b. increased risk of foodborne illness.
   c. gastrointestinal side effects of medications.
   d. altered appetite and taste perception from medications.

9. Regarding the major risk factors for gallstone disease:
   a. prevalence is much higher in men than in women.
   b. gallstone risk is increased during pregnancy.
   c. rapid weight loss can temporarily shrink gallstones.
   d. risk is generally similar among ethnic groups.

10. Nonsurgical approaches to gallstone treatment include:
    a. cholecystectomy.
    b. weight loss.
    c. dissolution and fragmentation.
    d. immunosuppressant drug therapy.

Answers to these questions appear in Appendix H.

Notes

1. D. E. Cohen and F. A. Anania, Nonalcoholic fatty liver disease, in N. J. Greenberger, ed., *Current Diagnosis and Treatment: Gastroenterology, Hepatology, and Endoscopy* (New York: McGraw-Hill Companies, 2012), pp. 502–508.

2. N. P. Chalasani, Alcoholic and nonalcoholic steatohepatitis, in L. Goldman and A. I. Schafer, eds., *Goldman's Cecil Medicine* (Philadelphia: Saunders, 2012), pp. 996–999.

3. J. M. Kneeman, J. Misdraji, and K. E. Corey, Secondary causes of nonalcoholic fatty liver disease, *Therapeutic Advances in Gastroenterology* 5 (2012): 199–207.

4. E. Franco and coauthors, Hepatitis B: Epidemiology and prevention in developing countries, *World Journal of Hepatology* 4 (2012): 74–80.

5. A. Rutherford and J. L. Dienstag, Viral hepatitis, in N. J. Greenberger, ed., *Current Diagnosis and Treatment: Gastroenterology, Hepatology, and Endoscopy* (New York: McGraw-Hill Companies, 2012), pp. 449–475.

6. Academy of Nutrition and Dietetics, *Nutrition Care Manual* (Chicago: Academy of Nutrition and Dietetics, 2014).

7. D. L. Hoyert and J. Xu, Deaths: Preliminary data for 2011, *National Vital Statistics Reports* 61 (October 2012).

8. G. Garcia-Tsao, Cirrhosis and its sequelae, in L. Goldman and A. I. Schafer, eds., *Goldman's Cecil Medicine* (Philadelphia: Saunders, 2012), pp. 999–1007.

9. N. J. Greenberger, Ascites and spontaneous bacterial peritonitis, in N. J. Greenberger, ed., *Current Diagnosis and Treatment: Gastroenterology, Hepatology, and Endoscopy* (New York: McGraw-Hill Companies, 2012), pp. 514–521.

10. N. J. Greenberger, Portal systemic encephalopathy and hepatic encephalopathy, in N. J. Greenberger, ed., *Current Diagnosis and Treatment: Gastroenterology, Hepatology, and Endoscopy* (New York: McGraw-Hill Companies, 2012), pp. 509–513.

11. K. Tajiri and Y. Shimizu, Branched-chain amino acids in liver diseases, *World Journal of Gastroenterology* 19 (2013): 7620–7629.

12. Greenberger, Portal systemic encephalopathy and hepatic encephalopathy, 2012.

13. T. M. Johnson and coauthors, Nutrition assessment and management in advanced liver disease, *Nutrition in Clinical Practice* 28 (2013): 15–29;

K. Cheung, S. S. Lee, and M. Raman, Prevalence and mechanisms of malnutrition in patients with advanced liver disease, and nutrition management strategies, *Clinical Gastroenterology and Hepatology* 10 (2012): 117–125.

14. Johnson and coauthors, 2013; Cheung, Lee, and Raman, 2012.

15. L. L. Gluud and coauthors, Oral branched-chain amino acids have a beneficial effect on manifestations of hepatic encephalopathy in a systematic review with meta-analyses of randomized controlled trials, *Journal of Nutrition* 143 (2013): 1263–1268.

16. Tajiri and Shimizu, 2013.

17. Cheung, Lee, and Raman, 2012.

18. Johnson and coauthors, 2013; B. A. Runyon, Management of adult patients with ascites due to cirrhosis: Update 2012, *Hepatology* 57 (2013): 1651–1653.

19. Academy of Nutrition and Dietetics, 2014.

20. Johnson and coauthors, 2013.

21. E. B. Keeffe, Hepatic failure and liver transplantation, in L. Goldman and A. I. Schafer, eds., *Goldman's Cecil Medicine* (Philadelphia: Saunders, 2012), pp. 1007–1011.

22. Keeffe, 2012.

23. A. A. Qamar, Liver transplantation, in N. J. Greenberger, ed., *Current Diagnosis and Treatment: Gastroenterology, Hepatology, and Endoscopy* (New York: McGraw-Hill Companies, 2012), pp. 555–566.

24. G. Paumgartner and N. J. Greenberger, Gallstone disease, in N. J. Greenberger, ed., *Current Diagnosis and Treatment: Gastroenterology, Hepatology, and Endoscopy* (New York: McGraw-Hill Companies, 2012), pp. 578–588.

25. Paumgartner and Greenberger, 2012.

26. N. H. Afdhal, Diseases of the gallbladder and bile ducts, in L. Goldman and A. I. Schafer, eds., *Goldman's Cecil Medicine* (Philadelphia: Saunders, 2012), pp. 1011–1020.

27. Afdhal, 2012.

28. Paumgartner and Greenberger, 2012.

29. Paumgartner and Greenberger, 2012.

30. Academy of Nutrition and Dietetics, 2014.

31. Paumgartner and Greenberger, 2012.

32. Paumgartner and Greenberger, 2012.

LO 20.5 Describe how alcohol is metabolized in the body and discuss the potential risks and benefits associated with its use.

As Chapter 20 described, excessive alcohol consumption is a primary cause of liver disease. Alcohol can be toxic to other organs as well, including the brain, gastrointestinal (GI) tract, and pancreas. In addition, **alcohol abuse** can lead to a number of nutrient deficiencies. Moderate use of alcohol, however, has been associated with some health benefits, such as lower heart disease risk in middle-aged and older adults. This Nutrition in Practice discusses current recommendations concerning alcohol and the health problems and benefits associated with its use. The Glossary in Box NP20-1 defines the relevant terms.

What are the current dietary guidelines for alcohol consumption?

For those who choose to drink alcoholic beverages, the *Dietary Guidelines for Americans* recommend that women and men limit their average daily intakes of alcohol to one drink and two drinks per day, respectively. In addition, women should avoid consuming more than three drinks in a single day, whereas men should consume no more than four drinks in one day.[1] One **drink** is defined as 12 ounces of beer, 5 ounces of wine, 10 ounces of wine cooler, or 1½ ounces of 80 proof distilled spirits such as gin, rum, vodka, and whiskey (see Figure NP20-1). Some individuals should not consume alcohol at all, such as pregnant and lactating women, women of childbearing age who may become pregnant, children and adolescents, people using medications that can interact with alcohol, and people who are unable to voluntarily restrict their alcohol intake. Alcohol should also be avoided by anyone who is involved in an activity that requires attention or coordination, such as driving or operating machinery.

BOX NP20-1 GLOSSARY

acetaldehyde (ah-set-AL-deh-hide): an intermediate in alcohol metabolism that, in excess, can damage the body's tissues and interfere with cellular functions.

acetate (AH-seh-tate): the product of alcohol metabolism that is used as a source of energy by many tissues in the body.

alcohol abuse: the continued use of alcohol despite the development of social, legal, or health problems. Individuals who abuse alcohol are called *alcoholics*.

alcoholic liver disease: liver disease that is related to excessive alcohol consumption. Disorders that may develop include fatty liver, hepatitis, and cirrhosis, which may lead to liver failure.

drink: an alcoholic beverage that contains about half an ounce of pure alcohol. One drink is equivalent to 12 ounces of beer, 5 ounces of wine, 10 ounces of wine cooler, or 1½ ounces of 80 proof distilled spirits.

FIGURE NP20-1 Each of the amounts shown is equivalent to one drink.

12 oz beer

10 oz wine cooler

1½ oz hard liquor (80 proof whiskey, gin, brandy, rum, vodka)

5 oz wine

Polara Studios, Inc

About 64 percent of adults in the United States drink alcoholic beverages.[2] The prevalence of alcohol abuse is estimated to be between 7.4 and 9.7 percent in the general population.

What happens to alcohol in the body?

Recall that alcohol is a source of food energy, providing 7 kcalories per gram. Although a small amount of alcohol is metabolized in the stomach, most of the alcohol consumed is quickly absorbed in the stomach or small intestine and passes readily into the body's cells, where alcohol concentrations reach levels similar to those in the blood. The liver is the site of most alcohol metabolism, although its ability to metabolize alcohol is somewhat limited: the average adult metabolizes only 7 to 10 grams of alcohol per hour, about the amount in one drink.[3] The main product of alcohol metabolism is **acetate,** which can be used as a source of energy by most tissues.

Because there is no storage pool for alcohol and it can be toxic to cells, the metabolism of alcohol in the liver takes priority over that of other substances. Thus, alcohol suppresses the breakdown of fat for energy, leading to fat accumulation in the liver and the increased release of triglyceride-carrying lipoproteins (very-low-density lipoproteins, or VLDL). An excessive alcohol intake inhibits both the storage of glycogen and the liver's production of glucose between meals. Heavy drinkers are at risk of developing hypoglycemia, an effect that is accentuated in people with diabetes who use insulin or medications to reduce glucose levels. Alcohol ingestion can also impair the synthesis and secretion of a number of liver proteins, including albumin and fibrinogen (a blood-clotting protein).

How is alcohol toxic to cells?

Alcohol can damage cells either directly, or indirectly via the metabolite **acetaldehyde** that is created during alcohol metabolism. High alcohol concentrations change the structure of cell membranes, increasing membrane permeability.

Cell membrane proteins may become damaged, interfering with the transport of substances across the membrane. The presence of alcohol also activates inflammatory responses in cells, which can eventually lead to cell death and tissue damage. Acetaldehyde can cause numerous adverse effects: it binds to proteins and interferes with their functions, alters immune responses, causes oxidative damage, inhibits DNA repair, and prevents the formation of microtubules within cells.

How does alcohol affect brain function?

Alcohol acts as a central nervous system depressant. It can cause sedation, slow reaction times, and relieve anxiety. In excess, it impairs judgment, reduces inhibitions, and impairs speech and motor functions. Extremely high blood alcohol levels can lead to coma, respiratory depression, and death.

Chronic heavy drinking can cause certain types of neurological damage. The most common abnormality is injury to the peripheral nerves, which is evidenced by tingling in the hands and feet, lack of muscular coordination, and changes in a person's manner of walking. Visual impairments, such as blurred vision and optic nerve degeneration, can also occur.

Chronic drinkers who are forced to discontinue their use of alcohol may experience withdrawal symptoms, which include anxiety, irritability, and palpitations. In severe cases, symptoms may include nausea and vomiting, delirium, and seizures.

What are some other long-term consequences of drinking too much alcohol?

Alcoholic liver disease is the most common complication of alcohol abuse, occurring in about 15 to 30 percent of chronic heavy drinkers.[4] The disease develops in a manner similar to the disease progression described in Chapter 20: fatty liver, hepatitis, and, eventually, cirrhosis and liver failure. In addition to liver damage, alcohol can cause damage to the GI tract, pancreas, and heart (see Figure NP20-2).

FIGURE NP20-2 Effects of Excessive Alcohol Intake on Organ Systems

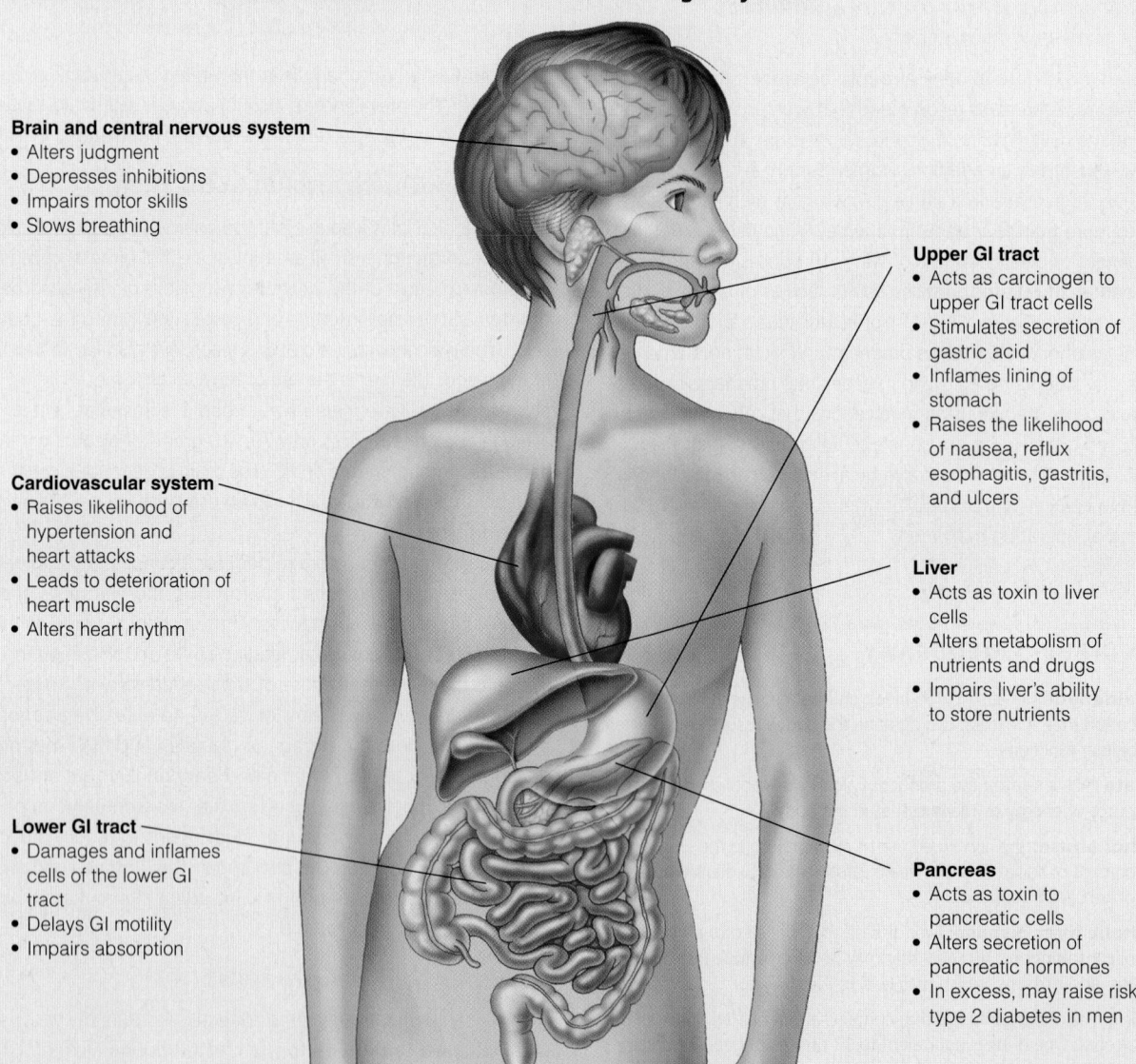

Brain and central nervous system
- Alters judgment
- Depresses inhibitions
- Impairs motor skills
- Slows breathing

Cardiovascular system
- Raises likelihood of hypertension and heart attacks
- Leads to deterioration of heart muscle
- Alters heart rhythm

Lower GI tract
- Damages and inflames cells of the lower GI tract
- Delays GI motility
- Impairs absorption

Upper GI tract
- Acts as carcinogen to upper GI tract cells
- Stimulates secretion of gastric acid
- Inflames lining of stomach
- Raises the likelihood of nausea, reflux esophagitis, gastritis, and ulcers

Liver
- Acts as toxin to liver cells
- Alters metabolism of nutrients and drugs
- Impairs liver's ability to store nutrients

Pancreas
- Acts as toxin to pancreatic cells
- Alters secretion of pancreatic hormones
- In excess, may raise risks of type 2 diabetes in men

In the GI tract, alcohol's eventual effects may include gastritis, ulcers, nutrient malabsorption, diarrhea, and GI cancers. Chronic alcohol ingestion frequently injures pancreatic tissue and may lead to chronic pancreatitis. Heavy drinking is also associated with heart arrhythmias, impaired heart muscle contractility, and hypertension.

What are the effects of excessive alcohol consumption on nutrition status?

An excessive intake of alcohol can lead to multiple nutrient deficiencies. Because alcohol supplies 7 kcalories per gram, it displaces other energy sources along with the essential nutrients such foods would provide. As mentioned earlier, alcohol consumption can cause nutrient malabsorption as a result of direct damage to the GI mucosa. Alcohol also interferes with the way the body processes nutrients. Examples of common deficiencies in persons who abuse alcohol include:[5]

▌ *Vitamin A.* Alcohol and vitamin A are metabolized by similar enzymes, so heavy drinking—which induces the enzymes that break down alcohol—increases the degradation of vitamin A.

▌ *Thiamin.* Alcohol abuse is the most common cause of thiamin deficiency in the United States. Heavy drinking is associated with low thiamin intakes, and alcohol ingestion dramatically reduces thiamin absorption.

▌ *Folate.* Alcohol reduces the absorption of folate in the small intestine and increases folate degradation. Because folate has a central role in cell division (and cells of the GI tract are rapidly dividing cells), folate deficiency contributes to the malabsorption of other nutrients as well.

Can alcohol have disruptive effects on the metabolism of medications?

Yes. Alcohol consumption activates enzymes that metabolize certain drugs, so alcohol ingestion can alter drug metabolism. For example, the consumption of several drinks daily activates enzymes that convert acetaminophen (Tylenol) to chemicals that are toxic to the liver; thus, alcohol drinkers should avoid combining alcohol and acetaminophen. In contrast, impaired drug metabolism is likely when the drugs and alcohol require similar enzymes for their metabolism. As an example, when alcohol is ingested at the same time that some sedative drugs are taken, drug metabolism is delayed until the alcohol is degraded, prolonging the drugs' effects.[6]

Does alcohol consumption have any beneficial effects on health?

Yes. Epidemiological studies in Western countries have consistently shown that a moderate alcohol intake reduces total mortality among middle-aged and older men and women. In addition, researchers have learned that moderate alcohol drinking can help reduce risks of developing the following chronic illnesses:[7]

▌ *Heart disease.* Individuals with a light to moderate intake of alcohol—from beer, wine, or liquor—have a lower risk of heart disease than nondrinkers. Alcohol helps to protect against the development of atherosclerosis, increases levels of high-density lipoproteins (HDL), and reduces the tendency for blood clotting. Its protective effects are seen mainly in older persons who have one or more classic risk factors for heart disease.

▌ *Stroke.* Moderate alcohol consumption may reduce the risk of stroke, especially ischemic stroke (caused by blood clotting in arteries that supply blood to the brain). Conversely, heavy drinking increases the risk of all forms of stroke.

▌ *Diabetes.* The risk of type 2 diabetes may be lower in moderate drinkers than in individuals who abstain from alcohol. In addition, some studies have found that a moderate alcohol intake may improve insulin sensitivity and reduce fasting glucose concentrations.

Note that unlike other recommendations for disease prevention, medical personnel rarely recommend that a nondrinker begin drinking to reduce disease risk, due to the potential for addiction and the adverse effects caused by excessive intakes.

The benefits or harm associated with alcohol consumption depend on a person's health status, age, and the amount consumed. Most people in the United States who consume alcoholic beverages are not heavy drinkers; however, health professionals should be alert to those who may be abusing alcohol and potentially endangering their health.

Notes

1. *Report of the Dietary Guidelines Advisory Committee on the Dietary Guidelines for Americans, 2010,* available at http://www.cnpp.usda.gov/DGAs2010-DGACReport.htm; site visited March 4, 2014.

2. P. G. O'Connor, Alcohol abuse and dependence, in L. Goldman and A. I. Schafer, eds., *Goldman's Cecil Medicine* (Philadelphia: Saunders, 2012), pp. 146–153.

3. S. B. Masters, The alcohols, in B. G. Katzung, ed., *Basic and Clinical Pharmacology* (New York: McGraw-Hill Companies, 2012), pp. 389–401.

4. Masters, 2012.

5. P. M. Suter, Alcohol: Its role in nutrition and health, in J. W. Erdman, I. A. Macdonald, and S. H. Zeisel, eds., *Present Knowledge in Nutrition* (Ames, IA: Wiley-Blackwell, 2012): pp. 912–938.

6. Masters, 2012.

7. *Report of the Dietary Guidelines Advisory Committee on the Dietary Guidelines for Americans, 2010.*

Carbohydrate-Controlled Diets for Diabetes Mellitus

21.1 Overview of Diabetes Mellitus

LO 21.1 Characterize type 1 and type 2 diabetes and describe the complications associated with these conditions.

21.2 Treatment of Diabetes Mellitus

LO 21.2 Describe how diabetes is managed using individualized dietary adjustments, medications, and physical activity plans.

21.3 Diabetes Management in Pregnancy

LO 21.3 Explain how diabetes can affect pregnancy outcomes and describe the approaches used to maintain glycemic control in pregnant women with diabetes.

21.4 Nutrition in Practice: The Metabolic Syndrome

LO 21.4 Identify the features and possible consequences of the metabolic syndrome and describe the current treatment approaches for this condition.

The incidence of **diabetes mellitus** is steadily increasing in the United States and many other countries. It now affects an estimated 12.3 percent of adults aged 20 and older in the United States, or about 29 million people.[1] About 28 percent of persons with diabetes are unaware that they have it,[2] a danger because its damaging effects often occur before symptoms develop. Diabetes ranks seventh among the leading causes of death in the United States. It also contributes to the development of other life-threatening diseases, including heart disease and kidney failure.

21.1 Overview of Diabetes Mellitus

LO 21.1 Characterize type 1 and type 2 diabetes and describe the complications associated with these conditions.

The term *diabetes mellitus* refers to metabolic disorders characterized by elevated blood glucose concentrations and disordered **insulin** metabolism. People with diabetes may be unable to produce sufficient insulin or to use insulin effectively, or they may have both types of abnormalities. These impairments result in defective glucose uptake and utilization in muscle and adipose cells and unrestrained glucose production in the liver. The result is **hyperglycemia,** a marked elevation in blood glucose levels that can ultimately cause damage to blood vessels, nerves, and tissues. Box 21-1 (p. 554) defines diabetes-related symptoms and complications.

Symptoms of Diabetes

Symptoms of diabetes are usually related to the degree of hyperglycemia present (see Table 21-1). When the plasma glucose level rises above about 200 milligrams per deciliter (mg/dL), it exceeds the **renal threshold,** the concentration at which the kidneys begin to pass glucose into the urine **(glycosuria).** The presence of glucose in the urine draws additional water from the blood, increasing the amount of urine produced. Thus, the symptoms that arise in diabetes may include frequent urination **(polyuria),** dehydration, and excessive thirst **(polydipsia).** Other possible symptoms include weight loss, excessive hunger **(polyphagia),** blurred vision (caused by the exposure of eye tissues to **hyperosmolar** fluids), increased infections (due to weakened immune responses and impaired circulation), and fatigue (due to altered energy metabolism, dehydration, or other effects of illness).

Diagnosis of Diabetes

The diagnosis of diabetes is based primarily on plasma glucose levels, which can be measured under fasting conditions or at random times during the day. In some cases, an **oral glucose tolerance test** is given: the individual ingests a 75-gram glucose load, and plasma glucose is measured at one or more time intervals following glucose ingestion. **Glycated hemoglobin (HbA$_{1c}$)** levels, which reflect hemoglobin's exposure to glucose over the preceding 2 to 3 months, are an indirect assessment of blood glucose levels. The following criteria are currently used to diagnose diabetes:[3]

- The plasma glucose concentration is 126 mg/dL or higher after a fast of at least eight hours (normal fasting plasma glucose levels are 75 to 100 mg/dL).

- In a person with classic symptoms of diabetes, the plasma glucose concentration of a random, or casual, blood sample (obtained from a non-fasting individual) is 200 mg/dL or higher.

- The plasma glucose concentration measured two hours after a 75-gram glucose load is 200 mg/dL or higher.

- The HbA$_{1c}$ level is 6.5 percent or higher.

TABLE 21-1 Symptoms of Diabetes Mellitus

- Frequent urination (polyuria)
- Dehydration, dry mouth
- Excessive thirst (polydipsia)
- Weight loss
- Excessive hunger (polyphagia)
- Blurred vision
- Increased infections
- Fatigue

© 2016 Cengage Learning®

diabetes (DYE-ah-BEE-teez) **mellitus:** a group of metabolic disorders characterized by hyperglycemia and disordered insulin metabolism.

- *diabetes* = siphon (in Greek), referring to the excessive passage of urine that is characteristic of untreated diabetes
- *mellitus* = sweet, honeylike

insulin: a pancreatic hormone that regulates glucose metabolism; its actions are countered mainly by the hormone *glucagon*.

renal threshold: the blood concentration of a substance that exceeds the kidneys' capacity for reabsorption, causing the substance to be passed into the urine.

hyperosmolar: having an abnormally high osmolarity; osmolarity refers to the concentration of osmotically active particles in solution. Hyperglycemia may cause some body fluids to become hyperosmolar.

oral glucose tolerance test: a test that evaluates a person's ability to tolerate an oral glucose load.

glycated hemoglobin (HbA$_{1c}$): hemoglobin that has nonenzymatically attached to glucose; the level of HbA$_{1c}$ in the blood helps to diagnose diabetes and evaluate long-term glycemic control. Also called *glycosylated hemoglobin*.

BOX 21-1 GLOSSARY OF DIABETES-RELATED SYMPTOMS AND COMPLICATIONS

acetone breath: a distinctive fruity odor on the breath of a person with ketosis.

albuminuria: the presence of albumin (a blood protein) in the urine, a sign of diabetic nephropathy.

claudication (CLAW-dih-KAY-shun)**:** pain in the legs while walking; usually due to an inadequate supply of blood to muscles.

diabetic coma: a coma that occurs in uncontrolled diabetes; may be due to diabetic ketoacidosis, the hyperosmolar hyperglycemic syndrome, or severe hypoglycemia. Diabetic coma was a frequent cause of death before insulin was routinely used to manage diabetes.

diabetic nephropathy (neh-FRAH-pah-thee)**:** damage to the kidneys that results from long-term diabetes.

diabetic neuropathy (nur-RAH-pah-thee)**:** nerve damage that results from long-term diabetes.

diabetic retinopathy (REH-tih-NAH-pah-thee)**:** retinal damage that results from long-term diabetes.

gangrene: death of tissue due to a deficient blood supply and/or infection.

gastroparesis (GAS-tro-pah-REE-sis)**:** delayed stomach emptying caused by nerve damage in stomach tissue.

glycosuria (GLY-co-SOOR-ee-ah)**:** the presence of glucose in the urine.

hyperglycemia: elevated blood glucose concentrations. Normal fasting plasma glucose levels are less than 100 mg/dL. Fasting plasma glucose levels between 100 and 125 mg/dL suggest prediabetes; values of 126 mg/dL and above suggest diabetes.

hyperosmolar hyperglycemic syndrome: a condition of extreme hyperglycemia associated with dehydration, hyperosmolar blood, and altered mental status; sometimes called the *hyperosmolar hyperglycemic nonketotic state.*

hypoglycemia: abnormally low blood glucose concentrations. In diabetes, hypoglycemia is treated when plasma glucose falls below 70 mg/dL.

ketoacidosis (KEY-to-ass-ih-DOE-sis)**:** an acidosis (lowering of blood pH) that results from the excessive production of ketone bodies.

ketonuria (KEY-to-NOOR-ee-ah)**:** the presence of ketone bodies in the urine.

ketosis (key-TOE-sis)**:** elevated levels of ketone bodies in the body.

macrovascular complications: disorders that affect large blood vessels, including the coronary arteries and arteries of the limbs.

microvascular complications: disorders that affect small blood vessels, including those in the retina and kidneys.

peripheral vascular disease: a condition characterized by impaired blood circulation in the limbs.

polydipsia (POL-ee-DIP-see-ah)**:** excessive thirst.

polyphagia (POL-ee-FAY-jee-ah)**:** excessive appetite or hunger.

polyuria (POL-ee-YOOR-ee-ah)**:** excessive urine production.

Overt symptoms of hyperglycemia help to confirm the diagnosis. Otherwise, a diagnosis of diabetes is confirmed only if a subsequent test yields similar results.

Individuals with **prediabetes** have blood glucose levels that are above normal but not high enough to be classified as diabetes; these individuals are at high risk of eventually developing type 2 diabetes (described in a later section) and cardiovascular diseases. Prediabetes affects approximately 37 percent of adults in the United States[4] and 23 percent of adolescents aged 12 to 19 years,[5] and it is especially prevalent among those who are overweight or obese.

Types of Diabetes

Table 21-2 lists features of the two main types of diabetes, type 1 and type 2 diabetes. Pregnancy can lead to abnormal glucose tolerance and the condition known as *gestational diabetes,* which often resolves after pregnancy but is a risk factor for type 2 diabetes. Diabetes can also be caused by medical conditions that damage the pancreas or interfere with insulin function.

Type 1 Diabetes **Type 1 diabetes** accounts for about 5 to 10 percent of diabetes cases. It is usually caused by **autoimmune** destruction of the pancreatic beta cells, which produce and secrete insulin (see Figure 21-1). By the time symptoms develop, the damage to the beta cells has progressed so far that insulin must be provided, most often by injection. Although the reason for the autoimmune attack is usually unknown, environmental toxins or infections are likely triggers. People with type 1 diabetes often have a genetic susceptibility for the disorder and are at increased risk of developing other autoimmune diseases.

Type 1 diabetes usually develops during childhood or adolescence, and symptoms may appear abruptly in previously healthy children.[6] Classic symptoms are polyuria,

prediabetes: the state of having plasma glucose levels that are higher than normal but not high enough to be diagnosed as diabetes (100–125 mg/dL when fasting or 140–199 mg/dL when measured two hours after ingesting 75 grams of glucose); occurs in individuals who have metabolic defects that often lead to type 2 diabetes.

type 1 diabetes: diabetes that is characterized by absolute insulin deficiency, usually resulting from the autoimmune destruction of pancreatic beta cells.

autoimmune: refers to an immune response directed against the body's own tissues.

❚ *auto* = self

TABLE 21-2 Features of Type 1 and Type 2 Diabetes Mellitus

Feature	Type 1 Diabetes	Type 2 Diabetes
Prevalence in diabetic population	5–10 percent of cases	90–95 percent of cases
Age of onset	<30 years	>40 years[a]
Associated conditions	Autoimmune diseases, viral infection, inherited factors	Obesity, aging, inactivity, inherited factors
Major defect	Destruction of pancreatic beta cells; insulin deficiency	Insulin resistance; insulin deficiency relative to needs
Insulin secretion	Little or none	Varies; may be normal, increased, or decreased
Requirement for insulin therapy	All cases	Some cases
Former names	Juvenile-onset diabetes Insulin-dependent diabetes	Adult-onset diabetes Noninsulin-dependent diabetes

[a]Incidence of type 2 diabetes is increasing in children and adolescents; in more than 90% of these cases, it is associated with overweight or obesity and a family history of type 2 diabetes.

FIGURE 21-1 Pancreatic Insulin Production
Cross-sections of the pancreas reveal small clusters of cells known as the islets of Langerhans; these regions contain the beta cells that produce insulin.

polydipsia, weight loss, and weakness or fatigue. **Ketoacidosis**—acidosis due to the excessive production of **ketone bodies**—is sometimes the first sign of disease. Disease onset tends to be more gradual in individuals who develop type 1 diabetes in later years. Blood tests that detect antibodies to insulin, pancreatic islet cells, and pancreatic enzymes can confirm the diagnosis and help to predict development of the disease in close relatives.

Type 2 Diabetes **Type 2 diabetes** is the most prevalent form of diabetes, accounting for 90 to 95 percent of cases. The defect in type 2 diabetes is **insulin resistance,** the reduced sensitivity to insulin in muscle, adipose, and liver cells, coupled with relative insulin deficiency, the lack of sufficient insulin to manage glucose effectively. Normally, the pancreatic beta cells secrete more insulin to compensate for insulin resistance. In type 2 diabetes, insulin levels are often abnormally high **(hyperinsulinemia)** but the additional insulin is insufficient to compensate for its diminished effect in cells. Thus, the hyperglycemia that develops represents a mismatch between the amount of insulin required and the amount produced by beta cells. Beta cell function tends to worsen over time in people with type 2 diabetes, and insulin production declines as the condition progresses.[7]

Although the precise causes of type 2 diabetes are unknown, risk is substantially increased by obesity (especially abdominal obesity), aging, and physical inactivity. The majority of individuals with type 2 diabetes are obese, and obesity itself can directly cause some degree of insulin resistance (see Nutrition in Practice 21).[8] Prevalence increases with age and probably exceeds 25 percent in persons older than 65 years; however, many cases remain undiagnosed.[9] Genetic factors strongly influence risk: type 2 diabetes is more prevalent in certain ethnic populations, including African Americans, Asian Americans, Hispanic populations, Native Americans, and Pacific Islanders.

Type 2 Diabetes in Children and Adolescents Although most cases of type 2 diabetes are diagnosed in individuals who are over 40 years of age, children and teenagers who are overweight or obese or have a family history of diabetes are at increased risk. Because type 2 diabetes is frequently asymptomatic, it is generally identified in youths only when high-risk groups are screened for the disease.

Increased rates of both type 1 and type 2 diabetes have been documented in children in past decades and correlate with the rise in childhood obesity. Type 1 and type 2 diabetes are sometimes difficult to distinguish in children, however, and a few studies

ketone bodies: products of fat metabolism that are produced in the liver; accumulate in the blood when abnormally high amounts of fatty acids are released from adipose tissue.

type 2 diabetes: diabetes that is characterized by insulin resistance coupled with insufficient insulin secretion.

insulin resistance: reduced sensitivity to insulin in muscle, adipose, and liver cells.

hyperinsulinemia: abnormally high levels of insulin in the blood.

suggest that some children diagnosed with type 1 diabetes may actually have had type 2 diabetes.[10] Type 2 diabetes is still extremely rare in children; for example, its estimated incidence in 10- to 19-year-old African-American and Hispanic-American youths—two groups at high risk—is about 27 and 17 cases per 100,000 individuals per year, respectively.[11] Its increasing prevalence, however, indicates that routine screening and diabetes prevention programs may be important safeguards for children at risk (see Box 21-2).

Acute Complications of Diabetes Mellitus

Untreated diabetes may result in life-threatening complications. Insulin deficiency can cause significant disturbances in energy metabolism, and severe hyperglycemia can lead to dehydration and electrolyte imbalances. In treated diabetes, **hypoglycemia** is a possible complication of inappropriate disease management. Figure 21-2 presents an overview of some of the effects of insulin insufficiency on energy metabolism.

Diabetic Ketoacidosis in Type 1 Diabetes A severe lack of insulin causes diabetic ketoacidosis. Without insulin, glucagon's effects become more pronounced, leading to the unrestrained breakdown of the triglycerides in adipose tissue and the protein in muscle. As a result, an increased supply of fatty acids and amino acids arrives in the liver, fueling the production of ketone bodies and glucose. Ketone bodies, which are acidic, can reach dangerously high levels in the blood (ketoacidosis) and spill into the urine **(ketonuria).** Blood pH typically falls below 7.30 (blood pH normally ranges between 7.35 and 7.45). Blood glucose levels usually exceed 250 mg/dL and rise

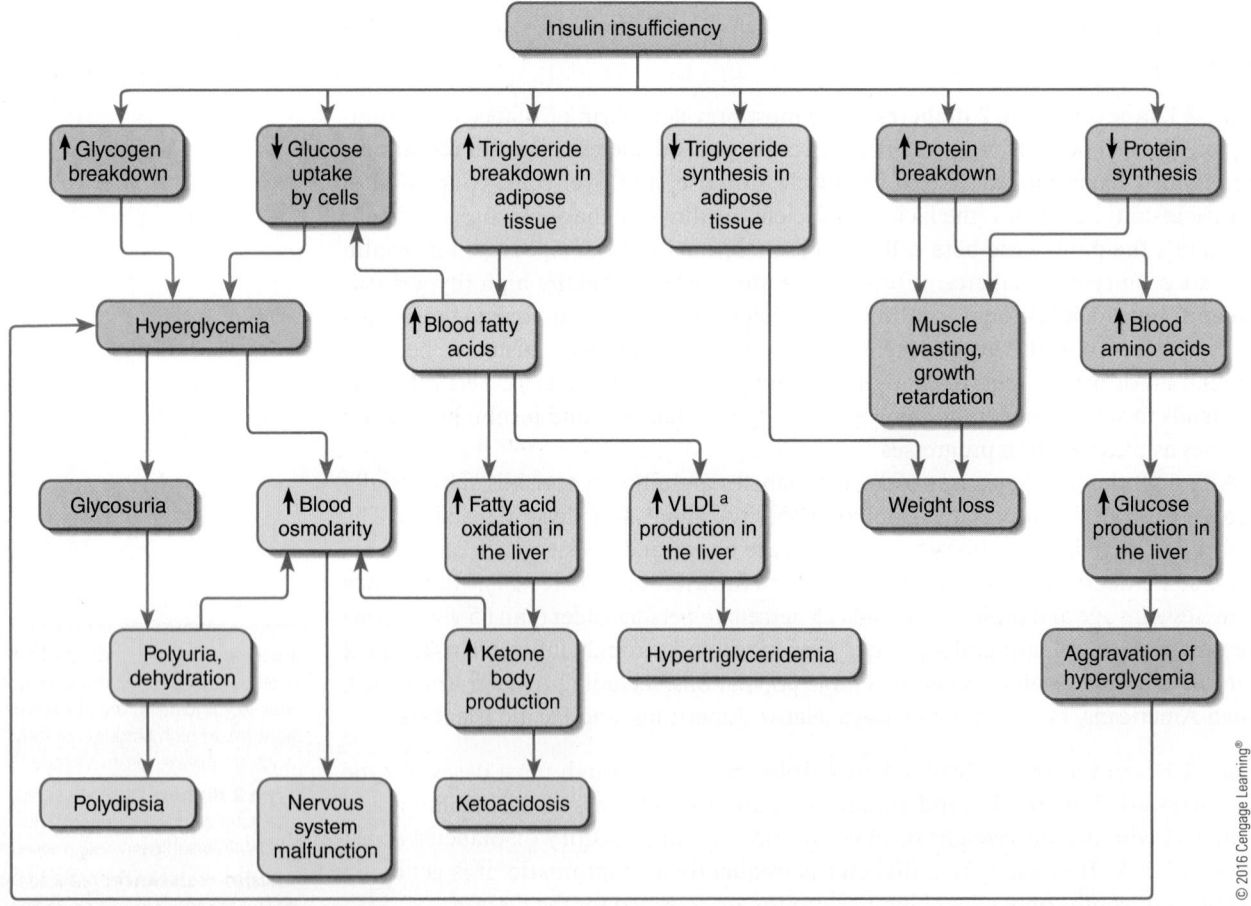

[a]Very low density lipoproteins; these lipoproteins transport triglycerides from the liver to other tissues.

FIGURE 21-2 Effects of Insulin Insufficiency
The effects of insulin insufficiency can be grouped according to its effects on carbohydrate, protein, and fat metabolism.

© 2016 Cengage Learning®

above 1,000 mg/dL in severe cases. The main features of diabetic ketoacidosis therefore include severe **ketosis,** acidosis, and hyperglycemia.[12]

Patients with ketoacidosis may exhibit symptoms of both acidosis and dehydration. Acidosis is partially corrected by exhalation of carbon dioxide, so rapid or deep breathing is characteristic.* Ketone accumulation is sometimes evident by a fruity odor on a person's breath **(acetone breath).** Significant urine loss (polyuria) accompanies the hyperglycemia, lowering blood volume and blood pressure and depleting electrolytes. In response, patients may demonstrate marked fatigue, lethargy, nausea, and vomiting. Mental state may vary from alert to comatose **(diabetic coma).** Treatment of diabetic ketoacidosis includes insulin therapy to correct the hyperglycemia, intravenous fluid and electrolyte replacement, and, in some cases, bicarbonate therapy to treat acidosis.

Diabetic ketoacidosis may result from inappropriate diabetes treatment (such as missed insulin injections), illness or infection, alcohol abuse, or other physiological stressors.[13] The condition usually develops quickly, within 1 to 2 days. Although diabetic ketoacidosis can occur in type 2 diabetes—usually due to severe stressors such as infection, trauma, or surgery—it rarely develops because even relatively low insulin concentrations suppress ketone body production.

Hyperosmolar Hyperglycemic Syndrome in Type 2 Diabetes The **hyperosmolar hyperglycemic syndrome** is a condition of severe hyperglycemia and dehydration that develops in the absence of significant ketosis. The condition often evolves slowly, over one week or longer. It is usually precipitated by a serious illness or infection that worsens hyperglycemia and results in substantial fluid losses due to polyuria or diarrhea; in addition, the patient is unable to recognize thirst or replace fluids adequately due to age, illness, sedation, or incapacity. The profound dehydration that eventually develops exacerbates the rise in blood glucose levels, which often exceed 600 mg/dL and may climb above 1000 mg/dL. Blood plasma may become so hyperosmolar as to cause neurological abnormalities, confusion, speech or vision impairments, muscle weakness, abnormal reflexes, and seizures; about 10 percent of patients lapse into coma.[14] Treatment includes intravenous fluid and electrolyte replacement and insulin therapy.

Hypoglycemia Hypoglycemia, or low blood glucose, is due to the inappropriate management of diabetes rather than the disease itself. It is usually caused by excessive dosages of insulin or antidiabetic drugs, prolonged exercise, skipped or delayed meals, inadequate food intake, or the consumption of alcohol without food. Hypoglycemia is the most frequent cause of coma in insulin-treated patients and is believed to account for 3 to 4 percent of deaths in this population.[15]

Symptoms of hypoglycemia include sweating, heart palpitations, shakiness, hunger, weakness, dizziness, and irritability. Mental confusion may prevent a person from recognizing the problem and taking such corrective action as ingesting glucose tablets, juice, or candy (see p. 567). If hypoglycemia occurs during the night, patients may be completely unaware of its presence.

Chronic Complications of Diabetes

Prolonged hyperglycemia can damage cells and tissues. Glucose nonenzymatically combines with proteins, producing molecules that eventually break down to form reactive compounds known as **advanced glycation end products (AGEs);** in diabetes, these AGEs accumulate to such high levels that they alter the structures of proteins and stimulate metabolic pathways that are damaging to tissues. Chronic complications of diabetes typically involve the large blood vessels **(macrovascular complications),** smaller vessels such as arterioles and capillaries **(microvascular complications),** and the nerves **(diabetic neuropathy).** Complications may appear 15 to 20 years after diabetes onset.

advanced glycation end products (AGEs): reactive compounds formed after glucose combines with protein; AGEs can damage tissues and lead to diabetic complications.

---

*Bicarbonate is a buffer in the blood that corrects acidosis. The acid (H^+) combines with bicarbonate (HCO_3^-) to form carbonic acid (H_2CO_3), which breaks down to water (H_2O) and carbon dioxide (CO_2). The carbon dioxide is then exhaled.

FIGURE 21-3 Diabetic Foot Ulcer
Foot ulcers are a common complication of diabetes because blood circulation is impaired, which slows healing, and nerve damage dampens foot pain, delaying recognition and treatment of cuts and bruises.

Macrovascular Complications The damage caused by diabetes accelerates the development of atherosclerosis in the arteries of the heart, brain, and limbs. Cardiovascular diseases are the leading cause of death in people with diabetes, accounting for up to 70 percent of deaths.[16] Moreover, type 2 diabetes is often accompanied by multiple risk factors for cardiovascular disease, including hypertension and blood lipid abnormalities. People with diabetes also have increased tendencies for thrombosis (blood clot formation) and abnormal ventricle function, both of which can worsen the clinical course of heart disease.

Peripheral vascular disease (impaired blood circulation in the limbs) increases the risk of **claudication** (pain while walking) and contributes to the development of foot ulcers (see Figure 21-3). Left untreated, foot ulcers can lead to **gangrene** (tissue death), and some patients require foot amputation, a major cause of disability in diabetes.

Microvascular Complications Long-term diabetes causes progressive damage to capillaries in the retina **(diabetic retinopathy),** leading to visual impairments and, in some cases, blindness. Damage to the kidneys' specialized capillaries **(diabetic nephropathy)** prevents adequate blood filtration, and kidney failure often develops, requiring the use of dialysis (artificial filtration of blood) for survival. Retinopathy and nephropathy progress most rapidly when diabetes is poorly controlled, and intensive diabetes management can help slow the progression of these conditions.

Diabetic Neuropathy Symptoms of diabetic neuropathy vary and may be experienced as deep pain or burning in the legs and feet, weakness of the arms and legs, or numbness and tingling in the hands and feet. Pain and cramping, especially in the legs, are often severe during the night and may interrupt sleep. Neuropathy also contributes to the development of foot ulcers because cuts and bruises may go unnoticed until wounds are severe. Other manifestations of neuropathy include sweating abnormalities, disturbances in bladder and bowel function, sexual dysfunction, constipation, and delayed stomach emptying **(gastroparesis).**

IN SUMMARY

▌ Diabetes mellitus is a chronic condition characterized by inadequate insulin secretion and/or impaired insulin action; diagnosis is based on indicators of hyperglycemia.

▌ In type 1 diabetes, the pancreas secretes little or no insulin, and insulin therapy is necessary for survival. Type 2 diabetes is characterized by insulin resistance coupled with relative insulin deficiency.

▌ Acute complications of poorly controlled diabetes include diabetic ketoacidosis, in which hyperglycemia is accompanied by ketosis and acidosis; the hyperosmolar hyperglycemic syndrome, characterized by severe hyperglycemia, dehydration, and mental impairments; and hypoglycemia, which most often results from inappropriate disease management.

▌ Chronic complications of diabetes include macrovascular disorders such as cardiovascular disease and peripheral vascular disease, microvascular conditions such as retinopathy and nephropathy, and neuropathy.

21.2 Treatment of Diabetes Mellitus

LO 21.2 Describe how diabetes is managed using individualized dietary adjustments, medications, and physical activity plans.

Diabetes is a chronic and progressive illness that requires lifelong treatment. Managing blood glucose levels is a delicate balancing act that involves meal planning, proper

TABLE 21-3 Comparison of Conventional and Intensive Therapies for Type 1 Diabetes[a]

	Conventional Therapy	Intensive Therapy
Blood glucose monitoring	Monitored daily	Monitored at least three times daily
Insulin therapy[b]	One or two daily injections; no daily adjustments	Three or more daily injections or use of an external insulin pump; dosage adjusted according to the results of blood glucose monitoring and expected carbohydrate intake
Advantages	Fewer incidences of severe hypoglycemia; less weight gain	Delayed progression of retinopathy, nephropathy, and neuropathy
Disadvantages	More rapid progression of retinopathy, nephropathy, and neuropathy	Twofold to threefold increase in severe hypoglycemia; weight gain; increased risk of becoming overweight

© 2016 Cengage Learning®

[a]The therapies shown here were compared in the *Diabetes Control and Complications Trial,* which was conducted in patients with type 1 diabetes.

[b]In the Diabetes Control and Complications Trial, insulin therapy was conducted using various mixtures of short-acting, intermediate-acting, and long-acting insulins. Since the study, a variety of other insulin therapies have been developed (including rapid-acting insulin and long-acting insulin analogs), allowing for treatments associated with less risk of hypoglycemia.

timing of medications, and physical exercise. Frequent adjustments in treatment are often necessary to establish good **glycemic** control. Individuals with type 1 diabetes require insulin therapy for survival. Type 2 diabetes may initially be treated with nutrition therapy and exercise, but most patients eventually need antidiabetic medications or insulin. Although the health care team must determine the appropriate therapy, the individual with diabetes ultimately assumes much of the responsibility for treatment and therefore requires education in self-management of the disease.

Treatment Goals

The main goal of diabetes treatment is to maintain blood glucose levels within a desirable range to prevent or reduce the risk of complications. Several multicenter clinical trials have shown that *intensive* diabetes treatment, which keeps blood glucose levels tightly controlled, can greatly reduce the incidence and severity of some chronic complications.*[17] Therefore, maintenance of near-normal glucose levels has become the fundamental objective of diabetes care plans (note that intensive treatment may be inappropriate for some individuals, including those with limited life expectancies, history of hypoglycemia, or previous heart disease). Other goals of treatment include maintaining healthy blood lipid concentrations, controlling blood pressure, and managing weight—measures that can help to prevent or delay diabetes complications as well. Table 21-3 provides examples of some major differences between conventional and intensive therapies for type 1 diabetes. Although intensive therapy is also associated with some risks, including an increased risk of hypoglycemia, its benefits for most people outweigh these disadvantages.

Diabetes education provides an individual with the knowledge and skills necessary to implement treatment. The primary instructor is often a **Certified Diabetes Educator (CDE),** a health care professional (often a nurse or dietitian) who has specialized knowledge about diabetes treatment and the health education process. To manage diabetes, patients must learn about appropriate meal planning, medication administration, blood glucose monitoring, weight management, appropriate physical activity, and prevention and treatment of diabetic complications.

glycemic (gly-SEE-mic)**:** pertaining to blood glucose.

Certified Diabetes Educator (CDE): a health care professional who specializes in diabetes management education; certification is obtained from the National Certification Board for Diabetes Educators.

*Studies that evaluated the benefits of intensive diabetes treatment include the *Diabetes Control and Complications Trial* and the *United Kingdom Prospective Diabetes Study.*

©Dmitry Lobanov/Shutterstock.com

FIGURE 21-4 Self-monitoring of blood glucose involves applying a drop of blood from a finger prick to a chemically treated paper strip, which is then analyzed for glucose.

BOX 21-3

Goals for glycemic control in adults (nonpregnant):

▪ Before meals: 70–130 mg/dL

▪ One to two hours after the start of a meal: <180 mg/dL

▪ HbA_{1c}: <7.0%

BOX 21-4

Comparison of HbA_{1c} and plasma glucose levels:

HbA_{1c} (%)	Average glucose levels (mg/dL)
6	126
7	154
8	183
9	212

self-monitoring of blood glucose: home monitoring of blood glucose levels using a glucose meter.

continuous glucose monitoring: continuous monitoring of tissue glucose levels using a small sensor placed under the skin.

Evaluating Diabetes Treatment

Diabetes treatment is largely evaluated by monitoring glycemic status. Good glycemic control requires frequent testing of blood glucose levels using a glucose meter, referred to as **self-monitoring of blood glucose** (see Figure 21-4 and Box 21-3). Glucose testing provides valuable feedback when the patient adjusts food intake, medications, and physical activity and is helpful for preventing hypoglycemia. Ideally, patients with type 1 diabetes should measure blood glucose levels prior to meals and snacks, at bedtime, prior to exercise, and whenever they suspect hypoglycemia.[18] Some patients may achieve better glycemic control by also using a **continuous glucose monitoring** system, which measures tissue glucose levels every few minutes using a tiny sensor placed under the skin. Although self-monitoring of blood glucose is also useful in type 2 diabetes, the recommended frequency varies according to the specific needs of individual patients.

Long-Term Glycemic Control Health care providers periodically evaluate long-term glycemic control by measuring glycated hemoglobin, or HbA_{1c}. The glucose in blood freely enters red blood cells and attaches to hemoglobin in direct proportion to the amount of glucose present (Box 21-4 shows how HbA_{1c} correlates with average plasma glucose levels). The percentage of HbA_{1c} reflects glycemic control over the preceding 2 to 3 months, the average age of circulating red blood cells.[19] The goal of diabetes treatment is usually an HbA_{1c} value less than 7 percent (HbA_{1c} is typically less than 6 percent in non-diabetics),[20] but the percentage is often markedly higher in people with diabetes, even those who are maintaining near-normal blood glucose levels. Less stringent HbA_{1c} goals (for example, an HbA_{1c} value less than 8 percent) may be suitable for some patients, including those with limited life expectancy, advanced diabetic complications, or a history of severe hypoglycemia. HbA_{1c} testing is typically conducted two to four times yearly.

Monitoring for Long-Term Complications Individuals with diabetes are routinely monitored for signs of long-term complications. Blood pressure is measured at each checkup. Annual lipid screening is suggested for adult patients. Routine checks for urinary protein **(albuminuria)** can determine if nephropathy has developed. Physical examinations generally screen for signs of retinopathy, neuropathy, and foot problems.

Ketone Testing Ketone testing, which checks for the development of ketoacidosis, should be performed if symptoms are present or if risk has increased due to acute illness, stress, or pregnancy. Both blood and urine tests are available for home use, although the blood tests are generally more reliable. Ketone testing is most useful for patients who have type 1 diabetes or gestational diabetes. Individuals with type 2 diabetes may produce excessive ketone bodies when severely stressed by infection or trauma.

Nutrition Therapy: Dietary Recommendations

Nutrition therapy can improve glycemic control and slow the progression of diabetic complications. As always, the nutrition care plan must consider personal preferences and lifestyle habits. In addition, dietary intakes must be modified to accommodate growth, lifestyle changes, aging, and any complications that develop. Although all members of the diabetes care team should understand the principles of dietary treatment, a registered dietitian is best suited to design and implement the nutrition therapy provided to diabetes patients.[21] This section presents the dietary recommendations for diabetes; a later section describes meal-planning strategies.

Macronutrient Intakes The recommended macronutrient distribution (percent of kcalories from carbohydrate, fat, and protein) depends on food preferences and metabolic factors (for example, insulin sensitivity, blood lipid levels, and kidney function).[22] Intakes suggested for the general population are often used as a guideline (see Box 21-5). Day-to-day consistency in carbohydrate intake is associated with better glycemic control, unless the patient is undergoing intensive insulin therapy that matches insulin doses to mealtime carbohydrate intakes.[23]

Total Carbohydrate Intake The amount of carbohydrate consumed has the greatest influence on blood glucose levels after meals—the more grams of carbohydrate ingested, the greater the glycemic response. The carbohydrate recommendation is based in part on the person's metabolic needs, the type of insulin or other medications used to manage the diabetes, and individual preferences. For optimal health, the carbohydrate sources should be whole grains, legumes, vegetables, fruits, and milk products, whereas foods made with refined grains and added sugars should be limited.[24]

Glycemic Index Different carbohydrate-containing foods have different effects on blood glucose levels after they are ingested; for example, consuming a portion of white rice causes blood glucose to increase more than would a similar portion of barley. A food's glycemic effect is influenced by the type of carbohydrate in a food, the food's fiber content, the preparation method, the other foods included in a meal, and individual tolerances. For individuals with diabetes, choosing foods with a low **glycemic index (GI)** over those with a high GI may modestly improve glycemic control.[25] A food's glycemic effect is not usually a primary consideration when treating diabetes, however, because clinical studies investigating the potential benefits of low-GI diets on glycemic control have had mixed results.[26] Nonetheless, high-fiber, minimally processed foods—which typically have lower glycemic effects than do highly processed, starchy foods—are among the foods frequently recommended for persons with diabetes.

Sugars A common misperception is that people with diabetes need to avoid sugar and sugar-containing foods. In reality, table sugar (sucrose), made up of glucose and fructose, has a lower glycemic effect than starch. Because moderate consumption of sugar has not been shown to adversely affect glycemic control,[27] sugar recommendations for people with diabetes are similar to those for the general population, which suggest minimizing foods and beverages that contain added sugars. However, sugars and sugary foods must be counted as part of the daily carbohydrate allowance.

Fructose, a naturally occurring monosaccharide in fruit, has minimal effects on blood glucose levels when compared with similar amounts of sucrose or starch. Although some food products marketed to people with diabetes are sweetened with fructose, intakes of fructose should be limited—to no more than 12 percent of total kcalories—to avoid excessive energy intakes or adverse effects on blood lipids (high fructose intakes may increase blood triglyceride levels in some individuals).[28] Sugar alcohols (such as sorbitol and maltitol) have lower glycemic effects than glucose or sucrose and may be used as sugar substitutes. Artificial sweeteners (such as aspartame, saccharin, and sucralose) contain no digestible carbohydrate and can be safely used in place of sugar.

Whole Grains and Fiber Recommendations for whole grain and fiber intakes are similar to those for the general population. People with diabetes are encouraged to include fiber-rich foods such as whole-grain cereals, legumes, fruits, and vegetables in their diet. Although some studies have suggested that very high intakes of fiber (more than 50 grams per day) may improve glycemic control, many individuals have difficulty enjoying or tolerating such large amounts of fiber.[29]

Dietary Fat In individuals with diabetes, a Mediterranean-style dietary pattern that emphasizes monounsaturated fats may benefit both glycemic control and cardiovascular disease (CVD) risk.[30] In addition, increased intakes of omega-3 fatty acids from fatty fish or plant sources may improve the lipoprotein profile and various other CVD risk factors (see Chapter 3). Other guidelines related to fat intake are similar to those suggested for the general population: saturated fat should be less than 10 percent of total kcalories, *trans* fats should be minimized, and cholesterol intake should be less than 300 milligrams daily.

BOX 21-5

Macronutrient DRI for adults:

Macronutrient ranges (% of total kcal):

- Carbohydrate: 45–65%
- Fat: 20–35%
- Protein: 10–35%

Carbohydrate RDA: 130 g/day

Fiber AI: 21–38 g/day

Protein RDA: 0.8 g/kg body weight

glycemic index (GI): a ranking of carbohydrate foods based on their effect on blood glucose levels after ingestion; low-GI foods are those with a lesser glycemic effect whereas high-GI foods have a greater glycemic effect. The website *www.glycemicindex.com* provides GI values for a wide variety of foods.

Protein Protein recommendations for people with diabetes are similar to those for the general population (see Box 21-5). In the United States, the average protein intake is about 15 percent of the energy intake. Although several small, short-term studies have suggested that protein intakes above 28 percent of total kcalories may improve glycemic control or lipoprotein levels in diabetic individuals, other studies did not show any benefit.[31] In addition, high protein intakes are sometimes discouraged because they may be detrimental to kidney function in patients with nephropathy.

Alcohol Use in Diabetes Guidelines for alcohol intake are similar to those for the general population, which recommend that women and men limit their average daily intakes of alcohol to one **drink** and two drinks per day, respectively. In addition, individuals using insulin or medications that promote insulin secretion should consume food when they ingest alcoholic beverages to avoid hypoglycemia (alcohol can cause hypoglycemia by interfering with glucose production in the liver).[32] Conversely, an excessive alcohol intake (three or more drinks per day) can worsen hyperglycemia and raise triglyceride levels in some individuals. People who should avoid alcohol include pregnant women and individuals with advanced neuropathy, abnormally high triglyceride levels, or a history of alcohol abuse.

Micronutrients Micronutrient recommendations for people with diabetes are the same as for the general population. Vitamin and mineral supplementation is not recommended unless nutrient deficiencies develop; those at risk include the elderly, pregnant or lactating women, strict vegetarians, and individuals on kcalorie-restricted diets.

Body Weight in Type 2 Diabetes Because excessive body fat can worsen insulin resistance, weight loss is recommended for overweight or obese individuals who have diabetes. Even moderate weight loss (5 to 10 percent of body weight) can help to improve insulin resistance, glycemic control, blood lipid levels, and blood pressure. Weight loss is most beneficial early in the course of diabetes, before insulin secretion has diminished.[33]

Not all persons with type 2 diabetes are overweight or obese. Older adults and those in long-term care facilities are often underweight and may need to gain weight. Low body weight increases risks of morbidity and mortality in these individuals.

Nutrition Therapy: Meal-Planning Strategies

Dietitians provide a number of meal-planning strategies to help people with diabetes maintain glycemic control. These strategies emphasize control of carbohydrate intake and portion sizes. Initial dietary instructions may include guidelines for maintaining a healthy diet, improving blood lipids, and reducing cardiovascular risk factors. Sample menus that include commonly eaten foods can help to illustrate general principles. People using intensive insulin therapy must learn to coordinate insulin injections with meals and to match insulin dosages to carbohydrate intake, as discussed later.

Carbohydrate Counting Carbohydrate-counting techniques are simpler and more flexible than other menu-planning approaches and are widely used for planning diabetes diets. Carbohydrate counting works as follows: After an interview in which the dietitian learns about the patient's usual food intake and calculates nutrient and energy needs, the patient is given a daily carbohydrate allowance, divided into a pattern of meals and snacks according to individual preferences. The carbohydrate allowance can be expressed in grams or as the number of carbohydrate portions allowed per meal (see Table 21-4). The user of the plan need only be concerned about meeting carbohydrate goals and can select from any of the carbohydrate-containing food groups when planning meals (see Table 21-5 and Figure 21-5 on p. 564). Although encouraged to make healthy food choices, the individual has the freedom to choose the foods desired at each meal without risking loss of glycemic control. Some people may also need guidance about consuming a diet that improves blood lipids or energy intakes. Box 21-6 shows how to implement carbohydrate counting in clinical practice.

drink: volume of an alcoholic beverage containing about ½ ounce of pure ethanol; equivalent to 12 oz of beer, 5 oz of wine, or 1½ oz of 80 proof distilled spirits such as gin, rum, vodka, and whiskey.

1. The first step in basic carbohydrate counting is to determine an appropriate carbohydrate allowance and suitable distribution pattern; an example is shown in Table 21-4. A nutrition assessment can help the dietitian estimate the usual carbohydrate intake and food habits of the person using the plan to ensure that the carbohydrate level will be acceptable. Frequent monitoring of blood glucose levels can help determine whether additional carbohydrate restriction would be helpful.

   The example given in Table 21-4 illustrates a meal pattern for a person consuming 2000 kcalories daily with a carbohydrate allowance of 50 percent of kcalories. This is calculated as follows:

   2000 kcal × 50% = 1000 kcal of carbohydrate

   $$\frac{1000 \text{ kcal carbohydrate}}{4 \text{ kcal/g carbohydrate}} = 250 \text{ g carbohydrate/day}$$

   $$\frac{250 \text{ g carbohydrate}}{15 \text{ g/1 carbohydrate portion}} = 16.7 \text{ carbohydrate portions/day}$$

2. The distribution of carbohydrates among meals and snacks is based on both individual preferences and metabolic needs. In type 1 diabetes, the insulin regimen must coordinate with the individual's dietary and lifestyle choices. People using conventional insulin therapy must maintain a consistent carbohydrate intake from day to day to match their particular insulin prescription, whereas those using intensive therapy can alter insulin dosages when carbohydrate intakes change. People with type 2 diabetes are encouraged to develop dietary patterns that suit their lifestyle and medication schedules. For all types of diabetes, the carbohydrate recommendation may need to be altered periodically to improve blood glucose control.

3. Carbohydrate counting can be done in one of two ways:
   - Count the grams of carbohydrate provided by foods.
   - Count carbohydrate portions, expressed in terms of servings that contain about 15 grams of carbohydrate each.

TABLE 21-4 Sample Carbohydrate Distribution for a 2000-kCalorie Diet

Meals	Carbohydrate Allowance	
	Grams	Portions[a]
Breakfast	60	4
Lunch	60	4
Afternoon snack	30	2
Dinner	75	5
Evening snack	30	2
Totals	**255 g**	**17**

Note: The carbohydrate allowance in this example is approximately 50% of total kcalories.

[a]1 portion = 15 g carbohydrate = 1 portion of starchy food, milk, or fruit.

Success with carbohydrate counting requires knowledge about the food sources of carbohydrates and an understanding of portion control. As shown in Table 21-5, food

TABLE 21-5 Carbohydrate-Containing Food Groups and Sample Portion Sizes

Bread, cereal, rice, and pasta: 1 portion = 15 g carbohydrate
- 1 slice of bread or 1 tortilla
- $\frac{1}{2}$ English muffin
- $\frac{3}{4}$ c unsweetened, ready-to-eat cereal
- $\frac{1}{2}$ c cooked oatmeal
- $\frac{1}{3}$ c cooked rice or pasta

Starchy vegetables: 1 portion = 15 g carbohydrate
- 1 small (3 oz) potato
- $\frac{1}{2}$ c canned or frozen corn
- $\frac{1}{2}$ c cooked beans
- 1 c winter squash, cubed

Fruit: 1 portion = 15 g carbohydrate
- 1 small apple or orange
- 1 medium peach
- $\frac{3}{4}$ c blueberries
- $\frac{1}{2}$ c apple or orange juice

Milk products: 1 portion = 12 g carbohydrate; may be rounded up to 15 g for ease in counting carbohydrate portions
- 1 c milk (whole, low-fat, or fat-free)
- 1 c buttermilk
- 6 oz plain yogurt

Sweets and desserts:[a] Carbohydrate content varies; portions listed contain approximately 15 g
- $\frac{1}{2}$ c ice cream
- 2 sandwich cookies (with cream filling)
- $\frac{1}{2}$ frosted cupcake
- 1 small granola bar (1 oz)
- 1 tbs honey

Nonstarchy vegetables: 1 portion = 3–6 g carbohydrate; 3 servings are equivalent to 1 carbohydrate portion; can be disregarded if fewer than 3 servings are consumed
- $\frac{1}{2}$ c cooked cauliflower
- $\frac{1}{2}$ c cooked cabbage, collards, or kale
- $\frac{1}{2}$ c cooked okra
- $\frac{1}{2}$ c diced or raw tomatoes

Note: Unprocessed meats, fish, and poultry contain negligible amounts of carbohydrate.

[a]Products sweetened with artificial sweeteners or sugar alcohols contain fewer grams of carbohydrate than products sweetened with sugar or honey.

© 2016 Cengage Learning®

(continued)

selections that contain about 15 grams of carbohydrate are interchangeable. The portions of foods that contain 15 grams may vary substantially, however, even among foods in a single food group. Accurate carbohydrate counting often requires instruction and practice in portion control using measuring cups, spoons, and a food scale. Food lists that indicate the carbohydrate contents of common foods are available from the American Diabetes Association and the Academy of Nutrition and Dietetics; these are helpful resources for learning carbohydrate-counting methods.

When using packaged foods, individuals should check the Nutrition Facts panel of food labels to find the carbohydrate content of a serving. If the fiber content is more than 5 grams per serving, it should be subtracted from the *Total Carbohydrate* value, as fiber does not contribute to blood glucose (some clinicians may suggest subtracting only half of the grams of fiber). If the sugar alcohol content is greater than 5 grams per serving, half of the grams of sugar alcohols can be subtracted from the *Total Carbohydrate* value.

4. Once they have learned the basic carbohydrate counting method, individuals can select whatever foods they wish as long as they do not exceed their carbohydrate goals. Figure 21-5 shows a day's menu that provides the carbohydrate allowance shown in Table 21-4. Although carbohydrate counting focuses on a single macronutrient, people using this technique should be encouraged to follow a healthy eating plan that meets other dietary objectives as well.

❋ SAMPLE MENU ❋

Breakfast:	Carbohydrate Portions	Afternoon snack:	Carbohydrate Portions
Carbohydrate goal = 4 portions or 60 g		**Carbohydrate goal = 2 portions or 30 g**	
3/4 c unsweetened, ready-to-eat cereal	1	2 sandwich cookies	1
1/2 c low-fat milk	1/2	1 c low-fat millk	1
1 scrambled egg	—	**Dinner:**	
1 slice whole-wheat toast (with margarine or butter)	1	**Carbohydrate goal = 5 portions or 75 g**	
6 oz orange juice	1 1/2	4 oz grilled steak	—
Coffee (without milk or sugar)	—	1 small baked potato (with margarine or butter)	1
Lunch:		Corn on cob, 1 large ear	2
Carbohydrate goal = 4 portions or 60 g		1/2 c steamed collard greens[a]	
1 tuna salad sandwich (includes 2 slices whole-grain bread, mayonnaise)	2	1 c sliced, raw tomatoes[a]	1
6 oz yogurt (plain) with 3/4 c blueberries and artificial sweetener	2	1/2 c ice cream	1
Diet cola	—	**Evening snack:**	
		Carbohydrate goal = 2 portions or 30 g	
		1 small apple	1
		1 oz granola bar	1

[a] Three servings of nonstarchy vegetables are equivalent to 1 carbohydrate portion.

FIGURE 21-5 Translating Carbohydrate Portions into a Day's Meals

© Cengage Learning®

Carbohydrate counting is taught at different levels of complexity depending on a person's needs and abilities. The basic carbohydrate-counting method just described can be helpful for most people, although it requires a consistent carbohydrate intake from day to day to match the medication or insulin regimen. Advanced carbohydrate counting allows more flexibility but is best suited for patients using intensive insulin therapy. With this method, a person can determine the specific dosage of insulin needed to cover the amount of carbohydrate consumed in a meal. The person is then free to choose the types and portions of food desired without sacrificing glycemic control. Advanced carbohydrate counting requires some training and should be attempted only after an individual has mastered more basic methods.

Food Lists for Diabetes A meal-planning system developed for persons with diabetes allows individuals to create an eating plan by choosing foods with specified portions from a variety of food lists. The different food lists group foods according to their proportions of carbohydrate, fat, and protein so that all items on a particular list have similar macronutrient and energy contents (see Appendix C, pp. C-1 to C-2). Thus, each food on a food list can be substituted for any other food on the same list without affecting the macronutrient balance in a day's meals. Although the food list system may be helpful for individuals who want to maintain a diet with specific macronutrient percentages, it is less flexible than carbohydrate counting and offers no advantages for maintaining glycemic control. However, the food lists may be helpful resources for individuals using carbohydrate-counting methods because the portions are similar to the portions used in carbohydrate counting, providing about 15 grams of carbohydrate per food item (see pp. C-3 to C-6; note that the carbohydrates in foods on the *Milk and Milk Substitutes* list can be rounded up to 15 grams).

Insulin Therapy

Insulin therapy is necessary for individuals who cannot produce enough insulin to meet their metabolic needs. It is therefore required by people with type 1 diabetes and those with type 2 diabetes who cannot maintain glycemic control with medications, diet, and exercise. The pancreas normally secretes insulin in relatively low amounts between meals and during the night (called *basal insulin*) and in much higher amounts when meals are ingested. Ideally, the insulin treatment should reproduce the natural pattern of insulin secretion as closely as possible.

Insulin Preparations The forms of insulin that are commercially available differ by their onset of action, timing of peak action, and duration of effects. Table 21-6 and Figure 21-6 (p. 566) show how insulin preparations are classified: they may be rapid acting (lispro, aspart, and glulisine), short acting (regular), intermediate acting (NPH), or long acting (glargine and detemir), thereby allowing substantial flexibility in establishing a suitable insulin regimen.[34] The rapid- and short-acting insulins are typically used at mealtimes, whereas the intermediate- and long-acting insulins provide basal insulin for the periods between meals and during the night. Thus, mixtures of several types of insulin can produce greater glycemic control than any one type alone. Several premixed formulations are also available; examples are listed in Table 21-6.

Insulin Delivery Insulin is most often administered by **subcutaneous** injection, either self-administered or provided by caregivers (note that insulin is a protein, and would be destroyed by digestive processes if taken orally). Disposable **syringes,** which are filled from vials that contain multiple doses of insulin, are the most common devices used for injecting insulin (see Figure 21-7, p. 566). Another option is to use

subcutaneous (sub-cue-TAY-nee-us): beneath the skin.

syringes: devices used for injecting medications. A syringe consists of a hypodermic needle attached to a hollow tube with a plunger inside.

TABLE 21-6 **Insulin Preparations**

Form of Insulin	Common Preparations	Onset of Action	Peak Action	Duration of Action
Rapid acting	Lispro (Humalog) Aspart (Novolog) Glulisine (Apidra)	5–15 minutes	60–90 minutes	3–5 hours
Short acting	Regular	30 minutes	2–3 hours	5–8 hours
Intermediate acting	NPH	2–4 hours	6–10 hours	10–16 hours
Long acting	Glargine (Lantus) Detemir (Levemir)	1–2 hours	Steady effects	24 hours
Insulin mixtures (with sample ratios)	NPH/regular (70:30) NPL (modified lispro)/lispro (50:50)	Variable; depends on formulation	Variable; depends on formulation	Variable; depends on formulation

© 2016 Cengage Learning®

FIGURE 21-6 **Effects of Insulin Preparations**

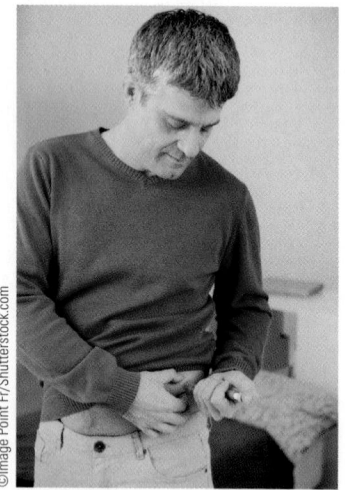

FIGURE 21-7 Insulin Injection
People with diabetes often become adept at administering the insulin they require.

FIGURE 21-8 Insulin Pump
An external insulin pump delivers a low dosage of insulin continuously and bolus doses at mealtimes.

carbohydrate-to-insulin ratio:
the amount of carbohydrate that can be handled per unit of insulin; on average, every 15 grams of carbohydrate requires about 1 unit of rapid- or short-acting insulin.

insulin pens, injection devices that resemble permanent marking pens. Disposable insulin pens are prefilled with insulin and used one time only, whereas reusable pens can be fitted with prefilled insulin cartridges and replaceable needles. Some individuals use insulin pumps, computerized devices that infuse insulin through thin, flexible tubing that remains in the skin; the pump can be attached to a belt or kept in a pocket (see Figure 21-8). Some of the newer insulin pumps include built-in continuous glucose monitoring systems.

Insulin Regimen for Type 1 Diabetes Type 1 diabetes is best managed with intensive insulin therapy, which typically involves three or four daily injections of several types of insulin or the use of an insulin pump. Insulin pumps are usually programmed to deliver low amounts of rapid-acting insulin continuously (to meet basal insulin needs) and bolus doses of rapid-acting insulin at mealtimes. In persons who inject insulin, intermediate- or long-acting insulin meets basal insulin needs, and rapid- or short-acting insulin is injected before meals. Simpler regimens involve twice-daily injections of a mixture of intermediate- and short-acting insulin. Regimens that include three or more injections allow for greater flexibility in carbohydrate intake and meal timing. With fewer injections, the timing of both meals and injections must be similar from day to day to avoid periods of insulin deficiency or excess.

A person using intensive therapy must learn to accurately determine the amount of insulin to inject before each meal. The amount required depends on the pre-meal blood glucose level, the carbohydrate content of the meal, and the person's body weight and sensitivity to insulin. To determine insulin sensitivity, the individual keeps careful records of food intake, insulin dosages, and blood glucose levels. Eventually, these records are analyzed by medical personnel to determine the appropriate **carbohydrate-to-insulin ratio** for that individual, which assists in calculating insulin dosages at mealtime. Intensive therapy allows for substantial variation in food intake and lifestyle, but it requires frequent testing of blood glucose levels and a good understanding of carbohydrate counting.

After insulin therapy is initiated, persons with type 1 diabetes may experience a temporary remission of disease symptoms and a reduced need for insulin, known as the *honeymoon period*. The remission is due to a temporary improvement in pancreatic beta-cell function and may last for several weeks or months. It is important to anticipate this period of remission to avoid insulin excess. In all cases, the honeymoon period eventually ends, and the patient must reinstate full insulin treatment.

Insulin Regimen for Type 2 Diabetes Approximately 30 percent of people diagnosed with type 2 diabetes can benefit from insulin therapy.[35] Although initial treatment of type 2 diabetes usually involves nutrition therapy, physical activity, and oral antidiabetic medications, long-term results with these treatments are often disappointing. As the disease progresses, pancreatic function worsens, and many individuals require insulin therapy to maintain glycemic control.

Many possible regimens can be used to control type 2 diabetes. Some persons may be treated with insulin alone, whereas others may use insulin in combination with other antidiabetic drugs. Many patients need only one or two daily injections. Some regimens involve a mixture of intermediate-acting and rapid- or short-acting insulin in the morning and an injection of intermediate- or long-acting insulin at dinner or before bedtime. In other cases, only a single injection of intermediate- or long-acting insulin may be needed at bedtime.[36] Doses and timing are adjusted according to the results of blood glucose self-monitoring.

Insulin Therapy and Hypoglycemia Hypoglycemia is the most common complication of insulin treatment, although it may also result from the use of some oral antidiabetic drugs. It most often results from intensive insulin therapy because the attempt to attain near-normal blood glucose levels increases the risk of overtreatment. Other potential causes include skipped meals or snacks or prolonged exercise.

Hypoglycemia can be corrected with the immediate intake of glucose or a glucose-containing food. Usually, 15 to 20 grams of carbohydrate (see Box 21-7) can relieve hypoglycemia in about 15 minutes, although patients should monitor their blood glucose levels in case additional treatment is necessary. Foods that provide pure glucose yield a better response than foods that contain other sugars, such as sucrose or fructose. Individuals who use insulin are usually advised to carry glucose tablets or a source of carbohydrate that can be easily ingested. After blood glucose normalizes, patients should consume a meal or snack to prevent recurrence. Those at risk of severe hypoglycemia are often given prescriptions for the hormone glucagon, which can be injected by caregivers in case of unconsciousness.

Insulin Therapy and Weight Gain Weight gain is sometimes an unintentional side effect of insulin therapy, especially in individuals undergoing intensive insulin treatment. Although the exact causes of the weight gain are unclear, it may partly be due to insulin's stimulatory effect on fat synthesis. Patients may be able to avoid weight gain by reducing the ratio of basal to mealtime insulin and improving carbohydrate-counting skills to obtain better estimates of mealtime insulin requirements.[37] Concerns about weight should not discourage the use of intensive therapy, which is associated with longer life expectancy and fewer complications than occur with conventional therapy.

Fasting Hyperglycemia Insulin therapy must sometimes be adjusted to prevent **fasting hyperglycemia,** which typically develops in the early morning after an overnight fast of at least eight hours. The usual cause is a waning of insulin action during the night due to insufficient insulin. A second possibility, known as the **dawn phenomenon,** is an increase of blood glucose in the morning due to the early morning secretion of growth hormone, which reduces insulin sensitivity. Less frequently, fasting hyperglycemia develops as a result of nighttime hypoglycemia, which increases the secretion of hormones that stimulate glucose production; the resulting condition is known as **rebound hyperglycemia** (also called the **Somogyi effect**). Whatever the cause, fasting hyperglycemia can be treated by adjusting the dosage or formulation of insulin administered in the evening.[38]

Antidiabetic Drugs

Treatment of type 2 diabetes often requires the use of oral medications and injectable drugs other than insulin. As shown in Table 21-7 (p. 568), these drugs can improve hyperglycemia by various modes of action. Treatment may involve the use of a single

BOX 21-7

Each of the following sources provides about 15 g of carbohydrate:

- Glucose tablets: 4 tablets
- Table sugar: 4 tsp
- Honey: 1 tbs
- Jelly beans: 15 small
- Orange juice: ½ c

fasting hyperglycemia: hyperglycemia that typically develops in the early morning after an overnight fast of at least eight hours.

dawn phenomenon: morning hyperglycemia that is caused by the early-morning release of growth hormone, which reduces insulin sensitivity.

rebound hyperglycemia: hyperglycemia that results from the release of counterregulatory hormones following nighttime hypoglycemia; also called the **Somogyi effect.**

TABLE 21-7 Antidiabetic Drugs

Drug Category	Common Examples	Mode of Action
Alpha-glucosidase inhibitors	Acarbose (Precose) Miglitol (Glyset)	Delay carbohydrate digestion and absorption
Amylin analogs (injected)	Pramlintide (Smylin)	Suppress glucagon secretion, delay stomach emptying, increase satiety
Biguanides	Metformin (Glucophage)	Inhibit liver glucose production, improve glucose utilization
Bile acid sequestrants	Colesevelam (Welchol)	Unknown; may inhibit liver glucose production
Dipeptidyl peptidase 4 (DPP-4) inhibitors	Saxagliptin (Onglyza) Sitagliptin (Januvia)	Improve insulin secretion, suppress glucagon secretion, delay stomach emptying
Dopamine D2 receptor agonists	Bromocriptine (Cycloset)	Increase insulin sensitivity
GLP-1 receptor agonists (injected)	Exenatide (Byetta) Liraglutide (Victoza)	Improve insulin secretion, suppress glucagon secretion, delay stomach emptying, increase satiety
Meglitinides	Nateglinide (Starlix) Repaglinide (Prandin)	Stimulate insulin secretion by the pancreas
Sulfonylureas	Glipizide (Glucotrol) Glyburide (Diabeta)	Stimulate insulin secretion by the pancreas
Thiazolidinediones	Pioglitazone (Actos) Rosiglitazone (Avandia)	Increase insulin sensitivity

medication (monotherapy) or a combination of several medications (combination therapy). By utilizing several mechanisms at once, combination therapy achieves more rapid and sustained glycemic control than is possible with monotherapy. Box 21-8 lists some nutrition-related effects of several antidiabetic drugs.

BOX 21-8 DIET-DRUG INTERACTIONS

Check this table for notable nutrition-related effects of the medications discussed in this chapter.

Alpha-glucosidase inhibitors	**Gastrointestinal effects:** Flatulence, abdominal cramps, diarrhea **Metabolic effects:** May decrease blood concentrations of calcium and vitamin B_6
Biguanides (metformin)	**Gastrointestinal effects:** Metallic taste, nausea, vomiting, anorexia, flatulence, abdominal cramps, diarrhea **Dietary interaction:** Excessive alcohol intake may cause lactic acidosis, which requires emergency treatment **Metabolic effects:** Decreased folate and vitamin B_{12} absorption, which may lead to deficiency
Meglitinides	**Metabolic effects:** Hypoglycemia, weight gain
Sulfonylureas	**Gastrointestinal effects:** Nausea, abdominal cramps, diarrhea, constipation **Dietary interaction:** Alcohol may delay drug absorption and prolong hypoglycemia (if hypoglycemia occurs) **Metabolic effects:** Hypoglycemia, weight gain, allergic skin reactions
Thiazolidinediones	**Metabolic effects:** Weight gain, fluid retention, edema, anemia, decreased bone density and increased risk of fractures (women)

Physical Activity and Diabetes Management

Regular physical activity can improve glycemic control considerably and is therefore a central feature of disease management. Physical activity also benefits other aspects of health, including cardiovascular risk factors and body weight. Children with diabetes or prediabetes should engage in at least 60 minutes of physical activity each day. Adults with diabetes are advised to perform at least 150 minutes of moderate-intensity aerobic activity per week, spread over at least 3 days of the week; they should also perform resistance exercise at least twice weekly unless contraindicated by a medical condition that increases risk of injury. Both aerobic and resistance exercise can improve insulin sensitivity.[39]

Medical Evaluation before Exercise Before a person with diabetes begins a new exercise program, a medical evaluation should screen for problems that may be aggravated by certain activities. Complications involving the heart and blood vessels, eyes, kidneys, feet, and nervous system may limit the types of activity recommended. For individuals with a low level of fitness who have been relatively inactive, only mild or moderate exercise may be prescribed at first; a short walk at a comfortable pace may be the first activity suggested. People with severe retinopathy should avoid vigorous aerobic or resistance exercise, which may lead to retinal detachment and damage to eye tissue. Individuals with peripheral neuropathy should ensure that they wear proper footwear during exercise; those with a foot injury or open sore should avoid weight-bearing activity. To prevent dehydration, proper hydration should be encouraged before and during exercise.

Maintaining Glycemic Control Individuals who use insulin or medications that increase insulin secretion must carefully adjust food intake and medication dosages to prevent hypoglycemia during physical activity. Medication dosages that precede exercise often need to be reduced substantially. Blood glucose levels should be checked both before and after an activity. If blood glucose is below 100 mg/dL, carbohydrate should be consumed before exercise begins.*[40] Additional carbohydrate may be needed during or after prolonged activity or even several hours after the activity is completed. Individuals with type 1 diabetes who have ketosis should avoid vigorous activity, which increases ketone body production and can worsen the ketosis.

Sick-Day Management

Illness, infection, or injury can cause hormonal changes that raise blood glucose levels and increase the risk of developing diabetic ketoacidosis or the hyperosmolar hyperglycemic syndrome. During illness, individuals with diabetes should measure blood glucose and ketone levels several times daily. They should continue to use antidiabetic drugs, including insulin, as prescribed; adjustments in dosages may be necessary if they alter their diet or have persistent hyperglycemia. If appetite is poor, patients should select easy-to-manage foods and beverages that provide the prescribed amount of carbohydrate at each meal. To prevent dehydration, especially if vomiting or diarrhea is present, patients should make sure they consume adequate amounts of liquids throughout the day.

IN SUMMARY

❚ Diabetes treatment includes nutrition therapy, the use of insulin or other antidiabetic medications, and appropriate physical activity. Glycemic control is evaluated by monitoring blood glucose levels and glycated hemoglobin.

❚ The quantity of carbohydrate consumed has the most significant influence on blood glucose levels after meals and is more important than the type of carbohydrate consumed.

*As an example, about 15 grams of carbohydrate may be needed for an activity equivalent to 30 minutes of brisk walking.

Nora is a 12-year-old girl who was diagnosed with type 1 diabetes 2 years ago. She practices intensive therapy and has had the support of her parents and an excellent diabetes management team. With their help, Nora has been able to assume the bulk of the responsibility for her diabetes care and has managed to control her blood glucose remarkably well. In the past few months, however, Nora has been complaining bitterly about the impositions diabetes has placed on her life and her interactions with friends. Sometimes she refuses to monitor her blood glucose levels, and she has skipped insulin injections a few times. Recently, Nora was admitted to the emergency room complaining of fever, nausea, vomiting, and intense thirst. The physician noted that Nora was confused and lethargic. A urine test was positive for ketones, and her blood glucose levels were 400 mg/dL. The diagnosis was diabetic ketoacidosis.

1. Describe the metabolic events that lead to ketoacidosis. Were Nora's symptoms and laboratory tests consistent with the diagnosis?

2. Review Table 21-3, and consider the advantages and disadvantages that intensive therapy might have for Nora. Describe the complications associated with long-term diabetes.

3. Discuss how Nora's age might influence her ability to cope with and manage her diabetes. Why might she feel that diabetes is disrupting her life? List suggestions that may help. How might you explain the importance of glycemic control to a 12-year-old girl?

▌ Carbohydrate counting is widely used in menu planning and can be taught at different levels of complexity depending on individual needs and abilities.

▌ Insulin therapy is required for patients who are unable to produce sufficient insulin and may be used in both type 1 and type 2 diabetes. Antidiabetic drugs prescribed for type 2 diabetes improve hyperglycemia by various modes of action.

▌ Physical activity can improve glycemic control and enhance various aspects of general health. Illness can worsen glycemic control and often requires medication adjustments.

The Case Study in Box 21-9 provides an opportunity to review the treatment for diabetes.

21.3 Diabetes Management in Pregnancy

LO 21.3 Explain how diabetes can affect pregnancy outcomes and describe the approaches used to maintain glycemic control in pregnant women with diabetes.

Women with diabetes face new challenges during pregnancy. Due to hormonal changes, pregnancy increases insulin resistance and the body's need for insulin, so maintaining glycemic control may be more difficult. In addition, 4 to 14 percent of nondiabetic women in the United States develop gestational diabetes (the prevalence depends on the patient population).[41] Women with gestational diabetes are at greater risk of developing type 2 diabetes later in life, and their children are at increased risk of developing obesity and type 2 diabetes as they enter adulthood.

A pregnancy complicated by diabetes increases health risks for both mother and fetus. Uncontrolled diabetes is linked with increased incidences of miscarriage, birth defects, and fetal deaths. Newborns are more likely to suffer from respiratory distress and to develop metabolic problems such as hypoglycemia, jaundice, and hypocalcemia. Women with diabetes often deliver babies with **macrosomia** (abnormally large bodies), which makes delivery more difficult and can result in birth trauma or the need for a cesarean section. Macrosomia results because maternal hyperglycemia induces excessive insulin production by the fetal pancreas, which stimulates growth and fat deposition.[42]

macrosomia (MAK-roh-SOH-mee-ah): the condition of having an abnormally large body; in infants, refers to birth weights of 4000 grams (8 pounds 13 ounces) and above.

Pregnancy in Type 1 or Type 2 Diabetes

Women with diabetes who achieve glycemic control at conception and during the first trimester of their pregnancy substantially reduce the risks of birth defects and spontaneous abortion (see Figure 21-9). For this reason, women contemplating pregnancy should receive preconception care to avoid complications due to uncontrolled diabetes. Maintaining glycemic control during the second and third trimesters minimizes the risks of macrosomia and morbidity in newborn infants.

Women with type 1 diabetes require intensive insulin therapy during pregnancy. Insulin adjustments may be necessary every few weeks due to changes in insulin sensitivity. Patients with type 2 diabetes may be switched from their usual medications to insulin therapy or medications considered safe to use during pregnancy (such as metformin or acarbose) to prevent possible toxicity to the fetus.[43]

Nutrient requirements during pregnancy are similar for women with and without diabetes. In women with diabetes, however, carbohydrate intakes must be balanced with insulin treatment and physical activity to avoid hypoglycemia and hyperglycemia. To help with this goal, women should consume meals and snacks at similar times each day, and select carbohydrate sources that facilitate glucose control after meals, such as whole grains, fruits, and vegetables. An evening snack is usually required to prevent overnight hypoglycemia and ketosis. When insulin dosages are adjusted, the diabetic woman will need to modify her carbohydrate intake as well.

FIGURE 21-9 Diabetic Pregnancy
Gycemic control during pregnancy offers the best chance of a safe delivery and a healthy infant.

Gestational Diabetes

Risk of gestational diabetes is highest in women who have a family history of diabetes, are obese, are in a high-risk ethnic group (African American, Asian American, Hispanic American, Native American, or Pacific Islander), or have previously given birth to an infant weighing over 9 pounds. To ensure that appropriate treatment is offered, physicians routinely test women for gestational diabetes between 24 and 28 weeks of gestation. In high-risk women, testing may begin prior to pregnancy or soon after conception; note that some women may be found to have undiagnosed type 2 diabetes at the earlier time points.

Weight loss is not recommended during pregnancy. For women with gestational diabetes who are overweight or obese, a modest caloric reduction (about 30 percent less than total energy needs) may improve glycemic control without increasing the risk of ketosis.[44] Limiting the carbohydrate intake to 40 to 45 percent of total energy intake may improve blood glucose levels after meals. Carbohydrate is usually poorly tolerated in the morning; therefore, restricting carbohydrate (to about 30 grams) at breakfast may be helpful. The remaining carbohydrate intake should be spaced throughout the day in several meals and snacks, including an evening snack to prevent ketosis during the night. Regular aerobic activity can help to improve glycemic control. Women who fail to achieve glycemic goals through diet and exercise alone may need to use insulin or an antidiabetic drug that is safe to use during pregnancy. The Case Study in Box 21-10 (p. 572) reviews the connections between gestational diabetes and type 2 diabetes.

IN SUMMARY

▌ Careful management of blood glucose levels before and during pregnancy may prevent complications in mother and infant. Women with diabetes who become pregnant may need to adjust their insulin therapy or medications, consume meals and snacks at similar times each day, and consume an evening snack to prevent overnight ketosis.

▌ Women with gestational diabetes may need to restrict energy and/or carbohydrate intakes to maintain appropriate glucose levels; insulin or an antidiabetic drug may be prescribed to help them maintain glycemic control.

Case Study

BOX 21-10 WOMAN WITH TYPE 2 DIABETES

Teresa Cordova is a 41-year-old Mexican-American woman recently diagnosed with type 2 diabetes. Mrs. Cordova developed gestational diabetes while she was pregnant with her second child. Her blood glucose levels returned to normal following pregnancy, and she was advised to get regular checkups, maintain a desirable weight, and engage in regular physical activity. Although she reports that she does not overeat and that she exercises regularly, she has been unable to maintain a healthy weight. At 5 feet 3 inches tall, Mrs. Cordova currently weighs 165 pounds. She has decided to lose weight and join a gym because she is concerned about the long-term effects of diabetes and the possibility that she may need insulin injections. She is also concerned about her husband and children because they are overweight and not very active. The physician refers Mrs. Cordova to a dietitian to help her with her weight-management goals.

1. What factors in Mrs. Cordova's medical history increase her risk for diabetes? Are her husband and children also at risk?

2. Describe the general characteristics of a diet and exercise program that would be appropriate for Mrs. Cordova. How might weight loss and physical activity benefit her diabetes?

3. If Mrs. Cordova is unable to control her blood glucose with diet and physical activity, what treatment might be suggested? Explain to Mrs. Cordova why she would probably not require insulin at this time.

4. What dietary and lifestyle changes may help to prevent diabetes in Mrs. Cordova's husband and children?

Nutrition Assessment Checklist FOR PEOPLE WITH DIABETES

Medical History

Check the medical record to determine:

- Type of diabetes
- Duration of diabetes
- Acute and chronic complications
- Conditions, including pregnancy, that may alter treatment

Medications

For people with preexisting diabetes who use antidiabetic drugs (including insulin), note:

- Type of medication
- Administration schedule

Check for use of other medications, including:

- Medications that affect blood glucose levels
- Cholesterol- and triglyceride-lowering medications
- Antihypertensive medications

Dietary Intake

To devise an acceptable meal plan and coordinate medications, obtain:

- An accurate and thorough record of food intake and meal patterns
- An account of usual physical activities

At medical checkups, reassess the person's ability to:

- Maintain an appropriate carbohydrate intake
- Maintain an appropriate energy intake

- Monitor blood glucose levels at home
- Adjust insulin and diet to accommodate sick days
- Use appropriate foods to treat hypoglycemia

Anthropometric Data

Take accurate baseline height and weight measurements as a basis for:

- Appropriate energy intake
- Initial insulin therapy

Periodically reassess height and weight for children and weight for adults and pregnant women to ensure that the meal plan provides an appropriate energy intake.

Laboratory Tests

Monitor the success of diabetes treatment using these tests:

- Blood lipid concentrations
- Blood or urinary ketones
- Glycated hemoglobin
- Urinary protein (albuminuria)

Physical Signs

Look for physical signs of:

- Dehydration, especially in older adults
- Foot ulcers
- Nerve damage
- Vision problems

Clinical Applications

1. Using the carbohydrate-counting method described in Box 21-6 on pp. 563–564, determine an appropriate carbohydrate intake (in both grams and portions) for a man with type 2 diabetes who requires approximately 2600 kcalories daily. Assume he would benefit from a carbohydrate allowance that is 50 percent of his energy intake. Using information from Tables 21-4 and 21-5, develop a 1-day sample menu that is likely to meet his carbohydrate goals. Use the food lists in Appendix C to find additional examples of foods to include in your menu.

2. A diabetes educator typically meets with patients who have a wide variety of problems, concerns, and abilities. What suggestions can be offered to patients who have the problems listed below?

▮ An 18-year-old college woman with type 1 diabetes has a date at an unfamiliar restaurant and is uncertain how she will calculate the correct dose of rapid-acting insulin before the meal.

▮ A 45-year-old man with an HbA$_{1c}$ value of 8.5 percent states that he is unable to improve his diet because his job keeps him busy all day and his wife handles the food shopping and meal preparations.

▮ A 75-year-old man with type 2 diabetes has developed retinopathy and can no longer read the digital display on his blood glucose monitor.

Self Check

1. Which of the following is characteristic of type 1 diabetes?
   a. Abdominal obesity increases risk.
   b. The pancreas makes little or no insulin.
   c. It is the predominant form of diabetes.
   d. It often arises during pregnancy.

2. Which of the following is true about type 2 diabetes?
   a. It is usually an autoimmune disease.
   b. The pancreas makes little or no insulin.
   c. Diabetic ketoacidosis is a common complication.
   d. Chronic complications may develop before it is diagnosed.

3. Most chronic complications associated with diabetes result from:
   a. altered kidney function.
   b. infections that deplete nutrient reserves.
   c. weight gain and hypertension.
   d. damage to blood vessels and nerves.

4. Long-term glycemic control is usually evaluated by:
   a. self-monitoring of blood glucose.
   b. testing urinary ketone levels.
   c. measuring glycated hemoglobin.
   d. testing urinary protein levels (albuminuria).

5. Regarding dietary carbohydrate, a patient with diabetes should be most concerned about:
   a. consuming an appropriate quantity of carbohydrate at each meal or snack.
   b. consuming the correct proportion of sugars, starches, and fiber in meals.
   c. avoiding added sugars and kcaloric sweeteners.
   d. choosing meals with ideal proportions of protein, carbohydrate, and fat.

6. Which of the following is true regarding the general use of alcohol in diabetes?
   a. A serving of alcohol is considered part of the carbohydrate allowance.
   b. Alcohol contributes to hyperglycemia and should be avoided completely.
   c. Alcohol can cause hypoglycemia and should therefore be consumed with food if patients use insulin or medications that stimulate insulin secretion.
   d. Patients can use alcohol in unlimited quantities unless they are pregnant.

7. The most effective meal-planning strategy for managing diabetes is:
   a. carbohydrate counting.
   b. an eating plan based on food lists created for persons with diabetes.
   c. following menus and recipes provided by a registered dietitian.
   d. the approach that best helps the patient control blood glucose levels.

8. A patient using intensive insulin therapy is likely to follow a regimen that involves:
   a. twice-daily injections that combine short-, intermediate-, and long-acting insulin in each injection.
   b. a mixture of intermediate- and long-acting insulin injected between meals.
   c. multiple daily injections that supply basal insulin and precise insulin doses at each meal and snack.
   d. the use of both insulin and oral antidiabetic agents.

9. In a person who has previously maintained good glycemic control, hyperglycemia can be precipitated by:
   a. infections or illnesses.
   b. chronic alcohol ingestion.
   c. undertreatment of hypoglycemia.
   d. prolonged exercise.

10. Which dietary adjustment may be helpful for women with gestational diabetes?
    a. Consuming most of the day's carbohydrate allotment in the morning
    b. Restricting carbohydrate to about 30 grams at breakfast
    c. Avoiding food intake after dinner
    d. Reducing energy intake to about 50 percent of the calculated requirement

Answers to these questions appear in Appendix H.

Notes

1. Centers for Disease Control and Prevention, National diabetes statistics report: Estimates of diabetes and its burden in the United States, 2014 (Atlanta, GA: U.S. Department of Health and Human Services, Centers for Disease Control and Prevention, 2014).

2. Centers for Disease Control and Prevention, 2014.

3. American Diabetes Association, Diagnosis and classification of diabetes mellitus, *Diabetes Care* 37 (2014): S81–S90.

4. Centers for Disease Control and Prevention, 2014.

5. A. L. May, E. V. Kuklina, and P. W. Yoon, Prevalence of cardiovascular disease risk factors among U.S. adolescents, 1999–2008, *Pediatrics* 129 (2012): 1035–1041.

6. S. E. Inzucchi and R. S. Sherwin, Type 1 diabetes mellitus, in L. Goldman and A. I. Schafer, eds., *Goldman's Cecil Medicine* (Philadelphia: Saunders, 2012), pp. 1475–1489.

7. U. Masharani and M. S. German, Pancreatic hormones and diabetes mellitus, in D. G. Gardner and D. Shoback, eds., *Greenspan's Basic and Clinical Endocrinology* (New York: McGraw-Hill/Lange, 2011), pp. 573–655.

8. T. Ota, Chemokine systems link obesity to insulin resistance, *Diabetes and Metabolism Journal* 37 (2013): 165–172; Masharani and German, 2011.

9. S. E. Inzucchi and R. S. Sherwin, Type 2 diabetes mellitus, in L. Goldman and A. I. Schafer, eds., *Goldman's Cecil Medicine* (Philadelphia: Saunders, 2012), pp. 1489–1499.

10. R. B. Lipton and coauthors, Onset features and subsequent clinical evolution of childhood diabetes over several years, *Pediatric Diabetes* 12 (2011): 326–334.

11. Centers for Disease Control and Prevention, 2014.

12. Masharani and German, 2011.

13. Inzucchi and Sherwin, Type 1 diabetes mellitus, 2012.

14. Inzucchi and Sherwin, Type 2 diabetes mellitus, 2012.

15. Inzucchi and Sherwin, Type 1 diabetes mellitus, 2012.

16. Inzucchi and Sherwin, Type 2 diabetes mellitus, 2012.

17. American Diabetes Association, Implications of the United Kingdom Prospective Diabetes Study, *Diabetes Care* 21 (1998): 2180–2184; Diabetes Control and Complications Trial Research Group, The effect of intensive treatment of diabetes on the development and progression of long-term complications in insulin-dependent diabetes mellitus, *New England Journal of Medicine* 329 (1993): 977–986.

18. American Diabetes Association, Standards of medical care in diabetes—2014, *Diabetes Care* 37 (2014): S14–S80.

19. Masharani and German, 2011.

20. American Diabetes Association, Standards of medical care in diabetes—2014, 2014.

21. American Diabetes Association, Standards of medical care in diabetes—2014, 2014.

22. American Diabetes Association, Nutrition therapy recommendations for the management of adults with diabetes, *Diabetes Care* 36 (2013): 3821–3842.

23. M. J. Franz and coauthors, The evidence for medical nutrition therapy for type 1 and type 2 diabetes in adults, *Journal of the American Dietetic Association* 110 (2010): 1852–1889.

24. American Diabetes Association, Standards of medical care in diabetes—2014, 2014; American Diabetes Association, 2013.

25. American Diabetes Association, 2013.

26. American Diabetes Association, 2013; Franz and coauthors, 2010.

27. American Diabetes Association, 2013; Franz and coauthors, 2010.

28. American Diabetes Association, 2013.

29. American Diabetes Association, 2013; Franz and coauthors, 2010.

30. American Diabetes Association, 2013.

31. American Diabetes Association, 2013.

32. American Diabetes Association, 2013.

33. American Diabetes Association, 2013.

34. M. S. N. Kennedy, Pancreatic hormones and antidiabetic drugs, in B. G. Katzung, ed., *Basic and Clinical Pharmacology* (New York: McGraw-Hill/Lange, 2012), pp. 743–768; Masharani and German, 2011.

35. Kennedy, 2012.

36. Inzucchi and Sherwin, Type 2 diabetes mellitus, 2012; Kennedy, 2012.

37. R. J. Brown and coauthors, Uncoupling intensive insulin therapy from weight gain and hypoglycemia in type 1 diabetes, *Diabetes Technology and Therapeutics* 13 (2011): 457–460.

38. Masharani and German, 2011.

39. American Diabetes Association, Standards of medical care in diabetes—2014, 2014.

40. American Diabetes Association, Standards of medical care in diabetes—2014, 2014.

41. K. Rosene-Montella, Common medical problems in pregnancy, in L. Goldman and A. I. Schafer, eds., *Goldman's Cecil Medicine* (Philadelphia: Saunders, 2012), pp. 1555–1565.

42. A. Maitra, Diseases of infancy and childhood, in V. Kumar and coeditors, *Robbins and Cotran Pathologic Basis of Disease* (Philadelphia: Saunders, 2010), pp. 447–483.

43. American Diabetes Association, Standards of medical care in diabetes—2014, 2014.

44. Academy of Nutrition and Dietetics, *Nutrition Care Manual* (Chicago: Academy of Nutrition and Dietetics, 2014).

LO 21.4 Identify the features and possible consequences of the metabolic syndrome and describe the current treatment approaches for this condition.

Chapter 21 described how insulin resistance—a reduced sensitivity to insulin in muscle, adipose, and liver cells—can contribute to hyperglycemia and hyperinsulinemia and, eventually, to type 2 diabetes. Insulin resistance is also a central feature of several other conditions, including the **metabolic syndrome,** a cluster of metabolic abnormalities that are associated with increased risk of developing cardiovascular diseases (CVD) and type 2 diabetes. This Nutrition in Practice describes how the metabolic syndrome is diagnosed, how and why it might develop, its potential consequences, and current treatment approaches. Box NP21-1 defines the relevant terms.

How is the metabolic syndrome diagnosed, and how common is it in the United States?

Table NP21-1 lists the laboratory values used to identify the metabolic syndrome, which is diagnosed when at least three of the following disorders are present: hyperglycemia, abdominal obesity, **hypertriglyceridemia** (elevated blood triglyceride levels), reduced high-density lipoprotein (HDL) cholesterol levels, and hypertension (high blood pressure). Although published values vary, an estimated 23 to 34 percent of adults in the United States may meet the criteria for the metabolic syndrome.[1] As Figure NP21-1 shows, prevalence increases with age. Risk also varies according to ethnicity and gender: Mexican-American women have the highest incidence of the metabolic syndrome in the United States, with an overall prevalence of nearly 41 percent.[2]

BOX NP21-1 GLOSSARY

adiponectin (AH-dih-poe-NECK-tin): a hormone produced by adipose cells that improves insulin sensitivity.

cytokines (SIGH-toe-kines): signaling proteins produced by the body's cells; many cytokines are produced by immune cells and regulate immune responses.

fibrinogen (fye-BRIN-oh-jen): a liver protein that promotes blood clot formation.

hypertriglyceridemia: high blood triglyceride levels. Blood triglycerides are transported in *very-low-density lipoproteins (VLDL).*

metabolic syndrome: a cluster of interrelated disorders, including abdominal obesity, insulin resistance, high blood pressure, and abnormal blood lipids, which together increase risk of diabetes and cardiovascular disease; also known as *insulin resistance syndrome* or *syndrome X.*

plasminogen activator inhibitor-1: a protein that promotes blood clotting by inhibiting blood clot degradation within blood vessels.

resistin (re-ZIST-in): a hormone produced by adipose cells that promotes insulin resistance.

TABLE NP21-1 Features of the Metabolic Syndrome

Metabolic syndrome is diagnosed when three or more of the following abnormalities are present.

Measure	Reference Value
Hyperglycemia	Fasting plasma glucose ≥100 mg/dL
Abdominal obesity	Waist circumference >40" in men, >35" in women
Hypertriglyceridemia	VLDLs ≥150 mg/dL
Reduced HDL cholesterol	HDLs <40 mg/dL in men, <50 mg/dL in women
Hypertension	Blood pressure ≥130/85 mm Hg

© 2016 Cengage Learning®

FIGURE NP21-1 Prevalence of the Metabolic Syndrome in the U.S. Population
Source: A. S. Go and coauthors, Heart disease and stroke statistics—2014 update: A report from the American Heart Association, *Circulation* 129 (2014): e28–e292.

Public Domain

Because the disorders that identify the metabolic syndrome are considered independent risk factors for heart disease or diabetes, some medical experts have questioned whether the diagnosis of metabolic syndrome is a useful one.[3] The main benefit of grouping the disorders may be to guide clinical management of these interrelated metabolic problems.[4] In addition, some studies indicate that heart disease risk actually varies substantially among individuals with the metabolic syndrome, suggesting that further screening is needed to identify those who may benefit from aggressive treatment.[5]

What causes the metabolic syndrome?

Both genetic and environmental factors probably contribute to the development of the metabolic syndrome. However, the close relationship between abdominal obesity and insulin resistance suggests that the current obesity crisis in the United States may be largely responsible for its high prevalence.[6] Visceral fat is thought to induce a number of metabolic changes that promote insulin resistance, which then leads to hyperglycemia and other abnormalities.

How does obesity lead to insulin resistance?

Various theories have been proposed to explain the relationship between obesity and insulin resistance. Some research indicates that the enlarged adipose cells of obese individuals have a reduced capacity to store triglyceride. Instead, these cells may increase their release of fatty acids into the bloodstream, resulting in the abnormal accumulation of triglycerides in the muscle and liver; the high fat content of these tissues may alter cellular responses to insulin that lead to insulin resistance.[7] In addition, obesity causes adipose cells to alter the hormones and proteins they release into the blood, promoting a state of insulin resistance.[8] For example, obesity is associated with the reduced secretion of **adiponectin,** a hormone that promotes insulin sensitivity and glucose tolerance. Conversely, the adipose cells release larger amounts of the hormone **resistin,** which promotes insulin resistance. Enlarged adipose cells also activate local macrophages (immune cells), which secrete a number of **cytokines** (signaling proteins) that induce inflammation; the inflammatory process leads to multiple metabolic changes that reduce insulin responsiveness.

Can obesity lead to other problems related to the metabolic syndrome?

Abdominal obesity is frequently associated with blood lipid abnormalities. Because the insulin-resistant adipose cells release more fatty acids into the blood, the liver must accelerate its production of very-low-density lipoproteins (VLDL), and hypertriglyceridemia develops.[9] At the same time, insulin resistance hinders the adipose cells' ability to extract and store triglycerides from chylomicrons and VLDL. Excessive body fatness is also associated with elevated low-density lipoprotein (LDL) cholesterol levels and reduced HDL levels.

Obesity heightens the risk of developing hypertension, although the underlying mechanisms are poorly understood. The elevated blood pressure may be due, in part, to the expanded blood volume that develops in obesity.[10] In addition, the insulin resistance and hyperinsulinemia that accompany obesity may stimulate the sympathetic nervous system, altering hormonal secretions and blood vessel activity in ways that favor a rise in blood pressure.[11] Hyperinsulinemia also promotes sodium reabsorption in the kidneys, resulting in fluid retention and increased blood volume.

How does the metabolic syndrome contribute to cardiovascular disease risk?

The disorders that characterize the metabolic syndrome—obesity, lipid abnormalities, and hypertension—are all independent risk factors for CVD. In addition, the condition is often associated with blood vessel dysfunction and the tendency to form blood clots, characteristics that favor the development of atherosclerosis and raise the risk of heart attack or stroke. For example, individuals with the metabolic syndrome exhibit reduced production of the vasodilator nitric oxide and increased secretion of the vasoconstrictor endothelin-1—changes that enhance vasoconstriction and stimulate the release of pro-inflammatory cytokines. These cytokines release factors that increase endothelial permeability, recruit immune cells, and increase oxidative stress, thereby promoting atherosclerosis. Inflammation of endothelial tissue, obesity, and insulin resistance may all promote the increased production of procoagulant proteins such as **fibrinogen** and **plasminogen activator inhibitor-1.**[12] Individuals with the metabolic syndrome are also at increased risk of developing diabetes, which is another major risk factor for CVD.

What is the usual treatment for the metabolic syndrome?

The main treatment goals are to correct the abnormalities that increase CVD and diabetes risk. In most individuals, a combination of weight loss and physical activity can improve insulin resistance, blood pressure, and blood lipid levels.[13] Even a moderate weight loss (5 to 10 percent of body weight) can improve symptoms, although many people find this difficult to achieve. Additional dietary strategies depend on a patient's specific symptoms. If dietary and lifestyle modifications are not successful, medications may be prescribed. Because effective treatment requires lifelong commitment, health care providers should work with patients to develop a treatment plan that they are willing to adopt.

What dietary strategies, other than weight loss, are suggested for people with the metabolic syndrome?

In individuals with hypertriglyceridemia, the general recommendations are to reduce intakes of added sugars and refined grain products (sugar-sweetened beverages, juices, white bread, sweetened cereal, and desserts) and increase servings of whole grains and foods high in fiber (whole-wheat bread, oatmeal, legumes, fruits, and vegetables).[14] In some people, carbohydrate restriction may help to reduce blood triglyceride levels and improve hyperglycemia. Including fish in the diet each week may also improve triglyceride levels. Individuals with hypertension are encouraged to reduce sodium intake and increase consumption of fruits and vegetables and low-fat milk products. A diet low in saturated fat, *trans* fats, and cholesterol can help to reduce LDL cholesterol levels. Chapter 22 describes additional dietary modifications that may reduce CVD risk.

Why is physical activity recommended for people with the metabolic syndrome?

Regular physical activity helps with weight management and may also improve blood lipid concentrations, hypertension, and insulin resistance—all changes that can reduce the risk of developing CVD.[15] A regular exercise program can also prevent or delay the onset of diabetes in persons at risk (see Figure NP21-2). About 150 minutes per week (about 30 minutes of activity on 5 days of the week) of moderate-intensity aerobic activity is often suggested, although longer periods (one hour daily) are recommended for

FIGURE NP21-2 Regular exercise can reduce the risks of developing the metabolic syndrome, cardiovascular diseases, and type 2 diabetes.

© Rolf Bruderer/Corbis

weight control. Resistance exercise, using free weights or weight machines, is beneficial for improving insulin sensitivity and should be performed at least twice weekly. A sedentary lifestyle can worsen the progression of metabolic syndrome and should be discouraged.

What types of medications are used to treat the metabolic syndrome?

If dietary and lifestyle changes are unsuccessful, medications may be prescribed to correct hypertriglyceridemia and hypertension (Chapter 22 provides details). At present, antidiabetic drugs are not routinely used to treat insulin resistance in patients with the metabolic syndrome due to insufficient evidence that the drugs can improve long-term outcomes better than lifestyle changes.

As explained in this Nutrition in Practice, the metabolic syndrome consists of a cluster of interrelated disorders that increase the risk of developing CVD and type 2 diabetes. Whereas most of the features of the metabolic syndrome are individual risk factors for CVD, in combination they may raise risk twofold to threefold. Treatment of the metabolic syndrome emphasizes dietary and lifestyle changes.

Notes

1. A. S. Go and coauthors, Heart disease and stroke statistics—2014 update: A report from the American Heart Association, *Circulation* 129 (2014): e28–e292; H. Beltrán-Sánchez and coauthors, Prevalence and trends of metabolic syndrome in the adult U.S. population, 1999–2010, *Journal of the American College of Cardiology* 62 (2013): 697–703.

2. Go and coauthors, 2014.

3. A. M. Kanaya and C. Vaisse, Obesity, in D. G. Gardner and D. Shoback, eds., *Greenspan's Basic and Clinical Endocrinology* (New York: McGraw-Hill/Lange, 2011), pp. 699–709.

4. U. Masharani and M. S. German, Pancreatic hormones and diabetes mellitus, in D. G. Gardner and D. Shoback, eds., *Greenspan's Basic and Clinical Endocrinology* (New York: McGraw-Hill/Lange, 2011), pp. 573–655.

5. S. Malik and coauthors, Impact of subclinical atherosclerosis on cardiovascular disease events in individuals with metabolic syndrome and diabetes, *Diabetes Care* 34 (2011): 2285–2290.

6. T. Ota, Chemokine systems link obesity to insulin resistance, *Diabetes and Metabolism Journal* 37 (2013): 165–172; B. Gustafson, Adipose tissue, inflammation, and atherosclerosis, *Journal of Atherosclerosis and Thrombosis* 17 (2010): 332–341.

7. D. N. Reeds, Metabolic syndrome: Definition, relationship with insulin resistance, and clinical utility, in A. C. Ross and coeditors, eds., *Modern Nutrition in Health and Disease* (Baltimore: Lippincott Williams & Wilkins, 2014), pp. 828–836; G. H. Goossens, The role of adipose tissue dysfunction in the pathogenesis of obesity-related insulin resistance, *Physiology and Behavior* 94 (2008): 208–218.

8. Ota, 2013; Kanaya and Vaisse, 2011; Gustafson, 2010.

9. Reeds, 2014.

10. R. G. Victor, Arterial hypertension, in L. Goldman and A. I. Schafer, eds., *Goldman's Cecil Medicine* (Philadelphia: Saunders, 2012): 373–389.

11. L. Duvnjak, T. Bulum, and Z. Metelko, Hypertension and the metabolic syndrome, *Diabetologia Croatica* 37 (2008): 83–89.

12. E. Kassi and coauthors, Metabolic syndrome: Definitions and controversies, *BMC Medicine* 9 (May 5 2011), available at doi:10.1186/1741-7015-9-48.

13. F. Magkos and coauthors, Management of the metabolic syndrome and type 2 diabetes through lifestyle modification, *Annual Review of Nutrition* 29 (2009): 223–256.

14. L. Berglund and coauthors, Evaluation and treatment of hypertriglyceridemia, *Journal of Clinical Endocrinology and Metabolism* 97 (2012): 2969–2989; M. Miller and coauthors, Triglycerides and cardiovascular disease: A scientific statement from the American Heart Association, *Circulation* 123 (2011): 2292–2333.

15. B. Strasser, Physical activity in obesity and metabolic syndrome, *Annals of the New York Academy of Sciences* 1281 (2013): 141–159.

22

Fat-Controlled, Mineral-Modified Diets for Cardiovascular Diseases

22.1 Atherosclerosis

LO 22.1 Identify the potential consequences of atherosclerosis and discuss the factors that contribute to its development.

22.2 Coronary Heart Disease

LO 22.2 Describe how CHD risk is evaluated and discuss strategies that can reduce risk or prevent future heart attacks.

22.3 Stroke

LO 22.3 Describe the different types of stroke, strategies that may prevent a stroke, and elements of treatment and rehabilitation following a stroke.

22.4 Hypertension

LO 22.4 Summarize the potential effects of hypertension, its risk factors, and current treatment approaches.

22.5 Heart Failure

LO 22.5 Identify the possible consequences of heart failure and describe the current treatment approaches for this condition.

22.6 Nutrition in Practice: Helping People with Feeding Disabilities

LO 22.6 Identify disabilities that may impair eating ability and give examples of strategies that may improve feeding skills.

Cardiovascular disease (CVD), a group of disorders involving the heart and blood vessels, is responsible for approximately 32 percent of deaths in the United States.[1] Although many people assume that heart conditions are men's diseases, more women than men die from CVD each year. Furthermore, CVD is a global health issue; it is the leading cause of death worldwide.[2] Figure 22-1 shows the percentages of deaths in the United States resulting from the various types of CVD.

The most common form of CVD is **coronary heart disease (CHD),** which is usually caused by **atherosclerosis** in the coronary arteries that supply blood to the heart muscle. If atherosclerosis restricts blood flow in these arteries, the resulting deprivation of oxygen and nutrients can destroy heart tissue and cause a **myocardial infarction (MI)**—a **heart attack.** When the blood supply to brain tissue is blocked, a **stroke** occurs. Both heart attack and stroke may result in disablement or death. Box 22-1 defines common terms related to CVD.

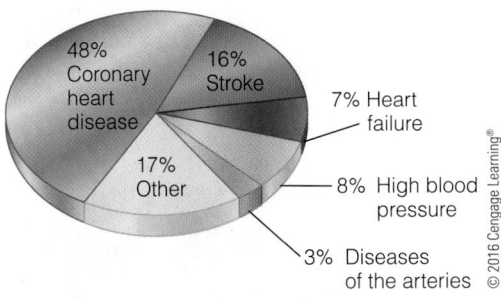

FIGURE 22-1 Percentage Breakdown of Deaths from Cardiovascular Diseases in the United States
Source: A. S. Go and coauthors, Heart disease and stroke statistics—2014 update: A report from the American Heart Association, *Circulation* 129 (2014): e28–e292.

22.1 Atherosclerosis

LO 22.1 Identify the potential consequences of atherosclerosis and discuss the factors that contribute to its development.

In atherosclerosis, the artery walls become progressively thickened due to an accumulation of fatty deposits, fibrous connective tissue, and smooth muscle cells, collectively known as **plaque.**[3] Atherosclerosis initially arises in response to minimal

BOX 22-1 GLOSSARY OF TERMS RELATED TO CARDIOVASCULAR DISEASES

aneurysm (AN-you-rih-zum)**:** an abnormal enlargement or bulging of a blood vessel (usually an artery) caused by weakness in the blood vessel wall.

angina (an-JYE-nah or AN-ji-nah) **pectoris:** a condition caused by ischemia in the heart muscle that results in discomfort or dull pain in the chest region. The pain often radiates to the left shoulder and arm or to the back, neck, and lower jaw.

atherosclerosis (ATH-er-oh-scler-OH-sis)**:** an arterial disease characterized by a buildup of lipids and fibrous scar tissue on the inner walls of arteries.

cardiovascular disease (CVD): a general term describing diseases of the heart and blood vessels.

▌ *cardio* = heart

▌ *vascular* = blood vessels

coronary heart disease (CHD): a chronic, progressive disease characterized by obstructed blood flow in the coronary arteries; also called *coronary artery disease.*

embolism (EM-boh-lizm)**:** the obstruction of a blood vessel by an embolus, causing sudden tissue death.

▌ *embol* = to insert, plug

embolus (EM-boh-lus)**:** an abnormal particle, such as a blood clot or air bubble, that travels in the blood.

fatty streaks: initial lesions of atherosclerosis that form on the artery wall, characterized by accumulations of foam cells, lipid material, and connective tissue.

foam cells: swollen cells in the artery wall that accumulate lipids.

ischemia (iss-KEE-mee-a)**:** inadequate blood supply within a tissue due to obstructed blood flow.

myocardial (MY-oh-CAR-dee-al) **infarction** (in-FARK-shun), or **MI:** death of heart muscle caused by a sudden reduction in coronary blood flow; also called a **heart attack** or *cardiac arrest.*

▌ *myo* = muscle

▌ *cardial* = heart

▌ *infarct* = tissue death

peripheral artery disease: impaired blood flow in the arteries of the legs; may cause pain or discomfort in the legs and feet.

plaque (PLACK)**:** an accumulation of fatty deposits, fibrous connective tissue, and smooth muscle cells in blood vessels.

stroke: a sudden injury to brain tissue resulting from impaired blood flow through an artery that supplies blood to the brain; also called a *cerebrovascular accident.*

▌ *cerebro* = brain

thrombosis (throm-BOH-sis)**:** the formation or presence of a blood clot in blood vessels. A *coronary thrombosis* occurs in a coronary artery, and a *cerebral thrombosis* occurs in an artery that supplies blood to the brain.

▌ *thrombo* = clot

thrombus: a blood clot formed within a blood vessel that remains attached to its place of origin.

① The coronary arteries deliver oxygen and nutrients to the heart muscle.

Plaque

② Plaque often develops at regions where arteries branch or bend.

③ When arteries become blocked by plaque or a blood clot, the part of the muscle that the arteries supply with blood may die.

© Cengage Learning®

FIGURE 22-2 **Plaque Formation in Atherosclerosis**

Plaque thickens and hardens as additional lipids, calcium + cellular debris accumulate.

but chronic injuries that damage the inner arterial wall. The first lesions tend to develop in regions where the arteries branch or bend due to the disturbed blood flow in those areas (see Figure 22-2). The subtle damage caused by disturbed blood flow or other factors elicits an inflammatory response, attracting immune cells and increasing the permeability of the artery walls. **Low-density lipoproteins (LDL)** slip under the artery's thin layer of **endothelial cells,** become oxidized by local enzymes, and accumulate. Arterial **macrophages** engulf this altered LDL and become **foam cells;** these fat-laden cells are visible as fatty deposits along artery walls, known as **fatty streaks** (see Figure 22-3). Eventually, the plaque thickens and hardens as additional lipids, calcium, and cellular debris accumulate. Atherosclerosis begins to develop as early as childhood or adolescence and typically progresses over several decades before symptoms develop.

Consequences of Atherosclerosis

As atherosclerosis worsens, it may eventually narrow the lumen of an artery and interfere with blood flow. Some types of plaque are highly susceptible to rupture, which promotes blood clotting within the artery **(thrombosis).** A blood clot **(thrombus)** may enlarge in time and ultimately obstruct blood flow. A portion of a clot can also break free **(embolus)** and travel through the circulatory system until it lodges in a narrowed artery and shuts off blood flow to the surrounding tissue **(embolism).** Most complications of atherosclerosis result from the deficiency of blood and oxygen within the tissue served by an obstructed artery **(ischemia).**

Monocytes

Fatty streaks

Site of injury
Foam cells

Plaque

Thin covering

Monocytes—phagocytic white blood cells—circulate in the bloodstream and respond to injury on the artery wall.

Monocytes slip under blood vessel cells and engulf LDL cholesterol, becoming foam cells. The thin layers of foam cells that develop on artery walls are known as *fatty streaks.*

A fatty streak thickens and forms plaque as it accumulates additional lipids, smooth muscle cells, connective tissue, and cellular debris.

The artery may expand to accommodate plaque. When this occurs, the plaque that develops often contains a large lipid core with a thin fibrous covering and is vulnerable to rupture and thrombosis.

© Cengage Learning®

FIGURE 22-3 **Stages of Plaque Progression**

Atherosclerosis can affect almost any organ or tissue in the body and, accordingly, is a major cause of disability or death. Obstructed blood flow in the coronary arteries can cause pain or discomfort in the chest and surrounding regions **(angina pectoris)** or lead to a heart attack. As mentioned earlier, obstructed blood flow to the brain can injure or destroy brain tissue, causing a stroke. Impaired blood flow in the arteries of the legs **(peripheral artery disease)** can cause pain and weakness in the legs and feet. Blockage of the arteries that supply the kidneys can result in kidney disease or even kidney failure.

Atherosclerosis is the most common cause of an **aneurysm**—the abnormal dilation of a blood vessel. Plaque can weaken the blood vessel wall, and eventually the pressure of blood flow can cause the damaged region to stretch and balloon outward. Aneurysms can rupture and lead to massive bleeding and death, particularly when a large vessel such as the aorta is affected. In the arteries of the brain, an aneurysm may lead to bleeding within the brain, coma, or a stroke.

Causes of Atherosclerosis

The factors that initiate atherosclerosis either cause direct damage to the artery wall or allow lipid materials to penetrate its surface. Factors that generally worsen atherosclerosis or lead to complications are those that cause plaque rupture or blood coagulation. The development of advanced atherosclerosis is a long-term process that involves recurrent plaque rupture, thrombosis, and healing at sites in the artery wall.

Shear Stress/Hypertension The stress of blood flow along artery walls—called **shear stress**—can cause physical damage to arteries.[4] Hypertension (high blood pressure) intensifies the stress of blood flow on arterial tissue, provoking a low-grade inflammatory state that may stimulate plaque formation or progression.[5]

Abnormal Blood Lipids When levels are high, LDL are actively taken up and retained in susceptible regions in the artery wall. Elevated levels of **very-low-density lipoproteins (VLDL)** can also promote atherosclerosis, either by influencing the production of other **atherogenic** lipoproteins or by causing molecular changes in endothelial cells and macrophages that promote inflammation or plaque development.[6] Because **high-density lipoproteins (HDL)** remove cholesterol from circulation and contain proteins that inhibit inflammation, LDL oxidation, and plaque accumulation, low HDL levels can contribute to the development of atherosclerosis as well.[7]

Elevated concentrations of a variant form of LDL called *lipoprotein(a)* have been found to speed the progression of atherosclerosis and to raise the risk of various types of CVD.[8] Lipoprotein(a) levels are primarily genetically determined and are influenced to only a minor degree by age and environmental factors.

Cigarette Smoking Chemicals in cigarette smoke (including nicotine) are toxic to endothelial cells and contribute to arterial injury. Other damaging effects of smoking include chronic inflammation, vasoconstriction, enhanced blood coagulation, increased LDL cholesterol, and decreased HDL cholesterol—all effects that can promote the progression of atherosclerosis.[9]

Diabetes Mellitus Chronic hyperglycemia leads to the accumulation of **advanced glycation end products (AGEs),** which promote inflammation and oxidative stress, induce the production of compounds that favor plaque progression, and disturb blood vessel function. By various other mechanisms, diabetes increases tendencies for vasoconstriction, blood clotting, and plaque rupture.[10]

Age and Gender As a person ages, arterial cells tend to degenerate, and risk factors for CVD accumulate. Risk of atherosclerosis increases significantly in men and women older than 45 and 55 years of age, respectively. After menopause, women's risk increases, in part, because the decline in estrogen has unfavorable effects on

low-density lipoproteins (LDL): lipoproteins that transport cholesterol in the blood.

endothelial cells: cells that line the inner surfaces of blood vessels, lymphatic vessels, and body cavities.

macrophages: immune cells that engulf pathogens and cellular debris; they are derived from white blood cells called *monocytes*.

shear stress: a stress that occurs sideways against a surface rather than perpendicular to a surface. In blood vessels, turbulent blood flow can be harmful to endothelial cells, whereas regular blood flow is protective against atherosclerosis.

very-low-density lipoproteins (VLDL): lipoproteins that transport triglycerides from the liver to other tissues; in clinical practice, VLDL are commonly referred to as *blood triglycerides*.

atherogenic: able to initiate or promote atherosclerosis.

high-density lipoproteins (HDL): lipoproteins that help to remove cholesterol from the bloodstream by transporting it to the liver for reuse or disposal.

advanced glycation end products (AGEs): reactive compounds formed after glucose combines with protein; AGEs can damage tissues and lead to diabetic complications.

© 2016 Cengage Learning®

TABLE 22-1 Risk Factors for CHD

Major Nonmodifiable Risk Factors

- Increasing age
- Male gender
- Family history of early heart disease

Major Modifiable Risk Factors

- High LDL cholesterol
- High blood triglyceride (VLDL) levels
- Low HDL cholesterol
- Hypertension (high blood pressure)
- Diabetes
- Obesity (especially abdominal obesity)
- Physical inactivity
- Cigarette smoking
- Alcohol overconsumption (≥3 drinks per day)
- An atherogenic diet (high in saturated fat and *trans* fats; low in fruits and vegetables)

Note: Risk factors highlighted in yellow have relationships with diet.

Sources: A. S. Go and coauthors, Heart disease and stroke statistics—2014 update: A report from the American Heart Association, *Circulation* 129 (2014): e28–e292; M. J. Klag, Epidemiology of cardiovascular disease, in L. Goldman and A. I. Schafer, eds., *Goldman's Cecil Medicine* (Philadelphia: Saunders, 2012), pp. 256–260.

homocysteine: an amino acid produced during the conversion of methionine to cysteine; blood homocysteine levels are influenced by intakes of folate, vitamin B_{12}, and vitamin B_6.

lipoprotein levels and arterial function.*[11] Levels of the amino acid **homocysteine,** which may impair endothelial cell function, rise with age and are generally higher in men; however, it is unclear whether the increased homocysteine levels directly contribute to the disease process or are merely an indicator of abnormal metabolism.[12]

IN SUMMARY

- Atherosclerosis, characterized by the buildup of arterial plaque, can lead to complications such as angina pectoris, heart attack, stroke, peripheral artery disease, kidney disease, and aneurysms.

- Leading causes of plaque development include disturbed blood flow, hypertension, elevated LDL and VLDL, cigarette smoking, diabetes, and aging.

22.2 Coronary Heart Disease

LO 22.2 Describe how CHD risk is evaluated and discuss strategies that can reduce risk or prevent future heart attacks.

Coronary heart disease (CHD), also called *coronary artery disease,* is the most common type of cardiovascular disease. As discussed earlier, CHD is most often caused by atherosclerosis, which leads to impaired blood flow through the coronary arteries; possible outcomes include angina pectoris, heart attack, or even sudden death.

The most common symptom of CHD is pain or discomfort in the chest region; the pain may radiate to the left neck and shoulder, arms, back, or jaw.[13] Other possible symptoms include shortness of breath, unusual weakness or fatigue, lightheadedness or dizziness, nausea, vomiting, and lower abdominal discomfort.

Evaluating Risk for Coronary Heart Disease

Because CHD develops over many years, prevention should begin well before symptoms appear. The American Heart Association (AHA) and American College of Cardiology (ACC) recommend an assessment of traditional risk factors for atherosclerotic CVD (including CHD) every 4 to 6 years in individuals who are 20 to 79 years of age.[14] The major risk factors for CHD are listed in Table 22-1; most of those listed can be modified by changes in diet and lifestyle. The AHA and ACC have developed an online calculator to predict 10-year and lifetime atherosclerotic CVD risk that includes some of these variables (available at *http://tools.cardiosource.org/ASCVD-Risk-Estimator/*).

Clinical Measures Risk assessment requires several key laboratory measures, as shown in Table 22-2. A typical lipoprotein profile (also called a *blood lipid profile*) includes measures of total cholesterol, LDL and HDL cholesterol, and blood triglycerides (VLDL). Some clinicians may use the ratio of total cholesterol to HDL cholesterol or LDL cholesterol to HDL cholesterol to help assess CHD risk. In persons with high blood triglycerides, the non-HDL cholesterol level (total cholesterol minus HDL) may be more accurate than the LDL level for predicting CHD risk.[15] Blood pressure and body weight measurements are also regularly included in risk assessment.

In some individuals, a CHD risk assessment may include tests that provide additional detail about blood lipids or suggest the presence of atherosclerosis.[16] Blood lipid status is sometimes evaluated by measuring LDL and HDL subclasses, the LDL particle number, lipoprotein(a) levels, or levels of proteins or enzymes associated with

*Estrogen replacement therapy after menopause has mixed effects on heart disease risk: it can improve endothelial function and reduce LDL levels, but it also promotes blood clotting.

TABLE 22-2 Laboratory Measures for CHD Risk Assessment

Clinical Measures	Desirable	Borderline Risk	High Risk
Total blood cholesterol (mg/dL)	<200	200–239	≥240
LDL cholesterol (mg/dL)	<100[a]	130–159	160–189[b]
HDL cholesterol (mg/dL)[c]	≥60	Men: 40–59 Women: 50–59	Men: <40 Women: <50
Triglycerides, fasting (mg/dL)	<150	150–199	200–499[d]
Blood pressure (systolic/diastolic)	<120/<80	120–139/80–89[e]	≥140/≥90[f]
Body mass index (BMI)[g]	18.5–24.9	25–29.9	≥30

[a]LDL levels of 100–129 mg/dL indicate a near-optimal level; <70 mg/dL is a desirable goal for very high-risk persons.

[b]LDL levels ≥190 mg/dL indicate a very high risk.

[c]To estimate non-HDL cholesterol, subtract the HDL level from the total cholesterol level; non-HDL cholesterol risk levels are 30 mg/dL higher than the LDL risk levels.

[d]Triglyceride levels ≥500 mg/dL indicate a very high risk.

[e]These values indicate prehypertension for most individuals.

[f]These values indicate stage 1 hypertension; ≥160/≥100 indicates stage 2 hypertension. Physicians use these classifications to determine medical treatment.

[g]Body mass index (BMI) was defined in Chapter 6; BMI standards are found on the inside back cover.

lipoproteins (especially apolipoprotein B—a component of LDL, lipoprotein(a), and VLDL). Atherosclerosis may be evaluated using the coronary artery calcium score, a value obtained from a computed tomography (CT) scan that analyzes the calcium content of plaque in the coronary arteries. Levels of C-reactive protein, a marker of inflammation, may identify some patients at risk for CHD. The ankle-brachial index, a ratio of blood pressure measurements taken at the ankle and the upper arms, can help to determine the presence or severity of peripheral artery disease.

Blood Cholesterol Levels and CHD Risk Once a person's level of risk has been identified, much of the treatment focuses on lowering LDL cholesterol. Elevated LDL levels are directly related to the development of atherosclerosis, and clinical studies have confirmed that LDL-lowering treatments can successfully reduce CHD mortality rates.[17] CHD is seldom seen in populations that maintain desirable LDL levels.

As mentioned earlier, HDL help to protect against atherosclerosis, and low HDL levels often coexist with other lipid abnormalities; thus, a low HDL level is highly predictive of CHD risk. In addition, low HDL levels are usually associated with other CHD risk factors, such as obesity, smoking, inactivity, and insulin resistance. Although having adequate HDL is beneficial, high HDL levels do not necessarily confer additional benefit.[18]

Lifestyle Management to Reduce CVD Risk

People at significant risk of heart attack, stroke, or other complications of atherosclerosis are typically advised to modify their health behaviors to reduce their risk. Table 22-3 (p. 584) summarizes the main features of lifestyle management, which include a healthy dietary pattern, regular physical activity, nonsmoking status, and maintaining a healthy body weight. The following sections describe adjustments that have been found to improve the lipoprotein profiles of individuals with elevated LDL levels.[19]

Healthy Dietary Pattern People with elevated LDL levels have been found to benefit from diets that emphasize vegetables, fruit, and whole grains; include low-fat milk products, poultry, fish, legumes, non-tropical vegetable oils, and nuts; and limit intakes of sweets, sugar-sweetened beverages, and red meats. Acceptable diets include the USDA Food Pattern (described in Chapter 1) and the DASH Eating Plan described later in this chapter (see p. 593).

TABLE 22-3 Lifestyle Management to Reduce CVD Risk

Ideal cardiovascular health is defined by the absence of CVD and presence of the following attributes: a healthy dietary pattern, appropriate physical activity, nonsmoking status, a healthy body weight, total blood cholesterol <200 mg/dL, blood pressure <120/<80 mm Hg, and fasting plasma glucose <100 mg/dL.[a] The strategies in this table may allow an individual at significant risk of CVD to achieve these goals.

Dietary Strategies

- Adopt a healthy dietary pattern such as the USDA Food Pattern or the DASH Eating Plan.

- Limit saturated fat to about 5 to 7 percent of total kcalories and cholesterol to less than 200 milligrams per day. Replace saturated fats with unsaturated fats from fish, vegetable oils, and nuts or with carbohydrates from whole grains, legumes, fruits, and vegetables.

- Avoid food products that contain *trans* fats. The *trans* fat content in packaged foods is shown on the Nutrition Facts panel.

- Choose foods high in soluble fibers, including oats, barley, legumes, and fruit. Food supplements that contain psyllium seed husks can be used to help lower LDL cholesterol levels.

- Regularly consume food products that contain added plant sterols or stanols.

- Fish can be consumed regularly as part of a CVD risk-reduction diet.

- If alcohol is consumed, it should be limited to one drink daily for women and two drinks daily for men.

- To reduce blood pressure, consume a low-sodium diet that is high in fruits and vegetables, whole grains, nuts, and low-fat milk products.

Lifestyle Choices

- Physical activity: Engage in moderate-to-vigorous aerobic activity, lasting about 40 minutes per session, at least 3 or 4 days per week.

- Tobacco avoidance: Exposure to any form of tobacco smoke should be minimized.

Weight Reduction

- In overweight or obese individuals, weight reduction may improve some CVD risk factors. The general goals of a weight-management program should be to prevent weight gain, reduce body weight, and maintain a lower body weight over the long term.

- The initial goal of a weight-loss program should be to lose no more than 5 to 10 percent of the original body weight.

[a]The concept of *ideal cardiovascular health* was defined and developed by the American Heart Association.

Saturated Fat Of the dietary lipids, saturated fat has the strongest effect on blood cholesterol levels, and replacing saturated fat with monounsaturated and polyunsaturated fats can generally lower LDL levels. For individuals with elevated LDL, current guidelines suggest limiting the saturated fat intake to about 5 to 7 percent of the total kcalories consumed.[20] The average saturated fat intake in the United States is about 11 percent of the energy intake.[21]

For most people, cutting down on saturated fat involves more than just switching from butter to vegetable oil, as the main sources of saturated fat in the United States are full-fat cheese, pizza, grain-based and dairy-based desserts, chicken dishes, sausages, frankfurters, and bacon.[22] Thus, choosing fat-free or low-fat milk products, selecting lean meat or fish, and avoiding certain types of desserts are usually more effective ways of reducing saturated fat. Some people may find that limiting their total fat intake can indirectly help them reduce their saturated fat intake.

Replacing saturated fats with carbohydrates can also lower LDL cholesterol, but such a change may raise blood triglyceride (VLDL) levels as well.[23] The effect on blood triglycerides can be minimized by limiting added sugars and including fiber-rich foods; ideally, the diet should include generous amounts of whole grains, legumes, fruits, and vegetables.

Trans Fats *Trans* fats can raise LDL levels, and when they replace saturated fats in the diet (as when stick margarine replaces butter), they may also reduce HDL levels.[24] Thus, the *trans* fat intake should be kept as low as possible.

Most sources of *trans* fats are products made with partially hydrogenated vegetable oils; examples include baked goods such as crackers, cookies, and doughnuts; snack foods such as potato chips and corn chips; and fried foods such as French fries and fried chicken. In recent years, food manufacturers have reformulated many food products so that they contain little or no *trans* fat. In some cases, however, the *trans* fats have been replaced with saturated fat sources, so consumers should read labels carefully to avoid both types of cholesterol-raising fats.

Dietary Cholesterol The influence of dietary cholesterol on CHD risk is somewhat unclear: although some research studies have found a relationship between dietary cholesterol and CHD risk, others have not.[25] Due to concerns about the potential adverse effects of excessive dietary cholesterol in some people, the general recommendation for high-risk individuals is a cholesterol intake of less than 200 milligrams per day.[26] Cholesterol intakes of women and men in the United States average about 261 and 333 milligrams per day, respectively.[27] Eggs contribute about one-quarter of the cholesterol in the U.S. diet, followed by chicken, beef, and cheese.[28]

The effect of eggs on CHD risk is controversial. While egg intakes have not been linked to CHD risk in healthy populations,[29] a number of observational studies have found an association in persons with diabetes.[30] Furthermore, a study that evaluated the effects of egg yolk intake on carotid artery plaque found that the individuals (both with and without diabetes) who had the highest egg intakes had the highest amounts of plaque.[31] Thus, the optimal number of eggs to include in a heart-healthy diet is undetermined, and different guidelines may be necessary for healthy and high-risk populations.

Soluble Fibers Soluble, viscous fibers can reduce LDL cholesterol levels by inhibiting cholesterol and bile absorption in the small intestine and reducing cholesterol synthesis in the liver. Good sources of soluble fibers include oats, barley, legumes, and fruits. The soluble fiber in psyllium seed husks, frequently used to treat constipation, is effective for lowering cholesterol levels when used as a dietary supplement.

Plant Sterols Foods or supplements that contain significant amounts of **plant sterols** (or *plant stanols*) can help to lower LDL cholesterol levels by interfering with cholesterol and bile absorption. These plant compounds are added to various food products, such as margarine and orange juice, or supplied in dietary supplements. About 2 grams of plant sterols daily (provided by 2 to 2½ tablespoons of sterol-enriched margarines) can lower LDL cholesterol by up to 10 percent.[32]

Fish and Omega-3 Fatty Acids The omega-3 fatty acids in fatty fish, known as EPA and DHA, may benefit people at risk of CHD by suppressing inflammation, lowering blood triglyceride levels, reducing blood clotting, and stabilizing heart rhythm. In addition, including fish in the diet can reduce CHD risk because fish is low in saturated fat and often replaces meat dishes that contain saturated fat. The American Heart Association recommends consuming two or more servings of fish per week, with an emphasis on fatty fish.[33] Of note, the use of fish oil supplements has not been shown to reduce heart attacks or heart disease-related deaths in most clinical trials.[34]

Alcohol Light to moderate consumption of alcohol—from beer, wine, or liquor—has favorable effects on atherosclerosis, HDL levels, blood-clotting activity, insulin resistance, and overall CHD risk.[35] Consumption should be limited to one drink daily for women and two for men, however, because higher intakes may promote plaque formation and increase blood triglyceride levels and blood pressure. Because alcohol consumption increases the risk of various cancers and may have other detrimental effects on health, nondrinkers are not encouraged to start drinking in an effort to decrease their risk for CHD.

Blood Pressure Reduction A low-sodium diet that contains generous amounts of fruits and vegetables, whole grains, nuts, and low-fat milk products has been found to substantially reduce blood pressure. Other lifestyle modifications that may reduce blood pressure are discussed in a later section (see pp. 592–594).

Handwritten note in right margin:

Reducing CVD risks
- healthy dietary plan
- ↓ saturated fats
- ↓ trans fats
- dietary cholesterol
- ↑ soluble fibers
- ↑ plant sterols
- ↑ fish omega 3
- ↓ alcohol
- ↓ blood pressure
- ↑ physical activity
- ↓ smoking
- weight reduction
- managing lifestyle change.

plant sterols: steroid compounds produced in plants; those added to commercial food products are extracted from soybeans and pine tree oils. Plant sterols can be hydrogenated to produce *plant stanols*, which have LDL-lowering effects similar to those of plant sterols.

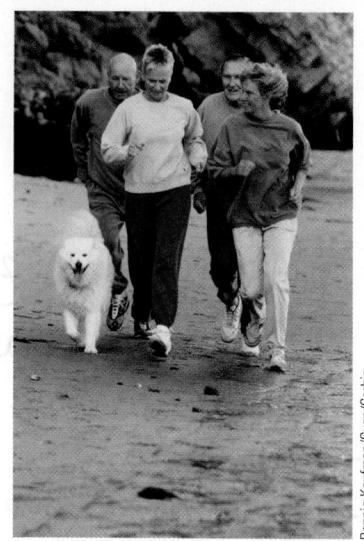

FIGURE 22-4 Regular aerobic activity can reduce CHD risk by strengthening the cardiovascular system, promoting weight loss, reducing blood pressure, and improving blood glucose and lipid levels.

Ronnie Kaufman/Cusp/Corbis

Regular Physical Activity Regular aerobic activity reverses a number of risk factors for CHD: it can lower LDL levels, reduce blood pressure, improve insulin sensitivity, promote weight loss, strengthen heart muscle, and increase coronary artery size and tone (see Figure 22-4). Current guidelines are to engage in moderate-to-vigorous aerobic activity, lasting about 40 minutes per session, at least 3 or 4 days per week.[36]

Smoking Cessation Smoking just one or two cigarettes daily—even low-tar, low-nicotine cigarettes—increases CHD risk. However, quitting smoking improves CHD risk quickly: the incidence of CHD drops to levels near those of nonsmokers within 3 years.[37] Currently, about 21 percent of men and 16 percent of women in the United States are cigarette smokers.[38] Although cigar and pipe smoking can also increase the risk of CHD, the risk may not be quite as great because the smoke is less likely to be inhaled.

Weight Reduction In persons who are obese, weight reduction can improve such CHD risk factors as hypertension, blood lipid abnormalities, and insulin resistance. However, individuals should focus on weight reduction only after they have adopted other dietary measures to lower LDL. This approach ensures that LDL reduction is given priority and that the individual does not receive a multitude of dietary suggestions at one time. For some, avoiding additional weight gain may be a desirable starting point.

Managing Lifestyle Changes Adopting multiple lifestyle changes at once is challenging. Health practitioners can help to motivate patients by explaining the reasons for each change, setting obtainable goals, and offering practical suggestions. In some individuals, high LDL levels may persist despite adjustments in health behaviors, and drug therapy may be the only effective treatment. Review Table 22-3 for a summary of the recommendations in this section. Box 22-2 offers suggestions for implementing a heart-healthy diet.

Vitamin Supplementation and CHD Risk

Patients are often interested in the potential benefits of using certain types of dietary supplements for reducing CHD risk, particularly B vitamin and antioxidant supplements. Most clinical trials have not been able to confirm any benefits from using these supplements, as described in this section.

B Vitamin Supplements and Homocysteine As mentioned earlier, elevated blood homocysteine is a risk factor for CHD, but whether homocysteine itself is directly damaging to arteries or is simply an indicator of other abnormalities remains unknown. Although increased intakes of folate, vitamin B_6, and vitamin B_{12} can lower homocysteine levels, clinical trials have not demonstrated that supplementation with these vitamins can reduce the incidence of heart attacks in those at risk.[39] Hence, B vitamin supplements are not currently recommended for patients at risk for CHD.

Antioxidant Supplements Because oxidative stress promotes atherosclerosis, researchers have hypothesized that antioxidant supplementation may inhibit atherosclerosis progression and reduce CHD risk. However, most studies that have tested supplementation with single antioxidants (such as vitamins C or E) or combinations of antioxidants have produced weak or inconsistent results, and several studies suggested possible harm.[40] Thus, the use of antioxidant supplements is not recommended for heart disease prevention.

Lifestyle Changes for Hypertriglyceridemia

Hypertriglyceridemia (see Box 22-3, p. 588) affects nearly one-third of adults in the United States.[41] It is common in people with diabetes mellitus, obesity, and the metabolic syndrome and may also result from other disorders. Elevated blood

hypertriglyceridemia: elevated blood triglyceride levels.

For many people, following a heart-healthy diet may require significant changes in food choices. It is often easier to adopt a new diet if only a few changes are made at a time. Discussing positive choices (what to eat) first, rather than negative ones (what not to eat), may improve compliance. These suggestions can help patients implement their diet:

Breads, Cereals, and Pasta

■ Choose whole-grain breads and cereals. Make sure the first ingredient on bread and cereal labels is "whole wheat flour" rather than "enriched wheat flour." Consume oats and barley regularly, as they are good sources of soluble fibers.

■ Bakery products and snack foods often contain *trans* fats. Buy only food products that list 0 grams of *trans* fat on the Nutrition Facts panel. Ingredient lists should not include any "partially hydrogenated vegetable oil," the main source of *trans* fatty acids.

Fruits and Vegetables

■ Incorporate at least one or two servings of fruits and vegetables into each meal. Keep the refrigerator stocked with a variety of ready-to-eat fruits and vegetables (baby carrots, blueberries, grapes) for snacks.

■ Purchase fruits that are canned in fruit juice rather than those canned in syrup. Avoid purchasing canned vegetables that are high in sodium (such as tomato-based products).

■ Avoid french fries from fast-food restaurants, which are often prepared with *trans* fats. Restrict high-sodium foods such as pickles, olives, sauerkraut, and kimchee.

Lunch and Dinner Entrées

■ Limit meat, fish, and poultry intake to 5 ounces per day. Plan to eat fish twice a week, preferably fatty fish such as salmon, tuna, and mackerel.

■ Select lean cuts of beef, such as sirloin tip and round steak; lean cuts of pork, such as loin chops and tenderloin; and skinless poultry pieces. Trim visible fat before cooking.

■ Select extra-lean ground meat and drain well after cooking. Use lean ground turkey, without skin added, in place of ground beef.

■ Prepare plant-based entrees whenever possible; use soybean products and other legumes as the main source of protein in soups, stews, and stir-fry dishes.

■ Limit cholesterol-rich organ meat (liver, brain, sweetbreads) and shrimp. Limit intake of whole eggs to two per week, as the yolks are high in cholesterol (about 210 milligrams per large egg). Replace whole eggs in recipes with egg whites or commercial egg substitutes.

■ Restrict these high-sodium foods: cured or smoked meat such as beef jerky, bologna, corned beef, frankfurters, ham, luncheon meat, salt pork, and sausage; salty or smoked fish such as anchovies, caviar, salted or dried cod, herring, and smoked salmon; and canned, frozen, or packaged soups, sauces, and entrées.

Milk Products

■ Select fat-free or low-fat milk products only. Use yogurt or fat-free sour cream to make dips or salad dressings. Substitute evaporated fat-free milk for heavy cream.

■ Limit products high in saturated fat or sodium, such as cheese, processed cheese, and ice cream or other milk-based desserts.

Fats and Oils

■ Prepare salad dressings and other foods with vegetable oils rich in omega-3 fatty acids, such as canola, soybean, flaxseed, and walnut oils. Select other unsaturated vegetable oils, such as corn, olive, peanut, sesame, and sunflower oils, instead of saturated fat sources such as butter and lard.

■ Select margarines that list 0 grams of *trans* fat on the Nutrition Facts panel; avoid products that list "partially hydrogenated vegetable oil" as an ingredient. To help lower LDL cholesterol levels, use margarines with added plant sterols or stanols.

■ Avoid products that contain tropical oils (coconut, palm, or palm kernel oil), which are high in saturated fat.

Spices and Seasonings

■ Use salt only at the end of cooking, and you will need to add much less. Use salt substitutes at the table. Spices and herbs can improve food flavor without adding sodium.

■ Check the sodium content on food labels. Flavorings and sauces that are usually high in sodium include bouillon cubes, soy sauce, steak and barbecue sauces, relishes, mustard, and catsup.

Snacks and Desserts

■ Select snacks that are low in sodium or saturated fat, such as pretzels and nuts, plain popcorn, and unsalted chips and crackers. Avoid products that include *trans* fats.

■ Select low-fat frozen desserts such as sherbet, sorbet, fruit bars, and some low-fat ice creams.

triglycerides may coexist with elevated LDL cholesterol or occur separately. Whereas mild or moderate hypertriglyceridemia is often associated with increased CHD risk, severe hypertriglyceridemia (blood triglycerides above 500 mg/dL) can cause additional complications, including fatty deposits in the skin and soft tissues and acute pancreatitis.[42]

BOX 22-3

Classification of elevated blood triglycerides:

- Borderline high: 150–199 mg/dL
- High: 200–499 mg/dL
- Very high: ≥500 mg/dL

Nutrition Therapy for Hypertriglyceridemia Dietary and lifestyle changes can improve most cases of mild hypertriglyceridemia.[43] Excessive weight gain and an inactive lifestyle may both raise triglyceride levels. Dietary factors that increase triglyceride levels include high intakes of alcohol and refined carbohydrates; sucrose and fructose are the carbohydrates with the strongest effect. Thus, controlling body weight, being physically active, restricting alcohol, and limiting intakes of refined carbohydrates (especially sweetened beverages and food items made with white flour and added sugars) are basic treatments for hypertriglyceridemia. As mentioned earlier, high triglyceride levels are often associated with low HDL, and the lifestyle changes listed here are likely to improve HDL levels as well.

Severe Hypertriglyceridemia In addition to dietary and lifestyle changes, medications are usually necessary for lowering blood triglyceride levels above 500 milligrams per deciliter. If blood triglycerides exceed 1000 milligrams per deciliter, a very low-fat diet, providing less than 15 percent of kcalories from fat, may be required. Patients must also eliminate consumption of alcoholic beverages.

Fish Oil Supplements and Hypertriglyceridemia Research studies suggest that fish oil supplements—containing 3 to 4 grams of EPA and DHA (combined)—can lower elevated triglyceride levels by 20 to 50 percent.[44] However, fish oil supplementation has not been shown to improve cardiovascular outcomes in patients with hypertriglyceridemia.[45]

Drug Therapies for CHD Prevention

Individuals who cannot improve CHD risk with dietary and lifestyle changes alone may be prescribed one or more medications. The drugs usually prescribed for lowering LDL levels are the *statins* (such as Lipitor and Crestor), which reduce cholesterol synthesis in the liver. Although less effective than the statins, *bile acid sequestrants* (such as Colestid or Questran) can reduce LDL levels by interfering with bile acid reabsorption in the small intestine. For lowering triglyceride levels and increasing HDL, both *fibrates* (such as Lopid) and *nicotinic acid* (a form of niacin) are effective; nicotinic acid can also reduce LDL and lipoprotein(a) levels. Individuals using these medications should continue their dietary and lifestyle modifications so that they can use the minimum effective doses of the drugs they require.

In addition to lipid-lowering medications, some people may require drugs that suppress blood clotting (such as anticoagulants and aspirin) or reduce blood pressure. Nitroglycerin (a vasodilator) may be given to alleviate angina as needed. Some medications may affect nutrition status or food intake (see Box 22-4); the interactions can be even more complicated when multiple medications are used.

Treatment for Heart Attack

As explained earlier, a heart attack occurs when the blood supply to heart muscle is blocked, causing damage to or death of heart tissue (see Figure 22-5). Drug therapies given immediately after a heart attack may include thrombolytic drugs (sometimes called *clot-busting drugs*), anticoagulants, aspirin, painkillers, and medications that regulate heart rhythm and reduce blood pressure.[46] Patients are not given food or beverages, except for sips of water or clear liquids, until their condition stabilizes. Once able to eat, they are initially offered small portions of foods that are low in sodium, saturated fat, and cholesterol. The sodium restriction helps to limit fluid retention but may be lifted after several days if the patient shows no signs of heart failure.

A heart attack patient needs to regain strength and learn strategies that can reduce the risk of a future heart attack; such strategies are similar to the lifestyle changes described earlier. Thus, the cardiac rehabilitation programs in hospitals and outpatient clinics include exercise therapy, instruction about heart-healthy food choices, help with smoking cessation, and medication counseling.

FIGURE 22-5 In a coronary artery narrowed by atherosclerotic plaque, as shown here, a blood clot may form and stop the flow of blood, resulting in a heart attack.

Dr. Gladden Willis/Encyclopedia/Corbis

BOX 22-4 DIET-DRUG INTERACTIONS

Check this table for notable nutrition-related effects of the medications discussed in this chapter.

Anticoagulants (warfarin)	**Dietary interactions:** Warfarin requires a consistent vitamin K intake to maintain effectiveness. Drug effects may be enhanced with supplementation of vitamin E, fish oils, garlic, ginkgo, and glucosamine. Drug effects may be reduced with coenzyme Q, St. John's wort, and green tea. Avoid alcohol.
Antihypertensives	
Calcium channel blockers	**Gastrointestinal effects:** Nausea, GI discomfort, flatulence, constipation, diarrhea **Dietary interactions:** Avoid herbal supplements that contain natural licorice. Avoid grapefruit juice, which may enhance drug effects (depends on specific drug used). Avoid alcohol. **Metabolic effects:** Edema, flushing
ACE inhibitors[a]	**Gastrointestinal effects:** Reduced taste sensation **Dietary interactions:** Food intake and certain mineral supplements may interfere with absorption (depends on specific drug used). Avoid herbal supplements that contain natural licorice. **Metabolic effects:** Elevated serum potassium levels
Antilipimics	
Statins	**Gastrointestinal effects:** Constipation, flatulence, GI discomfort **Dietary interactions:** Avoid grapefruit juice and red yeast rice, which may enhance drug effects, and St. John's wort, which may reduce drug effects (interactions depend on specific drug used). **Metabolic effects:** Elevated serum liver enzymes
Bile acid sequestrants	**Gastrointestinal effects:** Constipation, flatulence, GI discomfort **Dietary interactions:** May reduce absorption of fat, fat-soluble vitamins, and some minerals. **Metabolic effects:** Electrolyte imbalances, nutrient deficiencies
Nicotinic acid	**Gastrointestinal effects:** GI discomfort (unless taken with milk or food), nausea, diarrhea, flatulence **Dietary interactions:** Alcoholic beverages may increase side effects. **Metabolic effects:** Elevated serum liver enzymes, elevated uric acid levels, hyperglycemia, flushing
Digoxin	**Gastrointestinal effects:** Anorexia, nausea, vomiting, diarrhea **Dietary interactions:** Antacids or magnesium supplements can reduce drug absorption. St. John's wort may reduce drug efficacy. **Metabolic effects:** Electrolyte imbalances
Diuretics (furosemide, spironolactone)	**Gastrointestinal effects:** Dry mouth, anorexia, decreased taste perception **Dietary interactions:** Furosemide's bioavailability is reduced when taken with food. Licorice root may interfere with the effects of diuretics. **Metabolic effects:** Fluid and electrolyte imbalances,[b] hyperglycemia, hyperlipidemias, thiamin deficiency (furosemide), elevated uric acid levels (furosemide)

[a]ACE is an abbreviation for *angiotensin-converting enzyme*. An ACE inhibitor interferes with the conversion of angiotensin I to angiotensin II, a peptide that helps to regulate blood pressure.

[b]*Furosemide* is a potassium-wasting diuretic; patients should increase intakes of potassium-rich foods. *Spironolactone* is a potassium-sparing diuretic; patients should avoid supplemental potassium and potassium-containing salt substitutes.

IN SUMMARY

▮ Risk assessment for CHD involves periodic evaluation of traditional risk factors and relevant clinical measures, such as a lipoprotein profile.

▮ Dietary and lifestyle modifications help to correct blood lipid abnormalities and eliminate other risk factors. Dietary recommendations are to reduce saturated fat, *trans* fats, and cholesterol; increase soluble fiber; and incorporate plant sterols, plant stanols, and fish into the diet.

- Treatment for mild hypertriglyceridemia emphasizes weight control, regular physical activity, and restriction of refined carbohydrates (especially foods with added sugars) and alcohol. Severe hypertriglyceridemia requires drug therapies and dietary fat restriction.

- Medications given after a heart attack suppress blood clotting, regulate heart rhythm, and reduce blood pressure. To reduce the risk of a future heart attack, patients can use strategies similar to those recommended for CHD risk reduction.

22.3 Stroke

LO 22.3 Describe the different types of stroke, strategies that may prevent a stroke, and elements of treatment and rehabilitation following a stroke.

Stroke is the fourth most common cause of death in the United States and a leading cause of long-term disability in adults. About 87 percent of strokes are **ischemic strokes,**[47] caused by the obstruction of blood flow to brain tissue. **Hemorrhagic strokes** occur in 13 percent of cases and result from bleeding within the brain, which damages brain tissue. Most strokes are a consequence of atherosclerosis, hypertension, or both.

Strokes that occur suddenly and are short-lived (lasting several minutes to several hours) are called **transient ischemic attacks (TIAs).** These brief strokes are a warning sign that a more severe stroke may follow.

Stroke Prevention

Stroke is largely preventable by recognizing its risk factors and making lifestyle choices that reduce risk. Many of the risk factors are similar to those for heart disease and include hypertension, elevated LDL cholesterol, diabetes mellitus, cigarette smoking, and a history of cardiovascular disease. Medications that suppress blood clotting reduce the risk of ischemic stroke, especially in people who have suffered a first stroke or a TIA. The drugs typically prescribed include antiplatelet drugs (including aspirin) or anticoagulants such as warfarin (Coumadin). Anticoagulant therapy requires regular follow-up and occasional adjustments in dosage to prevent excessive bleeding.

Stroke Management

The effects of a stroke vary according to the area of the brain that has been injured. Body movements, senses, and speech are often impaired, and one side of the body may be weakened or paralyzed. Early diagnosis and treatment are necessary to preserve brain tissue and minimize long-term disability. Ideally, thrombolytic (clot-busting) drugs should be used within 4½ hours following an ischemic stroke to restore blood flow and prevent further brain damage.[48]

The focus of nutrition care is to help patients maintain nutrition status and overall health despite the disabilities caused by the stroke. The initial assessment should determine the nature of the patient's self-feeding difficulty (if any) and the adjustments required for appropriate food intake. Some patients may need to learn about dietary treatments that improve blood lipid levels and blood pressure. Dysphagia (difficulty swallowing) is a frequent complication and is associated with a poorer prognosis. Difficulty with speech may prevent patients from describing the problems they may be having with eating. Coordination problems can make it hard for patients to grasp utensils or bring food from table to mouth. In some cases, tube feedings may be necessary until the patient has regained these skills. Nutrition in Practice 22 describes additional options for people who have disabilities that impair eating ability as a result of a stroke or other condition.

ischemic strokes: strokes caused by the obstruction of blood flow to brain tissue.

hemorrhagic strokes: strokes caused by bleeding within the brain, which destroys or compresses brain tissue.

transient ischemic attacks (TIAs): brief ischemic strokes that cause short-term neurological symptoms.

CHAPTER TWENTY TWO

IN SUMMARY

- The two major types of stroke, ischemic and hemorrhagic stroke, may be a consequence of atherosclerosis, hypertension, or both. TIAs, which are short-lived ischemic strokes, are a warning sign that a more severe stroke may follow.

- Strokes are largely preventable by reversing modifiable risk factors. Treatment of an ischemic stroke includes the use of anticlotting drugs and anticoagulants. A patient who has had a major stroke may have problems eating normally due to lack of coordination and difficulty swallowing.

22.4 Hypertension

LO 22.4 Summarize the potential effects of hypertension, its risk factors, and current treatment approaches.

Although people cannot feel the physical effects of hypertension, it is a primary risk factor for atherosclerosis and cardiovascular diseases. In addition to hypertension's damaging effect on arteries, elevated blood pressure forces the heart to work harder to eject blood into the arteries; this effort weakens heart muscle and increases the risk of developing heart arrhythmias, heart failure, and even sudden death. Hypertension is also a primary cause of stroke and kidney failure, and reducing blood pressure can dramatically reduce the incidence of these diseases (see Box 22-5). Figure 22-6 shows a common technique for measuring blood pressure.

Hypertension affects about one-third of adults in the United States.[49] Prevalence is especially high in African Americans, who develop hypertension earlier in life and sustain higher average blood pressures throughout their lives than other ethnic groups. An estimated 18 percent of people with hypertension are unaware that they have it.[50]

Factors That Influence Blood Pressure

As shown in Figure 22-7 (p. 592), blood pressure depends on the volume of blood pumped by the heart (cardiac output) and the resistance the blood encounters in the arterioles (peripheral resistance). When either cardiac output or peripheral resistance increases, blood pressure rises. Cardiac output is raised when heart rate or blood volume increases; peripheral resistance is affected mostly by the diameters of the arterioles and blood viscosity. Blood pressure is therefore influenced by the nervous system, which regulates heart muscle contractions and arteriole diameters, and hormonal signals, which may cause fluid retention or blood vessel constriction. The kidneys also play a role in regulating blood pressure by controlling the secretion of the hormones involved in vasoconstriction and retention of sodium and water.

Factors That Contribute to Hypertension

In 90 to 95 percent of hypertension cases, the cause is unknown.[51] In other cases, hypertension is caused by a known physical or metabolic disorder, such as an abnormality in an organ or hormone involved in blood pressure regulation.

A number of risk factors for hypertension have been identified. These include the following:

- *Aging.* Hypertension risk increases with age. About two-thirds of persons older than 65 years have hypertension.[52] Moreover, individuals who have normal blood pressure at age 55 still have a 90 percent risk of developing high blood pressure during their lifetimes.[53]

BOX 22-5

Blood pressure is measured both when heart muscle contracts (*systolic* blood pressure) and when it relaxes (*diastolic* blood pressure). Measurements are expressed as millimeters of mercury (mm Hg).

	Systolic	Diastolic
Desirable	<120	<80
Prehypertension	120–139	80–89
Hypertension	≥140	≥90

FIGURE 22-6 Hypertension Screening
To determine blood pressure, the clinician restricts blood flow in the brachial artery using an inflatable cuff, and then slowly releases air from the cuff until blood flow resumes, indicating that blood pressure in the artery has matched or exceeded the air pressure in the cuff.

© Alexander Raths/Shutterstock.com

Cardiac output is the volume of blood pumped by the heart within a specified period of time.

Peripheral resistance refers to the resistance to pumped blood by the small arterial branches (arterioles) that carry blood to tissues.

© Cengage Learning®

FIGURE 22-7 Determinants of Blood Pressure
Blood pressure is influenced by both cardiac output and peripheral resistance as expressed by the formula *Blood Pressure = Cardiac Output × Peripheral Resistance.*

Genetic factors. Risk of hypertension is similar among family members. It is also more prevalent and severe in certain ethnic groups; for example, the prevalence in African-American adults is about 41 percent, compared with a prevalence of about 28 percent in both whites and Mexican Americans.[54]

Obesity. Numerous clinical studies have confirmed a strong relationship between excess body fat and increased blood pressure. Obesity raises blood pressure, in part, by stimulating the sympathetic nervous system and activating hormonal processes that promote sodium reabsorption and blood vessel constriction.[55]

Salt sensitivity. About 30 to 50 percent of those with hypertension have blood pressure that is sensitive to salt intake.[56] Salt sensitivity (also called *sodium sensitivity*) may worsen due to aging, obesity, diabetes, kidney disease, or hypertension itself.[57]

Alcohol. Heavy drinking (more than one drink daily for women or two drinks daily for men) increases the incidence and severity of hypertension. Reducing alcohol consumption reverses this effect.[58]

Dietary factors. A person's diet may influence hypertension risk. As explained later, diets that emphasize vegetables, fruit, and whole grains and include low-fat milk products have been shown to reduce blood pressure.

Treatment of Hypertension

Both lifestyle modifications and medications are used to treat hypertension. Table 22-4 lists lifestyle modifications that can reduce blood pressure and the expected reduction in systolic blood pressure for each change. The recommendations include weight reduction if overweight or obese, adopting a healthy dietary pattern, engaging in regular physical activity, and limiting alcohol intake, if one chooses to drink.[59] Combining two or more of these modifications can enhance results.

Weight Reduction In obese individuals, weight reduction may reduce blood pressure significantly. Clinical studies suggest that systolic blood pressure can be reduced by about 1 mm Hg for each kilogram of weight loss and that the blood pressure reduction may be sustained for several years.[60] In the long term, however (more than 3 years), blood pressure tends to revert to initial levels, even when weight loss is partially maintained. Thus, weight reduction appears to be most beneficial for blood pressure control during periods when the body weight is actually decreasing.[61]

Dietary Approaches for Blood Pressure Reduction Several studies have shown that a significant reduction in blood pressure can be achieved by following a diet that emphasizes fruits, vegetables, and whole grains and includes low-fat milk products, poultry, fish, and nuts.[62] The diet tested in these studies, now known as the *DASH Eating Plan* (see Table 22-5), provides more fiber, potassium, magnesium, and calcium than the typical American diet. The diet also limits red meat, sweets, sugar-containing beverages, saturated fat (to 7 percent of kcalories), and cholesterol (to 150 milligrams per day), so it is beneficial for reducing CHD risk as well.

The DASH Eating Plan is even more effective when accompanied by a low sodium intake. In a research study that tested the blood pressure–lowering effects of the DASH dietary pattern in combination with sodium restriction, the best results were achieved when sodium was reduced to 1500 milligrams daily—a level much

TABLE 22-4 Lifestyle Modifications for Blood Pressure Reduction

The goals of hypertension treatment are as follows:[a]

- For adults 18–59 years old: blood pressure <140/<90 mm Hg
- For adults ≥60 years old: blood pressure <150/<90 mm Hg

Lifestyle Modification	Recommendation	Expected Reduction in Systolic Blood Pressure
Weight reduction	Reduce weight to achieve a healthy body weight (BMI 18.5–24.9).	10 mm Hg per 10 kg weight loss
DASH Eating Plan[b]	Adopt a diet that emphasizes vegetables, fruit, and whole grains; includes low-fat milk products; and limits sugars and red meats.	5–6 mm Hg
Sodium restriction	Consume no more than 2400 mg sodium (<6 g salt) per day.	2 mm Hg
	For a greater reduction in blood pressure, consume no more than 1500 mg sodium (<4 g salt) per day.	7 mm Hg
	Reduce sodium intake by at least 1000 mg per day, even if the desired sodium intake is not achieved.	3–4 mm Hg
Physical activity	Engage in moderate-to-vigorous aerobic activity, lasting about 40 minutes per session, at least 3 or 4 days per week.	2–5 mm Hg
Moderate alcohol consumption	Men: Limit to two drinks per day. Women and lighter-weight men: Limit to one drink per day.	2–4 mm Hg

© 2016 Cengage Learning®

[a]These goals are recommended by panel members of the Eighth Joint National Committee (JNC 8), a group commissioned by the National Heart, Lung, and Blood Institute of the National Institutes of Health. Note that the treatment goals suggested by the American Society of Hypertension and International Society of Hypertension are <140/<90 mm Hg for adults 18–79 years old and <150/<90 mm Hg for adults ≥80 years old.

[b]The DASH Eating Plan was tested in a study called *Dietary Approaches to Stop Hypertension.*

Sources: R. H. Eckel and coauthors, 2013 AHA/ACC guideline on lifestyle management to reduce cardiovascular risk: A report of the American College of Cardiology American/Heart Association Task Force on Practice Guidelines, *Journal of the American College of Cardiology* (2013), doi: 10.1016/j.jacc.2013.11.003; C. C. Tyson and coauthors, Impact of 5-year weight change on blood pressure: Results from the weight loss maintenance trial, *Journal of Clinical Hypertension* 15 (2013): 458–464.

TABLE 22-5 The DASH Eating Plan

Food Group	Recommended Servings for Different Energy Intakes (servings per day except as noted)			
	1600 kcal	2000 kcal	2600 kcal	3100 kcal
Grains and grain products[a] (1 serving = 1 slice bread, 1 oz dry cereal,[b] or ½ c cooked rice, pasta, or cereal)	6	6–8	10–11	12–13
Vegetables (1 serving = ½ c cooked vegetables, 1 c raw leafy vegetables, or ½ c vegetable juice)	3–4	4–5	5–6	6
Fruits (1 serving = 1 medium fruit; ½ c fresh, frozen, or canned fruit; ¼ c dried fruit; or ½ c fruit juice)	4	4–5	5–6	6
Milk products (low fat or fat free) (1 serving = 1 c milk or yogurt, or 1½ oz cheese)	2–3	2–3	3	3–4
Meat, poultry, and fish (1 serving = 1 oz cooked lean meat, poultry, or fish; or 1 egg)	3–4 oz or less	6 oz or less	6 oz or less	6–9 oz or less
Nuts, seeds, and legumes (1 serving = ⅓ c nuts, 2 tbs peanut butter, 2 tbs seeds, or ½ c cooked dry beans or peas)	3–4 per week	4–5 per week	1	1
Fats and oils (1 serving = 1 tsp vegetable oil or soft margarine, ½ tbs mayonnaise, or 1 tbs salad dressing)	2	2–3	3	4
Sweets and added sugars (1 serving = 1 tbs sugar, jelly, or jam; ½ c sorbet; or 1 c lemonade)	3 or less per week	5 or less per week	≤2	≤2

© 2016 Cengage Learning®

[a]Whole grains are recommended for most servings consumed.
[b]One ounce of dry cereal may be equivalent to ½ to 1¼ cups, depending on the cereal. Check the food label for the portion size.

Source: U.S. Department of Agriculture and U.S. Department of Health and Human Services, *Dietary Guidelines for Americans, 2010* (Washington, D.C.: U.S. Government Printing Office, 2010).

- Select fresh, unprocessed foods. Packaged foods, canned goods, and frozen meals are often high in sodium.

- Do not use salt at the table or while cooking. Salt substitutes may be useful for some people. Salt substitutes often contain potassium, however, and are not appropriate for people using diuretics that promote potassium retention in the blood.

- Avoid eating in fast-food restaurants; most menu choices are very high in sodium.

- Check food labels. The labeling term *low sodium* is a better guide than the terms *reduced sodium* (contains 25 percent less sodium than the regular product) or *light in sodium* (contains 50 percent less sodium). To be labeled *low sodium,* a food product must contain less than 140 milligrams of sodium per serving. Keep your sodium goal in mind when you read labels.

- Recognize the high-sodium foods in each food category, and purchase only unsalted or low-sodium varieties of these products if they are available. High-sodium foods include the following:

  - Snack foods made with added salt, such as tortilla chips, popcorn, and nuts.

  - Processed meat, such as ham, corned beef, bologna, salami, sausage, bacon, frankfurters, and pastrami.

  - Processed fish, such as salted fish and canned fish.

  - Tomato-based products, such as tomato sauce, tomato juice, pizza, canned tomatoes, and catsup.

  - Canned soup or broth; note that even reduced-sodium varieties may contain excessive sodium.

  - Cheese, such as cottage cheese, American cheese, and Parmesan and most other hard cheeses.

  - Bakery products made with baking powder or baking soda (sodium bicarbonate), such as cake, cookies, doughnuts, and muffins.

  - Condiments and relishes, such as bouillon cubes, olives, and pickled vegetables.

  - Flavoring sauces, such as soy sauce, barbecue sauce, and steak sauce.

- Check for the word *sodium* on medication labels. Sodium is often an ingredient in some types of antacids and laxatives.

lower than the amounts typically consumed in the United States. These results suggest that the optimal sodium intake for people with hypertension may be far lower than the amounts typically recommended for the general population (less than 2300 or 2400 milligrams daily*). Box 22-6 lists practical suggestions for restricting sodium intake; additional detail is provided in Table 23-1 on p. 607.

Drug Therapies People with hypertension usually require two or more medications to meet their blood pressure goals. Using a combination of drugs with different modes of action can reduce the doses of each drug needed and minimize side effects. The drugs commonly prescribed include diuretics, calcium channel blockers, angiotensin-converting enzyme (ACE) inhibitors, and angiotensin-receptor blockers; some of these drugs are also used to treat various heart conditions. Drug dosages may need regular adjustment until the blood pressure goal is reached.

IN SUMMARY

- About one in three persons in the United States has hypertension, which increases the risk of developing CHD, stroke, heart failure, and kidney failure.

- Blood pressure is elevated by factors that increase blood volume, heart rate, or resistance to blood flow. Although the underlying cause of most hypertension cases is usually unknown, risk factors include aging, family history, ethnicity, obesity, and various dietary factors.

- Treatment of hypertension usually includes a combination of lifestyle modifications and drug therapies.

*The Tolerable Upper Intake Level (UL) for sodium was set at 2300 mg per day, whereas studies that evaluated the effects of the DASH diet tested sodium intakes of 2400 mg per day. The difference between these two values is minimal.

Robert Reid, a 48-year-old African-American computer programmer, is 5 feet 9 inches tall and weighs 240 pounds. He sits for long hours at work and is too tired to exercise when he gets home at night. His meals usually include fatty meat, eggs, and cheese, and he likes dairy desserts such as pudding and ice cream. He has a family history of CHD and hypertension. His recent laboratory tests show that his blood pressure is 160/100 mm Hg, and his LDL and HDL levels are 160 mg/dL and 35 mg/dL, respectively. He smokes a pack of cigarettes each day and usually has 2 glasses of wine at both lunch and dinner.

1. Identify Mr. Reid's major risk factors for CHD and hypertension. Which can be modified? What complications might occur if he delays treatment for his blood lipids and blood pressure?

2. What dietary changes would you recommend that could help to improve Mr. Reid's blood pressure and his LDL cholesterol? Explain the rationale for each dietary change. Prepare a day's menu for Mr. Reid using the DASH Eating Plan as an outline for your choices.

3. What other laboratory tests or measurements would you need to better assess Mr. Reid's condition? Why?

4. Describe several benefits that Mr. Reid might obtain from a program that includes weight reduction and regular physical activity. Explain why the use of alcohol can be both a protective and a damaging lifestyle habit.

5. Assuming that Mr. Reid does not make any changes in his diet and lifestyle and suffers a heart attack, identify the elements of a cardiac rehabilitation program that would be critical for his long-term survival.

The Case Study in Box 22-7 provides an opportunity to review the risk factors and treatments for CHD and hypertension.

22.5 Heart Failure

LO 22.5 Identify the possible consequences of heart failure and describe the current treatment approaches for this condition.

Heart failure, also called *congestive heart failure,* is characterized by the heart's inability to pump adequate blood, resulting in inadequate blood delivery and a buildup of fluids in the veins and tissues. Heart failure has various causes, but it is often a consequence of chronic disorders that create extra work for the heart muscle, such as hypertension or CHD. To accommodate the extra workload, the heart enlarges or pumps faster or harder, but it may eventually weaken enough to fail completely. Heart failure develops mostly in older adults and the elderly: the majority of cases occur in individuals 65 years or older.[63]

Consequences of Heart Failure

In heart failure, fluid may accumulate in the liver and abdomen and in the lower extremities, causing chest pain, difficulty with digestion and absorption, and swelling in the legs, ankles, and feet (see Figure 22-8, p. 596). Fluid can also build up in the lungs (called *pulmonary edema*), resulting in extreme shortness of breath and limited oxygen for activity; in severe cases, it can lead to respiratory failure. With inadequate blood flow, the functions of various organs, such as the liver and kidneys, may become impaired. The effects of heart failure depend on the severity of illness: mild cases may be asymptomatic, but severe cases may cause considerable damage to health.

Heart failure often affects a person's food intake and level of physical activity. In persons with abdominal bloating and liver enlargement, pain and discomfort may worsen with meals. Limb weakness and fatigue can limit physical activity. End-stage heart failure is often accompanied by **cardiac cachexia,** a condition of severe malnutrition characterized by significant weight loss and tissue wasting. Cardiac cachexia may develop due to increased levels of pro-inflammatory cytokines (which promote catabolism), elevated metabolic rate, reduced food intake, and malabsorption.[64] The resultant weakness further lowers the person's strength, functional capacity, and activity levels.

heart failure: a condition characterized by the heart's inability to pump adequate blood to the body's cells, resulting in fluid accumulation in the tissues; also called *congestive heart failure.*

cardiac cachexia: severe malnutrition that develops in heart failure patients; characterized by weight loss and tissue wasting.

FIGURE 22-8 Heart Failure
In heart failure, the overburdened heart enlarges in an effort to supply blood to the body's tissues.

Medical Management of Heart Failure

Heart failure is a chronic, progressive illness that may require frequent hospitalizations. Many patients face a combination of debilitating symptoms, complex treatments, and an uncertain outcome. Important goals of medical therapy are to slow disease progression and enhance the patient's quality of life.

The specific treatment for heart failure depends on the nature and severity of the illness. Medications help to manage fluid retention and improve heart function. Dietary sodium and fluid restrictions can help to prevent fluid accumulation. Vaccinations for influenza and pneumonia reduce the risk of developing respiratory infections. Treatment of CHD risk factors, such as hypertension and lipid disorders, can help to slow disease progression. Heart failure patients are also encouraged to participate in exercise programs to avoid becoming physically disabled and to improve endurance.

Nutrition Therapy for Heart Failure The main dietary recommendation for heart failure is a modest sodium restriction of 2000 milligrams or less daily to reduce the risk of fluid retention. In patients with persistent or recurrent fluid retention, fluid intakes may be restricted to 2 liters per day or less.[65] Individuals who have difficulty eating due to abdominal or chest pain may tolerate small, frequent meals better than large meals.

Patients with heart failure may be prone to constipation due to diuretic use and reduced physical activity. Maintaining an adequate fiber intake can help to minimize constipation problems. Because alcohol consumption may worsen heart function, some patients may need to restrict or avoid alcoholic beverages. Patients on diuretic therapy or restricted diets may benefit from daily multivitamin-mineral supplementation.[66]

No known therapies can reverse cardiac cachexia, and the prognosis is poor. For some patients, liquid supplements, tube feedings, or parenteral nutrition support can be supportive additions to treatment.

IN SUMMARY

▌ Heart failure is usually a chronic, progressive condition that results from other cardiovascular illnesses.

▌ In heart failure, the heart is unable to pump adequate blood to tissues. Consequences may include fluid accumulation in the veins, lungs, and other organs and impaired organ function.

▌ Drug therapies can reduce fluid accumulation and improve heart function. Nutrition therapy may include sodium, fluid, and alcohol restrictions and nutrient supplementation.

Nutrition Assessment Checklist FOR PEOPLE WITH CARDIOVASCULAR DISEASES

Medical History

Check the medical record for a diagnosis of:

- Coronary heart disease
- Stroke
- Hypertension
- Heart failure

Review the medical record for complications related to cardiovascular diseases:

- Heart attack
- Transient ischemic attack
- Cardiac cachexia

Note risk factors for CHD or stroke that are related to diet, including:

- Elevated LDL or triglyceride levels
- Obesity or overweight
- Diabetes
- Hypertension

Medications

For patients using drug treatments for cardiovascular diseases, note:

- Side effects that may alter food intake
- Medications that may interact with grapefruit juice
- Use of warfarin, which requires a consistent vitamin K intake
- Use of diuretics or other drugs associated with potassium imbalances
- Potential diet-drug or herb-drug interactions

Dietary Intake

For patients with CHD, a previous stroke, or hypertension, assess the diet for:

- Energy intake
- Saturated fat, *trans* fat, cholesterol, and sodium content
- Soluble fiber and plant sterol or plant stanol content
- Intake of fruit, vegetables, whole grains, legumes, and nuts
- Alcohol content

For patients with complications resulting from cardiovascular diseases:

- Check physical disabilities that may interfere with food preparation or consumption following a stroke.
- Check adequacy of food and nutrient intake in patients with heart failure.

Anthropometric Data

Measure baseline height and weight, and reassess weight at each medical checkup. Note whether patients are meeting weight goals, including:

- Weight loss or maintenance in patients who are overweight
- Weight maintenance in patients with advanced heart failure

Remember that weight may be deceptively high in people who are retaining fluids, especially individuals with heart failure.

Laboratory Tests

Monitor the following laboratory tests in people with cardiovascular diseases:

- LDL cholesterol, blood triglycerides, and HDL cholesterol
- Blood glucose in patients with diabetes
- Serum potassium in patients using diuretics, antihypertensive medications, or digoxin
- Blood-clotting times in patients using anticoagulants
- Indicators of fluid retention in patients with heart failure

Physical Signs

Blood pressure measurement is routine in physical exams but is especially important for people who:

- Have cardiovascular diseases
- Have experienced a heart attack or stroke
- Have risk factors for CHD or hypertension

Look for signs of:

- Potassium imbalances (muscle weakness, numbness and tingling, irregular heartbeat) in those using diuretics, antihypertensive medications, or digoxin
- Fluid overload in patients with heart failure

Clinical Applications

1. List risk factors for coronary heart disease, and identify possible interrelationships among the factors. For example, a woman over 55 years of age is also at risk for diabetes; a person with diabetes is more likely to have hypertension.

2. Review the DASH Eating Plan shown in Table 22-5. As the chapter describes, the DASH dietary pattern is helpful for lowering blood pressure and for reducing CHD risk as well.

- List elements of the DASH Eating Plan that are consistent with the dietary recommendations for CHD risk reduction.

- Suggest ways in which a person following the DASH Eating Plan might accomplish the following additional dietary modifications: consume a higher percentage of fat from monounsaturated sources, reduce intake of *trans* fats, and include EPA/DHA and plant sterols in the diet.

Self Check

1. Ischemia in the coronary arteries is a frequent cause of:
   a. angina pectoris.
   b. hemorrhagic stroke.
   c. aneurysm.
   d. hypertension.

2. Risk factors for atherosclerosis include all of the following *except:*
   a. smoking.
   b. hypertension.
   c. diabetes mellitus.
   d. elevated HDL cholesterol.

3. Which clinical test can help to diagnose peripheral artery disease?
   a. Lipoprotein profile
   b. Coronary artery calcium score
   c. Ankle-brachial index
   d. C-reactive protein levels

4. Dietary lipids with the strongest LDL cholesterol–raising effects are:
   a. monounsaturated fats.
   b. polyunsaturated fats.
   c. saturated fats.
   d. plant sterols.

5. Moderate alcohol consumption can improve heart disease risk, in part, because it:
   a. lowers blood pressure.
   b. increases HDL cholesterol levels.
   c. offsets the damage from smoking.
   d. improves nutrition status.

6. Patients with mild hypertriglyceridemia may improve their triglyceride levels by:
   a. reducing sodium intake.
   b. reducing cholesterol intake.
   c. consuming moderate amounts of alcohol.
   d. limiting intakes of refined carbohydrates.

7. Which medications reduce cholesterol synthesis in the liver?
   a. Bile acid sequestrants
   b. Statins
   c. ACE inhibitors
   d. Fibrates

8. Hemorrhagic stroke:
   a. is the most common type of stroke.
   b. results from obstructed blood flow within brain tissue.
   c. comes on suddenly and usually lasts for up to 30 minutes.
   d. results from bleeding within the brain, which damages brain tissue.

9. Hypertensive patients can benefit from all of the following dietary and lifestyle modifications *except:*
   a. including fat-free or low-fat milk products in the diet.
   b. reducing total fat intake.
   c. consuming generous amounts of fruit, vegetables, legumes, and nuts.
   d. reducing sodium intake.

10. Nutrition therapy for a patient with heart failure usually includes:
    a. weight loss.
    b. reducing total fat intake.
    c. sodium restriction.
    d. cholesterol restriction.

Answers to these questions appear in Appendix H.

Notes

1. A. S. Go and coauthors, Heart disease and stroke statistics 2014 update: A report from the American Heart Association, *Circulation* 129 (2014): e28–e292.

2. L. J. Laslett and coauthors, The worldwide environment of cardiovascular disease: Prevalence, diagnosis, therapy, and policy issues, *Journal of the American College of Cardiology* 60 (2012): S1–S49.

3. G. K. Hansson and A. Hamsten, Atherosclerosis, thrombosis, and vascular biology, in L. Goldman and A. I. Schafer, eds., *Goldman's Cecil Medicine* (Philadelphia: Saunders, 2012), pp. 409–412.

4. P. Nigro, J. Abe, and B. C. Berk, Flow shear stress and atherosclerosis: A matter of site specificity, *Antioxidants and Redox Signaling* 15 (2011): 1405–1414.

5. V. Cachofeiro and coauthors, Inflammation: A link between hypertension and atherosclerosis, *Current Hypertension Reviews* 5 (2009): 40–48.

6. M. Miller and coauthors, Triglycerides and cardiovascular disease: A scientific statement from the American Heart Association, *Circulation* 123 (2011): 2292–2333.

7. K. Mahdy Ali and coauthors, Cardiovascular disease risk reduction by raising HDL cholesterol—Current therapies and future opportunities, *British Journal of Pharmacology* 167 (2012): 1177–1194; D. Kothapalli and coauthors, Cardiovascular protection by apoE and apoE-HDL linked to suppression of ECM gene expression and arterial stiffening, *Cell Reports* 2 (2012): 1–13.

8. J. H. Wu, Lipoprotein(a) in vascular disease, cancer and longevity, *Chang Gung Medical Journal* 34 (2011): 555–564.

9. N. Chalouhi and coauthors, Cigarette smoke and inflammation: Role in cerebral aneurysm formation and rupture, *Mediators of Inflammation* 2012 (2012): 271582, doi: 10.1155/2012/271582.

10. C. E. Tabit and coauthors, Endothelial dysfunction in diabetes mellitus: Molecular mechanisms and clinical implications, *Reviews in Endocrine & Metabolic Disorders* 11 (2010): 61–74; G. Orasanu and J. Plutzky, Pathologic continuum of diabetic vascular disease, *Journal of the American College of Cardiology* 53 (2009): S35–S42.

11. F. Lenfant and coauthors, Timing of the vascular actions of estrogens in experimental and human studies: Why protective early, and not when delayed? *Maturitas* 68 (2011): 165–173.

12. K. L. Schalinske and A. L. Smazal, Homocysteine imbalance: A pathological metabolic marker, *Advances in Nutrition* 3 (2012): 755–762.

13. W. E. Boden, Angina pectoris and stable ischemic heart disease, in L. Goldman and A. I. Schafer, eds., *Goldman's Cecil Medicine* (Philadelphia: Saunders, 2012), pp. 412–425.

14. D. C. Goff and coauthors, 2013 ACC/AHA guideline on the assessment of cardiovascular risk, *Circulation* (2013): doi: 10.1161/01.cir.0000437741.48606.98.

15. P. S. Jellinger and coauthors, American Association of Clinical Endocrinologists' guidelines for management of dyslipidemia and prevention of atherosclerosis, *Endocrine Practice* 18 (2012): 269–293; J. S. Rana and coauthors, The role of non-HDL cholesterol in risk stratification for coronary artery disease. *Current Atherosclerosis Reports* 14 (2012): 130–134.

16. Jellinger and coauthors, 2012; M. H. Davidson and coauthors, Clinical utility of inflammatory markers and advanced lipoprotein testing, *Journal of Clinical Lipidology* 5 (2011): 338–367.

17. C. F. Semenkovich, Disorders of lipid metabolism, in L. Goldman and A. I. Schafer, eds., *Goldman's Cecil Medicine* (Philadelphia: Saunders, 2012), pp. 1346–1354.

18. B. F. Voight and coauthors, Plasma HDL cholesterol and risk of myocardial infarction: A mendelian randomization study, *Lancet* 380 (2012): 572–580.

19. R. H. Eckel and coauthors, 2013 AHA/ACC guideline on lifestyle management to reduce cardiovascular risk, *Journal of the American College of Cardiology* (2013), doi: 10.1016/j.jacc.2013.11.003.

20. Eckel and coauthors, 2013; J. M. Gonzalez-Campoy and coauthors, Clinical practice guidelines for healthy eating for the prevention and treatment of metabolic and endocrine diseases in adults, *Endocrine Practice* 19 (2013): S1–S82.

21. U.S. Department of Agriculture, Agricultural Research Service, *What We Eat in America, NHANES 2009–2010* (2012), available at www.ars.usda.gov/Services/docs.htm?docid=18349, site visited June 14, 2014.

22. U.S. Department of Agriculture and U.S. Department of Health and Human Services, *Dietary Guidelines for Americans, 2010* (Washington, DC: U.S. Government Printing Office, 2010).

23. Gonzalez-Campoy and coauthors, 2013.

24. D. Estadella and coauthors, Lipotoxicity: Effects of dietary saturated and trans fatty acids, *Mediators of Inflammation* 2013 (2013): doi: 10.1155/2013/137579.

25. M. L. Fernandez, Rethinking dietary cholesterol, *Current Opinion in Clinical Nutrition and Metabolic Care* 15 (2012): 117–121; J. D. Spence, D. J. A. Jenkins, and J. Davignon, Dietary cholesterol and egg yolks: Not for patients at risk of vascular disease, *Canadian Journal of Cardiology* 26 (2010): e336–e339.

26. M. M. Kanter and coauthors, Exploring the factors that affect blood cholesterol and heart disease risk, *Advances in Nutrition* 3 (2012): 711–717; Spence, Jenkins, and Davignon, 2010.

27. U.S. Department of Agriculture, Agricultural Research Service, 2012.

28. National Cancer Institute, Applied Research Program, *Sources of Cholesterol among the U.S. Population, 2005–06*, available at http://riskfactor.cancer.gov/diet/foodsources/cholesterol, site visited June 14, 2014.

29. Y. Rong and coauthors, Egg consumption and risk of coronary heart disease and stroke: Dose-response meta-analysis of prospective cohort studies, *British Medical Journal* 346 (2013): doi: 10.1136/bmj.e8539; Fernandez, 2012.

30. D. K. Houston and coauthors, Dietary fat and cholesterol and risk of cardiovascular disease in older adults, *Nutrition, Metabolism & Cardiovascular Diseases* 21 (2011): 430–437; Spence, Jenkins, and Davignon, 2010.

31. J. D. Spence, D. J. A. Jenkins, and J. Davignon, Egg yolk consumption and carotid plaque, *Atherosclerosis* 224 (2012): 469–473.

32. J. Plat and coauthors, Progress and prospective of plant sterol and plant stanol research, *Atherosclerosis* 225 (2012): 521–533.

33. D. M. Lloyd-Jones and coauthors, Defining and setting national goals for cardiovascular health promotion and disease reduction, *Circulation* 121 (2010): 586–613.

34. The Risk and Prevention Study Collaborative Group, n-3 fatty acids in patients with multiple cardiovascular risk factors, *New England Journal of Medicine* 368 (2013): 1800–1808; E. C. Rizos and coauthors, Association between omega-3 fatty acid supplementation and risk of major cardiovascular disease events, *Journal of the American Medical Association* 308 (2012): 1024–1033; S. M. Kwak and coauthors, Efficacy of omega-3 fatty acid supplements (eicosapentaenoic acid and docosahexaenoic acid) in the secondary prevention of cardiovascular disease, *Archives of Internal Medicine* 172 (2012): 686–694.

35. S. E. Brien and coauthors, Effect of alcohol consumption on biological markers associated with risk of coronary heart disease, *British Medical Journal* 342 (2011): doi:10.1136/bmj.d636; P. E. Ronksley and coauthors, Association of alcohol consumption with selected cardiovascular disease outcomes, *British Medical Journal* 342 (2011): doi:10.1136/bmj.d671.

36. Eckel and coauthors, 2013.

37. M. J. Klag, Epidemiology of cardiovascular disease, in L. Goldman and A. I. Schafer, eds., *Goldman's Cecil Medicine* (Philadelphia: Saunders, 2012), pp. 256–260.

38. Go and coauthors, 2014.

39. M. J. Jardine and coauthors, The effect of folic acid based homocysteine lowering on cardiovascular events in people with kidney disease, *British Medical Journal* 344 (2012): doi: http://dx.doi.org/10.1136/bmj.e3533; R. Clarke and coauthors, Homocysteine and vascular disease, *Journal of Inherited Metabolic Disease* 34 (2011): 83–91.

40. V. A. Moyer on behalf of the U.S. Preventive Services Task Force, Vitamin, mineral, and multivitamin supplements for the primary prevention of cardiovascular disease and cancer, *Annals of Internal Medicine* 160 (2014): 558–564.

41. Miller and coauthors, 2011.

42. M. J. Malloy and J. P. Kane, Disorders of lipoprotein metabolism, in D. G. Gardner and D. Shoback, eds., *Greenspan's Basic and Clinical Endocrinology* (New York: McGraw-Hill/Lange, 2011), pp. 675–698.

43. L. Berglund and coauthors, Evaluation and treatment of hypertriglyceridemia, *Journal of Clinical Endocrinology and Metabolism* 97 (2012): 2969–2989; Miller and coauthors, 2011.

44. Berglund and coauthors, 2012.

45. Berglund and coauthors, 2012; Miller and coauthors, 2011.

46. J. L. Anderson, ST segment elevation acute myocardial infarction and complications of myocardial infarction, in L. Goldman and A. I. Schafer, eds., *Goldman's Cecil Medicine* (Philadelphia: Saunders, 2012), pp. 434–448.

47. Go and coauthors, 2014.

48. E. C. Jauch and coauthors, Guidelines for the early management of patients with acute ischemic stroke, *Stroke* 44 (2013): 870–947.

49. Go and coauthors, 2014.

50. Go and coauthors, 2014.

51. R. G. Victor, Arterial hypertension, in L. Goldman and A. I. Schafer, eds., *Goldman's Cecil Medicine* (Philadelphia: Saunders, 2012), pp. 373–389.

52. G. L. Bakris, Arterial hypertension, in R. S. Porter and J. L. Kaplan, eds., *Merck Manual of Diagnosis and Therapy* (Whitehouse Station, NJ: Merck Sharp and Dohme Corp., 2011), pp. 2065–2081.

53. Bakris, 2011.

54. Go and coauthors, 2014; C. D. Fryar and coauthors, Trends in nutrient intakes and chronic health conditions among Mexican-American adults, a 25-year profile: United States, 1982–2006. *National Health Statistics Reports* 50 (Mar. 28, 2012).

55. L. Landsberg and coauthors, Obesity-related hypertension: Pathogenesis, cardiovascular risk, and treatment, *Journal of Clinical Hypertension* 15 (2013): 14–33.

56. V. Savica, G. Bellinghieri, and J. D. Kopple, The effect of nutrition on blood pressure, *Annual Review of Nutrition* 30 (2010): 365–401.

57. P. K. Whelton and coauthors, Sodium, blood pressure, and cardiovascular disease, *Circulation* 126 (2012): 2880–2889; Savica, Bellinghieri, and Kopple, 2010.

58. Victor, 2012.

59. Eckel and coauthors, 2013; Whelton and coauthors, 2012.

60. C. C. Tyson and coauthors, Impact of 5-year weight change on blood pressure, *Journal of Clinical Hypertension* 15 (2013): 458–464.

61. Tyson and coauthors, 2013; Savica, Bellinghieri, and Kopple, 2010.

62. F. M. Sacks and coauthors, Effects on blood pressure of reduced dietary sodium and the Dietary Approaches to Stop Hypertension (DASH) Diet, *New England Journal of Medicine* 344 (2001): 3–10; L. J. Appel and coauthors, A clinical trial on the effects of dietary patterns on blood pressure, *New England Journal of Medicine* 336 (1997): 1117–1124.

63. B. M. Massie, Heart failure: Pathophysiology and diagnosis, in L. Goldman and A. I. Schafer, eds., *Goldman's Cecil Medicine* (Philadelphia: Saunders, 2012), pp. 295–303.

64. Massie, 2012.

65. J. J. V. McMurray and M. A. Pfeffer, Heart failure: Management and prognosis, in L. Goldman and A. I. Schafer, eds., *Goldman's Cecil Medicine* (Philadelphia: Saunders, 2012), pp. 303–318.

66. J. Lindenfeld and coauthors, HFSA 1010 comprehensive heart failure practice guideline, *Journal of Cardiac Failure* 16 (2010): 475–539.

LO 22.6 Identify disabilities that may impair eating ability and give examples of strategies that may improve feeding skills.

Chapter 22 referred to difficulties following a stroke that can interfere with the ability to eat independently. This Nutrition in Practice discusses the problems faced by individuals who must cope with various disabilities that interfere with the process of eating, including those that interfere with chewing, swallowing, or bringing food to the mouth. These obstacles can arise at any time during a person's life and from any number of causes. An infant may be born with a physical impairment such as cleft palate; an adolescent may lose motor control following injuries sustained in an automobile accident; an older adult may struggle with the pain of arthritis or the mental deterioration of dementia. Table NP22-1 lists some of the conditions that may lead to feeding problems.

In what ways can disabilities impair a person's ability to eat?

Eating and drinking require a considerable number of individual coordinated motions. Consider an infant learning the skills required for feeding: each step—sitting, grasping cups and utensils, bringing food to the mouth, biting, chewing, and swallowing—requires coordinated movements. An injury or disability that interferes with any of these movements can lead to feeding problems and inadequate food intake. Total food intake is often significantly reduced when individuals with inefficient motor function take a long time to eat.[1] Difficulties that affect the procurement of food, such as the inability to drive, walk, or carry groceries, can also lower food intake and lead to malnutrition and weight loss.

Can disabilities alter a person's energy needs?

Yes, disabilities may either lower or raise energy requirements. Disabilities that affect muscle tension or mobility—such as cerebral

TABLE NP22-1 Conditions That May Lead to Feeding Problems

The following conditions may lead to feeding problems by interfering with a person's ability to suck, bite, chew, swallow, or coordinate hand-to-mouth movements.

▪ Accidents	▪ Huntington's chorea
▪ Amputations	▪ Language, visual, or hearing impairments
▪ Arthritis	▪ Multiple sclerosis
▪ Birth defects	▪ Muscle weakness
▪ Brain tumors	▪ Muscular dystrophy
▪ Cerebral palsy	▪ Parkinson's disease
▪ Cleft palate	▪ Polio
▪ Down syndrome	▪ Spinal cord injuries
▪ Head injuries	▪ Stroke

© 2016 Cengage Learning®

palsy—are typically associated with reduced muscle mass and physical activity; consequently, energy requirements tend to be lower.[2] Loss of a limb due to amputation reduces energy needs in proportion to the weight and metabolism represented by the missing limb, but energy needs may be higher if an individual increases activity to compensate for the loss, as is necessary when using a prosthesis.[3] Because the effects of disabilities are often unpredictable, the health care practitioner may find it difficult to assess energy requirements until weight gain or loss has occurred.

Overweight and obesity often accompany conditions that limit mobility or result in short stature; examples include Down syndrome and spina bifida. Obesity may also develop because the family or caregiver provides an inappropriate amount of food, sometimes out of sympathy for the disabled individual. In these cases, the health practitioner may need to counsel the family or caregiver about appropriate food choices and portion sizes.

Can disease symptoms cause problems with food intake and nutrition status?

Yes, physical symptoms of disease can sometimes create feeding problems; examples include difficulty with swallowing or breathing, frequent coughing or choking, and gastroesophageal reflux. Individuals with speech problems may have difficulty communicating with caregivers about thirst and hunger. Mobility problems and physical weakness can interfere with food preparation and the physical movements required for eating meals.

Which health professionals typically work with people who have feeding problems?

Evaluating and treating feeding problems may involve the joint efforts of health care professionals from a variety of disciplines, including dietitians, nurses, occupational therapists, speech-language pathologists, and gastroenterologists.[4] Together, these professionals can evaluate the patient's abilities to grasp and use utensils, bring foods from the plate to the mouth, chew, sip, and swallow. A speech-language pathologist or occupational therapist may evaluate chewing and swallowing abilities and self-feeding skills; these professionals can also demonstrate alternative feeding strategies, including changes in body position that improve feeding, techniques for handling utensils and food, and the use of special feeding devices (see Figure NP22-1). Gastroenterologists can use various noninvasive techniques to evaluate gastrointestinal function. Direct observation of the patient during mealtimes allows these health practitioners to assess current eating behaviors, demonstrate feeding techniques, monitor the patient's or caregiver's understanding of the techniques, and evaluate how well the care plan is working.

To illustrate one type of strategy used to treat feeding problems, consider a child with feeding difficulties caused by hypersensitivity to oral stimulation. The therapist may start by teaching the caregiver to gently stroke the child's face with a hand, washcloth, or soft toy. Once the child tolerates touch on less sensitive areas

FIGURE NP22-1 Adaptive feeding equipment can help patients with feeding disabilities gain independence.

JAECO Orthopedic

of the face, the therapist may encourage the caregiver to slowly begin to rub the child's lips, gums, palate, and tongue. With time, the child may be better able to tolerate the presence of food in the mouth. Examples of other strategies that can help feeding problems are listed in Table NP22-2.

Can special equipment be used to help people with certain feeding difficulties?

Yes. Adaptive feeding devices can make a remarkable difference in a person's ability to eat independently. Figure NP22-2 (p. 602) shows a few of the many special feeding devices that are available and describes their uses. Other examples of adaptive equipment include specialized chairs to improve posture, bolsters inserted under arms to improve elbow stability, and raised trays or eating surfaces to simplify hand-to-mouth movements.

Sometimes, despite the best efforts of all involved, a patient is unable to consume enough food by mouth. In these cases, tube feedings can help to improve nutrition status. Tube feedings are typically recommended for patients with severe dysphagia (difficulty swallowing), aspiration pneumonia, recurrent malnutrition, or failure to thrive.[5]

In what ways can feeding difficulties affect family life?

Mealtimes are a critical time for social interaction, and therefore individuals with feeding problems may encounter emotional and social problems if they are unable to participate. Children may fail to develop social skills, whereas adults may miss the social stimulation that mealtimes provide. Individuals should be encouraged to sit with family and friends during meals so that they are not deprived of the social and cultural aspects of eating.

The responsibility of caring for a person with a feeding problem can frequently overwhelm a caregiver.[6] Caring for a person with disabilities requires time and patience—and many new therapies to be learned and administered. The caregiver may spend many hours preparing special foods, monitoring the use of adaptive feeding equipment, and helping with feedings. Moreover, a person with disabilities may need help with other tasks as well, and all may require a considerable amount of time. In many cases, a caregiver receives little or no assistance. These conditions may lead to strained interactions between caregiver and patient and cause stress and frustration. Psychologists

TABLE NP22-2 Interventions for Feeding-Related Problems

Inability to Suck

- Use squeeze bottles, which do not require sucking, to express liquids into the mouth.
- Place a spoon on the center of the tongue and apply downward pressure to stimulate sucking.
- Apply rhythmic, slow strokes on the tongue to alter tongue position and improve the sucking response.

Inability to Chew

- Place foods between teeth to promote chewing.
- Improve chewing skills with foods of different textures; for example, fruit leathers stimulate jaw movements but dissolve quickly enough to minimize choking.
- Provide soft foods that require minimal chewing or are easily chewed.

Inability to Swallow

- Provide thickened liquids, pureed foods, and moist foods that form boluses easily.
- Provide cold formulas, frozen fruit juice bars, and ice; cold substances promote swallowing movements by the tongue and soft palate.
- Make sure the patient's jaw and lips are closed to facilitate swallowing action.
- Correct posture and head position if they interfere with swallowing ability.

Inability to Grasp or Coordinate Movements

- Provide utensils that have modified handles, or are smaller or larger as necessary.
- Encourage the use of hands for feeding if utensils are difficult to maneuver.
- Provide plates with food guards to prevent spilling.
- Supply clothing protection.

Impaired Vision

- Place foods (meats, vegetables) in similar locations on the plate at each meal.
- Provide plates with food guards to prevent spilling.

© 2016 Cengage Learning®

can offer counseling to patients or caregivers to help them adjust, and all members of the health care team can offer emotional support and practical suggestions to ease caregivers' responsibilities and frustrations.

Successful therapy for people with feeding disabilities requires the involvement of a number of different health professionals; these individuals should be able to accurately identify the feeding skills that are impaired and determine the appropriate interventions. Ideally, with training, people with disabilities can attain total independence: the ability to prepare, serve, and eat nutritionally adequate food daily without help. In some cases, these goals can be met with the help of caregivers. The combined efforts of the health care team can support both patients and caregivers in enhancing quality of life and in achieving independence to the greatest degree possible.

FIGURE NP22-2 **Examples of Adaptive Feeding Devices**

Utensils

Rocker knife

Roller knife

People with only one arm or hand may have difficulty cutting foods and may appreciate using a *rocker knife* or a *roller knife.*

People with a limited range of motion can feed themselves better when they use *flatware with built-up handles.*

People with extreme muscle weakness may be able to eat with a *utensil holder.*

For people with tremors, spasticity, and uneven jerky movements, *weighted utensils* can aid the feeding process.

Battery-powered feeding machines enable people with severe limitations to eat with less assistance from others.

Plates

People who have limited dexterity and difficulty maneuvering food find *scoop dishes* or *food guards* useful.

People with uncontrolled or excessive movements might move dishes around while eating and may benefit from using *unbreakable dishes with suction cups.*

Cups

People with limited neck motion can use a *cutout plastic cup.*

Two-handed cups enable people with moderate muscle weakness to lift a cup with two hands.

People with uncontrolled or excessive movements might prefer to drink liquids from a *covered cup* or glass with a *slotted opening* or *spout.*

A soft, flexible long plastic straw may also ease the task of drinking.

© Cengage Learning®

Notes

1. Position of the Canadian Paediatric Society: Nutrition in neurologically impaired children, *Paediatrics and Child Health* 14 (2009): 395–401.

2. K. L. Bell and L. Samson-Fang, Nutritional management of children with cerebral palsy, *European Journal of Clinical Nutrition* 67 (2013): S13–S16.

3. T. Chin and coauthors, Energy consumption during prosthetic walking and physical fitness in older hip disarticulation amputees, *Journal of Rehabilitation Research and Development* 49 (2012): 1255–1260.

4. R. M. Katz, J. K. Hyche, and E. K. Wingert, Pediatric feeding problems, in A. C. Ross and coeditors, eds., *Modern Nutrition in Health and Disease* (Baltimore: Lippincott Williams & Wilkins, 2014), pp. 887–893.

5. Position of the American Dietetic Association: Providing nutrition services for people with developmental disabilities and special health care needs, *Journal of the American Dietetic Association* 110 (2010): 296–307.

6. Katz, Hyche, and Wingert, 2014.

23

Protein-, Mineral-, and Fluid-Modified Diets for Kidney Diseases

The two kidneys sit just above the waist on each side of the spinal column. As part of the urinary system, they are responsible for filtering the blood and removing excess fluid and wastes for elimination in urine. Figure 23-1 shows the kidneys' placement and structure and one of their functional units, the **nephron**. Within each nephron, the **glomerulus**, a ball-shaped tuft of capillaries, serves as a gateway through which blood components must pass to form **filtrate**. The glomerulus and surrounding **Bowman's capsule** function like a sieve, retaining blood cells and most plasma proteins in the blood while allowing fluid and small solutes to enter the nephron's system of **tubules**. As the filtrate moves through the tubules, its composition continuously changes as some of its components are reabsorbed and returned to the blood via capillaries surrounding the tubules; the remaining substances contribute to the final urine product. By filtering blood and forming urine, the kidneys regulate the extracellular fluid volume and osmolarity, electrolyte concentrations, and acid-base balance. They also excrete metabolic waste products such as urea and **creatinine**, as well as various drugs and toxicants. Other roles of the kidneys include the following:

- Secretion of the enzyme *renin*, which helps to regulate blood pressure

- Production of the hormone **erythropoietin**, which stimulates the production of red blood cells in the bone marrow

- Conversion of vitamin D to its active form, thereby helping to regulate calcium balance and bone formation

Subsequent sections of this chapter explain how **renal** diseases can interfere with the kidneys' various functions and severely disrupt health.

A nephron (a working unit of the kidney). Each kidney contains about one million nephrons.

Blood vessel — Glomerulus

Capillaries of glomerulus

Tubule

1 Blood flows into the glomerulus, and some of its fluid, with dissolved substances, is absorbed into the tubule.

To the body

2 Then the fluid and substances needed by the body are returned to the blood in vessels alongside the tubule.

3 The tubule passes waste materials on to the bladder.

To the bladder

Kidney
Ureter
Pelvis
Bladder

Renal artery

Renal vein

Kidney, sectioned to show location of nephrons

© Cengage Learning®

FIGURE 23-1 The Kidneys and Nephron Function

23.1 Nephrotic Syndrome

LO 23.1 Identify the potential causes and consequences of the nephrotic syndrome and describe the medical and nutrition therapies used in treatment.

The **nephrotic syndrome** is not a specific disease; rather, the term refers to a syndrome caused by significant urinary protein losses (**proteinuria**) that result from severe glomerular damage. The condition arises because damage to the glomeruli increases their permeability to plasma proteins, allowing the proteins to escape into the urine. The loss of these proteins may cause serious consequences, including edema, blood lipid abnormalities, blood coagulation disorders, and infections. In some cases, the nephrotic syndrome can progress to renal failure.

Causes of the nephrotic syndrome include glomerular disorders, diabetic nephropathy, immunological and hereditary diseases, infections (involving the kidneys or elsewhere in the body), chemical damage (from medications or illicit drugs), and some cancers.[1] Depending on the underlying condition, some patients may experience one or more relapses and require additional treatment to prevent proteinuria from recurring.

Consequences of the Nephrotic Syndrome

In the nephrotic syndrome, urinary protein losses generally average about 8 grams daily.[2] The liver tries to compensate by increasing its synthesis of various plasma proteins, but some of the proteins are produced in excessive amounts. The imbalance in plasma protein concentrations contributes to a number of complications.

Edema Albumin is the most abundant plasma protein, and it is the protein with the most significant urinary losses as well. The **hypoalbuminemia** characteristic of the nephrotic syndrome contributes to a fluid shift from blood plasma to the interstitial spaces and, thus, edema. Impaired sodium excretion also contributes to edema: the nephrotic kidney tends to reabsorb sodium in greater amounts than usual, causing sodium and water retention within the body.

Blood Lipid and Blood Clotting Abnormalities Individuals with the nephrotic syndrome frequently have elevated levels of low-density lipoproteins (LDL), very-low-density lipoproteins (VLDL), and the more atherogenic LDL variant known as lipoprotein(a). Furthermore, blood clotting risk is increased due to urinary losses of proteins that inhibit blood clotting and elevated levels of plasma proteins that favor clotting. The blood clotting abnormalities increase the risk of **deep vein thrombosis** and similar disorders. The nephrotic syndrome is associated with accelerated atherosclerosis and a sharply increased risk of heart disease and stroke.

Other Effects of the Nephrotic Syndrome Proteins lost in urine include immunoglobulins (antibodies) and vitamin D-binding protein. Depletion of immunoglobulins increases risk of infection. Loss of vitamin D-binding protein lowers vitamin D and calcium levels and increases the risk of rickets in children. If proteinuria continues, protein-energy malnutrition (PEM) and muscle wasting may develop. Figure 23-2 (p. 606) summarizes the effects of urinary protein losses in the nephrotic syndrome.

Treatment of the Nephrotic Syndrome

Medical treatment of the nephrotic syndrome requires diagnosis and management of the underlying disorder responsible for the proteinuria. Complications are managed with medications and nutrition therapy. The drugs prescribed may include diuretics,

nephrotic (neh-FROT-ik) **syndrome:** a syndrome caused by significant urinary protein losses (more than 3 to 3½ grams daily), as a result of severe glomerular damage.

proteinuria (PRO-teen-NOO-ree-ah)**:** the presence of protein in the urine. When only urinary albumin is measured, the term used is *albuminuria*.

hypoalbuminemia: low plasma albumin concentrations. Plasma proteins such as albumin help to maintain fluid balance within the blood; thus, low levels contribute to edema.

deep vein thrombosis: formation of a stationary blood clot (thrombus) in a deep vein, usually in the leg, which causes inflammation, pain, and swelling, and is potentially fatal.

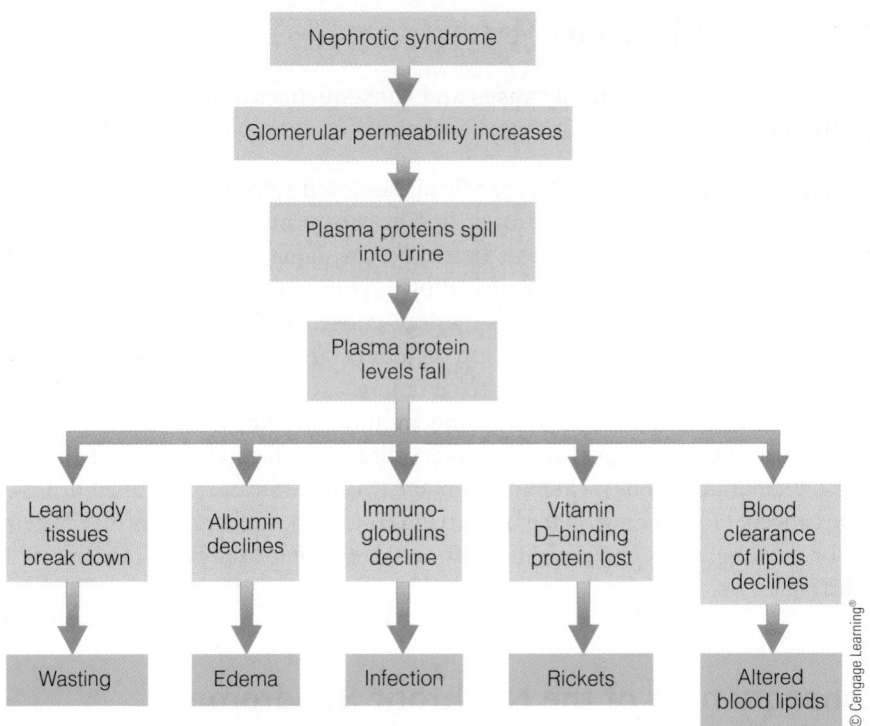

FIGURE 23-2 Effects of Urinary Protein Losses in the Nephrotic Syndrome

ACE inhibitors (which reduce protein losses), lipid-lowering drugs, anti-inflammatory drugs (usually corticosteroids), and immunosuppressants (such as cyclosporine).[3] Nutrition therapy can help to prevent PEM, correct lipid abnormalities, and alleviate edema.

Protein and Energy Meeting protein and energy needs helps to minimize losses of muscle tissue. High-protein diets are not advised, however, because they can exacerbate urinary protein losses and result in further damage to the kidneys. Instead, the protein intake should fall between 0.8 and 1.0 gram per kilogram of body weight per day; at least half of the protein consumed should be from high-quality protein sources.[4] An adequate energy intake (about 35 kcalories per kilogram of body weight daily) sustains weight and spares protein. Weight loss or infections suggest the need for additional energy.

Lipids As Chapter 22 explains, a diet low in saturated fat, *trans* fats, cholesterol, and refined sugars may help to control elevated LDL and VLDL levels. Dietary measures are usually inadequate for controlling blood lipids, however, so physicians may prescribe lipid-lowering medications as well. In some cases, treating the underlying cause of nephrotic syndrome is sufficient for correcting the lipid disorders.[5]

Sodium and Potassium Controlling sodium intake helps to control edema; therefore, the sodium intake is often limited to 1 to 2 grams daily.[6] Table 23-1 provides guidelines for following a diet restricted to 2 grams of sodium. If diuretics prescribed for the edema cause potassium losses, patients are encouraged to select foods rich in potassium (see Chapter 9).

Vitamins and Minerals Multivitamin/mineral supplementation can help patients avoid nutrient deficiencies; nutrients at risk include iron and vitamin D. To reduce risk of bone loss, calcium supplementation (1000 to 1500 milligrams per day) may also be advised.[7]

TABLE 23-1 Low-Sodium Diet

General Guidelines

About 75 percent of the sodium in a typical diet comes from processed foods, about 10 percent from unprocessed natural foods, and about 15 percent from table salt. With this in mind:

▮ Whenever possible, select fresh foods, which are usually low in sodium.

▮ Select frozen and canned food products that have been prepared without added salt.

▮ Avoid adding salt to foods while cooking or at the table.

▮ When dining in restaurants, ask that meals be prepared without salt.

Sodium in Foods

All foods contain sodium, but some contain more than others. Use the information in the table below to plan meals that are low in sodium.

Food Group	Portion	Sodium per Portion (mg)
Milk products	1 cup milk or yogurt, 1 oz hard cheese (cheddar, Swiss, jack)	150–200
	Avoid: buttermilk, cottage cheese, cheese spreads, processed cheese (such as American cheese)	
Meat, fish, poultry, and eggs	3 oz fresh meat, fish, or poultry; 1 large egg	60
	Avoid: luncheon meat, corned beef, salt pork, sausage, frankfurters, bacon, canned meat or fish, fresh meat or poultry prepared with injected broth	
Fruits and vegetables	$\frac{1}{2}$ cup fresh vegetables, $\frac{1}{2}$ cup fresh or frozen fruit, 6 oz fruit juice, 6 oz tomato or vegetable juice without added salt	10–20
	Avoid: pickled vegetables, olives, tomato or vegetable juices with added salt; dried fruit with added sodium sulfite	
Breads and cereals	$\frac{1}{2}$–$\frac{2}{3}$ cup dry or cooked cereal without added salt, $\frac{1}{2}$ cup cooked rice or pasta	0–10
	1 slice bread, 1 roll or tortilla, $\frac{1}{2}$–$\frac{2}{3}$ cup dry or cooked cereal prepared with salt	150
	Avoid: pancakes, waffles, muffins, biscuits, and quick breads made with baking powder or baking soda; instant or ready-to-eat cereals with >175 mg sodium; salted snack foods	
Condiments	$\frac{1}{2}$ tbs unsalted butter, 1 tsp no-salt mustard, 1 tbs no-salt ketchup, 1 tsp sodium-free bouillon	0–10
	Avoid: commercial salad dressings; gravy and soup mixes; barbeque sauce; steak sauce; soy sauce; spice, herb, or bouillon products made with salt, meat tenderizer, monosodium glutamate	

A Sample Diet Restricted to 2 Grams (2000 mg) of Sodium

Using the guidelines provided here, an individual can develop a variety of sample menus. A possible plan for a day might look like this:

Food Group	Sodium (mg)
Meat, 6 oz (2 servings × 60 mg)	120
Milk, 3 c (3 servings × 150 mg)	450
Fruit, 2 servings	negligible
Vegetables, 3 servings	45
Whole-grain bread, 4 slices (4 × 150 mg)	600
Salt, ¼ tsp (used lightly at meals)	600
Total	**1815**

Individuals can use the remainder of the sodium allowance for whatever foods they desire. The sodium content of most foods can be determined by reading food labels or using food composition tables (such as Appendix A). See additional information about reducing sodium intake in Chapter 22 (Box 22-6 on p. 594).

- The nephrotic syndrome is characterized by significant proteinuria due to glomerular damage. Complications include edema, lipid and blood clotting abnormalities, infections, and PEM.

- Medications treat the underlying cause of proteinuria and manage complications. Diets should provide sufficient protein and energy to maintain health, but patients should avoid consuming excess protein. Other dietary adjustments help to correct edema, lipid disorders, and nutrient deficiencies.

23.2 Acute Kidney Injury

LO 23.2 Discuss the potential causes and effects of acute kidney injury and describe the approaches to treatment for this condition.

In **acute kidney injury,** kidney function deteriorates rapidly, over hours or days. The loss of kidney function reduces urine output and allows nitrogenous wastes to build up in the blood. The degree of renal dysfunction varies from mild to severe. With prompt treatment, acute kidney injury is often reversible, although mortality rates are high, ranging from 40 to 70 percent in severe cases.[8] Most cases develop in the hospital, occurring in 5 to 7 percent of hospitalized patients.[9]

Causes of Acute Kidney Injury

Many disorders can lead to acute kidney injury, and it often develops as a consequence of critical illness, sepsis, or major surgery. To aid in diagnosis and treatment, its causes are classified as prerenal, intrarenal, or postrenal (see Table 23-2). *Prerenal* factors are conditions that cause a severe reduction in blood flow to the kidneys, such as heart failure, shock, or substantial blood loss. Factors that damage kidney tissue, such as infections, toxicants, drugs, or direct trauma, are classified as *intrarenal* causes of acute kidney injury. *Postrenal* factors are those that prevent urine excretion due to urinary tract obstructions.

Consequences of Acute Kidney Injury

A decline in renal function alters the composition of blood and urine. The kidneys become unable to regulate the levels of electrolytes, acid, and nitrogenous wastes in blood. Urine may be diminished in quantity **(oliguria)** or absent **(anuria),** leading to

acute kidney injury: the rapid decline of kidney function over a period of hours or days; potentially a cause of acute renal failure.

oliguria (OL-lih-GOO-ree-ah)**:** an abnormally low amount of urine, often less than 400 mL/day.

anuria (ah-NOO-ree-ah)**:** the absence of urine; clinically identified as urine output less than 50 mL/day.

TABLE 23-2 Causes of Acute Kidney Injury

Prerenal Factors (60 to 70% of cases)	Intrarenal Factors (25 to 40% of cases)	Postrenal Factors (5 to 10% of cases)
Low blood volume or pressure: hemorrhage, burns, sepsis or shock, anaphylactic reactions, nephrotic syndrome, gastrointestinal losses, diuretics, antihypertensive medications	**Vascular disorders:** sickle-cell disease, diabetes mellitus, transfusion reactions	**Obstructions (ureter or bladder):** strictures, tumors, stones, trauma
Renal artery disorders: blood clots or emboli, stenosis, aneurysm, trauma	**Obstructions (within kidney):** inflammation, tumors, stones, scar tissue	**Prostate disorders:** cancer or hyperplasia
Heart disorders: heart failure, heart attack, arrhythmias	**Renal injury:** infections, environmental contaminants, drugs, medications, *E. coli* food poisoning	**Renal vein thrombosis**
		Bladder disorders: neurological conditions, bladder rupture
		Pregnancy

© Cengage Learning®

fluid retention. Acute kidney injury is often identified by reduced urinary output coupled with a progressive rise in serum creatinine levels. Other laboratory findings may include abnormal levels of serum electrolytes, elevated blood urea nitrogen (BUN), and various changes in urine chemistry. Diagnosis is sometimes difficult, however, because the clinical effects can be subtle and vary according to the underlying cause of disease.

Fluid and Electrolyte Imbalances About half of patients with acute kidney injury experience oliguria, producing less than 400 milliliters of urine per day.[10] (Normal urine volume is about 1000 to 1500 milliliters daily.) The reduced excretion of fluids and electrolytes results in sodium retention and elevated levels of potassium, phosphate, and magnesium in the blood. Elevated potassium levels (**hyperkalemia**) are of particular concern because potassium imbalances can alter heart rhythm and lead to heart failure. Elevated serum phosphate levels (**hyperphosphatemia**) promote excessive secretion of parathyroid hormone, which leads to losses of bone calcium. Due to the sodium retention and reduced urine production, edema is a common symptom of acute kidney injury and may be apparent as puffiness in the face and hands and swelling of the feet and ankles.

Uremia As a result of impaired kidney function, nitrogen-containing compounds and various other waste products may accumulate in the blood—a condition referred to as **uremia**. The clinical outcome, called the **uremic syndrome,** includes a cluster of symptoms caused by impairments in multiple body systems. Complications may include hormonal imbalances, electrolyte and acid-base imbalances, disturbed heart and gastrointestinal (GI) functioning, neuromuscular disturbances, and depressed immunity, among other abnormalities. The uremic syndrome is described in more detail later in this chapter.

Treatment of Acute Kidney Injury

Treatment of acute kidney injury involves a combination of drug therapy, **dialysis** (see Nutrition in Practice 23), and nutrition therapy to restore fluid and electrolyte balances and minimize blood concentrations of toxic waste products. Both medical care and dietary measures are highly individualized to suit each patient's needs. Correcting the underlying illness is necessary to prevent further damage to the kidneys.

In oliguric patients (those with reduced urine production), recovery from kidney injury sometimes begins with a period of **diuresis,** in which large amounts of fluid (up to 3 liters daily) are excreted.[11] Because tubular function is minimal at this stage, electrolytes may not be sufficiently reabsorbed; consequently, both fluid and electrolyte replacement may be necessary in these cases.

Drug Treatment in Acute Kidney Injury Because kidney function is required for drug excretion, patients may need to use lower doses of their usual medications to compensate for limited urine output. Conversely, dialysis treatment may increase losses of some drugs, and doses may need to be increased. Drugs that are **nephrotoxic** (including some antibiotics and nonsteroidal anti-inflammatory drugs) must be avoided until kidney function improves.

The medications prescribed for acute kidney injury depend on the cause of illness and the complications that develop. Inflammatory conditions may require treatment with immunosuppressants. Edema is treated with diuretics; furosemide (Lasix) is the usual choice. Patients with hyperkalemia may be given potassium-exchange resins that bind potassium in the GI tract and reduce its absorption. Rapid correction of hyperkalemia may require the use of insulin, which drives extracellular potassium into cells; glucose must be coadministered to prevent hypoglycemia. To reduce serum phosphate levels, phosphate binders may be provided with meals to prevent phosphorus absorption. If acidosis is present, bicarbonate may be administered orally or intravenously.

hyperkalemia (HIGH-per-ka-LEE-me-ah)**:** elevated serum potassium levels.

hyperphosphatemia (HIGH-per-fos-fa-TEE-me-ah)**:** elevated serum phosphate levels. Note that the phosphorus in body fluids is present in a phosphate form; hence, the terms *serum phosphate* and *serum phosphorus* are often used interchangeably.

uremia (you-REE-me-ah)**:** the accumulation of nitrogenous and various other waste products in the blood (literally, "urine in the blood"); may also be used to indicate the toxic state that results when wastes are retained in the blood. The related term *azotemia* refers specifically to the accumulation of nitrogenous wastes in the blood.

uremic syndrome: the cluster of disorders caused by inadequate kidney function; complications include fluid, electrolyte, and hormonal imbalances; altered heart function; neuromuscular disturbances; and other metabolic derangements.

dialysis (dye-AH-lih-sis)**:** a treatment that removes wastes and excess fluid from the blood after the kidneys have stopped functioning.

diuresis (DYE-uh-REE-sis)**:** increased urine production.

nephrotoxic: toxic to the kidneys.

Energy and Protein Acute kidney injury is often associated with other critical illnesses, so patients may be hypermetabolic, catabolic, and at high risk of wasting. Furthermore, patients with acute kidney injury frequently develop hyperglycemia and hypertriglyceridemia because they are unable to metabolize energy nutrients efficiently. For these reasons, patients must ingest sufficient protein and energy to preserve muscle mass but should not be overfed. Protein recommendations are influenced by kidney function, the degree of catabolism, and the use of dialysis (dialysis removes nitrogenous wastes).

Although guidelines vary, patients are usually provided with 20 to 35 kcalories per kilogram of body weight per day, while body weight, nitrogen balance, blood glucose levels, and blood triglycerides are monitored to ensure that the energy intake is appropriate.[12] For noncatabolic patients who do not require dialysis, protein intakes should be limited to 0.8 to 1.0 grams per kilogram body weight per day.[13] Higher intakes (1.0 to 1.7 grams per kilogram daily) may be recommended if kidney function improves, the patient is catabolic, or the treatment includes dialysis. Patients who require higher amounts of protein (such as those with burns or large wounds) require more frequent dialysis to accommodate the nitrogen load.

Fluids Health practitioners can assess fluid status by monitoring weight fluctuations, blood pressure, pulse rates, and the appearance of the skin and mucous membranes. Another method is to measure serum sodium concentrations: a low sodium level often indicates excessive fluid intake, whereas a high sodium level suggests inadequate fluid intake.

Fluid balance must be restored in patients who are either overhydrated or dehydrated. Thereafter, fluid needs can be estimated by measuring urine output and adding 400 to 500 milliliters to account for the water lost from skin, lungs, and perspiration.[14] An individual with fever, vomiting, or diarrhea requires additional fluid. Patients undergoing dialysis can ingest fluids more freely.

Electrolytes Serum electrolyte levels are monitored closely to determine appropriate electrolyte intakes. Depending on the results of laboratory tests and the clinical assessment, restrictions may be necessary for potassium (2000 to 3000 milligrams per day), phosphorus (8 to 15 milligrams per kilogram body weight per day), and sodium (2000 to 3000 milligrams per day).[15] Patients undergoing dialysis may be allowed more liberal intakes.

Enteral and Parenteral Nutrition Many patients need nutrition support to obtain adequate energy and nutrients. Enteral support (tube feeding) is preferred over parenteral nutrition because it is less likely to cause infection and sepsis. Enteral formulas for patients with acute kidney injury are more kcalorically dense and may have lower protein and electrolyte concentrations than standard formulas. Total parenteral nutrition is necessary only if patients are severely malnourished or cannot consume food or tolerate tube feedings for an extended period.

IN SUMMARY

▌ Acute kidney injury is characterized by a rapid decline in kidney function, causing a buildup of waste products in the blood.

▌ Consequences of acute kidney injury may include fluid and electrolyte imbalances and uremia. If hyperkalemia develops, it can alter heart rhythm and lead to heart failure.

▌ Acute kidney injury is treated with medications, dialysis, and dietary modifications.

The Case Study in Box 23-1 checks your understanding of acute kidney injury.

Case Study BOX 23-1 WOMAN WITH ACUTE KIDNEY INJURY

Catherine Garber is a 42-year-old office manager admitted to the hospital's intensive care unit. She was first seen in the emergency room with severe edema, headache, nausea and vomiting, and a rapid heart rate. She reported an inability to pass more than minimal amounts of urine in the past 2 days. Her son, who drove her to the emergency room, reported that she had missed work for several days and seemed confused and unusually tired. Laboratory tests revealed elevated serum creatinine, BUN, and potassium levels. After learning from her medical history that Mrs. Garber had begun taking penicillin earlier in the week, the physician diagnosed acute kidney injury, probably caused by a reaction to the medication. Mrs. Garber is 5 feet 3 inches tall and weighs 125 pounds.

1. Describe the probable reason for Mrs. Garber's inability to produce urine. Is her reaction to penicillin considered a prerenal, intrarenal, or postrenal cause of kidney injury? Give examples of other medical problems that can cause acute kidney injury.

2. What medications may the physician prescribe to treat Mrs. Garber's edema and hyperkalemia? What recommendation is likely regarding her continued use of penicillin?

3. What concerns should be kept in mind when determining Mrs. Garber's energy, protein, fluid, and electrolyte needs during acute kidney injury? How would dialysis treatment alter recommendations?

4. After treatment begins, Mrs. Garber suddenly begins producing copious amounts of urine. How may this development alter dietary treatment?

As you read through the discussion of chronic kidney disease, consider how Mrs. Garber's diet would need to change if her kidney problems became chronic.

23.3 Chronic Kidney Disease

LO 23.3 Describe the potential causes and consequences of chronic kidney disease, its medical treatment, and nutrition therapy for this condition.

Unlike acute kidney injury, in which kidney function declines suddenly and rapidly, **chronic kidney disease** is characterized by gradual, irreversible deterioration. Because the kidneys have a large functional reserve—they are able to increase their workload to meet demands—chronic kidney disease typically progresses over many years without causing symptoms. Patients are often diagnosed late in the course of illness after most kidney function has been lost.[16]

The most common causes of chronic kidney disease are diabetes mellitus and hypertension, which are estimated to cause 45 and 27 percent of cases, respectively.[17] Other conditions that lead to chronic kidney disease include inflammatory, immunological, and hereditary diseases that directly involve the kidneys. Chronic kidney disease affects approximately 13 percent of the U.S. population.[18]

Consequences of Chronic Kidney Disease

In early stages of chronic kidney disease, the nephrons compensate by enlarging so that they can handle the extra workload. As the nephrons deteriorate, however, there is additional work for the remaining nephrons. The overburdened nephrons continue to degenerate until finally the kidneys are unable to function adequately, resulting in kidney failure. Once the extent of kidney damage necessitates active treatment—either dialysis or a kidney transplant—the condition is classified as **end-stage renal disease**. Table 23-3 (p. 612) lists common clinical effects of the early and advanced stages of chronic kidney disease.

Chronic kidney disease is evaluated based on the **glomerular filtration rate (GFR),** the rate at which the kidneys form filtrate, and the degree of albuminuria, the amount of albumin lost in urine daily.[19] GFR is considered the best index of overall kidney function, whereas albuminuria reflects the extent of kidney damage and correlates well with disease progression and health risks. Table 23-4 (p. 612) shows how kidney disease is classified according to estimated GFR.

chronic kidney disease: kidney disease characterized by gradual, irreversible deterioration of the kidneys; also called *chronic renal failure.*

end-stage renal disease: an advanced stage of chronic kidney disease in which dialysis or a kidney transplant is necessary to sustain life.

glomerular filtration rate (GFR): the rate at which filtrate is formed within the kidneys, normally about 125 mL/min in healthy young adults.

TABLE 23-3 Clinical Effects of Chronic Kidney Disease

Early Stages

- Anorexia
- Exercise intolerance
- Fatigue
- Headache
- Hypercoagulation
- Hypertension
- Proteinuria, hematuria (blood in urine)

Advanced Stages

- Anemia, bleeding tendency
- Cardiovascular disease
- Confusion, mental impairments
- Electrolyte imbalances
- Fluid retention, edema
- Hormonal abnormalities
- Itching
- Metabolic acidosis
- Nausea and vomiting
- Peripheral neuropathy
- Protein-energy malnutrition
- Reduced immunity
- Renal osteodystrophy

TABLE 23-4 Evaluation of Chronic Kidney Disease[a]

Stage of Disease	Description	GFR[b] (mL/min per 1.73 m²)
1	Kidney damage with normal or increased GFR	≥90
2	Mildly decreased GFR	60–89
3a	Mildly to moderately decreased GFR	45–59
3b	Moderately to severely decreased GFR	30–44
4	Severely decreased GFR	15–29
5	Kidney failure	<15 (or undergoing dialysis)

[a]A complete assessment of chronic kidney disease takes into account the likelihood of health risk, as indicated by the degree of albuminuria and other markers of kidney damage.

[b]Glomerular filtration rate, or GFR, is usually estimated using the Modification of Diet in Renal Disease study equation, which is based on serum creatinine levels, age, gender, body size, and ethnicity. Normal GFR averages 125 mL/min in young adults and declines with age.

Source: L. A. Inker and coauthors, KDOQI U.S. commentary on the 2012 KDIGO clinical practice guideline for the evaluation and management of CKD, *American Journal of Kidney Diseases* 63 (2014): doi: 10.1053/j.ajkd.2014.01.416; P.E. Stevens and A. Levin, Evaluation and management of chronic kidney disease: Synopsis of the kidney disease: improving global outcomes 2012 clinical practice guideline, *Annals of Internal Medicine* 158 (2013): 825–830.

Altered Electrolytes and Hormones As the GFR falls, the increased activity of the remaining nephrons is often sufficient to maintain electrolyte excretion. Thus, fluid and electrolyte disturbances may not develop until the third or fourth stage of chronic kidney disease. A number of hormonal adaptations also help to regulate electrolyte levels, but these changes may cause complications of their own. The increased secretion of **aldosterone** helps to prevent increases in serum potassium but contributes to fluid overload and the development of hypertension (in patients who were not previously hypertensive). Increased secretion of **parathyroid hormone** helps to prevent elevations in serum phosphate but contributes to bone loss and the development of **renal osteodystrophy,** a bone disorder common in renal patients. Electrolyte imbalances are likely when the GFR is very low (below 5 milliliters per minute), when hormonal adaptations are inadequate, or when intakes of water or electrolytes are either very restricted or excessive.

Because the kidneys are responsible for maintaining acid-base balance, acidosis often develops in chronic kidney disease. Although usually mild, the acidosis exacerbates renal bone disease because compounds in bone (for example, protein and phosphates) are released to buffer the acid in blood.

Uremic Syndrome Uremia may develop during the final stages of chronic kidney disease, when the GFR falls below about 15 milliliters per minute.[20] As mentioned previously, the many complications that result from uremia are collectively known as the *uremic syndrome*. Clinical effects may include the following:

- *Hormonal imbalances.* Diseased kidneys are unable to produce erythropoietin, causing anemia. Reduced production of active vitamin D contributes to bone disease.

- *Altered heart function/increased heart disease risk.* Fluid and electrolyte imbalances result in hypertension, arrhythmias, and eventual heart muscle enlargement. Excessive parathyroid hormone secretion leads to calcification of arteries and heart tissue.

- *Neuromuscular disturbances.* Initial symptoms may be mild, and include malaise, irritability, and altered thought processes. Later effects include muscle cramping, restless leg syndrome, sensory deficits, tremor, and seizures.

- *Other effects.* Defects in platelet function and clotting factors prolong bleeding time and contribute to bruising, GI bleeding, and anemia. Skin changes include increased pigmentation and severe pruritus (itchiness). Many patients have reduced immune responses.

aldosterone: a steroid hormone secreted by the adrenal cortex that promotes sodium (and therefore water) retention and potassium excretion.

parathyroid hormone: a protein hormone secreted by the parathyroid glands that helps to regulate serum concentrations of calcium and phosphate.

renal osteodystrophy: a bone disorder that develops in patients with chronic kidney disease as a result of increased secretion of parathyroid hormone, reduced serum calcium, acidosis, and impaired vitamin D activation in the kidneys.

Protein-Energy Malnutrition Patients with chronic kidney disease often eat poorly and develop PEM and wasting. Anorexia is common and may be caused by hormonal disturbances, restrictive diets, uremia, depression, or the effects of other illnesses. Nutrient losses contribute to malnutrition and may be a consequence of dialysis, frequent blood draws, or GI bleeding. The low-grade inflammation that accompanies chronic kidney disease can lead to the breakdown of body proteins and negative nitrogen balance.[21] A screening method sometimes used for assessing PEM risk is the *Subjective Global Assessment*, described in Chapter 14 (Table 14-2 on p. 394).

Treatment of Chronic Kidney Disease

The goals of treatment for patients with chronic kidney disease are to slow disease progression and prevent or alleviate complications. Dietary measures help to prevent PEM and weight loss. Once kidney disease reaches the final stages, dialysis or a kidney transplant is necessary to sustain life.

Drug Therapy Medications help to control some of the complications associated with chronic kidney disease. Treatment of hypertension is critical for preventing disease progression and reducing cardiovascular disease risk; thus, antihypertensive drugs are often prescribed (see Chapter 22). Some antihypertensive drugs (such as ACE inhibitors) can reduce proteinuria, helping to prevent additional kidney damage. Anemia is usually treated by injection or intravenous administration of erythropoietin (epoetin). Other drug treatments may include phosphate binders (taken with food) to reduce serum phosphate levels, sodium bicarbonate to reverse acidosis, and cholesterol-lowering medications.

Dialysis Dialysis replaces kidney function by removing excess fluid and wastes from the blood. In **hemodialysis,** the blood is circulated through a **dialyzer** (artificial kidney), where it is bathed by a **dialysate,** a solution that selectively removes fluid and wastes. In **peritoneal dialysis,** the dialysate is infused into a person's peritoneal cavity and blood is filtered by the peritoneum (the membrane surrounding the abdominal cavity). After several hours, the dialysate is drained, removing unneeded fluid and wastes. Nutrition in Practice 23 provides additional information about dialysis.

Nutrition Therapy for Chronic Kidney Disease The patient's diet strongly influences disease progression and the development of complications. Because the dietary measures for chronic kidney disease are complex and nutrient needs change frequently during the course of illness, a dietitian who specializes in renal disease is best suited to provide nutrition therapy. Table 23-5 (p. 614) summarizes the general dietary guidelines for patients in different stages of illness. Because patients' needs vary considerably, actual recommendations should be based on the results of a careful and complete nutrition assessment.

Energy Patients with chronic kidney disease should consume an energy intake that allows them to maintain a healthy body weight. Because obesity has been associated with disease progression, obese patients may benefit from weight loss.[22] Individuals at risk of PEM and wasting should consume foods with **high energy density;** some malnourished patients may require oral supplements or tube feedings to maintain an appropriate weight. Wasting is more prevalent during maintenance dialysis than in earlier stages of illness.[23]

The dialysate used in peritoneal dialysis contains glucose in order to draw fluid from the blood to the peritoneal cavity by osmosis; 40 to 60 percent of this glucose is absorbed.[24] The kcalories from glucose (as many as 800 kcalories daily) must be included in estimates of energy intake. Weight gain is sometimes a problem when peritoneal dialysis continues for a long period.

Protein A moderate protein restriction may be prescribed to slow disease progression and reduce nitrogenous wastes. Furthermore, low-protein diets supply

hemodialysis (HE-moe-dye-AL-ih-sis)**:** a treatment that removes fluids and wastes from the blood by passing the blood through a dialyzer.

dialyzer (DYE-ah-LYE-zer)**:** a machine used in hemodialysis to filter the blood; also called an *artificial kidney.*

dialysate (dye-AL-ih-sate)**:** the solution used in dialysis to draw wastes and fluids from the blood.

peritoneal (PEH-rih-toe-NEE-al) **dialysis:** a treatment that removes fluids and wastes from the blood by using the body's peritoneal membrane as a filter.

high energy density: a high number of kcalories per unit weight of food; foods of high energy density are generally high in fat and low in water content.

TABLE 23-5 Dietary Guidelines for Chronic Kidney Disease[a]

Nutrient	Predialysis (stages 3–4)[b]	Hemodialysis	Peritoneal Dialysis
Energy (kcal/kg body weight)	35 for <60 years old 30–35 for ≥60 years old (or as necessary to maintain a healthy weight)	35 for <60 years old 30–35 for ≥60 years old (or as necessary to maintain a healthy weight)	35 for <60 years old 30–35 for ≥60 years old (or as necessary to maintain a healthy weight) *Note:* The energy intake includes kcalories absorbed from the dialysate.
Protein (g/kg body weight)	0.6–0.75 (≥50% high-quality proteins)	1.2–1.4 (≥50% high-quality proteins)	1.2–1.3 (≥50% high-quality proteins)
Fat	As necessary to maintain a healthy lipid profile	As necessary to maintain a healthy lipid profile	As necessary to maintain a healthy lipid profile
Fluid (mL/day)	Unrestricted if urine output is normal	Urine output plus 500–1000 mL	2000–3000; unrestricted in some cases
Sodium (mg/day)	Varies; moderate restriction (2000–3000) often advised to improve hypertension	2000–3000	3000–4000; monitor fluid balance
Potassium (mg/day)	Varies; adjust according to serum potassium levels	2000–3000; adjust according to serum potassium levels	3000–4000; adjust according to serum potassium levels
Phosphorus (mg/day)	800–1000 if serum phosphate or parathyroid hormone is elevated	800–1000 if serum phosphate or parathyroid hormone is elevated	800–1000 if serum phosphate or parathyroid hormone is elevated
Calcium (mg/day)	800–1200; should not exceed 1500 from diet and medications	800–1200; should not exceed 1500 from diet and medications	800–1200; should not exceed 1500 from diet and medications

© 2016 Cengage Learning®

[a] Values listed in this table apply to adults; recommendations for children vary with age.

[b] The predialysis guidelines in this table apply to patients in stage 3 or 4 of disease; by stage 5, either hemodialysis or peritoneal dialysis is necessary.

Source: D. J. Goldstein-Fuchs and A. F. LaPierre, Nutrition and Kidney Disease, in S. J. Gilbert and D. E. Weiner, eds., *National Kidney Foundation's Primer on Kidney Diseases* (Philadelphia: Saunders, 2014), pp. 467–475; R. Filipowicz and S. Beddhu, Optimal nutrition for predialysis chronic kidney disease, *Advances in Chronic Kidney Disease* 20 (2013): 175–180.

less phosphorus than high-protein diets, reducing the risk of hyperphosphatemia. Because renal patients often develop PEM, however, their diet must provide enough protein to meet needs and prevent wasting. During the later stages of kidney disease, the recommended protein intake is 0.6 to 0.75 grams per kilogram of body weight per day, slightly below the protein RDA for adults (0.8 grams per kilogram).[25] To ensure appropriate intake of the essential amino acids, at least 50 percent of the protein consumed should come from high-quality protein sources (see Figure 23-3). Plant sources of protein should be included in the diet as they place less demand on the kidneys than animal proteins and are also low in phosphorus.[26] Low-protein breads, pastas, and other grain-based products are commercially available to help renal patients improve energy intakes without increasing protein consumption.

Due to the high risk of wasting and compliance difficulties associated with low-protein diets, some dietitians may suggest that patients consume higher amounts of protein to preserve health. Once dialysis has begun, protein restrictions can be relaxed because dialysis removes nitrogenous wastes and results in some amino acid losses as well.

Lipids To control elevated blood lipids and reduce heart disease risk, patients with chronic kidney disease may be advised to restrict intakes of saturated fat, *trans* fats, and cholesterol. Although patients are often encouraged to consume high-fat foods to improve their energy intakes, the foods they select

Craig M. Moore

To ensure adequate intake of the essential amino acids, people with chronic kidney disease should consume high-quality protein sources such as eggs, milk products, meat, poultry, fish, and soybeans.

Craig M. Moore

People with chronic kidney disease can consume most fruits and vegetables in limited amounts.

FIGURE 23-3 Diet and Kidney Disease

614

TABLE 23-6 Potassium Guide—Fruits and Vegetables

This table lists common fruits and vegetables according to their potassium content. One portion is ½ cup raw fruit or cooked vegetable unless otherwise noted. Keep in mind that the portion size may determine how a food is categorized. Check Appendix A for additional information about the potassium content of foods.

High Potassium (>250 mg per serving)	Medium Potassium (150–250 mg per serving)	Low Potassium (<150 mg per serving)
Avocado	Apple (1 medium)	Blueberries
Banana	Apricots (2 whole)	Cabbage
Beets	Asparagus	Carrots (1 medium)
Chard	Broccoli	Cauliflower
Dates (3 whole)	Cantaloupe	Cucumbers
Nectarine (1 small)	Celery	Eggplant
Orange (1 medium)	Corn	Grapes
Parsnips	Grapefruit (½ fruit)	Green beans
Potatoes	Honeydew melon	Green pepper
Pumpkin	Kale	Lettuce (4 leaves, raw)
Raisins	Peach (1 small)	Onions (1 small)
Spinach	Pear (1 medium)	Plum (1 small)
Sweet potatoes	Peas	Strawberries
Tomato	Zucchini	Watermelon

should provide mostly unsaturated fats. Good choices include nuts and seeds, oil-based salad dressings, mayonnaise, avocados, and soybean products.

Sodium and Fluids As kidney disease progresses, patients excrete less urine and become unable to handle normal amounts of sodium and fluids. Recommendations depend on the total urine output, changes in body weight and blood pressure, and serum sodium levels. A rise in body weight and blood pressure suggests that the person is retaining sodium and fluid; conversely, declines in these measurements indicate fluid loss. Most persons with kidney disease tend to retain sodium and may benefit from mild restriction; less often, a patient may have a salt-wasting condition that requires additional dietary sodium.

Fluids are not restricted until urine output decreases. For a person who is neither dehydrated nor overhydrated, the daily fluid intake should match the daily urine output. Once a person is on dialysis, sodium and fluid intakes should be controlled so that only about 2 pounds of water weight are gained daily—this excess fluid is then removed during the next dialysis treatment. Patients on fluid-restricted diets should be advised that foods such as flavored gelatin, soups, fruit ices, and frozen fruit juice bars contribute to the fluid allowance.

Potassium Most patients can handle typical intakes of potassium during stages 1 through 4 of illness. Restrictions are generally advised for patients who develop hyperkalemia, have diabetic nephropathy (which increases risk of hyperkalemia), or reach a later stage of illness. Conversely, potassium supplementation may be necessary for persons using potassium-wasting diuretics.

Dialysis patients must control potassium intakes to prevent hyperkalemia or, more rarely, **hypokalemia.** Restriction is necessary for persons treated with hemodialysis, whereas those undergoing peritoneal dialysis can consume potassium more freely. Recommended intakes are based on serum potassium levels, renal function, medications, and the dialysis procedure used.

All fresh foods provide potassium, but some fruits and vegetables contain such high amounts that some patients must limit intakes (see Figure 23-3). Table 23-6 shows the

hypokalemia (HIGH-po-ka-LEE-me-ah)**:** low serum potassium levels.

TABLE 23-7 **Foods High in Phosphorus**[a]

- Barley
- Bran (oat, wheat)
- Buckwheat groats
- Bulgur
- Canned iced tea
- Canned lemonade
- Coconut
- Cola beverages
- Cornmeal
- Couscous
- Dried peas and beans
- Fish
- Milk products
- Nuts and seeds
- Organ meats
- Peanut butter
- Processed meats
- Soybeans, tofu

© Cengage Learning®

[a]For a complete list, visit the USDA's Nutrient Database at *http://ndb.nal.usda.gov/*. Click on "Start your search here," then on "Nutrient Lists"; choose phosphorus as "First Nutrient" and choose to "Sort by" nutrient content, and then click "Go."

potassium content of some common fruits and vegetables. Foods in other food groups may be high in potassium as well; examples include dried beans, fish, milk and milk products, molasses, nuts and nut butters, and wheat bran. Note that salt substitutes and other low-sodium products often contain potassium chloride, which people on a potassium-restricted diet should avoid.

Calcium, Phosphorus, and Vitamin D To minimize the risk of bone disease, serum phosphate and calcium levels are monitored in renal patients and laboratory values help to guide recommendations. Elevated serum phosphate levels indicate the need for dietary phosphorus restriction and, if necessary, the use of phosphate binders (taken with meals). Because many phosphate binders are calcium salts, patients are at risk of developing **hypercalcemia** in response to simultaneous calcium and vitamin D supplementation. Vitamin D supplementation is recommended only for patients with suspected deficiency.[27]

High-protein foods are also high in phosphorus, so protein-restricted diets consumed by predialysis patients curb phosphorus intakes as well. After dialysis treatments begin and protein intakes are liberalized, phosphate binders become essential for phosphorus control. Because foods that are rich in calcium (such as milk and milk products) are usually high in phosphorus and are therefore restricted, patients may rely on calcium supplements (or calcium-based phosphate binders) to meet their calcium needs. Table 23-7 lists examples of foods that are high in phosphorus.

Vitamins and Minerals The restrictive renal diet interferes with vitamin and mineral intakes, increasing the risk of deficiencies. In addition, patients treated with dialysis lose water-soluble vitamins and some trace minerals into the dialysate. Thus, multivitamin/mineral supplements are typically recommended for all patients. Supplements prescribed for dialysis patients typically supply generous amounts of folic acid and vitamin B_6—about 1 milligram and 10 milligrams per day, respectively—along with recommended amounts of the other water-soluble vitamins.[28] Supplemental vitamin C should be limited to 70 milligrams per day because excessive intakes can contribute to kidney stone formation in those at risk (see p. 621). Vitamin A supplements are not recommended because vitamin A levels tend to rise as kidney function worsens.

Iron deficiency is common in hemodialysis patients and may be due to inadequate erythropoietin, gastrointestinal bleeding, reduced iron absorption, or blood losses associated with the dialysis treatment.[29] Intravenous administration of iron, in conjunction with erythropoietin therapy, is more effective than oral iron supplementation for improving iron status.

Enteral and Parenteral Nutrition Nutrition support is sometimes necessary for renal patients who cannot consume adequate amounts of food. The enteral formulas suitable for chronic kidney disease are more kcalorically dense and have lower protein and electrolyte concentrations than standard formulas. **Intradialytic parenteral nutrition** is an option for supplying supplemental nutrients to dialysis patients; this technique combines parenteral infusions with hemodialysis treatments. An advantage of this approach is that the volume of parenteral solution infused can be simultaneously removed (recall that fluid intake is controlled in dialysis patients). However, clinical studies have not shown intradialytic parenteral nutrition to be more successful than oral supplementation for improving nutrition status in malnourished dialysis patients.[30]

Dietary Compliance Adhering to a renal diet is probably the most challenging aspect of treatment for renal disease patients. Depending on the stage of illness and the patient's laboratory values, the renal diet may limit protein, fluids, sodium, potassium, and phosphorus, thereby affecting food selections from all major food groups. In addition, adjustments in nutrient intake are required as the disease progresses. If the kidney disease was caused by diabetes, patients must also continue the dietary changes necessary for controlling blood glucose levels. Because renal diets have so many restrictions, patient compliance is often a problem. Table 23-8 shows an example of a

hypercalcemia (HIGH-per-kal-SEE-me-ah): elevated serum calcium levels.

intradialytic parenteral nutrition: the infusion of nutrients during hemodialysis, often providing amino acids, dextrose, lipids, and some trace minerals.

TABLE 23-8 Chronic Kidney Disease—One-Day Menu

The menu below provides 2028 kcalories, 46 g protein, 784 mg phosphorus, 2190 mg potassium, and 1510 mg sodium.[a] The energy and protein content would be appropriate for a 135-pound predialysis patient. Note that the menu includes a number of refined and low-fiber foods due to the need to limit phosphorus and potassium.

Breakfast
- Corn flakes with milk (1 cup cereal, ½ cup whole milk)
- Apricot nectar (1 cup)
- Caffé latte (brewed coffee, 2 tsp sugar, ½ cup cream substitute)

Lunch
- Turkey sandwich (2 slices white bread, 1½ oz dark meat, 5 slices cucumber, 1 tbs mayonnaise)
- Grape juice (1 cup)
- Orange sherbet (½ cup)

Dinner
- Spaghetti with tomato sauce (1 cup cooked spaghetti, ½ cup bottled tomato sauce, ½ tbs grated cheese)
- Green beans with olive oil (1 cup cooked green beans, 1 tbs olive oil)
- Biscuit with margarine (2½-inch biscuit, ½ tbs margarine)
- Baked apple with nondairy sour cream (1 large apple, ¼ cup nondairy sour cream)

[a]Energy and nutrient values were obtained from the USDA National Nutrient Database for Standard Reference: http://ndb.nal.usda.gov/

© 2016 Cengage Learning®

1-day menu that includes some typical restrictions, and Box 23-2 (p. 618) provides suggestions to help patients comply with renal diets. The Case Study in Box 23-3 (p. 618) allows you to apply your knowledge about chronic kidney disease and hemodialysis.

Kidney Transplants

A preferred alternative to dialysis in patients with end-stage renal disease is kidney transplantation.[31] A successful kidney transplant restores kidney function, allows a more liberal diet, and frees the patient from routine dialysis. Given the choice, many patients would prefer transplants, but the demand for suitable kidneys far exceeds the supply. Other barriers to transplantation include advanced age, poor health, and financial difficulties. Approximately 30 percent of patients with end-stage renal disease receive a kidney transplant.[32]

Immunosuppressive Drug Therapy To prevent tissue rejection following transplant surgery, patients require high doses of immunosuppressive drugs (see Box 23-4). These drugs have multiple effects that can alter nutrition status, including nausea, vomiting, diarrhea, glucose intolerance, altered blood lipids, fluid retention, hypertension, and increased infection risk. Because immunosuppressive drug therapy increases the risk of foodborne infection, food safety guidelines should be provided to patients and caregivers. Box 23-5 (p. 619) summarizes the nutrition-related effects of immunosuppressants and other drugs mentioned in this chapter.

Nutrition Therapy after a Kidney Transplant After patients recover from transplant surgery, most nutrients can be consumed at levels recommended for the general population. Patients should attempt to maintain a healthy body weight and consume a diet that reduces their risk for cardiovascular diseases.

For most transplant patients, the side effects of drugs are the primary reason that dietary adjustments may be required. Although sodium, potassium, phosphorus, and fluid intakes are usually liberalized following a transplant, serum electrolyte levels must be monitored because some drug therapies can cause electrolyte imbalances

BOX 23-4

Examples of immunosuppressive drugs used after a kidney transplant:
- Corticosteroids (prednisone)
- Cyclosporine (Sandimmune)
- Mycophenolate mofetil (Cellcept)
- Tacrolimus (Prograf)

Patients with renal disease and their caregivers face considerable challenges as they learn to manage a renal diet. The following suggestions may help:

1. *To keep track of fluid intake:*

   ▮ Fill a container with an amount of water equal to your total fluid allowance. Each time you consume a liquid food or beverage, discard an equivalent amount of water from the container. The amount remaining in the container will show you how much fluid you have left for the day.

   ▮ Be sure to save enough fluid to take medications.

2. *To help control thirst:*

   ▮ Chew gum or suck hard candy.

   ▮ Suck on frozen grapes.

   ▮ Freeze allowed beverages to a semisolid state so that they take longer to consume. Or, fill an ice-cube tray with your favorite fruit-flavored beverage, and suck on flavored ice cubes during the day.

   ▮ Add lemon juice or crumpled mint leaves to water to make it more refreshing.

   ▮ Gargle with refrigerated mouthwash.

3. *To increase the energy content of meals:*

   ▮ Add extra margarine or a flavored oil to rice, noodles, breads, crackers, and cooked vegetables. Add extra salad dressing or mayonnaise to salads.

   ▮ Add nondairy whipped toppings to desserts.

   ▮ Include fried foods in your diet.

4. *To include more of your favorite vegetables in meals:*

   ▮ Consult your nurse or dietitian to learn whether you can safely use the process of leaching to remove some of the potassium from vegetables.

   ▮ To leach potassium from vegetables: Cut the vegetables into 1/8-inch slices and rinse. Soak the vegetables in a large amount of warm water for two hours—about 10 parts of water to 1 part of vegetables. Rinse vegetables well. Boil vegetables using 5 parts of water to 1 part of vegetables.

5. *To prevent the diet from becoming monotonous:*

   ▮ Experiment with new combinations of allowed foods.

   ▮ Substitute nondairy products for milk products. Nondairy products, which are lower in protein, phosphorus, and potassium, can substitute for milk and add energy to the diet.

   ▮ Add flavor to foods by seasoning with garlic, onion, chili powder, curry powder, oregano, mint, basil, parsley, pepper, or lemon juice.

   ▮ Consult a nurse or dietitian when you want to eat restricted foods. Many restricted foods can be used occasionally and in small amounts if the menu is carefully adjusted.

Case Study BOX 23-3 MAN WITH CHRONIC KIDNEY DISEASE

Thomas Stone is a 55-year-old banker who developed chronic kidney disease as a result of hypertension. His condition was discovered several years ago, when routine laboratory tests revealed elevated serum creatinine levels and persistent albuminuria. Since then, he has been taking antihypertensive medications and restricting dietary sodium, but he reported difficulty following the low-protein diet that was also prescribed. Mr. Stone recently visited his doctor with complaints of low urine output and reduced sensation in his hands and feet. He also reported feeling drowsy at work and mentioned that he was bruising more than usual. The examination revealed a 9-pound weight gain since his last visit and swelling in his ankles and feet. Tests revealed that his GFR had fallen to 10 milliliters per minute. Mr. Stone is 5 feet 8 inches tall and normally weighs 160 pounds.

1. Explain how chronic kidney disease progresses. What happens to GFR, serum creatinine levels, and albuminuria as renal function declines?

2. Describe the clinical effects you would expect during the final stage of disease, when kidney failure develops. Explain the significance of each of Mr. Stone's physical complaints.

3. Explain why a low-sodium, low-protein diet was prescribed for Mr. Stone at a former visit. What energy and protein intakes were probably recommended at that time?

4. The physician determines that Mr. Stone's kidney disease has reached the final stage and prescribes hemodialysis. How will dialysis alter Mr. Stone's diet? Calculate his new protein recommendation, and compare it to the amount of protein recommended before dialysis. What other changes in nutrient intake may be necessary?

or fluid retention. If corticosteroids are used as immunosuppressants, calcium supplementation is recommended because the medication increases urinary calcium losses. If drug treatment leads to hyperglycemia, patients should limit intakes of refined carbohydrates and concentrated sweets; for some individuals, oral medications or insulin therapy may be necessary. Patients should continue to follow food safety guidelines to avoid foodborne illness.

IN SUMMARY

▌ Chronic kidney disease is characterized by a gradual loss of kidney function and often results from long-standing diabetes mellitus or hypertension.

▌ Depending on the stage of illness, complications of chronic kidney disease may include fluid and electrolyte imbalances, hypertension, renal osteodystrophy, mental impairments, bleeding abnormalities, anemia, increased risk for cardiovascular disease, and reduced immunity.

▌ Treatment of chronic kidney disease can slow disease progression and correct complications and includes drug therapies, dialysis, and nutrition therapy. Dietary measures usually feature a low-protein diet, controlled fluid and sodium intakes, phosphorus restrictions, and nutrient supplementation; potassium restrictions are usually necessary after dialysis treatment begins.

▌ In patients with end-stage kidney disease, a kidney transplant can restore renal function and liberalize dietary restrictions.

23.4 Kidney Stones

LO 23.4 Compare the different types of kidney stones and explain how kidney stones can be prevented or treated.

Approximately 12 percent of men and 6 percent of women in the United States develop one or more **kidney stones** during their lifetimes.[33] A kidney stone is a crystalline mass that forms within the urinary tract. Although stones are often asymptomatic, their passage can cause severe pain or block the urinary tract. Stones tend to recur but can be prevented with dietary measures and medical treatment.

kidney stones: crystalline masses that form in the urinary tract; also called *renal calculi* or *nephrolithiasis*.

BOX 23-5 DIET-DRUG INTERACTIONS

Check this table for notable nutrition-related effects of the medications discussed in this chapter.

Immunosuppressants (cyclosporine, tacrolimus)	**Gastrointestinal effects:** Nausea, vomiting, abdominal discomfort, diarrhea, constipation, anorexia **Dietary interactions:** Limit alcohol intake due to the potential for toxic effects; the bioavailability of tacrolimus is reduced when the drug is taken with food; grapefruit juice can raise serum concentrations of these drugs to toxic levels **Metabolic effects:** Electrolyte imbalances, hyperglycemia, hyperlipidemias, anemia
Immunosuppressants (corticosteroids)	**Metabolic effects:** Fluid retention, hyperglycemia, hypocalcemia, hypokalemia, hypophosphatemia, increased appetite, protein catabolism
Phosphate binders (calcium-based)	**Gastrointestinal effect:** Constipation **Metabolic effects:** Electrolyte imbalances
Potassium-exchange resins (sodium polystyrene sulfonate)	**Gastrointestinal effects:** Anorexia, constipation **Dietary interactions:** Calcium and magnesium supplements must be taken separately **Metabolic effects:** Fluid and sodium retention, hypokalemia, hypocalcemia, hypomagnesemia
Potassium citrate	**Gastrointestinal effects:** Nausea, vomiting, abdominal pain, diarrhea **Metabolic effect:** Hyperkalemia

Formation of Kidney Stones

Kidney stones develop when stone constituents become concentrated in urine, allowing crystals to form and grow. Most kidney stones are made up primarily of calcium oxalate (see Figure 23-4). Less commonly, stones are composed of calcium phosphate, uric acid, the amino acid cystine, or magnesium ammonium phosphate (the latter are known as *struvite* stones). Stone formation is promoted by factors that reduce urine volume, block urine flow, or increase concentrations of stone-forming substances.

Calcium Oxalate Stones The most common abnormality in people with calcium oxalate stones is **hypercalciuria** (elevated urinary calcium levels). Hypercalciuria can result from excessive calcium absorption, impaired calcium reabsorption in kidney tubules, or elevated serum levels of parathyroid hormone or vitamin D. However, some people with calcium oxalate stones excrete normal amounts of calcium in the urine, and the reason they form stones is unknown.

Elevated urinary oxalate levels, or **hyperoxaluria,** also promote the formation of calcium oxalate crystals. Oxalate is a normal product of metabolism that readily binds to calcium. Hyperoxaluria reflects an increase in the body's synthesis of oxalate or increased absorption from dietary sources. Fat malabsorption can increase oxalate absorption: the malabsorbed fatty acids bind to minerals (such as calcium and magnesium) that would otherwise bind to oxalates and inhibit their absorption (see Chapter 19).

Uric Acid Stones Uric acid stones develop when the urine is abnormally acidic, contains excessive uric acid, or both. These stones are frequently associated with **gout,** a metabolic disorder characterized by elevated uric acid levels in the blood and urine. A diet rich in **purines** also contributes to high uric acid levels; purines are abundant in animal proteins (meat, poultry, seafood) and degrade to uric acid in the body. In addition, a high intake of animal protein increases urine acidity, which promotes the crystallization of uric acid.

Cystine and Struvite Stones Cystine stones can form in people with the inherited disorder **cystinuria,** in which the renal tubules are unable to reabsorb the amino acid cystine. This abnormality results in high concentrations of cystine in the urine, leading to subsequent crystallization and stone formation. **Struvite** stones, composed primarily of magnesium ammonium phosphate, form in alkaline urine; the urinary pH is sometimes elevated due to the bacterial degradation of urea to ammonia. Struvite stones can accompany chronic urinary infections or disorders that interfere with urinary flow.

Consequences of Kidney Stones

In most cases, kidney stones do not pose serious medical problems. Small stones can readily pass through the ureters and out of the body with minimal treatment.

Renal Colic A stone passing through the ureter can produce severe, stabbing pain, called **renal colic.** Generally, the pain begins in the back and intensifies as the stone travels toward the bladder. The pain can be severe enough to cause nausea and vomiting and sometimes requires medication. Blood may appear in the urine (**hematuria**) as a result of damage to the kidney or ureter lining.

Urinary Tract Complications Depending on the location of the stone, symptoms may include urination urgency, frequent urination, or inability to urinate. Stones that are unable to pass through the ureter can cause a urinary tract obstruction and possibly lead to infection or acute kidney injury.

Prevention and Treatment of Kidney Stones

Solutes are less likely to crystallize and form stones in dilute urine. Therefore, people who form kidney stones are advised to drink 12 to 16 cups of fluid daily to produce

FIGURE 23-4 Kidney Stones
The most common type of kidney stone is composed of calcium oxalate crystals, as shown here. Kidney stones may be as small as a bread crumb or as large as a golf ball.

hypercalciuria (HIGH-per-kal-see-YOO-ree-ah)**:** elevated urinary calcium levels.

hyperoxaluria (HIGH-per-ox-ah-LOO-ree-ah)**:** elevated urinary oxalate levels.

gout (GOWT)**:** a metabolic disorder characterized by elevated uric acid levels in the blood and urine and the deposition of uric acid in and around the joints, causing acute joint inflammation.

purines (PYOO-reens)**:** products of nucleotide metabolism that degrade to uric acid.

cystinuria (SIS-tin-NOO-ree-ah)**:** a genetic disorder characterized by the elevated urinary excretion of several amino acids, including cystine.

struvite (STROO-vite)**:** crystals of magnesium ammonium phosphate.

renal colic: the intense pain that occurs when a kidney stone passes through the ureter; the pain typically begins in the back and intensifies as the stone travels toward the bladder.

hematuria (HE-mah-TOO-ree-ah)**:** blood in the urine.

more than 2 to 2½ liters of urine per day (see Figure 23-5).[34] Additional fluid may be needed in hot weather or if an individual is extremely active.

Calcium Oxalate Stones Most dietary strategies and drug treatments for calcium oxalate stones aim to reduce urinary calcium and oxalate levels. Dietary measures may include adjustments in calcium, oxalate, protein, and sodium intakes.[35] Patients should consume adequate calcium from food sources (about 800 to 1200 milligrams per day) because dietary calcium combines with oxalate in the intestines, reducing oxalate absorption and helping to control hyperoxaluria.* Conversely, low-calcium diets promote oxalate absorption and higher urinary oxalate levels. Some individuals with hyperoxaluria may benefit from dietary oxalate restriction (see Table 23-9). High intakes of protein (especially from meat, fish, poultry, or eggs) and sodium increase urinary calcium excretion, so moderate protein consumption (0.8 to 1.0 gram per kilogram of body weight per day) and a controlled sodium intake (no more than about 2300 milligrams daily) are also advised. Vitamin C intakes should not exceed the RDA (90 and 75 milligrams for men and women, respectively) because vitamin C degrades to oxalate.[36] Medications used to prevent calcium oxalate stones include thiazide diuretics, which reduce urinary calcium levels by enhancing calcium reabsorption; potassium citrate (a base), which inhibits crystal formation; and allopurinol (Zyloprim), which reduces uric acid production in the body and may have other effects.[37]

Uric Acid Stones Although diets restricted in purines may help to control urinary uric acid levels, the effects on stone formation are unclear. Moreover, because all animal proteins contain purines, long-term restriction can be difficult to achieve. Drug treatments for uric acid stones include allopurinol to reduce uric acid levels and potassium citrate to reduce urine acidity.

FIGURE 23-5 Diet and Kidney Stones
Drinking plenty of fluids throughout the day is the most important measure for preventing kidney stones. Acceptable fluid sources include water, tea, coffee, wine, and beer, but sugar-sweetened soft drinks should be limited because they may increase the risk of stone formation.

James Darell/Getty Images

TABLE 23-9 Foods High in Oxalate

Vegetables	Fruit	Other
Asparagus	Avocados	Buckwheat
Bamboo shoots	Dates	Chocolate
Beets	Figs, dried	Cocoa powder
Carrots	Grapefruit	Cornmeal, grits
Celery, cooked	Kiwis	Millet
Chard	Lemons	Miso
Collard greens	Oranges, orange peel	Nuts, nut butters
Dried beans	Pineapple, canned	Peanut butter
Okra	Prunes	Pumpkin seeds
Parsnips	Raspberries	Rice
Potatoes	Rhubarb	Sesame seeds, tahini
Rutabagas	Tangerines	Soybean products
Spinach		Sunflower seeds
Sweet potatoes		Tea
Tomato sauce		Wheat bran
Turnips		Whole-wheat flour
Yams		

© 2016 Cengage Learning®

Note: The oxalate content of many foods has not been analyzed, and few studies have been conducted to determine which foods raise urinary oxalate levels.

*Note that calcium supplements can elevate urinary calcium levels, so they are not as helpful as dietary sources of calcium.

Cystine and Struvite Stones High fluid intakes may prevent the formation of cystine stones in some patients, whereas other individuals require drug therapy to reduce cystine production in the body. Medications frequently prescribed include penicillamine (Cuprimine) and tiopronin (Thiola), which increase the solubility of cystine, and potassium citrate, which reduces urine acidity. For preventing struvite stones, preventing or promptly treating urinary tract infections is a central strategy.

Medical Treatment for Kidney Stones Medical treatment may be necessary for a kidney stone that is too large to pass, blocks urine flow, or causes severe pain or bleeding. Medications that relax the ureter and increase urine flow may be given to facilitate stone passage; examples include alpha-receptor blockers and calcium channel blockers. Sometimes a *stent* (a thin, flexible tube) is placed in the ureter to promote stone passage. Some kidney stones can be fragmented via high-amplitude sound waves so they are small enough to pass in the urine. Surgical methods that involve physical removal of kidney stones have a higher success rate but are also more invasive.

IN SUMMARY

- Kidney stones form when stone constituents—calcium oxalate, calcium phosphate, uric acid, cystine, or magnesium ammonium phosphate—crystallize in urine. Complications include renal colic, difficulty with urination, and obstruction.

- Kidney stones may be prevented by drinking enough fluid to maintain urine volumes of at least 2 to 2½ liters daily. Other dietary measures include the consumption of appropriate amounts of calcium, oxalates, protein, sodium, and purines.

- Symptomatic kidney stones may be treated with medications or treatments that facilitate stone passage or surgeries that fragment or remove stones.

Nutrition Assessment Checklist FOR PEOPLE WITH KIDNEY DISEASES

Medical History

Check the medical record to determine:

- Degree of kidney function
- Cause of the nephrotic syndrome or kidney disease
- Type of dialysis, if appropriate
- Whether the patient has received a kidney transplant
- Type of kidney stone

Review the medical record for complications that may alter nutritional needs:

- Anemia
- Diabetes mellitus
- Edema or oliguria
- Hyperlipidemia
- Hypertension
- Metabolic stress or infection
- Protein-energy malnutrition

Medications

Assess risks for medication-related malnutrition related to:

- Long-term use of medications
- Multiple medication use, especially if medications affect nutrition status

For all patients with kidney diseases, note:

- Whether medications or supplements contain electrolytes that must be controlled
- Use of drugs or herbs that may be toxic to the kidneys

Dietary Intake

For patients with the nephrotic syndrome, kidney disease, or a kidney transplant, assess intakes of:

- Protein and energy
- Fluid
- Vitamins, especially vitamin D
- Minerals, especially calcium, phosphorus, iron, and electrolytes

For patients with kidney stones or a history of kidney stones:

- Stress the need to drink plenty of fluids throughout the day.
- Assess intake of calcium, oxalate, sodium, protein, purines, or vitamin C, as appropriate for the type of stone.

Anthropometric Data

Take accurate baseline height and weight measurements. Keep in mind that:

- Fluid retention due to the nephrotic syndrome or kidney failure can mask malnutrition.

- For dialysis patients, the weight measured immediately after the dialysis treatment (called the *dry weight*) most accurately reflects the person's true weight. Rapid weight gain between dialysis treatments reflects fluid retention. If fluid retention is excessive, review the fluid intake to determine if the patient understands and is complying with diet recommendations.

Laboratory Tests

Note that serum protein levels are often low in patients with nephrotic syndrome or advanced kidney disease. Review the following laboratory test results to assess the degree of kidney function and response to treatments:

- Albuminuria
- Creatinine
- Glomerular filtration rate (GFR)
- Serum electrolytes

Check laboratory test results for complications associated with kidney disease, including:

- Anemia
- Hyperglycemia
- Hyperlipidemia
- Hyperparathyroidism (related to bone disease)

Physical Signs

For patients with nephrotic syndrome or kidney disease, look for physical signs of:

- Bone disease
- Dehydration or fluid retention
- Hyperkalemia
- Iron deficiency
- Uremia

Clinical Applications

1. A person with chronic kidney disease may need multiple medications to control disease progression and treat symptoms and complications. For people with diabetes and hyperlipidemias who develop chronic kidney disease, medications might include insulin, oral hypoglycemic drugs, antihypertensives, diuretics, lipid-lowering medications, and phosphate binders. Review the nutrition-related side effects of these medications. Describe the ways in which these medications may make it harder for people to maintain nutrition status.

2. Identify the recommended energy, protein, and sodium intakes for a 65-year-old hemodialysis patient who weighs 60 kilograms (use the guidelines shown in Table 23-5). Then, consider the type of diet that would be appropriate for this patient by following these steps:

   - Create a one-day menu that provides appropriate amounts of energy, protein, and sodium for this patient (use the energy and nutrient values in Appendix A or an online database).

   - Assuming that the patient's laboratory test results suggest that potassium and phosphorus restrictions are necessary, would the day's intake of these nutrients be within the ranges suggested in Table 23-5? If not, adjust the food list to better match the guidelines.

   - If this patient were to begin peritoneal dialysis, which nutrient recommendations would change? Explain why the diet would be easier to follow than the diet required during hemodialysis.

Self Check

1. Which of the following is *not* a function of the kidneys?
   a. Activation of vitamin K
   b. Maintenance of acid-base balance
   c. Elimination of metabolic waste products
   d. Maintenance of fluid and electrolyte balances

2. The nephrotic syndrome frequently results in:
   a. the uremic syndrome.
   b. oliguria.
   c. edema.
   d. renal colic.

3. Dietary recommendations for patients with the nephrotic syndrome include:
   a. a high protein intake.
   b. sodium restriction.
   c. calcium and potassium restrictions.
   d. fluid restriction.

4. What is a common treatment for hyperkalemia?
   a. Eliminating potassium from the diet.
   b. Using potassium-wasting diuretics to increase potassium losses.
   c. Increasing fluid intake to maintain a high urine volume.
   d. Using potassium-exchange resins, which bind potassium in the GI tract.

5. If a patient with acute kidney injury should require a high protein intake, which additional treatment may be necessary?
   a. Frequent dialysis
   b. Use of diuretics
   c. Enteral nutrition support
   d. Fluid restrictions

6. The most common cause of chronic kidney disease is:
   a. diabetes mellitus.
   b. hypertension.
   c. autoimmune disease.
   d. exposure to toxins.

7. A person with chronic kidney disease who has been following a renal diet for several years begins hemodialysis treatment. An appropriate dietary adjustment would be to:
   a. reduce protein intake.
   b. consume protein more liberally.
   c. increase intakes of sodium and water.
   d. consume potassium and phosphorus more liberally.

8. Which of the following nutrients may be unintentionally restricted when a patient restricts phosphorus intake?
   a. Water
   b. Calcium
   c. Potassium
   d. Sodium

9. Most kidney stones are made primarily from:
   a. struvite.
   b. uric acid.
   c. calcium oxalate.
   d. cystine.

10. Treatment for all kidney stones includes:
   a. dietary oxalate restriction.
   b. dietary protein restriction.
   c. vitamin C supplementation.
   d. a fluid intake that produces more than 2 to 2½ liters of urine daily.

Answers to these questions appear in Appendix H.

Notes

1. G. B. Appel and J. Radhakrishnan, Glomerular disorders and nephrotic syndromes, in L. Goldman and A. I. Schafer, eds., *Goldman's Cecil Medicine* (Philadelphia: Saunders, 2012), pp. 761–771.

2. B. R. Don and G. A. Kaysen, Proteinuria and nephrotic syndrome, in R. W. Schrier, ed., *Renal and Electrolyte Disorders* (Philadelphia: Lippincott Williams & Wilkins, 2010), pp. 519–558.

3. Appel and Radhakrishnan, 2012; Don and Kaysen, 2010.

4. Academy of Nutrition and Dietetics, *Nutrition Care Manual* (Chicago: Academy of Nutrition and Dietetics, 2014); Don and Kaysen, 2010.

5. Don and Kaysen, 2010.

6. Academy of Nutrition and Dietetics, 2014.

7. Academy of Nutrition and Dietetics, 2014.

8. P. M. Palevsky and coauthors, KDOQI U.S. commentary on the 2012 KDIGO clinical practice guideline for acute kidney injury, *American Journal of Kidney Diseases* 61 (2013): 649–672.

9. B. A. Molitoris, Acute kidney injury, in L. Goldman and A. I. Schafer, eds., *Goldman's Cecil Medicine* (Philadelphia: Saunders, 2012), pp. 756–761.

10. R. W. Schrier and C. L. Edelstein, Acute kidney injury: Pathogenesis, diagnosis, and management, in R. W. Schrier, ed., *Renal and Electrolyte Disorders* (Philadelphia: Lippincott Williams & Wilkins, 2010), pp. 325–388.

11. C. E. Alpers, The kidney, in V. Kumar and coeditors, *Robbins and Cotran Pathologic Basis of Disease* (Philadelphia: Saunders, 2010), pp 905–969.

12. J. D. Kopple, Nutrition, diet, and the kidney, in A. C. Ross and coeditors, eds., *Modern Nutrition in Health and Disease* (Baltimore: Lippincott Williams & Wilkins, 2014), pp. 1330–1371; Kidney Disease: Improving Global Outcomes (KDIGO)

Acute Kidney Injury Work Group, KDIGO clinical practice guideline for acute kidney injury, *Kidney International Supplements* 2 (2012):1–138.

13. Kidney Disease: Improving Global Outcomes (KDIGO) Acute Kidney Injury Work Group, 2012.

14. Kopple, 2014; Academy of Nutrition and Dietetics, 2014.

15. Academy of Nutrition and Dietetics, 2014.

16. M. Chonchol and L. Chan, Chronic kidney disease: Manifestations and pathogenesis, in R. W. Schrier, ed., *Renal and Electrolyte Disorders* (Philadelphia: Lippincott Williams & Wilkins, 2010), pp. 389–425.

17. W. E. Mitch, Chronic kidney disease, in L. Goldman and A. I. Schafer, eds., *Goldman's Cecil Medicine* (Philadelphia: Saunders, 2012), pp. 810–818.

18. Mitch, 2012.

19. L. A. Inker and coauthors, KDOQI U.S. commentary on the 2012 KDIGO clinical practice guideline for the evaluation and management of CKD, *American Journal of Kidney Diseases* 63 (2014): doi: 10.1053/j.ajkd.2014.01.416; P.E. Stevens and A. Levin, Evaluation and management of chronic kidney disease: Synopsis of the kidney disease: improving global outcomes 2012 clinical practice guideline, *Annals of Internal Medicine* 158 (2013): 825–830.

20. J. A. Kraut, Chronic renal failure, in E. T. Bope and R. D. Kellerman, eds., *Conn's Current Therapy 2012* (Philadelphia: Saunders, 2012), pp. 883–888.

21. Kopple, 2014; T. G. Axelsson, M. Chmielewski, and B. Lindholm, Kidney disease, in J. W. Erdman, I. A. Macdonald, and S. H. Zeisel, eds., *Present Knowledge in Nutrition* (Ames, IA: Wiley-Blackwell, 2012), pp. 874–888.

22. R. Filipowicz and S. Beddhu, Optimal nutrition for predialysis chronic kidney disease, *Advances in Chronic Kidney Disease* 20 (2013): 175–180.

23. Kopple, 2014; T. A. Ikizler, Optimal nutrition in hemodialysis patients, *Advances in Chronic Kidney Disease* 20 (2013): 181–189.

24. Academy of Nutrition and Dietetics, 2014.

25. Filipowicz and Beddhu, 2013.

26. Filipowicz and Beddhu, 2013.

27. Inker and coauthors, 2014.

28. Kopple, 2014.

29. N. Tolkoff-Rubin, Treatment of irreversible renal failure, in L. Goldman and A. I. Schafer, eds., *Goldman's Cecil Medicine* (Philadelphia: Saunders, 2012), pp. 818–826.

30. Ikizler, 2013.

31. Tolkoff-Rubin, 2012.

32. U.S. Renal Data System, *USRDS 2013 Annual Data Report: Atlas of Chronic Kidney Disease and End-Stage Renal Disease in the United States* (Bethesda, MD: National Institutes of Health, 2013).

33. G. C. Curhan, Nephrolithiasis, in L. Goldman and A. I. Schafer, eds., *Goldman's Cecil Medicine* (Philadelphia: Saunders, 2012), pp. 789–794.

34. I. P. Heilberg and D. S. Goldfarb, Optimum nutrition for kidney stone disease, *Advances in Chronic Kidney Disease* 20 (2013): 165–174; Curhan, 2012.

35. Heilberg and Goldfarb, 2013.

36. J. Lamarche and coauthors, Vitamin C-induced oxalate nephropathy, *International Journal of Nephrology* 2011 (2011), available at doi:10.4061/2011/146927.

37. Curhan, 2012.

LO 23.5 Explain how dialysis removes fluids and wastes from the blood and compare the different types of dialysis procedures.

Although there is no perfect substitute for one's own kidneys, dialysis offers a life-sustaining treatment option for people with chronic kidney disease who develop renal failure. Dialysis can serve as a long-term treatment or as a temporary measure to sustain life until a suitable kidney donor can be found. Dialysis can also restore fluid and electrolyte balances in patients with acute kidney injury. Clinicians who routinely work with renal patients should understand how dialysis procedures work. This Nutrition in Practice describes the process of dialysis and outlines the various types of procedures that are available. The glossary in Box NP23-1 defines the relevant terms.

How does dialysis work?

Dialysis removes excess fluids and wastes from the blood by employing the processes of **diffusion, osmosis,** and **ultrafiltration** (see Figure NP23-1). The dialysate, a solution similar in composition to normal blood plasma, is carried through a compartment beside a **semipermeable membrane**; the person's blood flows in the opposite direction along the other side of the membrane. The semipermeable membrane acts like a filter: small molecules such as urea and glucose can pass through microscopic pores in the membrane, whereas large molecules are unable to cross.

In *hemodialysis*, the tiny tubes that carry blood through the dialyzer are made of materials that serve as semipermeable membranes. In *peritoneal dialysis*, the body's peritoneal membrane, rich with blood vessels, is used to filter the blood.

How are solutes separated from the blood in dialysis?

The chemical composition of the dialysate affects the movement of solutes across the semipermeable membrane. When the concentration of a substance is lower in the dialysate than in the blood,

---

BOX NP23-1 GLOSSARY

continuous ambulatory peritoneal dialysis (CAPD): the most common method of peritoneal dialysis; involves frequent exchanges of dialysate, which remains in the peritoneal cavity throughout the day.

continuous renal replacement therapy (CRRT): a slow, continuous method of removing solutes and/or fluids from the blood by gently pumping the blood across a filtration membrane over a prolonged time period.

diffusion: movement of solutes from an area of high concentration to one of low concentration.

hemofiltration: removal of fluid and solutes from the blood by pumping the blood across a membrane; no osmotic gradients are created during the process.

oncotic pressure: the pressure exerted by fluid on one side of a membrane as a result of osmosis.

osmosis: movement of water across a membrane toward the side where solutes are more concentrated.

peritonitis: inflammation of the peritoneal membrane.

pressure gradient: the change in pressure over a given distance. In dialysis, a pressure gradient is created between the blood and the dialysate.

semipermeable membrane: a membrane that allows some, but not all, particles to pass through.

ultrafiltration: removal of fluids and solutes from the blood by using pressure to transfer the blood across a semipermeable membrane.

urea kinetic modeling: a method of determining the adequacy of dialysis treatment by calculating the urea clearance from blood.

---

the substance—provided it can cross the membrane—will diffuse out of the blood. For example, the goal is to remove as much as possible of the waste product urea from the blood, so the dialysate contains no urea. For many other solutes, the dialysate is adjusted so that only excesses will be removed. Potassium can be removed from the blood, for example, by providing a dialysate that has a

---

FIGURE NP23-1
Diffusion, Osmosis, and Ultrafiltration

© Cengage Learning®

Diffusion	Osmosis	Ultrafiltration
Small molecules (electrolytes and waste products) move from an area of high concentration to an area of low concentration by diffusion.	Water moves from an area of high water concentration to an area of low water concentration. In other words, water moves toward the side where solutes are more concentrated.	Pressure squeezes water and small molecules through the pores of a semipermeable membrane during ultrafiltration.

625

lower concentration of potassium than is found in the person's blood. The dialysate must contain some potassium, however; otherwise, the blood potassium would fall too low.

The dialysate can also be used to add needed components back into the blood. For a person with acidosis, for example, bases such as bicarbonate are added to the dialysate; the bases then move by diffusion into the blood to alleviate the acidosis.

How is fluid removed from the blood?

Because albumin and other plasma proteins are so adept at retaining fluids in blood, osmosis alone is not an efficient process for removing fluid. In hemodialysis, a **pressure gradient** is created between the blood and the dialysate. Most modern dialyzers produce *positive* pressure in the blood compartment and *negative* pressure in the dialysate compartment, establishing a pressure gradient that "pushes" water (and accompanying solutes) through the pores of the membrane. This process, called ultrafiltration, relies on pumps to establish an appropriate flow rate between the blood and the dialysate.

How often do patients require hemodialysis, and how long do treatments last?

Most patients undergo hemodialysis three times weekly and the treatments last three to five hours (see Figure NP23-2). Other options include short daily dialysis, performed for about two hours each day, and daily nocturnal hemodialysis, in which dialysis is done at home five or six nights a week while the patient is sleeping.[1] Although some studies have reported improved outcomes in patients who undergo more frequent dialysis, these approaches have not been widely adopted.[2] Note that most patients must visit dialysis centers to obtain treatment, as few patients have access to a dialysis machine at home.

How does the health practitioner know if the dialysis treatment has been effective?

A number of methods have been devised for gauging the adequacy of dialysis treatment. The most common method is **urea kinetic modeling**, a technique that evaluates the amount of urea cleared from the blood. The formula used most often is Kt/V, where K is the amount of urea cleared, t is the time spent on dialysis, and V is the blood volume. The value obtained indicates whether the patient has undergone sufficient dialysis; the goal is a Kt/V result of

FIGURE NP23-2 During hemodialysis, blood passes through a dialyzer, where wastes are extracted, and the cleansed blood is returned to the body.

approximately 1.2. Because technical data (such as dialyzer clearance data, blood flow rate, and dialysate flow rate) need to be incorporated into the calculation, the computation is usually done by computer analysis. Current treatment guidelines recommend that hemodialysis adequacy be evaluated at least monthly, or more often if problems develop or patients are noncompliant.[3]

Are any complications associated with hemodialysis?

Yes. Although lifesaving, hemodialysis is associated with a substantial number of complications.[4] Problems at the vascular access site include infections and blood clotting. Hypotension can develop while blood is circulated through the dialyzer. Muscle cramping often occurs during the procedure, especially in the hands, legs, and feet. Blood losses can worsen anemia, which is already severe in two-thirds of patients beginning hemodialysis treatment.[5] Patients may also experience headaches, weakness, nausea, vomiting, restlessness, and agitation. Many patients are extremely fatigued after a hemodialysis treatment, and some may require rest or sleep.

How does peritoneal dialysis work?

In peritoneal dialysis, the peritoneal membrane surrounding the abdominal organs serves as a semipermeable membrane. The dialysate is infused into a catheter that empties into the peritoneal space—the space within the abdomen near the intestines (see Figure NP23-3). In the most common procedure, **continuous ambulatory peritoneal dialysis (CAPD),** the dialysate remains in the peritoneal cavity for four to six hours, after which it is drained and replaced with fresh dialysate (about 2 to 3 liters in adults). Generally, the dialysate solution is exchanged four times daily and requires only about 30 minutes to drain and replace.

Because a pressure gradient cannot be created in the peritoneal cavity as it can in a dialyzer, the glucose concentration in the dialysate must be high enough to create sufficient **oncotic pressure** to draw fluid from the blood. As indicated in Chapter 23, a substantial amount of glucose can be absorbed into the patient's blood and may contribute to weight gain over time. The high glucose load may also cause hyperglycemia and hypertriglyceridemia in some patients.

What are the advantages and disadvantages of peritoneal dialysis?

Peritoneal dialysis offers a number of advantages over hemodialysis: vascular access is not required, dietary restrictions are fewer, and the procedure can be scheduled when convenient. The most common complication is infection, which can occur at the catheter site or within the peritoneal cavity (**peritonitis**). Other problems that may arise include blood clotting in the catheter, catheter migration, and abdominal hernia due to the dialysate volume.

What are the features of continuous renal replacement therapy?

In most people with acute kidney injury, **continuous renal replacement therapy (CRRT)** removes fluids and wastes. CRRT uses the process of **hemofiltration,** in which blood is gently pumped across a filtration membrane over a prolonged time period. (This process differs from dialysis treatments that rely on the diffusion of wastes across a membrane into the dialysate.) Either a pump or the patient's own

FIGURE NP23-3 Peritoneal Dialysis

In peritoneal dialysis, dialysate is infused into the peritoneal cavity.

Peritoneum
Peritoneal cavity
Catheter
Dialysate
Internal organs
Dialysate in
Drain line
Waste solution

Four to six hours later, the fluid is drained and replaced with new dialysate. This process is repeated several times daily.

Waste out

© Cengage Learning®

blood pressure moves the blood across the membrane. The procedure can be used to remove fluids, solutes, or both. Some patients require fluid replacement during the procedure to maintain adequate blood volume, so hydration status must be closely monitored.

The use of CRRT is advantageous in acute care situations because it corrects imbalances without causing sudden shifts in blood volume, which are poorly tolerated in acute care patients. In addition, replacement fluids can include parenteral feedings without upsetting fluid balance. Complications include clotting problems, damage to arteries, and inadequate blood flow rates in hypotensive patients.

Dialysis and CRRT help to remove the wastes and fluids that are normally removed by healthy kidneys. Although these procedures cannot restore the kidneys' hormonal functions, they provide a lifesaving means of alleviating symptoms of uremia, hypertension, and edema.

Notes

1. J. I. McMillan, Renal replacement therapy, in R. S. Porter and J. L. Kaplan, eds., *Merck Manual of Diagnosis and Therapy* (Whitehouse Station, NJ: Merck Sharp and Dohme Corp., 2011), pp. 2447–2453.

2. E. D. Weinhandl and coauthors, Survival in daily home hemodialysis and matched thrice-weekly in-center hemodialysis patients, *Journal of the American Society of Nephrology* 23 (2012): 895–904; P. Susantitaphong and coauthors, Effect of frequent or extended hemodialysis on cardiovascular parameters: A meta-analysis, *American Journal of Kidney* Diseases 59 (2012): 689–699.

3. National Kidney Foundation, KDOQI Clinical practice guidelines and clinical practice recommendations for 2006 updates: Hemodialysis adequacy, peritoneal dialysis adequacy and vascular access, *American Journal of Kidney Diseases* 48 (2006): S1–S322 (suppl 1).

4. N. Tolkoff-Rubin, Treatment of irreversible renal failure, in L. Goldman and A. I. Schafer, eds., *Goldman's Cecil Medicine* (Philadelphia: Saunders, 2012), pp. 818–826.

5. Tolkoff-Rubin, 2012.

24

Energy- and Protein-Modified Diets for Metabolic and Respiratory Stress

The body's response to severe stress can alter metabolism enough to threaten survival. Stress also raises nutritional needs considerably—increasing the risk of malnutrition even in previously healthy individuals. **Metabolic stress,** a disruption in the body's internal chemical environment, can result from uncontrolled infections or extensive tissue damage. As the first part of this chapter explains, the body's stress response is an attempt to restore balance, but it can have both helpful and harmful effects. Later sections of this chapter describe **respiratory stress,** characterized by inadequate oxygen and excessive carbon dioxide in the blood and tissues. Both metabolic and respiratory stress can lead to **hypermetabolism** (above-normal metabolic rate), **wasting** (loss of muscle tissue), and, in severe circumstances, life-threatening complications.

24.1 The Body's Responses to Stress and Injury

LO 24.1 Describe the stress and inflammatory responses and discuss the potentially damaging effects of these processes.

The **stress response** is the body's *nonspecific* response to a variety of stressors, such as burns, fractures, infection, surgery, and wounds. During stress, the metabolic processes that support immediate survival are given priority, while those of lesser consequence are delayed. Energy is of primary importance, and therefore the energy nutrients are mobilized from storage and made available in the blood. Heart rate and respiration (breathing rate) increase to deliver oxygen and nutrients to cells more quickly, and blood pressure rises. Meanwhile, energy is diverted from processes that are not life sustaining, such as growth, reproduction, and long-term immunity. If stress continues for a long period, interference with these processes may begin to cause damage or illness.

Hormonal Responses to Stress

The stress response is mediated by several hormones, which are released into the blood soon after the onset of injury (see Table 24-1, p. 630).[1] The catecholamines (epinephrine and norepinephrine)—often called the *fight-or-flight hormones*—stimulate heart muscle, raise blood pressure, and increase metabolic rate. Epinephrine also promotes glucagon secretion from the pancreas, prompting the release of nutrients from storage. The steroid hormone cortisol enhances muscle protein degradation, raising amino acid levels in the blood and making amino acids available for conversion to glucose. All of these hormones have similar effects on glucose and fat metabolism, causing the breakdown of glycogen, the production of glucose from amino acids, and the breakdown of triglycerides in adipose tissue. Thus, the combined effects of these hormones contribute to hyperglycemia, which often accompanies critical illness. Two other hormones induced by stress, aldosterone and antidiuretic hormone, help to maintain blood volume by stimulating the kidneys to reabsorb more sodium and water, respectively.

Cortisol's effects can be detrimental when stress is prolonged. In excess, cortisol causes the depletion of protein in muscle, bone, connective tissue, and skin. It impairs wound healing, so high cortisol levels may be especially dangerous for a patient with severe injuries. Because cortisol inhibits protein synthesis, consuming more protein cannot easily reverse tissue losses. Excess cortisol also leads to insulin resistance, contributing to hyperglycemia, and suppresses immune responses, increasing susceptibility to infection. Note that pharmaceutical forms of cortisol (such as *cortisone* and *prednisone*) are common anti-inflammatory medications; their long-term use can cause undesirable side effects such as muscle wasting, thinning of the skin, diabetes, and early osteoporosis.

metabolic stress: a disruption in the body's chemical environment due to the effects of disease or injury. Metabolic stress is characterized by changes in metabolic rate, heart rate, blood pressure, hormonal status, and nutrient metabolism.

respiratory stress: a condition characterized by abnormal oxygen and carbon dioxide levels in body tissues due to abnormal gas exchange between the air and blood.

hypermetabolism: a higher-than-normal metabolic rate.

wasting: the breakdown of muscle tissue that results from disease or malnutrition.

stress response: the chemical and physical changes that occur within the body during stress.

TABLE 24-1 Metabolic Effects of Hormones Released during the Stress Response

Hormone	Metabolic Effects
Catecholamines	▪ Increase in metabolic rate ▪ Glycogen breakdown in the liver and muscle ▪ Glucose production from amino acids ▪ Release of fatty acids from adipose tissue ▪ Glucagon secretion from the pancreas
Glucagon	▪ Glycogen breakdown in the liver ▪ Glucose production from amino acids ▪ Release of fatty acids from adipose tissue
Cortisol	▪ Protein degradation ▪ Enhancement of glucagon's action on liver glycogen ▪ Glucose production from amino acids ▪ Release of fatty acids from adipose tissue
Aldosterone	▪ Sodium reabsorption in the kidneys
Antidiuretic hormone	▪ Water reabsorption in the kidneys

© 2016 Cengage Learning®

Note: The catecholamines, glucagon, and cortisol have actions that oppose those of insulin and are therefore referred to as *counterregulatory hormones.*

The Inflammatory Response

Cells of the immune system mount a quick, nonspecific response to infection or tissue injury. This so-called **inflammatory response** serves to contain and destroy infectious agents (and their products) and prevent further tissue damage; it also triggers various events that promote healing. As in the stress response, however, there is a delicate balance between a response that protects tissues from further injury and an excessive response that can cause additional damage to tissue.

The Inflammatory Process The inflammatory response begins with the dilation of arterioles and capillaries at the site of injury, which increases the blood flow to the affected area. The capillaries within the damaged tissue become more permeable, allowing some blood plasma to escape into the tissue and cause local edema (see Figure 24-1

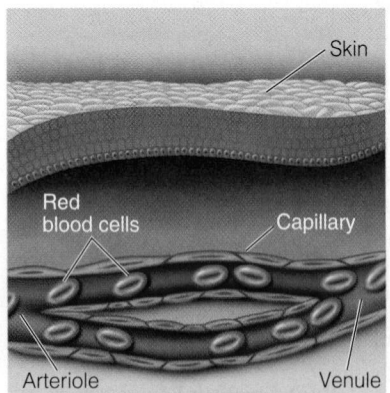

Cells lining the blood vessels lie close together, and normally do not allow the contents to cross into tissue.

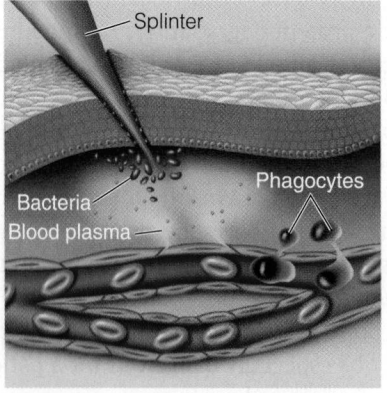

When tissues are damaged, immune cells release histamine, which dilates some blood vessels, increasing blood flow to the damaged area. Fluid leaks out of capillaries (causing swelling), and phagocytes escape between the small gaps in the blood vessel walls.

Phagocytes engulf bacteria and disable them with hydrolytic enzymes and reactive forms of oxygen.

© Cengage Learning®

FIGURE 24-1 The Inflammatory Process

and Box 24-1). The various changes in blood vessels attract immune cells that can destroy foreign agents and clear cellular debris. Among the first cells to arrive are the **phagocytes,** which slip through gaps between the endothelial cells that form the vessel walls. The phagocytes engulf microorganisms and destroy them with reactive forms of oxygen and hydrolytic enzymes. When inflammation becomes chronic, these normally useful products of phagocytes can damage healthy tissue.

Mediators of Inflammation Numerous chemical substances control the inflammatory process. These *mediators* are released from damaged tissue, blood vessel cells, and activated immune cells. Many of them help to regulate more than one step in the process. Histamine, a small molecule similar to an amino acid in structure, is released from granules within **mast cells,** causing vasodilation and capillary permeability.* Other compounds that participate in the inflammatory process include **cytokines,** produced by white blood cells (and various other cells), and **eicosanoids,** which are derived from dietary fatty acids. Note that most anti-inflammatory medications, including steroidal drugs (such as cortisone and prednisone) and nonsteroidal anti-inflammatory drugs (such as aspirin and ibuprofen), act by blocking eicosanoid synthesis.

Changing dietary fat sources may have subtle effects on the inflammatory process.[2] The major precursor for the eicosanoids is arachidonic acid, which derives from the omega-6 fatty acids in vegetable oils. Some omega-3 fatty acids compete with arachidonic acid and may inhibit the production of the most powerful inflammatory mediators. Although health professionals sometimes recommend replacing some of the omega-6 fatty acids in the diet with omega-3 fatty acids to reduce inflammation, most clinical studies conducted thus far have not confirmed this benefit.[3]

Systemic Effects of Inflammation The cytokines released during acute inflammation produce a number of **systemic** effects, which are collectively known as the **acute-phase response.**[4] Within hours after inflammation, infection, or severe injury, the liver steps up its production of certain plasma proteins (called *acute-phase proteins*) including **C-reactive protein, complement, hepcidin,** blood-clotting proteins such as fibrinogen and prothrombin, and others. At the same time, plasma concentrations of albumin, iron, and zinc fall. The acute-phase response is accompanied by muscle catabolism to make amino acids available for glucose production, tissue repair, and immune protein synthesis; consequently, negative nitrogen balance (and wasting) frequently results. Other clinical features of the acute-phase response may include fever, an elevated metabolic rate, increased pulse rate and blood pressure, increased blood neutrophil levels, lethargy, and anorexia.

If inflammation does not resolve, the continued production of pro-inflammatory cytokines may lead to the **systemic inflammatory response syndrome (SIRS),** which is diagnosed when the patient's symptoms include substantial increases in heart rate and respiratory rate, abnormal white blood cell counts, and/or fever. If these problems result from a severe infection, the condition is called **sepsis.** Complications associated with severe cases of SIRS or sepsis include fluid retention and tissue edema, low blood pressure, and impaired blood flow. If the reduction in blood flow is severe enough to deprive the body's tissues of oxygen and nutrients (a condition known as **shock**), multiple organs may fail simultaneously, as discussed in Nutrition in Practice 24.

IN SUMMARY

▪ The stress and inflammatory responses are nonspecific responses to stressors that cause infection and injury.

▪ The stress response is mediated by the catecholamine hormones, cortisol, and glucagon, which together raise nutrient levels in blood, stimulate heart rate, raise blood pressure, and increase metabolic rate.

Antihistamines are medications taken to reduce the effects of histamine.

BOX 24-1

Classic signs of inflammation that accompany altered blood flow:

▪ *Heat*—from the influx of warm arterial blood

▪ *Redness*—from the increase in blood in the injured area

▪ *Swelling*—from the accumulation of fluid and immune cells at the site of injury

▪ *Pain*—from the swelling and the actions of chemical mediators that stimulate pain receptors

systemic (sih-STEM-ic)**:** relating to the entire body.

acute-phase response: changes in body chemistry resulting from infection, inflammation, or injury; characterized by alterations in plasma proteins.

C-reactive protein: an acute-phase protein produced in substantial amounts during acute inflammation; it binds dead or dying cells to activate certain immune responses. C-reactive protein is considered the best clinical indicator of the acute-phase response although it is elevated during many chronic illnesses.

complement: a group of plasma proteins that assist the activities of antibodies.

hepcidin: an acute-phase protein involved in the regulation of iron metabolism.

systemic inflammatory response syndrome (SIRS): a whole-body inflammatory response caused by severe illness or trauma; characterized by raised heart and respiratory rates, abnormal white blood cell counts, and fever.

sepsis: a whole-body inflammatory response caused by infection; characterized by signs and symptoms similar to those of SIRS.

shock: a severe reduction in blood flow that deprives the body's tissues of oxygen and nutrients; characterized by reduced blood pressure, raised heart and respiratory rates, and muscle weakness.

FIGURE 24-2 Pressure Sores
Pressure sores, wounds that develop when prolonged pressure cuts off blood circulation to the skin and underlying tissues, are a frequent source of metabolic stress in bedridden and wheelchair-bound patients. Some patients with pressure sores may be prescribed a high-protein, high-kcalorie diet to prevent malnutrition.

■ The inflammatory process is characterized by changes in acute-phase proteins and increases in body temperature, pulse, blood pressure, metabolic rate, and blood neutrophil levels.

24.2 Nutrition Treatment of Acute Stress

LO 24.2 Describe the features of nutrition care of acutely stressed patients.

As described earlier, an excessive response to metabolic stress can worsen illness and even threaten survival. Therefore, medical personnel must manage both the acute medical condition that initiated stress and the complications that arise as a result of the stress and inflammatory responses (see Figure 24-2). Immediate concerns during severe stress are to restore lost fluids and electrolytes and remove underlying stressors. Thus, initial treatments include administering intravenous solutions to correct fluid and electrolyte imbalances, treating infections, repairing wounds, draining **abscesses** (pus), and removing dead tissue (**debridement**). After stabilization, nutrient needs can be estimated and nutrition therapy provided.

Determining Nutritional Requirements

Notable metabolic changes in patients undergoing metabolic stress include hypermetabolism, negative nitrogen balance, insulin resistance, and hyperglycemia. Hypermetabolism and negative nitrogen balance can lead to wasting, which may impair organ function and delay recovery. Hyperglycemia increases the risk of infection. Therefore, the principal goals of nutrition therapy are to preserve lean (muscle) tissue, maintain immune defenses, and promote healing.

Feeding an acutely stressed patient is often challenging. Underfeeding can worsen negative nitrogen balance and increase lean tissue losses. Overfeeding increases the risk of **refeeding syndrome** and its associated hyperglycemia. Assessing nutritional needs can be complicated, however, because fluid imbalances prevent accurate weight measurements, and laboratory data may reflect the metabolic alterations of illness rather than the person's nutrition status.

The amounts of protein and energy to provide during acute illness are controversial and still under investigation. Research results have been mixed, in part because various conditions are associated with metabolic stress and each patient's situation is somewhat different. Moreover, protein and energy needs can vary substantially over the course of illness. Clinicians need to closely observe patients' responses to feedings and readjust nutrient intakes as necessary.

Estimating Energy Needs in Acute Stress In critical-care and intensive-care patients, **indirect calorimetry**—which is typically used to measure the resting metabolic rate (RMR)—can be used to determine energy requirements. This is because the RMR closely reflects total energy expenditure in bedridden, non-fasting patients. If indirect calorimetry cannot be conducted, the RMR may be estimated using a predictive equation, such as those introduced in Chapter 14 (see pp. 405–406). In some cases, the RMR value may be multiplied by a "stress factor" to account for the increased energy requirements of stress and healing. Box 24-2 reviews the use of stress factors and provides examples (note that stress factors vary among institutions, as

abscesses (AB-sess-es): accumulations of pus.

debridement: the surgical removal of dead, damaged, or contaminated tissue resulting from burns or wounds; helps to prevent infection and hasten healing.

refeeding syndrome: a group of metabolic abnormalities that may result from aggressive refeeding in severely malnourished persons; characterized by shifts in fluid and electrolyte levels that can lead to organ failure and other complications.

indirect calorimetry: a method of estimating resting energy expenditure by measuring a person's oxygen consumption and carbon dioxide production.

To estimate the appropriate energy intake for a patient with an acute illness, the health practitioner may measure or calculate the patient's resting metabolic rate (RMR), and, in some cases, apply a "stress factor" to accommodate the additional energy needs imposed by the illness.

Method

Step 1. Estimate the RMR using indirect calorimetry or a predictive equation (see Table 14-9, p. 406).[a]

Step 2. Multiply the estimated RMR by an appropriate stress factor for acute illness (see Box 14-5 on p. 406; note that patients with acute illnesses are usually bedridden and do not require additional energy for activity).

Examples of stress factors[b]

- Intensive care: 1.0 to 1.1
- Acute kidney injury: 1.3
- Burns (more than 20 percent of body surface): 1.3 to 1.5
- Repletion after acute inflammation: 1.3 to 1.5
- Acute pancreatitis: 1.4 to 1.8

[a]In overweight and obese individuals, the Mifflin–St. Jeor equation estimates RMR more accurately than other currently used equations.

[b]Published values vary; energy intakes should be adjusted if the patient fails to maintain body weight at the energy level provided.

Sources: Academy of Nutrition and Dietetics, *Nutrition Care Manual* (Chicago: Academy of Nutrition and Dietetics, 2014); A. Skipper, ed., *Dietitian's Handbook of Enteral and Parenteral Nutrition* (Sudbury, MA: Jones & Bartlett Learning, 2012).

few have been adequately validated in research studies). Several predictive equations used for estimating energy needs in critically ill patients include "built-in" stress factors to account for stress, injury, or intensive treatment.*

Another common method for estimating energy needs during acute illness is to multiply a person's body weight by a factor considered appropriate for the medical problem. As an example, many critical care patients require between 25 and 30 kcalories per kilogram per day;[5] a patient weighing 160 pounds (72.7 kilograms) may therefore require between 1818 and 2182 kcalories per day. For critically ill obese patients (BMI > 30), **hypocaloric feedings** may improve patient outcome; the suggested energy intake is 11 to 14 kcalories per kilogram of actual body weight (or 22 to 25 kcalories per kilogram of ideal body weight) daily.[6]

Protein Requirements in Acute Stress To maintain lean tissue, the protein intakes recommended during acute stress are higher than DRI values (the adult RDA is 0.8 grams per kilogram body weight). For example, the protein needs of nonobese critically ill patients may range between 1.2 and 2.0 grams per kilogram body weight per day.[7] Obese patients given hypocaloric feedings may require 2.0 to 2.5 grams per kilogram ideal body weight per day to maintain nitrogen balance.[8] Despite high intakes, however, nitrogen balance is difficult to achieve during acute stress because hormonal changes encourage the degradation of body protein. The bed rest required during critical illness also contributes substantially to muscle breakdown.

The amino acids glutamine and arginine are sometimes added to the diets of acutely stressed and immune-compromised patients. Although some studies have shown that glutamine supplementation may improve infection, muscle mass, and mortality rates in some critically ill patients,[9] other studies suggest that the treatment may increase mortality risk in patients with multiple organ failure and renal dysfunction.[10] Arginine supplementation has been shown to improve infection rates and wound healing in surgical patients but may have adverse effects in patients with sepsis.[11] Thus, supplementation with glutamine and arginine may be beneficial for some patient populations but harmful in others.

Carbohydrate and Fat Intakes in Acute Stress Most of the energy required is supplied by carbohydrate and fat. Carbohydrate is usually the main source of energy,

---

*One example is the Penn State equation, developed for ventilator-dependent patients: Energy needs (kcal/day) = $[RMR \times 0.96] + [V_E \times 31] + [T_{max} \times 167] - 6212$ where RMR is calculated using the Mifflin–St. Jeor equation (see Table 14-9, p. 406), V_E is minute ventilation in liters per minute (reading taken from the ventilator), and T_{max} is the patient's maximum body temperature (in degrees Celsius) in the preceding 24 hours.

hypocaloric feedings: reduced-kcalorie feedings that usually include sufficient protein and micronutrients to maintain nitrogen balance and prevent malnutrition.

providing 50 to 60 percent of total energy requirements. When parenteral nutrition is necessary for critically ill patients, dextrose is usually limited to 5 milligrams per kilogram body weight per minute to prevent hyperglycemia (see Chapter 16). In patients with severe hyperglycemia, fat may supply up to 50 percent of kcalories, although high fat intakes may suppress immune function and increase the risks of developing infections and hypertriglyceridemia. Patients with blood triglyceride levels above 500 milligrams per deciliter may require fat restriction.[12]

Micronutrient Needs in Acute Stress Acutely stressed patients are believed to have increased micronutrient needs, but specific requirements remain unknown.[13] In hypermetabolic patients, the need for B vitamins may be higher to support the increase in energy metabolism. Several micronutrients, such as vitamin A, vitamin C, and zinc, have critical roles in immunity and wound healing; thus, their supplementation may speed recovery under certain circumstances. Patients with burns and tissue injuries may have increased requirements for trace minerals due to tissue losses.

The acute-phase response causes a redistribution in the tissue content of some micronutrients that either raises or lowers their blood levels (for example, plasma levels of iron and zinc fall, whereas copper levels rise). Therefore, micronutrient status is sometimes difficult to interpret. Blood concentrations of trace minerals are monitored in patients receiving parenteral nutrition support to ensure that excessive amounts are not given intravenously.

Approaches to Nutrition Care in Acute Stress

As mentioned earlier, the initial care following acute stress focuses on maintaining fluid and electrolyte balances. Simple intravenous solutions often contain dextrose, providing minimal kcalories. Once patients are stable, nutrition support may be necessary if poor appetite, the medical condition, or a medical procedure (such as mechanical ventilation) interferes with food intake. For acutely ill patients with a functional GI tract, early enteral feedings—started in the first 24 to 48 hours after hospitalization—are associated with fewer complications and shorter hospital stays compared with delayed feedings.[14] If enteral nutrition is not possible, malnourished patients may receive parenteral nutrition support soon after admission to the hospital. In previously healthy patients, however, parenteral nutrition support may be withheld during the first seven days of hospitalization to avoid the risk of infectious complications.

Once patients can tolerate oral feedings, a high-kcalorie, high-protein diet is often prescribed, although care must be taken not to overfeed patients who are at risk of developing refeeding syndrome or hyperglycemia. Because meeting protein and energy needs may be difficult, nutrient-dense formulas or other supplements may be added to the diet. Some supplements may contain extra amounts of nutrients believed to promote healing or benefit immune function, such as the amino acids arginine and glutamine, omega-3 fatty acids, and the antioxidant nutrients. Nutrient needs should be reassessed frequently as the patient's condition improves. The Case Study in Box 24-3 reviews the nutrition care of a patient undergoing acute metabolic stress.

chronic obstructive pulmonary disease (COPD): a group of lung diseases characterized by persistent obstructed airflow through the lungs and airways; includes chronic bronchitis and emphysema.

bronchi (BRON-key), **bronchioles** (BRON-key-oles)**:** the main airways of the lungs. The singular form of bronchi is *bronchus*.

alveoli (al-VEE-oh-lie)**:** air sacs in the lungs. One air sac is an *alveolus*.

IN SUMMARY

▮ The objectives of nutrition care during acute stress are to preserve muscle tissue, maintain immune defenses, and promote healing.

▮ To determine the energy needs of patients with acute illness, indirect calorimetry is recommended; otherwise, predictive equations may be used to estimate RMR or energy requirements. Protein recommendations are higher than DRI levels to help prevent tissue losses and allow healing of damaged tissue.

▮ Enteral or parenteral nutrition support or oral supplements may be used to meet the high nutrient needs of acutely stressed patients.

Case Study BOX 24-3 PATIENT WITH A SEVERE BURN

David Bray, a 42-year-old man, has been admitted to intensive care. He suffered a severe burn covering 35 percent of his body when he was trapped inside a burning building. His wife told the nurse that Mr. Bray's height is 6 feet and that he usually weighs about 175 pounds. The physician ordered lab work, including serum protein concentrations, but the results are not yet available.

1. Identify Mr. Bray's immediate needs after the injury. Describe the initial concerns of the health care team and the measures they might take soon after Mr. Bray's arrival at the hospital.

2. Considering Mr. Bray's condition, what problems might the health care team encounter when they attempt to obtain information that can help them assess his nutrition status? What additional concerns might they have if Mr. Bray was malnourished before he experienced the burn?

3. Estimate Mr. Bray's energy and protein needs (use a protein factor of 2.0 grams per kilogram). What problems may interfere with Mr. Bray's ability to meet his nutrient needs?

4. After Mr. Bray transitions to oral feedings, he is able to obtain only 65 percent of his energy requirements. What other feeding options may be considered?

24.3 Nutrition and Respiratory Stress

LO 24.3 Identify medical conditions that may lead to respiratory stress and describe their causes, potential consequences, and treatments.

Some medical problems upset the process of gas exchange between the air and blood and result in respiratory stress, which is characterized by a reduction in the blood's oxygen supply and an increase in carbon dioxide levels. Excessive carbon dioxide in the blood may disturb the breathing pattern enough to interfere with food intake. Moreover, the labored breathing caused by many respiratory disorders entails a higher energy cost than normal breathing does, raising energy needs and increasing carbon dioxide production further. Lung diseases make physical activity difficult and can lead to muscle wasting. Weight loss and malnutrition therefore become dangerous outcomes of some types of respiratory illnesses.

Chronic Obstructive Pulmonary Disease

Chronic obstructive pulmonary disease (COPD) refers to a group of conditions characterized by the persistent obstruction of airflow through the lungs. Figure 24-3 illustrates the main airways (**bronchi** and **bronchioles**) and air sacs (**alveoli**) of the normal respiratory system, and Figure 24-4 (p. 636) shows

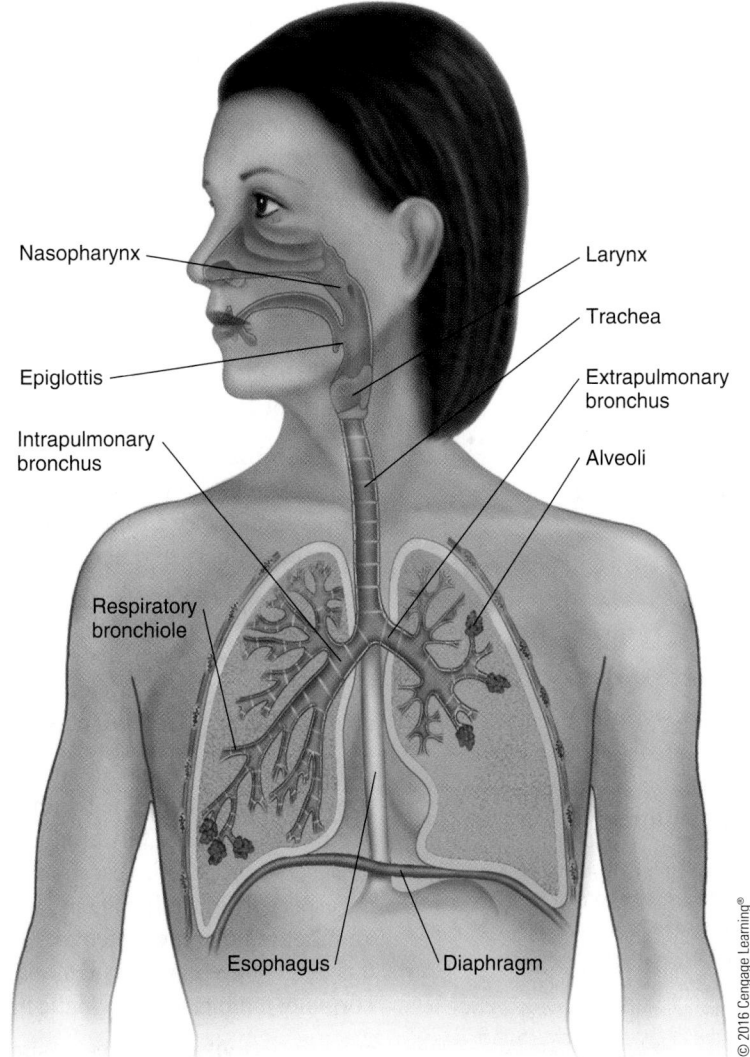

FIGURE 24-3 The Respiratory System
Inhaled air travels via the trachea to the bronchi and bronchioles, the major airways of the lungs. Oxygen and carbon dioxide are exchanged across the thin-walled alveoli, which are surrounded by capillaries.

© 2016 Cengage Learning®

Chronic bronchitis is characterized by inflammation, excessive secretion of mucus, and narrowing of the airways—factors that reduce normal airflow.

Emphysema is characterized by gradual destruction of the walls separating the alveoli and reduced lung elasticity.

© Cengage Learning®

Bronchus (plural: bronchi)

Alveolus (plural: alveoli)

Bronchiole

Healthy bronchi provide an open passageway for air. Healthy alveoli permit gas exchange between the air and blood.

FIGURE 24-4 Chronic Obstructive Pulmonary Disease

how they are altered in COPD. The two main types of COPD are **chronic bronchitis** and **emphysema,** and many patients display features of both conditions:[15]

▌ *Chronic bronchitis* is characterized by persistent inflammation and excessive secretions of mucus in the airways of the lungs, which may ultimately thicken and become too narrow for adequate mucus clearance. Chronic bronchitis is diagnosed when a chronic, productive cough persists for at least 3 months of the year for 2 consecutive years.

▌ *Emphysema* is characterized by the breakdown of the lungs' elastic structure and destruction of the walls of the bronchioles and alveoli, changes that significantly reduce the surface area available for respiration. Emphysema is diagnosed on the basis of clinical signs and the results of lung function tests.

Both chronic bronchitis and emphysema are associated with abnormal levels of oxygen and carbon dioxide in the blood and shortness of breath (**dyspnea**). COPD may eventually lead to respiratory or heart failure, and, together with other chronic respiratory illnesses, ranks as the third leading cause of death in the United States.[16]

COPD is a debilitating condition. Generally, dyspnea worsens as the disease progresses, resulting in dramatic reductions in physical activity and quality of life. Activities of daily living such as bathing or dressing may cause exhaustion or breathlessness. Weight loss and wasting are common in the advanced stages of disease and may result from hypermetabolism, poor food intake, and the actions of various inflammatory proteins.

Causes of COPD Cigarette smoking is the primary risk factor for COPD and is especially damaging when combined with respiratory infections or an occupational exposure to dusts or chemicals. Only a minority of smokers (about 25 percent[17]) develops COPD, however; thus, genetic susceptibility also contributes to its development. Genetic factors are especially likely in patients with early-onset COPD. Alpha-1-antitrypsin deficiency, an inherited disorder, accounts for 1 to 2 percent of COPD cases.[18] Individuals with this defect have inadequate blood levels of a plasma protein (alpha-1-antitrypsin) that normally inhibits the enzymatic breakdown of lung tissue.

Treatment of COPD The primary objectives of COPD treatment are to prevent the disease from progressing and relieve major symptoms (dyspnea and coughing). Individuals with COPD are encouraged to quit smoking to prevent disease progression and to get vaccinated against influenza and pneumonia to avoid complications. The most frequently prescribed medications are bronchodilators, which improve

chronic bronchitis (bron-KYE-tis)**:** a lung disorder characterized by persistent inflammation and excessive secretions of mucus in the main airways of the lungs.

emphysema (EM-fih-ZEE-mah)**:** a progressive lung disease characterized by the breakdown of the lungs' elastic structure and destruction of the walls of the bronchioles and alveoli, reducing the surface area involved in respiration.

dyspnea (DISP-nee-ah)**:** shortness of breath.

airflow, and corticosteroids (anti-inflammatory medications), which help to relieve symptoms and prevent exacerbations; note that corticosteroids promote catabolic processes and can exacerbate muscle loss. For people with severe COPD, supplemental oxygen therapy (12 hours daily) can maintain normal oxygen levels in the blood and reduce mortality risk (see Figure 24-5). Box 24-4 lists nutrition-related effects of the medications used to treat COPD.

Nutrition Therapy for COPD The main goals of nutrition therapy for COPD are to correct malnutrition (which affects up to 60 percent of COPD patients[19]), promote the maintenance of a healthy body weight, and prevent muscle wasting. Energy needs of COPD patients are usually raised due to hypermetabolism (about 20 percent above normal), which results from chronic inflammation and the increased workload of respiratory muscles.[20] Because underweight COPD patients have higher mortality rates, encouraging adequate food intake is generally the main focus of the nutrition care plan. Conversely, excess body weight places an additional strain on the respiratory system, and so COPD patients who are overweight or obese may benefit from energy restriction and gradual weight reduction.

FIGURE 24-5 Oxygen Therapy
Patients who need supplemental oxygen can use lightweight, portable equipment that allows them to move around freely.

Food intake often declines as COPD progresses, although the causes of poor intake vary among patients. Dyspnea may interfere with chewing or swallowing. Physical changes in the lungs and diaphragm may reduce abdominal volume, leading to early satiety. Appetite may be reduced by medications, depression, or altered taste perception (which may be due to the use of bronchodilators or the mouth dryness caused by chronic mouth breathing). Some patients may become too disabled to shop or prepare food or may lack adequate support at home. The clinician must assess the unique needs of a COPD patient before proposing a nutrition care plan.

Some patients may benefit from eating small, frequent meals spaced throughout the day rather than two or three large ones. The lower energy content of small meals reduces the carbon dioxide load, and the smaller meals may produce less abdominal discomfort and dyspnea. Some individuals may eat better if they receive supplemental oxygen at mealtimes. Consuming adequate fluids should be encouraged to help prevent the secretion of overly thick mucus; however, some patients should consume liquids between meals so as not to interfere with food intake. For undernourished persons, a high-kcalorie, high-protein diet may be helpful, but excessive energy intakes increase the amount of carbon dioxide produced and can increase respiratory stress. Oral supplements may be recommended as between-meal snacks to improve weight gain or endurance, but patients should be cautioned not to consume amounts that reduce energy intake at mealtime.

Pulmonary Formulas Enteral formulas designed for use in COPD provide more kcalories from fat and fewer from carbohydrate than standard formulas. The ratio of carbon dioxide production to oxygen consumption is lower when fat is consumed, so

BOX 24-4 DIET-DRUG INTERACTIONS

Check this table for notable nutrition-related effects of the medications discussed in this chapter.

Bronchodilators (albuterol, salmeterol, ipratropium, tiotropium)	**Gastrointestinal effect:** dry mouth (ipratropium, tiotropium) **Metabolic effect:** mild hypokalemia (albuterol, salmeterol)
Corticosteroids (inhaled) (fluticasone, beclomethasone)	**Gastrointestinal effect:** decreased taste sensation **Metabolic effect:** low bone density

John Todaro is an 84-year-old man who has severe emphysema that affects both lungs. He is 5 feet 9 inches tall and currently weighs 150 pounds, about 20 pounds less than his weight in earlier years. He lives with a daughter and son-in-law and eats meals with their family. He becomes breathless when eating and when walking around the house, and he feels tired much of the time. A medical clinic recently ordered oxygen therapy for home use, but supplies have not yet arrived. Mr. Todaro's daughter is concerned about her father's recent weight loss and breathlessness.

1. Assess Mr. Todaro's risk of malnutrition, using information from Table 14-6 in Chapter 14 (p. 401). What factors may have contributed to his weight loss?

2. What are possible reasons for Mr. Todaro's difficulty with eating? List some dietary suggestions that may help to improve his appetite and food intake. How might the use of oxygen therapy help?

3. Based on the history given, what factors may account for Mr. Todaro's tiredness? What suggestions would you give Mr. Todaro and his daughter regarding physical activity?

---

theoretically these formulas should lower respiratory requirements. However, research studies have not confirmed that the reduced-carbohydrate formulas improve clinical outcomes more than moderate energy intakes.[21]

Incorporating an Exercise Program Loss of muscle can be more readily prevented or reversed if the treatment plan includes an effective exercise program. With exercise, patients are likely to see improvements in their strength, endurance, and ability to perform activities of daily living. Both aerobic training and resistance exercise can be beneficial.[22] Some patients may need to increase activity gradually over a period of 4 to 6 weeks before reaching exercise goals.[23] The Case Study in Box 24-5 allows you to review the nutrition care for a patient with COPD.

Respiratory Failure

In **respiratory failure,** the gas exchange between the air and circulating blood is severely impaired, resulting in abnormal levels of tissue gases that can be life threatening. Any of a large number of conditions that cause lung injury or impair lung function can be the underlying cause of failure; examples include infection (such as pneumonia or sepsis), physical trauma, neuromuscular disorders, smoke inhalation, and airway obstruction.[24]

If an acute lung injury causes enough damage that emergency care is required to restore normal oxygen and carbon dioxide levels, the condition is known as **acute respiratory distress syndrome (ARDS)**. In ARDS, the lungs exhibit extensive inflammation and fluid buildup (called *pulmonary edema*) that interfere with lung ventilation and damage the alveoli. Later stages are associated with a proliferation of lung cells, which results in fibrosis and disrupts lung structure. A dangerous complication of ARDS is the progression to multiple organ dysfunction syndrome, described in the Nutrition in Practice following this chapter.

Consequences of Respiratory Failure Respiratory failure is characterized by severe **hypoxemia** (low oxygen levels in the blood) and **hypercapnia** (excessive carbon dioxide in the blood). The low oxygen content of tissues (**hypoxia**) impedes cellular function and may lead to cell death. Severe hypercapnia can cause **acidosis,** which interferes with normal functioning of the central nervous system. To compensate for respiratory failure, a person breathes more rapidly, and the heart rate increases. The skin may become sweaty and develop a bluish cast (**cyanosis**). Headache, confusion, and drowsiness may occur. Severe cases of respiratory failure can cause heart arrhythmias, and, ultimately, coma.

Treatment of Respiratory Failure The treatment of respiratory failure focuses on supporting lung function and correcting the underlying disorder. Because respiratory failure can be caused by a number of different conditions, treatment plans vary

---

respiratory failure: a potentially life-threatening condition in which inadequate respiratory function impairs gas exchange between the air and circulating blood, resulting in abnormal levels of tissue gases.

acute respiratory distress syndrome (ARDS): respiratory failure triggered by severe lung injury; a medical emergency that causes dyspnea and pulmonary edema and usually requires mechanical ventilation.

hypoxemia (high-pock-SEE-me-ah)**:** a low level of oxygen in the blood.

hypercapnia (high-per-CAP-nee-ah)**:** excessive carbon dioxide in the blood.

hypoxia (high-POCK-see-ah)**:** a low amount of oxygen in body tissues.

acidosis: acid accumulation in body tissues; depresses the central nervous system and may lead to disorientation and, eventually, coma.

cyanosis (sigh-ah-NOH-sis)**:** a bluish cast in the skin due to the color of deoxygenated hemoglobin. Cyanosis is most evident in individuals with lighter, thinner skin; it is mostly seen on lips, cheeks, and ears and under the nails.

considerably. Individuals with chronic lung disorders may be provided with oxygen therapy via a face mask or nasal tubing to relieve symptoms, whereas patients with ARDS receive mechanical ventilation until they are able to breathe independently (see Figure 24-6). Diuretics may be prescribed to help remove the fluid that has accumulated in lung tissue; other medications are provided to treat infections, keep airways open, or relieve inflammation. Complications are common in ARDS and must be forestalled to prevent multiple organ dysfunction.

Nutrition Therapy for Respiratory Failure Patients with lung injuries or ARDS are frequently hypermetabolic and/or catabolic and at high risk of muscle wasting. The primary concerns are therefore to provide enough energy and protein to sustain muscle mass and lung function without overtaxing the respiratory system. Specific recommendations include the following:

FIGURE 24-6 Mechanical ventilation controls the rate and amount of oxygen supplied to a person's airways.

- *Energy.* Energy needs typically range from 25 to 35 kilocalories per kilogram body weight per day; intakes may be started within this range and adjusted according to patient response.[25] The body weight used for determining energy needs may need to be corrected for pulmonary edema. Energy needs can also be estimated using either indirect calorimetry or predictive equations such as those described earlier. Overfeeding should be avoided because it can cause excessive carbon dioxide production and worsen respiratory function.

- *Protein.* Protein needs are increased in patients with lung inflammation or ARDS. For mild or moderate lung injury, protein recommendations range from 1.0 to 1.5 grams of protein per kilogram body weight per day. Patients with ARDS may require 1.5 to 2.0 grams of protein per kilogram body weight daily.

- *Fluids.* Although most patients have normal fluid requirements, fluid status should be monitored daily to prevent fluid imbalance. Some patients may require fluid restriction to prevent edema in lung tissue, whereas others may become dehydrated due to diuretic therapy or increased bronchial secretions.

Nutrition Support in Respiratory Failure Patients with severe cases of respiratory failure may be unable to eat meals and may require nutrition support. Enteral nutrition is used if the intestine is functional, and intestinal feedings may be preferred over gastric feedings because they reduce the risk of aspiration. Patients with acute lung injuries or ARDS may benefit from enteral formulas designed to reduce inflammation and promote healing; these formulas are typically fortified with omega-3 fatty acids and antioxidant nutrients.[26] Nutrient-dense formulas (1.5 to 2.0 kcalories per milliliter) are prescribed for patients with fluid restrictions. If the risk of aspiration is too high to continue enteral feedings, parenteral nutrition support may be considered.

IN SUMMARY

- Chronic obstructive pulmonary diseases are debilitating, progressive illnesses that can lead to malnutrition, muscle wasting, and activity intolerance. The goals of nutrition therapy are to improve food intake, maintain proper weight, preserve muscle tissue, and improve exercise endurance.

- Respiratory failure can result from conditions that cause lung injury or impair lung function. Acute respiratory distress syndrome is a severe form of respiratory failure that requires emergency care. Goals of nutrition therapy are to provide enough energy and protein to support lung function without burdening the respiratory system.

Nutrition Assessment Checklist FOR PEOPLE UNDERGOING METABOLIC OR RESPIRATORY STRESS

Medical History

Check the medical record to determine:

- Cause of stress
- Severity of stress
- Whether any organ system is compromised
- Whether nutrition support is required

For patients with COPD, check to determine:

- Degree of breathing difficulty
- Use of oxygen therapy
- Activity tolerance

Review the medical record for complications related to underfeeding or overfeeding, such as:

- Dehydration or fluid overload
- Electrolyte imbalances
- Fatty liver
- Hyperglycemia
- Hypertriglyceridemia

Medications

Record all medications and note:

- Side effects that may alter food intake or nutrition status

Dietary Intake

If the patient is not meeting nutrition goals:

- Monitor intakes to ensure that the patient is receiving the diet prescribed.
- Investigate appetite problems or difficulties with eating.
- Consider interventions to improve food intake.
- Consider the need for oral supplements.
- In patients with COPD, consider problems that may hamper the patient's ability to prepare or consume foods.

Anthropometric Data

Measure baseline height and weight, and monitor daily weights. Remember that body weight can fluctuate in acutely ill patients

who undergo fluid resuscitation. After the patient's weight has stabilized:

- Reevaluate protein and energy needs.
- Consider the need to alter the energy prescription to meet weight goals.

Laboratory Tests

Laboratory tests that may be affected by stress and therefore require careful interpretation include:

- Albumin
- C-reactive protein
- Serum iron and zinc
- Transferrin
- Transthyretin
- White blood cell count

Monitor laboratory tests for signs of:

- Dehydration or fluid overload
- Electrolyte and acid-base imbalances
- Hyperglycemia
- Hypertriglyceridemia
- Nutrient deficiencies
- Negative nitrogen balance
- Organ dysfunction or organ function that has normalized

Physical Signs

Regularly assess vital signs, including:

- Blood pressure
- Body temperature
- Pulse
- Respiratory rate

Look for physical signs of:

- Protein-energy malnutrition
- Dehydration or fluid overload
- Nutrient deficiencies and excesses

Clinical Applications

1. Adam is a 29-year-old male who is 6 feet 2 inches tall and has a usual body weight of 180 pounds. He underwent emergency surgery following a serious injury and is now being cared for in the intensive care unit. Using the method described in Box 24-2 on p. 633, estimate Adam's energy requirement. Estimate his protein requirement, using the factor 1.5 grams per kilogram of body weight.

2. Ayesha is a 23-year-old law student who was admitted to the hospital following an automobile accident in which she broke several bones and ruptured part of her small intestine. She has been in the hospital for several weeks and has just begun eating table foods. Her brother, who was driving the vehicle, was also seriously injured and nearly lost his life. Aside from the increased nutritional needs imposed by the stress of the

accident, discuss how the following factors might interfere with Ayesha's ability to improve her nutrition status:

▮ Ayesha's injuries are painful.

▮ Ayesha's medications cause drowsiness.

▮ Ayesha is depressed.

▮ Ayesha is often out of her room for X-rays and other diagnostic tests when the menus and food trays arrive.

▮ Ayesha's food intake is sometimes restricted due to the procedures she is undergoing.

How might these problems be resolved to improve Ayesha's food intake?

Self Check

1. Which of the following metabolic changes accompanies acute stress?
   a. Hypoglycemia
   b. Reduced heart and respiratory rates
   c. Elevated immune responses
   d. Muscle protein catabolism

2. After an injury occurs, typical changes in the damaged tissue include all of the following *except:*
   a. reduced capillary permeability.
   b. increased blood flow.
   c. warmth.
   d. fluid accumulation.

3. How do nonsteroidal anti-inflammatory drugs suppress inflammatory processes?
   a. They interfere with histamine secretion.
   b. They inhibit eicosanoid synthesis.
   c. They impair the actions of certain cytokines.
   d. They inhibit the absorption of omega-6 fatty acids.

4. Examples of acute-phase proteins include all of the following *except:*
   a. C-reactive protein.   c. albumin.
   b. hepcidin.   d. fibrinogen.

5. Which of the following statements concerning protein and energy recommendations during acute metabolic stress is true?
   a. Protein and energy recommendations are similar to those for healthy people.
   b. Protein and energy recommendations are reduced because a stressed individual cannot metabolize nutrients normally.
   c. Acutely stressed individuals can benefit from as much protein and energy as can be provided.
   d. Protein and energy recommendations are often increased to minimize muscle tissue losses.

6. Hypocaloric feedings may benefit critical care patients who are:
   a. elderly.
   b. obese.
   c. receiving mechanical ventilation.
   d. accumulating fluid.

7. The primary risk factor for COPD is:
   a. alpha-1 antitrypsin deficiency.
   b. occupational exposure to dusts or chemicals.
   c. cigarette smoking.
   d. frequent respiratory infections.

8. A primary feature of emphysema is:
   a. obstruction within the bronchi.
   b. obstruction within the bronchioles.
   c. destruction of the walls separating the alveoli.
   d. excessive lung elasticity.

9. The weight loss and wasting that often occur in COPD can be caused by:
   a. reduced food intake.
   b. increased metabolic rate.
   c. reduced exercise tolerance.
   d. all of the above.

10. Nutrition therapy for a person with respiratory failure includes:
    a. careful attention to providing enough, but not too much, energy.
    b. a generous fluid intake to facilitate mucus clearance.
    c. a high fat intake to prevent weight loss and wasting.
    d. a high carbohydrate intake to increase carbon dioxide production.

Answers to these questions can be found in Appendix H.

Notes

1. P. A. Fitzgerald, Adrenal medulla and paraganglia, in D. G. Gardner and D. Shoback, eds., *Greenspan's Basic & Clinical Endocrinology* (New York: McGraw-Hill, 2011), pp. 345–393; T. B. Carroll and coauthors, Glucocorticoids and adrenal androgens, in D. G. Gardner and D. Shoback, eds., *Greenspan's Basic & Clinical Endocrinology* (New York: McGraw-Hill, 2011), pp. 285–327.

2. P. C. Calder, Mechanisms of action of (n-3) fatty acids, *Journal of Nutrition* 142 (2012): 592S–599S.

3. G. H. Johnson and K. Fritsche, Effect of dietary linoleic acid on markers of inflammation in healthy persons: A systematic review of randomized controlled trials, *Journal of the Academy of Nutrition and Dietetics* 112 (2012): 1029–1041.

4. D. S. Pisetsky, Laboratory testing in the rheumatic diseases, in L. Goldman and A. I. Schafer, eds., *Goldman's Cecil Medicine* (Philadelphia: Saunders, 2012), pp. 1651–1656; V. Kumar and coauthors, Acute and chronic inflammation, in V. Kumar and coeditors, *Robbins and Cotran Pathologic Basis of Disease* (Philadelphia: Saunders, 2010), pp. 43–77.

5. S. A. McClave and coauthors, Guidelines for the provision and assessment of nutrition support therapy in the adult critically ill patient: Society of Critical Care Medicine (SCCM) and American Society for Parenteral and Enteral Nutrition (A.S.P.E.N.), *Journal of Parenteral and Enteral Nutrition* 33 (2009): 277–316.

6. P. Choban and coauthors and the American Society for Parenteral and Enteral Nutrition, A.S.P.E.N. clinical guidelines: Nutrition support of hospitalized adult patients with obesity, *Journal of Parenteral and Enteral Nutrition* (2013): 714–744; McClave and coauthors, 2009.

7. Academy of Nutrition and Dietetics, *Nutrition Care Manual* (Chicago: Academy of Nutrition and Dietetics, 2014).

8. P. Choban and coauthors and the American Society for Parenteral and Enteral Nutrition, 2013; McClave and coauthors, 2009.

9. L. Bollhalder and coauthors, A systematic literature review and meta-analysis of randomized clinical trials of parenteral glutamine supplements, *Clinical Nutrition* 32 (2013): 213–223.

10. D. K. Heyland and coauthors, Glutamine and antioxidants in the critically ill patient: A post hoc analysis of a large-scale randomized trial, *Journal of Parenteral and Enteral Nutrition* 38 (2014): *in press*.

11. P. E. Wischmeyer, Evolution of nutrition in critical care: How much, how soon? *Critical Care* 17 (2013): S7, doi: 10.1186/cc11505.

12. K. A. Kudsk, Nutrition support for the patient with surgery, trauma, or sepsis, in A. C. Ross and coeditors, eds., *Modern Nutrition in Health and Disease* (Baltimore: Lippincott Williams & Wilkins, 2014), pp. 1273–1288.

13. Kudsk, 2014.

14. Academy of Nutrition and Dietetics, 2014; McClave and coauthors, 2009.

15. D. E. Niewoehner, Chronic obstructive pulmonary disease, in L. Goldman and A. I. Schafer, eds., *Goldman's Cecil Medicine* (Philadelphia: Saunders, 2012), pp. 537–544; A. N. Husain, The lung, in V. Kumar and coeditors, *Robbins and Cotran Pathologic Basis of Disease* (Philadelphia: Saunders, 2010), pp. 677–737.

16. A. M. Miniño, Death in the United States, 2011, *NCHS Data Brief* 115 (Hyattsville, MD: National Center for Health Statistics, 2013).

17. N. M. Patel and M. M. Johnson, Nutrition in respiratory diseases, in A. C. Ross and coeditors, eds., *Modern Nutrition in Health and Disease* (Baltimore: Lippincott Williams & Wilkins, 2014), pp. 1385–1395.

18. Niewoehner, 2012.

19. Patel and Johnson, 2014.

20. R. A. Wise, Chronic obstructive pulmonary disease, in R. S. Porter and J. L. Kaplan, eds., *Merck Manual of Diagnosis and Therapy* (Whitehouse Station, NJ: Merck Sharp and Dohme Corp., 2011), pp. 1889–1902; C. C. Kao, Resting energy expenditure and protein turnover are increased in patients with severe chronic obstructive pulmonary disease, *Metabolism* 60 (2011): 1449–1455.

21. A. Malone, Enteral formula selection, in P. Charney and A. Malone, eds., *Pocket Guide to Enteral Nutrition* (Chicago: Academy of Nutrition and Dietetics, 2013), pp. 120–152.

22. W. D. Reid and coauthors, Exercise prescription for hospitalized people with chronic obstructive pulmonary disease and comorbidities: A synthesis of systematic reviews, *International Journal of COPD* 7 (2012): 297–320.

23. Wise, 2011.

24. L. D. Hudson and A. S. Slutsky, Acute respiratory failure, in L. Goldman and A. I. Schafer, eds., *Goldman's Cecil Medicine* (Philadelphia: Saunders, 2012), pp. 629–638.

25. Academy of Nutrition and Dietetics, 2014.

26. K. L. Coughlin, S. I. Austhof, and C. Hamilton, Nutrition support: Indication and efficacy, in A. Skipper, ed., *Dietitian's Handbook of Enteral and Parenteral Nutrition* (Sudbury, MA: Jones & Bartlett Learning, 2012), pp. 22–45; McClave and coauthors, 2009.

LO 24.4 Describe the development of multiple organ dysfunction syndrome and identify major risk factors and approaches to treatment for this condition.

Multiple organ dysfunction syndrome (MODS), also called *multiple organ failure,* is a frequent cause of death in intensive care patients. Described as the progressive dysfunction of two or more of the body's organ systems, MODS most often involves the lungs, kidneys, and liver. MODS is not a disease *per se,* but rather a late stage of severe illness or injury that results from a severe inflammatory response (discussed in Chapter 24). MODS can be initiated by a number of very different critical illnesses and conditions, including respiratory failure, sepsis, burn injuries, trauma, and pancreatitis. This Nutrition in Practice discusses how MODS develops, the manner in which it is treated, and the importance of its prevention.

How long has MODS been a major clinical problem?

MODS was recognized as a clinical entity only after World War II. Prior to the mid-20th century, patients with severe illnesses or multiple injuries frequently died of shock or circulatory failure. After fluid replacement and blood transfusions became standard treatments, the kidneys became the organs at highest risk, and kidney failure became the most common cause of death. Eventually, physicians learned to better support kidney function by providing appropriate electrolyte solutions and improving urine output. With improved kidney care, the lungs became the most vulnerable organ after severe injury. Improved treatment of respiratory failure eventually led to the current situation: advances in critical care allow patients to survive severe illnesses and injuries, but the body's defenses often overburden organs that were not originally injured.

Why does critical illness sometimes lead to MODS?

As discussed earlier in Chapter 24, injury and infection cause the release of chemical mediators that have systemic (whole-body) effects. A severe, persistent inflammatory response can lead to the systemic inflammatory response syndrome (SIRS), which is associated with a constellation of symptoms including fever, raised heart and respiratory rates, and abnormal white blood cell counts. SIRS is a normal adaptive response to a severe insult, but if not reversed quickly enough it can progress to shock, which is characterized by extremely low blood pressure and an inadequate blood supply for the tissues and organs of the body.[1]

As might be expected from a systemic reduction in blood availability, shock can impair numerous organ systems. The abnormal delivery of oxygen and nutrients to tissues and insufficient removal of wastes result in irreversible injury to cells and tissues. Although each organ system is affected differently, ultimately one or more organs may begin to fail. The failure of one organ may place excessive demands on another, causing the second to fail as well. The progression of SIRS to MODS reflects the inability of the

body's defenses and medical treatments to counter the detrimental effects of a sustained and potent inflammatory response.

The specific pathophysiology of MODS is poorly understood. Although early reports attempted to link the development of MODS directly to sepsis, sepsis is not present in all cases. Infection often results from impaired immune function and therefore is a frequent consequence of MODS, but it is not necessarily the underlying trigger of organ dysfunction. Recall from this chapter that sepsis gives rise to symptoms identical to those seen in SIRS. Figure NP24-1 illustrates the relationships among SIRS, infection, sepsis, and MODS.

Do organs fail in a specific pattern?

Although the clinical course of MODS differs substantially among patients, the sequence of organ dysfunction often follows a similar pattern: first the lungs fail, then the heart, and finally the liver, kidneys, and gastrointestinal tract.[2] Other organs or systems may also become involved, and each additional failure reduces the likelihood of survival. Table NP24-1 (p. 644) lists the organs and systems most often involved in MODS and the potential consequences of their failure.

Are there any risk factors for MODS?

Epidemiological studies have identified a number of factors that increase risk. For example, people who develop MODS are often older, have multiple or severe injuries, or are obese.[3] Table NP24-2

FIGURE NP24-1 Relationships among SIRS, Sepsis, and Multiple Organ Dysfunction Syndrome

*After critical injury, shock may sometimes precede and be the cause of SIRS.

© Cengage Learning®

TABLE NP24-1 Physiological Effects of Organ or System Failure

Organ or System	Effects of Failure
Lungs	Inability to maintain gas exchange
Heart	Low cardiac output, low blood pressure, inadequate circulation, shock
Liver	Altered metabolic processes
Kidneys	Inability to regulate blood volume, maintain electrolytes, remove wastes
GI tract	Impaired digestion and absorption, abnormal bleeding, bacterial translocation
Immune system	Infection, sepsis
Coagulation system	Excessive bleeding or blood clotting
Central nervous system	Decreased perceptions, brain injury, coma

© 2016 Cengage Learning®

lists the major risk factors associated with MODS, some of which are discussed below:

■ *Age.* Patients over 55 years old are several times more likely to develop MODS than are younger patients. In elderly patients, the increased risk may be due to the presence of chronic illnesses that directly affect organ function, such as heart disease, lung disease, diabetes, or liver damage. Aging also decreases the functional reserve of organs, thereby reducing an older patient's ability to deal with the additional stress that arises during critical illness.

■ *Severity of SIRS.* The length of time that SIRS persists is related to the development of MODS. Patients who have SIRS that persists for more than three days are more likely to develop MODS than patients who have SIRS for less than two days.

■ *Infection.* Prolonged SIRS can suppress immune function and increase the risk of developing an infection. During hospital stays, critically ill patients often contract pneumonia—the principal infection associated with MODS. The risks of infection and sepsis greatly increase with the use of invasive catheters, which are frequently needed during intensive care to provide oxygen support, intravenous fluid resuscitation, nutrition support, and urine clearance.

■ *Blood transfusions.* Blood transfusions are immunosuppressive and may increase a patient's risks of developing infection or sepsis. Blood transfusions frequently have adverse effects that can add

TABLE NP24-2 Factors That Influence Risk of Multiple Organ Dysfunction Syndrome

■ Age over 55 years
■ Obesity
■ Prior chronic disease
■ Persistent SIRS
■ Major infection
■ Blood transfusions
■ Severity of tissue injury
■ Length of time between injury and arrival at hospital
■ Malnutrition

© 2016 Cengage Learning®

further stress: they may cause acute lung injury, allergic reactions, red blood cell hemolysis (breakdown), and other complications.

What is the treatment for MODS?

Once MODS has developed, extensive medical support is needed until the inflammatory response has abated. Unfortunately, aggressive treatments can have damaging effects of their own and may cause further injury to organs that are already weakened by illness. Health practitioners must therefore be aware of the adverse effects of aggressive therapies and remain alert to a patient's responses to treatments. Therapies that are often used to manage MODS include the following:[4]

■ *Lung support.* Mechanical ventilation is used to assist injured lungs and sustain gas exchange.

■ *Fluid resuscitation.* Fluids and electrolytes are supplied to restore blood volume and maintain electrolyte balance.

■ *Support of heart and blood vessel function.* Medications help to sustain or increase cardiac output and maintain adequate blood pressure.

■ *Kidney support.* Hemofiltration or dialysis helps to prevent the buildup of toxic metabolites in the blood.

■ *Protection against infection.* Antibiotic therapy may reverse or prevent infections.

■ *Nutrition support.* Enteral and parenteral nutrition support provide nutrients, help to prevent excessive wasting, and promote recovery.

What can be done to reduce the incidence of MODS?

Because mortality rates for MODS are so high, prevention must be considered at the earliest stages of injury and treatment, before an excessive inflammatory response can cause further damage. Health practitioners have learned to identify the conditions that can increase organ stress whether they are due to a disease process, an inflammatory response, or an aggressive treatment that is intended to provide organ support. Although improvements in care over the past few decades have reduced some of the complications that arise during intensive care, rates of mortality from MODS have not changed. Thus, a focus on prevention is critical until a better understanding of the pathophysiology of MODS is achieved, which may lead to additional therapeutic options.

Notes

1. J. A. Russell, Shock syndromes related to sepsis, in L. Goldman and A. I. Schafer, eds., *Goldman's Cecil Medicine* (Philadelphia: Saunders, 2012), pp. 658–666.

2. D. C. Dewar and coauthors, Post-injury multiple organ failure, *Trauma* 13 (2011): 81–91.

3. Dewar and coauthors, 2011.

4. Russell, 2012; D. J. Cook, Approach to the patient in a critical care setting, in L. Goldman and A. I. Schafer, eds., *Goldman's Cecil Medicine* (Philadelphia: Saunders, 2012), pp. 624–626.

25

Energy- and Protein-Modified Diets for Cancer and HIV Infection

25.1 Cancer

LO 25.1 Explain how cancer develops, and discuss the factors that influence cancer risk, the effects of cancer on nutrition status, and the main approaches to cancer treatment.

25.2 HIV Infection

LO 25.2 Describe the potential consequences of HIV infection, its medical treatment, and nutrition therapy for this condition.

25.3 Nutrition in Practice: Ethical Issues in Nutrition Care

LO 25.3 Identify the ethical principles that guide treatment decisions, and compare the responsibilities of physicians and patients in determining the appropriate care during medical emergencies.

Although **cancers** and **human immunodeficiency virus (HIV)** infections are distinct disorders, from a nutritional standpoint they share some similarities. Both disorders have debilitating effects that influence nutritional needs, and both can lead to severe wasting in advanced cases. These illnesses require nutrition therapy that is highly individualized based on the symptoms manifested and the organ systems involved.

BOX 25-1

Cancers are classified by the tissues or cells from which they develop:

- *Adenocarcinomas* arise from glandular tissues.
- *Carcinomas* arise from epithelial tissues.
- *Leukemias* arise from white blood cell precursors.
- *Lymphomas* arise from lymphoid tissue.
- *Melanomas* arise from pigmented skin cells.
- *Myelomas* arise from plasma cells in the bone marrow.
- *Sarcomas* arise from connective tissues, such as muscle or bone.

25.1 Cancer

LO 25.1 Explain how cancer develops, and discuss the factors that influence cancer risk, the effects of cancer on nutrition status, and the main approaches to cancer treatment.

Cancer, the growth of **malignant** tissue, is the second most common cause of death in the United States, ranking just below cardiovascular disease. Cancer is not a single disorder, however; there are many different kinds of malignant growths. The various types of cancer have different characteristics, occur in different locations in the body, progress differently, and require different treatments (see Box 25-1). Whereas an isolated, non-spreading type of skin cancer may be removed in a physician's office with no effect on nutrition status, advanced cancers—especially those of the gastrointestinal (GI) tract and pancreas—can seriously impair nutrition status. In the United States, the most common cancers are breast cancer (in women), prostate cancer (in men), lung cancer, and colorectal cancers.[1]

How Cancer Develops

The development of cancer, called **carcinogenesis,** often proceeds slowly and continues for several decades. A cancer usually arises from either genetic mutations or the altered expression of genes that regulate cell division in a single cell.[2] These changes may promote cellular growth, interfere with growth restraint, or prevent cellular death. The affected cell thereby loses its built-in capacity for halting cell division and produces daughter cells with the same genetic defects. As the abnormal mass of cells, called a **tumor** (or *neoplasm*), grows, a network of blood vessels forms to supply the tumor with the nutrients it needs to support its growth. The tumor can disrupt the functioning of the normal tissue around it, and some tumor cells may **metastasize,** spreading to other regions in the body. In leukemia (cancer affecting the white blood cells), the abnormal cells do not form a tumor; they accumulate in the blood and other tissues. Figure 25-1 illustrates the steps in cancer development.

Normal cells → Initiation → Genetic mutations or changes in gene expression induce abnormal division of a single cell. → Promotion → Proliferation of the altered cells results in formation of a tumor. → Further tumor development →

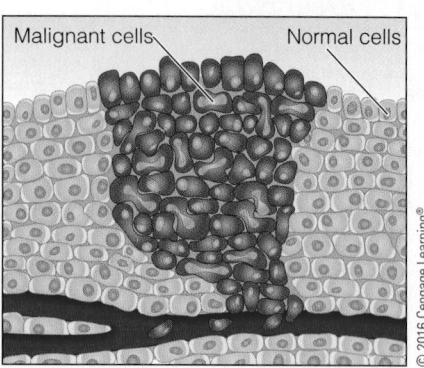

Malignant cells   Normal cells

The cancerous tumor releases cells into the bloodstream or lymphatic system (metastasis).

© 2016 Cengage Learning®

FIGURE 25-1 **Cancer Development**

TABLE 25-1 Environmental Factors That Increase Cancer Risk

Environmental Factors	Cancer Sites
Aflatoxins (toxins in moldy peanuts or grains)	Liver
Arsenic	Skin, lung, bladder, kidney
Asbestos[a]	Larynx, lung, pleura, ovary, peritoneum
Chromium (hexavalent) compounds	Nasal cavity, lung
Estrogen-progesterone menopausal therapy	Endometrium, breast
Immunosuppressive drugs	Lymphoid tissues, liver, skin
Infection with *Helicobacter pylori*	Stomach
Infection with hepatitis B and hepatitis C viruses	Liver
Infection with human papillomavirus (HPV)	Cervix, vulva, vagina, penis, anus, oropharynx
Ionizing radiation (X-rays, radon, radioactive isotopes, and other sources)	White blood cells (leukemia), thyroid, lung, salivary glands, esophagus, stomach, colon, rectum, skin, bladder, breast, bone, liver, kidney, brain
Tobacco[b]	Lip, oral cavity, nasal cavity, pharynx, larynx, lung, esophagus, stomach, colon, rectum, liver, pancreas, kidney, bladder
Ultraviolet radiation (sun exposure)	Skin

© 2016 Cengage Learning®

[a] Risk is greatly increased in cigarette smokers.

[b] A combined exposure to tobacco and alcohol multiplies the risks of developing cancers of the oral cavity, pharynx, larynx, and esophagus.

Sources: M. J. Thun and A. Jemel, Epidemiology of cancer, in L. Goldman and A. I. Schafer, eds., *Goldman's Cecil Medicine* (Philadelphia: Saunders, 2012), pp. 1177–1182; World Cancer Research Fund/American Institute for Cancer Research, *Food, Nutrition, Physical Activity, and the Prevention of Cancer: A Global Perspective* (Washington, DC: American Institute for Cancer Research, 2007), pp. 157–171.

The reasons why cancers develop are numerous and varied. Vulnerability to cancer is sometimes inherited: a genetic defect may alter DNA structure, function, or repair. Some metabolic processes may initiate carcinogenesis, as when phagocytes (immune cells) produce oxidants that cause DNA damage, or when chronic inflammation increases the rate of cell division and the risk of a damaging mutation. More often, cancers are caused by interactions between a person's genes and the environment. Exposure to cancer-causing substances, or **carcinogens,** may induce genetic mutations that lead to cancer; other substances may stimulate division or proliferation of the altered cells. Table 25-1 provides examples of environmental factors that increase cancer risk.

Nutrition and Cancer Risk

Like other environmental factors, diet and lifestyle strongly influence cancer risk. Various food components can alter processes of DNA repair, gene expression, or cell differentiation in ways that affect cancer development.[3] Moreover, some food compounds can directly damage DNA, alter carcinogen metabolism in the liver, or inhibit the formation of carcinogens in the body. Energy balance and growth rate can both influence cancer risk due to their effects on cell division rates (and therefore, mutation risk) and hormones that regulate cell growth. Table 25-2 (p. 648) includes examples of nutrition-related factors that may increase or decrease the risk of developing cancer.

Nutrition and Increased Cancer Risk As shown in Table 25-2, obesity is a risk factor for a number of different cancers, including some relatively common cancers such as colon cancer and postmenopausal breast cancer. Obesity increases cancer risk, in part, by altering the levels of hormones that influence cell growth, such as insulin, the sex hormones, and several kinds of growth factors.[4] For example, in the case of breast cancer in postmenopausal women, the hormone estrogen is likely involved: obese

cancers: diseases characterized by the uncontrolled growth of a group of abnormal cells, which can destroy adjacent tissues and spread to other areas of the body via the lymph or blood.

human immunodeficiency virus (HIV): the virus that causes acquired immune deficiency syndrome (AIDS). HIV destroys immune cells and progressively impedes the body's ability to fight infections and certain cancers.

malignant (ma-LIG-nent)**:** describes a cancerous cell or tumor, which can injure healthy tissue and spread cancer to other regions of the body.

carcinogenesis (CAR-sin-oh-JEN-eh-sis)**:** the process of cancer development.

tumor: an abnormal tissue mass that has no physiological function; also called a *neoplasm* (NEE-oh-plazm). Tumors may be malignant (cancerous) or benign (noncancerous).

metastasize (meh-TAS-tah-size)**:** to spread from one part of the body to another; refers to cancer cells.

carcinogens (CAR-sin-oh-jenz or car-SIN-oh-jenz)**:** substances that can cause cancer (the adjective is *carcinogenic*).

TABLE 25-2 Nutrition-Related Factors That Influence Cancer Risk

Nutrition-Related Factors[a]	Cancer Sites
Factors that may increase cancer risk	
Obesity	Esophagus, colon, rectum, pancreas, gallbladder, kidney, breast (postmenopausal), endometrium
Red meat, processed meats	Colon, rectum
Salted and salt-preserved foods	Stomach
Beta-carotene supplements	Lung[b]
High-calcium diets (over 1500 mg daily)	Prostate
Alcohol[c]	Mouth, pharynx, larynx, esophagus, colon, rectum, liver, breast
Low level of physical activity[d]	Colon, rectum, breast (postmenopausal), endometrium
Factors that may decrease cancer risk	
Fruits and nonstarchy vegetables	Lung, mouth, pharynx, larynx, esophagus, stomach
Carotenoid-containing foods	Lung, mouth, pharynx, larynx, esophagus
Tomato products	Prostate
Allium vegetables (onion, garlic)	Stomach, colon, rectum
Vitamin C–containing foods	Esophagus
Folate-containing foods	Pancreas, colon, rectum
Fiber-containing foods	Colon, rectum
Milk and calcium supplements	Colon, rectum
High level of physical activity[d]	Colon, rectum, breast (postmenopausal), endometrium

[a] Altered cancer risk is associated with high intakes of the dietary substances listed.

[b] Cancer risk is increased in tobacco smokers and may not apply to other groups.

[c] A combined exposure to alcohol and tobacco multiplies the risks of developing cancers of the oral cavity, pharynx, larynx, and esophagus.

[d] Physical activity may influence cancer risk by altering body fatness, intestinal transit time, insulin sensitivity, hormone levels, enzyme activities, and immune responses.

Sources: W. C. Willett and coauthors, Diet, obesity, and physical activity, in B. W. Stewart and C. B. Wild, eds., *World Cancer Report 2014* (Lyon, France: International Agency for Research on Cancer; 2014), pp. 171–184; World Cancer Research Fund/American Institute for Cancer Research, *Food, Nutrition, Physical Activity, and the Prevention of Cancer: A Global Perspective* (Washington, DC: American Institute for Cancer Research, 2007).

women have higher estrogen levels than lean women do because adipose tissue is the primary source of estrogen after menopause. The increase in circulating estrogen may create an environment that encourages carcinogenesis in breast tissue.[5]

About 1 in 30 cancer deaths can be attributed to alcohol consumption, which correlates strongly with cancers of the head and neck, liver, colon, rectum, and breast.[6] For head and neck cancers, the risk is multiplied when alcohol drinkers also smoke tobacco. These findings illustrate why the potential benefits of moderate alcohol consumption on cardiovascular disease risk must be weighed against the potential dangers.

Food preparation methods can influence carcinogen production (see Box 25-2). Cooking meat, poultry, and fish at high temperatures (by frying or broiling, for example) may cause carcinogens to form in these foods.[7]* Carcinogens also accompany the smoke that adheres to foods during grilling and are present in the charred surfaces of grilled meat and fish.** However, the cancer risk from eating such foods is unclear because the biological effects of these carcinogens are modulated by other dietary components, including compounds in vegetables and other plant foods.

*These carcinogens are *heterocyclic amines,* formed when amino acids, sugars, and creatine react at high temperatures.

**These carcinogens are *polycyclic aromatic hydrocarbons,* formed from the incomplete combustion of organic compounds.

BOX 25-2

To minimize carcinogen formation during cooking:

■ Marinate meats before cooking.

■ Use lower-heat options such as roasting, stewing, or microwaving.

■ Choose lean meats for grilling, and take care not to blacken surfaces.

■ To reduce smoke formation, prevent fat from dripping onto the heat source.

Nutrition and Decreased Cancer Risk Consuming fruits and vegetables may reduce the risks of some cancers (see Table 25-2 and Figure 25-2).[8] Possible benefit has been attributed, in part, to nutrients and phytochemicals with antioxidant activity, as these substances may prevent or reduce the oxidative reactions in cells that cause DNA damage. In addition, phytochemicals may inhibit carcinogen production in the body, enhance immune responses that protect against cancer development, or promote enzyme reactions that inactivate carcinogens. The B vitamin folate (provided by certain fruits and vegetables) functions in DNA synthesis and repair; thus, inadequate folate intakes may allow DNA damage to accumulate. Fruits and vegetables also contribute dietary fiber, which may help to protect against colon and rectal cancers by diluting potential carcinogens in fecal matter and accelerating their removal from the GI tract. Table 25-3 summarizes dietary and lifestyle practices that may help to reduce cancer risk.

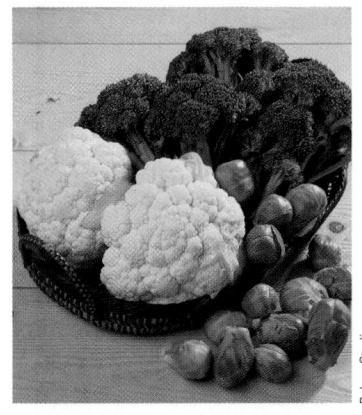

FIGURE 25-2 Cruciferous Vegetables and Cancer Risk
Cruciferous vegetables, such as cauliflower, broccoli, and brussels sprouts, may inhibit several types of cancer, including cancers of the prostate, bladder, and lung.

Polara Studios

Consequences of Cancer

Once cancer develops, its consequences depend on the location of the cancer, its severity, and the treatment. The complications that develop are often due to the tumor's impingement on surrounding tissues. Nonspecific effects of cancer include

TABLE 25-3 Guidelines for Reducing Cancer Risk

Achieve and maintain a healthy body weight throughout life.

▪ Be as lean as possible within the normal range of body weight for your height.

▪ Avoid weight gain and increases in waist circumference throughout adulthood.

Be physically active as part of everyday life.

▪ For adults: engage in moderate physical activity (equivalent to brisk walking) for at least 30 minutes each day; increase duration or intensity of activity as fitness improves.

▪ For children and adolescents: engage in moderate to vigorous activity for at least 60 minutes each day.

▪ Limit sedentary habits such as watching television.

Choose a healthy diet that emphasizes plant sources.

▪ Limit consumption of energy-dense foods (>225 kcal per 100 g food) and sugary drinks that contribute to weight gain.

▪ Consume relatively unprocessed grains and/or legumes with every meal. Choose whole-grain products instead of processed (refined) grains.

▪ Consume at least 2½ cups of nonstarchy vegetables and fruits every day.

Limit consumption of foods that may increase cancer risk.

▪ Limit consumption of red meats (beef, pork, or lamb) to 18 ounces per week.

▪ Limit consumption of processed meats (those preserved by smoking, curing, or salting).

▪ Avoid salt-preserved, salted, and salty foods.

▪ Avoid moldy grains and legumes.

Limit consumption of alcoholic beverages.

▪ For women: consume no more than one drink daily.

▪ For men: consume no more than two drinks daily.

Aim to meet nutritional needs through the diet.

▪ Obtain necessary nutrients from the diet. Dietary supplements are not recommended for cancer prevention, and they may have unexpected adverse effects.

Avoid using tobacco in any form.

© 2016 Cengage Learning®

Sources: L. H. Kushi and coauthors, American Cancer Society guidelines on nutrition and physical activity for cancer prevention: Reducing the risk of cancer with healthy food choices and physical activity, *CA: A Cancer Journal for Clinicians* 62 (2012): 30–67; World Cancer Research Fund/American Institute for Cancer Research, *Food, Nutrition, Physical Activity, and the Prevention of Cancer: A Global Perspective* (Washington, D.C.: American Institute for Cancer Research, 2007).

anorexia, malaise, weight loss, night sweats, and fever.[9] During the early stages, many cancers produce no symptoms, and the person may be unaware of the threat to health.

Anorexia and Reduced Food Intake Anorexia is a major contributor to the weight loss often associated with cancer. Some factors that contribute to anorexia or otherwise reduce food intake include the following:

▮ *Mental stress.* A cancer diagnosis can cause distress, anxiety, and depression, all of which may reduce appetite. Facing and undergoing cancer treatments induces additional psychological stress.

▮ *Chronic nausea and early satiety.* People with cancer frequently experience nausea and a premature feeling of fullness after eating small amounts of food.

▮ *Fatigue.* People with cancer may tire easily and lack the energy to prepare and eat meals. If severe weight loss occurs, these tasks become even more difficult.

▮ *Pain.* People in pain may have little interest in eating, particularly if eating makes the pain worse.

▮ *Gastrointestinal obstructions.* A tumor may partially or completely obstruct a portion of the GI tract, causing complications such as nausea and vomiting, early satiety, delayed gastric emptying, and bacterial overgrowth. Some patients with obstructions are unable to tolerate oral diets.

▮ *Effects of cancer therapies.* Chemotherapy and radiation treatments for cancer frequently have side effects that make food consumption difficult, such as nausea, vomiting, dry mouth, altered taste perceptions, **oral mucositis** (inflamed oral mucosa), esophagitis, dysphagia, abdominal pain, and diarrhea.

Metabolic Changes The metabolic changes that arise in cancer contribute to weight loss and nutrient depletion.[10] **Cytokines,** released by both tumor cells and immune cells, induce an inflammatory and catabolic state. Cancer patients exhibit an increased rate of **protein turnover,** but reduced muscle protein synthesis. Muscle contributes amino acids for gluconeogenesis (glucose production), further depleting the body's supply of protein. Triglyceride breakdown increases, elevating serum lipids. Many patients develop insulin resistance. These metabolic abnormalities help to explain why people with cancer fail to regain lean tissue or maintain healthy body weights even when they are consuming adequate energy and nutrients.

Cancer Cachexia The combined effects of a poor appetite, accelerated and abnormal metabolism, and the diversion of nutrients to support tumor growth result in a lower supply of energy and nutrients at a time when demands are high. **Cancer cachexia**—characterized by anorexia, weight loss, muscle wasting, anemia, and fatigue—develops in up to 50 percent of cancer patients and is responsible for as many as 20 percent of cancer deaths.[11] Cachexia may be indicated by an involuntary weight loss of more than five percent of body weight; care must be taken not to overlook unintentional weight loss in patients who are overweight or obese. Unlike in starvation, nutrition intervention alone is unable to reverse cachexia.[12]

Treatments for Cancer

The primary medical treatments for cancer—surgery, chemotherapy, radiation therapy, or any combination of the three—aim to remove cancer cells, prevent further tumor growth, and alleviate symptoms.[13] The likelihood of effective treatment is highest with early detection and intervention. Because treatment decisions are difficult and cancer therapies have considerable side effects, patients rely on health care providers to help them make informed decisions.

anorexia: lack of appetite.

oral mucositis: inflammation of the oral mucosa; signs may include swelling, redness, mouth sores, bleeding, or ulcerations in mucosal tissue.

cytokines: signaling proteins produced by the body's cells; the cytokines that promote inflammation and catabolism include tumor necrosis factor-α, interleukin-1, interleukin-6, and γ-interferon.

protein turnover: the continuous degradation and synthesis of the body's proteins.

cancer cachexia (ka-KEK-see-ah): a wasting syndrome associated with cancer that is characterized by anorexia, weight loss, muscle wasting, and fatigue.

Surgery Surgery is performed to remove tumors, determine the extent of cancer, and protect nearby tissues. Often, surgery must be followed by other cancer treatments to prevent the growth of new tumors. The acute metabolic stress caused by surgery raises protein and energy needs and can exacerbate wasting. Surgery also contributes to pain, fatigue, and anorexia, all of which can reduce food intake at a time when nutritional needs are substantial. Blood loss contributes to nutrient losses and further exacerbates malnutrition. Some surgeries can have long-term effects on nutritional status (see Table 25-4).

Chemotherapy **Chemotherapy** relies on the use of drugs to treat cancer, and is used to inhibit tumor growth, shrink tumors before surgery, and prevent or suppress metastasis. Some cancer drugs (such as **methotrexate**) interfere with the process of cell division; others sterilize cells that are in a resting phase and are not actively dividing. Unfortunately, most of these drugs have toxic effects on normal cells as well and are especially damaging to rapidly dividing cells, such as those of the GI tract, skin, and bone marrow. The bone marrow damage can impair the production of red blood cells (causing anemia) and white blood cells (causing **neutropenia**). Some of the newer drugs target properties specific to cancer cells and are better tolerated by the body's tissues. Table 25-5 describes some nutrition-related side effects that may result from chemotherapy.

Radiation Therapy **Radiation therapy** treats cancer by bombarding cancer cells with X-rays, gamma rays, or various atomic particles. These treatments generate reactive forms of oxygen, such as superoxide and hydroxyl radicals, which can damage cellular DNA and cause cell death. Newer techniques can focus the radiation directly at tumors and minimize damage to nearby tissues. An advantage of radiation therapy

TABLE 25-4 Nutrition-Related Side Effects of Cancer Surgeries

Head and Neck Surgeries
- Aspiration
- Dry or sore mouth
- Reduced chewing or swallowing ability
- Reduced sense of taste or smell

Esophageal Resection
- Acid reflux
- Altered gastric motility
- Reduced swallowing ability

Gastric Resection
- Dumping syndrome
- Early satiety
- Inadequate gastric acid secretion
- Malabsorption of iron, folate, and vitamin B_{12}

Intestinal Resection
- Bile insufficiency
- Diarrhea
- Fluid and electrolyte imbalances
- General malabsorption

Pancreatic Resection
- Diabetes mellitus
- General malabsorption

© 2016 Cengage Learning®

TABLE 25-5 Nutrition-Related Side Effects of Chemotherapy and Radiation Therapy

	Reduced Nutrient Intake	Increased Nutrient Losses	Altered Metabolism
Chemotherapy	Abdominal pain	Diarrhea	Anemia, neutropenia
	Anorexia	Gastrointestinal inflammation	Fluid and electrolyte imbalances as a consequence of vomiting, diarrhea, or malabsorption
	Nausea and vomiting	Malabsorption	
	Oral mucositis	Vomiting	
	Reduced taste sensation		Hyperglycemia
			Interference with vitamins or body compounds
			Negative nitrogen and micronutrient balances
			Secondary effects of malnutrition, infection, or inflammation
Radiation therapy	Anorexia	Blood loss from intestine and bladder	Fluid and electrolyte imbalances as a consequence of vomiting, diarrhea, or malabsorption
	Damage to teeth, jaws, or salivary glands	Diarrhea	
	Dysphagia	Fistulas	
	Esophagitis	Intestinal obstructions	Secondary effects of malnutrition, infection, or inflammation
	Nausea and vomiting	Malabsorption	
	Oral mucositis	Radiation enteritis	
	Reduced salivary secretions	Vomiting	
	Reduced taste sensation		

chemotherapy: the use of drugs to arrest or destroy cancer cells; these drugs are called *antineoplastic agents.*

methotrexate: an anticancer drug that inhibits cell division. Methotrexate closely resembles the B vitamin folate, which is needed for DNA synthesis; the drug works by blocking activity of the enzyme that converts folate to its active form (see Figure 15-3, p. 426).

neutropenia: a low white blood cell (neutrophil) count, which increases susceptibility to infection.

radiation therapy: the use of X-rays, gamma rays, or atomic particles to destroy cancer cells.

over surgery is that it can shrink tumors while preserving organ structure and function. Compared with chemotherapy, radiation therapy is better able to target specific regions of the body, rather than involving all body cells. Nonetheless, radiation therapy can damage healthy tissues and sometimes has long-term detrimental effects on nutrition status (see Table 25-5). Radiation to the head and neck can damage the salivary glands and taste buds, causing inflammation, dry mouth, and a reduced sense of taste; in severe cases, the damage may be permanent. Radiation treatment in the lower abdomen can cause **radiation enteritis,** an inflammatory condition of the small intestine that causes nausea, vomiting, and diarrhea; the condition may persist for months or years and lead to chronic malabsorption in some individuals.

Hematopoietic Stem Cell Transplantation **Hematopoietic stem cell transplantation** replaces the blood-forming stem cells that have been destroyed by high-dose chemotherapy or radiation therapy. These procedures may be used to treat leukemia, lymphomas, and multiple myeloma.[14] If possible, stem cells are collected from the patient's bone marrow or circulating blood before chemotherapy or radiation treatment begins so that a separate donor is not required. If another person's cells are used, the patient must take immunosuppressant drugs to prevent **graft-versus-host disease,** in which the donor's immune cells attack the recipient's tissues, and **graft rejection,** in which the recipient's immune system rejects the donor cells. Graft-versus-host disease often damages tissues of the GI tract, leading to severe intestinal inflammation, profuse diarrhea, and bleeding.

The high-dose chemotherapy or radiation therapy preceding stem cell transplants and the immunosuppressant drugs often required afterward can impair immune function substantially, increasing the risk of infection and foodborne illness. Patients are often unable to consume adequate food during or after these procedures and usually require nutrition support.

Biological Therapies Newer therapies for cancer include the use of biological molecules that stimulate immune responses against cancer cells (also called *immunotherapy*). These substances include antibodies, cytokines, and other proteins that strengthen the body's immune defenses, enable the destruction of cancer cells, or interfere with cancer development in some way. Although side effects vary, many of these treatments can cause anorexia, GI symptoms, and general discomfort, reducing a person's ability or desire to consume adequate amounts of food.

Medications to Combat Anorexia and Wasting Medications prescribed to stimulate the appetite and promote weight gain include megestrol acetate (Megace), a synthetic compound similar in structure to the hormone progesterone, and dronabinol (Marinol), which resembles the psychoactive ingredient in marijuana and stimulates the appetite at doses that have minimal mental effects. Under investigation are medications that promote muscle protein synthesis, induce the secretion of growth hormone or growth factors, or reduce catabolism.[15]

Alternative Therapies Many patients turn to **complementary and alternative medicine (CAM)** to assist them in their fight against cancer. Although few abandon conventional medicine, up to 80 percent of cancer patients combine one or more CAM approaches with standard treatment.[16] Many patients do not discuss their use of CAM with physicians.

Multivitamin and herbal supplements are among the most frequently used CAM therapies. Although many supplements can be used without risk, some may have adverse effects or interfere with conventional treatments. Use of the herb St. John's wort, for example, can reduce the effectiveness of some anticancer drugs.[17] As another example, some studies suggest that antioxidant supplements interfere with chemotherapy and radiation treatments.[18] Most current research suggests that dietary supplements (including multivitamins) are unable to improve outcomes or survival after a cancer diagnosis and may actually increase mortality rates.[19]

radiation enteritis: inflammation of intestinal tissue caused by radiation therapy.

hematopoietic stem cell transplantation: transplantation of the stem cells that produce red blood cells and white blood cells; the stem cells are obtained from bone marrow (*bone marrow transplantation*) or circulating blood.

▮ *haima* = blood

▮ *poiesis* = to make

graft-versus-host disease: a condition in which the immune cells in transplanted tissue (the graft) attack recipient (host) cells, leading to widespread tissue damage.

graft rejection: destruction of donor tissue by the recipient's immune system, which recognizes the donor cells as foreign.

complementary and alternative medicine (CAM): health care practices that have not been proved to be effective and consequently are not included as part of conventional treatment (see Nutrition in Practice 15).

CHAPTER TWENTY FIVE

Nutrition Therapy for Cancer

The goals of nutrition therapy for cancer patients are to maintain a healthy weight, preserve muscle tissue, prevent or correct nutrient deficiencies, and provide a diet that patients can tolerate and enjoy despite the complications of illness.[20] Appropriate nutrition care helps patients preserve their strength and improves recovery after stressful cancer treatments. Moreover, malnourished cancer patients develop more complications and have shorter survival times than patients who maintain good nutrition status.

Because there are many forms of cancer and a variety of potential treatments, nutritional needs among cancer patients vary considerably. Furthermore, a person's needs may change at different stages of illness. Patients should be screened for malnutrition when cancer is diagnosed and reassessed during the treatment and recovery periods.

Protein and Energy For patients at risk of weight loss and wasting, the focus of nutrition care is to ensure appropriate intakes of protein and energy. Protein requirements are often between 1.0 and 1.6 grams per kilogram of body weight daily.[21] Patients should consume adequate energy to prevent weight loss; those who cannot eat enough food may be able to meet their needs by supplementing the diet with nutrient-dense oral supplements.[22] Box 25-3 provides suggestions that can help to increase the energy and protein content of meals.

How To BOX 25-3 INCREASE KCALORIES AND PROTEIN IN MEALS

To increase the energy content of a meal, try these suggestions:

- *Meat.* Choose high-fat meat instead of lean meat. Sauté or pan-fry meat instead of baking or roasting it, and use sauces or gravies liberally. Sprinkle bacon bits or sausage pieces on vegetable dishes.

- *Cheese.* Include cheese slices or cream cheese in sandwiches made with luncheon meat. Spread cream cheese on raw vegetables, toast, and crackers or mix into dishes that contain chopped fruit.

- *Half-and-half and cream.* Replace milk or water with half-and-half or cream in breakfast cereals, soups, mashed potatoes, sauces, hot chocolate, and desserts. Add sour cream or cream sauce to soup, vegetable dishes, and potato dishes. Add whipped cream to fruit salad and desserts.

- *Breads and cereals.* Choose high-fat grain products such as granola, pancakes, waffles, French toast, and biscuits. Prepare hot cereal with whole milk or cream, or added fat.

- *Fruit.* Mash avocados to make guacamole, or use mashed avocado as a sandwich spread. Add chopped dried fruit to salads and baked goods. Snack on dried fruit between meals.

- *Nuts.* Add chopped nuts to stir-fried vegetables, pasta dishes, fruit salad, and green salad. Use nut meats in baked products. Spread nut butters on bread or crackers.

- *Butter or margarine.* Melt on pasta, potatoes, rice, and cooked vegetables. Add to hot cereal, soup, and casseroles. Spread liberally on bread, crackers, and rolls.

- *Mayonnaise or salad dressing.* Add to pasta, tuna, and potato salads. Use as a dressing for raw or cooked vegetables.

- *Beverages.* Replace water and non-kcaloric beverages with sweetened drinks, fruit juice, and milk shakes. Drink whole milk instead of low-fat or nonfat milk. Add strawberry or chocolate syrup to plain milk to boost kcalories.

These suggestions can help to add protein to a meal:

- *Meat.* Add small chunks of meat to soup, potato salad, egg dishes, bean dishes, and casseroles. Add chunks of chicken or turkey to green salads. Add minced meat to pasta sauce and vegetable dishes.

- *Eggs.* Add raw eggs when preparing casseroles, meatballs, and hamburgers. Add chopped hard-cooked eggs to salads, vegetable dishes, sandwich fillings, and pasta and potato salads.

- *Cheese.* Melt on scrambled eggs, vegetable dishes, potatoes, hamburgers, meat loaf, and casseroles. Add cottage cheese to egg dishes, pasta recipes, and salad dressing. Grate hard cheese and sprinkle on soup, salad, and cooked vegetables. Avoid using reduced-fat cheese.

- *Milk.* Use in place of water when preparing cereal or soup. Use cream sauces (which are made with milk) to flavor vegetable and pasta dishes.

- *Powdered milk (use full-fat milk powder if available).* Add to recipes that include milk. Dissolve extra milk powder into milk-containing beverages. Stir into hot cereal, potato dishes, casseroles, and sauces. Add to scrambled eggs, hamburgers, and meat loaf.

- *Protein supplements.* Snack on protein bars between meals. Add protein powder to beverages and shakes. Drink meal replacement formulas, such as Ensure or Boost, instead of juice or soda.

TABLE 25-6 Dietary Considerations for Specific Cancers

Cancer Sites	Common Complications[a]	Possible Dietary Measures
Brain and nervous system	Chewing or swallowing difficulty, headache, altered taste or smell sensation, difficulty feeding oneself	Mechanically altered diet, use of adaptive feeding devices (see Nutrition in Practice 22)
Head and neck[b]	Chewing or swallowing difficulty, aspiration, dry mouth, altered taste or smell sensation, inflamed mucosa	Tube feeding, mechanically altered diet
Esophagus	Swallowing difficulty, aspiration, obstruction, acid reflux, inflamed mucosa	Tube feeding, mechanically altered diet
Stomach	Anorexia, early satiety, reduced secretion of gastric acid and intrinsic factor, delayed stomach emptying, dumping syndrome, malabsorption, nutrient deficiencies	Tube feeding (for obstruction or unmanageable dumping syndrome); postgastrectomy diet; small, frequent meals; limited sugar intake; modified fiber intake (see Chapter 17); nutrient supplementation
Intestine	Inflamed mucosa, bacterial overgrowth, obstruction, lactose intolerance, general malabsorption, bile insufficiency, nutrient deficiencies, short bowel syndrome (if resected), altered bowel function, fluid and electrolyte imbalances	Tube feeding or total parenteral nutrition for obstruction, enteritis, or short bowel syndrome; fat- and lactose-restricted diet (see Chapter 19); nutrient supplementation
Pancreas	Reduced secretion of digestive enzymes, bile insufficiency, general malabsorption, nutrient deficiencies, hyperglycemia	Enzyme replacement (see Chapter 19); small, frequent meals; fat-restricted diet; carbohydrate-controlled diet (Chapter 21); nutrient supplementation

© 2016 Cengage Learning®

[a] Actual complications depend on the exact location of the cancer and the specific methods used for treating the cancer.

[b] Includes cancers of the salivary glands, oral and nasal cavities, pharynx, and larynx.

Although weight loss is a problem for many cancer patients, breast cancer patients often gain weight.[23] The weight gain occurs during the first 2 years after breast cancer diagnosis and is associated with an increase in total body fat. By discussing weight maintenance soon after diagnosis and encouraging physical activity, health practitioners can help patients avoid unnecessary weight gain.

Managing Symptoms and Complications A thorough nutrition assessment often uncovers specific problems or symptoms that interfere with food consumption. Table 25-6 lists dietary considerations related to cancers affecting different sites in the body. Box 25-4 describes dietary strategies that may alleviate symptoms and improve food intake. Patients' responses to these strategies can vary considerably, and in some cases, a number of adjustments may be necessary.

Low-Microbial Diet Patients with suppressed immunity or neutropenia (such as those who have undergone hematopoietic stem cell transplants or are taking immunosuppressant drugs) may be prescribed a **low-microbial diet** (sometimes called a *neutropenic diet*), which includes only foods that are unlikely to be contaminated with bacteria or other microbes.[24] Acceptable foods include well-cooked meats and eggs, pasteurized milk products, well-washed fruits and vegetables, and shelf-stable packaged foods. Foods that must be avoided include unwashed raw fruits and vegetables, unpasteurized juices and milk products, leftover luncheon meats, and foods from salad bars or street vendors. In addition, patients should follow safe food-handling practices to minimize the risk of foodborne illness (see Nutrition in Practice 5 for details).

Enteral and Parenteral Nutrition Support Tube feedings or parenteral nutrition may be necessary for patients who are experiencing complications that interfere with food intake or have long-term or permanent gastrointestinal impairment.[25] For example, many patients who undergo radiation therapy for head and neck cancers develop dysphagia or oral mucositis and may benefit from tube feeding. Parenteral nutrition is reserved for patients who have inadequate GI function, such as those with severe radiation enteritis. Whenever possible, enteral nutrition is strongly preferred over parenteral nutrition, to preserve GI function and avoid infection.

low-microbial diet: a diet that contains foods that are unlikely to be contaminated with bacteria or other microbes.

BOX 25-4 HELP PATIENTS HANDLE FOOD-RELATED PROBLEMS

In people with cancer or HIV infection, various complications can interfere with food intake. Health care providers can try to identify a patient's specific problems and offer appropriate solutions. Not every suggestion will work for each person; encourage patients to experiment and find strategies that work best.

I just don't have an appetite.

▪ Eat small meals and snacks at regular times each day.

▪ Eat the largest meal at the time of day when you feel the best.

▪ Include nutrient-dense foods in meals, and consume them before other foods.

▪ Indulge in favorite foods throughout the day. Serve foods attractively.

▪ Avoid drinking large amounts of liquids before or with meals.

▪ Eat in a pleasant and relaxed environment. Eat with family and friends when possible.

▪ Listen to your favorite music or enjoy a TV or radio program while you eat.

▪ Ask your doctor about appetite-enhancing medications.

I am too tired to fix meals and eat.

▪ Let family members and friends prepare food for you.

▪ Obtain foods that are easy to prepare and easy to eat, such as sandwiches, ready-to-eat soups and entrees, ready-made foods from the deli counter, frozen dinners, instant breakfast drinks, and energy bars.

▪ Find time to rest before you attempt to prepare a large meal.

▪ Prepare soups, stews, and casserole dishes in sufficient quantity to provide enough for several meals, so that you will have enough to eat at times when you are too tired to cook.

Foods just don't taste right.

▪ Brush your teeth or use mouthwash before you eat.

▪ Consume foods chilled or at room temperature. Use plastic, rather than metal, eating utensils.

▪ Choose eggs, fish, poultry, and milk products instead of meat dishes.

▪ Experiment with sauces, seasonings, herbs, spices, and sweeteners to improve food taste and flavor.

▪ Save your favorite foods for times when you are not feeling nauseated.

I am nauseated a lot of the time, and sometimes I need to vomit.

▪ Consume liquids throughout the day to replace fluids.

▪ If you become nauseated from chemotherapy treatments, avoid eating for at least two hours before treatments.

▪ Consume your largest meal at a time when you are least likely to feel nauseous.

▪ Try consuming smaller meals, and eat slowly. Experiment with foods to see if some foods cause nausea more than others.

▪ Avoid foods and meals that have strong odors or are fatty, greasy, or gas forming.

I have problems chewing and swallowing food.

▪ Experiment with food consistencies to find the ones you can manage best. Thin liquids, dry foods, and sticky foods (such as peanut butter) are often difficult to swallow.

▪ Add sauces and gravies to dry foods.

▪ Drink fluids during meals to ease chewing and swallowing.

▪ Try using a straw to drink liquids. Experiment with beverage thickeners if you cannot tolerate thin beverages.

▪ Tilt your head forward and backward to see if you can swallow more easily when your head is positioned differently.

I have sores in my mouth, and they hurt when I eat.

▪ Try eating chilled or frozen foods; they are often soothing.

▪ Try soft foods such as ice cream, milk shakes, bananas, applesauce, mashed potatoes, cottage cheese, and macaroni and cheese. Mix dry foods with sauces or gravies.

▪ Cut foods into smaller pieces, so they are less likely to irritate the mouth.

▪ Avoid foods that irritate mouth sores, such as citrus fruits and juices, tomatoes and tomato-based products, spicy foods, foods that are very salty, foods with seeds (such as poppy seeds and sesame seeds) that can scrape the sores, and coarse foods such as raw vegetables, crackers, corn chips, and toast.

▪ Ask your doctor about using a local anesthetic solution such as lidocaine before eating to reduce the pain.

▪ Use a straw for drinking liquids, in order to bypass the sores.

My mouth is really dry.

▪ Rinse your mouth with warm salt water or mouthwash frequently. Avoid using mouthwash that contains alcohol.

▪ Drink small amounts of liquid frequently between meals.

▪ Ask your doctor or pharmacist about medications or saliva substitutes that can help a dry mouth condition.

▪ Use sour candy or chewing gum to stimulate the flow of saliva.

▪ Sip fluids frequently while eating. Add broth, sauces, gravies, mayonnaise, butter, or margarine to dry foods.

▪ Make sure you brush your teeth and floss regularly to prevent tooth decay and oral infections.

I am having trouble with constipation.

▪ Drink plenty of fluids. Try warm fluids, especially in the morning.

▪ Eat whole-grain breads and cereals, nuts, fresh fruits and vegetables, prunes, and prune juice. Avoid refined carbohydrate foods such as white bread, white rice, and enriched pasta.

▪ Engage in physical activity regularly.

(continued)

- Try an over-the-counter bulk-forming agent, such as methylcellulose (Citrucel), psyllium (Metamucil or Fiberall), or polycarbophil (Fiber-Lax).

I am having trouble with diarrhea.

- To avoid dehydration, drink plenty of fluids throughout the day. Diluted fruit juices, sports drinks, and salty broths and soups are good choices. Avoid caffeine- and alcohol-containing beverages. For severe diarrhea, try oral rehydration formulas that are commercially prepared.

- Avoid foods and beverages that increase gas, such as legumes, onions, vegetables of the cabbage family, foods that contain sorbitol or mannitol, and carbonated beverages.

- Try using lactase enzyme replacements when you use milk products in case you are experiencing lactose intolerance. Yogurt and aged cheeses may be easier to tolerate than milk and fresh cheeses.

- Avoid fatty foods if you are fat intolerant. Try reducing your intake of whole-grain breads and cereals if they worsen the diarrhea.

- Eat small, frequent meals instead of large ones. Try consuming cool or lukewarm foods instead of very cold or hot foods.

- Ask your doctor about using a bulk-forming agent or antidiarrheal medication.

IN SUMMARY

- Cancer arises from mutations in (or altered expression of) the genes that control cell division. Some dietary substances promote carcinogenesis, while others may help to prevent cancer.

- Cancer's effects on nutrition status depend on the type of cancer a person has, its severity, and the methods used to treat the cancer. Cancer cachexia is a frequent complication of cancer and may be a consequence of anorexia, altered metabolism, and responses to cancer treatment.

- Medical treatments for most cancers include surgery, chemotherapy, and/or radiation therapy. Nutrition therapy aims to minimize weight loss and wasting, correct deficiencies, and manage complications that impair food intake.

The Case Study in Box 25-5 allows you to apply information about nutrition and cancer to a clinical situation.

Case Study BOX 25-5 WOMAN WITH CANCER

Sheri Nixon is a 58-year-old public relations consultant who was recently diagnosed with colon cancer after a routine colonoscopy, a procedure in which the colon is examined using a flexible tube attached to an optical device. Mrs. Nixon is scheduled to have surgery to remove the segment of colon that contains the tumor and to determine if the cancer has spread to the surrounding lymph nodes and, possibly, other organs. The nurse completing the nutrition assessment finds that Mrs. Nixon is 5 feet 5 inches tall and weighs 178 pounds. Mrs. Nixon usually spends most of the day sitting and has little time to engage in recreational exercise. Her diet typically includes red meat at both lunch and dinner, and she consumes one or two glasses of wine with both meals. She eats two or three servings of fruits and vegetables each day, although she does not like green leafy vegetables very much. She rarely drinks milk or consumes milk products.

1. Review Table 25-2 on p. 648, and describe the factors in Mrs. Nixon's diet and lifestyle that may have contributed to the development of colon cancer.

2. What symptoms and complications may arise after colon surgery and impair nutrition status? If the cancer team decides that Mrs. Nixon needs follow-up chemotherapy, how might the chemotherapy affect her nutrition status?

3. If Mrs. Nixon is unresponsive to treatment and her cancer progresses, she may develop cancer cachexia. Describe this syndrome, its causes, and its consequences.

4. Provide suggestions that may help Mrs. Nixon handle the following problems should they develop: poor appetite, fatigue, taste alterations, nausea and vomiting, chewing and swallowing difficulties, mouth sores, dry mouth, diarrhea, constipation, and weight loss.

TABLE 25-7 The HIV and AIDS Epidemic at a Glance, 2012

Stage of Epidemic	World	Sub-Saharan Africa	North America
Individuals living with HIV infection or AIDS	35,300,000	25,000,000	1,300,000
Individuals newly infected with HIV	2,300,000	1,600,000	48,000
AIDS-related deaths	1,600,000	1,200,000	20,000

Source: Joint United Nations Programme on HIV/AIDS (UNAIDS), *2013 Global Fact Sheet,* available at www.unaids .org/en/media/unaids/contentassets/documents/epidemiology/2013/gr2013/20130923_FactSheet_Global_en.pdf; site visited May 7, 2014.

© 2016 Cengage Learning®

25.2 HIV Infection

LO 25.2 Describe the potential consequences of HIV infection, its medical treatment, and nutrition therapy for this condition.

Possibly the most infamous infectious disease today is **acquired immune deficiency syndrome (AIDS).** AIDS develops from infection with human immunodeficiency virus (HIV), which attacks the immune system and disables a person's defenses against other diseases, including infections and certain cancers. Then these diseases—which would produce mild, if any, illness in people with healthy immune systems—destroy health and life.

Although the global incidence of HIV infection has been declining in recent years, its prevalence continues to be high in sub-Saharan Africa, where it affects about 4.7 percent of the adult population (see Table 25-7).[26] Fortunately, remarkable progress has been made in understanding and treating HIV infection. Access to antiretroviral drugs continues to increase throughout the world, reducing AIDS-related deaths and the risk of HIV transmission.

As there is still no cure for AIDS, the best course is prevention. HIV is most often sexually transmitted and can be spread by direct contact with contaminated body fluids, such as blood, semen, vaginal secretions, and breast milk. Because many people remain symptom-free during the early stages of infection, they may not realize that they can pass the infection to others. To reduce the spread of HIV infection, individuals at risk (see Table 25-8) are encouraged to undergo testing. A blood test can usually detect HIV antibodies within several months after exposure and, often, after 2 or 3 weeks. An estimated 21 percent of persons in the United States who have HIV infection are unaware that they are infected.[27]

Consequences of HIV Infection

HIV infection destroys immune cells that have a protein called CD4 on their surfaces.[28] The cells most affected are the **helper T cells,** also called *CD4+ T cells* because the presence of CD4 is a primary characteristic. Other cells that have the CD4 protein (and can be infected by HIV) include tissue macrophages and certain cells of the central nervous system. Early symptoms of HIV infection are nonspecific and may include fever, sore throat, malaise, swollen lymph nodes, skin rashes, muscle and joint pain, and diarrhea. After these symptoms subside, many people remain symptom-free for 5 to 10 years or even longer. If the HIV infection is not treated, however, the depletion of T cells eventually increases the person's susceptibility to **opportunistic infections**—that is, infections caused by microorganisms that normally do not cause disease in healthy individuals.

The term *AIDS* applies to the advanced stages of HIV infection, in which the inability to fight illness allows a number of serious diseases and complications to develop; such **AIDS-defining illnesses** include severe infections, certain cancers, and

TABLE 25-8 Risk Factors for HIV Infection

- History of receiving blood transfusions or blood components before 1985
- Infant born to mother with HIV infection
- Intravenous drug use in which syringes are shared among users
- Sexual contact with intravenous drug users, prostitutes, or individuals with a history of HIV or other sexually transmitted diseases
- Sexual contact with multiple partners
- Unsafe sexual practices

© Cengage Learning®

acquired immune deficiency syndrome (AIDS): the late stage of illness caused by infection with the human immunodeficiency virus (HIV); characterized by severe damage to immune function.

helper T cells: lymphocytes that have a specific protein called CD4 on their surfaces and therefore are also known as *CD4+ T cells;* these are the cells most affected in HIV infection.

opportunistic infections: infections caused by microorganisms that normally do not cause disease in healthy people but are damaging to persons with compromised immune function.

AIDS-defining illnesses: diseases and complications associated with the later stages of an HIV infection, including wasting, recurrent bacterial pneumonia, opportunistic infections, and certain cancers.

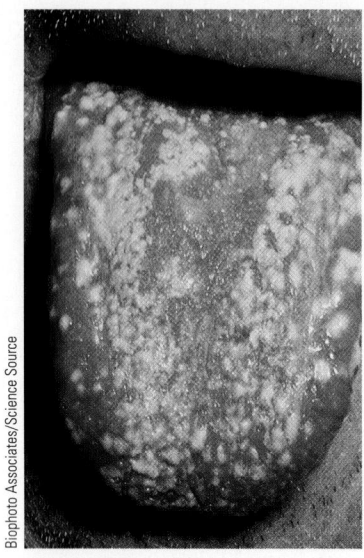

FIGURE 25-3 **Oral Candidiasis**

Oral candidiasis (also known as *thrush*) is characterized by a milky white coating or individual white patches on the tongue and other oral tissues.

candidiasis: a fungal infection on the mucous membranes of the oral cavity and elsewhere; usually caused by *Candida albicans.*

herpes simplex virus: a common virus that can cause blisterlike lesions on the lips and in the mouth.

Kaposi's (kah-POH-seez) **sarcoma:** a common cancer in HIV-infected persons that is characterized by lesions in the skin, lungs, and GI tract.

wasting of muscle tissue. Without treatment, AIDS develops in 26 to 36 percent of HIV-infected persons within 7 years.[29] Health practitioners evaluate disease progression by measuring the concentrations of helper T cells and circulating virus (called the *viral load*) and by monitoring clinical symptoms. Although drug therapies can dramatically slow the progression of HIV infection, the drugs' side effects may make it difficult for some patients to adhere to treatments.

Weight Loss and Wasting Even with effective treatment of HIV infection, weight loss and wasting remain common problems among HIV-infected patients. The wasting has been linked with accelerated disease progression, reduced strength, and fatigue. In the later stages of AIDS, the wasting is severe and increases the risk of death. Much as in cancer, the wasting associated with HIV infection has many causes: anorexia and inadequate food intake, nutrient malabsorption, altered metabolism, and various diet-drug interactions. *HIV-associated wasting* is diagnosed in patients who unintentionally lose 5 percent of body weight within 3 months, 7.5 percent within 6 months, or 10 percent within 12 months.[30]

Reduced Food Intake As mentioned, inadequate food intake is a key factor in the development of wasting. Poor food intake may result from various factors, including the following:

- *Oral infections.* The oral infections associated with HIV infection may cause discomfort and interfere with food consumption. Common infections include **candidiasis** and **herpes simplex virus** infection. Oral candidiasis (commonly called *thrush;* see Figure 25-3) can cause mouth pain, dysphagia (difficulty swallowing), and altered taste sensation; an oral infection with herpes simplex virus may cause painful lesions around the lips and in the mouth.

- *Cancer.* As described earlier in this chapter, cancer leads to anorexia for numerous reasons. In addition, **Kaposi's sarcoma,** a type of cancer frequently associated with HIV infection, can cause lesions in the mouth and throat that make eating painful.

- *Medications.* The medications given to treat HIV infection, other infections, and cancer often cause anorexia, nausea and vomiting, altered taste sensation, food aversions, and diarrhea.

- *Respiratory disorders.* Respiratory infections, including pneumonia and tuberculosis, are common in people with HIV infection. Symptoms may include chest pain, shortness of breath, and cough, which interfere with eating and contribute to anorexia.

- *Emotional distress, pain, and fatigue.* The physical and social problems that accompany chronic illness may cause fear, anxiety, and depression, which contribute to anorexia. Pain and fatigue, which are often associated with some disease complications, can lead to anorexia and difficulty with eating.

GI Complications GI complications in HIV-infected patients may result from opportunistic infections, medications, or the HIV infection itself.[31] In addition to the oral infections described previously, infections may develop in the esophagus, stomach, and intestines. The medications that treat some of these infections may promote bacterial overgrowth. In addition, many patients develop nausea, vomiting, and diarrhea from the medications used to suppress HIV. As a result of these multiple problems, HIV-infected patients using standard treatments face an extremely high risk of malnutrition due to the combination of GI discomfort, bacterial overgrowth, malabsorption, and nutrient losses from vomiting, steatorrhea, and diarrhea.

Patients in the advanced stages of HIV infection often develop pathological changes in the small intestine referred to as *AIDS enteropathy*.[32] The condition is characterized by villus atrophy and blunting, intestinal cell losses, and inflammation. The result is a substantial reduction in the intestinal absorptive area, causing malabsorption, diarrhea, and weight loss.

Lipodystrophy Many patients who use drug therapies to suppress HIV infection develop abnormalities in body fat and fat metabolism known as **lipodystrophy**.[33] Patients may lose fat from the face and extremities, accumulate abdominal fat, or both. Also observed are breast enlargement (in both men and women), fat accumulation at the base of the neck (sometimes called a **buffalo hump;** see Figure 25-4), and benign growths composed of fat tissue (called **lipomas**). The changes in body composition are often disfiguring and may cause physical discomfort; moreover, patients often develop hypertriglyceridemia, elevated low-density lipoprotein (LDL) cholesterol levels, reduced high-density lipoprotein (HDL) cholesterol levels, insulin resistance, and hyperinsulinemia. The specific reasons for the development of lipodystrophy are unknown.

Other Complications Patients with HIV infection can develop anemia due to nutrient malabsorption, blood loss, disturbed bone marrow function, or medication side effects. HIV infection may also lead to neurological complications (dementia, muscle weakness, gait disturbances), skin disorders (rashes, infections, cancers), kidney diseases (nephrotic syndrome, chronic kidney disease), eye disorders (retinal infection or detachment), and coronary heart disease.

Treatments for HIV Infection

Although there is no cure for HIV infection, treatments can help to slow its progression, reduce complications, and alleviate pain. The standard drug treatment for suppressing HIV infection is a combination of at least three antiretroviral drugs.[34] Table 25-9 lists the

FIGURE 25-4 HIV Lipodystrophy
HIV-associated lipodystrophy is sometimes evident by the accumulation of fatty tissue at the base of the neck, referred to as *buffalo hump.*

lipodystrophy (LIP-oh-DIS-tro-fee)**:** abnormalities in body fat and fat metabolism that may result from drug treatments for HIV infection. The accumulation of abdominal fat is sometimes called *protease paunch.*

buffalo hump: the accumulation of fatty tissue at the base of the neck.

lipomas (lih-POE-muz)**:** benign tumors composed of fatty tissue.

TABLE 25-9 Antiretroviral Drugs for Treatment of HIV Infection

Category	Examples	Mode of Action
CCR5 antagonists	Maraviroc	CCR5 antagonists prevent HIV from entering cells by blocking a membrane receptor on the host cell.
Fusion inhibitors	Enfuvirtide	Fusion inhibitors prevent HIV from entering cells by binding a viral protein needed for its entry.
Integrase inhibitors	Raltegravir	Integrase inhibitors impair the function of HIV's integrase enzyme, which incorporates viral DNA into the host cell's genome.
Non-nucleoside reverse transcriptase inhibitors (NNRTIs)	Efavirenz, etravirine, nevirapine	NNRTIs bind active sites on HIV's reverse transcriptase enzyme, blocking the ability of HIV to produce DNA copies of its genetic material.
Nucleoside reverse transcriptase inhibitors (NRTIs)	Didanosine, lamivudine, zidovudine	As analogs of the nucleosides needed for DNA synthesis, NRTIs impair the ability of HIV's reverse transcriptase enzyme to produce usable copies of DNA.
Protease inhibitors (PIs)	Ritonavir, saquinavir, tipranavir	PIs inhibit HIV's protease enzyme, which cleaves HIV's gene products into usable structural proteins.

Sources: U.S. Department of Health and Human Services, Panel on Antiretroviral Guidelines for Adults and Adolescents, *Guidelines for the Use of Antiretroviral Agents in HIV-1-Infected Adults and Adolescents*, pp. P1–P23 (updated February 12, 2013), available at www.aidsinfo.nih.gov/contentfiles/lvguidelines/adultandadolescentgl .pdf, site visited May 1, 2014; S. Safrin, Antiviral agents, in B. G. Katzung, ed., *Basic and Clinical Pharmacology* (New York: Lange/McGraw-Hill, 2012), pp. 861–890.

BOX 25-6 DIET-DRUG INTERACTIONS

Check this table for notable nutrition-related effects of the medications discussed in this chapter.

Appetite stimulants (megestrol acetate, dronabinol)	**Gastrointestinal effects:** Nausea, vomiting, diarrhea **Dietary interaction:** Dronabinol potentiates the effects of alcohol **Metabolic effect:** Hyperglycemia (megestrol acetate)
Didanosine	**Gastrointestinal effects:** Nausea, vomiting, anorexia, dry mouth, altered taste sensation, abdominal pain, diarrhea **Dietary interactions:** Take medication either one-half hour before or two hours after a meal; avoid magnesium supplements and alcohol while taking the drug **Metabolic effects:** Pancreatitis, anemia, increased serum uric acid and liver enzyme levels
Methotrexate	**Gastrointestinal effects:** Nausea, vomiting, gingivitis, diarrhea **Dietary interaction:** Reduces folate absorption **Metabolic effects:** Liver toxicity, increased serum uric acid levels, anemia
Ritonavir	**Gastrointestinal effects:** Nausea, vomiting, altered taste sensation, anorexia, diarrhea **Dietary interaction:** Must be taken with food; avoid using alcohol while taking the drug **Metabolic effects:** Hyperglycemia, liver toxicity, jaundice, hyperlipidemias (especially hypertriglyceridemia)
Zidovudine	**Gastrointestinal effects:** Nausea, vomiting, anorexia **Dietary interactions:** Do not take with a high-fat meal, which may decrease drug absorption **Metabolic effects:** Insulin resistance, diabetes, anemia, hyperlipidemias

Note: Most antiretroviral drugs that treat HIV infection have gastrointestinal and metabolic side effects; only a few are listed here as examples.

major drug categories included in antiretroviral therapy and describes the drugs' modes of action. These antiretroviral agents have multiple adverse effects that make their long-term use difficult to tolerate. In addition to the GI effects discussed previously, side effects include skin rashes, headache, anemia, tingling and numbness, hepatitis, pancreatitis, and kidney stones. Thus, although antiretroviral therapy has improved the life span and quality of life for many patients, the drug regimens are difficult to adhere to and cause complications that require continual management. Box 25-6 summarizes the nutrition-related effects of some of the antiretroviral agents and other drugs mentioned in this chapter.

Control of Anorexia and Wasting Anabolic hormones, appetite stimulants, and regular physical activity have been successful in reversing unintentional weight loss and increasing muscle mass in HIV-infected patients. Testosterone and human growth hormone have demonstrated positive effects on muscle tissue, especially in combination with resistance training. A regular program of resistance exercise (see Figure 25-5) improves muscle mass and strength and corrects some of the metabolic abnormalities (altered blood lipids and insulin resistance) that are common in HIV-infected patients. The medications megestrol acetate and dronabinol (described on p. 652) are sometimes prescribed to stimulate appetite and improve weight gain, although much of the weight increase is attributable to a gain of fat rather than lean tissue.[35]

Control of Lipodystrophy Treatment strategies for lipodystrophy are under investigation. Both aerobic activity and resistance training may help to reduce abdominal fat, although some patients opt for cosmetic surgery. An alternative antiretroviral drug regimen may improve the condition. Medications may be prescribed to treat abnormal blood lipids and insulin resistance.

Ken Kaminesky/Take 2 Productions/Corbis

FIGURE 25-5 Resistance Training

Resistance exercises involve moving objects of weight to improve muscle mass and strength; examples include weight lifting, use of weight machines or stretchable bands, push-ups, chin-ups, arm raises, and leg lifts.

Alternative Therapies Like cancer patients, people with HIV infection and AIDS are frequently tempted to try unconventional methods of treatment. Although many alternative therapies are harmless, some may have side effects that worsen complications or interfere with treatment. For example, herbal preparations that contain St. John's wort, echinacea, or garlic may reduce the effectiveness of some antiretroviral drugs.[36] Monitoring patients' use of dietary supplements is essential to reduce the likelihood of adverse effects or diet-drug interactions.

Nutrition Therapy for HIV Infection

HIV-infected individuals must learn how to maintain a healthy body weight, preserve muscle mass, prevent malnutrition, and cope with nutrition-related side effects of medications. Therefore, nutrition assessment and counseling should begin soon after a patient is diagnosed with HIV infection. The initial assessment should include an evaluation of body weight and body composition. Follow-up measurements may indicate the need to adjust dietary measures and drug therapies.

Weight Management Since the development of successful drug therapies for HIV infection, obesity and overweight have become more prevalent than wasting among HIV-infected individuals in the United States.[37] Because excessive body weight can increase the risk of cardiovascular disease and diabetes, moderate weight loss may be recommended for patients with HIV infection who are overweight or obese.

Individuals who experience weight loss and wasting may benefit from a high-kcalorie, high-protein diet. If food consumption is difficult, small, frequent meals may be better tolerated than several large ones. The addition of nutrient-dense snacks, protein or energy bars, and oral supplements can improve intakes. Liquid formulas may be useful for the person who is too tired to eat or prepare meals. Review Box 25-3 on p. 653 for additional suggestions for adding energy and protein to the diet.

Metabolic Complications To improve insulin resistance and blood lipid abnormalities, patients are advised to achieve or maintain a desirable weight, replace saturated fats with monounsaturated and polyunsaturated fats, increase fiber intake, and limit intakes of *trans* fats, cholesterol, added sugars, and alcohol. Regular physical activity can improve both insulin resistance and blood lipid levels. If problems persist, alternative antiretroviral medications may be prescribed in an attempt to improve the metabolic abnormalities.

Vitamins and Minerals Micronutrient recommendations for patients with HIV infection are similar to those for the general population. Because nutrient deficiencies may result from reduced food intake, malabsorption, diet-drug interactions, and nutrient losses, multivitamin-mineral supplements are often recommended. Patients should avoid taking high-dose supplements, however, due to the potential for adverse effects.[38]

Symptom Management The discomfort associated with antiretroviral therapy, opportunistic GI infections, and symptoms of malabsorption can make food consumption difficult, and problems such as vomiting and diarrhea contribute to fluid and electrolyte losses. Box 25-4 on pp. 655–656 describes measures for improving food and fluid intakes in individuals with these problems.

Food Safety The depressed immunity of people with HIV infections places them at extremely high risk of developing foodborne illnesses. Health practitioners should caution patients about their high susceptibility to foodborne illness and provide detailed instructions about the safe handling of foods; for some individuals, a low-microbial diet may be suggested (see p. 654). Water can also be a source of foodborne illness and is a common cause of **cryptosporidiosis** in HIV-infected individuals. In places where water quality is questionable, patients should consult their local health departments to determine whether the tap water is safe to drink. If not, water used for drinking and making ice cubes should be boiled for one minute.

Enteral and Parenteral Nutrition Support In later stages of illness, people with HIV infections may be unable to consume enough food and may need aggressive nutrition support. Tube feedings are preferred whenever the GI tract is functional; they can be provided at night as a supplement to the usual diet. Parenteral nutrition is reserved for patients who are unable to tolerate enteral nutrition, such as those with GI obstructions that prevent food intake.

IN SUMMARY

▌ By attacking immune cells, HIV causes progressive damage to immune function and may eventually lead to AIDS.

▌ Improved drug therapies have slowed the progression of HIV infection; however, the drugs may promote the development of lipodystrophy, characterized by body fat redistribution, abnormal blood lipid levels, and insulin resistance.

▌ HIV infection may lead to weight loss and wasting, anorexia, and complications that affect food intake. Dietary adjustments, resistance training, and medications can help patients maintain their weight and prevent wasting.

▌ People with HIV infections must pay strict attention to food safety guidelines to prevent foodborne illnesses.

cryptosporidiosis (KRIP-toe-spor-ih-dee-OH-sis): a foodborne illness caused by the parasite *Cryptosporidium parvum.*

The Case Study in Box 25-7 provides an opportunity to review the nutrition concerns of a person with HIV infection.

Case Study BOX 25-7 MAN WITH HIV INFECTION

Three years ago, George Judd, a 37-year-old financial planner, sought medical help when he began feeling run-down and developed a painful white fungal infection over his mouth and tongue. The presence of thrush, recent weight loss, and anemia alerted Mr. Judd's physician to the possibility of an HIV infection. When Mr. Judd tested positive for HIV, he and his family and friends were devastated by the news, but those close to him have remained supportive. During the 3 years since Mr. Judd began antiretroviral drug therapy, he has maintained his weight but has also developed lipodystrophy and hypertriglyceridemia. Mr. Judd is 6 feet tall and currently weighs 185 pounds. He occasionally develops diarrhea and sometimes anorexia.

1. Describe lipodystrophy, and discuss its typical pattern in people who have an HIV infection. What adjustments in treatment and lifestyle may be helpful for Mr. Judd?

2. Describe an appropriate diet for Mr. Judd. What strategies may improve his problems with diarrhea and anorexia?

Suggest reasons why diarrhea and anorexia may develop in people with HIV infections.

3. Explain why an HIV infection can lead to wasting as the disease progresses to the later stages. What recommendations may be helpful for maintaining weight and health if wasting becomes a problem?

Nutrition Assessment Checklist FOR PEOPLE WITH CANCER OR HIV INFECTIONS

Medical History

Check the medical record to determine:

- Type and stage of cancer
- Stage of HIV infection

Review the medical record for complications that may alter nutrition therapy, including:

- Altered organ function
- Altered taste perception
- Anorexia
- Dry mouth and oral infections
- GI symptoms and infections
- Hyperlipidemias
- Insulin resistance
- Malnutrition and wasting

Medications

For patients with cancer or HIV infections:

- Check medications to identify potential diet-drug interactions.
- Recommend the use of antinauseants, if needed.
- Ask about the use of dietary supplements, including herbal products.

For cancer patients who require chemotherapy:

- Recommend strategies to prevent food aversions.
- Offer suggestions for managing drug-related complications.

For HIV-infected patients using antiretroviral drug therapy:

- Remind patients that some drugs are better absorbed with foods and that others must be taken on an empty stomach.
- Help patients work out a medication schedule that suits their lifestyle and is timed appropriately in regard to food intake.
- Offer suggestions for managing drug-related complications.

Dietary Intake

For patients with poor food intakes and weight loss:

- Determine the reasons for reduced food intake.
- Offer appropriate suggestions to improve food intake.
- Provide interventions before weight loss progresses further.

For patients with HIV infections who experience weight gain, elevated triglyceride or LDL cholesterol levels, or hyperglycemia:

- Assess intakes of energy, total fat, saturated fat, cholesterol, fiber, and sugars.
- For patients with hyperlipidemias, recommend a diet low in saturated fat, *trans* fats, cholesterol, and sugars.
- For patients with hyperglycemia, recommend a consistent carbohydrate intake at meals and snacks that emphasizes complex carbohydrates and limits concentrated sweets.
- Recommend regular physical activity for weight control and for improving blood lipid levels and insulin resistance.

Anthropometric Data

Take baseline height and weight measurements, monitor weight regularly, and suggest dietary adjustments for weight maintenance, if necessary. Remember that body composition may change without affecting body weight. Perform baseline and periodic body composition measurements in HIV-infected patients who are using antiretroviral drug therapy.

Laboratory Tests

Note that albumin and other serum proteins may be reduced in patients with cancer or HIV infections, especially in those experiencing wasting. Check laboratory tests for indications of:

- Anemia
- Dehydration
- Elevated LDL cholesterol levels
- Elevated triglyceride levels
- Hyperglycemia

For patients with HIV infections, evaluate disease progression by checking:

- Helper T cell counts
- Viral load

Physical Signs

Look for physical signs of:

- Dehydration (especially in patients with fever, vomiting, or diarrhea)
- Kaposi's sarcoma
- Oral infections
- Protein-energy malnutrition and wasting

Clinical Applications

1. Consider the nutrition problems that may develop in a 36-year-old woman with a malignant brain tumor that affects her ability to move the right side of her body (including the tongue) and to speak coherently. She is taking a pain medication that makes her nauseated and sleepy. Her expected survival time is only about 6 months.

   - If she is right-handed, how might her impairment interfere with eating? What suggestions do you have for overcoming this problem?

- How might her nutrition status be affected by her inability to communicate effectively? What suggestions may help?

- In what ways might the pain medication she is taking affect her nutrition status?

2. Various types of chronic conditions can lead to weight loss and wasting. For some of these conditions, such as Crohn's disease and celiac disease (Chapters 18 and 19), diet is a cornerstone of treatment. For others, such as cancer and HIV infection, nutrition plays a supportive role. What determines whether nutrition plays a primary role or a supportive role in the treatment of disease?

Self Check

1. Which of these dietary substances may help to protect against cancer?
   a. Alcoholic beverages
   b. Well-cooked meats, poultry, and fish
   c. Animal fats
   d. Compounds in fruits and vegetables

2. The metabolic changes that often accompany cancer include all of the following *except:*
   a. increased triglyceride breakdown.
   b. increased protein turnover.
   c. increased muscle protein synthesis.
   d. insulin resistance.

3. An advantage of radiation therapy over chemotherapy is that:
   a. radiation is not damaging to rapidly dividing cells.
   b. side effects of radiation therapy do not include malnutrition.
   c. radiation can be directed toward the regions affected by cancer.
   d. the radiation used is too weak to damage GI tissues.

4. Although many cancer patients lose weight, which type of cancer is often associated with weight gain?
   a. Kidney cancer
   b. Breast cancer
   c. Colon cancer
   d. Lung cancer

5. Which food below should be avoided by a patient consuming a low-microbial diet?
   a. Baked potato
   b. Pasteurized yogurt
   c. Banana
   d. Leftover luncheon meat

6. HIV can enter and destroy:
   a. epithelial cells.
   b. helper T cells.
   c. liver cells.
   d. intestinal cells.

7. In patients who develop lipodystrophy, which abnormality is unlikely?
   a. Increased abdominal fat
   b. Increased fat in the arms and legs
   c. Fat accumulation at the base of the neck
   d. Hypertriglyceridemia

8. In people with HIV infection, mouth sores may be caused by all of the following *except:*
   a. cryptosporidiosis.
   b. Kaposi's sarcoma.
   c. herpes simplex virus.
   d. candidiasis.

9. Megestrol acetate and dronabinol are:
   a. medications used to promote weight gain.
   b. protease inhibitors that fight HIV infection.
   c. medications that treat common opportunistic infections.
   d. anabolic hormones that promote gain of muscle tissue.

10. To prevent cryptosporidiosis, a person with HIV infection may need to:
    a. wash his or her hands carefully before meals.
    b. avoid consuming undercooked meat, poultry, and eggs.
    c. consume a high-kcalorie, high-protein diet.
    d. boil drinking water for one minute.

Answers to these questions can be found in Appendix H.

Notes

1. R. Siegel and coauthors, Cancer statistics, 2014, *CA: A Cancer Journal for Clinicians* 64 (2014): 9–29.

2. H. T. Lynch and C. R. Boland, Cancer genetics, in L. Goldman and A. I. Schafer, eds., *Goldman's Cecil Medicine* (Philadelphia: Saunders, 2012), pp. 1182–1184; J. A. Moscow and K. H. Cowan, Biology of cancer, in L. Goldman and A. I. Schafer, eds., *Goldman's Cecil Medicine* (Philadelphia: Saunders, 2012), pp. 1184–1187.

3. J. L. Freudenheim, Nutrition and genetic factors in carcinogenesis, in A. M. Coulston, C. J. Boushey, and M. G. Ferruzzi, eds., *Nutrition in the Prevention and Treatment of Disease* (London: Academic Press/Elsevier, 2013), pp. 645–656.

4. K. Robien, C. L. Rock, and W. Demark-Wahnefried, Nutrition and cancers of the breast, endometrium, and ovary, in A. M. Coulston, C. J. Boushey, and M. G. Ferruzzi, eds., *Nutrition in the Prevention and Treatment of Disease* (London: Academic Press/Elsevier, 2013), pp. 657–672.

5. S. D. Hursting and coauthors, Obesity, energy balance, and cancer: New opportunities for prevention, *Cancer Prevention Research* 5 (2012): 1260–1272.

6. D. E. Nelson and coauthors, Alcohol-attributable cancer deaths and years of potential life lost in the United States, *American Journal of Public Health* 103 (2013): 641–648.

7. R. J. Turesky and L. Le Marchand, Metabolism and biomarkers of heterocyclic aromatic amines in molecular epidemiology studies: Lessons learned from aromatic amines, *Chemical Research in Toxicology* 24 (2011): 1169–1214.

8. W. C. Willett and coauthors, Diet, obesity, and physical activity, in B. W. Stewart and C. B. Wild, eds., *World Cancer Report 2014* (Lyon, France: International Agency for Research on Cancer; 2014), pp. 171–184.

9. H. S. Rugo, Paraneoplastic syndromes and other non-neoplastic effects of cancer, in L. Goldman and A. I. Schafer, eds., *Goldman's Cecil Medicine* (Philadelphia: Saunders, 2012), pp. 1192–1200.

10. V. C. Vaughan, P. Martin, and P. A. Lewandowski, Cancer cachexia: Impact, mechanisms and emerging treatments, *Journal of Cachexia, Sarcopenia, and Muscle* 4 (2013): 95–109; K. C. H. Fearon, The 2011 ESPEN Arvid Wretlind lecture: Cancer cachexia: The potential impact of translational research on patient-focused outcomes, *Clinical Nutrition* 31 (2012): 577–582.

11. Vaughan, Martin, and Lewandowski, 2013.

12. S. Dodson and coauthors, Muscle wasting in cancer cachexia: Clinical implications, diagnosis, and emerging treatment strategies, *Annual Review of Medicine* 62 (2011): 8.1–8.15.

13. M. C. Perry, Approach to the patient with cancer, in L. Goldman and A. I. Schafer, eds., *Goldman's Cecil Medicine* (Philadelphia: Saunders, 2012), pp. 1164–1177.

14. J. M. Vose, Hematopoietic stem cell transplantation, in L. Goldman and A. I. Schafer, eds., *Goldman's Cecil Medicine* (Philadelphia: Saunders, 2012), pp. 1158–1162.

15. Dodson and coauthors, 2011.

16. M. Charlson, Complementary and alternative medicine, in L. Goldman and A. I. Schafer, eds., *Goldman's Cecil Medicine* (Philadelphia: Saunders, 2012), pp. 177–181.

17. A. Agins, *ADA Quick Guide to Drug-Supplement Interactions* (Chicago: American Dietetic Association, 2011), pp. 19–20.

18. Agins, 2011; M. L. Heaney and coauthors, Vitamin C antagonizes the cytotoxic effects of antineoplastic drugs, *Cancer Research* 68 (2008): 8031–8038.

19. C. L. Rock and coauthors, Nutrition and physical activity guidelines for cancer survivors, *CA: A Cancer Journal for Clinicians* 62 (2012): 242–274.

20. Rock and coauthors, 2012.

21. J. Doley, HIV and cancer, in A. Skipper, ed., *Dietitian's Handbook of Enteral and Parenteral Nutrition* (Sudbury, MA: Jones and Bartlett Learning, 2012), pp. 199–216.

22. Academy of Nutrition and Dietetics, *Nutrition Care Manual* (Chicago: Academy of Nutrition and Dietetics, 2014.

23. Rock and coauthors, 2012.

24. Academy of Nutrition and Dietetics, 2014.

25. Doley, 2012.

26. Joint United Nations Programme on HIV/AIDS (UNAIDS), *Global summary of the AIDS epidemic, 2012,* available at www.unaids.org/en/media /unaids/contentassets/documents/epidemiology /2013/gr2013/201309_epi_core_en.pdf; site visited May 7, 2014.

27. E. M. Gardner and coauthors, The spectrum of engagement in HIV care and its relevance to test-and-treat strategies for prevention of HIV infection, *Clinical Infectious Diseases* 52 (2011): 793–800.

28. G. M. Shaw, Biology of human immunodeficiency viruses, in L. Goldman and A. I. Schafer, eds., *Goldman's Cecil Medicine* (Philadelphia: Saunders, 2012), pp. 2177–2181.

29. Shaw, 2012.

30. J. L. Gerrior, Unintentional weight loss and wasting in HIV infection, in K. M. Hendricks, K. R. Dong, and J. L. Gerrior, eds., *Nutrition Management of HIV and AIDS* (Chicago: American Dietetic Association, 2009), pp. 41–55.

31. T. A. Knox and C. Wanke, Gastrointestinal manifestations of HIV and AIDS, in L. Goldman and A. I. Schafer, eds., *Goldman's Cecil Medicine* (Philadelphia: Saunders, 2012), pp. 2196–2199.

32. F. Maingat and coauthors, Inflammation and epithelial cell injury in AIDS enteropathy: Involvement of endoplasmic reticulum stress, *FASEB Journal* 25 (2011): 2211–2220, doi:10.1096/ fj.10-175992.

33. H. Masur, L. Healey, and C. Hadigan, Treatment of human immunodeficiency virus infection and acquired immunodeficiency syndrome, in L. Goldman and A. I. Schafer, eds., *Goldman's Cecil Medicine* (Philadelphia: Saunders, 2012), pp. 2185–2196.

34. U.S. Department of Health and Human Services, Panel on Antiretroviral Guidelines for Adults and Adolescents, *Guidelines for the Use of Antiretroviral Agents in HIV-1-Infected Adults and Adolescents*, pp. P1–P23 (updated February 12, 2013), available at www.aidsinfo.nih.gov /contentfiles/lvguidelines/adultandadolescentgl. pdf, site visited July 20, 2013; S. Safrin, Antiviral agents, in B. G. Katzung, ed., *Basic and Clinical Pharmacology* (New York: Lange/McGraw-Hill, 2012), pp. 861–890.

35. Gerrior, 2009.

36. C. E. Dennehy and C. Tsourounis, Dietary supplements and herbal medications, in B. G. Katzung, ed., *Basic and Clinical Pharmacology* (New York: McGraw-Hill, 2012), pp. 1125–1137.

37. N. Crum-Cianflone and coauthors, Increasing rates of obesity among HIV-infected persons during the HIV epidemic, *PLoS One* 5 (Apr 9 2010): e10106, doi: 10.1371/journal .pone.0010106.

38. Doley, 2012; J. E. Forrester and K. A. Sztam, Micronutrients in HIV/AIDS: Is there evidence to change the WHO 2003 recommendations? *American Journal of Clinical Nutrition* 94 (2011): 1683S–1689S.

25.3 ETHICAL ISSUES IN NUTRITION CARE

LO 25.3 Identify the ethical principles that guide treatment decisions, and compare the responsibilities of physicians and patients in determining the appropriate care during medical emergencies.

As with other medical technologies, the availability of specialized nutrition support forces health care professionals and members of our society to face difficult **ethical** issues. When medical treatments prolong life by merely delaying death, the lifetime that remains may be of extremely low quality. This Nutrition in Practice examines the ethical dilemmas that clinicians must face when dealing with patients in critical care. Box NP25-1 defines the relevant terms.

If providing nutrition care can do little to promote recovery, is it appropriate to withhold or withdraw nutrition support?

In attempting to answer questions such as these, health professionals must consider the following ethical principles:[1]

■ A patient has the right to make decisions concerning his or her own well-being (**patient autonomy**), even if refusing treatment could result in death. It is generally accepted that a patient's preferences should take precedence over those of his or her health care providers.

■ A patient should be fully informed of a treatment's benefits and risks in a fair and honest manner (**disclosure**). A patient's acceptance of a treatment that has been adequately disclosed is considered **informed consent.**

■ A patient must have the mental capacity to make appropriate health care decisions (**decision-making capacity**). If a patient is mentally incapable of doing so, a person designated by the patient should serve as a **surrogate** decision maker.

■ The potential benefits (**beneficence**) of any treatment should outweigh its potential harm (**maleficence**).

■ Health care providers must determine whether the provision of health care to one patient would unfairly limit the care of other patients (**distributive justice**).

Although these principles may seem simple and obvious, it is often difficult to determine the appropriate action to take during intensive care. When clinicians and families disagree, the courts may be asked to decide.

What kinds of treatments can help to sustain a patient's life?

Nutrition support and hydration are both considered life-sustaining treatments because withholding or withdrawing either can result

---

BOX NP25-1 GLOSSARY

advance health care directive: written or oral instructions regarding one's preferences for medical treatment to be used in the event of becoming incapacitated; also called an *advance medical directive* or a *living will*.

beneficence (be-NEF-eh-sense)**:** the act of performing beneficial services rather than harmful ones.

cardiopulmonary resuscitation (CPR): life-sustaining treatment that supplies oxygen and restores a person's ability to breathe and pump blood.

decision-making capacity: the ability to understand pertinent information and make appropriate decisions; known as *decision-making competency* within the legal system.

defibrillation: life-sustaining treatment in which an electronic device is used to shock the heart and reestablish a pattern of normal contractions. Defibrillation is used when the heart has arrhythmias or has experienced cardiac arrest.

dialysis: life-sustaining treatment in which a patient's blood is filtered using selective diffusion through a semipermeable membrane; substitutes for kidney function.

disclosure: the act of revealing pertinent information. For example, clinicians should accurately describe proposed tests and procedures, their benefits and risks, and alternative approaches.

distributive justice: the equitable distribution of resources.

do-not-resuscitate (DNR) order: a request by a patient or surrogate to withhold cardiopulmonary resuscitation.

durable power of attorney: a legal document (sometimes called a *health care proxy*) that gives legal authority to another (a *health care agent*) to make medical decisions in the event of incapacitation.

ethical: in accordance with accepted principles of right and wrong.

futile: describes medical care that will not improve the medical circumstances of a patient.

health care agent: a person given legal authority to make medical decisions for another in the event of incapacitation.

informed consent: a patient's or caregiver's agreement to undergo a treatment that has been adequately disclosed. Persons must be mentally competent in order to make the decision.

maleficence (mah-LEF-eh-sense)**:** the act of doing evil or harm.

mechanical ventilation: life-sustaining treatment in which a mechanical ventilator is used to substitute for a patient's failing lungs.

patient autonomy: a principle of self-determination, such that patients (or surrogate decision makers) are free to choose the medical interventions that are acceptable to them, even if they choose to refuse interventions that may extend their lives.

persistent vegetative state: a vegetative mental state resulting from brain injury that persists for at least 1 month. Individuals lose awareness and the ability to think but retain noncognitive brain functions, such as motor reflexes and normal sleep patterns.

surrogate: a substitute; a person who takes the place of another.

Is it ever morally or legally appropriate to withhold or withdraw nutrition support?

Carolyn A. McKeone/Science Source

in death (see Figure NP25-1). Other life-sustaining treatments include **cardiopulmonary resuscitation (CPR),** which supplies oxygen and restores a person's ability to breathe and pump blood; **defibrillation,** in which an electronic device shocks the heart and reestablishes normal contractions; **mechanical ventilation,** which substitutes for lung function; and **dialysis,** which substitutes for kidney function.[2]

Do patients have a right to life-sustaining treatments?

Although life-sustaining treatments are readily provided to patients who have a reasonable chance of recovering from illness, it may be difficult to determine the best course of action for patients who are dying or who are unlikely to regain consciousness. Under such circumstances, such treatments may be considered **futile** because they are unable to improve the outcome of disease or increase the patient's comfort and well-being.[3] If patients or caregivers demand treatment that health practitioners have determined to be useless, a legal resolution may be required. Conversely, medical personnel may find it objectionable to withdraw life support when they know that the inevitable consequence will be the patient's death.

How have the courts resolved conflicts involving nutrition support?

One of the landmark cases involving nutrition support concerned Nancy Cruzan, who suffered permanent and irreversible brain damage after a car crash in 1983 when she was 26 years of age.[4] After she had been in a **persistent vegetative state** for 5 years, her parents requested permission to discontinue tube feeding, but hospital staff refused to honor the request and the matter was taken to court. The Missouri Supreme Court determined that Nancy had never definitively stated her "right to die" wishes and that her parents were unable to make such a request for her. The court also stated that preserving life, no matter what its quality, should take

precedence over all other considerations. Nancy's parents appealed the ruling, but in 1990, the U.S. Supreme Court upheld the Missouri Supreme Court in a 5–4 decision. Three witnesses were eventually found who could testify that Nancy would not have desired life-sustaining treatment under the circumstances, and the Court finally granted permission to remove the feeding tube. This case illustrates the importance of having an **advance health care directive** (discussed in a later section) that specifies one's preferences for medical treatment in the event of incapacitation.

In a more recent case that received widespread media attention, the spouse and parents of a patient in a persistent vegetative state fought a 10-year legal battle over her medical care. In 1990, at the age of 25, Terri Schiavo suffered a full cardiac arrest.[5] She initially fell into a coma, but her condition evolved into a persistent vegetative state that was considered irreversible. Despite the neurologists' diagnosis and a series of computed tomography (CT) and magnetic resonance imaging (MRI) scans showing extensive brain atrophy, her parents maintained that she was minimally conscious and could improve somewhat with rigorous treatment. Her husband, who was legally responsible for her care, insisted that she would never have wanted to be kept alive in a vegetative state. Like Nancy Cruzan, Terri had never expressed her wishes in an advance directive.

In 1998, Terri's husband filed a petition to have her feeding tube removed, and a Florida court approved the motion in February 2000. Although Terri's parents appealed, an appeals court affirmed the decision, and the Florida Supreme Court declined to review the case. In April 2001, Terri's physicians removed her feeding tube, but within days, a federal circuit court judge ordered it to be reinserted and reopened the case. Eventually, the various motions filed by the parents were dismissed and Terri's feeding tube was removed for the second time in October 2003. Within days, the Florida legislature passed a bill known as *Terri's Law* that gave the governor the authority to intervene, and Governor Jeb Bush ordered the feeding tube reinserted. A year later, Florida's Supreme Court declared Terri's Law to be unconstitutional. Although the governor appealed the decision, his appeal was rejected in January 2005. Terri's feeding tube was removed for the third and final time in March 2005. Despite emergency petitions by her parents and an attempt by the U.S. Congress to have her case reconsidered, the courts refused to grant a restraining order, and Terri died 13 days after her feeding tube was removed.

How can people ensure that their wishes will be considered in the event that they become incapacitated?

A person can declare preferences about medical treatments in an advance health care directive, sometimes called a *living will*. These directives include detailed instructions about life-sustaining procedures that a person does or does not want. The documents are incorporated into the medical record and updated when appropriate; they take effect only if a physician determines that a patient lacks the ability to understand and make decisions about available treatments. If a person's preferences are unknown, decisions are based on a patient's best interests as determined by a caregiver or family member.[6]

Another important directive is a **durable power of attorney** (sometimes called a *health care proxy*), in which another person (a **health care agent**) is appointed to act as decision maker in the event of incapacitation. The agent should understand one's medical preferences and be absolutely trustworthy. Only one person can be designated, although one or two alternates may also be listed. If an agent is given comprehensive power to supervise care, he or she may make decisions about medical staff, health care facilities, and medical procedures.

Laws regarding advance directives vary from state to state. In some states, nutrition and hydration are not considered life-sustaining treatments, and a person's instructions about them may need to be indicated separately. Some states restrict the use of advance directives to terminal illness or disallow them during pregnancy. Generally, advance directives created in one state are honored in another.

How does a "do-not-resuscitate" order differ from other advance directives?

A **do-not-resuscitate (DNR) order** is frequently used to withhold CPR in the event of cardiopulmonary arrest, which occurs too suddenly for deliberate decision making. A DNR order is written in the medical record as other directives are, but it does not exclude the use of other life-prolonging measures. The DNR order is most often used in patients for whom death is expected and unavoidable, such as those with serious illnesses or advanced age. Some institutions allow a physician to write a DNR order for a patient who has a poor prognosis, but the physician must inform the patient or surrogate if this is done.

Have advance directives changed the way that medical care is provided?

Not really. Despite the availability of advance directives, only about 20 percent of people in the United States have completed one.[7] Among older adults (60 years of age and older), up to 70 percent of individuals have an advance directive.[8] However, advance directives are sometimes too general or vague to guide specific treatment decisions. Furthermore, patients' preferences often change as their medical conditions evolve or they learn more about their prognosis.[9]

Physicians must often provide patient care before they have a chance to discuss treatments with patients or caregivers. In many cases, life-sustaining treatments are begun without the prior knowledge of patients or their decision makers, or the treatments continue even if patients want them stopped. Patients who are fully aware of treatment options and clearly state their preferences are more likely to be successful at obtaining the care they desire.

What resources are available to individuals who have difficulty making decisions about life-sustaining medical treatments?

Many medical institutions have ethics committees that meet regularly to update patient care policies pertaining to end-of-life treatments; these committees provide guidelines to help families and hospital staff who face difficult treatment decisions. Medical staff may also provide referrals for hospice care to dying patients who prefer comfort and palliation over invasive procedures in their final days.

Notes

1. E. J. Emanuel, Bioethics in the practice of medicine, in L. Goldman and A. I. Schafer, eds., *Goldman's Cecil Medicine* (Philadelphia: Saunders, 2012), pp. 4–9; J. M. Luce and D. B. White, A history of ethics and law in the intensive care unit, *Critical Care Clinics* 25 (2009): 221–237.

2. Luce and White, 2009.

3. Emanuel, 2012; J. M. Luce, End-of-life decision making in the intensive care unit, *American Journal of Respiratory and Critical Care Medicine* 182 (2010): 6–11.

4. M. R. Andrews and J. O. Maillet, An ethics primer, in A. Skipper, ed., *Dietitian's Handbook of Enteral and Parenteral Nutrition* (Sudbury, MA: Jones and Bartlett Learning, 2012), pp. 46–56; Luce and White, 2009.

5. R. Cranford, Facts, lies, and videotapes: The permanent vegetative state and the sad case of Terri Schiavo, *Journal of Law, Medicine, and Ethics* 33 (2005): 363–372.

6. L. Snyder, American College of Physicians ethics manual, *Annals of Internal Medicine* (2012): 73–104.

7. E. Wheatley and M. K. Huntington, Advanced directives and code status documentation in an academic practice, *Family Medicine* 44 (2012): 574–578.

8. M. J. Silveira, S. Y. H. Kim, and K. M. Langa, Advance directives and outcomes of surrogate decision making before death, *New England Journal of Medicine* 362 (2010): 1211–1218.

9. Luce and White, 2009.

Appendices

Table of Food Composition

This edition of the table of food composition (Table A-2) includes a wide variety of foods. It is updated with each edition to reflect current nutrient data for foods, to remove outdated foods, and to add foods that are new to the marketplace.* The nutrient database for this appendix is compiled from a variety of sources, including the USDA Nutrient Database and manufacturers' data. The USDA database provides data for a wider variety of foods and nutrients than other sources. Because laboratory analysis for each nutrient can be quite costly, manufacturers tend to provide data only for those nutrients mandated on food labels. Consequently, data for their foods are often incomplete; any missing information on this table is designated as a dash. Keep in mind that a dash means only that the information is unknown and should not be interpreted as a zero. A zero means that the nutrient is not present in the food.

Whenever using nutrient data, remember that many factors influence the nutrient contents of foods. These factors include the mineral content of the soil, the diet fed to the animal or the fertilizer used on the plant, the season of harvest, the method of processing, the length and method of storage, the method of cooking, the method of analysis, and the moisture content of the sample analyzed. With so many influencing factors, users should view nutrient data as a close approximation of the actual amount.

▮ *Fats* Total fats, as well as the breakdown of total fats to saturated, monounsaturated, and polyunsaturated, are listed in the table. The fatty acids seldom add up to the total in part due to rounding but also because values may include some non-fatty acids, such as glycerol, phosphate, or sterols. *Trans*-fatty acids are not listed separately in this edition because newer hydrogenated fats generally add less than 0.5 g *trans* fat to a serving of food, an amount often reported as 0.

▮ *Vitamin A, Vitamin E, and Folate* In keeping with the RDA for vitamin A, this appendix presents data for vitamin A in micrograms (μg) RAE. Similarly, because the RDA for vitamin E is based only on the alpha-tocopherol form of vitamin E, this appendix reports vitamin E data in milligrams (mg) alpha-tocopherol, listed in the table as Vit E (mg α). Folate is reported as micrograms (μg) DFE, listed in the table as Fola (μg). This measure adjusts for lower bioavailability of naturally occurring folate from foods compared to that from fortified foods or supplements.

▮ *Bioavailability* Keep in mind that the availability of nutrients from foods depends not only on the quantity provided by a food, but also on the amount absorbed and used by the body—the bioavailability. The bioavailability of folate from fortified foods, for example, is greater than from naturally occurring sources. Similarly, the body can make niacin from the amino acid tryptophan, but niacin values in this table (and most databases) report preformed niacin only. Chapter 8 provides conversion factors and additional details.

*This food composition table has been prepared by Cengage Learning. The nutritional data are supplied by Axxya Systems.

▌ *Using the Table*   The foods and beverages in this table are organized into several categories, which are listed at the head of each right-hand page. Page numbers are provided, and each group is color-coded to make it easier to find individual foods.

▌ *Caffeine Sources*   Caffeine occurs in several plants, including the familiar coffee bean, the tea leaf, and the cocoa bean from which chocolate is made. Most human societies use caffeine regularly, most often in beverages, for its stimulant effect and flavor. Caffeine contents of beverages vary depending on the plants they are made from, the climates and soils where the plants are grown, the grind or cut size, the method and duration of brewing, and the amounts served. Table A-1 shows that, in general, a cup of coffee contains the most caffeine; a cup of tea, less than half as much; and cocoa or chocolate, less still. As for cola beverages, they are made from kola nuts, which contain caffeine, but most of their caffeine is added, using the purified compound obtained from decaffeinated coffee beans. The FDA lists caffeine as a multipurpose GRAS ("generally recognized as safe") substance that may be added to foods and beverages. Drug manufacturers also use caffeine in many products.

TABLE A-1 Caffeine Content of Selected Beverages, Foods, and Medications

Beverages and Foods	Serving Size	Average (mg)	Beverages and Foods	Serving Size	Average (mg)
Coffee			**Soft Drinks**		
Brewed	8 oz	95	A&W Creme Soda	12 oz	29
Decaffeinated	8 oz	2	Braq's Root Beer	12 oz	18
Espresso	1 oz	64	Coca-Cola	12 oz	30
Instant	8 oz	64	Dr. Pepper, Mr. Pibb, Sunkist Orange	12 oz	36
Tea			A&W Root Beer, club soda, Fresca, ginger ale, 7-Up, Sierra Mist, Sprite, Squirt, tonic water, caffeine-free soft drinks	12 oz	0
Brewed, green	8 oz	30			
Brewed, herbal	8 oz	0			
Brewed, leaf or bag	8 oz	47	Mello Yello	12 oz	51
Instant	8 oz	26	Mountain Dew	12 oz	45
Lipton Brisk iced tea	12 oz	7	Pepsi	12 oz	32
Nestea Cool iced tea	12 oz	12			
Snapple iced tea (all flavors)	16 oz	42			

TABLE A-1 **Caffeine Content of Selected Beverages, Foods, and Medications** (continued)

Beverages and Foods	Serving Size	Average (mg)	Beverages and Foods	Serving Size	Average (mg)
Energy Drinks			**Foods**		
AMP	16 oz	145	Frozen yogurt, Ben & Jerry's coffee fudge	1 cup	85
Full Throttle	16 oz	200	Frozen yogurt, Häagen-Dazs coffee	1 cup	40
Monster	16 oz	160	Ice cream, Starbucks coffee	1 cup	50
NOS	16 oz	160			
Red Bull	8.3 oz	75	Ice cream, Starbucks Frappuccino bar	1 bar	15
Rockstar	16 oz	160	Pudding, chocolate	1 cup	5
Xyience Xenergy	16 oz	185	Yogurt, Dannon coffee flavored	1 cup	45

Beverages and Foods	Serving Size	Average (mg)	Drugs[a]	Serving Size	Average (mg)
Other Beverages			**Cold Remedies**		
Chocolate milk or hot cocoa	8 oz	5	Coryban-D, Dristan	1 tablet	30
Starbucks Frappuccino Mocha	9.5 oz	72	**Diuretics**		
Starbucks Frappuccino Vanilla	9.5 oz	64	Aqua-Ban	1 tablet	100
Yoohoo chocolate drink	9 oz	3	Pre-Mens Forte	1 tablet	100
Candies			**Pain Relievers**		
Baker's chocolate	1 oz	26	Anacin, BC Fast Pain Reliever	1 tablet	32
Dark chocolate covered coffee beans	1 oz	235	Excedrin, Midol, Midol Max Strength	1 tablet	65
Dark chocolate, semisweet	1 oz	18	**Stimulants**		
Milk chocolate	1 oz	6	Awake, NoDoz	1 tablet	100
Milk chocolate covered coffee beans	1 oz	224	Awake Maximum Strength, Caffedrine, NoDoz Maximum Strength, Stay Awake, Vivarin	1 tablet	200
White chocolate	1 oz	0	**Weight-Control Aids**		
			Dexatrim	1 tablet	200

[a]A pharmacologically active dose of caffeine is defined as 200 milligrams.

Note: The FDA suggests a maximum of 65 milligrams per 12-ounce cola beverage but does not regulate the caffeine contents of other beverages. Because products change, contact the manufacturer for an update on products you use regularly.

Source: Adapted from USDA database Release 18 (www.nal.usda.gov/fnic/foodcomp/Data/), Caffeine content of foods, drugs, and energy drinks, Center for Science and the Public Interest (www.cspinet.org/new/cafchart.htm), and R. R. McCusker, B. A. Goldberger, and E. J. Cone, Caffeine content of carbonated sodas and other beverages, *Journal of Analytical Toxicology* 30 (2006): 112–114.

TABLE A-2 Table of Food Composition   (Computer code is for Cengage Diet Analysis program)   (For purposes of calculations, use "0" for t, <1, <0.1, <0.01)

DA+ Code	Food Description	Quantity	Measure	Wt (g)	H₂O (g)	Ener (kcal)	Prot (g)	Carb (g)	Fiber (g)	Fat (g)	Fat Breakdown (g) Sat	Mono	Poly
Breads, Baked Goods, Cakes, Cookies, Crackers, Chips, Pies													
	Bagels												
8534	Cinnamon and raisin	1	item(s)	71	22.7	195	7.0	39.2	1.6	1.2	0.2	0.1	0.5
8538	Oat bran	1	item(s)	71	23.4	181	7.6	37.8	2.6	0.9	0.1	0.2	0.3
4910	Plain, enriched	1	item(s)	71	25.8	182	7.1	35.9	1.6	1.2	0.3	0.4	0.5
4911	Plain, enriched, toasted	1	item(s)	66	18.7	190	7.4	37.7	1.7	1.1	0.2	0.3	0.6
72275	Whole wheat	1	item(s)	94	—	210	10.0	41.0	6.0	1.5	0	0	0.5
	Biscuits												
25008	Biscuits	1	item(s)	41	15.8	121	2.6	16.4	0.5	4.9	1.4	1.4	1.8
16729	Scone	1	item(s)	42	11.5	149	3.8	19.0	0.6	6.3	2.0	2.5	1.4
25166	Wheat biscuits	1	item(s)	55	21.0	162	3.6	21.9	1.4	6.7	1.9	1.9	2.5
	Bread												
325	Boston brown, canned	1	slice(s)	45	21.2	88	2.3	19.5	2.1	0.7	0.1	0.1	0.3
8716	Bread sticks, plain	4	item(s)	24	1.5	99	2.9	16.4	0.7	2.3	0.3	0.9	0.9
25176	Cornbread	2	piece(s)	55	25.9	141	4.6	18.4	0.6	5.4	2.1	1.5	1.4
327	Cracked wheat	1	slice(s)	25	8.9	65	2.2	12.4	1.4	1.0	0.2	0.5	0.2
9079	Croutons, plain	¼	cup(s)	8	0.4	31	0.9	5.5	0.4	0.5	0.1	0.2	0.1
8582	Egg	1	slice(s)	40	13.9	115	3.8	19.1	0.9	2.4	0.6	0.9	0.4
8585	Egg, toasted	1	slice(s)	37	10.5	117	3.9	19.5	0.9	2.4	0.6	1.1	0.4
329	French	1	slice(s)	32	8.9	92	3.8	18.1	0.8	0.6	0.2	0.1	0.3
8591	French, toasted	1	slice(s)	23	4.7	73	3.0	14.2	0.7	0.5	0.1	0.1	0.2
42096	Indian fry, made with lard (Navajo)	3	ounce(s)	85	26.9	281	5.7	41.0	—	10.4	3.9	3.8	0.9
332	Italian	1	slice(s)	30	10.7	81	2.6	15.0	0.8	1.0	0.3	0.2	0.4
1393	Mixed grain	1	slice(s)	26	9.6	69	3.5	11.3	1.9	1.1	0.2	0.2	0.5
8604	Mixed grain, toasted	1	slice(s)	24	7.6	69	3.5	11.3	1.9	1.1	0.2	0.2	0.5
8605	Oat bran	1	slice(s)	30	13.2	71	3.1	11.9	1.4	1.3	0.2	0.5	0.5
8608	Oat bran, toasted	1	slice(s)	27	10.4	70	3.1	11.8	1.3	1.3	0.2	0.5	0.5
8609	Oatmeal	1	slice(s)	27	9.9	73	2.3	13.1	1.1	1.2	0.2	0.4	0.5
8613	Oatmeal, toasted	1	slice(s)	25	7.8	73	2.3	13.2	1.1	1.2	0.2	0.4	0.5
1409	Pita	1	item(s)	60	19.3	165	5.5	33.4	1.3	0.7	0.1	0.1	0.3
7905	Pita, whole wheat	1	item(s)	64	19.6	170	6.3	35.2	4.7	1.7	0.3	0.2	0.7
338	Pumpernickel	1	slice(s)	32	12.1	80	2.8	15.2	2.1	1.0	0.1	0.3	0.4
334	Raisin, enriched	1	slice(s)	26	8.7	71	2.1	13.6	1.1	1.1	0.3	0.6	0.2
8625	Raisin, toasted	1	slice(s)	25	6.9	74	2.1	14.2	1.2	1.2	0.3	0.6	0.2
10168	Rice, white, gluten-free, wheat-free	1	slice(s)	38	—	100	1.0	17.0	1.0	3.5	0	—	—
8653	Rye	1	slice(s)	32	11.9	83	2.7	15.5	1.9	1.1	0.2	0.4	0.3
74338	Rye, light	1	slice(s)	43	—	100	3.0	20.0	1.0	0.5	0	—	—
8654	Rye, toasted	1	slice(s)	29	9.0	82	2.7	15.4	1.9	1.0	0.2	0.4	0.3
8588	Sourdough	1	slice(s)	25	7.0	72	2.9	14.1	0.6	0.5	0.1	0.1	0.2
8592	Sourdough, toasted	1	slice(s)	23	4.7	73	3.0	14.2	0.7	0.5	0.1	0.1	0.2
8596	Vienna, toasted	1	slice(s)	23	4.7	73	3.0	14.2	0.7	0.5	0.1	0.1	0.2
8670	Wheat	1	slice(s)	25	8.6	68	2.6	12.4	1.0	0.9	0.2	0.2	0.4
8671	Wheat, toasted	1	slice(s)	23	5.6	72	3.0	12.8	1.1	1.0	0.2	0.2	0.4
340	White	1	slice(s)	25	9.1	66	2.3	12.3	0.7	0.8	0.2	0.1	0.4
1395	Whole wheat	1	slice(s)	46	15.0	128	3.9	23.6	2.8	2.5	0.4	0.5	1.4
	Cakes												
386	Angel food, prepared from mix	1	piece(s)	50	16.5	129	3.0	29.4	0.1	0.2	0	0	0.1
8772	Butter pound, ready to eat, commercially prepared	1	slice(s)	75	18.5	291	4.1	36.6	0.4	14.9	8.7	4.4	0.8
28517	Carrot	1	slice(s)	131	56.4	340	4.8	56.8	1.8	11.1	1.0	6.1	3.6
4931	Chocolate with chocolate icing, commercially prepared	1	slice(s)	64	14.7	235	2.6	34.9	1.8	10.5	3.1	5.6	1.2
8756	Chocolate, prepared from mix	1	slice(s)	95	23.2	352	5.0	50.7	1.5	14.3	5.2	5.7	2.6
8757	Fruitcake, ready to eat, commercially prepared	1	piece(s)	43	10.9	139	1.2	26.5	1.6	3.9	0.5	1.8	1.4
14284	Lemon, prepared from mix	1	slice(s)	80	—	250	3.0	36.0	0.5	11.1	2.6	—	—
1397	Pineapple upside down, prepared from mix	1	slice(s)	115	37.1	367	4.0	58.1	0.9	13.9	3.4	6.0	3.8
411	Sponge, prepared from mix	1	slice(s)	63	18.5	187	4.6	36.4	0.3	2.7	0.8	1.0	0.4

PAGE KEY: A-6 = Breads/Baked Goods A-12 = Cereal/Rice/Pasta A-16 = Fruit A-22 = Vegetables/Legumes A-32 = Nuts/Seeds A-34 = Vegetarian A-36 = Dairy A-44 = Eggs A-44 = Seafood A-46 = Meats A-50 = Poultry
A-52 = Processed Meats A-54 = Beverages A-58 = Fats/Oils A-60 = Sweets A-62 = Spices/Condiments/Sauces A-66 = Mixed Foods/Soups/Sandwiches A-72 = Fast Food A-90 = Convenience A-92 = Baby Foods

Chol (mg)	Calc (mg)	Iron (mg)	Magn (mg)	Pota (mg)	Sodi (mg)	Zinc (mg)	Vit A (µg)	Thia (mg)	Vit E (mg α)	Ribo (mg)	Niac (mg)	Vit B$_6$ (mg)	Fola (µg)	Vit C (mg)	Vit B$_{12}$ (µg)	Sele (µg)
0	13	2.70	19.9	105.1	244.2	0.80	14.9	0.27	0.22	0.20	2.19	0.04	123.5	0.5	0	22.0
0	9	2.19	22.0	81.7	418.9	0.64	0.7	0.24	0.23	0.24	2.10	0.03	95.1	0.1	0	24.3
0	63	4.30	15.6	53.3	338.7	1.35	0	0.43	0.07	0.18	2.82	0.05	160.5	0.7	0	16.2
0	65	2.97	15.8	56.1	354.4	0.86	0	0.40	0.08	0.18	2.89	0.05	134.0	0	0	16.6
0	40	2.70	—	—	420.0	—	0	—	—	—	—	—	—	0	—	—
0	37	0.94	6.0	45.9	204.5	0.20	0	0.16	0.05	0.13	1.20	0.01	59.3	0	0.1	7.3
43	79	1.34	7.1	49.1	281.8	0.31	66.4	0.15	0.55	0.16	1.20	0.03	49.1	0.1	0.1	10.8
0	57	1.22	16.1	81.2	321.2	0.42	0	0.20	0.12	0.15	1.65	0.04	63.2	0.1	0.1	12.2
0	32	0.94	28.4	143.1	284.0	0.22	11.3	0.01	0.14	0.05	0.50	0.04	6.3	0	0	9.9
0	5	1.03	7.7	29.8	171.1	0.21	0	0.14	0.24	0.13	1.27	0.02	61.2	0	0	9.0
21	94	0.94	10.1	69.2	208.8	0.49	0	0.14	0.40	0.16	1.06	0.04	61.7	1.5	0.2	6.8
0	11	0.70	13.0	44.3	134.5	0.31	0	0.09	—	0.06	0.92	0.08	19.0	0	0	6.3
0	6	0.31	2.3	9.3	52.3	0.07	0	0.05	—	0.02	0.41	0	15.7	0	0	2.8
20	37	1.22	7.6	46.0	152.0	0.32	25.2	0.18	0.10	0.17	1.94	0.03	52.0	0	0	12.0
21	38	1.24	7.8	46.6	154.3	0.32	25.5	0.14	0.11	0.16	1.77	0.02	47.4	0	0	12.2
0	14	1.16	9.0	41.0	164.2	0.30	0	0.14	0.06	0.09	1.52	0.03	73.6	0.1	0	8.7
0	11	0.89	7.1	32.2	165.6	0.24	0	0.10	0.04	0.09	1.24	0.02	49.9	0	0	6.8
6	48	3.44	15.3	65.5	279.8	0.30	—	0.37	0	0.18	3.91	0.03	166.7	—	0	15.8
0	23	0.88	8.1	33.0	183.9	0.26	0	0.14	0.09	0.09	1.31	0.01	91.2	0	0	8.2
0	27	0.65	20.3	59.8	99.1	0.44	0	0.07	0.10	0.03	1.05	0.07	19.5	0	0	8.6
0	27	0.65	20.4	60.0	99.4	0.44	0	0.06	0.10	0.03	1.05	0.07	16.8	0	0	8.6
0	20	0.94	10.5	44.1	105.9	0.27	0.6	0.15	0.13	0.10	1.45	0.02	36.0	0	0	9.0
0	19	0.93	9.2	33.2	104.5	0.28	0.5	0.12	0.13	0.09	1.29	0.01	28.1	0	0	8.9
0	18	0.73	10.0	38.3	120.7	0.28	1.4	0.11	0.13	0.06	0.85	0.02	23.5	0	0	6.6
0	18	0.74	10.3	38.5	121.5	0.28	1.3	0.09	0.13	0.06	0.77	0.02	18.8	0.1	0	6.8
0	52	1.57	15.6	72.0	321.6	0.50	0	0.36	0.18	0.20	2.78	0.02	99.0	0	0	16.3
0	10	1.96	44.2	108.8	284.2	0.97	0	0.22	0.39	0.05	1.82	0.17	22.4	0	0	28.2
0	22	0.92	17.3	66.6	190.7	0.47	0	0.10	0.13	0.10	0.99	0.04	42.9	0	0	7.8
0	17	0.75	6.8	59.0	90.2	0.19	0	0.09	0.07	0.10	0.90	0.02	40.6	0	0	5.2
0	18	0.79	7.0	61.5	94.3	0.19	0	0.07	0.08	0.10	0.85	0.02	37.0	0.1	0	5.4
0	20	0.72	—	—	120.0	—	0	0.15	—	0.07	1.20	—	—	0	—	—
0	23	0.91	12.8	53.1	193.0	0.36	0	0.14	0.11	0.11	1.22	0.02	48.3	0.1	0	9.9
0	0	1.08	—	—	220.0	—	0	—	—	—	—	—	—	1.2	—	—
0	23	0.90	12.5	53.1	192.6	0.36	0	0.11	0.11	0.10	1.09	0.02	42.9	0.1	0	9.9
0	11	0.91	7.0	32.0	128.3	0.23	0	0.11	0.05	0.07	1.19	0.03	57.5	0.1	0	6.8
0	11	0.89	7.1	32.2	165.6	0.24	0	0.10	0.04	0.09	1.24	0.02	49.9	0	0	6.8
0	11	0.89	7.1	32.2	165.6	0.24	0	0.10	0.04	0.09	1.24	0.02	49.9	0	0	6.8
0	35	0.88	11.5	45.5	129.8	0.29	0	0.12	0.05	0.07	1.48	0.03	24.8	0.1	0	7.2
0	38	0.94	13.6	51.3	138.2	0.34	0	0.10	0.06	0.09	1.44	0.04	23.0	0	0	7.7
0	65	0.90	6.3	28.8	122.8	0.21	0	0.13	0.05	0.06	1.20	0.02	42.8	0	0	5.5
0	15	1.43	37.3	144.4	159.2	0.69	0	0.14	0.35	0.10	1.83	0.09	35.9	0	0	17.8
0	42	0.12	4.0	67.5	255.5	0.06	0	0.05	0	0.10	0.09	0	14.5	0	0	7.7
166	26	1.03	8.3	89.3	298.5	0.34	111.8	0.10	—	0.17	0.98	0.03	46.5	0	0.2	6.6
0	64	1.87	19.2	250.5	370.2	0.44	0	0.24	1.96	0.21	1.74	0.11	77.7	4.8	0	14.6
27	28	1.41	21.8	128.0	213.8	0.44	16.6	0.02	0.63	0.09	0.37	0.03	14.9	0.1	0.1	2.1
55	57	1.53	30.4	133.0	299.3	0.66	38.0	0.13	—	0.20	1.08	0.04	37.0	0.2	0.2	11.3
2	14	0.89	6.9	65.8	43.4	0.12	3.0	0.02	0.39	0.04	0.34	0.02	13.8	0.2	0	0.9
54	40	0.72	—	—	312.0	—	0	0.12	—	0.14	0.80	—	—	0	—	—
25	138	1.70	14.9	128.8	366.9	0.36	71.3	0.18	—	0.18	1.37	0.04	44.8	1.4	0.1	10.8
107	26	1.00	5.7	88.8	143.6	0.37	48.5	0.10	—	0.19	0.76	0.04	33.4	0	0.2	11.7

TABLE A-2 Table of Food Composition *(continued)*   (Computer code is for Cengage Diet Analysis program)   (For purposes of calculations, use "0" for t, <1, <0.1, <0.01)

DA+ Code	Food Description	Quantity	Measure	Wt (g)	H₂O (g)	Ener (kcal)	Prot (g)	Carb (g)	Fiber (g)	Fat (g)	Sat	Mono	Poly
											Fat Breakdown (g)		

Breads, Baked Goods, Cakes, Cookies, Crackers, Chips, Pies—*continued*

DA+ Code	Food Description	Quantity	Measure	Wt (g)	H₂O (g)	Ener (kcal)	Prot (g)	Carb (g)	Fiber (g)	Fat (g)	Sat	Mono	Poly
8817	White with coconut frosting, prepared from mix	1	slice(s)	112	23.2	399	4.9	70.8	1.1	11.5	4.4	4.1	2.4
8819	Yellow with chocolate frosting, ready to eat, commercially prepared	1	slice(s)	64	14.3	243	2.0	35.4	1.0	11.4	3.7	4.6	3.0
8822	Yellow with vanilla frosting, ready to eat, commercially prepared	1	slice(s)	64	14.1	239	2.2	37.6	0.2	9.3	1.5	3.9	3.3
	Snack cakes												
8791	Chocolate snack cake, creme filled, with frosting	1	item(s)	50	9.3	200	1.8	30.2	1.6	8.0	2.4	4.3	0.9
25010	Cinnamon coffee cake	1	piece(s)	72	22.6	231	3.6	35.9	0.7	8.3	2.2	2.6	3.0
16777	Funnel cake	1	item(s)	90	37.7	275	7.3	29.2	0.9	14.3	2.7	5.5	5.4
8794	Sponge snack cake, creme filled	1	item(s)	43	8.3	159	1.5	27.2	0.4	4.9	1.8	2.1	0.8
	Snacks, chips, pretzels												
57179	Bagel chips, plain	1	ounce(s)	28	—	132	4.1	19.2	1.0	4.6	0.5	3.5	0.5
57180	Bagel chips, toasted garlic	1	ounce(s)	28	—	132	4.1	19.2	1.0	4.6	0.5	3.5	0.5
38192	Chex traditional snack mix	1	cup(s)	52	—	220	4.0	38.0	1.0	6.0	1.0	—	—
654	Potato chips, salted	1	ounce(s)	28	0.6	154	1.9	14.4	1.2	10.3	1.1	4.5	4.5
8816	Potato chips, unsalted	1	ounce(s)	28	0.5	152	2.0	15.0	1.4	9.8	3.1	2.8	3.5
5096	Pretzels, plain, hard, twists	5	item(s)	30	1.0	114	3.1	23.9	0.9	0.8	0.2	0.4	0.3
4632	Pretzels, whole wheat	1	ounce(s)	28	1.1	103	3.1	23.0	2.2	0.7	0.2	0.3	0.2
4641	Tortilla chips, plain	6	item(s)	11	0.2	53	0.8	7.1	0.6	2.5	0.3	0.7	1.2
	Cookies												
8859	Animal crackers	12	item(s)	30	1.2	134	2.1	22.2	0.3	4.1	1.0	2.3	0.6
8876	Brownie, prepared from mix	1	item(s)	24	3.0	112	1.5	12.0	0.5	7.0	1.8	2.6	2.3
25207	Chocolate chip cookies	1	item(s)	30	3.7	140	2.0	16.2	0.6	7.9	2.1	3.3	2.1
8915	Chocolate sandwich cookie with extra creme filling	1	item(s)	13	0.2	65	0.6	8.9	0.4	3.2	0.7	2.1	0.3
14145	Fig Newtons cookies	1	item(s)	16	—	55	0.5	11.0	0.5	1.0	0	—	—
8920	Fortune cookie	1	item(s)	8	0.6	30	0.3	6.7	0.1	0.2	0.1	0.1	0.0
25208	Oatmeal cookies	1	item(s)	69	12.5	234	5.4	45.3	3.2	4.2	0.7	1.3	1.8
25213	Peanut butter cookies	1	item(s)	35	4.1	162	4.2	16.9	0.9	9.2	1.7	4.7	2.4
33095	Sugar cookies	1	item(s)	16	4.1	61	1.1	7.4	0.1	3.0	0.6	1.4	0.8
9002	Vanilla sandwich cookie with creme filling	1	item(s)	10	0.2	48	0.5	7.2	0.1	2.0	0.3	0.8	0.8
	Crackers												
9012	Cheese cracker sandwich with peanut butter	4	item(s)	28	0.9	139	3.5	15.9	1.0	7.0	1.2	3.6	1.4
9008	Cheese crackers (mini)	30	item(s)	30	1.1	147	3.3	17.8	0.7	6.8	1.6	1.7	3.0
33362	Cheese crackers, low sodium	1	serving(s)	30	0.9	151	3.0	17.5	0.7	7.6	2.9	3.6	0.7
8928	Honey graham crackers	4	item(s)	28	1.2	118	1.9	21.5	0.8	2.8	0.4	1.1	1.1
9016	Matzo crackers, plain	1	item(s)	28	1.2	112	2.8	23.8	0.9	0.4	0.1	0	0.2
9024	Melba toast	3	item(s)	15	0.8	59	1.8	11.5	0.9	0.5	0.1	0.1	0.2
9028	Melba toast, rye	3	item(s)	15	0.7	58	1.7	11.6	1.2	0.5	0.1	0.1	0.2
14189	Ritz crackers	5	item(s)	16	0.5	80	1.0	10.0	0	4.5	1.0	1.0	1.7
9014	Rye crispbread crackers	1	item(s)	10	0.6	37	0.8	8.2	1.6	0.1	0	0	0.1
9040	Rye wafer	1	item(s)	11	0.6	37	1.1	8.8	2.5	0.1	0	0	0
432	Saltine crackers	5	item(s)	15	0.6	63	1.4	11.2	0.4	1.3	0.3	0.3	0.6
9046	Saltine crackers, low salt	5	item(s)	15	0.6	63	1.4	11.2	0.4	1.3	0.3	0.3	0.6
9052	Snack cracker sandwich with cheese filling	4	item(s)	28	1.1	134	2.6	17.3	0.5	5.9	1.7	3.2	0.7
9054	Snack cracker sandwich with peanut butter filling	4	item(s)	28	0.8	138	3.2	16.3	0.6	6.9	1.4	3.9	1.3
9048	Snack crackers, round	10	item(s)	30	1.0	151	2.0	18.4	0.6	7.7	1.6	2.0	3.8
9050	Snack crackers, round, low salt	10	item(s)	30	1.0	151	2.2	18.3	0.5	7.6	1.1	3.2	2.9
9044	Soda crackers	5	item(s)	15	0.6	63	1.4	11.2	0.4	1.3	0.3	0.3	0.6
9059	Wheat cracker sandwich with cheese filling	4	item(s)	28	0.9	139	2.7	16.3	0.9	7.0	1.2	2.9	2.6
9061	Wheat cracker sandwich with peanut butter filling	4	item(s)	28	1.0	139	3.8	15.1	1.2	7.5	1.3	3.3	2.5
9055	Wheat crackers	10	item(s)	30	1.0	137	2.7	20.2	1.1	5.2	0.8	1.3	2.8
9057	Wheat crackers, low salt	10	item(s)	30	0.9	142	2.6	19.5	1.4	6.2	1.6	3.4	0.8
9022	Whole wheat crackers	7	item(s)	28	0.8	120	3.0	19.5	2.9	4.0	0.6	0.9	1.9

PAGE KEY: A-6 5 Breads/Baked Goods A-12 = Cereal/Rice/Pasta A-16 = Fruit A-22 = Vegetables/Legumes A-32 = Nuts/Seeds A-34 = Vegetarian A-36 = Dairy A-44 = Eggs A-44 = Seafood A-46 = Meats A-50 = Poultry A-52 = Processed Meats A-54 = Beverages A-58 = Fats/Oils A-60 = Sweets A-62 = Spices/Condiments/Sauces A-66 = Mixed Foods/Soups/Sandwiches A-72 = Fast Food A-90 = Convenience A-92 = Baby Foods

Chol (mg)	Calc (mg)	Iron (mg)	Magn (mg)	Pota (mg)	Sodi (mg)	Zinc (mg)	Vit A (µg)	Thia (mg)	Vit E (mg α)	Ribo (mg)	Niac (mg)	Vit B6 (mg)	Fola (µg)	Vit C (mg)	Vit B12 (µg)	Sele (µg)
1	101	1.30	13.4	110.9	318.1	0.37	13.4	0.14	0.13	0.21	1.19	0.03	57.1	0.1	0.1	12.0
10	20	1.30	12.8	119.7	198.4	0.27	21.1	0.03	2.88	0.06	0.51	0	20.5	0	0	3.8
35	40	0.68	3.8	33.9	220.2	0.16	12.2	0.06	—	0.04	0.32	0.02	25.6	0	0.1	3.5
0	58	1.80	18.0	88.0	166.0	0.52	0.5	0.02	0.55	0.04	0.46	0.07	17.5	0.9	0	1.7
26	54	1.20	8.3	72.6	275.8	0.30	0	0.18	0.35	0.17	1.30	0.03	66.1	0	0.1	9.8
55	127	1.90	16.2	147.6	271.8	0.69	56.7	0.24	1.58	0.33	1.86	0.05	75.6	0	0.3	17.5
17	10	0.58	3.4	30.2	199.8	0.25	2.1	0.08	0.26	0.07	0.66	0	23.0	0	0.1	1.5
0	0	1.09	—	—	313.9	—	0	—	—	—	—	—	—	0	—	—
0	0	1.09	—	—	303.8	—	0	—	—	—	—	—	—	0	—	—
0	0	0.72	—	—	480.0	—	0	—	—	—	—	—	—	0	—	—
0	7	0.46	19.8	465.5	136.1	0.68	0	0.02	1.91	0.07	1.19	0.20	21.3	5.3	0	2.3
0	7	0.46	19.0	361.5	2.3	0.31	0	0.05	2.58	0.06	1.08	0.19	12.8	8.8	0	2.3
0	5	1.56	8.7	40.8	407.1	0.43	0	0.15	0.10	0.10	1.54	0.01	85.6	0	0	1.8
0	8	0.76	8.5	121.9	57.6	0.18	0	0.12	—	0.08	1.85	0.08	15.3	0.3	0	
0	19	0.25	15.8	23.2	45.5	0.27	0	0	0.46	0.01	0.14	0.02	2.2	0	0	0.7
0	13	0.82	5.4	30.0	122.1	0.19	0	0.10	0.04	0.10	1.04	0.01	49.5	0	0	2.1
18	14	0.44	12.7	42.2	82.3	0.23	42.2	0.03	—	0.05	0.24	0.02	9.4	0.1	0	2.8
13	11	0.64	11.4	51.3	108.6	0.24	0	0.08	0.60	0.06	0.87	0.02	29.8	0	0	4.2
0	2	1.01	4.7	17.8	45.6	0.10	0	0.01	0.25	0.02	0.25	0	9.0	0	0	1.1
0	10	0.36	—	—	62.5	—	—	—	—	—	—	—	—	0	—	—
0	1	0.12	0.6	3.3	2.5	0.01	0.1	0.01	0	0.01	0.15	0	8.4	0	0	0.2
0	26	1.83	45.5	157.5	310.3	1.49	0	0.23	1.02	0.13	1.40	0.09	46.4	0.3	0	16.7
13	27	0.65	20.3	107.2	153.7	0.46	0	0.09	1.45	0.09	1.86	0.06	34.7	0.1	0.1	4.7
18	5	0.32	1.7	12.8	50.0	0.08	0	0.04	0.32	0.05	0.31	0.01	17.1	0	0	3.1
0	3	0.22	1.4	9.1	34.9	0.04	0	0.03	0.16	0.02	0.27	0	8.2	0	0	0.3
0	14	0.76	15.7	61.0	232.1	0.29	0.3	0.15	0.66	0.08	1.63	0.04	39.8	0	0.1	2.3
1	41	1.46	7.5	46.8	291.9	0.36	5.1	0.17	0.66	0.10	1.83	0.05	72.3	0	0.1	4.1
4	45	1.43	10.8	31.8	137.4	0.34	5.1	0.17	0.09	0.13	1.40	0.17	40.2	0	0.1	2.6
0	7	1.04	8.4	37.8	133.6	0.23	0	0.06	0.09	0.09	1.15	0.02	18.5	0	0	2.9
0	4	0.90	7.1	31.8	0	0.19	0	0.11	0.02	0.08	1.11	0.03	4.8	0	0	10.5
0	14	0.56	8.9	30.3	89.7	0.30	0	0.06	0.06	0.04	0.62	0.01	29.0	0	0	5.2
0	12	0.55	5.8	29.0	134.9	0.20	0	0.07	—	0.04	0.71	0.01	19.4	0	0	5.8
0	20	0.36	3.0	19.0	135.0	0.10	—	0.07	0.56	0.04	0.78	0.01	17.8	0	—	0.7
0	3	0.24	7.8	31.9	41.0	0.24	0	0.02	0.08	0.01	0.10	0.02	6.5	0	0	3.7
0	4	0.65	13.3	54.5	61.3	0.31	0	0.05	0.09	0.03	0.17	0.03	4.9	0	0	2.6
0	3	0.77	3.8	23.9	153.1	0.12	0	0.09	0.17	0.05	0.79	0.01	33.2	0	0	1.0
0	18	0.77	3.8	108.6	29.7	0.12	0	0.09	0.17	0.05	0.79	0.01	33.2	0	0	1.0
1	72	0.67	10.1	120.1	273.8	0.17	4.8	0.12	0.06	0.19	1.05	0.01	44.8	0	0	6.0
0	23	0.78	15.4	60.2	224.3	0.32	0.3	0.14	0.58	0.08	1.71	0.04	34.2	0	0	3.0
0	29	1.14	5.4	33.3	224.4	0.17	0	0.13	1.07	0.07	1.25	0.02	55.8	0	0	1.1
0	36	1.08	8.1	106.5	64.8	0.20	0	0.12	0.61	0.10	1.21	0.02	42.6	0	0	2.0
0	3	0.77	3.8	23.9	153.1	0.12	0	0.09	0.17	0.05	0.79	0.01	33.2	0	0	1.0
2	57	0.73	15.1	85.7	234.9	0.24	5.9	0.10	—	0.12	0.89	0.07	26.9	0.4	0	6.8
0	48	0.75	10.6	83.2	226.0	0.23	0	0.11	—	0.08	1.65	0.04	26.0	0	0	6.1
0	24	1.41	13.8	62.1	236.1	0.52	0	0.18	0.33	0.09	1.49	0.04	56.1	0	0.1	3.8
0	15	1.32	18.6	60.9	57.0	0.48	0	0.15	0.15	0.10	1.49	0.04	21.6	0	0	10.1
0	10	0.94	30.8	96.6	197.1	0.74	0	0.05	0.39	0.01	1.30	0.05	7.8	0	0	2.8

TABLE A-2 Table of Food Composition (*continued*)   (Computer code is for Cengage Diet Analysis program)   (For purposes of calculations, use "0" for t, <1, <0.1, <0.01)

DA+ Code	Food Description	Quantity	Measure	Wt (g)	H₂O (g)	Ener (kcal)	Prot (g)	Carb (g)	Fiber (g)	Fat (g)	Fat Breakdown (g)		
											Sat	Mono	Poly
Breads, Baked Goods, Cakes, Cookies, Crackers, Chips, Pies—*continued*													
	Pastry												
16754	Apple fritter	1	item(s)	17	6.4	61	1.0	5.5	0.2	3.9	1.0	1.6	1.1
41565	Cinnamon rolls with icing, refrigerated dough	1	serving(s)	44	12.3	145	1.9	23.5	0.6	5.0	1.4	—	—
4945	Croissant, butter	1	item(s)	57	13.2	231	4.7	26.1	1.5	12.0	6.6	3.1	0.6
9096	Danish, nut	1	item(s)	65	13.3	280	4.6	29.7	1.3	16.4	3.8	8.9	2.8
9115	Doughnut with creme filling	1	item(s)	85	32.5	307	5.4	25.5	0.7	20.8	4.6	10.3	2.6
9117	Doughnut with jelly filling	1	item(s)	85	30.3	289	5.0	33.2	0.8	15.9	4.1	8.7	2.0
4947	Doughnut, cake	1	item(s)	47	10.8	196	2.8	21.4	0.8	11.1	3.3	6.0	1.2
9105	Doughnut, cake, chocolate glazed	1	item(s)	42	6.8	175	1.9	24.1	0.9	8.4	2.2	4.7	1.0
437	Doughnut, glazed	1	item(s)	60	15.2	242	3.8	26.6	0.7	13.7	3.5	7.7	1.7
10617	Toaster pastry, brown sugar cinnamon	1	item(s)	50	5.3	210	2.0	34.0	0.5	8.0	2.5	—	—
30928	Toaster pastry, cream cheese	1	item(s)	54	—	200	3.0	24.0	0.5	11.0	4.0	—	—
	Muffins												
25015	Blueberry	1	item(s)	63	29.8	160	3.4	23.0	0.8	6.0	0.9	1.6	3.0
9189	Corn, ready to eat	1	item(s)	57	18.6	174	3.4	29.0	1.9	4.8	0.8	1.2	1.8
9121	English muffin, plain, enriched	1	item(s)	57	24.0	134	4.4	26.2	1.5	1.0	0.1	0.2	0.5
29582	English muffin, toasted	1	item(s)	50	16.5	135	5.2	26.3	1.4	1.0	0.3	0.2	0.5
9145	English muffin, wheat	1	item(s)	57	24.1	127	5.0	25.5	2.6	1.1	0.2	0.2	0.5
8894	Oat bran	1	item(s)	57	20.0	154	4.0	27.5	2.6	4.2	0.6	1.0	2.4
	Granola bars												
34783	Kudos milk chocolate with M&Ms granola bar	1	item(s)	24	—	100	1.0	17.0	1.0	2.5	1.5	—	—
38187	Nature Valley fruit 'n' nut trail mix bar	1	item(s)	35	—	140	3.0	25.0	2.0	4.0	0.5	—	—
3436	Nature Valley oats 'n honey crunchy granola bars	2	item(s)	42	—	180	4.0	29.0	2.0	6.0	0.5	—	—
1383	Plain, hard	1	item(s)	25	1.0	115	2.5	15.8	1.3	4.9	0.6	1.1	3.0
4606	Plain, soft	1	item(s)	28	1.8	126	2.1	19.1	1.3	4.9	2.1	1.1	1.5
	Pies												
454	Apple pie, prepared from home recipe	1	slice(s)	155	73.3	411	3.7	57.5	2.3	19.4	4.7	8.4	5.2
470	Pecan pie, prepared from home recipe	1	slice(s)	122	23.8	503	6.0	63.7	—	27.1	4.9	13.6	7.0
33356	Pie crust mix, prepared, baked	1	slice(s)	20	2.1	100	1.3	10.1	0.4	6.1	1.5	3.5	0.8
9007	Pie crust, ready to bake, frozen, enriched, baked	1	slice(s)	16	1.1	81	1.0	9.0	0.5	4.6	1.5	2.2	0.6
472	Pumpkin pie, prepared from home recipe	1	slice(s)	155	90.7	316	7.0	40.9	—	14.4	4.9	5.7	2.8
	Rolls												
8555	Crescent dinner roll	1	item(s)	28	9.6	78	2.8	14.0	0.6	1.1	0.2	0.3	0.4
489	Hamburger roll or bun, plain	1	item(s)	43	14.7	120	4.2	21.6	0.9	1.6	0.4	0.4	0.7
490	Hard roll	1	item(s)	57	17.7	167	5.6	30.0	1.3	2.5	0.3	0.6	1.0
5127	Kaiser roll	1	item(s)	57	17.7	167	5.6	30.0	1.3	2.5	0.3	0.6	1.0
5130	Whole wheat roll or bun	1	item(s)	28	9.4	75	2.5	14.5	2.1	1.3	0.2	0.3	0.6
	Sport bars												
37026	Balance original chocolate bar	1	item(s)	50	—	200	14.0	21.0	2.0	7.0	4.0	—	—
37024	Balance original peanut butter bar	1	item(s)	50	—	200	15.0	21.0	0.5	7.0	3.0	—	—
36580	Clif Bar chocolate brownie energy bar	1	item(s)	68	—	240	10.0	44.0	5.0	5.0	1.5	—	—
36583	Clif Bar crunchy peanut butter energy bar	1	item(s)	68	—	250	11.0	42.0	5.0	6.0	1.0	—	—
36589	Clif Luna Nutz over Chocolate energy bar	1	item(s)	48	—	180	9.0	25.0	4.0	6.0	2.0	—	—
12005	PowerBar apple cinnamon	1	item(s)	65	—	230	8.0	45.0	2.0	3.5	0.5	—	—
16078	PowerBar banana	1	item(s)	65	—	240	8.0	46.0	1.0	3.5	0.5	—	—
16080	PowerBar chocolate	1	item(s)	65	—	240	8.0	45.0	3.0	3.0	1.0	—	—
29092	PowerBar peanut butter	1	item(s)	65	—	240	9.0	44.0	1.0	4.0	1.0	—	—
	Tortillas												
1391	Corn tortillas, soft	1	item(s)	24	11.0	52	1.4	10.7	1.5	0.7	0.1	0.2	0.3
1669	Flour tortilla	1	item(s)	30	9.5	90	2.4	15.4	0.7	2.0	0.5	1.1	0.4
1390	Taco shells, hard	1	item(s)	13	0.9	63	0.9	8.5	0.9	2.8	0.8	0.8	0.9

PAGE KEY: A-6 5 Breads/Baked Goods A-12 = Cereal/Rice/Pasta A-16 = Fruit A-22 = Vegetables/Legumes A-32 = Nuts/Seeds A-34 = Vegetarian A-36 = Dairy A-44 = Eggs A-44 = Seafood A-46 = Meats A-50 = Poultry A-52 = Processed Meats A-54 = Beverages A-58 = Fats/Oils A-60 = Sweets A-62 = Spices/Condiments/Sauces A-66 = Mixed Foods/Soups/Sandwiches A-72 = Fast Food A-90 = Convenience A-92 = Baby Foods

Chol (mg)	Calc (mg)	Iron (mg)	Magn (mg)	Pota (mg)	Sodi (mg)	Zinc (mg)	Vit A (µg)	Thia (mg)	Vit E (mg α)	Ribo (mg)	Niac (mg)	Vit B_6 (mg)	Fola (µg)	Vit C (mg)	Vit B_{12} (µg)	Sele (µg)
13	9	0.26	2.2	22.3	7.3	0.10	8.2	0.03	0.25	0.04	0.23	0.01	9.2	0.2	0	2.6
0	12	0.85	—	—	343.2	—	0	—	—	—	—	—	—	0	—	—
38	21	1.16	9.1	67.3	424.1	0.43	117.4	0.22	0.48	0.14	1.25	0.03	74.1	0.1	0.1	12.9
30	61	1.17	20.8	61.8	193.7	0.57	5.8	0.14	0.53	0.16	1.50	0.07	79.3	1.1	0.1	9.2
20	21	1.56	17.0	68.0	262.8	0.68	9.4	0.29	0.25	0.13	1.91	0.06	92.7	0	0.1	9.2
22	21	1.50	17.0	67.2	387.0	0.64	14.5	0.27	0.37	0.12	1.82	0.09	88.5	0	0.2	10.6
4	12	1.41	7.5	53.1	261.8	0.32	1.4	0.11	0.89	0.07	0.93	0.01	54.0	0.6	0	4.8
24	89	0.95	14.3	44.5	90.3	0.24	5.0	0.02	0.09	0.03	0.20	0.01	26.9	0	0	1.7
4	26	0.36	13.2	64.8	205.2	0.46	2.4	0.53	—	0.04	0.39	0.03	13.2	0.1	0.1	5.0
0	0	1.80	8.0	67.5	190.0	0.61	150.1	0.15	—	0.17	2.00	0.20	—	0	0	—
10	0	0.72	—	—	210.0	—	0	—	—	—	—	—	—	0	—	—
20	56	1.04	7.9	68.6	287.8	0.29	0	0.17	0.85	0.16	1.26	0.03	62.5	0.2	0.2	9.0
15	42	1.60	18.2	39.3	118.6	0.31	29.6	0.16	0.46	0.19	1.16	0.05	63.8	0	0.1	8.7
0	30	1.42	12.0	74.7	264.5	0.40	0	0.25	—	0.16	2.21	0.02	57.0	0	0	
0	99	2.33	14.0	64.5	238.5	0.70	0	0.27	0.18	0.14	2.49	0.03	90.0	0.9	0	13.1
0	101	1.64	21.1	106.0	201.2	0.61	0	0.25	0.26	0.17	1.91	0.05	46.2	0	0	16.6
0	36	2.39	89.5	289.0	224.0	1.05	0	0.15	0.38	0.05	0.24	0.09	79.2	0	0	6.3
0	300	0.36	—	—	105.0	—	0	—	—	—	—	—	—	0	—	—
0	0	0.36	—	—	100.0	—	0	—	—	—	—	—	—	0	—	—
0	0	1.08	—	95.0	160.0	—	0	—	—	—	—	—	—	0	—	—
0	15	0.72	23.8	82.3	72.0	0.50	0.5	0.06	0.51	0.03	0.39	0.02	5.6	0.2	0	4.0
0	30	0.73	21.0	92.3	79.0	0.43	0	0.08	—	0.05	0.15	0.03	6.8	0	0.1	4.6
0	11	1.74	10.9	122.4	327.0	0.29	17.0	0.23	—	0.17	1.91	0.05	58.9	2.6	0	12.1
106	39	1.81	31.7	162.3	319.6	1.24	100.0	0.23	—	0.22	1.03	0.07	41.5	0.2	0.2	14.6
0	12	0.43	3.0	12.4	145.8	0.08	0	0.06	—	0.04	0.47	0.01	22.2	0	0	4.4
0	3	0.45	2.7	18.2	74.7	0.08	0	0.05	0.09	0.02	0.55	0.01	16.3	0	0	1.1
65	146	1.97	29.5	288.3	348.8	0.71	660.3	0.14	—	0.31	1.21	0.07	43.4	2.6	0.1	11.0
0	48	0.96	6.7	35.6	140.0	0.24	0	0.18	0.02	0.06	1.33	0.02	47.9	0.4	0.1	6.4
0	74	1.47	10.3	54.6	215.0	0.37	0	0.28	0.03	0.09	2.05	0.03	73.5	0.6	0.1	9.8
0	54	1.87	15.4	61.6	310.1	0.54	0	0.27	0.24	0.19	2.42	0.02	86.1	0	0	22.3
0	54	1.87	15.4	61.6	310.1	0.54	0	0.27	0.24	0.19	2.42	0.02	86.1	0	0	22.3
0	30	0.69	24.1	77.1	135.5	0.57	0	0.07	0.26	0.04	1.04	0.06	8.5	0	0	14.0
0	150	2.70	—	260.0	160.0	2.25	—	0.22	—	0.25	3.00	0.30	102.0	60.0	0.9	10.5
0	150	2.70	—	150.0	170.0	2.25	—	0.22	—	0.25	3.00	0.30	102.0	60.0	0.9	10.5
0	250	4.50	100.0	340.0	150.0	3.00	—	0.38	—	0.25	3.00	0.40	—	60.0	0.9	14.0
0	250	4.50	100.0	270.0	230.0	3.00	—	0.38	—	0.25	3.00	0.40	—	60.0	0.9	14.0
0	350	5.40	40.0	160.0	190.0	5.25	—	0.15	—	0.68	8.00	1.50	—	12.0	4.5	24.5
0	250	4.50	—	105.0	200.0	—	0	0.22	—	0.17	—	0.50	—	42.0	—	—
0	150	2.70	—	105.0	200.0	—	0	0.22	—	0.17	—	0.50	—	42.0	—	—
0	150	2.70	—	260.0	200.0	—	0	0.22	—	0.17	—	0.50	—	42.0	—	—
0	20	0.72	—	105.0	200.0	—	0	—	—	—	—	—	—	0	—	—
0	19	0.30	17.3	44.6	10.8	0.31	0	0.02	0.07	0.02	0.36	0.05	1.2	0	0	1.5
0	32	1.00	6.0	45.9	205.8	0.16	0	0.15	0.06	0.04	1.09	0.01	60.3	0	0	7.2
0	13	0.24	11.4	31.0	32.3	0.21	0.1	0.03	0.09	0.01	0.25	0.03	11.3	0	0	0.6

TABLE A-2 Table of Food Composition *(continued)*   (Computer code is for Cengage Diet Analysis program)   (For purposes of calculations, use "0" for t, <1, <0.1, <0.01)

DA+ Code	Food Description	Quantity	Measure	Wt (g)	H₂O (g)	Ener (kcal)	Prot (g)	Carb (g)	Fiber (g)	Fat (g)	Sat	Mono	Poly

Breads, Baked Goods, Cakes, Cookies, Crackers, Chips, Pies—continued

Pancakes, waffles

8926	Pancakes, blueberry, prepared from recipe	3	item(s)	114	60.6	253	7.0	33.1	0.8	10.5	2.3	2.6	4.7
13402	Pancakes, frozen	3	item(s)	105	—	240	5.0	41.0	1.0	6.0	1.0	—	—
9221	Waffle plain, frozen, toasted	1	item(s)	33	10.1	103	2.4	16.3	0.8	3.2	0.5	1.6	0.7
30311	Waffle, 100% whole-grain	1	item(s)	182	85.2	426	16.1	60.7	4.2	14.2	3.5	5.5	4.1
500	Waffle, plain, prepared from recipe	1	item(s)	75	31.5	218	5.9	24.7	1.7	10.6	2.1	2.6	5.1

Cereal, Flour, Grain, Pasta, Noodles, Popcorn

Grain

2861	Amaranth, dry	½	cup(s)	98	11.0	362	13.2	63.6	6.5	6.8	1.4	1.6	2.7
1953	Barley, pearled, cooked	½	cup(s)	79	54.0	97	1.8	22.2	3.0	0.3	0.1	0	0.2
1956	Buckwheat groats, cooked, roasted	½	cup(s)	84	63.5	77	2.8	16.7	2.3	0.5	0.1	0.2	0.2
1957	Bulgur, cooked	½	cup(s)	91	70.8	76	2.8	16.9	4.1	0.2	0	0	0.1
1963	Couscous, cooked	½	cup(s)	79	57.0	88	3.0	18.2	1.1	0.1	0	0	0.1
1967	Millet, cooked	½	cup(s)	120	85.7	143	4.2	28.4	1.6	1.2	0.2	0.2	0.6
1969	Oat bran, dry	½	cup(s)	47	3.1	116	8.1	31.1	7.2	3.3	0.6	1.1	1.3
1972	Quinoa, dry	½	cup(s)	85	11.3	313	12.0	54.6	6.0	5.2	0.6	1.4	2.8

Rice

129	Brown, long grain, cooked	½	cup(s)	98	71.3	108	2.5	22.4	1.8	0.9	0.2	0.3	0.3
2863	Brown, medium grain, cooked	½	cup(s)	98	71.1	109	2.3	22.9	1.8	0.8	0.2	0.3	0.3
37488	Jasmine, saffroned, cooked	½	cup(s)	79	—	85	2.0	19.5	0	0	0	0	0
30280	Pilaf, cooked	½	cup(s)	103	73.4	135	2.1	22.2	0.6	4.1	0.6	1.6	1.7
28066	Spanish, cooked	½	cup(s)	113	85.2	114	2.9	23.5	1.5	1.0	0.2	0.3	0.3
2867	White glutinous, cooked	½	cup(s)	87	66.7	84	1.8	18.3	0.9	0.2	0	0.1	0.1
484	White, long grain, boiled	½	cup(s)	79	54.1	103	2.1	22.3	0.3	0.2	0.1	0.1	0.1
482	White, long grain, enriched, instant, boiled	½	cup(s)	83	59.4	97	1.8	20.7	0.5	0.4	0	0.1	0
486	White, long grain, enriched, parboiled, cooked	½	cup(s)	79	55.6	97	2.3	20.6	0.7	0.3	0.1	0.1	0.1
1994	Wild brown, cooked	½	cup(s)	82	60.6	83	3.3	17.5	1.5	0.3	0	0	0.2

Flour & grain fractions

505	All-purpose flour, self-rising, enriched	½	cup(s)	63	6.6	221	6.2	46.4	1.7	0.6	0.1	0.1	0.3
503	All-purpose flour, white, bleached, enriched	½	cup(s)	63	7.4	228	6.5	47.7	1.7	0.6	0.1	0.1	0.3
53271	Barley flour	½	cup(s)	74	9.0	255	7.8	55.1	7.5	1.2	0.2	0.2	0.6
383	Buckwheat flour, whole groat	½	cup(s)	60	6.7	201	7.6	42.4	6.0	1.9	0.4	0.6	0.6
504	Cake wheat flour, enriched	½	cup(s)	69	8.6	248	5.6	53.5	1.2	0.6	0.1	0.1	0.3
426	Cornmeal, degermed, enriched	½	cup(s)	69	7.7	255	4.9	54.8	2.7	1.2	0.1	0.2	0.4
424	Cornmeal, yellow whole grain	½	cup(s)	61	6.3	221	5.0	46.9	4.5	2.2	0.3	0.6	1.0
1978	Dark rye flour	½	cup(s)	64	6.9	208	10.2	43.9	15.2	1.4	0.2	0.2	0.7
1644	Masa corn flour, enriched	½	cup(s)	57	5.2	208	5.3	43.5	3.6	2.2	0.3	0.6	1.0
1976	Rice flour, brown	½	cup(s)	79	9.5	287	5.7	60.4	3.6	2.2	0.4	0.8	0.8
1645	Rice flour, white	½	cup(s)	79	9.4	289	4.7	63.3	1.9	1.1	0.3	0.3	0.3
1980	Semolina, enriched	½	cup(s)	84	10.6	301	10.6	60.8	3.3	0.9	0.1	0.1	0.4
2827	Soy flour, raw	½	cup(s)	42	2.2	185	14.7	14.9	4.1	8.8	1.3	1.9	4.9
1990	Wheat germ, crude	2	tablespoon(s)	14	1.6	52	3.3	7.4	1.9	1.4	0.2	0.2	0.9
506	Whole-wheat flour	½	cup(s)	60	6.4	204	7.9	43.2	6.4	1.5	0.3	0.2	0.7

Breakfast bars

39230	Atkins Day Break apple crisp bar	1	item(s)	35	—	130	10.0	17.0	7.0	5.0	2.0	—	—
10571	Nutri-Grain apple cinnamon cereal bar	1	item(s)	37	—	130	2.0	24.0	2.0	3.0	0.5	—	—
10647	Nutri-Grain blueberry cereal bar	1	item(s)	37	—	130	2.0	24.0	2.0	3.0	0.5	—	—
10648	Nutri-Grain raspberry cereal bar	1	item(s)	37	—	130	2.0	24.0	2.0	3.0	0.5	—	—
10649	Nutri-Grain strawberry cereal bar	1	item(s)	37	—	130	2.0	24.0	2.0	3.0	0.5	—	—

Breakfast cereals, hot

| 41046 | Cream of Wheat, instant, prepared | ½ | cup(s) | 121 | 101.8 | 75 | 2.2 | 15.8 | 0.7 | 0.3 | 0 | 0 | 0.2 |
| 365 | Farina, enriched, cooked with water and salt | ½ | cup(s) | 117 | 100.8 | 62 | 2.1 | 12.7 | 0.9 | 0.4 | 0.1 | 0 | 0.1 |

PAGE KEY: A-6 5 Breads/Baked Goods A-12 = Cereal/Rice/Pasta A-16 = Fruit A-22 = Vegetables/Legumes A-32 = Nuts/Seeds A-34 = Vegetarian A-36 = Dairy A-44 = Eggs A-44 = Seafood A-46 = Meats A-50 = Poultry A-52 = Processed Meats A-54 = Beverages A-58 = Fats/Oils A-60 = Sweets A-62 = Spices/Condiments/Sauces A-66 = Mixed Foods/Soups/Sandwiches A-72 = Fast Food A-90 = Convenience A-92 = Baby Foods

Chol (mg)	Calc (mg)	Iron (mg)	Magn (mg)	Pota (mg)	Sodi (mg)	Zinc (mg)	Vit A (µg)	Thia (mg)	Vit E (mg α)	Ribo (mg)	Niac (mg)	Vit B$_6$ (mg)	Fola (µg)	Vit C (mg)	Vit B$_{12}$ (µg)	Sele (µg)
64	235	1.96	18.2	157.3	469.7	0.62	57.0	0.22	—	0.31	1.74	0.06	60.4	2.5	0.2	16.0
35	40	1.80	—	—	500.0	—	0	0.30	—	0.17	2.00	—	—	0	—	—
5	101	2.28	7.9	47.5	240.9	0.17	131.3	0.17	0.32	0.23	2.93	0.34	39.3	0	1.0	4.2
4	460	3.15	69.2	424.1	910.0	1.60	3.6	0.38	1.04	0.60	3.20	0.17	80.1	0	0.6	41.3
52	191	1.73	14.3	119.3	383.3	0.51	48.8	0.20	—	0.26	1.55	0.04	51.0	0.3	0.2	34.7
0	155	7.42	241.8	495.3	3.9	2.80	0	0.11	1.16	0.19	0.90	0.58	79.9	4.1	0	18.2
0	9	1.04	17.3	73.0	2.4	0.64	0	0.07	0.01	0.05	1.62	0.09	12.6	0	0	6.8
0	6	0.67	42.8	73.9	3.4	0.51	0	0.03	0.08	0.03	0.79	0.06	11.8	0	0	1.8
0	9	0.87	29.1	61.9	4.6	0.52	0	0.05	0.01	0.03	0.91	0.08	16.4	0	0	0.5
0	6	0.30	6.3	45.5	3.9	0.20	0	0.05	0.10	0.02	0.77	0.04	11.8	0	0	21.6
0	4	0.76	52.8	74.4	2.4	1.09	0	0.13	0.02	0.10	1.60	0.13	22.8	0	0	1.1
0	27	2.54	110.4	266.0	1.9	1.46	0	0.55	0.47	0.10	0.44	0.08	24.4	0	0	21.2
0	40	3.89	167.5	478.8	4.3	2.64	0.9	0.31	2.08	0.27	1.29	0.41	156.5	—	0	7.2
0	10	0.41	41.9	41.9	4.9	0.61	0	0.09	0.03	0.02	1.49	0.14	3.9	0	0	9.6
0	10	0.52	42.9	77.0	1.0	0.60	0	0.10	—	0.01	1.30	0.15	3.9	0	0	38.0
0	—	0.54	—	—	195.0	—	—	—	—	—	—	—	—	—	—	—
0	12	1.15	9.3	53.6	366.7	0.37	0	0.13	0.50	0.02	1.24	0.06	73.1	0.4	0	4.3
0	17	0.73	44.1	157.6	14.7	0.65	126.7	0.13	0.28	0.03	1.72	0.18	8.8	6.3	0	6.8
0	2	0.12	4.3	8.7	4.3	0.36	0	0.02	0.03	0.01	0.25	0.02	0.9	0	0	4.9
0	8	0.95	9.5	27.6	0.8	0.39	0	0.13	0.03	0.01	1.17	0.07	76.6	0	0	5.9
0	7	1.46	4.1	7.4	3.3	0.40	0	0.06	0.01	0.01	1.43	0.04	97.3	0	0	4.0
0	15	1.43	7.1	44.2	1.6	0.29	0	0.17	0.01	0.02	1.82	0.12	107.4	0	0	7.3
0	2	0.49	26.2	82.8	2.5	1.10	0	0.04	0.20	0.07	1.06	0.11	21.3	0	0	0.7
0	211	2.92	11.9	77.5	745.6	0.39	0	0.42	0.03	0.26	3.64	0.03	191.9	0	0	21.5
0	9	2.90	13.8	66.9	1.3	0.44	0	0.49	0.04	0.31	3.69	0.03	181.9	0	0	21.2
0	24	1.98	71.0	228.6	3.0	1.48	0	0.27	0.42	0.08	4.64	0.29	5.9	0	0	27.9
0	25	2.44	150.6	346.2	6.6	1.87	0	0.25	0.19	0.11	3.69	0.35	32.4	0	0	3.4
0	10	5.01	11.0	71.9	1.4	0.42	0	0.61	0.01	0.29	4.65	0.02	193.2	0	0	3.4
0	2	3.01	22.1	98.0	4.8	0.46	7.6	0.38	0.08	0.26	3.43	0.13	231.1	0	0	7.2
0	4	2.10	77.5	175.1	21.4	1.11	6.7	0.23	0.26	0.12	2.22	0.19	15.3	0	0	9.5
0	24	3.18	102.4	458.9	1.3	3.23	0.6	0.20	1.75	0.16	2.73	0.28	21.1	0	0	11.5
0	78	4.27	53.0	149.9	2.8	1.03	0	0.84	0.07	0.46	5.66	0.27	190.9	0	0	8.0
0	9	1.56	88.5	228.3	6.3	1.94	0	0.35	0.95	0.06	5.01	0.58	12.6	0	0	—
0	8	0.28	27.6	60.0	0.0	0.63	0	0.11	0.09	0.02	2.05	0.34	3.2	0	0	11.9
0	14	3.64	39.2	155.3	0.8	0.88	0	0.68	0.22	0.48	5.00	0.09	217.9	0	0	74.6
0	87	2.70	182.0	1066.9	5.5	1.66	2.5	0.25	0.83	0.49	1.83	0.20	146.3	0	0	3.2
0	6	0.90	34.4	128.3	1.7	1.77	0	0.27	—	0.07	0.98	0.19	40.4	0	0	11.4
0	20	2.16	82.2	217.8	1.2	1.56	0	0.30	0.43	0.10	2.97	0.24	26.4	0	0	37.1
0	200	1.44	—	35.0	140.0	—	—	0.15	—	0.17	2.00	—	68.0	12.0	—	—
0	200	1.80	—	—	105.0	1.50	225.0	0.22	—	0.43	5.00	0.50	—	0	—	—
0	200	1.80	—	—	105.0	1.50	225.0	0.22	—	0.43	5.00	0.50	—	0	—	—
0	200	1.80	—	—	100.0	1.50	225.0	0.22	—	0.43	5.00	0.50	—	0	—	—
0	200	1.80	—	—	120.0	1.50	225.0	0.22	—	0.43	5.00	0.50	—	0	—	—
0	77	5.99	7.2	24.1	123.1	0.21	280.0	0.28	0.02	0.25	3.73	0.37	121.9	0	0	4.2
0	113	6.21	8.2	26.8	146.8	0.27	0	0.15	0.05	0.08	1.74	0.11	138.6	0	0	3.5

TABLE A-2 Table of Food Composition (continued)　　(Computer code is for Cengage Diet Analysis program)　(For purposes of calculations, use "0" for t, <1, <0.1, <0.01)

DA+ Code	Food Description	Quantity	Measure	Wt (g)	H₂O (g)	Ener (kcal)	Prot (g)	Carb (g)	Fiber (g)	Fat (g)	Fat Breakdown (g) Sat	Mono	Poly
Cereal, Flour, Grain, Pasta, Noodles, Popcorn—*continued*													
363	Grits, white corn, regular and quick, enriched, cooked with water and salt	½	cup(s)	121	100.3	86	2.1	17.9	1.0	0.6	0.1	0.1	0.2
8636	Grits, yellow corn, regular and quick, enriched, cooked with salt	½	cup(s)	121	102.1	79	1.5	16.8	0.8	0.5	0.1	0.1	0.2
8657	Oatmeal, cooked with water	½	cup(s)	117	97.8	83	3.0	14.0	2.0	1.8	0.4	0.5	0.7
5500	Oatmeal, maple and brown sugar, instant, prepared	1	item(s)	198	147.3	208	4.8	41.9	3.7	2.5	0.4	0.7	0.9
5510	Oatmeal, ready to serve, packet, prepared	1	item(s)	186	152.2	143	4.8	25.2	3.8	2.5	0.4	0.8	0.9
	Breakfast cereals, ready to eat												
1197	All-Bran	1	cup(s)	62	1.3	160	8.0	46.0	20.0	2.0	0	0.4	—
1200	All-Bran Buds	1	cup(s)	91	2.7	242	9.1	72.7	39.4	3.0	0	0.5	1.1
1199	Apple Jacks	1	cup(s)	28	0.8	100	1.0	25.0	3.0	0.5	0	0.1	0.2
1204	Cap'n Crunch	1	cup(s)	36	0.9	147	1.3	30.7	1.3	2.0	1.3	0	0
1205	Cap'n Crunch Crunchberries	1	cup(s)	35	0.9	133	1.3	29.3	1.3	2.0	1.3	0.2	0.3
1206	Cheerios	1	cup(s)	28	1.1	100	3.0	20.0	3.0	2.0	0	0.5	0.5
3415	Cocoa Puffs	1	cup(s)	36	0.6	147	1.3	30.7	1.3	2.0	0	0.7	0.7
1207	Cocoa Rice Krispies	1	cup(s)	41	1.2	160	1.3	36.0	0.7	1.3	0.7	0.2	0.1
5522	Complete wheat bran flakes	1	cup(s)	39	1.1	120	4.0	30.7	6.7	0.7	0	0	0
1211	Corn Flakes	1	cup(s)	28	1.1	100	2.0	24.0	1.0	0	0	0	0
1247	Corn Pops	1	cup(s)	32	1.0	120	1.0	29.0	3.0	0	0	0	0
1937	Cracklin' Oat Bran	1	cup(s)	65	1.8	267	5.3	46.7	8.0	9.3	4.0	3.1	2.0
58208	Fiber One Honey Clusters	1	cup(s)	52	—	160	5.0	42.0	13.0	1.5	0	0	0.5
1220	Froot Loops	1	cup(s)	29	0.9	110	1.0	25.0	3.0	1.0	0.5	0.1	0.2
38214	Frosted Cheerios	1	cup(s)	37	0.8	147	2.7	30.7	2.7	1.3	0	0	0.7
372	Frosted Flakes	1	cup(s)	40	1.3	147	1.3	36.0	1.3	0	0	0	0
1221	Frosted Mini-Wheats	1	cup(s)	47	2.6	158	4.7	37.9	4.7	0.8	0	0	0.4
1223	Granola, prepared	½	cup(s)	61	3.3	298	9.1	32.5	5.5	14.7	2.5	5.8	5.6
2415	Honey Bunches of Oats honey roasted	1	cup(s)	40	1.2	160	2.7	33.3	2.7	2.0	0	1.3	0
1227	Honey Nut Cheerios	1	cup(s)	37	0.8	147	2.7	29.3	2.7	2.0	0	0.7	0.7
1248	Honey Smacks	1	cup(s)	36	0.6	133	2.7	32.0	1.3	0.7	0	0.2	0.3
2424	Honeycomb	1	cup(s)	21	0.3	87	1.3	18.7	0.7	0.7	0	0	0
10286	Kashi Whole Grain Puffs	1	cup(s)	19	0.6	70	2.0	15.0	1.0	0.5	0	0.2	0.2
41142	Kellogg's Mueslix	1	cup(s)	82	7.2	294	7.5	60.2	6.8	4.5	0.5	2.1	1.1
1231	Kix	1	cup(s)	24	0.7	88	1.6	20.0	2.4	0.8	0	0	0
30569	Life	1	cup(s)	43	1.8	160	4.0	33.3	2.7	2.0	0	0.7	0.7
1233	Lucky Charms	1	cup(s)	36	1.1	147	2.7	29.3	1.3	1.3	0	0	0
38220	Multi Grain Cheerios	1	cup(s)	29	0.7	110	2.0	24.0	3.0	1.0	0	0	0.5
1201	Multi-Bran Chex	1	cup(s)	63	1.6	213	4.0	52.0	8.0	2.0	0	0	0.7
13633	Post Bran Flakes	1	cup(s)	40	1.1	133	4.0	32.0	6.7	0.7	0	0	0
1241	Product 19	1	cup(s)	30	0.9	100	2.0	25.0	1.0	0	0	0	0
32432	Puffed rice, fortified	1	cup(s)	14	0.4	56	0.9	12.6	0.2	0.1	0	—	—
32433	Puffed wheat, fortified	1	cup(s)	12	0.4	44	1.8	9.6	0.5	0.1	0	—	—
5584	Quaker Oatmeal Squares, brown sugar	1	cup(s)	55	1.1	210	6.0	44.0	5.0	2.5	0.5	1.0	1.0
41095	Quaker Oatmeal Squares, cinnamon	1	cup(s)	60	1.6	227	6.7	46.8	5.2	2.9	0.5	1.0	0.9
2420	Raisin Bran	1	cup(s)	59	4.8	190	4.0	46.0	8.0	1.0	0	0	0.5
1244	Rice Chex	1	cup(s)	27	0.7	100	2.0	23.0	0.0	0.5	0	0	0
1245	Rice Krispies	1	cup(s)	26	0.9	104	1.6	23.2	0.4	0	0	0	0
13648	Shredded Wheat	1	cup(s)	54	0.9	184	5.7	46.0	6.9	1.1	0	0	0.6
1246	Special K	1	cup(s)	31	0.9	120	6.0	23.0	0.5	0.5	0	0.1	0.2
41119	Total Raisin Bran	1	cup(s)	55	4.6	172	3.1	42.2	5.0	0.9	0.2	0.2	0.4
1253	Total whole grain	1	cup(s)	40	1.1	133	2.7	30.7	4.0	0.7	0	0	0
1254	Trix	1	cup(s)	32	0.6	120	1.0	28.0	1.0	1.5	0	0.5	0.5
41030	Wheat Chex	1	cup(s)	30	0.8	104	2.9	24.7	3.7	0.5	0.1	0.1	0.3
382	Wheat germ, toasted	2	tablespoon(s)	14	0.8	54	4.1	7.0	2.1	1.5	0.3	0.2	0.9
1257	Wheaties	1	cup(s)	36	0.9	133	4.0	29.3	4.0	0.7	0	0	0

PAGE KEY: A-6 5 Breads/Baked Goods A-12 = Cereal/Rice/Pasta A-16 = Fruit A-22 = Vegetables/Legumes A-32 = Nuts/Seeds A-34 = Vegetarian A-36 = Dairy A-44 = Eggs A-44 = Seafood A-46 = Meats A-50 = Poultry
A-52 = Processed Meats A-54 = Beverages A-58 = Fats/Oils A-60 = Sweets A-62 = Spices/Condiments/Sauces A-66 = Mixed Foods/Soups/Sandwiches A-72 = Fast Food A-90 = Convenience A-92 = Baby Foods

Chol (mg)	Calc (mg)	Iron (mg)	Magn (mg)	Pota (mg)	Sodi (mg)	Zinc (mg)	Vit A (μg)	Thia (mg)	Vit E (mg α)	Ribo (mg)	Niac (mg)	Vit B$_6$ (mg)	Fola (μg)	Vit C (mg)	Vit B$_{12}$ (μg)	Sele (μg)
0	1	0.69	8.5	32.7	269.8	0.22	0	0.10	0.04	0.07	0.97	0.06	46.0	0	0	3.8
0	1	0.69	6.1	26.6	269.8	0.17	0	0.12	0.02	0.07	0.92	0.04	44.8	0	0	3.3
0	11	1.05	31.6	81.9	4.7	1.17	0	0.09	0.09	0.02	0.26	0.01	7.0	0	0	6.3
0	99	7.40	48.1	136.7	272.2	1.09	0	1.12	—	0.05	2.55	0.33	56.5	0	0	11.1
0	109	4.79	48.9	138.5	242.7	1.11	0	0.78	—	0.05	1.78	0.22	40.2	0	0	3.8
0	200	9.00	200.0	700.0	160.0	3.00	300.5	0.75	0.77	0.85	10.00	4.00	1362.8	12.4	12.0	5.8
0	0	13.64	186.4	—	636.4	4.55	455.0	1.14	0.65	1.27	15.15	6.06	2052.7	18.2	18.2	26.3
0	0	4.50	5.9	35.0	130.0	1.50	146.8	0.38	0.04	0.43	5.00	0.50	184.5	15.0	1.5	1.6
0	0	6.00	19.4	66.7	266.7	5.00	0	0.51	0.26	0.57	6.68	0.67	906.7	0	0	2.3
0	0	6.00	18.7	66.7	253.4	5.00	0	0.51	0.22	0.57	6.68	0.67	906.8	0	0	0
0	100	8.10	40.0	170.0	190.0	3.75	150.1	0.38	0.19	0.43	5.00	0.50	460.3	6.0	1.5	8.0
0	133	6.00	10.7	80.0	200.0	5.00	23.8	0.50	0.28	0.57	6.67	0.67	199.1	8.0	2.0	2.3
0	53	6.00	15.7	80.0	200.0	1.98	203.3	0.50	0.11	0.57	6.61	0.67	446.4	20.0	2.0	6.7
0	0	24.00	53.3	226.7	280.0	20.00	300.5	2.00	17.92	2.27	26.67	2.67	901.4	80.0	8.0	4.1
0	0	8.12	2.5	25.0	200.0	0.05	127.3	0.38	0.04	0.43	5.00	0.50	221.8	6.0	1.5	2.3
0	0	1.80	2.2	45.0	125.0	1.57	143.1	0.38	0.02	0.43	5.00	0.50	174.7	6.0	1.5	2.1
0	27	2.40	80.0	293.3	200.0	2.03	300.5	0.50	0.37	0.57	6.66	0.65	218.2	20.0	2.0	7.0
0	100	4.50	32.0	320.0	280.0	3.75	0	0.38	—	0.43	5.00	0.50		0	1.5	—
0	0	4.50	6.7	35.0	135.0	1.50	144.7	0.38	0.03	0.43	5.00	0.50	150.5	15.0	1.5	1.7
0	133	6.00	19.9	73.3	226.6	5.00	200.1	0.50	0.16	0.57	6.67	0.67	448.3	8.0	2.0	5.8
0	0	6.00	2.8	26.7	186.7	0.06	200.2	0.50	0.04	0.57	6.67	0.67	254.0	8.0	2.0	1.8
0	0	12.80	47.4	158.1	4.0	1.19	0	0.30	0	0.34	3.95	0.40	149.2	0	1.2	1.9
0	48	2.58	106.8	329.4	15.3	2.46	0.6	0.45	6.78	0.18	1.31	0.18	50.0	0.7	0	17.0
0	0	14.40	21.3	73.3	200.0	0.40	300.3	0.50	0.59	0.57	6.67	0.67	549.6	0	2.0	3.3
0	133	6.00	42.7	153.3	253.3	5.00	200.1	0.50	0.36	0.57	6.67	0.67	448.3	8.0	2.0	8.8
0	0	0.48	21.2	53.3	66.7	0.47	200.2	0.50	0.17	0.58	6.66	0.67	224.6	8.0	2.0	17.5
0	0	1.80	10.7	33.3	120.0	1.00	150.1	0.25	0.04	0.28	3.33	0.33	122.2	0	1.0	4.3
0	0	0.36	29.3	60.0	0	0.58	0	0.02	0.17	0.03	0.61	0.06	6.1	0	0	6.8
0	48	6.76	73.4	256.5	207.8	5.61	135.2	0.66	5.94	0.66	8.25	3.05	1023.3	0.3	9.1	14.3
0	120	6.48	12.2	36.0	168.0	3.00	116.3	0.30	0.06	0.34	4.00	0.40	317.8	4.8	1.2	2.0
0	133	10.80	40.5	120.0	213.4	5.00	0	0.50	0.26	0.57	6.67	0.67	544.0	0	2.0	1.4
0	133	6.00	10.7	60.0	253.3	5.00	201.2	0.50	0.10	0.57	6.67	0.67	451.1	8.0	2.0	5.9
0	97	18.00	16.0	85.0	200.0	15.00	150.2	1.50	13.50	1.70	20.00	2.00	676.3	15.0	6.0	4.9
0	133	21.60	80.0	253.3	413.4	5.00	184.2	0.50	0.19	0.57	6.67	0.67	888.7	8.0	2.0	5.0
0	0	10.80	80.0	240.0	293.3	2.00	300.3	0.50	0.93	0.57	6.67	0.67	453.3	0	2.0	3.2
0	0	18.00	15.9	50.0	210.0	15.00	225.0	1.50	20.10	1.70	20.01	2.00	675.9	60.0	6.0	3.6
0	1	4.44	3.5	15.8	0.4	0.14	0	0.36	—	0.25	4.94	0.01	2.7	0	0	1.5
0	3	3.80	17.4	41.8	0.5	0.28	0	0.31	—	0.22	4.24	0.02	3.8	0	0	14.8
0	100	16.20	60.0	210.0	250.0	3.75	150.4	0.38	1.35	0.43	5.00	0.50	680.0	6.0		3.8
0	127	17.71	69.6	218.4	204.6	4.51	180.6	0.45	1.85	0.51	6.01	0.60	732.6	7.2	0	3.8
0	20	10.80	100.0	310.0	250.0	2.25	225.2	0.38	0.48	0.43	5.00	0.50	333.9	0	1.5	3.5
0	100	9.00	24.0	45.0	250.0	3.75	150.1	0.38	0.18	0.43	5.00	0.50	339.1	6.0	1.5	1.1
0	0	7.20	6.9	24.0	176.0	0.33	300.2	0.30	0.03	0.34	4.00	0.40	241.0	12.0	1.2	4.8
0	23	1.24	68.9	218.3	0	1.72	0	0.14	0	0.07	3.45	0.62	23.2	0	0	1.5
0	0	8.10	19.2	50.0	220.0	0.60	225.2	0.53	4.74	0.59	7.00	2.00	675.8	21.0	6.0	7.0
0	1038	18.70	33.0	277.2	186.4	15.56	154.6	1.54	14.01	1.76	20.74	2.08	698.5	0	6.2	3.8
0	1333	24.00	42.7	120.0	253.3	20.00	200.4	2.00	18.00	2.27	26.67	2.67	901.2	80.0	8.0	1.6
0	100	4.50	8.0	40.0	180.0	3.75	150.1	0.38	0.38	0.43	5.00	0.50	165.8	6.0	1.5	2.1
0	64	9.18	25.5	110.7	171.0	3.36	95.1	0.24	0.20	0.27	3.18	0.32	429.9	3.8	1.0	1.5
0	6	1.28	45.2	133.7	0.6	2.35	0.7	0.24	2.26	0.12	0.79	0.14	49.7	0.8	0	9.2
0	27	10.80	32.0	126.7	253.3	10.00	200.4	1.00	0.43	1.13	13.33	1.33	403.6	8.0	4.0	1.7

TABLE A-2 Table of Food Composition *(continued)*   (Computer code is for Cengage Diet Analysis program)   (For purposes of calculations, use "0" for t, <1, <0.1, <0.01)

DA+ Code	Food Description	Quantity	Measure	Wt (g)	H₂O (g)	Ener (kcal)	Prot (g)	Carb (g)	Fiber (g)	Fat (g)	Sat	Mono	Poly
											Fat Breakdown (g)		

Cereal, Flour, Grain, Pasta, Noodles, Popcorn—*continued*

Pasta, noodles

DA+ Code	Food Description	Quantity	Measure	Wt (g)	H₂O (g)	Ener (kcal)	Prot (g)	Carb (g)	Fiber (g)	Fat (g)	Sat	Mono	Poly
449	Chinese chow mein noodles, cooked	½	cup(s)	23	0.3	103	2.4	15.1	0.6	4.0	0.4	1.2	2.4
1995	Corn pasta, cooked	½	cup(s)	70	47.8	88	1.8	19.5	3.4	0.5	0.1	0.1	0.2
448	Egg noodles, enriched, cooked	½	cup(s)	80	54.2	110	3.6	20.1	1.0	1.7	0.3	0.5	0.4
1563	Egg noodles, spinach, enriched, cooked	½	cup(s)	80	54.8	106	4.0	19.4	1.8	1.3	0.3	0.4	0.3
440	Macaroni, enriched, cooked	½	cup(s)	70	43.5	111	4.1	21.6	1.3	0.7	0.1	0.1	0.2
2000	Macaroni, tricolor vegetable, enriched, cooked	½	cup(s)	67	45.8	86	3.0	17.8	2.9	0.1	0	0	0
1996	Plain pasta, fresh-refrigerated, cooked	½	cup(s)	64	43.9	84	3.3	16.0		0.7	0.1	0.1	0.3
1725	Ramen noodles, cooked	½	cup(s)	114	90.9	104	3.0	15.4	1.0	4.3	0.2	0.2	0.2
2878	Soba noodles, cooked	½	cup(s)	95	69.4	94	4.8	20.4	—	0.1	0	0	0
2879	Somen noodles, cooked	½	cup(s)	88	59.8	115	3.5	24.2	—	0.2	0	0	0.1
2881	Spaghetti, enriched, cooked	½	cup(s)	70	43.5	111	4.1	21.6	1.3	0.7	0.1	0.1	0.2
2884	Spaghetti, whole wheat, cooked	½	cup(s)	70	47.0	87	3.7	18.6	3.2	0.4	0.1	0.1	0.1

Popcorn

DA+ Code	Food Description	Quantity	Measure	Wt (g)	H₂O (g)	Ener (kcal)	Prot (g)	Carb (g)	Fiber (g)	Fat (g)	Sat	Mono	Poly
476	Air popped	1	cup(s)	8	0.3	31	1.0	6.2	1.2	0.4	0	0.1	0.2
4619	Caramel	1	cup(s)	35	1.0	152	1.3	27.8	1.8	4.5	1.3	1.0	1.6
4620	Cheese flavored	1	cup(s)	35	0.9	185	3.3	18.2	3.5	11.7	2.3	3.4	5.4
477	Popped in oil	1	cup(s)	11	0.1	64	0.8	5.0	0.9	4.8	0.8	1.1	2.6

Fruit and Fruit Juices

Apples

DA+ Code	Food Description	Quantity	Measure	Wt (g)	H₂O (g)	Ener (kcal)	Prot (g)	Carb (g)	Fiber (g)	Fat (g)	Sat	Mono	Poly
226	Applesauce, sweetened, canned	½	cup(s)	123	100.8	84	0.2	21.5	1.5	0.2	0	0	0.1
227	Applesauce, unsweetened, canned	½	cup(s)	122	107.6	51	0.2	13.7	1.3	0.1	0	0	0
38492	Crabapples	1	item(s)	35	27.6	27	0.1	7.0	0.9	0.1	0	0	0
948	Dried, sulfured	¼	cup(s)	22	6.8	52	0.2	14.2	1.9	0.1	0	0	0
952	Juice, prepared from frozen concentrate	½	cup(s)	120	105.0	56	0.2	13.8	0.1	0.1	0	0	0
225	Juice, unsweetened, canned	½	cup(s)	124	109.4	57	0.1	14.0	0.2	0.2	0	0	0
223	Raw medium, with peel	1	item(s)	182	155.7	95	0.5	25.1	4.4	0.3	0.1	0	0.1
224	Slices	½	cup(s)	55	46.6	28	0.1	7.5	1.3	0.1	0	0	0
946	Slices without skin, boiled	½	cup(s)	86	73.1	45	0.2	11.7	2.1	0.3	0	0	0.1

Apricot

DA+ Code	Food Description	Quantity	Measure	Wt (g)	H₂O (g)	Ener (kcal)	Prot (g)	Carb (g)	Fiber (g)	Fat (g)	Sat	Mono	Poly
228	Fresh without pits	4	item(s)	140	120.9	67	2.0	15.6	2.8	0.5	0	0.2	0.1
229	Halves with skin, canned in heavy syrup	½	cup(s)	129	100.1	107	0.7	27.7	2.1	0.1	0	0	0
230	Halves, dried, sulfured	¼	cup(s)	33	10.1	79	1.1	20.6	2.4	0.2	0	0	0

Avocado

DA+ Code	Food Description	Quantity	Measure	Wt (g)	H₂O (g)	Ener (kcal)	Prot (g)	Carb (g)	Fiber (g)	Fat (g)	Sat	Mono	Poly
233	California, whole, without skin or pit	½	cup(s)	115	83.2	192	2.3	9.9	7.8	17.7	2.4	11.3	2.1
234	Florida, whole, without skin or pit	½	cup(s)	115	90.6	138	2.6	9.0	6.4	11.6	2.3	6.3	1.9
2998	Pureed	½	cup(s)	115	84.2	184	2.3	9.8	7.7	16.9	2.4	11.3	2.1

Banana

DA+ Code	Food Description	Quantity	Measure	Wt (g)	H₂O (g)	Ener (kcal)	Prot (g)	Carb (g)	Fiber (g)	Fat (g)	Sat	Mono	Poly
4580	Dried chips	¼	cup(s)	18	0.8	93	0.4	10.5	1.4	6.0	5.2	0.4	0.1
235	Fresh whole, without peel	1	item(s)	118	88.4	105	1.3	27.0	3.1	0.4	0.1	0	0.1

Blackberries

DA+ Code	Food Description	Quantity	Measure	Wt (g)	H₂O (g)	Ener (kcal)	Prot (g)	Carb (g)	Fiber (g)	Fat (g)	Sat	Mono	Poly
958	Frozen, unsweetened	½	cup(s)	76	62.1	48	0.9	11.8	3.8	0.3	0	0	0.2
237	Raw	½	cup(s)	72	63.5	31	1.0	6.9	3.8	0.4	0	0	0.2

Blueberries

DA+ Code	Food Description	Quantity	Measure	Wt (g)	H₂O (g)	Ener (kcal)	Prot (g)	Carb (g)	Fiber (g)	Fat (g)	Sat	Mono	Poly
959	Canned in heavy syrup	½	cup(s)	128	98.3	113	0.8	28.2	2.0	0.4	0	0.1	0.2
960	Frozen, unsweetened	½	cup(s)	78	67.1	40	0.3	9.4	2.1	0.5	0	0.1	0.2
238	Raw	½	cup(s)	74	62.3	42	0.5	10.7	1.8	0.2	0	0	0.1

Boysenberries

DA+ Code	Food Description	Quantity	Measure	Wt (g)	H₂O (g)	Ener (kcal)	Prot (g)	Carb (g)	Fiber (g)	Fat (g)	Sat	Mono	Poly
961	Canned in heavy syrup	½	cup(s)	128	97.6	113	1.3	28.6	3.3	0.2	0	0	0.1
962	Frozen, unsweetened	½	cup(s)	66	56.7	33	0.7	8.0	3.5	0.2	0	0	0.1
35576	Breadfruit	1	item(s)	384	271.3	396	4.1	104.1	18.8	0.9	0.2	0.1	0.3

Appendix A

PAGE KEY: A-6 5 Breads/Baked Goods A-12 = Cereal/Rice/Pasta A-16 = Fruit A-22 = Vegetables/Legumes A-32 = Nuts/Seeds A-34 = Vegetarian A-36 = Dairy A-44 = Eggs A-44 = Seafood A-46 = Meats A-50 = Poultry
A-52 = Processed Meats A-54 = Beverages A-58 = Fats/Oils A-60 = Sweets A-62 = Spices/Condiments/Sauces A-66 = Mixed Foods/Soups/Sandwiches A-72 = Fast Food A-90 = Convenience A-92 = Baby Foods

Chol (mg)	Calc (mg)	Iron (mg)	Magn (mg)	Pota (mg)	Sodi (mg)	Zinc (mg)	Vit A (µg)	Thia (mg)	Vit E (mg α)	Ribo (mg)	Niac (mg)	Vit B$_6$ (mg)	Fola (µg)	Vit C (mg)	Vit B$_{12}$ (µg)	Sele (µg)
0	5	1.06	11.7	27.0	190.6	0.31	0	0.13	0.53	0.09	1.34	0.03	38.0	0	0	9.7
0	1	0.17	25.2	21.7	0	0.44	2.1	0.04	—	0.02	0.39	0.04	4.2	0	0	2.0
23	10	1.18	16.8	30.4	4.0	0.52	4.8	0.23	0.14	0.11	1.66	0.04	110.4	0	0.1	19.1
26	15	0.87	19.2	29.6	9.6	0.50	8.0	0.20	0.44	0.10	1.18	0.09	75.2	0	0.1	17.4
0	5	0.90	12.6	30.8	0.7	0.36	0	0.19	0.04	0.10	1.18	0.03	83.3	0	0	18.5
0	7	0.33	12.7	20.8	4.0	0.29	3.3	0.08	0.14	0.04	0.72	0.02	71.0	0	0	13.3
21	4	0.73	11.5	15.4	3.8	0.36	3.8	0.13	—	0.10	0.63	0.02	66.6	0	0.1	—
18	9	0.89	8.5	34.5	414.5	0.31	—	0.08	0.11	0.05	0.71	0.03	—	0.1	0	—
0	4	0.46	8.5	33.3	57.0	0.11	0	0.09	—	0.02	0.48	0.04	6.7	0	0	
0	7	0.46	1.8	25.5	141.7	0.19	0	0.02	—	0.03	0.09	0.01	1.8	0	0	
0	5	0.90	12.6	30.8	0.7	0.36	0	0.19	0.04	0.10	1.18	0.03	83.3	0	0	18.5
0	11	0.74	21.0	30.8	2.1	0.57	0	0.08	0.21	0.03	0.49	0.06	3.5	0	0	18.1
0	1	0.26	11.5	26.3	0.6	0.25	0.8	0.01	0.02	0.01	0.18	0.01	2.5	0	0	0
2	15	0.61	12.3	38.4	72.5	0.20	0.7	0.02	0.42	0.02	0.77	0.01	1.8	0	0	1.3
4	40	0.79	32.0	91.9	312.9	0.71	13.4	0.04	—	0.08	0.51	0.08	3.9	0.2	0.2	4.2
0	0	0.22	8.7	20.0	116.4	0.34	0.9	0.01	0.27	0.01	0.13	0.01	2.8	0	0	0.2
0	4	0.15	3.7	92.3	2.5	0.04	0	0.02	0.22	0.03	0.09	0.03	1.2	2.1	0	0.4
0	5	0.28	3.7	90.3	2.4	0.04	1.2	0.03	0.20	0.04	0.10	0.03	3.7	1.2	0	0.4
0	6	0.13	2.5	67.9	0.3	—	0.7	0.01	0.21	0.01	0.04	—	2.0	2.8	0	—
0	3	0.30	3.4	96.8	18.7	0.04	0	0	0.11	0.03	0.20	0.03	0	0.8	0	0.3
0	7	0.31	6.0	150.6	8.4	0.05	0	0	0.01	0.02	0.05	0.04	0	0.7	0	0.1
0	10	0.15	6.2	125.2	5.0	0.02	0	0.03	0.01	0.01	0.09	0.02	0	1.1	0	0.1
0	11	0.22	9.1	194.7	1.8	0.07	5.5	0.03	0.33	0.05	0.17	0.07	5.5	8.4	0	0
0	3	0.07	2.7	58.3	0.5	0.02	1.6	0.01	0.10	0.01	0.05	0.02	1.6	2.5	0	0
0	4	0.16	2.6	75.2	0.9	0.03	1.7	0.01	0.04	0.01	0.08	0.04	0.9	0.2	0	0.3
0	18	0.55	14.0	362.6	1.4	0.28	134.4	0.04	1.25	0.06	0.84	0.08	12.6	14.0	0	0.1
0	12	0.39	9.0	180.6	5.2	0.14	80.0	0.03	0.77	0.03	0.49	0.07	2.6	4.0	0	0.1
0	18	0.87	10.5	381.5	3.3	0.13	59.1	0	1.42	0.02	0.85	0.05	3.3	0.3	0	0.7
0	15	0.70	33.4	583.1	9.2	0.78	8.1	0.09	2.27	0.16	2.20	0.33	102.4	10.1	0	0.5
0	12	0.20	27.6	403.7	2.3	0.46	8.1	0.02	3.06	0.06	0.77	0.09	40.2	20.0	0	—
0	14	0.63	33.4	557.8	8.1	0.74	8.0	0.08	2.38	0.15	2.00	0.30	93.2	11.5	0	0.5
0	3	0.22	13.7	96.4	1.1	0.13	0.7	0.02	0.04	0	0.13	0.05	2.5	1.1	0	0.3
0	6	0.31	31.9	422.4	1.2	0.18	3.5	0.04	0.12	0.09	0.78	0.43	23.6	10.3	0	1.2
0	22	0.60	16.6	105.7	0.8	0.19	4.5	0.02	0.88	0.03	0.91	0.05	25.7	2.3	0	0.3
0	21	0.45	14.4	116.6	0.7	0.38	7.9	0.01	0.84	0.02	0.47	0.02	18.0	15.1	0	0.3
0	6	0.42	5.1	51.2	3.8	0.09	2.6	0.04	0.49	0.07	0.14	0.05	2.6	1.4	0	0.1
0	6	0.14	3.9	41.8	0.8	0.05	1.5	0.02	0.37	0.03	0.40	0.05	5.4	1.9	0	0.1
0	4	0.21	4.4	57.0	0.7	0.12	2.2	0.03	0.42	0.03	0.31	0.04	4.4	7.2	0	0.1
0	23	0.55	14.1	115.2	3.8	0.24	2.6	0.03	—	0.04	0.29	0.05	43.5	7.9	0	0.5
0	18	0.56	10.6	91.7	0.7	0.15	2.0	0.03	0.57	0.02	0.51	0.04	41.6	2.0	0	0.1
0	65	2.07	96.0	1881.6	7.7	0.46	7.7	0.42	0.38	0.12	3.46	0.38	53.8	111.4	0	2.3

TABLE A-2 Table of Food Composition *(continued)*   (Computer code is for Cengage Diet Analysis program)   (For purposes of calculations, use "0" for t, <1, <0.1, <0.01)

DA+ Code	Food Description	Quantity	Measure	Wt (g)	H₂O (g)	Ener (kcal)	Prot (g)	Carb (g)	Fiber (g)	Fat (g)	Fat Breakdown (g) Sat	Mono	Poly
Fruit and Fruit Juices—*continued*													
	Cherries												
967	Sour red, canned in water	½	cup(s)	122	109.7	44	0.9	10.9	1.3	0.1	0	0	0
3000	Sour red, raw	½	cup(s)	78	66.8	39	0.8	9.4	1.2	0.2	0.1	0.1	0.1
3004	Sweet, canned in heavy syrup	½	cup(s)	127	98.2	105	0.8	26.9	1.8	0.2	0	0.1	0.1
969	Sweet, canned in water	½	cup(s)	124	107.9	57	1.0	14.6	1.9	0.2	0	0	0
240	Sweet, raw	½	cup(s)	77	63.3	49	0.8	12.3	1.6	0.2	0	0	0
	Cranberries												
3007	Chopped, raw	½	cup(s)	55	47.9	25	0.2	6.7	2.5	0.1	0	0	0
1717	Cranberry apple juice drink	½	cup(s)	123	102.6	77	0	19.4	0	0.1	0	0	0.1
1638	Cranberry juice cocktail	½	cup(s)	127	109.0	68	0	17.1	0	0.1	0	0	0
241	Cranberry juice cocktail, low calorie, with saccharin	½	cup(s)	119	112.8	23	0	5.5	0	0	0	0	0
242	Cranberry sauce, sweetened, canned	¼	cup(s)	69	42.0	105	0.1	26.9	0.7	0.1	0	0	0
	Dates												
244	Domestic, chopped	¼	cup(s)	45	9.1	125	1.1	33.4	3.6	0.2	0	0	0
243	Domestic, whole	¼	cup(s)	45	9.1	125	1.1	33.4	3.6	0.2	0	0	0
	Figs												
975	Canned in heavy syrup	½	cup(s)	130	98.8	114	0.5	29.7	2.8	0.1	0	0	0.1
974	Canned in water	½	cup(s)	124	105.7	66	0.5	17.3	2.7	0.1	0	0	0.1
973	Raw, medium	2	item(s)	100	79.1	74	0.8	19.2	2.9	0.3	0.1	0.1	0.1
	Fruit cocktail & salad												
245	Fruit cocktail, canned in heavy syrup	½	cup(s)	124	99.7	91	0.5	23.4	1.2	0.1	0	0	0
978	Fruit cocktail, canned in juice	½	cup(s)	119	103.6	55	0.5	14.1	1.2	0	0	0	0
977	Fruit cocktail, canned in water	½	cup(s)	119	107.6	38	0.5	10.1	1.2	0.1	0	0	0
979	Fruit salad, canned in water	½	cup(s)	123	112.1	37	0.4	9.6	1.2	0.1	0	0	0
	Gooseberries												
982	Canned in light syrup	½	cup(s)	126	100.9	92	0.8	23.6	3.0	0.3	0	0	0.1
981	Raw	½	cup(s)	75	65.9	33	0.7	7.6	3.2	0.4	0	0	0.2
	Grapefruit												
251	Juice, pink, sweetened, canned	½	cup(s)	125	109.1	57	0.7	13.9	0.1	0.1	0	0	0
249	Juice, white	½	cup(s)	124	111.2	48	0.6	11.4	0.1	0.1	0	0	0
3022	Pink or red, raw	½	cup(s)	114	100.8	48	0.9	12.2	1.8	0.2	0	0	0
247	Raw, white	½	cup(s)	115	104.1	38	0.8	9.7	1.3	0.1	0	0	0
248	Sections, canned in light syrup	½	cup(s)	127	106.2	76	0.7	19.6	0.5	0.1	0	0	0
983	Sections, canned in water	½	cup(s)	122	109.6	44	0.7	11.2	0.5	0.1	0	0	0
	Grapes												
255	American, slip skin	½	cup(s)	46	37.4	31	0.3	7.9	0.4	0.2	0.1	0	0
256	European, red or green, adherent skin	½	cup(s)	76	60.8	52	0.5	13.7	0.7	0.1	0	0	0
3159	Juice drink, canned	½	cup(s)	125	106.6	71	0	18.2	0.1	0	0	0	0
259	Juice, sweetened, with added vitamin C, prepared from frozen concentrate	½	cup(s)	125	108.6	64	0.2	15.9	0.1	0.1	0	0	0
3060	Raisins, seeded, packed	¼	cup(s)	41	6.8	122	1.0	32.4	2.8	0.2	0.1	0	0.1
987	**Guava, raw**	1	item(s)	55	44.4	37	1.4	7.9	3.0	0.5	0.1	0	0.2
35593	**Guava, strawberry**	1	item(s)	6	4.8	4	0	1.0	0.3	0	0	0	0
3027	**Jackfruit**	½	cup(s)	83	60.6	78	1.4	19.2	1.2	0.5	0.2	0.1	0.1
990	**Kiwi fruit or Chinese gooseberries**	1	item(s)	76	63.1	46	0.9	11.1	2.3	0.4	0	0	0.2
	Lemon												
262	Juice	1	tablespoon(s)	15	14.1	3	0.1	1.1	0	0	0	0	0
993	Peel	1	teaspoon(s)	2	1.6	1	0	0.3	0.2	0	0	0	0
992	Raw	1	item(s)	108	94.4	22	1.3	11.6	5.1	0.3	0	0	0.1
	Lime												
269	Juice	1	tablespoon(s)	15	14.0	4	0.1	1.3	0.1	0	0	0	0
994	Raw	1	item(s)	67	59.1	20	0.5	7.1	1.9	0.1	0	0	0
995	**Loganberries, frozen**	½	cup(s)	74	62.2	40	1.1	9.6	3.9	0.2	0	0	0.1
	Mandarin orange												
1038	Canned in juice	½	cup(s)	125	111.4	46	0.8	11.9	0.9	0	0	0	0
1039	Canned in light syrup	½	cup(s)	126	104.7	77	0.6	20.4	0.9	0.1	0	0	0

PAGE KEY: A-6 5 Breads/Baked Goods A-12 = Cereal/Rice/Pasta A-16 = Fruit A-22 = Vegetables/Legumes A-32 = Nuts/Seeds A-34 = Vegetarian A-36 = Dairy A-44 = Eggs A-44 = Seafood A-46 = Meats A-50 = Poultry
A-52 = Processed Meats A-54 = Beverages A-58 = Fats/Oils A-60 = Sweets A-62 = Spices/Condiments/Sauces A-66 = Mixed Foods/Soups/Sandwiches A-72 = Fast Food A-90 = Convenience A-92 = Baby Foods

Chol (mg)	Calc (mg)	Iron (mg)	Magn (mg)	Pota (mg)	Sodi (mg)	Zinc (mg)	Vit A (µg)	Thia (mg)	Vit E (mg α)	Ribo (mg)	Niac (mg)	Vit B$_6$ (mg)	Fola (µg)	Vit C (mg)	Vit B$_{12}$ (µg)	Sele (µg)
0	13	1.67	7.3	119.6	8.5	0.09	46.4	0.02	0.28	0.05	0.22	0.05	9.8	2.6	0	0
0	12	0.25	7.0	134.1	2.3	0.08	49.6	0.02	0.05	0.03	0.31	0.03	6.2	7.8	0	0
0	11	0.44	11.4	183.4	3.8	0.13	10.1	0.03	0.22	0.05	0.50	0.03	5.1	4.6	0	0
0	14	0.45	11.2	162.4	1.2	0.10	9.9	0.03	0.29	0.05	0.51	0.04	5.0	2.7	0	0
0	10	0.28	8.5	170.9	0	0.05	2.3	0.02	0.05	0.03	0.12	0.04	3.1	5.4	0	0
0	4	0.14	3.3	46.8	1.1	0.05	1.6	0.01	0.66	0.01	0.06	0.03	0.6	7.3	0	0.1
0	4	0.09	1.2	20.8	2.5	0.02	0	0	0.15	0	0	0	0	48.4	0	0
0	4	0.13	1.3	17.7	2.5	0.04	0	0	0.28	0	0.05	0	0	53.5	0	0.3
0	11	0.05	2.4	29.6	3.6	0.02	0	0	0.06	0	0	0	0	38.2	0	0
0	3	0.15	2.1	18.0	20.1	0.03	1.4	0.01	0.57	0.01	0.07	0.01	0.7	1.4	0	0.2
0	17	0.45	19.1	291.9	0.9	0.13	0	0.02	0.02	0.03	0.57	0.07	8.5	0.2	0	1.3
0	17	0.45	19.1	291.9	0.9	0.13	0	0.02	0.02	0.03	0.57	0.07	8.5	0.2	0	1.3
0	35	0.36	12.9	128.2	1.3	0.14	2.6	0.03	0.16	0.05	0.55	0.09	2.6	1.3	0	0.3
0	35	0.36	12.4	127.7	1.2	0.15	2.5	0.03	0.10	0.05	0.55	0.09	2.5	1.2	0	0.1
0	35	0.37	17.0	232.0	1.0	0.15	7.0	0.06	0.11	0.05	0.40	0.11	6.0	2.0	0	0.2
0	7	0.36	6.2	109.1	7.4	0.10	12.4	0.02	0.50	0.02	0.46	0.06	3.7	2.4	0	0.6
0	9	0.25	8.3	112.6	4.7	0.11	17.8	0.01	0.47	0.02	0.48	0.06	3.6	3.2	0	0.6
0	6	0.30	8.3	111.4	4.7	0.11	15.4	0.02	0.47	0.01	0.43	0.06	3.6	2.5	0	0.6
0	9	0.37	6.1	95.6	3.7	0.10	27.0	0.02	—	0.03	0.46	0.04	3.7	2.3	0	1.0
0	20	0.42	7.6	97.0	2.5	0.14	8.8	0.03	—	0.07	0.19	0.02	3.8	12.6	0	0.5
0	19	0.23	7.5	148.5	0.8	0.09	11.3	0.03	0.28	0.02	0.22	0.06	4.5	20.8	0	0.4
0	10	0.45	12.5	202.2	2.5	0.07	0	0.05	0.05	0.03	0.40	0.02	12.5	33.6	0	0.1
0	11	0.25	14.8	200.1	1.2	0.06	1.2	0.05	0.27	0.02	0.25	0.05	12.4	46.9	0	0.1
0	25	0.09	10.3	154.5	0	0.08	66.4	0.05	0.15	0.04	0.23	0.06	14.9	35.7	0	0.1
0	14	0.07	10.3	170.2	0	0.08	2.3	0.04	0.15	0.02	0.31	0.05	11.5	38.3	0	1.6
0	18	0.51	12.7	163.8	2.5	0.10	0	0.05	0.11	0.03	0.31	0.03	11.4	27.1	0	1.1
0	18	0.50	12.2	161.0	2.4	0.11	0	0.05	0.11	0.03	0.30	0.02	11.0	26.6	0	1.1
0	6	0.13	2.3	87.9	0.9	0.02	2.3	0.04	0.09	0.03	0.14	0.05	1.8	1.8	0	0
0	8	0.27	5.3	144.2	1.5	0.05	2.3	0.05	0.14	0.05	0.14	0.06	1.5	2.4	0	0.1
0	9	0.16	7.5	41.3	11.3	0.04	0	0.28	0	0.44	0.18	0.04	1.3	33.1	0	0.1
0	5	0.13	5.0	26.3	2.5	0.05	0	0.02	0	0.03	0.16	0.05	1.3	29.9	0	0.1
0	12	1.07	12.4	340.3	11.6	0.07	0	0.05	—	0.08	0.46	0.08	1.2	2.2	0	0.2
0	10	0.14	12.1	229.4	1.1	0.13	17.0	0.04	0.40	0.02	0.60	0.06	27.0	125.6	0	0.3
0	1	0.01	1.0	17.5	2.2	—	0.3	0	0	0	0.04	0.00	—	2.2	0	0
0	20	0.19	23.9	369.6	1.6	0.11	4.1	0.09	0.28	0.05	0.76	0.27	19.8	11.3	0	0.5
0	26	0.24	12.9	237.1	2.3	0.11	3.0	0.02	1.11	0.02	0.26	0.05	19.0	70.5	0	0.2
0	1	0.01	0.9	15.7	0.2	0.01	0	0	0.02	0	0.01	0.01	3.0	5.9	0	0
0	3	0.02	0.3	3.2	0.1	0	0.1	0	0	0	0.01	0.0	0.3	2.6	0	0
0	66	0.76	13.0	156.6	3.2	0.11	2.2	0.05	—	0.04	0.22	0.12	—	83.2	0	1.0
0	2	0.01	1.2	18.0	0.3	0.01	0.3	0	0.03	0	0.02	0.01	1.5	4.6	0	0
0	22	0.40	4.0	68.3	1.3	0.07	1.3	0.02	0.15	0.01	0.13	0.03	5.4	19.5	0	0.3
0	19	0.47	15.4	106.6	0.7	0.25	1.5	0.04	0.64	0.02	0.62	0.05	19.1	11.2	0	0.1
0	14	0.34	13.7	165.6	6.2	0.63	53.5	0.10	0.12	0.04	0.55	0.05	6.2	42.6	0	0.5
0	9	0.47	10.1	98.3	7.6	0.30	52.9	0.07	0.13	0.06	0.56	0.05	6.3	24.9	0	0.5

TABLE A-2 Table of Food Composition (continued) (Computer code is for Cengage Diet Analysis program) (For purposes of calculations, use "0" for t, <1, <0.1, <0.01)

DA+ Code	Food Description	Quantity	Measure	Wt (g)	H₂O (g)	Ener (kcal)	Prot (g)	Carb (g)	Fiber (g)	Fat (g)	Fat Breakdown (g) Sat	Mono	Poly
Fruit and Fruit Juices—*continued*													
999	**Mango**	½	cup(s)	83	68.9	49	0.7	12.4	1.3	0.3	0.1	0.1	0.1
1005	**Nectarine, raw, sliced**	½	cup(s)	69	60.4	30	0.7	7.3	1.2	0.2	0	0.1	0.1
	Melons												
271	Cantaloupe	½	cup(s)	80	72.1	27	0.7	6.5	0.7	0.2	0	0	0.1
1000	Casaba melon	½	cup(s)	85	78.1	24	0.9	5.6	0.8	0.1	0	0	0
272	Honeydew	½	cup(s)	89	79.5	32	0.5	8.0	0.7	0.1	0	0	0.1
318	Watermelon	½	cup(s)	76	69.5	23	0.5	5.7	0.3	0.1	0	0	0
	Orange												
14412	Juice with calcium and vitamin D	½	cup(s)	120	105.5	55	1.0	13.0	0	0	0	0	0
29630	Juice, fresh squeezed	½	cup(s)	124	109.5	56	0.9	12.9	0.2	0.2	0	0	0
14411	Juice, not from concentrate	½	cup(s)	120	105.5	55	1.0	13.0	0	0	0	0	0
278	Juice, unsweetened, prepared from frozen concentrate	½	cup(s)	125	109.7	56	0.8	13.4	0.2	0.1	0	0	0
3040	Peel	1	teaspoon(s)	2	1.5	2	0	0.5	0.2	0	0	0	0
273	Raw	1	item(s)	131	113.6	62	1.2	15.4	3.1	0.2	0	0	0
274	Sections	½	cup(s)	90	78.1	42	0.8	10.6	2.2	0.1	0	0	0
	Papaya												
16830	Dried, strips	2	item(s)	46	9.6	131	1.4	33.0	5.2	0.8	0.2	0.2	0.2
282	Raw	½	cup(s)	70	61.6	30	0.3	7.6	1.2	0.2	0.1	0.1	0
35640	**Passion fruit, purple**	1	item(s)	18	13.1	17	0.4	4.2	1.9	0.1	0	0	0.1
	Peach												
285	Halves, canned in heavy syrup	½	cup(s)	131	103.9	97	0.6	26.1	1.7	0.1	0	0	0.1
286	Halves, canned in water	½	cup(s)	122	113.6	29	0.8	7.5	1.6	0.1	0	0	0
283	Raw, medium	1	item(s)	150	133.3	59	1.4	14.3	2.3	0.4	0	0.1	0.1
290	Slices, sweetened, frozen	½	cup(s)	125	93.4	118	0.8	30.0	2.3	0.2	0	0.1	0.1
	Pear												
8672	Asian	1	item(s)	122	107.7	51	0.6	13.0	4.4	0.3	0	0.1	0.1
80684	Bartlett	1	item(s)	177	148.9	112	0.7	26.6	5.5	0.3	—	—	—
294	Halves, canned in heavy syrup	½	cup(s)	133	106.9	98	0.3	25.5	2.1	0.2	0	0	0
1012	Halves, canned in juice	½	cup(s)	124	107.2	62	0.4	16.0	2.0	0.1	0	0	0
291	Raw	1	item(s)	166	139.4	95	0.6	25.3	5.1	0.2	0	0.1	0.2
1017	**Persimmon**	1	item(s)	25	16.1	32	0.2	8.4	—	0.1	0	0	0
	Pineapple												
3053	Canned in extra heavy syrup	½	cup(s)	130	101.0	108	0.4	28.0	1.0	0.1	0	0	0
1019	Canned in juice	½	cup(s)	125	104.0	75	0.5	19.5	1.0	0.1	0	0	0
296	Canned in light syrup	½	cup(s)	126	108.0	66	0.5	16.9	1.0	0.2	0	0	0.1
1018	Canned in water	½	cup(s)	123	111.7	39	0.5	10.2	1.0	0.1	0	0	0
299	Juice, unsweetened, canned	½	cup(s)	125	108.0	66	0.4	16.1	0.3	0.2	0	0	0.1
295	Raw, diced	½	cup(s)	78	66.7	39	0.4	10.2	1.1	0.1	0	0	0
1024	**Plantain, cooked**	½	cup(s)	77	51.8	89	0.6	24.0	1.8	0.1	0.1	0	0
300	**Plum, raw, large**	1	item(s)	66	57.6	30	0.5	7.5	0.9	0.2	0	0.1	0
1027	**Pomegranate**	1	item(s)	282	219.8	234	4.7	52.7	11.3	3.3	0.3	0.3	0.2
	Prunes												
5644	Dried	2	item(s)	17	5.2	40	0.4	10.7	1.2	0.1	0	0	0
305	Dried, stewed	½	cup(s)	124	86.5	133	1.2	34.8	3.8	0.2	0	0.1	0
306	Juice, canned	1	cup(s)	256	208.0	182	1.6	44.7	2.6	0.1	0	0.1	0
	Raspberries												
309	Raw	½	cup(s)	62	52.7	32	0.7	7.3	4.0	0.4	0	0	0.2
310	Red, sweetened, frozen	½	cup(s)	125	90.9	129	0.9	32.7	5.5	0.2	0	0	0.1
39793	**Rhubarb, frozen, cooked with sugar**	½	cup(s)	120	81.3	139	0.5	37.4	2.4	0.1	0	0	0
	Strawberries												
313	Raw	½	cup(s)	72	65.5	23	0.5	5.5	1.4	0.2	0	0	0.1
315	Sweetened, frozen, thawed	½	cup(s)	128	99.5	99	0.7	26.8	2.4	0.2	0	0	0.1
16828	**Tangelo**	1	item(s)	95	82.4	45	0.9	11.2	2.3	0.1	0	0	0
	Tangerine												
1040	Juice	½	cup(s)	124	109.8	53	0.6	12.5	0.2	0.2	0	0	0
316	Raw	1	item(s)	88	74.9	47	0.7	11.7	1.6	0.3	0	0.1	0.1

PAGE KEY: A-6 5 Breads/Baked Goods A-12 = Cereal/Rice/Pasta A-16 = Fruit A-22 = Vegetables/Legumes A-32 = Nuts/Seeds A-34 = Vegetarian A-36 = Dairy A-44 = Eggs A-44 = Seafood A-46 = Meats A-50 = Poultry A-52 = Processed Meats A-54 = Beverages A-58 = Fats/Oils A-60 = Sweets A-62 = Spices/Condiments/Sauces A-66 = Mixed Foods/Soups/Sandwiches A-72 = Fast Food A-90 = Convenience A-92 = Baby Foods

Chol (mg)	Calc (mg)	Iron (mg)	Magn (mg)	Pota (mg)	Sodi (mg)	Zinc (mg)	Vit A (µg)	Thia (mg)	Vit E (mg α)	Ribo (mg)	Niac (mg)	Vit B$_6$ (mg)	Fola (µg)	Vit C (mg)	Vit B$_{12}$ (µg)	Sele (µg)
0	9	0.13	8.3	138.6	0.8	0.07	44.5	0.02	0.74	0.03	0.55	0.10	35.5	30.0	0	0.5
0	4	0.19	6.2	138.7	0	0.12	11.7	0.02	0.53	0.02	0.78	0.02	3.5	3.7	0	0
0	7	0.17	9.6	213.6	12.8	0.14	135.2	0.03	0.04	0.02	0.59	0.06	16.8	29.4	0	0.3
0	9	0.29	9.4	154.8	7.7	0.06	0.0	0.01	0.04	0.03	0.20	0.14	6.8	18.5	0	0.3
0	5	0.15	8.8	201.8	15.9	0.08	2.7	0.03	0.02	0.01	0.37	0.08	16.8	15.9	0	0.6
0	5	0.18	7.6	85.1	0.8	0.08	21.3	0.03	0.04	0.02	0.14	0.03	2.3	6.2	0	0.3
0	175	0	12.0	225.0	0	0.06	0	0.08	0.24	0.03	0.40	0.06	—	36.0	0	0.1
0	14	0.25	13.6	248.0	1.2	0.06	12.4	0.11	0.05	0.04	0.50	0.05	37.2	62.0	0	0.1
0	10	0	12.4	225.0	0	0.06	0	0.08	0.24	0.03	0.40	0.06	—	36.0	0	0.1
0	11	0.12	12.4	236.6	1.2	0.06	6.2	0.10	0.25	0.02	0.25	0.05	54.8	48.4	0	0.1
0	3	0.02	0.4	4.2	0.1	0	0.4	0	0	0	0.02	0.00	0.6	2.7	0	0
0	52	0.13	13.1	237.1	0	0.09	14.4	0.11	0.24	0.05	0.37	0.08	39.3	69.7	0	0.7
0	36	0.09	9.0	162.9	0	0.06	9.9	0.08	0.16	0.04	0.25	0.05	27.0	47.9	0	0.5
0	61	0.76	63.9	554.3	24.4	0.24	71.8	0.05	0.92	0.07	0.98	0.10	56.6	37.1	0	1.8
0	14	0.17	14.7	127.4	5.6	0.06	32.9	0.02	0.21	0.02	0.25	0.03	25.9	42.6	0	0.4
0	2	0.29	5.2	62.6	5.0	0.02	11.5	0	0	0.02	0.27	0.02	2.5	5.4	0	0.1
0	4	0.35	6.6	120.5	7.9	0.12	22.3	0.01	0.64	0.03	0.80	0.02	3.9	3.7	0	0.4
0	2	0.39	6.1	120.8	3.7	0.11	32.9	0.01	0.60	0.02	0.64	0.02	3.7	3.5	0	0.4
0	9	0.38	13.5	285.0	0	0.25	24.0	0.04	1.10	0.05	1.21	0.04	6.0	9.9	0	0.2
0	4	0.46	6.3	162.5	7.5	0.06	17.5	0.02	0.77	0.04	0.82	0.02	3.8	117.8	0	0.5
0	5	0	9.8	147.6	0	0.02	0	0.01	0.15	0.01	0.27	0.03	9.8	4.6	0	0.1
—	16	0.34	10.6	178.8	1.8	0.14	1.8	0.02	0.21	0.05	0.29	0.05	—	7.8	—	0.2
0	7	0.29	5.3	86.4	6.7	0.11	0	0.01	0.11	0.03	0.32	0.02	1.3	1.5	0	0
0	11	0.36	8.7	119.0	5.0	0.11	0	0.01	0.10	0.01	0.25	0.02	1.2	2.0	0	0
0	15	0.30	11.6	192.6	1.7	0.17	1.7	0.02	0.20	0.04	0.27	0.05	11.6	7.1	0	0.2
0	7	0.63	—	77.5	0.3	—	—	—	—	—	—	—	—	16.5	0	—
0	18	0.49	19.5	132.6	1.3	0.14	1.3	0.12	—	0.03	0.37	0.10	6.5	9.5	0	—
0	17	0.35	17.4	151.9	1.2	0.12	2.5	0.12	0.01	0.02	0.35	0.09	6.2	11.8	0	0.5
0	18	0.49	20.2	132.3	1.3	0.15	2.5	0.11	0.01	0.03	0.37	0.09	6.3	9.4	0	0.5
0	18	0.49	22.1	156.2	1.2	0.15	2.5	0.11	0.01	0.03	0.37	0.09	6.2	9.5	0	0.5
0	16	0.39	15.0	162.5	2.5	0.14	0	0.07	0.03	0.03	0.25	0.13	22.5	12.5	0	0.1
0	10	0.22	9.3	84.5	0.8	0.09	2.3	0.06	0.02	0.02	0.39	0.09	13.9	37.0	0	0.1
0	2	0.45	24.6	358.0	3.8	0.10	34.7	0.04	0.10	0.04	0.58	0.18	20.0	8.4	0	1.1
0	4	0.11	4.6	103.6	0	0.07	11.2	0.02	0.17	0.02	0.28	0.02	3.3	6.3	0	0
0	28	0.85	33.8	665.5	8.5	0.99	0	0.19	1.69	0.15	0.83	0.21	107.2	28.8	0	1.4
0	7	0.16	6.9	123.0	0.3	0.07	6.6	0.01	0.07	0.03	0.32	0.03	0.7	0.1	0	0.1
0	24	0.51	22.3	398.0	1.2	0.24	21.1	0.03	0.24	0.12	0.90	0.27	0	3.6	0	0.1
0	31	3.02	35.8	706.6	10.2	0.54	0	0.04	0.31	0.18	2.01	0.56	0	10.5	0	1.5
0	15	0.42	13.5	92.9	0.6	0.26	1.2	0.02	0.54	0.02	0.37	0.03	12.9	16.1	0	0.1
0	19	0.81	16.3	142.5	1.3	0.22	3.8	0.02	0.90	0.06	0.29	0.04	32.5	20.6	0	0.4
0	174	0.25	14.4	115.2	1.2	0.10	4.8	0.02	0.23	0.03	0.24	0.02	6.0	4.0	0	1.1
0	12	0.30	9.4	110.2	0.7	0.10	0.7	0.02	0.21	0.02	0.28	0.03	17.3	42.3	0	0.3
0	14	0.60	7.7	124.9	1.3	0.06	1.3	0.02	0.31	0.10	0.37	0.04	5.1	50.4	0	0.9
0	38	0.09	9.5	171.9	0	0.07	10.4	0.08	0.17	0.04	0.27	0.06	28.5	50.5	0	0.5
0	22	0.25	9.9	219.8	1.2	0.04	16.1	0.07	0.16	0.02	0.12	0.05	6.2	38.3	0	0.1
0	33	0.13	10.6	146.1	1.8	0.06	29.9	0.05	0.18	0.03	0.33	0.07	14.1	23.5	0	0.1

TABLE A-2 **Table of Food Composition** *(continued)*   (Computer code is for Cengage Diet Analysis program)   (For purposes of calculations, use "0" for t, <1, <0.1, <0.01)

DA+ Code	Food Description	Quantity	Measure	Wt (g)	H$_2$O (g)	Ener (kcal)	Prot (g)	Carb (g)	Fiber (g)	Fat (g)	Fat Breakdown (g) Sat	Mono	Poly
Vegetables, Legumes													
	Amaranth												
1043	Leaves, boiled, drained	½	cup(s)	66	60.4	14	1.4	2.7	—	0.1	0	0	0.1
1042	Leaves, raw	1	cup(s)	28	25.7	6	0.7	1.1	—	0.1	0	0	0
8683	**Arugula leaves, raw**	1	cup(s)	20	18.3	5	0.5	0.7	0.3	0.1	0	0	0.1
	Artichoke												
1044	Boiled, drained	1	item(s)	120	100.9	64	3.5	14.3	10.3	0.4	0.1	0	0.2
2885	Hearts, boiled, drained	½	cup(s)	84	70.6	45	2.4	10.0	7.2	0.3	0.1	0.0	0.1
	Asparagus												
566	Boiled, drained	½	cup(s)	90	83.4	20	2.2	3.7	1.8	0.2	0	0	0.1
568	Canned, drained	½	cup(s)	121	113.7	23	2.6	3.0	1.9	0.8	0.2	0	0.3
40162	Frozen, boiled, drained	½	cup(s)	90	84.7	16	2.7	1.7	1.4	0.4	0.1	0	0.2
	Bamboo shoots												
1048	Boiled, drained	½	cup(s)	60	57.6	7	0.9	1.2	0.6	0.1	0	0	0.1
1049	Canned, drained	½	cup(s)	66	61.8	12	1.1	2.1	0.9	0.3	0.1	0	0.1
	Beans												
1801	Adzuki beans, boiled	½	cup(s)	87	57.7	111	6.5	21.5	6.4	0.1	0	0	0
511	Baked beans with franks, canned	½	cup(s)	130	89.8	184	8.7	19.9	8.9	8.5	3.0	3.7	1.1
513	Baked beans with pork in sweet sauce, canned	½	cup(s)	127	89.5	140	6.6	26.7	5.4	1.7	0.4	0.4	0.7
512	Baked beans with pork in tomato sauce, canned	½	cup(s)	127	93.0	119	6.5	23.6	5.1	1.2	0.4	0.4	0.2
1805	Black beans, boiled	½	cup(s)	86	56.5	114	7.6	20.4	7.5	0.5	0.1	0	0.2
14597	Chickpeas, garbanzo beans or bengal gram, boiled	½	cup(s)	82	49.4	134	7.3	22.5	6.2	2.1	0.2	0.5	0.9
569	Fordhook lima beans, frozen, boiled, drained	½	cup(s)	85	62.1	88	5.2	16.4	4.9	0.3	0.1	0	0.1
1806	French beans, boiled	½	cup(s)	89	58.9	114	6.2	21.3	8.3	0.7	0.1	0	0.4
2773	Great northern beans, boiled	½	cup(s)	89	61.1	104	7.4	18.7	6.2	0.4	0.1	0	0.2
2736	Hyacinth beans, boiled, drained	½	cup(s)	44	37.8	22	1.3	4.0	—	0.1	0.1	0.1	0
570	Lima beans, baby, frozen, boiled, drained	½	cup(s)	90	65.1	95	6.0	17.5	5.4	0.3	0.1	0	0.1
515	Lima beans, boiled, drained	½	cup(s)	85	57.1	105	5.8	20.1	4.5	0.3	0.1	0	0.1
579	Mung beans, sprouted, boiled, drained	½	cup(s)	62	57.9	13	1.3	2.6	0.5	0.1	0	0	0
510	Navy beans, boiled	½	cup(s)	91	58.1	127	7.5	23.7	9.6	0.6	0.1	0.1	0.4
32816	Pinto beans, boiled, drained, no salt added	½	cup(s)	63	58.8	14	1.2	2.6	—	0.2	0	0	0.1
1052	Pinto beans, frozen, boiled, drained	½	cup(s)	47	27.3	76	4.4	14.5	4.0	0.2	0	0	0.1
514	Red kidney beans, canned	½	cup(s)	128	99.8	104	6.7	19.0	6.8	0.5	0.1	0.1	0.3
71879	Red kidney beans, canned, reduced sodium	½	cup(s)	130	—	105	7.0	22.0	8.0	0.0	0	—	—
1810	Refried beans, canned	½	cup(s)	119	90.6	108	6.4	18.2	6.1	1.4	0.5	0.5	0.4
1053	Shell beans, canned	½	cup(s)	123	111.1	37	2.2	7.6	4.2	0.2	0	0	0.1
1670	Soybeans, boiled	½	cup(s)	86	53.8	149	14.3	8.5	5.2	7.7	1.1	1.7	4.4
1108	Soybeans, green, boiled, drained	½	cup(s)	90	61.7	127	11.1	9.9	3.8	5.8	0.7	1.1	2.7
1807	White beans, small, boiled	½	cup(s)	90	56.6	127	8.0	23.1	9.3	0.6	0.1	0.1	0.2
575	Yellow snap, string or wax beans, boiled, drained	½	cup(s)	63	55.8	22	1.2	4.9	2.1	0.2	0	0	0.1
576	Yellow snap, string or wax beans, frozen, boiled, drained	½	cup(s)	68	61.7	19	1.0	4.4	2.0	0.1	0	0	0.1
	Beets												
584	Beet greens, boiled, drained	½	cup(s)	72	64.2	19	1.9	3.9	2.1	0.1	0	0	0.1
2730	Pickled, canned with liquid	½	cup(s)	114	92.9	74	0.9	18.5	3.0	0.1	0	0	0
581	Sliced, boiled, drained	½	cup(s)	85	74.0	37	1.4	8.5	1.7	0.2	0	0	0.1
583	Sliced, canned, drained	½	cup(s)	85	77.4	26	0.8	6.1	1.5	0.1	0	0	0.1
580	Whole, boiled, drained	2	item(s)	100	87.1	44	1.7	10.0	2.0	0.2	0	0	0.1
585	**Cowpeas or black-eyed peas, boiled, drained**	½	cup(s)	83	62.3	80	2.6	16.8	4.1	0.3	0.1	0	0.1
	Broccoli												
588	Chopped, boiled, drained	½	cup(s)	78	69.6	27	1.9	5.6	2.6	0.3	0.1	0	0.1
590	Frozen, chopped, boiled, drained	½	cup(s)	92	83.5	26	2.9	4.9	2.8	0.1	0	0	0.1
587	Raw, chopped	½	cup(s)	46	40.6	15	1.3	3.0	1.2	0.2	0	0	0

PAGE KEY: A-6 5 Breads/Baked Goods A-12 = Cereal/Rice/Pasta A-16 = Fruit A-22 = Vegetables/Legumes A-32 = Nuts/Seeds A-34 = Vegetarian A-36 = Dairy A-44 = Eggs A-44 = Seafood A-46 = Meats A-50 = Poultry
A-52 = Processed Meats A-54 = Beverages A-58 = Fats/Oils A-60 = Sweets A-62 = Spices/Condiments/Sauces A-66 = Mixed Foods/Soups/Sandwiches A-72 = Fast Food A-90 = Convenience A-92 = Baby Foods

Chol (mg)	Calc (mg)	Iron (mg)	Magn (mg)	Pota (mg)	Sodi (mg)	Zinc (mg)	Vit A (µg)	Thia (mg)	Vit E (mg α)	Ribo (mg)	Niac (mg)	Vit B$_6$ (mg)	Fola (µg)	Vit C (mg)	Vit B$_{12}$ (µg)	Sele (µg)
0	138	1.49	36.3	423.1	13.9	0.58	91.7	0.01	—	0.09	0.37	0.12	37.6	27.1	0	0.6
0	60	0.65	15.4	171.1	5.6	0.25	40.9	0.01	—	0.04	0.18	0.05	23.8	12.1	0	0.3
0	32	0.29	9.4	73.8	5.4	0.09	23.8	0.01	0.09	0.02	0.06	0.01	19.4	3.0	0	0.1
0	25	0.73	50.4	343.2	72.0	0.48	1.2	0.06	0.23	0.11	1.33	0.10	106.8	8.9	0	0.2
0	18	0.51	35.3	240.2	50.4	0.34	0.8	0.04	0.16	0.07	0.93	0.07	74.8	6.2	0	0.2
0	21	0.82	12.6	201.6	12.6	0.54	45.0	0.15	1.35	0.13	0.98	0.07	134.1	6.9	0	5.5
0	19	2.21	12.1	208.1	347.3	0.48	49.6	0.07	1.48	0.12	1.15	0.13	116.2	22.3	0	2.1
0	16	0.50	9.0	154.8	2.7	0.37	36.0	0.06	1.08	0.09	0.93	0.02	121.5	22.0	0	3.5
0	7	0.14	1.8	319.8	2.4	0.28	0	0.01	—	0.03	0.18	0.06	1.2	0	0	0.2
0	5	0.21	2.6	52.4	4.6	0.43	0.7	0.02	0.41	0.02	0.09	0.09	2.0	0.7	0	0.3
0	24	1.74	45.2	462.8	7.0	1.54	0	0.10	—	0.06	0.62	0.08	105.3	0	0	1.0
8	62	2.24	36.3	304.3	556.8	2.42	5.2	0.08	0.21	0.07	1.17	0.06	38.8	3.0	0.4	8.4
1	72	2.09	40.5	322.6	426.3	1.02	1.3	0.06	0.06	0.07	0.44	0.07	10.1	3.4	0	6.3
9	71	4.10	43.0	373.2	552.8	6.93	5.1	0.07	0.13	0.06	0.62	0.08	19.0	3.8	0	5.9
0	23	1.81	60.2	305.3	0.9	0.96	0	0.21	—	0.05	0.43	0.06	128.1	0	0	1.0
0	40	2.37	39.4	238.6	5.7	1.25	0.8	0.10	0.29	0.05	0.43	0.11	141.0	1.1	0	3.0
0	26	1.55	35.7	258.6	58.7	0.63	8.5	0.06	0.25	0.05	0.91	0.10	17.9	10.9	0	0.5
0	56	0.96	49.6	327.5	5.3	0.57	0	0.12	—	0.05	0.48	0.09	66.4	1.1	0	1.1
0	60	1.89	44.3	346.0	1.8	0.78	0	0.14	—	0.05	0.60	0.10	90.3	1.2	0	3.6
0	18	0.33	18.3	114.0	0.9	0.17	3.0	0.02	—	0.04	0.21	0.01	20.4	2.2	0	0.7
0	25	1.76	50.4	369.9	26.1	0.50	7.2	0.06	0.58	0.05	0.69	0.10	14.4	5.2	0	1.5
0	27	2.08	62.9	484.8	14.5	0.67	12.8	0.12	0.12	0.08	0.88	0.16	22.1	8.6	0	1.7
0	7	0.40	8.7	62.6	6.2	0.29	0.6	0.03	0.04	0.06	0.51	0.03	18.0	7.1	0	0.4
	63	2.15	48.2	354.0	0	0.94	0	0.22	0.01	0.06	0.59	0.13	127.4	0.8	0	2.6
0	9	0.42	11.3	61.7	32.1	0.11	0	0.04	—	0.04	0.46	0.03	18.3	3.8	0	0.4
0	24	1.27	25.4	303.6	39.0	0.32	0	0.13	—	0.05	0.30	0.09	16.0	0.3	0	0.7
0	37	1.60	38.4	332.8	327.7	0.79	0	0.14	0.03	0.09	0.63	0.10	33.3	1.0	0	1.4
0	80	1.80	—	400.0	130.0	—	0	—	—	—	—	—	—	0	0	—
0	39	1.99	45.2	399.8	534.3	0.77	0	0.04	0.06	0.02	0.50	0.13	13.1	7.1	0	7.7
0	36	1.21	18.4	133.5	409.1	0.33	13.5	0.04	0.04	0.07	0.25	0.06	22.0	3.8	0	2.6
0	88	4.42	74.0	442.9	0.9	0.99	0	0.13	0.30	0.25	0.34	0.20	46.4	1.5	0	6.3
0	131	2.25	54.0	485.1	12.6	0.82	7.2	0.23	—	0.14	1.13	0.05	99.9	15.3	0	1.3
0	65	2.54	60.9	414.4	1.8	0.98	0	0.21	—	0.05	0.24	0.11	122.6	0	0	1.2
0	29	0.80	15.6	186.9	1.9	0.22	2.5	0.05	0.28	0.06	0.38	0.04	20.6	6.1	0	0.3
0	33	0.59	16.2	85.1	6.1	0.32	4.1	0.02	0.03	0.06	0.26	0.04	15.5	2.8	0	0.3
0	82	1.37	49.0	654.5	173.5	0.36	275.8	0.08	1.30	0.21	0.36	0.10	10.1	17.9	0	0.6
0	12	0.47	17.0	168.0	299.6	0.30	2.3	0.01	0.07	0.05	0.28	0.06	30.6	2.6	0	1.1
0	14	0.67	19.6	259.4	65.5	0.30	1.7	0.02	0.03	0.03	0.28	0.06	68.0	3.1	0	0.6
0	13	1.55	14.5	125.9	165.0	0.18	0.9	0.01	0.03	0.03	0.13	0.05	25.5	3.5	0	0.4
0	16	0.79	23.0	305.0	77.0	0.35	2.0	0.03	0.04	0.04	0.33	0.07	80.0	3.6	0	0.7
0	106	0.92	42.9	344.9	3.3	0.85	33.0	0.08	0.18	0.12	1.16	0.05	104.8	1.8	0	2.1
0	31	0.52	16.4	228.5	32.0	0.35	60.1	0.05	1.13	0.10	0.43	0.16	84.2	50.6	0	1.2
0	30	0.56	12.0	130.6	10.1	0.26	46.9	0.05	1.21	0.07	0.42	0.12	51.5	36.9	0	0.6
0	21	0.33	9.6	143.8	15.0	0.19	14.1	0.03	0.35	0.05	0.29	0.08	28.7	40.6	0	1.1

TABLE A-2 Table of Food Composition *(continued)*   (Computer code is for Cengage Diet Analysis program)   (For purposes of calculations, use "0" for t, <1, <0.1, <0.01)

DA+ Code	Food Description	Quantity	Measure	Wt (g)	H₂O (g)	Ener (kcal)	Prot (g)	Carb (g)	Fiber (g)	Fat (g)	Fat Breakdown (g) Sat	Mono	Poly
Vegetables, Legumes—*continued*													
16848	**Broccoflower, raw, chopped**	½	cup(s)	32	28.7	10	0.9	1.9	1.0	0.1	0	0	0
	Brussels sprouts												
591	Boiled, drained	½	cup(s)	78	69.3	28	2.0	5.5	2.0	0.4	0.1	0	0.2
592	Frozen, boiled, drained	½	cup(s)	78	67.2	33	2.8	6.4	3.2	0.3	0.1	0	0.2
	Cabbage												
595	Boiled, drained, no salt added	1	cup(s)	150	138.9	35	1.9	8.3	2.8	0.1	0	0	0
35611	Chinese (pak choi or bok choy), boiled with salt, drained	1	cup(s)	170	162.4	20	2.7	3.0	1.7	0.3	0	0	0.1
16869	Kim chee	1	cup(s)	150	137.6	32	2.4	5.9	1.8	0.3	0	0	0.2
594	Raw, shredded	1	cup(s)	70	64.5	18	0.9	4.1	1.8	0.1	0	0	0
596	Red, shredded, raw	1	cup(s)	70	63.3	22	1.0	5.2	1.5	0.1	0	0	0.1
597	Savoy, shredded, raw	1	cup(s)	70	63.7	19	1.4	4.3	2.2	0.1	0	0	0
35417	**Capers**	1	teaspoon(s)	4	—	2	0	0	0	0	0	0	0.0
	Carrots												
8691	Baby, raw	8	item(s)	80	72.3	28	0.5	6.6	2.3	0.1	0	0	0.1
601	Grated	½	cup(s)	55	48.6	23	0.5	5.3	1.5	0.1	0	0	0.1
1055	Juice, canned	½	cup(s)	118	104.9	47	1.1	11.0	0.9	0.2	0	0	0.1
600	Raw	½	cup(s)	61	53.9	25	0.6	5.8	1.7	0.1	0	0	0.1
602	Sliced, boiled, drained	½	cup(s)	78	70.3	27	0.6	6.4	2.3	0.1	0	0	0.1
32725	**Cassava or manioc**	½	cup(s)	103	61.5	165	1.4	39.2	1.9	0.3	0.1	0.1	
	Cauliflower												
606	Boiled, drained	½	cup(s)	62	57.7	14	1.1	2.5	1.4	0.3	0	0	0.1
607	Frozen, boiled, drained	½	cup(s)	90	84.6	17	1.4	3.4	2.4	0.2	0	0	0.1
605	Raw, chopped	½	cup(s)	50	46.0	13	1.0	2.5	1.0	0.1	0	0	0
	Celery												
609	Diced	½	cup(s)	51	48.2	8	0.3	1.5	0.8	0.1	0	0	0
608	Stalk	2	item(s)	80	76.3	13	0.6	2.4	1.3	0.1	0	0	0.1
	Chard												
1057	Swiss chard, boiled, drained	½	cup(s)	88	81.1	18	1.6	3.6	1.8	0.1	0	0	0.1
1056	Swiss chard, raw	1	cup(s)	36	33.4	7	0.6	1.3	0.6	0.1	0	0	0
	Collard greens												
610	Boiled, drained	½	cup(s)	95	85.7	31	2.6	5.4	3.8	0.7	0	0	0.2
611	Frozen, chopped, boiled, drained	½	cup(s)	85	75.2	31	2.5	6.0	2.4	0.3	0.1	0	0.2
	Corn												
29614	Yellow corn, fresh, cooked	1	item(s)	100	73.0	95	3.4	20.9	2.4	1.5	0.2	0.4	0.6
615	Yellow creamed sweet corn, canned	½	cup(s)	128	100.8	92	2.2	23.2	1.5	0.5	0.1	0.2	0.3
612	Yellow sweet corn, boiled, drained	½	cup(s)	82	60.2	79	2.8	17.2	2.0	1.2	0.2	0.3	0.5
614	Yellow sweet corn, frozen, boiled, drained	½	cup(s)	82	63.2	66	2.1	15.8	2.0	0.5	0.1	0.2	0.3
	Cucumber												
703	Pickled, dill	¼	cup(s)	39	36.6	5	0.2	1.0	0.4	0.1	0	0	0
2755	Pickled, dill, low sodium	¼	cup(s)	39	35.5	7	0.2	1.6	0.5	0.1	0	0	0
618	Raw	¼	item(s)	75	71.7	11	0.5	2.7	0.4	0.1	0	0	0
	Dandelion greens												
620	Chopped, boiled, drained	½	cup(s)	53	47.1	17	1.0	3.4	1.5	0.3	0.1	0	0.1
2734	Raw	1	cup(s)	55	47.1	25	1.5	5.1	1.9	0.4	0.1	0	0.2
1066	**Eggplant, boiled, drained**	½	cup(s)	50	44.4	17	0.4	4.3	1.2	0.1	0	0	0
621	**Endive or escarole, chopped, raw**	1	cup(s)	50	46.9	9	0.6	1.7	1.6	0.1	0	0	0
8784	**Jicama or yambean**	½	cup(s)	67	60.1	25	0.5	5.9	3.3	0.1	0	0	0.0
	Kale												
623	Frozen, chopped, boiled, drained	½	cup(s)	65	58.8	20	1.8	3.4	1.3	0.3	0	0	0.2
29313	Raw	1	cup(s)	67	56.3	33	2.9	5.9	1.3	0.6	0.1	0	0.2
	Kohlrabi												
1072	Boiled, drained	½	cup(s)	83	74.5	24	1.5	5.5	0.9	0.1	0	0	0
1071	Raw	1	cup(s)	135	122.8	36	2.3	8.4	4.9	0.1	0	0	0
	Leeks												
1074	Boiled, drained	½	cup(s)	52	47.2	16	0.4	4.0	0.5	0.1	0	0	0.1
1073	Raw	1	cup(s)	89	73.9	54	1.3	12.6	1.6	0.3	0	0	0.1

Chol (mg)	Calc (mg)	Iron (mg)	Magn (mg)	Pota (mg)	Sodi (mg)	Zinc (mg)	Vit A (µg)	Thia (mg)	Vit E (mg α)	Ribo (mg)	Niac (mg)	Vit B$_6$ (mg)	Fola (µg)	Vit C (mg)	Vit B$_{12}$ (µg)	Sele (µg)
0	11	0.23	6.4	96.0	7.4	0.20	2.6	0.03	0.01	0.03	0.23	0.07	18.2	28.2	0	0.2
0	28	0.94	15.6	247.3	16.4	0.26	30.4	0.08	0.34	0.06	0.47	0.14	46.8	48.4	0	1.2
0	20	0.37	13.9	224.8	11.6	0.19	35.7	0.08	0.40	0.09	0.42	0.22	78.3	35.4	0	0.5
0	72	0.25	22.5	294.0	12.0	0.30	6.0	0.09	0.21	0.06	0.37	0.17	45.0	56.3	0	0.9
0	158	1.77	18.7	630.7	459.0	0.29	360.4	0.05	0.15	0.11	0.73	0.28	69.7	44.2	0	0.7
0	137	1.23	27.0	367.5	936.0	0.36	274.5	0.07	0.41	0.10	0.78	0.33	85.5	68.1	0	1.5
0	28	0.33	8.4	119.0	12.6	0.13	3.5	0.04	0.10	0.03	0.16	0.09	30.1	25.6	0	0.2
0	32	0.56	11.2	170.1	18.9	0.15	39.2	0.04	0.08	0.05	0.29	0.15	12.6	39.9	0	0.4
0	25	0.28	19.6	161.0	19.6	0.19	35.0	0.05	0.12	0.02	0.21	0.13	56.0	21.7	0	0.6
0	0	0	—	—	140.0	—	0	—	—	—	—	—	—	0	—	—
0	26	0.71	8.0	189.6	62.4	0.14	552.0	0.02	—	0.03	0.44	0.08	21.6	2.1	0	0.7
0	18	0.17	6.6	176.0	37.9	0.13	459.3	0.04	0.36	0.03	0.54	0.08	10.5	3.2	0	0.1
0	28	0.54	16.5	344.6	77.9	0.21	1128.1	0.11	1.37	0.06	0.46	0.26	4.7	10.0	0	0.7
0	20	0.18	7.3	195.2	42.1	0.15	509.4	0.04	0.40	0.04	0.60	0.08	11.6	3.6	0	0.1
0	23	0.27	7.8	183.3	45.2	0.16	664.6	0.05	0.80	0.03	0.50	0.12	10.9	2.8	0	0.5
0	16	0.28	21.6	279.1	14.4	0.35	1.0	0.09	0.20	0.05	0.88	0.09	27.8	21.2	0	0.7
0	10	0.20	5.6	88.0	9.3	0.11	0.6	0.03	0.04	0.03	0.25	0.11	27.3	27.5	0	0.4
0	15	0.37	8.1	125.1	16.2	0.12	0	0.03	0.05	0.05	0.28	0.08	36.9	28.2	0	0.5
0	11	0.21	7.5	149.5	15.0	0.14	0	0.03	0.04	0.03	0.25	0.09	28.5	24.1	0	0.3
0	20	0.10	5.6	131.3	40.4	0.07	11.1	0.01	0.14	0.03	0.16	0.04	18.2	1.6	0	0.2
0	32	0.16	8.8	208.0	64.0	0.10	17.6	0.02	0.22	0.05	0.26	0.06	28.8	2.5	0	0.3
0	51	1.98	75.3	480.4	156.6	0.29	267.8	0.03	1.65	0.08	0.31	0.07	7.9	15.8	0	0.8
0	18	0.65	29.2	136.4	76.7	0.13	110.2	0.01	0.68	0.03	0.14	0.04	5.0	10.8	0	0.3
0	134	1.07	20.0	111.2	14.3	0.22	361.0	0.04	0.84	0.10	0.55	0.12	15.2	17.3	0	0.5
0	179	0.95	25.5	213.5	42.5	0.23	489.0	0.04	1.06	0.10	0.54	0.10	64.6	22.5	0	1.3
0	3	0.45	26.0	217.0	227.0	0.62	13.0	0.09	0.09	0.06	1.67	0.14	23.0	5.5	0	0.2
0	4	0.49	21.8	171.5	364.8	0.68	5.1	0.03	0.09	0.07	1.23	0.08	57.6	5.9	0	0.5
0	2	0.37	21.3	178.8	0.8	0.51	10.7	0.08	0.07	0.05	1.38	0.11	18.9	4.5	0	0.2
0	2	0.39	23.0	191.1	0.8	0.52	8.2	0.02	0.06	0.05	1.08	0.08	28.7	2.9	0	0.6
0	16	0.14	2.7	35.7	339.1	0.04	3.5	0.01	0.03	0.01	0.04	0.01	0.4	0.3	0	0
0	3	0.21	4.3	45.0	7.0	0.05	5.0	0.01	—	0.01	0.02	0.01	0.4	0.7	0	0
0	12	0.21	9.8	110.6	1.5	0.15	3.8	0.02	0.02	0.02	0.07	0.03	5.3	2.1	0	0.2
0	74	0.94	12.6	121.8	23.1	0.15	179.6	0.07	1.28	0.09	0.27	0.08	6.8	9.4	0	0.2
0	103	1.70	19.8	218.3	41.8	0.23	279.4	0.10	1.89	0.14	0.44	0.14	14.8	19.3	0	0.3
0	3	0.12	5.4	60.9	0.5	0.06	1.0	0.04	0.20	0.01	0.30	0.04	6.9	0.6	0	0
0	26	0.41	7.5	157.0	11.0	0.40	54.0	0.04	0.22	0.04	0.20	0.01	71.0	3.3	0	0.1
0	8	0.40	8.0	100.0	2.7	0.11	0.7	0.01	0.31	0.02	0.13	0.03	8.0	13.5	0	0.5
0	90	0.61	11.7	208.6	9.8	0.12	477.8	0.03	0.60	0.07	0.44	0.06	9.1	16.4	0	0.6
0	101	0.98	31.5	329.0	25.5	0.38	335.0	0.07	—	0.09	0.67	0.18	20.8	80.4	0	0.6
0	21	0.33	15.7	280.5	17.3	0.26	1.6	0.03	0.43	0.02	0.32	0.13	9.9	44.5	0	0.7
0	32	0.54	25.6	472.5	27.0	0.04	2.7	0.07	0.65	0.03	0.54	0.20	21.6	83.7	0	0.9
0	16	0.57	7.3	45.2	5.2	0.03	21.3	0.01	0.26	0.01	0.10	0.06	12.5	2.2	0	0.3
0	53	1.87	24.9	160.2	17.8	0.11	73.9	0.05	0.82	0.03	0.36	0.21	57.0	10.7	0	0.9

TABLE A-2 Table of Food Composition *(continued)* (Computer code is for Cengage Diet Analysis program) (For purposes of calculations, use "0" for t, <1, <0.1, <0.01)

DA+ Code	Food Description	Quantity	Measure	Wt (g)	H₂O (g)	Ener (kcal)	Prot (g)	Carb (g)	Fiber (g)	Fat (g)	Fat Breakdown (g) Sat	Mono	Poly
Vegetables, Legumes—*continued*													
	Lentils												
522	Boiled	¼	cup(s)	50	34.5	57	4.5	10.0	3.9	0.2	0	0	0.1
1075	Sprouted	1	cup(s)	77	51.9	82	6.9	17.0	—	0.4	0	0.1	0.2
	Lettuce												
625	Butterhead leaves	11	piece(s)	83	78.9	11	1.1	1.8	0.9	0.2	0	0	0.1
624	Butterhead, Boston or Bibb	1	cup(s)	55	52.6	7	0.7	1.2	0.6	0.1	0	0	0.1
626	Iceberg	1	cup(s)	72	68.9	10	0.6	2.1	0.9	0.1	0	0	0.1
628	Iceberg, chopped	1	cup(s)	55	52.6	8	0.5	1.6	0.7	0.1	0	0	0
629	Looseleaf	1	cup(s)	36	34.2	5	0.5	1.0	0.5	0.1	0	0	0
1665	Romaine, shredded	1	cup(s)	47	44.5	8	0.6	1.5	1.0	0.1	0	0	0.1
	Mushrooms												
15585	Crimini (about 6)	3	ounce(s)	85	—	28	3.7	2.8	1.9	0	0	0	0.1
8700	Enoki	30	item(s)	90	79.5	33	2.4	7.0	2.4	0.3	0	0	0.1
1079	Mushrooms, boiled, drained	½	cup(s)	78	71.0	22	1.7	4.1	1.7	0.4	0	0	0.1
1080	Mushrooms, canned, drained	½	cup(s)	78	71.0	20	1.5	4.0	1.9	0.2	0	0	0.1
630	Mushrooms, raw	½	cup(s)	48	44.4	11	1.5	1.6	0.5	0.2	0	0	0.1
35465	Portabella, raw	1	item(s)	84	78.0	18	1.8	3.3	1.1	0.3	0.1	0	0.1
2743	Shiitake, cooked	½	cup(s)	73	60.5	41	1.1	10.4	1.5	0.2	0	0.1	0
	Mustard greens												
2744	Frozen, boiled, drained	½	cup(s)	75	70.3	14	1.7	2.3	2.1	0.2	0	0.1	0
29319	Raw	1	cup(s)	56	50.8	15	1.6	2.6	1.8	0.2	0	0.1	0
	Okra												
16866	Batter coated, fried	11	piece(s)	83	50.3	159	4.0	20.1	2.3	7.1	1.4	2.8	2.4
32742	Frozen, boiled, drained, no salt added	½	cup(s)	92	83.8	27	1.5	5.9	1.9	0.2	0.1	0	0.1
632	Sliced, boiled, drained	½	cup(s)	80	74.1	18	1.5	3.6	2.0	0.2	0	0	0
	Onions												
635	Chopped, boiled, drained	½	cup(s)	105	92.3	46	1.4	10.7	1.5	0.2	0	0	0.1
2748	Frozen, boiled, drained	½	cup(s)	106	97.8	30	0.8	7.0	1.9	0.1	0	0	0
1081	Onion rings, breaded and pan fried, frozen, heated	10	piece(s)	71	20.2	289	3.8	27.1	0.9	19.0	6.1	7.7	3.6
633	Raw, chopped	½	cup(s)	80	71.3	32	0.9	7.5	1.4	0.1	0	0	0
16850	Red onions, sliced, raw	½	cup(s)	58	51.2	23	0.6	5.4	1.0	0.1	0	0	0
636	Scallions, green or spring onions	2	item(s)	30	26.9	10	0.5	2.2	0.8	0.1	0	0	0
16860	**Palm hearts, cooked**	½	cup(s)	73	50.7	84	2.0	18.7	1.1	0.1	0	0	0.1
637	**Parsley, chopped**	1	tablespoon(s)	4	3.3	1	0.1	0.2	0.1	0	0	0	0
638	**Parsnips, sliced, boiled, drained**	½	cup(s)	78	62.6	55	1.0	13.3	2.8	0.2	0	0.1	0
	Peas												
639	Green peas, canned, drained	½	cup(s)	88	72.0	60	3.9	9.9	4.3	0.7	0.1	0.1	0.3
641	Green peas, frozen, boiled, drained	½	cup(s)	80	63.6	62	4.1	11.4	4.4	0.2	0	0	0.1
35694	Pea pods, boiled with salt, drained	½	cup(s)	80	71.1	32	2.6	5.2	2.2	0.2	0	0	0.1
1082	Peas and carrots, canned with liquid	½	cup(s)	128	112.4	48	2.8	10.8	2.5	0.3	0.1	0	0.2
1083	Peas and carrots, frozen, boiled, drained	½	cup(s)	80	68.6	38	2.5	8.1	2.5	0.3	0.1	0	0.2
2750	Snow or sugar peas, frozen, boiled, drained	½	cup(s)	80	69.3	42	2.8	7.2	2.5	0.3	0.1	0	0.1
640	Snow or sugar peas, raw	½	cup(s)	32	28.0	13	0.9	2.4	0.8	0.1	0	0	0
29324	Split peas, sprouted	½	cup(s)	60	37.4	74	5.3	16.3	—	0.4	0.1	0	0.2
	Peppers												
644	Green bell or sweet, boiled, drained	½	cup(s)	68	62.5	19	0.6	4.6	0.8	0.1	0	0	0
643	Green bell or sweet, raw	½	cup(s)	75	69.9	15	0.6	3.5	1.3	0.1	0	0	0
1664	Green hot chili	1	item(s)	45	39.5	18	0.9	4.3	0.7	0.1	0	0	0
1663	Green hot chili, canned with liquid	½	cup(s)	68	62.9	14	0.6	3.5	0.9	0.1	0	0	0
1086	Jalapeño, canned with liquid	½	cup(s)	68	60.4	18	0.6	3.2	1.8	0.6	0.1	0	0.3
8703	Yellow bell or sweet	1	item(s)	186	171.2	50	1.9	11.8	1.7	0.4	0.1	0	0.2
1087	**Poi**	½	cup(s)	120	86.0	134	0.5	32.7	0.5	0.2	0	0	0.1

PAGE KEY: A-6 5 Breads/Baked Goods A-12 = Cereal/Rice/Pasta A-16 = Fruit A-22 = Vegetables/Legumes A-32 = Nuts/Seeds A-34 = Vegetarian A-36 = Dairy A-44 = Eggs A-44 = Seafood A-46 = Meats A-50 = Poultry A-52 = Processed Meats A-54 = Beverages A-58 = Fats/Oils A-60 = Sweets A-62 = Spices/Condiments/Sauces A-66 = Mixed Foods/Soups/Sandwiches A-72 = Fast Food A-90 = Convenience A-92 = Baby Foods

Chol (mg)	Calc (mg)	Iron (mg)	Magn (mg)	Pota (mg)	Sodi (mg)	Zinc (mg)	Vit A (µg)	Thia (mg)	Vit E (mg α)	Ribo (mg)	Niac (mg)	Vit B$_6$ (mg)	Fola (µg)	Vit C (mg)	Vit B$_{12}$ (µg)	Sele (µg)
0	9	1.65	17.8	182.7	1.0	0.63	0	0.08	0.05	0.04	0.52	0.09	89.6	0.7	0	1.4
0	19	2.47	28.5	247.9	8.5	1.16	1.5	0.18	—	0.10	0.87	0.15	77.0	12.7	0	0.5
0	29	1.02	10.7	196.4	4.1	0.17	136.9	0.05	0.15	0.05	0.29	0.07	60.2	3.1	0	0.5
0	19	0.68	7.2	130.9	2.8	0.11	91.3	0.03	0.10	0.03	0.20	0.05	40.1	2.0	0	0.3
0	13	0.30	5.0	101.5	7.2	0.11	18.0	0.03	0.13	0.02	0.09	0.03	20.9	2.0	0	0.1
0	10	0.23	3.9	77.5	5.5	0.08	13.8	0.02	0.10	0.01	0.07	0.02	15.9	1.5	0	0.1
0	13	0.31	4.7	69.8	10.1	0.06	133.2	0.03	0.08	0.03	0.14	0.03	13.7	3.3	0	0.2
0	16	0.46	6.6	116.1	3.8	0.11	204.9	0.03	0.06	0.03	0.15	0.03	63.9	1.9	0	0.2
0	0	0.67	—	—	32.6	—	0	—	—	—	—	—	—	0	0	—
0	0	1.03	14.4	323.1	2.7	0.58	—	0.20	0.01	0.18	6.33	0.09	43.2	0	0	2.0
0	5	1.36	9.4	277.7	1.6	0.68	0	0.06	0.01	0.23	3.48	0.07	14.0	3.1	0	9.3
0	9	0.62	11.7	100.6	331.5	0.56	0	0.07	0.01	0.02	1.24	0.05	9.4	0	0	3.2
0	1	0.24	4.3	152.6	2.4	0.25	0	0.04	0	0.19	1.73	0.05	8.2	1.0	0	4.5
0	3	0.26	9.2	305.8	7.6	0.45	0	0.05	0.02	0.11	3.77	0.12	23.5	0	0	15.6
0	2	0.32	10.1	84.8	2.9	0.96	0	0.03	0	0.12	1.09	0.12	15.2	0.2	0	18.0
0	76	0.84	9.8	104.3	18.8	0.15	265.5	0.03	1.01	0.04	0.19	0.08	52.5	10.4	0	0.4
0	64	0.92	17.9	215.0	11.2	0.14	84.6	0.04	1.13	0.06	0.45	0.10	6.7	39.2	0	0.5
40	47	1.54	34.7	190.6	142.7	0.57	28.9	0.21	0.69	0.16	1.52	0.14	95.7	8.6	0.1	7.3
0	68	0.48	36.8	169.3	2.8	0.45	13.8	0.07	0.29	0.09	0.57	0.03	92.0	8.8	0	0.6
0	62	0.22	28.8	108.0	4.8	0.34	11.2	0.11	0.22	0.04	0.70	0.15	36.8	13.0	0	0.3
0	23	0.25	11.5	174.3	3.1	0.22	0	0.04	0.02	0.02	0.17	0.14	15.8	5.5	0	0.6
0	17	0.32	6.4	114.5	12.7	0.07	0	0.02	0.01	0.03	0.15	0.07	13.8	2.8	0	0.4
0	22	1.20	13.5	91.6	266.3	0.30	7.8	0.20	—	0.10	2.56	0.05	73.1	1.0	0	2.5
0	18	0.17	8.0	116.8	3.2	0.14	0	0.04	0.02	0.02	0.09	0.10	15.2	5.9	0	0.4
0	13	0.12	5.8	83.9	2.3	0.10	0	0.03	0.01	0.02	0.07	0.07	10.9	4.3	0	0.3
0	22	0.44	6.0	82.8	4.8	0.12	15.0	0.02	0.17	0.02	0.16	0.02	19.2	5.6	0	0.2
0	13	1.23	7.3	1318.4	10.2	2.72	2.2	0.03	0.37	0.13	0.62	0.53	14.6	5.0	0	0.5
0	5	0.24	1.9	21.1	2.1	0.04	16.0	0	0.03	0	0.05	0	5.8	5.1	0	0
0	29	0.45	22.6	286.3	7.8	0.20	0	0.06	0.78	0.04	0.56	0.07	45.2	10.1	0	1.3
0	20	1.03	15.8	92.8	238.9	0.58	37.6	0.09	0.33	0.05	0.86	0.05	27.1	3.7	0	1.5
0	19	1.22	17.6	88.0	57.6	0.54	84.0	0.23	0.02	0.08	1.18	0.09	47.2	7.9	0	0.8
0	34	1.58	20.8	192.0	192.0	0.30	41.6	0.10	0.31	0.06	0.43	0.12	23.2	38.3	0	0.6
0	29	0.96	17.9	127.5	331.5	0.74	368.5	0.09	—	0.07	0.74	0.11	23.0	8.4	0	1.1
0	18	0.75	12.8	126.4	54.4	0.36	380.8	0.18	0.42	0.05	0.92	0.07	20.8	6.5	0	0.9
0	47	1.92	22.4	173.6	4.0	0.39	52.8	0.05	0.38	0.10	0.45	0.14	28.0	17.6	0	0.6
0	14	0.66	7.6	63.0	1.3	0.09	17.0	0.05	0.12	0.03	0.19	0.05	13.2	18.9	0	0.2
0	22	1.36	33.6	228.6	12.0	0.63	4.8	0.14	—	0.09	1.85	0.16	86.4	6.2	0	0.4
0	6	0.31	6.8	112.9	1.4	0.08	15.6	0.04	0.34	0.02	0.32	0.16	10.9	50.6	0	0.2
0	7	0.25	7.4	130.4	2.2	0.10	13.4	0.04	0.28	0.02	0.36	0.17	7.4	59.9	0	0
0	8	0.54	11.3	153.0	3.2	0.14	26.5	0.04	0.31	0.04	0.43	0.13	10.4	109.1	0	0.2
0	5	0.34	9.5	127.2	797.6	0.12	24.5	0.01	0.47	0.03	0.54	0.10	6.8	46.2	0	0.2
0	16	1.28	10.2	131.2	1136.3	0.23	57.8	0.03	0.47	0.03	0.27	0.13	9.5	6.8	0	0.3
0	20	0.86	22.3	394.3	3.7	0.32	18.6	0.05	—	0.05	1.66	0.31	48.4	341.3	0	0.6
0	19	1.06	28.8	219.6	14.4	0.26	3.6	0.16	2.76	0.05	1.32	0.33	25.2	4.8	0	0.8

TABLE A-2 Table of Food Composition (*continued*)   (Computer code is for Cengage Diet Analysis program)   (For purposes of calculations, use "0" for t, <1, <0.1, <0.01)

DA+ Code	Food Description	Quantity	Measure	Wt (g)	H₂O (g)	Ener (kcal)	Prot (g)	Carb (g)	Fiber (g)	Fat (g)	Fat Breakdown (g) Sat	Mono	Poly
Vegetables, Legumes—*continued*													
	Potatoes												
1090	Au gratin mix, prepared with water, whole milk and butter	½	cup(s)	122	96.3	113	2.8	15.7	1.1	5.0	3.2	1.4	0.2
1089	Au gratin, prepared with butter	½	cup(s)	123	90.7	162	6.2	13.8	2.2	9.3	5.8	2.6	0.3
5791	Baked, flesh and skin	1	item(s)	202	151.3	188	5.1	42.7	4.4	0.3	0.1	0	0.1
645	Baked, flesh only	½	cup(s)	61	46.0	57	1.2	13.1	0.9	0.1	0	0	0
1088	Baked, skin only	1	item(s)	58	27.4	115	2.5	26.7	4.6	0.1	0	0	0
5795	Boiled in skin, flesh only, drained	1	item(s)	136	104.7	118	2.5	27.4	2.1	0.1	0	0	0.1
5794	Boiled, drained, skin and flesh	1	item(s)	150	115.9	129	2.9	29.8	2.5	0.2	0	0	0.1
647	Boiled, flesh only	½	cup(s)	78	60.4	67	1.3	15.6	1.4	0.1	0	0	0
648	French fried, deep fried, prepared from raw	14	item(s)	113	47.9	335	4.6	39.5	5.0	18.3	2.4	7.3	7.9
649	French fried, frozen, heated	14	item(s)	70	43.7	115	1.9	19.4	2.0	3.7	0.7	2.3	0.2
1091	Hashed brown	½	cup(s)	78	36.9	207	2.3	27.4	2.5	9.8	1.5	4.1	3.7
652	Mashed with margarine and whole milk	½	cup(s)	105	79.0	119	2.1	17.8	1.6	4.4	1.0	2.0	1.2
653	Mashed, prepared from dehydrated granules with milk, water, and margarine	½	cup(s)	105	79.8	122	2.2	16.9	1.4	5.0	1.2	2.2	1.4
2759	Microwaved	1	item(s)	202	145.5	212	4.9	49.0	4.6	0.2	0.1	0	0.1
2760	Microwaved in skin, flesh only	½	cup(s)	78	57.1	78	1.6	18.1	1.2	0.1	0	0	0
5804	Microwaved, skin only	1	item(s)	58	36.8	77	2.5	17.2	4.2	0.1	0	0	0
1097	Potato puffs, frozen, heated	½	cup(s)	64	38.2	122	1.3	17.8	1.6	5.5	1.2	3.9	0.3
1094	Scalloped mix, prepared with water, whole milk and butter	½	cup(s)	124	98.6	116	2.6	15.9	1.4	5.4	3.3	1.5	0.2
1093	Scalloped, prepared with butter	½	cup(s)	123	99.2	108	3.5	13.2	2.3	4.5	2.8	1.3	0.2
	Pumpkin												
656	Canned	½	cup(s)	123	110.2	42	1.3	9.9	3.6	0.3	0.2	0	0
1773	Boiled, drained	½	cup(s)	123	114.8	25	0.9	6.0	1.3	0.1	0	0	0
	Radicchio												
8731	Leaves, raw	1	cup(s)	40	37.3	9	0.6	1.8	0.4	0.1	0	0	0
2498	Raw	1	cup(s)	40	37.3	9	0.6	1.8	0.4	0.1	0	0	0
657	**Radishes**	6	item(s)	27	25.7	4	0.2	0.9	0.4	0	0	0	0
1099	**Rutabaga, boiled, drained**	½	cup(s)	85	77.9	26	0.8	5.8	1.5	0.2	0	0	0.1
658	**Sauerkraut, canned**	½	cup(s)	118	109.2	22	1.1	5.1	3.4	0.2	0	0	0.1
	Seaweed												
1102	Kelp	½	cup(s)	40	32.6	17	0.7	3.8	0.5	0.2	0.1	0	0
1104	Spirulina, dried	½	cup(s)	56	2.6	162	32.2	13.4	2.0	4.3	1.5	0.4	1.2
1106	**Shallots**	3	tablespoon(s)	30	23.9	22	0.8	5.0	1.0	0	0	0	0
	Soybeans												
1670	Boiled	½	cup(s)	86	53.8	149	14.3	8.5	5.2	7.7	1.1	1.7	4.4
2825	Dry roasted	½	cup(s)	86	0.7	388	34.0	28.1	7.0	18.6	2.7	4.1	10.5
2824	Roasted, salted	½	cup(s)	86	1.7	405	30.3	28.9	15.2	21.8	3.2	4.8	12.3
8739	Sprouted, stir fried	½	cup(s)	62	41.7	77	8.1	5.8	0.5	4.4	0.6	1.0	2.5
	Soy products												
1813	Soy milk	1	cup(s)	240	211.3	130	7.8	15.1	1.4	4.2	0.5	1.0	2.3
2838	Tofu, dried, frozen (koyadofu)	3	ounce(s)	85	4.9	408	40.8	12.4	6.1	25.8	3.7	5.7	14.6
13844	Tofu, extra firm	3	ounce(s)	85	68.8	86	8.6	2.2	1.1	4.3	0.5	1.1	2.7
13843	Tofu, firm	3	ounce(s)	85	70.9	75	7.5	2.2	0.5	3.2	0	1.1	2.2
1816	Tofu, firm, with calcium sulfate and magnesium chloride (nigari)	3	ounce(s)	85	72.2	60	7.0	1.4	0.8	3.5	0.7	1.0	1.5
1817	Tofu, fried	3	ounce(s)	85	43.0	230	14.6	8.9	3.3	17.2	2.5	3.8	9.7
13841	Tofu, silken	3	ounce(s)	85	77.0	42	3.7	0.9	0	1.9	0	0.5	0.9
13842	Tofu, soft	3	ounce(s)	85	73.0	65	6.5	1.1	0.5	3.2	0	0.5	2.2
1671	Tofu, soft, with calcium sulfate and magnesium chloride (nigari)	3	ounce(s)	85	74.2	52	5.6	1.5	0.2	3.1	0.5	0.7	1.8
	Spinach												
663	Canned, drained	½	cup(s)	107	98.2	25	3.0	3.6	2.6	0.5	0.1	0	0.2
660	Chopped, boiled, drained	½	cup(s)	90	82.1	21	2.7	3.4	2.2	0.2	0	0	0.1
661	Chopped, frozen, boiled, drained	½	cup(s)	95	84.5	32	3.8	4.6	3.5	0.8	0.1	0	0.4
662	Leaf, frozen, boiled, drained	½	cup(s)	95	84.5	32	3.8	4.6	3.5	0.8	0.1	0	0.4
659	Raw, chopped	1	cup(s)	30	27.4	7	0.9	1.1	0.7	0.1	0	0	0

PAGE KEY: A-6 5 Breads/Baked Goods A-12 = Cereal/Rice/Pasta A-16 = Fruit A-22 = Vegetables/Legumes A-32 = Nuts/Seeds A-34 = Vegetarian A-36 = Dairy A-44 = Eggs A-44 = Seafood A-46 = Meats A-50 = Poultry A-52 = Processed Meats A-54 = Beverages A-58 = Fats/Oils A-60 = Sweets A-62 = Spices/Condiments/Sauces A-66 = Mixed Foods/Soups/Sandwiches A-72 = Fast Food A-90 = Convenience A-92 = Baby Foods

Chol (mg)	Calc (mg)	Iron (mg)	Magn (mg)	Pota (mg)	Sodi (mg)	Zinc (mg)	Vit A (µg)	Thia (mg)	Vit E (mg α)	Ribo (mg)	Niac (mg)	Vit B$_6$ (mg)	Fola (µg)	Vit C (mg)	Vit B$_{12}$ (µg)	Sele (µg)
18	101	0.39	18.3	267.2	535.5	0.29	63.4	0.02	—	0.10	1.15	0.05	8.5	3.8	0	3.3
28	146	0.78	24.5	485.1	530.4	0.85	78.4	0.08	—	0.14	1.22	0.21	15.9	12.1	0	3.3
0	30	2.18	56.6	1080.7	20.2	0.73	2.0	0.13	0.08	0.10	2.85	0.63	56.6	19.4	0	0.8
0	3	0.21	15.3	238.5	3.0	0.18	0	0.06	0.02	0.01	0.85	0.18	5.5	7.8	0	0.2
0	20	4.08	24.9	332.3	12.2	0.28	0.6	0.07	0.02	0.06	1.78	0.36	12.8	7.8	0	0.4
0	7	0.42	29.9	515.4	5.4	0.41	0	0.14	0.01	0.03	1.96	0.41	13.6	17.7	0	0.4
0	13	1.27	34.1	572.0	7.4	0.47	0	0.15	0.01	0.03	2.13	0.44	15.0	18.4	0	—
0	6	0.24	15.6	255.8	3.9	0.21	0	0.08	0.01	0.01	1.02	0.21	7.0	5.8	0	0.2
0	27	1.78	52.2	952.6	276.7	0.66	0	0.15	2.25	0.07	2.27	0.63	27.2	35.6	0	0.7
0	8	0.52	18.2	315.7	271.6	0.27	0	0.09	0.08	0.02	1.55	0.13	19.6	9.3	0	0.1
0	11	0.43	27.3	449.3	266.8	0.37	0	0.13	0.01	0.03	1.80	0.37	12.5	10.1	0	0.4
1	22	0.27	20.0	342.3	349.6	0.31	46.2	0.10	0.44	0.04	1.23	0.26	9.5	11.0	0.1	0.8
2	37	0.21	21.0	162.7	180.6	0.25	53.5	0.09	0.54	0.09	0.90	0.17	8.4	6.8	0.1	5.9
0	22	2.50	54.5	902.9	16.2	0.73	0	0.24	—	0.06	3.46	0.69	24.2	30.5	0	0.8
0	4	0.32	19.4	319.0	5.4	0.26	0	0.10	—	0.02	1.26	0.25	9.3	11.7	0	0.3
0	27	3.45	21.5	377.0	9.3	0.30	0	0.04	0.01	0.04	1.29	0.29	9.9	8.9	0	0.3
0	9	0.41	10.9	199.7	295.7	0.20	0	0.08	0.15	0.02	0.97	0.08	9.0	4.0	0	0.4
14	45	0.47	17.4	252.7	424.5	0.31	43.6	0.02	—	0.07	1.28	0.05	12.4	4.1	0	2.0
15	70	0.70	23.3	463.0	410.4	0.49	—	0.08	—	0.11	1.29	0.22	15.9	13.0	0	2.0
0	32	1.70	28.2	252.4	6.1	0.21	953.0	0.03	1.30	0.07	0.45	0.07	14.7	5.1	0	0.5
0	18	0.70	11.0	281.8	1.2	0.28	352.8	0.04	0.98	0.10	0.51	0.05	11.0	5.8	0	0.2
0	8	0.23	5.2	120.8	8.8	0.25	0.4	0.01	0.90	0.01	0.10	0.02	24.0	3.2	0	0.4
0	8	0.23	5.2	120.8	8.8	0.25	0.4	0.01	0.90	0.01	0.10	0.02	24.0	3.2	0	0.4
0	7	0.09	2.7	62.9	10.5	0.08	0	0	0.00	0.01	0.07	0.02	6.8	4.0	0	0.2
0	15	0.15	8.5	183.7	4.3	0.10	0	0.07	0.20	0.03	0.61	0.09	12.8	16.0	0	0.6
0	35	1.73	15.3	200.6	780.0	0.22	1.2	0.02	0.17	0.03	0.17	0.15	28.3	17.3	0	0.7
0	67	1.14	48.4	35.6	93.2	0.49	2.4	0.02	0.35	0.06	0.19	0	72.0	1.2	0	0.3
0	67	15.96	109.2	763.3	586.9	1.12	16.2	1.33	2.80	2.06	7.18	0.20	52.6	5.7	0	4.0
0	11	0.36	6.3	100.2	3.6	0.12	0	0.02	0.01	0.01	0.06	0.10	10.2	2.4	0	0.4
0	88	4.42	74.0	442.9	0.9	0.99	0	0.13	0.30	0.25	0.34	0.20	46.4	1.5	0	6.3
0	120	3.40	196.1	1173.0	1.7	4.10	0	0.37	—	0.65	0.91	0.19	176.3	4.0	0	16.6
0	119	3.35	124.7	1264.2	140.2	2.70	8.6	0.09	0.78	0.12	1.21	0.18	181.5	1.9	0	16.4
0	51	0.25	59.5	351.5	8.7	1.30	0.6	0.26	—	0.12	0.68	0.10	78.7	7.4	0	2.4
0	60	1.54	60.0	283.2	122.4	0.29	0	0.14	0.26	0.17	1.23	0.18	43.2	0	0	11.5
0	310	8.27	50.2	17.0	5.1	4.17	22.1	0.42	—	0.27	1.01	0.24	78.2	0.6	0	46.2
0	65	1.55	—	—	0	—	0	—	—	—	—	—	—	0	—	—
0	108	1.16	—	—	0	—	0	—	—	—	—	—	—	0	—	—
0	171	1.37	31.5	125.9	10.2	0.71	0	0.05	0.01	0.05	0.09	0.06	16.2	0.2	0	8.4
0	316	4.14	51.0	124.2	13.6	1.69	0.9	0.14	0.03	0.04	0.09	0.08	23.0	0	0	24.2
0	56	0.67	—	—	0	—	0	—	—	—	—	—	—	0	—	—
0	108	1.16	—	—	0	—	0	—	—	—	—	—	—	0	—	—
0	94	0.94	23.0	102.0	6.8	0.54	0	0.04	0.01	0.03	0.45	0.04	37.4	0.2	0	7.6
0	136	2.46	81.3	370.2	344.5	0.49	524.3	0.02	2.08	0.15	0.42	0.11	104.9	15.3	0	1.5
0	122	3.21	78.3	419.4	63.0	0.68	471.6	0.09	1.87	0.21	0.44	0.22	131.4	8.8	0	1.4
0	145	1.86	77.9	286.9	92.2	0.47	572.8	0.07	3.36	0.17	0.42	0.13	114.9	2.1	0	5.2
0	145	1.86	77.9	286.9	92.2	0.47	572.8	0.07	3.36	0.17	0.42	0.13	114.9	2.1	0	5.2
0	30	0.81	23.7	167.4	23.7	0.16	140.7	0.02	0.61	0.06	0.22	0.06	58.2	8.4	0	0.3

TABLE A-2 Table of Food Composition (*continued*)   (Computer code is for Cengage Diet Analysis program)   (For purposes of calculations, use "0" for t, <1, <0.1, <0.01)

DA+ Code	Food Description	Quantity	Measure	Wt (g)	H₂O (g)	Ener (kcal)	Prot (g)	Carb (g)	Fiber (g)	Fat (g)	Fat Breakdown (g) Sat	Mono	Poly
Vegetables, Legumes—*continued*													
	Squash												
1662	Acorn winter, baked	½	cup(s)	102	87.0	58	1.2	15.3	4.6	0.1	0	0	0.1
29702	Acorn winter, boiled, mashed	½	cup(s)	170	152.5	58	1.1	14.9	4.4	0.1	0	0	0.1
1661	Butternut winter, baked	½	cup(s)	103	90.0	41	0.9	10.8	3.3	0.1	0	0	0
32773	Butternut winter, frozen, boiled, mashed, no salt added	½	cup(s)	121	106.4	47	1.5	12.2	—	0.1	0	0	0
29451	Butternut, frozen, boiled	½	cup(s)	120	105.4	47	1.5	12.1	1.8	0.1	0	0	0
29700	Crookneck and straightneck summer, boiled, drained	½	cup(s)	65	61.0	12	0.7	2.5	0.6	0.2	0.1	0	0.1
29703	Hubbard winter, baked	½	cup(s)	102	86.8	51	2.5	11.0	5.0	0.6	0.1	0	0.3
1660	Hubbard winter, boiled, mashed	½	cup(s)	118	107.5	35	1.7	7.6	3.4	0.4	0.1	0	0.2
29704	Spaghetti winter, boiled, drained, or baked	½	cup(s)	78	71.5	21	0.5	5.0	1.1	0.2	0	0	0.1
664	Summer, all varieties, sliced, boiled, drained	½	cup(s)	90	84.3	18	0.8	3.9	1.3	0.3	0.1	0	0.1
665	Winter, all varieties, baked, mashed	½	cup(s)	103	91.4	38	0.9	9.1	2.9	0.4	0.1	0	0.2
1112	Zucchini summer, boiled, drained	½	cup(s)	90	85.7	14	1.0	2.4	0.9	0.3	0.1	0	0.1
1113	Zucchini summer, frozen, boiled, drained	½	cup(s)	112	105.6	19	1.3	4.0	1.4	0.1	0	0	0.1
	Sweet potatoes												
666	Baked, peeled	½	cup(s)	100	75.8	90	2.0	20.7	3.3	0.2	0	0	0.1
667	Boiled, mashed	½	cup(s)	164	131.4	125	2.2	29.1	4.1	0.2	0.1	0	0.1
668	Candied, home recipe	½	cup(s)	91	57.3	150	0.8	29.3	1.9	3.2	2.0	0.8	0.2
670	Canned, vacuum pack	½	cup(s)	100	76.0	91	1.6	21.1	1.8	0.2	0	0	0.1
2765	Frozen, baked	½	cup(s)	88	64.5	88	1.5	20.5	1.6	0.1	0	0	0.1
1136	Yams, baked or boiled, drained	½	cup(s)	68	47.7	79	1.0	18.7	2.7	0.1	0	0	0
32785	**Taro shoots, cooked, no salt added**	½	cup(s)	70	66.7	10	0.5	2.2	—	0.1	0	0	0
	Tomatillo												
8774	Raw	2	item(s)	68	62.3	22	0.7	4.0	1.3	0.7	0.1	0.1	0.3
8777	Raw, chopped	½	cup(s)	66	60.5	21	0.6	3.9	1.3	0.7	0.1	0.1	0.3
	Tomato												
16846	Cherry, fresh	5	item(s)	85	80.4	15	0.7	3.3	1.0	0.2	0	0	0.1
671	Fresh, ripe, red	1	item(s)	123	116.3	22	1.1	4.8	1.5	0.2	0	0	0.1
675	Juice, canned	½	cup(s)	122	114.1	21	0.9	5.2	0.5	0.1	0	0	0.1
75	Juice, no salt added	½	cup(s)	122	114.1	21	0.9	5.2	0.5	0.1	0	0	0
1699	Paste, canned	2	tablespoon(s)	33	24.1	27	1.4	6.2	1.3	0.2	0	0	0.1
1123	Paste, canned, no salt added	2	tablespoon(s)	32	23.5	26	1.4	6.1	1.3	0.2	0	0	0.1
1700	Puree, canned	¼	cup(s)	63	54.9	24	1.0	5.6	1.2	0.1	0	0	0.1
1124	Puree, canned, no salt added	¼	cup(s)	63	54.9	24	1.0	5.6	1.2	0.1	0	0	0.1
1118	Red, boiled	½	cup(s)	120	113.2	22	1.1	4.8	0.8	0.1	0	0	0.1
3952	Red, diced	½	cup(s)	90	85.1	16	0.8	3.5	1.1	0.2	0	0	0.1
1120	Red, stewed, canned	½	cup(s)	128	116.7	33	1.2	7.9	1.3	0.2	0	0	0.1
1125	Sauce, canned	¼	cup(s)	61	55.6	15	0.8	3.3	0.9	0.1	0	0	0
8778	Sun dried	½	cup(s)	27	3.9	70	3.8	15.1	3.3	0.8	0.1	0.1	0.3
8783	Sun dried in oil, drained	¼	cup(s)	28	14.8	59	1.4	6.4	1.6	3.9	0.5	2.4	0.6
	Turnips												
678	Turnip greens, chopped, boiled, drained	½	cup(s)	72	67.1	14	0.8	3.1	2.5	0.2	0	0	0.1
679	Turnip greens, frozen, chopped, boiled, drained	½	cup(s)	82	74.1	24	2.7	4.1	2.8	0.3	0.1	0	0.1
677	Turnips, cubed, boiled, drained	½	cup(s)	78	73.0	17	0.6	3.9	1.6	0.1	0	0	0
	Vegetables, mixed												
1132	Mixed vegetables, canned, drained	½	cup(s)	82	70.9	40	2.1	7.5	2.4	0.2	0	0	0.1
680	Mixed vegetables, frozen, boiled, drained	½	cup(s)	91	75.7	59	2.6	11.9	4.0	0.1	0	0	0.1
7489	V8 100% vegetable juice	½	cup(s)	122	114.1	25	1.0	5.0	1.0	0	0	0	0
7490	V8 low-sodium vegetable juice	½	cup(s)	122	114.1	25	1.0	5.0	1.0	0	0	0	0
7491	V8 Spicy Hot vegetable juice	½	cup(s)	122	114.2	25	1.0	5.0	1.0	0	0	0	0

PAGE KEY: A-6 5 Breads/Baked Goods A-12 = Cereal/Rice/Pasta A-16 = Fruit A-22 = Vegetables/Legumes A-32 = Nuts/Seeds A-34 = Vegetarian A-36 = Dairy A-44 = Eggs A-44 = Seafood A-46 = Meats A-50 = Poultry
A-52 = Processed Meats A-54 = Beverages A-58 = Fats/Oils A-60 = Sweets A-62 = Spices/Condiments/Sauces A-66 = Mixed Foods/Soups/Sandwiches A-72 = Fast Food A-90 = Convenience A-92 = Baby Foods

Chol (mg)	Calc (mg)	Iron (mg)	Magn (mg)	Pota (mg)	Sodi (mg)	Zinc (mg)	Vit A (µg)	Thia (mg)	Vit E (mg α)	Ribo (mg)	Niac (mg)	Vit B$_6$ (mg)	Fola (µg)	Vit C (mg)	Vit B$_{12}$ (µg)	Sele (µg)
0	46	0.98	45.2	459.0	4.2	0.18	22.1	0.18	—	0.01	0.93	0.20	20.0	11.4	0	0.7
0	44	0.95	44.2	447.1	5.1	0.19	69.7	0.17	—	0.01	0.90	0.20	18.7	11.1	0	0.7
0	42	0.62	29.7	291.1	4.1	0.13	572.0	0.07	1.32	0.02	0.99	0.13	19.5	15.5	0	0.5
0	23	0.70	10.9	161.2	2.4	0.15	202.4	0.06	—	0.05	0.56	0.08	19.4	4.2	0	0.6
0	23	0.70	10.8	159.6	2.4	0.14	200.4	0.06	0.14	0.05	0.56	0.08	19.2	4.2	0	0.6
0	14	0.28	12.9	143.6	1.3	0.19	5.2	0.03	0.08	0.03	0.29	0.07	12.3	12.5	0	0.1
0	17	0.48	22.4	365.1	8.2	0.15	341.7	0.08	0.20	0.05	0.57	0.18	16.3	9.7	0	0.6
0	12	0.33	15.3	252.5	5.9	0.12	236.0	0.05	0.14	0.03	0.39	0.12	11.8	7.7	0	0.4
0	16	0.26	8.5	90.7	13.9	0.16	4.7	0.03	0.09	0.02	0.63	0.08	6.2	2.7	0	0.2
0	24	0.32	21.6	172.8	0.9	0.35	9.9	0.04	0.13	0.04	0.46	0.07	18.0	4.9	0	0.2
0	23	0.45	13.3	247.0	1.0	0.23	267.5	0.02	0.12	0.07	0.51	0.17	20.5	9.8	0	0.4
0	16	0.33	17.1	237.6	2.7	0.30	50.4	0.03	0.11	0.02	0.46	0.07	25.2	11.6	0	0.2
0	19	0.54	14.5	216.3	2.2	0.22	10.0	0.05	0.13	0.04	0.43	0.05	8.9	4.1	0	0.2
0	38	0.69	27.0	475.0	36.0	0.32	961.0	0.11	0.71	0.11	1.49	0.29	6.0	19.6	0	0.2
0	44	1.18	29.5	377.2	44.3	0.33	1290.7	0.09	1.54	0.08	0.88	0.27	9.8	21.0	0	0.3
8	24	0.72	11.9	162.6	108.7	0.15	318.7	0.02	0.82	0.04	0.37	0.05	5.5	8.2	0	0.7
0	22	0.89	22.0	312.0	53.0	0.18	399.0	0.04	1.00	0.06	0.74	0.19	17.0	26.4	0	0.7
0	31	0.47	18.4	330.1	7.0	0.26	913.3	0.06	0.67	0.05	0.49	0.16	19.3	8.0	0	0.5
0	10	0.35	12.2	455.6	5.4	0.14	4.1	0.06	0.23	0.02	0.38	0.16	10.9	8.2	0	0.5
0	10	0.29	5.6	240.8	1.4	0.38	2.1	0.03	—	0.04	0.57	0.08	2.1	13.2	0	0.7
0	5	0.42	13.6	182.2	0.7	0.15	4.1	0.03	0.26	0.02	1.26	0.04	4.8	8.0	0	0.3
0	5	0.41	13.2	176.9	0.7	0.15	4.0	0.03	0.25	0.02	1.22	0.04	4.6	7.7	0	0.3
0	9	0.23	9.4	201.6	4.3	0.15	35.7	0.03	0.46	0.02	0.51	0.07	12.8	11.7	0	0
0	12	0.33	13.5	291.5	6.2	0.21	51.7	0.05	0.66	0.02	0.73	0.10	18.5	16.9	0	0
0	12	0.52	13.4	278.2	326.8	0.18	27.9	0.06	0.39	0.04	0.82	0.13	24.3	22.2	0	0.4
0	12	0.52	13.4	278.2	12.1	0.18	27.9	0.06	0.39	0.04	0.82	0.13	24.3	22.2	0	0.4
0	12	0.98	13.8	332.6	259.1	0.21	24.9	0.02	1.41	0.05	1.01	0.07	3.9	7.2	0	1.7
0	12	0.95	13.4	324.5	18.9	0.20	24.3	0.02	1.38	0.05	0.98	0.07	3.8	7.0	0	1.7
0	11	1.11	14.4	274.4	249.4	0.22	16.3	0.02	1.23	0.05	0.92	0.08	6.9	6.6	0	0.4
0	11	1.11	14.4	274.4	17.5	0.22	16.3	0.02	1.23	0.05	0.92	0.08	6.9	6.6	0	0.4
0	13	0.82	10.8	261.6	13.2	0.17	28.8	0.04	0.67	0.03	0.64	0.09	15.6	27.4	0	0.6
0	9	0.24	9.9	213.3	4.5	0.15	37.8	0.03	0.49	0.02	0.53	0.07	13.5	12.3	0	0
0	43	1.70	15.3	263.9	281.8	0.22	11.5	0.06	1.06	0.04	0.91	0.02	6.4	10.1	0	0.8
0	8	0.62	9.8	201.9	319.6	0.12	13.4	0.01	0.87	0.04	0.59	0.06	6.7	4.3	0	0.1
0	30	2.45	52.4	925.3	66.7	0.54	11.9	0.14	0	0.13	2.44	0.09	18.4	10.6	0	1.5
0	13	0.74	22.3	430.4	73.2	0.21	17.6	0.05	—	0.11	1.00	0.09	6.3	28.0	0	0.8
0	99	0.58	15.8	146.2	20.9	0.10	274.3	0.03	1.35	0.05	0.30	0.13	85.0	19.7	0	0.6
0	125	1.59	21.3	183.7	12.3	0.34	441.2	0.04	2.18	0.06	0.38	0.05	32.0	17.9	0	1.0
0	26	0.14	7.0	138.1	12.5	0.09	0	0.02	0.02	0.02	0.23	0.05	7.0	9.0	0	0.2
0	22	0.86	13.0	237.2	121.4	0.33	475.1	0.04	0.24	0.04	0.47	0.06	19.6	4.1	0	0.2
0	23	0.75	20.0	153.8	31.9	0.45	194.7	0.06	0.35	0.11	0.77	0.07	17.3	2.9	0	0.3
0	20	0.36	—	235.0	210.0	—	50.0	0	0	0	0	0	—	36.0	0	—
0	10	0.18	—	450.0	70.0	—	50.0	0	—	0	0	0	—	36.0	0	—
0	20	0.54	—	325.0	240.0	—	31.3	—	—	—	—	—	—	36.0	0	—

TABLE A-2 Table of Food Composition *(continued)*   (Computer code is for Cengage Diet Analysis program)   (For purposes of calculations, use "0" for t, <1, <0.1, <0.01)

DA+ Code	Food Description	Quantity	Measure	Wt (g)	H₂O (g)	Ener (kcal)	Prot (g)	Carb (g)	Fiber (g)	Fat (g)	Fat Breakdown (g)		
											Sat	Mono	Poly
Vegetables, Legumes—*continued*													
	Water chestnuts												
31073	Sliced, drained	½	cup(s)	75	—	20	0	5.0	1.0	0	0	0	0
31087	Whole	½	cup(s)	75	—	20	0	5.0	1.0	0	0	0	0
1135	Watercress	1	cup(s)	34	32.3	4	0.8	0.4	0.2	0	0	0	0
Nuts, Seeds, and Products													
	Almonds												
32940	Almond butter with salt added	1	tablespoon(s)	16	0.3	98	3.4	3.0	1.6	8.9	1.0	5.2	2.2
1137	Almond butter, no salt added	1	tablespoon(s)	16	0.3	98	3.4	3.0	1.6	8.9	0.7	5.2	2.2
32886	Blanched	¼	cup(s)	36	1.6	214	7.8	6.8	3.6	19.0	1.4	12.1	4.5
32887	Dry roasted, no salt added	¼	cup(s)	35	0.9	205	7.3	7.3	3.8	18.0	1.4	11.2	4.5
29724	Dry roasted, salted	¼	cup(s)	35	0.9	205	7.3	7.3	3.8	18.0	1.4	11.2	4.5
29725	Oil roasted, salted	¼	cup(s)	39	1.1	238	8.3	6.9	4.1	21.7	1.7	13.7	5.3
508	Slivered	¼	cup(s)	27	1.3	155	5.7	5.9	3.3	13.3	1.0	8.3	3.3
1138	**Beechnuts, dried**	¼	cup(s)	57	3.8	328	3.5	19.1	5.3	28.5	3.3	12.5	11.5
517	**Brazil nuts, dried, unblanched**	¼	cup(s)	33	1.2	218	4.8	4.1	2.5	22.1	5.0	8.2	6.8
1166	**Breadfruit seeds, roasted**	¼	cup(s)	57	28.3	118	3.5	22.9	3.4	1.5	0.4	0.2	0.8
1139	**Butternuts, dried**	¼	cup(s)	30	1.0	184	7.5	3.6	1.4	17.1	0.4	3.1	12.8
	Cashews												
32931	Cashew butter with salt added	1	tablespoon(s)	16	0.5	94	2.8	4.4	0.3	7.9	1.6	4.7	1.3
32889	Cashew butter, no salt added	1	tablespoon(s)	16	0.5	94	2.8	4.4	0.3	7.9	1.6	4.7	1.3
1140	Dry roasted	¼	cup(s)	34	0.6	197	5.2	11.2	1.0	15.9	3.1	9.4	2.7
518	Oil roasted	¼	cup(s)	32	1.1	187	5.4	9.6	1.1	15.4	2.7	8.4	2.8
	Coconut												
32896	Dried, not sweetened	¼	cup(s)	23	0.7	150	1.6	5.4	3.7	14.6	13.0	0.6	0.2
1153	Dried, shredded, sweetened	¼	cup(s)	23	2.9	116	0.7	11.1	1.0	8.3	7.3	0.4	0.1
520	Shredded	¼	cup(s)	20	9.4	71	0.7	3.0	1.8	6.7	5.9	0.3	0.1
	Chestnuts												
1152	Chinese, roasted	¼	cup(s)	71	28.7	171	3.2	37.4	—	0.9	0.1	0.4	0.2
32895	European, boiled and steamed	¼	cup(s)	45	30.9	59	0.9	12.6		0.6	0.1	0.2	0.2
32911	European, roasted	¼	cup(s)	36	14.5	88	1.1	18.9	1.8	0.8	0.1	0.3	0.3
32922	Japanese, boiled and steamed	¼	cup(s)	35	30.5	20	0.3	4.5	—	0.1	0	0	0
32923	Japanese, roasted	¼	cup(s)	36	17.8	72	1.1	16.1	—	0.3	0	0.1	0.1
4958	**Flax seeds or linseeds**	¼	cup(s)	28	2.2	150	5.5	8.1	7.8	11.6	1.0	2.1	8.0
32904	**Ginkgo nuts, dried**	¼	cup(s)	39	4.8	134	4.0	27.9	—	0.8	0.1	0.3	0.3
	Hazelnuts or filberts												
32901	Blanched	¼	cup(s)	45	2.6	285	6.2	7.7	5.0	27.7	2.1	21.9	2.5
32902	Dry roasted, no salt added	¼	cup(s)	29	0.7	185	4.3	5.0	2.7	17.8	1.3	13.3	2.4
1156	**Hickorynuts, dried**	¼	cup(s)	30	0.8	197	3.8	5.5	1.9	19.3	2.1	9.8	6.6
	Macadamias												
32905	Dry roasted, no salt added	¼	cup(s)	34	0.5	241	2.6	4.5	2.7	25.5	4.0	19.9	0.5
32932	Dry roasted, with salt added	¼	cup(s)	34	0.5	240	2.6	4.3	2.7	25.5	4.0	19.9	0.5
1157	Raw	¼	cup(s)	34	0.5	241	2.6	4.6	2.9	25.4	4.0	19.7	0.5
	Mixed nuts												
1159	With peanuts, dry roasted	¼	cup(s)	34	0.6	203	5.9	8.7	3.1	17.6	2.4	10.8	3.7
32933	With peanuts, dry roasted, with salt added	¼	cup(s)	34	0.6	203	5.9	8.7	3.1	17.6	2.2	10.8	3.7
32906	Without peanuts, oil roasted, no salt added	¼	cup(s)	36	1.1	221	5.6	8.0	2.0	20.2	3.3	11.9	4.1
	Peanuts												
2807	Dry roasted	¼	cup(s)	37	0.6	214	8.6	7.9	2.9	18.1	2.5	9.0	5.7
2806	Dry roasted, salted	¼	tablespoon(s)	37	0.6	214	8.6	7.9	2.9	18.1	2.5	9.0	5.7
1763	Oil roasted, salted	¼	cup(s)	36	0.5	216	10.1	5.5	3.4	18.9	3.1	9.4	5.5
1884	Peanut butter, chunky	1	tablespoon(s)	16	0.2	94	3.8	3.5	1.3	8.0	1.2	3.7	2.2
30303	Peanut butter, low sodium	1	tablespoon(s)	16	0.3	94	4.0	3.1	1.0	8.1	1.6	3.8	2.2
30421	Peanut butter, natural	1	tablespoon(s)	16	—	100	3.5	3.0	1.0	8.0	1.3	4.0	2.3
30422	Peanut butter, natural, no salt added	1	tablespoon(s)	16	—	105	3.5	3.0	1.0	8.0	1.3	—	—
30305	Peanut butter, reduced fat	1	tablespoon(s)	18	0.2	94	4.7	6.4	0.9	6.1	1.0	2.9	1.7
524	Peanut butter, smooth	1	tablespoon(s)	16	0.3	94	4.0	3.1	1.0	8.1	1.7	3.9	2.3
2804	Raw	¼	cup(s)	37	2.4	207	9.4	5.9	3.1	18.0	2.5	8.9	5.7

PAGE KEY: A-6 5 Breads/Baked Goods A-12 = Cereal/Rice/Pasta A-16 = Fruit A-22 = Vegetables/Legumes A-32 = Nuts/Seeds A-34 = Vegetarian A-36 = Dairy A-44 = Eggs A-44 = Seafood A-46 = Meats A-50 = Poultry
A-52 = Processed Meats A-54 = Beverages A-58 = Fats/Oils A-60 = Sweets A-62 = Spices/Condiments/Sauces A-66 = Mixed Foods/Soups/Sandwiches A-72 = Fast Food A-90 = Convenience A-92 = Baby Foods

Chol (mg)	Calc (mg)	Iron (mg)	Magn (mg)	Pota (mg)	Sodi (mg)	Zinc (mg)	Vit A (µg)	Thia (mg)	Vit E (mg α)	Ribo (mg)	Niac (mg)	Vit B6 (mg)	Fola (µg)	Vit C (mg)	Vit B12 (µg)	Sele (µg)
0	0	0	—	—	5.0	—	0	—	—	—	—	—	—	2.4	—	—
0	7	0	—	—	5.0	—	0	—	—	—	—	—	—	2.0	—	—
0	41	0.07	7.1	112.2	13.9	0.04	54.4	0.03	0.34	0.04	0.07	0.04	3.1	14.6	0	0.3
0	56	0.56	44.6	119.7	36.3	0.53	0	0.01	3.87	0.15	0.50	0.02	8.5	0	0	0.4
0	56	0.56	44.6	119.7	1.1	0.53	0	0.01	3.87	0.15	0.50	0.02	8.5	0	0	0.4
0	86	1.19	97.2	238.9	6.9	1.08	0	0.07	8.61	0.26	1.27	0.04	17.8	0	0	1.2
0	92	1.32	96.9	245.6	1.0	1.14	0	0.03	8.21	0.33	1.23	0.04	18.3	0	0	0.8
0	92	1.32	96.9	245.6	226.3	1.14	0	0.03	8.21	0.33	1.23	0.04	18.3	0	0	0.8
0	114	1.44	107.5	274.4	133.1	1.20	0	0.04	10.19	0.31	1.44	0.05	10.6	0	0	1.1
0	71	1.00	72.4	190.4	0.3	0.83	0	0.06	7.08	0.27	0.91	0.04	13.5	0	0	0.7
0	1	1.40	0	579.7	21.7	0.21	0	0.17	—	0.21	0.50	0.39	64.4	8.8	0	4.0
0	53	0.81	125.0	219.1	1.0	1.35	0	0.21	1.91	0.01	0.10	0.03	7.3	0.2	0	637.4
0	49	0.51	35.3	616.7	16.0	0.59	8.6	0.23	—	0.14	4.22	0.24	33.6	4.3	0	8.0
0	16	1.21	71.1	126.3	0.3	0.94	1.8	0.11	—	0.04	0.31	0.17	19.8	1.0	0	5.2
0	7	0.80	41.3	87.4	65.0	0.83	0	0.05	0.15	0.03	0.26	0.04	10.9	0	0	1.8
0	7	0.80	41.3	87.4	2.4	0.83	0	0.05	—	0.03	0.26	0.04	10.9	0	0	1.8
0	15	2.06	89.1	193.5	5.5	1.92	0	0.07	0.32	0.07	0.48	0.09	23.6	0	0	4.0
0	14	1.95	88.0	203.8	4.2	1.73	0	0.12	0.30	0.07	0.56	0.10	8.1	0.1	0	6.5
0	6	0.75	20.4	123.2	8.4	0.46	0	0.01	0.10	0.02	0.14	0.07	2.0	0.3	0	4.2
0	3	0.45	11.6	78.4	60.9	0.42	0	0.01	0.09	0	0.11	0.06	1.9	0.2	0	3.9
0	3	0.49	6.4	71.2	4.0	0.22	0	0.01	0.05	0	0.11	0.01	5.2	0.7	0	2.0
0	14	1.07	64.3	341.0	2.9	0.66	0	0.11	—	0.06	1.07	0.31	51.5	27.5	0	5.0
0	21	0.78	24.5	324.3	12.2	0.11	0.5	0.07	—	0.05	0.33	0.11	17.2	12.1	0	—
0	10	0.33	11.8	211.6	0.7	0.20	0.4	0.09	0.18	0.06	0.48	0.18	25.0	9.3	0	0.4
0	4	0.19	6.4	42.2	1.8	0.14	0.4	0.04	—	0.02	0.19	0.04	6.0	3.4	0	—
0	13	0.75	22.9	152.7	6.8	0.51	1.4	0.16	—		0.25	0.15	21.1	10.0	0	—
0	94	1.40	102.6	232.7	7.8	1.20	0	0.46	0.09	0.05	0.86	0.13	24.4	0.2	0	7.1
0	8	0.62	20.4	384.7	5.0	0.26	21.2	0.17	—	0.07	4.52	0.25	40.9	11.3	0	—
0	68	1.50	72.6	298.4	0	1.00	0.9	0.22	7.94	0.05	0.70	0.27	35.4	0.9	0	1.9
0	35	1.25	49.4	215.8	0	0.71	0.9	0.10	4.37	0.04	0.59	0.18	25.2	1.1	0	1.2
0	18	0.64	51.9	130.8	0.3	1.29	2.1	0.26	—	0.04	0.27	0.06	12.0	0.6	0	2.4
0	23	0.89	39.5	121.6	1.3	0.43	0	0.24	0.19	0.03	0.76	0.12	3.3	0.2	0	3.9
0	23	0.89	39.5	121.6	118.3	0.43	0	0.24	0.19	0.03	0.76	0.12	3.3	0.2	0	3.9
0	28	1.24	43.5	123.3	1.7	0.44	0	0.40	0.18	0.05	0.83	0.09	3.7	0.4	0	1.2
0	24	1.27	77.1	204.5	4.1	1.30	0.3	0.07	—	0.07	1.61	0.10	17.1	0.1	0	1.0
0	24	1.27	77.1	237.4	118.2	1.30	0	0.07	3.75	0.07	1.61	0.10	17.1	0.1	0	2.6
0	38	0.93	90.4	195.8	4.0	1.68	0.4	0.18	—	0.17	0.71	0.06	20.2	0.2	0	—
0	20	0.82	64.2	240.2	2.2	1.21	0	0.16	2.53	0.04	4.94	0.09	52.9	0	0	2.7
0	20	0.82	64.2	240.2	247.8	1.21	0	0.16	2.85	0.04	4.94	0.09	52.9	0	0	2.7
0	22	0.55	63.4	261.4	115.2	1.18	0	0.03	2.50	0.03	4.98	0.17	43.2	0.3	0	1.2
0	7	0.30	25.6	119.2	77.8	0.45	0	0.02	1.01	0.02	2.19	0.07	14.7	0	0	1.3
0	7	0.30	24.6	103.8	2.7	0.47	0	0.01	1.44	0.02	2.14	0.09	11.8	0	0	0.9
0	0	0.18	—	—	52.5	—	0	—	—	—	—	—	—	0	—	—
0	0	0.18	—	—	0	—	0	—	—	—	—	—	—	0	—	—
0	6	0.34	30.6	120.4	97.2	0.50	0	0.05	1.63	0.01	2.63	0.06	10.8	0	0	1.4
0	7	0.30	24.6	103.8	73.4	0.47	0	0.01	1.44	0.02	2.14	0.09	11.8	0	0	0.9
0	34	1.67	61.3	257.3	6.6	1.19	0	0.23	3.04	0.05	4.40	0.13	87.6	0	0	2.6

TABLE A-2 **Table of Food Composition** (continued)   (Computer code is for Cengage Diet Analysis program)   (For purposes of calculations, use "0" for t, <1, <0.1, <0.01)

DA+ Code	Food Description	Quantity	Measure	Wt (g)	H₂O (g)	Ener (kcal)	Prot (g)	Carb (g)	Fiber (g)	Fat (g)	Fat Breakdown (g) Sat	Mono	Poly
Nuts, Seeds, and Products—*continued*													
	Pecans												
32907	Dry roasted, no salt added	¼	cup(s)	28	0.3	195	2.6	3.7	2.6	20.4	1.7	12.1	5.7
32936	Dry roasted, with salt added	¼	cup(s)	28	0.3	195	2.6	3.7	2.6	20.4	1.7	12.1	5.7
1162	Oil roasted	¼	cup(s)	28	0.3	197	2.5	3.6	2.6	20.7	2.0	11.3	6.5
526	Raw	¼	cup(s)	27	1.0	188	2.5	3.8	2.6	19.6	1.7	11.1	5.9
12973	**Pine nuts or pignolia, dried**	1	tablespoon(s)	9	0.2	58	1.2	1.1	0.3	5.9	0.4	1.6	2.9
	Pistachios												
1164	Dry roasted	¼	cup(s)	31	0.6	174	6.4	9.0	3.0	13.8	1.7	7.3	4.1
32938	Dry roasted, with salt added	¼	cup(s)	32	0.6	180	6.7	9.2	3.2	14.3	1.7	7.6	4.3
1167	**Pumpkin or squash seeds, roasted**	¼	cup(s)	57	1.2	326	16.9	8.3	3.7	27.8	4.8	8.9	11.3
	Sesame												
32912	Sesame butter paste	1	tablespoon(s)	16	0.3	94	2.9	3.8	0.9	8.1	1.1	3.1	3.6
32941	Tahini or sesame butter	1	tablespoon(s)	15	0.4	89	2.6	3.2	0.7	8.0	1.1	3.0	3.5
1169	Whole, roasted, toasted	3	tablespoon(s)	27	0.9	153	4.6	6.9	3.8	13.0	1.8	4.9	5.7
	Soy nuts												
34173	Deep sea salted	¼	cup(s)	28	—	130	11.0	9.0	6.0	6.0	1.0	1.0	3.5
34174	Unsalted	¼	cup(s)	28	—	130	11.0	9.0	6.0	6.0	1.0	1.0	3.5
	Sunflower seeds												
528	Kernels, dried	1	tablespoon(s)	9	0.4	53	1.9	1.8	0.8	4.6	0.4	1.7	2.1
29721	Kernels, dry roasted, salted	1	tablespoon(s)	8	0.1	47	1.5	1.9	0.7	4.0	0.4	0.8	2.6
29723	Kernels, toasted, salted	1	tablespoon(s)	8	0.1	52	1.4	1.7	1.0	4.8	0.5	0.9	3.1
32928	Sunflower seed butter with salt added	1	tablespoon(s)	16	0.1	99	2.8	3.7	0.9	8.8	0.7	6.2	1.6
	Trail mix												
4646	Trail mix	¼	cup(s)	38	3.5	173	5.2	16.8	2.0	11.0	2.1	4.7	3.6
4647	Trail mix with chocolate chips	¼	cup(s)	38	2.5	182	5.3	16.8	—	12.0	2.3	5.1	4.2
4648	Tropical trail mix	¼	cup(s)	35	3.2	155	2.2	23.0	—	6.0	3.0	0.9	1.8
	Walnuts												
529	Dried black, chopped	¼	cup(s)	31	1.4	193	7.5	3.1	2.1	18.4	1.1	4.7	11.0
531	English or Persian	¼	cup(s)	29	1.2	191	4.5	4.0	2.0	19.1	1.8	2.6	13.8
Vegetarian Foods													
	Prepared												
34222	Brown rice and tofu stir-fry (vegan)	8	ounce(s)	227	183.7	227	12.3	12.6	2.8	16.3	1.3	4.0	9.5
34368	Cheese enchilada casserole (lacto)	8	ounce(s)	227	88.3	400	17.6	37.3	3.8	19.5	10.3	6.6	1.5
34247	Five bean casserole (vegan)	8	ounce(s)	227	164.0	224	4.8	40.3	4.6	5.0	0.9	2.3	1.6
34261	Lentil stew (vegan)	8	ounce(s)	227	150.6	127	7.3	24.2	7.3	0.5	0.1	0.1	0.2
34397	Macaroni and cheese (lacto)	8	ounce(s)	227	163.3	182	8.2	17.3	0.6	8.8	4.5	3.0	0.9
34238	Steamed rice and vegetables (vegan)	8	ounce(s)	227	99.7	263	4.9	39.2	2.5	10.3	1.8	4.2	3.9
34308	Tofu rice burgers (ovo-lacto)	1	piece(s)	218	78.2	446	22.5	67.0	6.0	10.4	2.2	2.5	4.7
34276	Vegan spinach enchiladas (vegan)	1	piece(s)	80	59.1	86	4.8	12.7	2.1	2.3	0.4	0.6	1.0
34243	Vegetable chow mein (vegan)	8	ounce(s)	227	163.5	164	6.3	22.2	2.0	6.2	0.7	2.8	2.4
34454	Vegetable lasagna (lacto)	8	ounce(s)	227	154.8	178	11.6	25.4	2.3	3.6	2.0	0.9	0.3
34339	Vegetable marinara (vegan)	8	ounce(s)	227	180.6	93	2.8	14.9	1.4	2.8	0.4	1.3	0.9
34356	Vegetable rice casserole (lacto)	8	ounce(s)	227	172.6	222	9.0	23.5	3.8	11.3	4.4	3.4	2.0
34311	Vegetable strudel (ovo-lacto)	8	ounce(s)	227	99.9	754	18.8	50.9	3.9	53.5	18.2	26.4	6.1
34371	Vegetable taco (lacto)	1	item(s)	85	54.6	140	4.9	16.7	3.0	6.3	2.9	1.8	1.3
34282	Vegetarian chili (vegan)	8	tablespoon(s)	227	195.6	115	5.6	21.3	6.8	1.5	0.3	0.3	0.7
34367	Vegetarian vegetable soup (vegan)	8	ounce(s)	227	204.6	92	2.5	13.6	2.5	4.0	0.7	1.8	1.2
	Boca												
68284	All American Classic patty w/ organic soy	1	item(s)	71	—	140	15.0	9.0	4.0	5.0	1.5	—	—
32072	Breakfast links	2	item(s)	45	—	70	8.0	5.0	2.0	3.0	1.0	—	—
68285	Bruschetta tomato basil parmesan patty	1	item(s)	71	—	70	10.0	9.0	3.5	1.5	0.5	0.5	—
35780	Cheeseburger meatless burger patty	1	item(s)	71	—	100	13.0	6.0	4.0	4.5	1.5	—	—
68290	Chik'n nuggets	1	item(s)	22	—	45	3.5	4.3	0.8	1.8	0.1	1.3	—

PAGE KEY: A-6 5 Breads/Baked Goods A-12 = Cereal/Rice/Pasta A-16 = Fruit A-22 = Vegetables/Legumes A-32 = Nuts/Seeds A-34 = Vegetarian A-36 = Dairy A-44 = Eggs A-44 = Seafood A-46 = Meats A-50 = Poultry
A-52 = Processed Meats A-54 = Beverages A-58 = Fats/Oils A-60 = Sweets A-62 = Spices/Condiments/Sauces A-66 = Mixed Foods/Soups/Sandwiches A-72 = Fast Food A-90 = Convenience A-92 = Baby Foods

Chol (mg)	Calc (mg)	Iron (mg)	Magn (mg)	Pota (mg)	Sodi (mg)	Zinc (mg)	Vit A (µg)	Thia (mg)	Vit E (mg α)	Ribo (mg)	Niac (mg)	Vit B$_6$ (mg)	Fola (µg)	Vit C (mg)	Vit B$_{12}$ (µg)	Sele (µg)
0	20	0.77	36.3	116.6	0.3	1.39	1.9	0.12	0.36	0.03	0.32	0.05	4.4	0.2	0	1.1
0	20	0.77	36.3	116.6	105.4	1.39	1.9	0.12	0.36	0.03	0.32	0.05	4.4	0.2	0	1.1
0	18	0.68	33.3	107.8	0.3	1.23	1.4	0.13	0.70	0.03	0.33	0.05	4.1	0.2	0	1.6
0	19	0.69	33.0	111.7	0	1.23	0.8	0.18	0.38	0.04	0.32	0.06	6.0	0.3	0	1.0
0	1	0.48	21.6	51.3	0.2	0.55	0.1	0.03	0.80	0.02	0.38	0.01	2.9	0.1	0	0.1
0	33	1.24	33.5	309.7	1.8	0.72	4.0	0.21	0.74	0.07	0.42	0.35	15.7	0.9	0	3.1
0	34	1.29	34.9	322.2	137.0	0.75	4.2	0.22	0.77	0.07	0.44	0.36	16.3	1.0	0	3.2
0	30	4.58	312.1	447.2	10.2	4.34	0	0.04	0.32	0.09	2.51	0.06	32.3	1.0	0	5.3
0	154	3.07	57.9	93.1	1.9	1.17	0.5	0.04	—	0.03	1.07	0.13	16.0	0	0	5.7
0	21	0.66	14.3	68.8	5.3	0.69	0.4	0.24	—	0.02	0.85	0.02	14.7	0.6	0	5.2
0	267	3.99	96.1	128.3	3.0	1.93	0	0.22	—	0.07	1.24	0.22	26.5	0	0	9.3
0	40	1.80	—	—	95.0	—	0	—	—	—	—	—	—	1.2	—	—
0	40	1.80	—	—	2.0	—	0	—	—	—	—	—	—	1.2	—	—
0	7	0.47	29.3	58.0	0.8	0.45	0.3	0.13	3.17	0.03	0.75	0.12	20.4	0.1	0	4.8
0	6	0.30	10.3	68.0	29.4	0.42	0	0.01	2.09	0.02	0.56	0.06	19.0	0.1	0	6.3
0	5	0.57	10.8	41.1	51.3	0.44	0	0.03	—	0.02	0.35	0.07	19.9	0.1	0	5.2
0	10	0.66	49.8	92.2	53.0	0.78	0.5	0.01	3.66	0.03	1.08	0.09	37.9	0.4	0	16.7
0	29	1.14	59.3	256.9	85.9	1.21	0.4	0.17	—	0.07	1.77	0.11	26.6	0.5	0	—
2	41	1.27	60.4	243.0	45.4	1.18	0.8	0.15	—	0.08	1.65	0.10	24.4	0.5	0	—
0	20	0.92	33.6	248.1	33.3	0.41	0.7	0.16	—	0.04	0.52	0.11	14.7	2.7	0	—
0	19	0.98	62.8	163.4	0.6	1.05	0.6	0.02	0.56	0.04	0.15	0.18	9.7	0.5	0	5.3
0	29	0.85	46.2	129.0	0.6	0.90	0.3	0.10	0.20	0.04	0.33	0.16	28.7	0.4	0	1.4
0	268	4.67	88.0	379.7	111.4	1.53	0	0.13	0.68	0.11	1.07	0.28	39.0	15.5	0	10.9
43	478	2.52	34.7	215.7	1350.3	1.87	0	0.33	0.48	0.36	2.28	0.12	128.6	22.2	0.4	20.7
0	45	1.25	37.2	376.6	776.2	0.73	0	0.08	1.01	0.08	0.67	0.10	64.5	4.6	0	4.0
0	25	2.09	33.9	388.5	288.8	1.08	0	0.18	1.05	0.09	1.47	0.16	134.2	12.3	0	8.9
22	193	0.68	20.4	126.3	772.5	1.14	0	0.14	0.29	0.24	0.98	0.05	75.4	0.1	0.5	15.6
0	42	1.40	67.5	355.8	1397.4	0.92	175.8	0.16	1.66	0.11	2.75	0.29	31.3	13.1	0	8.3
51	528	5.83	96.8	426.9	1800.8	2.46	0	0.85	0.64	0.45	5.83	0.31	167.7	3.2	0.2	35.1
0	106	1.12	37.2	161.3	104.4	0.68	0	0.06	0.21	0.05	0.54	0.11	19.8	1.4	0	5.3
0	187	3.47	28.5	305.1	367.0	0.75	0	0.13	0.85	0.12	1.37	0.14	76.8	8.1	0	6.4
10	146	1.82	34.5	396.7	647.7	1.12	0	0.19	1.03	0.26	2.02	0.22	107.4	15.2	0.4	19.1
0	17	0.77	17.1	182.0	376.5	0.38	18.2	0.12	0.86	0.08	1.20	0.11	71.6	17.7	0	10.0
16	172	2.01	29.4	393.3	579.0	1.28	0	0.17	1.70	0.28	2.33	0.20	148.5	53.2	0.2	11.6
46	317	3.36	39.0	298.5	815.8	1.98	0	0.45	1.47	0.50	4.51	0.16	175.8	27.1	0.3	31.1
8	79	0.85	26.5	205.7	331.4	0.68	0	0.09	0.26	0.07	0.60	0.08	32.7	4.2	0.1	2.3
0	68	2.42	40.9	531.0	358.9	1.23	0	0.14	1.43	0.13	1.25	0.22	48.6	16.6	0	3.6
0	38	1.32	27.9	444.6	504.1	0.45	0	0.11	0.73	0.08	1.55	0.21	39.7	23.8	0	1.0
5	150	1.44	—	—	500.0	—	0	—	—	—	—	—	—	0	—	—
0	20	1.44	—	—	330.0	—	0	—	—	—	—	—	—	0	—	—
5	150	2.70	—	—	290.0	—	0	—	—	—	—	—	—	0	—	—
10	100	1.44	—	—	320.0	—	—	—	—	—	—	—	—	0	—	—
0	10	0.36	—	—	125.0	—	—	—	—	—	—	—	—	0	—	—

TABLE A-2 Table of Food Composition (continued) (Computer code is for Cengage Diet Analysis program) (For purposes of calculations, use "0" for t, <1, <0.1, <0.01)

DA+ Code	Food Description	Quantity	Measure	Wt (g)	H₂O (g)	Ener (kcal)	Prot (g)	Carb (g)	Fiber (g)	Fat (g)	Sat	Mono	Poly
Vegetarian Foods—*continued*													
68289	Chik'n patty, original	1	item(s)	71	—	160	11.0	15.0	2.0	6.0	0	—	—
68291	Chik'n patty, spicy	1	item(s)	71	—	160	11.0	15.0	2.0	6.0	0	—	—
35781	Grilled vegetable patty	1	item(s)	71	—	80	12.0	7.0	4.0	1.0	0	—	—
68287	Meatless ground crumbles	½	cup(s)	57	—	60	13.0	6.0	3.0	0.5	0	—	—
68282	Original vegan patty	1	item(s)	71	—	70	13.0	6.0	4.0	0.5	0	—	—
	Gardenburger												
39661	Black bean chipotle burger	1	item(s)	71	45.8	100	5.0	16.0	5.0	3.0	0	1.6	0.8
29913	Original	1	item(s)	71	43.7	100	5.0	18.0	5.0	3.0	1.0	1.2	0.7
29920	Portabella veggie burger	1	item(s)	71	44.9	100	4.0	17.0	5.0	2.5	1.0	0.7	0.5
39662	Sun-dried tomato basil burger	1	item(s)	71	46.3	100	4.0	17.0	4.0	2.5	0.5	0.9	0.6
29915	Veggie medley	1	item(s)	71	46.5	100	3.0	17.0	5.0	2.5	0	1.0	1.0
	Loma Linda												
9311	Big franks, canned	1	item(s)	51	30.1	110	11.0	3.0	2.0	6.0	1.0	1.5	3.5
9323	Fried Chik'n with gravy	2	piece(s)	80	—	150	12.0	5.0	2.0	10.0	1.5	2.5	5.0
9326	Linketts, canned	1	item(s)	35	21.4	70	7.0	1.0	1.0	4.0	0.5	1.0	2.5
9336	Redi-Burger patties, canned	1	slice(s)	85	55.1	120	18.0	7.0	4.0	2.5	0.5	0.5	1.5
9354	Tender Rounds meatball substitute, canned in gravy	6	piece(s)	80	55.3	120	13.0	6.0	1.0	4.5	0.5	1.5	2.5
9356	Vege-Burger, canned	¼	cup(s)	55	39.6	60	12.0	2.0	2.0	0.5	0	0	0.5
	Morningstar Farms												
9371	Breakfast bacon strips	2	item(s)	16	6.7	60	2.0	1.0	1.0	4.5	0.5	1.0	3.0
9368	Breakfast sausage links	2	item(s)	45	28.3	80	9.0	3.0	2.0	3.0	0.5	1.0	1.5
33705	Chik'n nuggets	4	piece(s)	86	43.5	190	12.0	19.0	4.0	9.0	1.5	2.5	4.5
11587	Chik patties	1	item(s)	71	38.3	140	8.0	16.0	2.0	5.0	0.5	1.0	3.5
2531	Garden veggie patties	1	item(s)	67	40.1	110	10.0	9.0	3.0	3.5	0.5	0.5	1.5
9376	Grillers patties, original	1	item(s)	64	35.6	130	15.0	5.0	2.0	6.0	1.0	2.0	3.0
50552	Meal Starters Chik'n strips	12	piece(s)	85	50.6	140	23.0	6.0	1.0	3.5	0.5	1.5	1.5
33715	Meal Starters Grillers recipe crumbles	½	cup(s)	42	26.9	61	7.6	3.8	2.3	1.9	0	0.4	1.1
33702	Spicy black bean veggie burger	1	item(s)	67	37.7	120	11.0	13.0	4.0	4.0	0.5	1.0	2.0
	Worthington												
9418	Chic-ketts, frozen	2	slice(s)	55	31.7	110	14.0	3.0	2.0	5.0	1.0	1.0	3.0
9424	Chili, canned	1	cup(s)	230	167.1	280	24.0	25.0	8.0	10.0	1.5	1.5	7.0
9436	Diced Chik, canned	¼	cup(s)	55	43.0	50	9.0	2.0	1.0	0	0	0	0.0
9440	Dinner roast, frozen	1	slice(s)	85	52.4	180	14.0	6.0	3.0	11.0	1.5	4.5	5.0
9446	Fripats patties, frozen	1	item(s)	64	36.4	130	15.0	5.0	3.0	6.0	1.0	1.5	3.5
9452	Leanies links, frozen	1	item(s)	40	21.6	100	8.0	2.0	1.0	7.0	1.0	1.5	4.5
36702	Meatless chicken style roll, frozen	1	slice(s)	55	—	90	9.0	2.0	1.0	4.5	0.5	1.0	2.5
9428	Meatless corned beef, sliced, frozen	3	slice(s)	57	30.8	145	10.4	5.2	0	8.3	1.0	2.1	5.2
9462	Prosage links	2	item(s)	45	28.9	80	9.0	3.0	2.0	3.0	0.5	0.5	2.0
9484	Stakelets patty beef steak substitute, frozen	1	piece(s)	71	40.8	150	14.0	7.0	2.0	7.0	1.0	2.5	3.5
9486	Stripples bacon substitute	2	item(s)	16	6.7	60	2.0	2.0	0.5	4.5	0.5	1.0	3.0
9496	Vegetable Skallops meat substitute, canned	½	cup(s)	85	61.8	90	17.0	4.0	3.0	1.0	0	0	0.5
Dairy													
	Cheese												
1433	Blue, crumbled	1	ounce(s)	28	12.0	100	6.1	0.7	0	8.1	5.3	2.2	0.2
884	Brick	1	ounce(s)	28	11.7	105	6.6	0.8	0	8.4	5.3	2.4	0.2
885	Brie	1	ounce(s)	28	13.7	95	5.9	0.1	0	7.8	4.9	2.3	0.2
34821	Camembert	1	ounce(s)	28	14.7	85	5.6	0.1	0	6.9	4.3	2.0	0.2
888	Cheddar or colby	1	ounce(s)	28	10.8	112	6.7	0.7	0	9.1	5.7	2.6	0.3
32096	Cheddar or colby, low-fat	1	ounce(s)	28	17.9	49	6.9	0.5	0	2.0	1.2	0.6	0.1
32121	Cheddar or colby, low-sodium	1	ounce(s)	28	11.1	113	6.9	0.5	0	9.2	5.9	2.6	0.3
5	Cheddar, shredded	¼	cup(s)	28	10.4	114	7.0	0.4	0	9.4	6.0	2.7	0.3
889	Edam	1	ounce(s)	28	11.8	101	7.1	0.4	0	7.9	5.0	2.3	0.2
890	Feta	1	ounce(s)	28	15.7	75	4.0	1.2	0	6.0	4.2	1.3	0.2
891	Fontina	1	ounce(s)	28	10.8	110	7.3	0.4	0	8.8	5.4	2.5	0.5
8527	Goat cheese, soft	1	ounce(s)	28	17.2	75	5.3	0	0	6.0	4.1	1.4	0.1

PAGE KEY: A-6 5 Breads/Baked Goods A-12 = Cereal/Rice/Pasta A-16 = Fruit A-22 = Vegetables/Legumes A-32 = Nuts/Seeds A-34 = Vegetarian A-36 = Dairy A-44 = Eggs A-44 = Seafood A-46 = Meats A-50 = Poultry A-52 = Processed Meats A-54 = Beverages A-58 = Fats/Oils A-60 = Sweets A-62 = Spices/Condiments/Sauces A-66 = Mixed Foods/Soups/Sandwiches A-72 = Fast Food A-90 = Convenience A-92 = Baby Foods

Chol (mg)	Calc (mg)	Iron (mg)	Magn (mg)	Pota (mg)	Sodi (mg)	Zinc (mg)	Vit A (µg)	Thia (mg)	Vit E (mg α)	Ribo (mg)	Niac (mg)	Vit B$_6$ (mg)	Fola (µg)	Vit C (mg)	Vit B$_{12}$ (µg)	Sele (µg)
0	40	1.80	—	—	430.0	—	—	—	—	—	—	—	—	0	—	—
0	40	1.80	—	—	560.0	—	—	—	—	—	—	—	—	0	—	—
0	60	1.80	—	—	300.0	—	—	—	—	—	—	—	—	0	—	—
0	60	1.80	—	—	270.0	—	0	—	—	—	—	—	—	0	—	—
0	60	1.80	—	—	280.0	—	—	—	—	—	—	—	—	0	—	—
0	20	1.44	18.5	140.0	390.0	0.35	10.0	—	—	—	—	—	—	6.0	—	—
10	40	1.08	2.8	110.2	400.7	0.78	—	—	—	—	—	—	—	3.6	—	—
3	40	0.72	6.4	105.2	490.9	0.07	—	—	—	—	—	—	—	1.2	—	—
3	20	0.72	2.8	55.0	270.0	0.07	—	—	—	—	—	—	—	2.4	—	—
0	20	0.72	12.8	125.2	380.7	0.21	62.6	—	—	—	—	—	—	12.0	0	—
0	0	0.77	—	50.0	220.0	1.17	0	0.22	—	0.10	2.00	0.70	—	0	2.4	—
0	20	1.80	—	70.0	430.0	—	0	1.05	—	0.34	4.00	0.30	—	0	2.4	—
0	0	0.36	—	20.0	160.0	0.52	0	0.12	—	0.20	0.80	0.16	—	0	0.9	—
0	0	1.06	—	140.1	450.3	1.45	0	0.15	—	0.26	4.00	0.40	—	0	1.2	—
0	20	1.08	—	80.0	340.0	0.64	0	0.75	—	0.17	2.00	0.16	—	0	1.2	—
0	0	0.36	—	40.0	130.0	0.71	0	0.12	—	0.10	0.78	0.30	—	0	2.4	—
0	0	0.36	—	15.0	230.0	0.10	0	0.75	—	0.04	1.20	0.07	—	0	0.2	—
0	0	1.80	—	50.0	300.0	—	0	0.38	—	0.17	7.00	0.50	—	0	3.0	—
0	60	1.80	3.4	320.0	600.0	0.69	0	0.38	—	0.10	4.00	0.20	—	0	1.8	—
0	20	1.80	—	280.0	590.0	0.35	0	0.22	—	0.10	3.00	0.16	—	0	1.2	—
0	40	0.72	—	180.0	350.0	0.67	—	7.50	—	0.20	0.94	0.60	—	0	—	—
0	43	1.80	—	130.0	260.0	0.77	0	1.80	—	0.17	4.00	0.40	—	0	2.7	—
0	40	5.40	24.0	109.9	499.8	4.50	0	0.45	—	0.25	7.00	0.40	—	0	1.8	—
0	0	1.36	—	75.8	174.2	0.46	0	0.23	—	0.08	3.03	0.23	0	0	2.3	—
0	60	1.44	34.2	250.0	350.0	0.67	0	9.11	—	0.20	1.21	0.11	32.8	0	0	—
0	0	1.80	—	85.0	390.0	0.88	0	0.22	—	0.14	2.00	0.11	3.8	0	1.2	—
0	40	3.60	—	330.0	1130.0	1.84	0	0.30	—	0.14	2.00	0.70	—	0	1.5	—
0	0	1.08	—	100.0	220.0	0.38	0	0.06	—	0.10	4.00	0.08	—	0	0.2	—
0	20	1.80	—	120.1	580.3	0.77	0	1.80	—	0.26	6.00	0.60	—	0	1.5	—
0	60	1.80	—	120.0	320.0	0.77	0	1.80	—	0.17	3.00	0.60	—	0	1.2	—
0	20	0.72	—	40.0	430.0	0.32	0	0.22	—	0.14	0.80	0.20	—	0	0.9	—
0	100	1.08	—	240.0	240.0	—	0	0.38	—	0.14	4.00	0.30	—	0	1.8	—
0	0	1.87	—	134.7	466.4	0.46	0	1.87	—	0.18	5.18	0.31	—	0	1.9	—
0	0	1.44	—	50.0	320.0	0.45	0	1.80	—	0.17	2.00	0.30	—	0	3.0	—
0	40	1.08	—	130.0	480.0	0.85	0	1.20	—	0.14	3.00	0.30	—	0	1.5	—
0	0	0.36	—	15.0	220.0	0.10	0	0.75	—	0.03	0.40	0.08	—	0	0.2	—
0	0	0.36	—	10.0	390.2	0.85	0	—	—	—	—	—	—	0	0	—
21	150	0.09	6.5	72.6	395.5	0.75	56.1	0.01	0.07	0.11	0.29	0.05	10.2	0	0.3	4.1
27	191	0.12	6.8	38.6	158.8	0.74	82.8	0	0.07	0.10	0.03	0.02	5.7	0	0.4	4.1
28	52	0.14	5.7	43.1	178.3	0.67	49.3	0.02	0.07	0.15	0.11	0.07	18.4	0	0.5	4.1
20	110	0.09	5.7	53.0	238.7	0.67	68.3	0.01	0.06	0.14	0.18	0.06	17.6	0	0.4	4.1
27	194	0.22	7.4	36.0	171.2	0.87	74.8	0	0.08	0.11	0.03	0.02	5.1	0	0.2	4.1
6	118	0.12	4.5	18.7	173.5	0.52	17.0	0	0.02	0.06	0.01	0.01	3.1	0	0.1	4.1
28	199	0.20	7.7	31.8	6.0	0.88	74.8	0.01	0.08	0.11	0.02	0.02	5.1	0	0.2	4.1
30	204	0.19	7.9	27.7	175.4	0.88	74.9	0.01	0.08	0.11	0.02	0.02	5.1	0	0.2	3.9
25	207	0.12	8.5	53.3	273.6	1.06	68.9	0.01	0.07	0.11	0.02	0.02	4.5	0	0.4	4.1
25	140	0.18	5.4	17.6	316.4	0.82	35.4	0.04	0.05	0.24	0.28	0.12	9.1	0	0.5	4.3
33	156	0.07	4.0	18.1	226.8	0.99	74.0	0.01	0.08	0.06	0.04	0.02	1.7	0	0.5	4.1
13	40	0.54	4.5	7.4	104.3	0.26	81.6	0.02	0.05	0.11	0.12	0.07	3.4	0	0.1	0.8

TABLE A-2 **Table of Food Composition** *(continued)*   (Computer code is for Cengage Diet Analysis program)   (For purposes of calculations, use "0" for t, <1, <0.1, <0.01)

DA+ Code	Food Description	Quantity	Measure	Wt (g)	H₂O (g)	Ener (kcal)	Prot (g)	Carb (g)	Fiber (g)	Fat (g)	Fat Breakdown (g) Sat	Mono	Poly
Dairy—*continued*													
893	Gouda	1	ounce(s)	28	11.8	101	7.1	0.6	0	7.8	5.0	2.2	0.2
894	Gruyere	1	ounce(s)	28	9.4	117	8.5	0.1	0	9.2	5.4	2.8	0.5
895	Limburger	1	ounce(s)	28	13.7	93	5.7	0.1	0	7.7	4.7	2.4	0.1
896	Monterey jack	1	ounce(s)	28	11.6	106	6.9	0.2	0	8.6	5.4	2.5	0.3
42324	Mozarella, low-sodium	1	ounce(s)	28	14.1	79	7.8	0.9	0	4.8	3.1	1.4	0.1
13	Mozzarella, part skim milk	1	ounce(s)	28	15.2	72	6.9	0.8	0	4.5	2.9	1.3	0.1
12	Mozzarella, whole milk	1	ounce(s)	28	14.2	85	6.3	0.6	0	6.3	3.7	1.9	0.2
897	Muenster	1	ounce(s)	28	11.8	104	6.6	0.3	0	8.5	5.4	2.5	0.2
898	Neufchatel	1	ounce(s)	28	17.9	72	2.6	1.0	0	6.5	3.6	1.6	0.3
14	Parmesan, grated	1	tablespoon(s)	5	1.0	22	1.9	0.2	0	1.4	0.9	0.4	0.1
17	Provolone	1	ounce(s)	28	11.6	100	7.3	0.6	0	7.5	4.8	2.1	0.2
19	Ricotta, part skim milk	¼	cup(s)	62	45.8	85	7.0	3.2	0	4.9	3.0	1.4	0.2
18	Ricotta, whole milk	¼	cup(s)	62	44.1	107	6.9	1.9	0	8.0	5.1	2.2	0.2
20	Romano	1	tablespoon(s)	5	1.5	19	1.6	0.2	0	1.3	0.9	0.4	0
900	Roquefort	1	ounce(s)	28	11.2	105	6.1	0.6	0	8.7	5.5	2.4	0.4
21	Swiss	1	ounce(s)	28	10.5	108	7.6	1.5	0	7.9	5.0	2.1	0.3
53952	Swiss, low-sodium	1	ounce(s)	28	10.7	106	8.1	1.0	0	7.8	5.0	2.1	0.3
	Imitation cheese												
42245	Imitation American cheddar	1	ounce(s)	28	15.1	68	4.7	3.3	0	4.0	2.5	1.2	0.1
53914	Imitation cheddar	1	ounce(s)	28	15.1	68	4.7	3.3	0	4.0	2.5	1.2	0.1
	Cottage cheese												
9	Low fat, 1% fat	½	cup(s)	113	93.2	81	14.0	3.1	0	1.2	0.7	0.3	0
42265	Low fat, 1% fat, no sodium added	½	cup(s)	113	94.4	81	14.0	3.1	0	1.1	0.7	0.3	0
8	Low fat, 2% fat	½	cup(s)	113	91.2	97	13.4	4.1	0	2.8	1.1	0.5	0.1
	Cream cheese												
11	Cream cheese	2	tablespoon(s)	29	15.8	99	1.7	1.2	0	9.9	5.6	2.5	0.4
17366	Cream cheese, fat-free	2	tablespoon(s)	30	21.6	32	4.7	2.3	0	0.3	0.2	0.1	0
10438	Tofutti Better than Cream Cheese	2	tablespoon(s)	30	—	85	1.0	9.0	0	5.0	2.0	—	—
	Processed cheese												
24	American cheese food, processed	1	ounce(s)	28	12.5	94	4.8	2.4	0	7.3	4.3	1.9	0.3
25	American cheese spread, processed	1	ounce(s)	28	13.5	82	4.7	2.5	0	6.0	3.8	1.8	0.2
22	American cheese, processed	1	ounce(s)	28	11.2	104	5.1	1.4	0	8.7	5.1	2.3	0.4
42285	Cheddar or American, pasteurized process, low-sodium	1	ounce(s)	28	12.1	107	6.3	0.5	0	8.8	5.6	2.5	0.3
9110	Kraft Deluxe Singles pasteurized process American cheese	1	ounce(s)	28	—	108	5.4				9.5	5.4	—	—
23	Swiss cheese, processed	1	ounce(s)	28	12.0	95	7.0	0.6	0	7.1	4.5	2.0	0.2
	Soy cheese												
65625	Galaxy Foods vegan American cheese slices alternative	1	slice(s)	19	—	40	1.0	5.0	0	2.0	0	0.5	1.5
10437	Galaxy Foods vegan grated parmesan cheese alternative	1	tablespoon(s)	8	—	23	3.0	1.5	0	0	0	0	0
	Cream												
26	Half and half cream	1	tablespoon(s)	15	12.2	20	0.4	0.7	0	1.7	1.1	0.5	0.1
32	Heavy whipping cream, liquid	1	tablespoon(s)	15	8.7	52	0.3	0.4	0	5.6	3.5	1.6	0.2
28	Light coffee or table cream, liquid	1	tablespoon(s)	15	11.1	29	0.4	0.5	0	2.9	1.8	0.8	0.1
30	Light whipping cream, liquid	1	tablespoon(s)	15	9.5	44	0.3	0.4	0	4.6	2.9	1.4	0.1
34	Whipped cream topping, pressurized	1	tablespoon(s)	3	1.8	8	0.1	0.4	0	0.7	0.4	0.2	0
	Sour cream												
36	Sour cream	2	tablespoon(s)	24	17.9	46	0.5	0.7	0	4.7	2.8	1.2	0.1
30556	Sour cream, fat free	2	tablespoon(s)	32	25.8	24	1.0	5.0	0	0	0	0	0
	Imitation cream												
3659	Coffeemate nondairy creamer, liquid	1	tablespoon(s)	15	—	20	0	2.0	0	1.0	0	0	0
40	Cream substitute, powder	1	teaspoon(s)	2	0	11	0.1	1.1	0	0.7	0.7	0	0
904	Imitation sour cream	2	tablespoon(s)	29	20.5	60	0.7	1.9	0	5.6	5.1	0.2	0
35972	Nondairy coffee whitener, liquid, frozen	1	tablespoon(s)	15	11.5	20	0.1	1.7	0	1.5	0.3	1.1	0

Chol (mg)	Calc (mg)	Iron (mg)	Magn (mg)	Pota (mg)	Sodi (mg)	Zinc (mg)	Vit A (µg)	Thia (mg)	Vit E (mg α)	Ribo (mg)	Niac (mg)	Vit B$_6$ (mg)	Fola (µg)	Vit C (mg)	Vit B$_{12}$ (µg)	Sele (µg)
32	198	0.07	8.2	34.3	232.2	1.11	46.8	0.01	0.07	0.09	0.02	0.02	6.0	0	0.4	4.1
31	287	0.05	10.2	23.0	95.3	1.11	76.8	0.02	0.08	0.08	0.03	0.02	2.8	0	0.5	4.1
26	141	0.04	6.0	36.3	226.8	0.60	96.4	0.02	0.07	0.14	0.04	0.02	16.4	0	0.3	4.1
25	211	0.20	7.7	23.0	152.0	0.85	56.1	0	0.07	0.11	0.03	0.02	5.1	0	0.2	4.1
15	207	0.07	7.4	26.9	4.5	0.89	38.8	0.01	0.04	0.10	0.03	0.02	2.6	0	0.3	4.5
18	222	0.06	6.5	23.8	175.5	0.78	36.0	0.01	0.04	0.09	0.03	0.02	2.6	0	0.2	4.1
22	143	0.12	5.7	21.5	177.8	0.83	50.7	0.01	0.05	0.08	0.03	0.01	2.0	0	0.6	4.8
27	203	0.12	7.7	38.0	178.0	0.80	84.5	0	0.07	0.09	0.03	0.02	3.4	0	0.4	4.1
21	33	0.04	2.8	43.1	94.7	0.23	68.3	0.01	0.11	0.04	0.06	0.01	4.0	0	0.1	0.9
4	55	0.05	1.9	6.3	76.4	0.19	11.4	0	0.01	0.02	0.01	0	0.5	0	0.1	0.9
20	214	0.15	7.9	39.1	248.3	0.92	66.9	0.01	0.07	0.09	0.04	0.02	2.8	0	0.4	4.1
19	167	0.27	9.2	76.9	76.9	0.82	65.8	0.01	0.04	0.11	0.05	0.01	8.0	0	0.2	10.3
31	127	0.23	6.8	64.6	51.7	0.71	73.8	0.01	0.07	0.12	0.06	0.03	7.4	0	0.2	8.9
5	53	0.04	2.0	4.3	60.0	0.13	4.8	0	0.01	0.02	0	0	0.3	0	0.1	0.7
26	188	0.16	8.5	25.8	512.9	0.59	83.3	0.01	—	0.17	0.21	0.04	13.9	0	0.2	4.1
26	224	0.06	10.8	21.8	54.4	1.24	62.4	0.02	0.11	0.08	0.03	0.02	1.7	0	0.9	5.2
26	272	0.05	10.2	31.5	4.0	1.11	61.2	0.01	0.10	0.10	0.03	0.02	1.7	0	0.5	3.5
10	159	0.09	8.2	68.6	381.3	0.73	32.3	0.01	0.08	0.12	0.04	0.03	2.0	0	0.1	4.3
10	159	0.09	8.2	68.6	381.3	0.73	32.3	0.01	0.08	0.12	0.04	0.03	2.0	0	0.1	4.3
5	69	0.16	5.7	97.2	458.8	0.43	12.4	0.02	0.01	0.19	0.14	0.08	13.6	0	0.7	10.2
5	69	0.16	5.7	97.2	14.7	0.43	12.4	0.02	0.01	0.18	0.15	0.08	13.6	0	0.7	9.5
11	103	0.17	7.9	94.9	372.9	0.46	22.6	0.05	0.05	0.22	0.12	0.02	11.3	0	0.5	11.2
32	28	0.11	2.6	40.0	93.1	0.15	106.1	0.01	0.08	0.04	0.04	0.01	3.2	0	0.1	0.7
4	105	0.06	6.6	83.4	210.6	0.45	3.3	0.01	0.01	0.08	0.07	0.01	10.5	0	0.3	1.5
0	0	0	—	—	160.0	—	—	—	—	—	—	—	—	0	—	—
28	193	0.07	7.7	72.3	364.0	0.65	57.0	0.01	0.18	0.10	0.04	0.03	2.0	0	0.4	5.6
16	159	0.09	8.2	68.6	460.7	0.73	49.0	0.01	0.05	0.12	0.04	0.03	2.0	0	0.1	3.2
28	296	0.18	7.4	37.4	473.7	0.71	89.9	0	0.23	0.07	0.02	0.01	2.3	0	0.4	5.7
27	175	0.11	6.2	45.9	2.0	0.85	72.0	0.01	0.08	0.10	0.02	0.02	2.3	0	0.2	3.6
27	338	0	—	33.8	459.0	—	—	—	—	—	—	—	—	0	—	—
24	219	0.17	8.2	61.2	388.4	1.02	56.1	0	0.10	0.08	0.01	0.01	1.7	0	0.3	4.5
0	200	0	—	—	120.0	—	0	—	—	—	—	—	—	0	—	—
0	60	0	—	75.0	97.5	—	15.0	—	—	—	—	—	—	0	—	—
6	16	0.01	1.5	19.7	6.2	0.08	14.7	0.01	0.05	0.02	0.01	0.01	0.5	0.1	0	0.3
21	10	0	1.0	11.3	5.7	0.03	61.7	0	0.16	0.02	0.01	0	0.6	0.1	0	0.1
10	14	0.01	1.4	18.3	6.0	0.04	27.1	0	0.08	0.02	0.01	0	0.3	0.1	0	0.1
17	10	0	1.0	14.6	5.1	0.04	41.8	0	0.13	0.02	0.01	0	0.6	0.1	0	0.1
2	3	0	0.3	4.4	0.2	0.01	5.6	0	0.02	0	0	0	0.1	0	0	0
12	26	0.04	2.4	33.8	19.2	0.09	42.2	0.01	0.11	0.04	0.03	0.01	1.7	0.2	0.1	0.6
3	40	0	3.2	41.3	45.1	0.16	23.4	0.01	0	0.05	0.02	0.01	3.5	0	0.1	1.7
0	0	0	—	—	0	—	0	—	—	—	—	—	—	0	—	—
0	0	0.02	0.1	16.2	3.6	0.01	0	0	0.01	0	0	0	0	0	0	0
0	1	0.11	1.7	46.3	29.3	0.34	0	0	0.21	0	0	0	0	0	0	0.7
0	1	0	0	28.5	11.8	0.0	0.1	0	0.12	0	0	0	0	0	0	0.2

TABLE A-2 **Table of Food Composition** (continued)   (Computer code is for Cengage Diet Analysis program)   (For purposes of calculations, use "0" for t, <1, <0.1, <0.01)

DA+ Code	Food Description	Quantity	Measure	Wt (g)	H₂O (g)	Ener (kcal)	Prot (g)	Carb (g)	Fiber (g)	Fat (g)	Fat Breakdown (g) Sat	Mono	Poly
Dairy—continued													
35976	Nondairy dessert topping, frozen	1	tablespoon(s)	5	2.4	15	0.1	1.1	0	1.2	1.0	0.1	0
35975	Nondairy dessert topping, pressurized	1	tablespoon(s)	4	2.6	12	0	0.7	0	1.0	0.8	0.1	0
	Fluid milk												
60	Buttermilk, low-fat	1	cup(s)	245	220.8	98	8.1	11.7	0	2.2	1.3	0.6	0.1
54	Low-fat, 1%	1	cup(s)	244	219.4	102	8.2	12.2	0	2.4	1.5	0.7	0.1
55	Low-fat, 1%, with nonfat milk solids	1	cup(s)	245	220.0	105	8.5	12.2	0	2.4	1.5	0.7	0.1
57	Nonfat, skim or fat-free	1	cup(s)	245	222.6	83	8.3	12.2	0	0.2	0.1	0.1	0
58	Nonfat, skim or fat-free with nonfat milk solids	1	cup(s)	245	221.4	91	8.7	12.3	0	0.6	0.4	0.2	0
51	Reduced fat, 2%	1	cup(s)	244	217.7	122	8.1	11.7	0	4.8	3.1	1.4	0.2
52	Reduced fat, 2%, with nonfat milk solids	1	cup(s)	245	217.7	125	8.5	12.2	0	4.7	2.9	1.4	0.2
50	Whole, 3.3%	1	cup(s)	244	215.0	149	7.7	11.7	0	7.9	4.6	2.0	0.5
	Canned milk												
62	Nonfat or skim evaporated	2	tablespoon(s)	32	25.3	25	2.4	3.6	0	0.1	0	0	0
63	Sweetened condensed	2	tablespoon(s)	38	10.4	123	3.0	20.8	0	3.3	2.1	0.9	0.1
61	Whole evaporated	2	tablespoon(s)	32	23.3	42	2.1	3.2	0	2.4	1.4	0.7	0.1
	Dried milk												
64	Buttermilk	¼	cup(s)	30	0.9	117	10.4	14.9	0	1.8	1.1	0.5	0.1
65	Instant nonfat with added vitamin A	¼	cup(s)	17	0.7	61	6.0	8.9	0	0.1	0.1	0	0
5234	Skim milk powder	¼	cup(s)	17	0.7	61	6.0	8.9	0	0.1	0.1	0	0
907	Whole	¼	cup(s)	32	0.8	159	8.4	12.3	0	8.5	5.4	2.5	0.2
909	**Goat milk**	1	cup(s)	244	212.4	168	8.7	10.9	0	10.1	6.5	2.7	0.4
	Chocolate milk												
33155	Chocolate syrup, prepared with milk	1	cup(s)	282	227.0	254	8.7	36.0	0.8	8.3	4.7	2.1	0.5
33184	Cocoa mix with aspartame, added sodium and vitamin A, no added calcium or phosphorus, prepared with water	1	cup(s)	192	177.4	56	2.3	10.8	1.2	0.4	0.3	0.1	0
908	Hot cocoa, prepared with milk	1	cup(s)	250	206.1	193	8.8	26.9	2.5	5.8	3.6	1.7	0.2
69	Low-fat	1	cup(s)	250	205.9	178	8.1	31.5	1.3	2.5	1.5	0.8	0.1
68	Reduced fat	1	cup(s)	250	205.4	190	7.5	30.3	1.8	4.8	2.9	1.1	0.2
67	Whole	1	cup(s)	250	205.8	208	7.9	25.9	2.0	8.5	5.3	2.5	0.3
70	**Eggnog**	1	cup(s)	254	209.7	224	11.6	20.4	0	10.6	6.6	3.3	0.5
	Breakfast drinks												
10089	Carnation Breakfast Essentials classic chocolate malt, prepared with skim milk	1	cup(s)	273	—	220	12.5	39.0	0.8	1.0	0.8	—	—
10092	Carnation Breakfast Essentials classic French vanilla, prepared with skim milk, no sugar added	1	cup(s)	257	—	150	12.9	24.0	3.0	0.6	0.2	—	—
57630	Carnation Breakfast Essentials milk chocolate, ready to drink, no sugar added	1	cup(s)	237	—	109	9.5	11.6	1.5	3.6	1.1	—	—
10091	Carnation Breakfast Essentials Strawberry Sensation, prepared with skim milk	1	cup(s)	273	—	220	12.5	39.0	0	0.6	0.4	—	—
1417	Ovaltine rich chocolate flavor, prepared with skim milk	1	cup(s)	258	—	170	8.5	31.0	0	0	0	0	0
8539	**Malted milk, chocolate mix, fortified, prepared with milk**	1	cup(s)	265	215.3	231	8.7	29.7	1.1	8.6	5.0	2.2	0.5
	Milkshakes												
73	Chocolate	1	cup(s)	227	164.0	270	6.9	48.1	0.7	6.1	3.8	1.8	0.2
3163	Strawberry	1	cup(s)	226	167.8	256	7.7	42.8	0.9	6.3	3.9	—	—
74	Vanilla	1	cup(s)	227	169.2	254	8.8	40.3	0	6.9	4.3	2.0	0.3
	Ice cream												
4776	Chocolate	½	cup(s)	66	36.8	143	2.5	18.6	0.8	7.3	4.5	2.1	0.3
12137	Chocolate fudge, no sugar added	½	cup(s)	71	—	100	3.0	16.0	2.0	3.0	1.5	—	—
16514	Chocolate, soft serve	½	cup(s)	87	51.7	192	3.5	19.2	0.6	11.2	6.5	3.0	0.4

PAGE KEY: A-6 5 Breads/Baked Goods A-12 = Cereal/Rice/Pasta A-16 = Fruit A-22 = Vegetables/Legumes A-32 = Nuts/Seeds A-34 = Vegetarian A-36 = Dairy A-44 = Eggs A-44 = Seafood A-46 = Meats A-50 = Poultry
A-52 = Processed Meats A-54 = Beverages A-58 = Fats/Oils A-60 = Sweets A-62 = Spices/Condiments/Sauces A-66 = Mixed Foods/Soups/Sandwiches A-72 = Fast Food A-90 = Convenience A-92 = Baby Foods

Chol (mg)	Calc (mg)	Iron (mg)	Magn (mg)	Pota (mg)	Sodi (mg)	Zinc (mg)	Vit A (µg)	Thia (mg)	Vit E (mg α)	Ribo (mg)	Niac (mg)	Vit B_6 (mg)	Fola (µg)	Vit C (mg)	Vit B_{12} (µg)	Sele (µg)
0	0	0.01	0.1	0.8	1.2	0.0	0.3	0	0.05	0	0	0	0	0	0	0.1
0	0	0	0	0.8	2.7	0.0	0.2	0	0.04	0	0	0	0	0	0	0.1
10	284	0.12	27.0	370.0	257.3	1.03	34.3	0.08	0.12	0.38	0.14	0.08	12.3	2.5	0.5	4.9
12	305	0.07	26.8	366.0	107.4	1.02	141.5	0.05	0.02	0.45	0.23	0.09	12.2	0	1.1	8.1
10	314	0.12	34.3	396.9	127.4	0.98	144.6	0.10		0.42	0.22	0.11	12.3	2.5	0.9	5.6
5	299	0.07	27.0	382.2	102.9	1.03	149.4	0.11	0.02	0.45	0.23	0.09	12.3	0	1.2	7.6
5	316	0.12	36.8	419.0	129.9	1.00	156.8	0.10	0.02	0.43	0.22	0.11	12.3	2.5	1.0	5.4
20	293	0.05	26.8	341.6	114.7	1.17	134.2	0.10	0.07	0.45	0.22	0.09	12.2	0.5	1.3	6.1
20	314	0.12	34.3	396.9	127.4	0.98	137.2	0.10	—	0.42	0.22	0.11	12.3	2.5	0.9	5.6
24	276	0.07	24.4	322.1	104.9	0.90	112.2	0.11	0.17	0.41	0.22	0.09	12.2	0	1.1	9.0
1	93	0.09	8.6	105.9	36.7	0.29	37.6	0.01	0	0.10	0.06	0.02	2.9	0.4	0.1	0.8
13	109	0.07	9.9	141.9	48.6	0.36	28.3	0.03	0.06	0.16	0.08	0.02	4.2	1.0	0.2	5.7
9	82	0.06	7.6	95.4	33.4	0.24	20.5	0.01	0.04	0.10	0.06	0.02	2.5	0.6	0.1	0.7
21	359	0.09	33.3	482.5	156.7	1.22	14.9	0.12	0.03	0.48	0.27	0.10	14.2	1.7	1.2	6.2
3	209	0.05	19.9	289.9	93.3	0.75	120.5	0.07	0	0.30	0.15	0.06	8.5	1.0	0.7	4.6
3	211	0.05	20.0	291.9	94.0	0.75	114.5	0.07	0	0.30	0.15	0.06	8.6	1.0	0.7	4.7
31	292	0.15	27.2	425.6	118.7	1.07	82.6	0.09	0.19	0.39	0.21	0.10	11.8	2.8	1.0	5.2
27	327	0.12	34.2	497.8	122.0	0.73	139.1	0.12	0.17	0.34	0.68	0.11	2.4	3.2	0.2	3.4
25	251	0.90	50.8	408.9	132.5	1.21	70.5	0.11	0.14	0.47	0.39	0.09	14.1	0	1.1	9.6
0	92	0.75	32.6	405.1	138.2	0.52	0	0.04	0	0.21	0.16	0.05	1.9	0	0.2	2.5
20	285	1.05	57.5	492.5	110.0	1.58	127.5	0.10	0.08	0.46	0.33	0.10	12.5	0.5	1.2	6.8
8	290	0.68	32.5	425.0	152.5	1.02	145.0	0.09	0.05	0.41	0.32	0.10	12.5	2.3	0.8	4.8
20	273	0.60	35.0	422.5	165.0	0.98	160.0	0.11	0.10	0.46	0.41	0.06	5.0	0	0.8	8.5
30	280	0.60	32.5	417.5	150.0	1.02	67.5	0.09	0.17	0.41	0.31	0.10	12.5	2.3	0.8	4.8
150	330	0.51	48.3	419.1	137.2	1.17	149.9	0.09	0.53	0.48	0.27	0.13	2.5	3.8	1.1	10.7
6	500	4.47	100.0	665.0	240.0	3.75	675.7	0.38	3.38	0.51	5.07	0.50	—	30.0	1.5	—
9	500	4.50	100.0	595.0	168.0	3.75	675.7	0.38	3.38	0.51	5.00	0.50	—	30.0	1.5	—
7	364	3.28	87.4	393.1	174.7	2.73	491.9	0.27	2.46	0.31	3.64	0.36	—	21.8	1.1	—
9	500	4.47	100.0	665.0	288.0	3.75	675.7	0.38	3.38	0.51	5.07	0.50	—	30.0	1.5	8.8
5	350	3.60	100.0	—	240.0	3.75	—	0.38	—	0.43	4.00	0.40	—	12.0	1.2	—
27	368	3.76	45.0	575.0	230.6	1.14	946.0	0.76	0.19	1.28	11.03	1.01	13.3	31.8	1.1	9.5
25	300	0.70	36.4	508.9	252.2	1.09	40.9	0.11	0.11	0.50	0.28	0.06	11.4	0	0.7	4.3
25	256	0.25	29.4	412.0	187.9	0.82	58.9	0.10	—	0.44	0.40	0.10	6.8	1.8	0.7	4.8
27	332	0.23	27.3	415.8	215.8	0.89	56.8	0.07	0.11	0.44	0.33	0.10	15.9	0	1.2	5.2
22	72	0.61	19.1	164.3	50.2	0.38	77.9	0.03	0.20	0.13	0.15	0.04	10.6	0.5	0.2	1.6
10	100	0.36	—	—	65.0	—	—	—	—	—	—	—	—	0	—	—
79	113	0.18	10.4	153.1	52.8	0.45	140.1	0.04	0.53	0.16	0.08	0.04	7.8	0.7	0.4	2.6

TABLE A-2 Table of Food Composition *(continued)*   (Computer code is for Cengage Diet Analysis program)   (For purposes of calculations, use "0" for t, <1, <0.1, <0.01)

DA+ Code	Food Description	Quantity	Measure	Wt (g)	H₂O (g)	Ener (kcal)	Prot (g)	Carb (g)	Fiber (g)	Fat (g)	Fat Breakdown (g) Sat	Mono	Poly
Dairy—*continued*													
16523	Sherbet, all flavors	½	cup(s)	97	63.8	139	1.1	29.3	1.3	1.9	1.1	0.5	0.1
4778	Strawberry	½	cup(s)	66	39.6	127	2.1	18.2	0.6	5.5	3.4	—	—
76	Vanilla	½	cup(s)	72	43.9	149	2.5	17.0	0.5	7.9	4.9	2.1	0.3
12146	Vanilla chocolate swirl, fat-free, no sugar added	½	cup(s)	71	—	100	3.0	14.0	2.0	3.0	2.0	—	—
82	Vanilla, light	½	cup(s)	76	45.5	137	3.6	22.4	0.2	3.7	2.2	1.0	0.2
78	Vanilla, light, soft serve	½	cup(s)	88	61.2	111	4.3	19.2	0	2.3	1.4	0.7	0.1
	Soy desserts												
15726	Tofutti premium Better Pecan nondairy frozen dessert	½	cup(s)	70	—	210	1.0	21.0	0	13.0	2.0	—	—
15721	Tofutti premium Chocolate Supreme nondairy frozen dessert	½	cup(s)	70	—	180	3.0	18.0	0	11.0	2.0	—	—
15720	Tofutti premium vanilla non-dairy frozen dessert	½	cup(s)	70	—	210	2.0	21.0	0	13.0	2.0	—	—
	Ice milk												
16517	Chocolate	½	cup(s)	74	45.5	138	3.7	19.0	0.6	5.3	3.2	1.5	0.2
16516	Flavored, not chocolate	½	cup(s)	74	44.3	133	3.5	21.8	0.2	3.6	2.2	0.9	0.2
	Pudding												
25032	Chocolate	½	cup(s)	144	109.8	153	5.2	22.7	0.8	5.3	3.1	2.2	0.3
1923	Chocolate, sugar-free, prepared with 2% milk	½	cup(s)	133	—	100	5.0	14.0	0.3	3.0	1.5	—	—
1722	Rice	½	cup(s)	113	75.5	151	4.1	30.0	0.4	1.9	1.1	0.5	0.1
4747	Tapioca, ready to eat	1	item(s)	142	102.0	185	2.8	30.8	0	5.5	1.4	3.6	0.1
25031	Vanilla	½	cup(s)	136	109.7	116	4.6	17.6	0	2.9	1.7	1.5	0.3
1924	Vanilla, sugar-free, prepared with 2% milk	½	cup(s)	133	—	90	4.0	12.0	0.2	2.0	1.5	—	—
	Frozen yogurt												
4785	Chocolate, soft serve	½	cup(s)	72	45.9	115	2.9	17.9	1.6	4.3	2.6	1.3	0.2
29649	Flavors other than chocolate, nonfat	½	cup(s)	80	52.1	103	3.5	22.2	5.9	0	0	0	0
4786	Vanilla, soft serve	½	cup(s)	72	47.0	114	2.9	17.4	0	4.0	2.5	1.1	0.2
	Milk substitutes												
	Lactose-free												
16081	Fat-free, calcium fortified milk	1	cup(s)	240	—	90	8.0	13.0	0	0	0	0	0
36486	Low-fat milk	1	cup(s)	240	—	110	8.0	13.0	0	2.5	1.5	—	—
36487	Reduced fat milk	1	cup(s)	240	—	130	8.0	13.0	0	5.0	3.0	—	—
36488	Whole milk	1	cup(s)	240	—	160	8.0	13.0	0	8.0	5.0	—	—
	Rice												
10083	Rice Dream carob rice beverage	1	cup(s)	240	—	150	1.0	30.0	0.5	2.5	0	1.5	0.5
17089	Rice Dream original rice beverage, enriched	1	cup(s)	240	—	120	1.0	23.0	0	2.5	0	1.5	0.5
10087	Rice Dream vanilla enriched rice beverage	1	cup(s)	240	—	130	1.0	26.0	0	2.5	0	1.5	0.5
	Soy												
66705	Silk chocolate soymilk	1	cup(s)	243	209.9	140	5.0	23.0	2.0	3.0	0.5	1.0	1.5
66710	Silk DHA omega-3 enriched soymilk	1	cup(s)	243	221.4	110	7.0	8.0	1.0	5.0	0.5	1.0	3.0
66703	Silk soymilk, unsweetened	1	cup(s)	243	226.4	80	7.0	4.0	1.0	4.0	0.5	1.0	2.5
66704	Silk vanilla soymilk	1	cup(s)	243	221.9	100	6.0	10.0	1.0	3.5	0.5	1.0	2.0
34750	Soy Dream chocolate enriched soy beverage	1	cup(s)	240	205.5	150	7.0	21.0	3.0	4.0	0.5	1.0	2.5
34749	Soy Dream vanilla enriched soy beverage	1	cup(s)	240	213.5	120	7.0	14.0	2.0	4.0	0.5	1.0	2.5
	Yogurt												
3615	Custard style, fruit flavors	6	ounce(s)	170	—	180	7.0	31.0	0	2.5	1.5	—	—
3617	Custard style, vanilla	6	ounce(s)	170	—	180	7.0	31.0	0	2.5	1.5	—	—
32101	Fruit, low-fat	1	cup(s)	245	184.5	243	9.8	45.7	0	2.8	1.8	0.8	0.1
29638	Fruit, nonfat, sweetened with low calorie sweetener	1	cup(s)	241	210.3	108	9.0	19.0	1.0	0.4	0.2	0.1	0
68613	Greek style, vanilla	1	cup(s)	245	—	173	23.0	18.7	0	0	0	0	0
93	Plain, low-fat	1	cup(s)	245	208.4	154	12.9	17.2	0	3.8	2.5	1.0	0.1
94	Plain, nonfat	1	cup(s)	245	208.8	137	14.0	18.8	0	0.4	0.3	0.1	0

PAGE KEY: A-6 5 Breads/Baked Goods A-12 = Cereal/Rice/Pasta A-16 = Fruit A-22 = Vegetables/Legumes A-32 = Nuts/Seeds A-34 = Vegetarian A-36 = Dairy A-44 = Eggs A-44 = Seafood A-46 = Meats A-50 = Poultry
A-52 = Processed Meats A-54 = Beverages A-58 = Fats/Oils A-60 = Sweets A-62 = Spices/Condiments/Sauces A-66 = Mixed Foods/Soups/Sandwiches A-72 = Fast Food A-90 = Convenience A-92 = Baby Foods

Chol (mg)	Calc (mg)	Iron (mg)	Magn (mg)	Pota (mg)	Sodi (mg)	Zinc (mg)	Vit A (µg)	Thia (mg)	Vit E (mg α)	Ribo (mg)	Niac (mg)	Vit B$_6$ (mg)	Fola (µg)	Vit C (mg)	Vit B$_{12}$ (µg)	Sele (µg)
1	52	0.14	7.7	92.6	44.4	0.46	11.6	0.03	0.01	0.09	0.06	0.02	3.9	2.2	0.1	1.4
19	79	0.14	9.2	124.1	39.6	0.22	63.4	0.03	—	0.17	0.11	0.03	7.9	5.1	0.2	1.3
32	92	0.06	10.1	143.3	57.6	0.50	85.0	0.03	0.22	0.17	0.08	0.03	3.6	0.4	0.3	1.3
10	100	0	—	—	65.0	—	—	—	—	—	—	—	—	0	—	—
21	122	0.14	10.6	158.1	56.2	0.55	97.3	0.04	0.09	0.19	0.10	0.03	4.6	0.9	0.4	1.5
11	138	0.05	12.3	194.5	61.6	0.47	25.5	0.05	0.05	0.17	0.10	0.04	4.4	0.8	0.4	3.2
0	0	0	—	22.0	220.0	—	—	—	—	—	—	—	—	0	—	—
0	0	0	—	—	180.0	—	—	—	—	—	—	—	—	0	—	—
0	0	0	—	—	130.0	—	—	—	—	—	—	—	—	0	—	—
21	118	0.51	14.8	125.8	52.5	0.32	52.5	0.02	0.15	0.09	0.09	0.02	3.0	0.9	0.1	1.6
20	119	0.14	10.4	153.9	54.8	0.54	94.7	0.04	0.09	0.19	0.10	0.03	4.4	0.9	0.3	1.5
35	149	0.95	28.6	211.0	134.8	1.07	0	0.06	0.11	0.25	0.18	0.05	9.9	0.2	0.7	5.4
10	150	0.72	—	330.0	310.0	—	—	0.06	—	0.26	—	—	—	0	—	—
7	115	0.27	15.8	194.6	72.0	0.58	24.8	0.04	0.05	0.18	0.34	0.06	4.5	0.2	0.3	4.3
1	101	0.16	8.5	130.6	205.9	0.31	0	0.03	0.21	0.14	0.09	0.03	4.3	0.4	0.3	0
35	144	0.16	13.8	173.2	133.7	0.63	0	0.05	0.09	0.24	0.11	0.05	8.7	0.2	0.7	5.0
10	150	0	—	190.0	380.0	—	—	0.03	—	0.17	—	—	—	0	—	—
4	106	0.90	19.4	187.9	70.6	0.35	31.7	0.03	—	0.15	0.22	0.05	7.9	0.2	0.2	1.7
0	117	0	7.2	155.8	87.4	0.25	105.7	0.02	0	0.10	0.06	0.02	3.2	0	0.4	1.5
1	103	0.22	10.1	151.9	62.6	0.30	42.5	0.03	0.08	0.16	0.21	0.06	4.3	0.6	0.2	2.4
3	500	0	—	410.0	125.0	—	150.1	—	—	0.43	—	—	—	0	0.9	—
15	300	0	—	410.0	125.0	—	150.1	—	—	0.43	—	—	—	0	0.9	—
20	300	0	—	410.0	125.0	—	150.1	—	—	0.43	—	—	—	0	0.9	—
35	300	0	—	410.0	125.0	—	90.1	—	—	0.43	—	—	—	0	0.9	—
0	0	0	—	0	80.0	—	0	—	0.80	—	—	—	—	0	—	—
0	300	0.72	—	0	100.0	—	25.0	—	—	—	—	—	—	0	1.5	—
0	300	0.36	—	0	105.0	—	25.0	—	—	—	—	—	—	0	1.5	—
0	300	1.44	40.0	350.0	100.0	0.60	25.0	—	—	0.51	—	—	—	0	3.0	4.2
0	350	1.08	40.0	350.0	120.0	1.50	50.0	—	—	0.51	—	0.60	—	21.0	3.0	5.6
0	300	1.08	40.0	300.0	85.0	0.60	25.0	—	—	0.51	—	—	—	0	3.0	5.6
0	300	1.08	40.0	300.0	95.0	0.60	25.0	—	—	0.51	—	—	—	0	3.0	5.6
0	400	1.80	60.0	290.0	125.0	0.75	25.0	0.15	5.03	0.63	1.20	0.20	—	0	3.0	11.2
0	350	8.10	60.0	250.0	135.0	0.62	25.0	0.15	5.03	0.44	1.02	0.20	21.6	0	3.0	5.5
15	300	0	—	290.0	110.0	—	—	—	—	—	—	—	—	0	—	—
15	300	0	—	290.0	110.0	—	—	—	—	—	—	—	—	0	—	—
12	338	0.15	31.9	433.6	129.9	1.64	27.0	0.08	0.05	0.40	0.21	0.09	22.0	1.5	1.1	6.9
5	323	0.58	33.7	470.0	127.7	1.57	4.8	0.09	0.14	0.38	0.42	0.10	26.5	21.9	1.0	6.7
0	288	0	—	—	108.0	—	—	—	—	—	—	—	—	0	—	—
15	448	0.20	41.7	573.3	171.5	2.18	34.3	0.11	0.07	0.52	0.28	0.12	27.0	2.0	1.4	8.1
5	488	0.22	46.5	624.8	188.6	2.38	4.9	0.12	0	0.57	0.30	0.13	29.4	2.2	1.5	8.8

TABLE A-2 **Table of Food Composition** *(continued)*   (Computer code is for Cengage Diet Analysis program)   (For purposes of calculations, use "0" for t, <1, <0.1, <0.01)

DA+ Code	Food Description	Quantity	Measure	Wt (g)	H₂O (g)	Ener (kcal)	Prot (g)	Carb (g)	Fiber (g)	Fat (g)	Sat	Mono	Poly
											\multicolumn{3} Fat Breakdown (g)		

DA+ Code	Food Description	Quantity	Measure	Wt (g)	H₂O (g)	Ener (kcal)	Prot (g)	Carb (g)	Fiber (g)	Fat (g)	Sat	Mono	Poly
Dairy—*continued*													
32100	Vanilla, low-fat	1	cup(s)	245	193.6	208	12.1	33.8	0	3.1	2.0	0.8	0.1
5242	Yogurt beverage	1	cup(s)	245	199.8	172	5.9	28.7	0	3.7	2.5	0.6	0.1
	Soy yogurt												
29767	Silk blueberry cultured soy yogurt	5.3	ounce(s)	150	117.5	132	3.5	25.6	0.9	1.8	0	0.4	0.9
34617	Stonyfield Farm O'Soy strawberry-peach pack organic cultured soy yogurt	1	item(s)	113	—	100	5.0	15.0	1.0	2.0	0	—	—
34616	Stonyfield Farm O'Soy vanilla organic cultured soy yogurt	1	item(s)	170	—	150	7.0	24.0	1.0	3.0	0	—	—
Eggs													
	Eggs												
99	Fried	1	item(s)	46	32.0	90	6.3	0.4	0	6.8	2.0	2.8	1.5
100	Hard boiled	1	item(s)	50	37.3	78	6.3	0.6	0	5.3	1.6	2.0	0.7
101	Poached	1	item(s)	50	37.9	72	6.3	0.4	0	4.7	1.6	1.8	1.0
97	Raw, white	1	item(s)	33	28.9	17	3.6	0.2	0	0.1	0	0	0
96	Raw, whole	1	item(s)	50	38.1	72	6.3	0.4	0	4.8	1.6	1.8	1.0
98	Raw, yolk	1	item(s)	17	8.9	55	2.7	0.6	0	4.5	1.6	2.0	0.7
102	Scrambled, prepared with milk and butter	2	item(s)	122	93.2	182	12.2	2.0	0	13.4	4.1	5.4	3.0
	Egg substitutes												
4028	Egg Beaters	¼	cup(s)	61	—	30	6.0	1.0	0	0	0	0	0
920	Frozen	¼	cup(s)	60	43.9	96	6.8	1.9	0	6.7	1.2	1.5	3.7
918	Liquid	¼	cup(s)	63	51.9	53	7.5	0.4	0	2.1	0.4	0.6	1.0
Seafood													
	Cod												
1573	Atlantic cod, cooked, dry heat	3	ounce(s)	85	64.6	89	19.4	0	0	0.7	0.1	0.1	0.2
6040	Atlantic cod or scrod, baked or broiled	3	ounce(s)	85	64.6	89	19.4	0	0	0.7	0.1	0.1	0.2
2905	**Eel, raw**	3	ounce(s)	85	58.0	156	15.7	0	0	9.9	2.0	6.1	0.8
	Fish fillets												
25079	Baked	3	ounce(s)	85	79.9	99	21.7	0	0	0.7	0.1	0.1	0.3
8615	Batter coated or breaded, fried	3	ounce(s)	85	45.6	197	12.5	14.4	0.4	10.5	2.4	2.2	5.3
25082	Broiled fish steaks	3	ounce(s)	85	68.1	128	24.2	0	0	2.6	0.4	0.9	0.8
25083	Poached fish steaks	3	ounce(s)	85	67.1	111	21.1	0	0	2.3	0.3	0.8	0.7
25084	Steamed	3	ounce(s)	85	72.2	79	17.2	0	0	0.6	0.1	0.1	0.2
25089	**Flounder, baked**	3	ounce(s)	85	64.4	113	14.8	0.4	0.1	5.5	1.1	2.2	1.4
1825	**Grouper, cooked, dry heat**	3	ounce(s)	85	62.4	100	21.1	0	0	1.1	0.3	0.2	0.3
	Haddock												
6049	Baked or broiled	3	ounce(s)	85	63.1	95	20.6	0	0	0.8	0.1	0.1	0.3
1578	Cooked, dry heat	3	ounce(s)	85	67.7	77	17.0	0	0	0.5	0.1	0.1	0.2
1886	**Halibut, Atlantic and Pacific, cooked, dry heat**	3	ounce(s)	85	64.7	94	19.2	0	0	1.4	0.3	0.5	0.3
1582	**Herring, Atlantic, pickled**	4	piece(s)	60	33.1	157	8.5	5.8	0	10.8	1.4	7.2	1.0
1587	**Jack mackerel, solids, canned, drained**	2	ounce(s)	57	39.2	88	13.1	0	0	3.6	1.1	1.3	0.9
8580	**Octopus, common, cooked, moist heat**	3	ounce(s)	85	51.4	139	25.4	3.7	0	1.8	0.4	0.3	0.4
1831	**Perch, mixed species, cooked, dry heat**	3	ounce(s)	85	62.3	99	21.1	0	0	1.0	0.2	0.2	0.4
1592	**Pacific rockfish, cooked, dry heat**	3	ounce(s)	85	63.5	93	18.9	0	0	1.4	0.4	0.4	0.4
	Salmon												
1594	Broiled or baked with butter	3	ounce(s)	85	53.9	155	22.9	0	0	6.3	1.2	2.3	2.3
2938	Coho, farmed, raw	3	ounce(s)	85	59.9	136	18.1	0	0	6.5	1.5	2.8	1.6
75533	Pink, canned, boneless, drained	3	ounce(s)	85	60.1	116	20.9	0	0	3.6	0.6	0.6	1.1
50124	Pink, canned, with bones, drained	3	ounce(s)	85	60.1	117	19.6	0.0	0	4.3	0.8	1.0	1.3
75532	Red (sockeye), canned, boneless, drained	3	ounce(s)	85	57.6	134	22.4	0	0	5.0	1.0	1.6	1.3
33210	Red (sockeye), canned, with bones, no salt, drained	3	ounce(s)	85	58.4	130	17.4	0	0	6.2	1.4	2.4	1.9
29727	Smoked chinook (lox)	2	ounce(s)	57	40.8	66	10.4	0	0.0	2.4	0.5	1.1	0.6

PAGE KEY: A-6 5 Breads/Baked Goods A-12 = Cereal/Rice/Pasta A-16 = Fruit A-22 = Vegetables/Legumes A-32 = Nuts/Seeds A-34 = Vegetarian A-36 = Dairy A-44 = Eggs A-44 = Seafood A-46 = Meats A-50 = Poultry
A-52 = Processed Meats A-54 = Beverages A-58 = Fats/Oils A-60 = Sweets A-62 = Spices/Condiments/Sauces A-66 = Mixed Foods/Soups/Sandwiches A-72 = Fast Food A-90 = Convenience A-92 = Baby Foods

Chol (mg)	Calc (mg)	Iron (mg)	Magn (mg)	Pota (mg)	Sodi (mg)	Zinc (mg)	Vit A (µg)	Thia (mg)	Vit E (mg α)	Ribo (mg)	Niac (mg)	Vit B$_6$ (mg)	Fola (µg)	Vit C (mg)	Vit B$_{12}$ (µg)	Sele (µg)
12	419	0.17	39.2	536.5	161.7	2.03	29.4	0.10	0.05	0.49	0.26	0.11	27.0	2.0	1.3	12.0
15	225	0.22	27.0	303.8	95.6	1.10	14.7	0.11	0	0.27	0.30	0.15	29.4	2.1	0.7	—
0	265	0.95	—	—	22.1	—	—	—	—	—	—	—	—	26.5	—	—
0	100	1.08	32.0	220.0	25.0	—	—	0.22	—	0.10	—	0.08	—	0	0	—
0	150	1.44	40.0	310.0	40.0	—	—	0.38	—	0.17	—	0.08	—	0	0	—
184	29	0.87	6.0	69.9	95.2	0.64	100.7	0.02	0.60	0.23	0.04	0.08	23.5	0	0.4	15.2
187	25	0.60	5.0	63.0	62.0	0.52	74.5	0.03	0.51	0.26	0.03	0.06	22.0	0	0.6	15.4
185	28	0.88	6.0	69.0	148.5	0.64	80.0	0.02	0.52	0.19	0.03	0.07	17.5	0	0.4	15.3
0	2	0.03	3.6	53.8	54.8	0.01	0.0	0	0	0.14	0.03	0	1.3	0	0	6.6
186	28	0.88	6.0	69.0	71.0	0.64	80.0	0.02	0.52	0.23	0.04	0.09	23.5	0	0.4	15.4
184	22	0.46	0.9	18.5	8.2	0.39	64.8	0.03	0.44	0.09	0.00	0.06	24.8	0	0.3	9.5
338	81	1.60	13.4	161.0	176.9	1.27	196.4	0.05	1.40	0.46	0.09	0.16	43.9	0	0.9	28.7
0	20	1.08	—	95.0	115.0	0.60	225.0	0.15	—	0.85	—	0.08	—	0	1.2	
1	44	1.19	9.0	127.8	119.4	0.59	6.6	0.07	0.95	0.23	0.08	0.08	9.6	0.3	0.2	24.8
1	33	1.32	5.6	207.1	111.1	0.82	11.3	0.07	0.17	0.19	0.07	0	9.4	0	0.2	15.6
47	12	0.42	35.7	207.5	66.3	0.49	11.9	0.07	0.69	0.07	2.14	0.24	6.8	0.9	0.9	32.0
47	12	0.42	35.7	207.5	66.3	0.49	11.9	0.07	0.69	0.07	2.14	0.24	6.8	0.9	0.9	32.0
107	17	0.43	17.0	231.3	43.4	1.38	886.9	0.13	3.40	0.03	2.98	0.06	12.8	1.5	2.6	5.5
44	8	0.32	29.1	489.0	86.1	0.49	0	0.03	0.78	0.05	2.48	0.46	8.5	3.0	1.0	44.3
29	15	1.79	20.4	272.1	452.4	0.37	9.4	0.09	—	0.09	1.79	0.09	17.0	0	0.9	7.7
37	55	0.98	96.7	524.3	62.9	0.49	0	0.06	0.99	0.08	6.81	0.36	14.0	0	1.2	42.5
32	48	0.85	84.0	455.6	54.7	0.43	0	0.06	0.86	0.08	5.92	0.33	12.1	0	1.1	37.0
41	12	0.29	24.7	319.3	41.8	0.35	0	0.07	0.62	0.06	1.89	0.21	6.8	0.8	0.8	32.0
44	19	0.35	47.3	224.7	280.2	0.21	0	0.06	0.42	0.08	2.03	0.19	7.8	2.8	1.6	33.5
40	18	0.97	31.5	403.9	45.1	0.43	42.5	0.07	—	0.01	0.32	0.30	8.5	0	0.6	39.8
63	36	1.15	42.5	339.3	74.0	0.41	16.2	0.03	0.43	0.04	3.94	0.29	6.8	0	1.2	34.4
56	12	0.18	22.1	298.5	222.0	0.34	17.9	0.02	0.47	0.06	3.50	0.28	11.1	0	1.8	27.0
51	8	0.17	23.8	449.0	69.7	0.37	20.4	0.05	0.63	0.03	6.73	0.54	11.9	0	1.1	47.1
8	46	0.73	4.8	41.4	522.0	0.32	154.8	0.02	1.03	0.08	1.98	0.10	1.2	0	2.6	35.1
45	137	1.16	21.0	110.0	214.9	0.58	73.7	0.02	0.58	0.12	3.50	0.12	2.8	0.5	3.9	21.4
82	90	8.11	51.0	535.8	391.2	2.86	76.5	0.05	1.02	0.06	3.21	0.55	20.4	6.8	30.6	76.2
98	87	0.99	32.3	292.5	67.2	1.22	8.5	0.07	—	0.10	1.62	0.12	5.1	1.4	1.9	13.7
52	14	0.31	28.1	397.1	75.7	0.37	4.3	0.02	0.37	0.19	2.46	0.20	8.5	0	1.4	64.8
40	15	1.02	26.9	376.5	98.6	0.56		0.14	1.15	0.05	8.33	0.19	—	1.8	2.3	41.0
43	10	0.29	26.4	382.7	40.0	0.37	47.6	0.08	—	0.09	5.79	0.56	11.1	0.9	2.3	10.7
71	51	0.48	20.4	277.3	321.5	0.55	17.0	0.02	1.09	0.17	6.32	0.09	3.4	0	4.2	33.7
71	241	0.65	27.2	283.2	324.0	0.82	17.0	0.02	1.09	0.17	6.30	0.09	3.4	0	4.2	33.6
56	31	0.41	20.4	265.4	328.3	0.49	47.6	0.03	1.78	0.18	6.54	0.10	3.4	0	4.7	29.4
37	203	0.90	24.7	320.6	63.8	0.87	45.1	0.01	—	0.16	4.66	0.26	8.5	0	0.3	30.1
13	6	0.48	10.2	99.2	1133.8	0.18	14.7	0.01	—	0.06	2.68	0.16	1.1	0	1.8	21.6

TABLE A-2 Table of Food Composition (continued)   (Computer code is for Cengage Diet Analysis program)   (For purposes of calculations, use "0" for t, <1, <0.1, <0.01)

DA+ Code	Food Description	Quantity	Measure	Wt (g)	H₂O (g)	Ener (kcal)	Prot (g)	Carb (g)	Fiber (g)	Fat (g)	Fat Breakdown (g) Sat	Mono	Poly
Seafood—*continued*													
154	**Sardines, Atlantic with bones, canned in oil**	3	ounce(s)	85	50.7	177	20.9	0	0	9.7	1.3	3.3	4.4
	Scallops												
155	Mixed species, breaded, fried	3	item(s)	47	27.2	100	8.4	4.7	—	5.1	1.2	2.1	1.3
1599	Steamed	3	ounce(s)	85	69.7	59	10.2	2.7	0	0.4	0.1	0	0.1
1839	**Snapper, mixed species, cooked, dry heat**	3	ounce(s)	85	59.8	109	22.4	0	0	1.5	0.3	0.3	0.5
	Squid												
1868	Mixed species, fried	3	ounce(s)	85	54.9	149	15.3	6.6	0	6.4	1.6	2.3	1.8
16617	Steamed or boiled	3	ounce(s)	85	63.3	89	15.2	3.0	0	1.3	0.3	0.1	0.5
1570	**Striped bass, cooked, dry heat**	3	ounce(s)	85	62.4	105	19.3	0	0	2.5	0.6	0.7	0.9
1601	**Sturgeon, steamed**	3	ounce(s)	85	59.6	111	17.0	0	0	4.3	1.0	2.0	0.7
1840	**Surimi, formed**	3	ounce(s)	85	64.9	84	12.9	5.8	0	0.8	0.2	0.1	0.4
1842	**Swordfish, cooked, dry heat**	3	ounce(s)	85	58.0	146	19.9	0	0	6.7	1.6	3.0	1.2
1846	**Tuna, yellowfin or ahi, raw**	3	ounce(s)	85	63.0	93	20.7	0	0	0.4	0.1	0.1	0.1
	Tuna, canned												
159	Light, canned in oil, drained	2	ounce(s)	57	33.9	112	16.5	0	0	4.7	0.9	1.7	1.6
355	Light, canned in water, drained	2	ounce(s)	57	44.3	49	11.0	0	0	0.5	0.1	0.1	0.2
33211	Light, no salt, canned in oil, drained	2	ounce(s)	57	33.9	112	16.5	0	0	4.7	0.9	1.7	1.6
33212	Light, no salt, canned in water, drained	2	ounce(s)	57	42.6	66	14.5	0	0	0.5	0.1	0.1	0.2
2961	White, canned in oil, drained	2	ounce(s)	57	36.3	105	15.0	0	0	4.6	0.7	1.8	1.7
351	White, canned in water, drained	2	ounce(s)	57	41.5	73	13.4	0	0	1.7	0.4	0.4	0.6
33213	White, no salt, canned in oil, drained	2	ounce(s)	57	36.3	105	15.0	0	0	4.6	0.9	1.4	1.9
33214	White, no salt, canned in water, drained	2	ounce(s)	57	42.0	73	13.4	0	0	1.7	0.4	0.4	0.6
	Yellowtail												
8548	Mixed species, cooked, dry heat	3	ounce(s)	85	57.3	159	25.2	0	0	5.7	1.4	2.2	1.5
2970	Mixed species, raw	2	ounce(s)	57	42.2	83	13.1	0	0	3.0	0.7	1.1	0.8
	Shellfish, meat only												
1857	Abalone, mixed species, fried	3	ounce(s)	85	51.1	161	16.7	9.4	0	5.8	1.4	2.3	1.4
16618	Abalone, steamed or poached	3	ounce(s)	85	40.7	177	28.9	10.1	0	1.3	0.3	0.2	0.2
	Crab												
1851	Blue crab, canned	2	ounce(s)	57	45.2	47	10.1	0	0	0.4	0.1	0.1	0.1
1852	Blue crab, cooked, moist heat	3	ounce(s)	85	67.8	71	15.2	0	0	0.6	0.2	0.1	0.2
8562	Dungeness crab, cooked, moist heat	3	ounce(s)	85	62.3	94	19.0	0.8	0	1.1	0.1	0.2	0.3
1860	**Clams, cooked, moist heat**	3	ounce(s)	85	54.1	126	21.7	4.4	0	1.7	0.2	0.1	0.5
1853	**Crayfish, farmed, cooked, moist heat**	3	ounce(s)	85	68.7	74	14.9	0	0	1.1	0.2	0.2	0.4
	Oysters												
8720	Baked or broiled	3	ounce(s)	85	71.6	77	4.5	2.2	0	5.4	1.1	2.1	1.6
152	Eastern, farmed, raw	3	ounce(s)	85	73.3	50	4.4	4.7	0	1.3	0.4	0.1	0.5
8715	Eastern, wild, cooked, moist heat	3	ounce(s)	85	66.5	87	9.7	4.6	0	2.9	0.8	0.4	0.9
8584	Pacific, cooked, moist heat	3	ounce(s)	85	54.5	139	16.1	8.4	0	3.9	0.9	0.7	1.5
1865	Pacific, raw	3	ounce(s)	85	69.8	69	8.0	4.2	0	2.0	0.4	0.3	0.8
1854	**Lobster, northern, cooked, moist heat**	3	ounce(s)	85	66.4	76	16.2	0	0	0.7	0.2	0.2	0.3
1862	**Mussels, blue, cooked, moist heat**	3	ounce(s)	85	52.0	146	20.2	6.3	0	3.8	0.7	0.9	1.0
	Shrimp												
158	Mixed species, breaded, fried	3	ounce(s)	85	45.0	206	18.2	9.8	0.3	10.4	1.8	3.2	4.3
1855	Mixed species, cooked, moist heat	3	ounce(s)	85	60.9	101	19.4	1.3	0	1.4	0.4	0.3	0.5
Beef, Lamb, Pork													
	Beef												
4450	Breakfast strips, cooked	2	slice(s)	23	5.9	101	7.1	0.3	0	7.8	3.2	3.8	0.4
174	Corned beef, canned	3	ounce(s)	85	49.1	213	23.0	0	0	12.7	5.3	5.1	0.5
33147	Cured, thin siced	2	ounce(s)	57	32.9	100	15.9	3.2	0	2.2	0.9	1.0	0.1
4581	Jerky	1	ounce(s)	28	6.6	116	9.4	3.1	0.5	7.3	3.1	3.2	0.3

PAGE KEY: A-6 5 Breads/Baked Goods A-12 = Cereal/Rice/Pasta A-16 = Fruit A-22 = Vegetables/Legumes A-32 = Nuts/Seeds A-34 = Vegetarian A-36 = Dairy A-44 = Eggs A-44 = Seafood A-46 = Meats A-50 = Poultry
A-52 = Processed Meats A-54 = Beverages A-58 = Fats/Oils A-60 = Sweets A-62 = Spices/Condiments/Sauces A-66 = Mixed Foods/Soups/Sandwiches A-72 = Fast Food A-90 = Convenience A-92 = Baby Foods

Chol (mg)	Calc (mg)	Iron (mg)	Magn (mg)	Pota (mg)	Sodi (mg)	Zinc (mg)	Vit A (µg)	Thia (mg)	Vit E (mg α)	Ribo (mg)	Niac (mg)	Vit B_6 (mg)	Fola (µg)	Vit C (mg)	Vit B_{12} (µg)	Sele (µg)
121	325	2.48	33.2	337.6	429.5	1.11	27.2	0.07	1.74	0.19	4.46	0.14	8.5	0	7.6	44.8
25	20	0.38	27.4	154.8	215.8	0.49	10.2	0.02	—	0.05	0.70	0.07	23.3	1.1	0.6	12.5
20	5	0.29	18.7	155.6	547.7	0.76	0.8	0.01	0	0.01	0.53	0.06	10.2	0	1.1	10.8
40	34	0.20	31.5	443.9	48.5	0.37	29.8	0.05	—	0	0.29	0.39	5.1	1.4	3.0	41.7
221	33	0.86	32.3	237.3	260.2	1.48	9.4	0.05	—	0.39	2.21	0.05	17.0	3.6	1.0	44.1
227	31	0.63	28.9	192.2	356.3	1.50	8.5	0.01	1.17	0.32	1.70	0.04	3.4	3.2	1.0	43.7
88	16	0.92	43.4	278.9	74.8	0.43	26.4	0.10	—	0.03	2.18	0.29	8.5	0	3.8	39.8
64	11	0.59	29.8	239.8	316.3	0.36	199.8	0.07	0.53	0.07	8.33	0.19	14.5	0	2.2	13.3
26	8	0.22	36.6	95.2	121.6	0.28	17.0	0.02	0.54	0.02	0.19	0.03	1.7	0	1.4	23.9
66	5	0.38	29.8	424.3	82.5	0.66	36.6	0.08	2.05	0.05	7.87	0.52	1.7	0	1.4	58.3
33	3	0.65	29.8	375.0	38.3	0.31	15.3	0.10	0.20	0.10	15.71	0.79	1.7	0	1.8	77.0
10	7	0.79	17.6	117.3	200.6	0.51	13.0	0.02	0.49	0.07	7.03	0.06	2.8	0	1.2	43.1
20	10	0.92	13.0	101.4	140.0	0.39	9.6	0.02	0.19	0.05	5.74	0.18	2.3	0	1.4	40.0
10	7	0.79	17.6	117.3	28.3	0.51	—	0.02	—	0.07	7.03	0.06	2.8	0	1.2	43.1
17	6	0.87	15.3	134.4	28.3	0.44	—	0.02	—	0.04	7.53	0.20	2.3	0	1.7	45.6
18	2	0.37	19.3	188.8	224.5	0.27	2.8	0.01	1.30	0.04	6.63	0.24	2.8	0	1.2	34.1
24	8	0.55	18.7	134.3	213.6	0.27	3.4	0	0.48	0.02	3.29	0.12	1.1	0	0.7	37.2
18	2	0.37	19.3	188.8	28.3	0.27	—	0.01	—	0.04	6.63	0.24	2.8	0	1.2	34.1
24	8	0.55	18.7	134.4	28.3	0.27	3.4	0	—	0.02	3.29	0.12	1.1	0	0.7	37.2
60	25	0.54	32.3	457.5	42.5	0.57	26.4	0.15		0.04	7.41	0.16	3.4	2.5	1.1	39.8
31	13	0.28	17.0	238.1	22.1	0.29	16.4	0.08	—	0.02	3.85	0.09	2.3	1.6	0.7	20.7
80	31	3.23	47.6	241.5	502.6	0.81	1.7	0.19	—	0.11	1.62	0.13	17.0	1.5	0.6	44.1
144	50	4.85	68.9	295.1	980.6	1.39	3.4	0.29	6.74	0.13	1.90	0.22	6.0	2.6	0.7	75.6
55	52	0.28	20.4	146.8	223.9	2.16	0.6	0.01	1.04	0.05	1.56	0.09	28.9	1.9	1.9	24.3
82	77	0.43	30.6	220.3	335.9	3.24	0.9	0.02	1.56	0.08	2.34	0.13	43.4	2.8	2.8	36.5
65	50	0.37	49.3	347.0	321.5	4.65	26.4	0.05	—	0.17	3.08	0.15	35.7	3.1	8.8	40.5
57	78	23.78	15.3	534.1	1022.2	2.32	145.4	0.13	—	0.36	2.85	0.09	24.7	18.8	84.1	54.4
117	43	0.94	28.1	202.4	82.5	1.26	12.8	0.04	—	0.07	1.42	0.11	9.4	0.4	2.6	29.1
31	48	3.67	14.5	125.0	308.7	31.26	49.3	0.01	1.12	0.06	0.70	0.02	5.1	0	6.6	15.6
21	37	4.92	28.1	105.5	151.4	32.25	6.8	0.09	—	0.06	1.08	0.05	15.3	4.0	13.8	54.2
67	99	7.83	29.8	118.2	141.2	66.84	22.1	0.03	1.45	0.15	1.57	0.05	11.9	0	14.9	33.6
85	14	7.82	37.4	256.8	180.3	28.27	124.2	0.11	0.72	0.38	3.08	0.08	12.8	10.9	24.5	131.0
43	7	4.35	18.7	142.9	90.1	14.13	68.9	0.06	—	0.20	1.71	0.04	8.5	6.8	13.6	65.5
124	82	0.25	36.6	195.6	413.3	3.44	0.8	0.02	0.85	0.01	1.56	0.10	9.4	0	1.2	62.2
48	28	5.71	31.5	227.9	313.8	2.27	77.4	0.26	—	0.36	2.55	0.09	64.6	11.6	20.4	76.2
117	57	1.07	34.0	191.4	292.6	1.17	47.6	0.11	1.11	0.12	2.61	0.08	33.2	1.3	1.6	35.5
179	77	0.27	31.5	144.6	805.3	1.39	76.5	0.03	1.87	0.02	2.28	0.21	20.4	0	1.4	42.1
27	2	0.71	6.1	93.1	509.2	1.44	0	0.02	0.07	0.06	1.46	0.07	1.8	0	0.8	6.1
73	10	1.77	11.9	115.7	762.8	3.04	0	0.02	0.13	0.13	2.07	0.11	7.7	0	1.4	36.5
23	6	1.53	10.8	243.2	815.8	2.26	0	0.05	0	0.11	2.99	0.19	6.2	0	1.5	16.0
14	6	1.54	14.5	169.2	590.0	2.30	0	0.04	0.14	0.04	0.49	0.05	38.0	0	0.3	3.0

TABLE A-2 Table of Food Composition *(continued)*   (Computer code is for Cengage Diet Analysis program)   (For purposes of calculations, use "0" for t, <1, <0.1, <0.01)

DA+ Code	Food Description	Quantity	Measure	Wt (g)	H₂O (g)	Ener (kcal)	Prot (g)	Carb (g)	Fiber (g)	Fat (g)	Sat	Mono	Poly
	Beef, Lamb, Pork—*continued*												
	Ground beef												
5898	Lean, broiled, medium	3	ounce(s)	85	50.4	202	21.6	0	0	12.2	4.8	5.3	0.5
5899	Lean, broiled, well done	3	ounce(s)	85	48.4	214	23.8	0	0	12.5	5.0	5.7	0.3
5914	Regular, broiled, medium	3	ounce(s)	85	46.1	246	20.5	0	0	17.6	6.9	7.7	0.7
5915	Regular, broiled, well done	3	ounce(s)	85	43.8	259	21.6	0	0	18.4	7.5	8.5	0.5
	Beef rib												
4241	Rib, small end, separable lean, 0" fat, broiled	3	ounce(s)	85	53.2	164	25.0	0.0	0	6.4	2.4	2.6	0.2
4183	Rib, whole, lean and fat, 1/4" fat, roasted	3	ounce(s)	85	39.0	320	18.9	0.0	0	26.6	10.7	11.4	0.9
	Beef roast												
16981	Bottom round, choice, separable lean and fat, 1/8" fat, braised	3	ounce(s)	85	46.2	216	27.9	0	0	10.7	4.1	4.6	0.4
16979	Bottom round, separable lean and fat, 1/8" fat, roasted	3	ounce(s)	85	52.4	185	22.5	0	0	9.9	3.8	4.2	0.4
16924	Chuck, arm pot roast, separable lean and fat, 1/8" fat, braised	3	ounce(s)	85	42.9	257	25.6	0	0	16.3	6.5	7.0	0.6
16930	Chuck, blade roast, separable lean and fat, 1/8" fat, braised	3	ounce(s)	85	40.5	290	22.8	0	0	21.4	8.5	9.2	0.8
5853	Chuck, blade roast, separable lean, 0" trim, pot roasted	3	ounce(s)	85	47.4	202	26.4	0	0	10.0	3.9	4.3	0.3
4296	Eye of round, choice, separable lean, 0" fat, roasted	3	ounce(s)	85	56.5	138	24.4	0.0	0	3.7	1.3	1.5	0.1
16989	Eye of round, separable lean and fat, 1/8" fat, roasted	3	ounce(s)	85	52.2	180	24.2	0	0	8.5	3.2	3.6	0.3
	Beef steak												
4348	Short loin, t-bone steak, lean and fat, 1/4" fat, broiled	3	ounce(s)	85	43.2	274	19.4	0.0	0	21.2	8.3	9.6	0.8
4349	Short loin, t-bone steak, lean, 1/4" fat, broiled	3	ounce(s)	85	52.3	174	22.8	0.0	0	8.5	3.1	4.2	0.3
4360	Top loin, prime, lean and fat, 1/4" fat, broiled	3	ounce(s)	85	42.7	275	21.6	0.0	0	20.3	8.2	8.6	0.7
	Beef variety												
188	Liver, pan-fried	3	ounce(s)	85	52.7	149	22.6	4.4	0	4.0	1.3	0.6	0.5
4447	Tongue, simmered	3	ounce(s)	85	49.2	242	16.4	0.0	0	19.0	6.9	8.6	0.6
	Lamb chop												
3275	Loin, domestic, lean and fat, 1/4" fat, broiled	3	ounce(s)	85	43.9	269	21.4	0	0	19.6	8.4	8.2	1.4
	Lamb leg												
3264	Domestic, lean and fat, 1/4" fat, cooked	3	ounce(s)	85	45.7	250	20.9	0	0	17.8	7.5	7.5	1.3
	Lamb rib												
182	Domestic, lean and fat, 1/4" fat, broiled	3	ounce(s)	85	40.0	307	18.8	0	0	25.2	10.8	10.3	2.0
183	Domestic, lean, 1/4" fat, broiled	3	ounce(s)	85	50.0	200	23.6	0	0	11.0	4.0	4.4	1.0
	Lamb shoulder												
186	Shoulder, arm and blade, domestic, choice, lean and fat, 1/4" fat, roasted	3	ounce(s)	85	47.8	235	19.1	0	0	17.0	7.2	6.9	1.4
187	Shoulder, arm and blade, domestic, choice, lean, 1/4" fat, roasted	3	ounce(s)	85	53.9	174	21.2	0	0	9.2	3.5	3.7	0.8
3287	Shoulder, arm, domestic, lean and fat, 1/4" fat, braised	3	ounce(s)	85	37.6	294	25.8	0	0	20.4	8.4	8.7	1.5
3290	Shoulder, arm, domestic, lean, 1/4" fat, braised	3	ounce(s)	85	41.9	237	30.2	0	0	12.0	4.3	5.2	0.8
	Lamb variety												
3375	Brain, pan-fried	3	ounce(s)	85	51.6	232	14.4	0	0	18.9	4.8	3.4	1.9
3406	Tongue, braised	3	ounce(s)	85	49.2	234	18.3	0	0	17.2	6.7	8.5	1.1
	Pork, cured												
29229	Bacon, Canadian style, cured	2	ounce(s)	57	37.9	89	11.7	1.0	0	4.0	1.3	1.8	0.4
161	Bacon, cured, broiled, pan-fried or roasted	2	slice(s)	16	2.0	87	5.9	0.2	0	6.7	2.2	3.0	0.7
42274	Bacon, cured, broiled, pan-fried or roasted, reduced sodium	2	slice(s)	16	2.0	87	5.9	0.2	0	6.7	2.2	3.0	0.7

Chol (mg)	Calc (mg)	Iron (mg)	Magn (mg)	Pota (mg)	Sodi (mg)	Zinc (mg)	Vit A (µg)	Thia (mg)	Vit E (mg α)	Ribo (mg)	Niac (mg)	Vit B$_6$ (mg)	Fola (µg)	Vit C (mg)	Vit B$_{12}$ (µg)	Sele (µg)
58	6	2.00	17.9	266.2	59.5	4.64	0	0.05	—	0.23	4.22	0.23	7.7	0	1.8	16.0
69	12	2.21	18.5	250.0	62.4	5.87	0	0.09	—	0.24	5.10	0.16	9.4	0	1.7	19.1
62	9	2.08	17.0	248.3	70.6	4.41	0	0.03	—	0.16	4.91	0.23	7.7	0	2.5	16.2
71	12	2.30	18.5	242.4	72.4	5.19	0	0.09	—	0.23	4.93	0.18	8.5	0	1.6	18.0
77	16	1.59	21.3	319.8	51.9	4.64	0	0.07	0.34	0.13	7.16	0.54	8.5	0	1.4	29.2
72	9	1.96	16.2	251.7	53.6	4.46	0	0.06	—	0.14	2.86	0.20	6.0	0	2.1	18.7
86	6	2.30	17.9	223.7	35.7	4.59	0	0.06	0.42	0.16	5.05	0.37	8.5	0	1.7	29.3
72	5	1.84	14.5	182.0	29.8	3.77	0	0.05	0.35	0.12	3.93	0.30	6.8	0	1.3	23.0
102	14	2.15	17.0	205.8	42.5	5.94	0	0.05	0.45	0.15	3.63	0.25	7.7	0	1.9	24.1
88	11	2.66	16.2	198.1	55.3	7.15	0	0.06	0.17	0.20	2.07	0.22	4.3	0	1.9	20.9
73	11	3.13	19.6	223.7	60.4	8.73	0	0.07	—	0.24	2.27	0.25	5.1	0	2.1	22.7
63	5	2.17	16.2	200.7	32.3	4.29	0	0.05	0.31	0.15	4.70	0.34	8.5	0	1.4	28.0
73	5	1.98	15.3	193.0	31.5	3.95	0	0.05	0.35	0.14	4.38	0.32	7.7	0	1.5	25.2
58	7	2.56	17.9	233.9	57.8	3.56	0	0.08	0.19	0.18	3.29	0.28	6.0	0	1.8	10.0
50	5	3.11	22.1	278.1	65.5	4.35	0	0.09	0.12	0.21	3.94	0.33	6.8	0	1.9	8.5
67	8	1.89	19.6	294.2	53.6	3.85	0	0.07	—	0.15	3.96	0.31	6.0	0	1.6	19.5
324	5	5.25	18.7	298.5	65.5	4.45	6586.3	0.15	0.39	2.91	14.86	0.87	221.1	0.6	70.7	27.9
112	4	2.22	12.8	156.5	55.3	3.48	0	0.02	0.26	0.25	2.97	0.13	6.0	1.1	2.7	11.2
85	17	1.54	20.4	278.1	65.5	2.96	0	0.09	0.11	0.21	6.04	0.11	15.3	0	2.1	23.3
82	14	1.60	19.6	263.6	61.2	3.79	0	0.09	0.12	0.21	5.66	0.11	15.3	0	2.2	22.5
84	16	1.60	19.6	229.6	64.6	3.40	0	0.08	0.10	0.19	5.95	0.09	11.9	0	2.2	20.3
77	14	1.88	24.7	266.2	72.3	4.48	0	0.09	0.15	0.21	5.57	0.13	17.9	0	2.2	26.4
78	17	1.68	19.6	213.5	56.1	4.45	0	0.08	0.12	0.20	5.23	0.11	17.9	0	2.2	22.3
74	16	1.81	21.3	225.4	57.8	5.14	0	0.08	0.15	0.22	4.90	0.13	21.3	0	2.3	24.2
102	21	2.03	22.1	260.2	61.2	5.17	0	0.06	0.13	0.21	5.66	0.09	15.3	0	2.2	31.6
103	22	2.30	24.7	287.4	64.6	6.21	0	0.06	0.15	0.23	5.38	0.11	18.7	0	2.3	32.1
2129	18	1.73	18.7	304.4	133.5	1.70	0	0.14	—	0.31	3.87	0.20	6.0	19.6	20.5	10.2
161	9	2.24	13.6	134.4	57.0	2.54	0	0.07	—	0.36	3.14	0.14	2.6	6.0	5.4	23.8
28	5	0.39	9.6	195.0	512.5	0.79	0	0.43	0.12	0.10	3.53	0.22	2.3	0	0.4	14.2
18	2	0.23	5.3	90.4	274.7	0.56	1.8	0.06	0.05	0.04	1.78	0.06	0.3	0	0.2	9.9
18	2	0.23	5.3	90.4	164.8	0.56	1.8	0.06	0.05	0.04	1.78	0.06	0.3	0	0.2	9.9

TABLE A-2 Table of Food Composition *(continued)* (Computer code is for Cengage Diet Analysis program) (For purposes of calculations, use "0" for t, <1, <0.1, <0.01)

DA+ Code	Food Description	Quantity	Measure	Wt (g)	H₂O (g)	Ener (kcal)	Prot (g)	Carb (g)	Fiber (g)	Fat (g)	Fat Breakdown (g) Sat	Mono	Poly
Beef, Lamb, Pork—*continued*													
35422	Breakfast strips, cured, cooked	3	slice(s)	34	9.2	156	9.8	0.4	0	12.5	4.3	5.6	1.9
189	Ham, cured, boneless, 11% fat, roasted	3	ounce(s)	85	54.9	151	19.2	0	0	7.7	2.7	3.8	1.2
29215	Ham, cured, extra lean, 4% fat, canned	2	ounce(s)	57	41.7	68	10.5	0	0	2.6	0.9	1.3	0.2
1316	Ham, cured, extra lean, 5% fat, roasted	3	ounce(s)	85	57.5	123	17.8	1.3	0	4.7	1.5	2.2	0.5
16561	Ham, smoked or cured, lean, cooked	1	slice(s)	42	28.8	58	9.1	0.4	0	2.1	0.7	1.0	0.3
42257	Ham, smoked or cured, lean, cooked, low-sodium	1	slice(s)	42	28.4	61	8.8	0.6	0	2.3	0.8	1.1	0.2
	Pork chop												
32671	Loin, blade, chops, lean and fat, pan-fried	3	ounce(s)	85	49.3	218	21.3	0	0	14.1	3.8	4.3	1.7
32672	Loin, center cut, chops, lean and fat, pan-fried	3	ounce(s)	85	49.7	202	23.5	0	0	11.3	4.1	4.7	1.8
32682	Loin, center rib, chops, boneless, lean and fat, braised	3	ounce(s)	85	49.5	217	22.4	0	0	13.4	5.2	6.1	1.1
32603	Loin, center rib, chops, lean, broiled	3	ounce(s)	85	55.4	158	21.9	0	0	7.1	2.4	3.0	0.8
32478	Loin, whole, lean and fat, braised	3	ounce(s)	85	49.6	203	23.2	0	0	11.6	4.3	5.2	1.0
32481	Loin, whole, lean, braised	3	ounce(s)	85	52.2	173	24.3	0	0	7.8	2.9	3.5	0.6
	Pork leg or ham												
32471	Rump portion, lean and fat, roasted	3	ounce(s)	85	52.7	178	23.0	0	0	8.8	2.9	3.7	1.9
32468	Whole, lean and fat, roasted	3	ounce(s)	85	46.8	232	22.8	0	0	15.0	5.5	6.7	1.4
	Pork ribs												
32693	Loin, country style, lean and fat, roasted	3	ounce(s)	85	41.1	305	18.5	0	0	25.1	9.1	10.9	2.5
32696	Loin, country style ribs, lean, roasted	3	ounce(s)	85	49.9	193	24.8	0	0	9.7	3.2	3.7	1.2
	Pork shoulder												
32626	Shoulder, arm picnic, lean and fat, roasted	3	ounce(s)	85	44.3	270	20.0	0	0	20.4	7.5	9.1	2.0
32629	Shoulder, arm picnic, lean, roasted	3	ounce(s)	85	51.3	194	22.7	0	0	10.7	3.7	5.1	1.0
	Rabbit												
3366	Domesticated, roasted	3	ounce(s)	85	51.5	168	24.7	0	0	6.8	2.0	1.8	1.3
3367	Domesticated, stewed	3	ounce(s)	85	50.0	175	25.8	0	0	7.2	2.1	1.9	1.4
	Veal												
3391	Liver, braised	3	ounce(s)	85	50.9	163	24.2	3.2	0	5.3	1.7	1.0	0.9
3319	Rib, lean only, roasted	3	ounce(s)	85	55.0	151	21.9	0	0	6.3	1.8	2.3	0.6
1732	Deer or venison, roasted	3	ounce(s)	85	55.5	134	25.7	0	0	2.7	1.1	0.7	0.5
Poultry													
	Chicken												
29562	Flaked, canned	2	ounce(s)	57	39.3	97	10.3	0.1	0	5.8	1.6	2.3	1.3
	Chicken, fried												
73336	Breast, meat and skin, breaded, fried, fast food	3	ounce(s)	85	45.1	214	18.6	6.6	0.4	12.6	3.3	4.7	3.4
36413	Broiler breast, meat and skin, flour coated, fried	3	ounce(s)	85	48.1	189	27.1	1.4	0.1	7.5	2.1	3.0	1.7
35327	Broiler breast, meat only, fried	3	ounce(s)	85	51.2	159	28.4	0.4	0	4.0	1.1	1.5	0.9
36414	Broiler drumstick, meat and skin, flour coated, fried	3	ounce(s)	85	48.2	208	22.9	1.4	0.1	11.7	3.1	4.6	2.7
35389	Broiler drumstick, meat only, fried	3	ounce(s)	85	52.9	166	24.3	0	0	6.9	1.8	2.5	1.7
35406	Broiler leg, meat only, fried	3	ounce(s)	85	51.5	177	24.1	0.6	0	7.9	2.1	2.9	1.9
35484	Broiler wing, meat only, fried	3	ounce(s)	85	50.9	179	25.6	0	0	7.8	2.1	2.6	1.8
29580	Patty, fillet or tenders, breaded, cooked	3	ounce(s)	85	39.1	246	15.9	13.4	0.7	14.2	2.3	5.4	5.8
	Chicken, roasted, meat only												
35409	Broiler leg, meat only, roasted	3	ounce(s)	85	55.0	162	23.0	0	0	7.2	1.9	2.6	1.7
35486	Broiler wing, meat only, roasted	3	ounce(s)	85	53.4	173	25.9	0	0	6.9	1.9	2.2	1.5
35138	Roasting chicken, dark meat, meat only, roasted	3	ounce(s)	85	57.0	151	19.8	0	0	7.4	2.1	2.8	1.7

PAGE KEY: A-6 5 Breads/Baked Goods A-12 = Cereal/Rice/Pasta A-16 = Fruit A-22 = Vegetables/Legumes A-32 = Nuts/Seeds A-34 = Vegetarian A-36 = Dairy A-44 = Eggs A-44 = Seafood A-46 = Meats A-50 = Poultry
A-52 = Processed Meats A-54 = Beverages A-58 = Fats/Oils A-60 = Sweets A-62 = Spices/Condiments/Sauces A-66 = Mixed Foods/Soups/Sandwiches A-72 = Fast Food A-90 = Convenience A-92 = Baby Foods

Chol (mg)	Calc (mg)	Iron (mg)	Magn (mg)	Pota (mg)	Sodi (mg)	Zinc (mg)	Vit A (μg)	Thia (mg)	Vit E (mg α)	Ribo (mg)	Niac (mg)	Vit B$_6$ (mg)	Fola (μg)	Vit C (mg)	Vit B$_{12}$ (μg)	Sele (μg)
36	5	0.67	8.8	158.4	713.7	1.25	0	0.25	0.09	0.13	2.58	0.12	1.4	0	0.6	8.4
50	7	1.14	18.7	347.9	1275.8	2.10	0	0.62	0.26	0.28	5.23	0.26	2.6	0	0.6	16.8
22	3	0.53	9.6	206.4	711.5	1.09	0	0.47	0.10	0.13	3.01	0.26	3.4	0	0.5	8.2
45	7	1.26	11.9	244.1	1023.0	2.45	0	0.64	0.21	0.17	3.42	0.34	2.6	0	0.6	16.6
22	3	0.37	8.4	131.5	540.1	0.94	2.5	0.23	0.10	0.09	2.18	0.18	1.3	0	0.2	11.9
22	3	0.62	5.9	120.5	407.0	1.21	0	0.31	0.11	0.08	1.69	0.17	1.3	0	0.3	8.2
70	41	0.71	17.0	270.4	72.3	2.45	4.3	0.41	0.17	0.28	7.07	0.40	0	0	0.6	31.2
67	45	0.79	19.6	300.2	79.9	2.72	4.3	0.46	0.17	0.31	7.81	0.45	0	0	0.7	34.7
62	4	0.78	14.5	329.1	34.0	1.76	1.7	0.45	—	0.21	3.67	0.26	3.4	0.3	0.4	28.4
56	22	0.58	21.3	291.7	48.5	1.91	0	0.48	0.09	0.19	6.68	0.57	0	0	0.4	38.6
68	18	0.91	16.2	318.0	40.8	2.02	1.7	0.54	0.20	0.22	3.76	0.31	2.6	0.5	0.5	38.5
67	15	0.96	17.0	329.1	42.5	2.11	1.7	0.56	0.18	0.23	3.90	0.33	3.4	0.5	0.5	41.0
72	14	0.77	21.3	353.8	65.5	1.96	2.6	0.42	0.23	0.32	6.33	0.43	0	0	0.6	21.3
80	12	0.86	18.7	299.3	51.0	2.52	2.6	0.54	0.19	0.27	3.89	0.34	8.5	0.3	0.6	38.5
77	21	0.85	18.7	273.8	44.2	1.87	1.7	0.70	0	0.28	3.57	0.36	3.4	0.3	0.6	29.3
84	26	0.83	18.7	331.7	77.4	3.35	0.9	0.49	0.23	0.39	6.65	0.44	0	0	0.8	40.5
80	16	1.00	14.5	276.4	59.5	2.93	1.7	0.44	—	0.26	3.33	0.30	3.4	0.2	0.6	28.6
81	8	1.21	17.0	298.5	68.0	3.46	0	0.49	—	0.30	3.67	0.35	4.3	0.3	0.7	32.7
70	16	1.93	17.9	325.7	40.0	1.93	0	0.08	—	0.18	7.17	0.40	9.4	0	7.1	32.7
73	17	2.02	17.0	255.1	31.5	2.02	0	0.05	0.37	0.14	6.09	0.29	7.7	0	5.5	32.7
435	5	4.35	17.0	279.8	66.3	9.55	17981.7	0.15	0.58	2.43	11.18	0.78	281.5	0.9	71.9	16.4
98	10	0.82	20.4	264.5	82.5	3.82	0	0.05	0.31	0.25	6.38	0.23	11.9	0	1.3	9.4
95	6	3.80	20.4	284.9	45.9	2.34	0	0.15	—	0.51	5.71		—	0	—	11.0
35	8	0.90	6.8	147.4	408.2	0.80	19.3	0.01	—	0.07	3.59	0.20	2.3	0	0.2	—
75	23	0.56	21.3	232.2	468.6	0.66	16.2	0.06	0.22	0.12	7.55	0.31	25.3	0	0.3	21.9
76	14	1.01	25.5	220.3	64.6	0.94	12.8	0.07	0.39	0.11	11.69	0.49	6.3	0	0.3	20.3
77	14	0.97	26.4	234.7	67.2	0.92	6.0	0.07	0.36	0.11	12.57	0.54	3.4	0	0.3	22.3
77	10	1.14	19.6	194.7	75.7	2.46	21.3	0.07	0.66	0.19	5.13	0.30	9.7	0	0.3	15.6
80	10	1.12	20.4	211.7	81.6	2.74	15.3	0.07	—	0.20	5.23	0.33	7.7	0	0.3	16.7
84	11	1.19	21.3	216.0	81.6	2.53	17.0	0.07	0.38	0.21	5.69	0.33	7.7	0	0.3	16.0
71	13	0.97	17.9	176.9	77.4	1.80	15.4	0.04	0.41	0.11	6.16	0.50	3.4	0	0.2	21.6
38	20	0.55	23.8	265.3	728.8	0.51	4.3	0.06	0.76	0.06	7.22	0.42	37.4	0	0.2	15.4
80	10	1.11	20.4	205.8	77.4	2.43	16.2	0.06	0.23	0.20	5.37	0.31	6.8	0	0.3	18.8
72	14	0.99	17.9	178.6	78.2	1.82	15.3	0.04	0.23	0.11	6.22	0.50	3.4	0	0.3	21.0
64	9	1.13	17.0	190.5	80.8	1.81	13.6	0.05	—	0.16	4.88	0.26	6.0	0	0.2	16.7

TABLE A-2 Table of Food Composition *(continued)*   (Computer code is for Cengage Diet Analysis program)   (For purposes of calculations, use "0" for t, <1, <0.1, <0.01)

DA+ Code	Food Description	Quantity	Measure	Wt (g)	H₂O (g)	Ener (kcal)	Prot (g)	Carb (g)	Fiber (g)	Fat (g)	Fat Breakdown (g) Sat	Mono	Poly
Poultry—*continued*													
35136	Roasting chicken, light meat, meat only, roasted	3	ounce(s)	85	57.7	130	23.1	0	0	3.5	0.9	1.3	0.8
35132	Roasting chicken, meat only, roasted	3	ounce(s)	85	57.3	142	21.3	0	0	5.6	1.5	2.1	1.3
	Chicken, stewed												
1268	Gizzard, simmered	3	ounce(s)	85	57.8	131	25.8	0.0	0	2.3	0.6	0.4	0.3
1270	Liver, simmered	3	ounce(s)	85	56.8	142	20.8	0.7	0	5.5	1.8	1.2	1.7
3174	Meat only, stewed	3	ounce(s)	85	56.8	151	23.2	0	0	5.7	1.6	2.0	1.3
	Duck												
1286	Domesticated, meat and skin, roasted	3	ounce(s)	85	44.1	287	16.1	0	0	24.1	8.2	11.0	3.1
1287	Domesticated, meat only, roasted	3	ounce(s)	85	54.6	171	20.0	0	0	9.5	3.4	3.3	1.3
	Goose												
35507	Domesticated, meat and skin, roasted	3	ounce(s)	85	44.2	259	21.4	0	0	18.6	5.8	8.7	2.1
35524	Domesticated, meat only, roasted	3	ounce(s)	85	48.7	202	24.6	0	0	10.8	3.9	3.7	1.3
1297	Liver pate, smoked, canned	4	tablespoon(s)	52	19.3	240	5.9	2.4	0	22.8	7.5	13.3	0.4
	Turkey												
3256	Ground, cooked	3	ounce(s)	85	52.8	173	23.3	0	0	8.8	2.3	2.9	2.5
3263	Patty, batter-coated, breaded, fried	1	item(s)	94	46.7	266	13.2	14.8	0.5	16.9	4.4	7.0	4.4
219	Roasted, dark meat, meat only	3	ounce(s)	85	55.5	147	23.6	0	0	5.1	1.5	1.8	1.4
222	Roasted, fryer roaster breast, meat only	3	ounce(s)	85	58.2	115	25.6	0	0	0.6	0.2	0.1	0.2
220	Roasted, light meat, meat only	3	ounce(s)	85	57.7	125	25.6	0	0	1.8	0.5	0.5	0.4
1303	Turkey roll, light and dark meat	2	slice(s)	57	39.8	84	10.3	1.2	0	4.0	1.2	1.3	1.0
1302	Turkey roll, light meat	2	slice(s)	57	42.9	56	9.2	1.4	0	1.2	0.3	0.3	0.3
Processed Meats													
	Beef												
1331	Corned beef loaf, jellied, sliced	2	slice(s)	57	39.2	87	13.0	0	0	3.5	1.5	1.5	0.2
	Bologna												
13459	Beef	1	slice(s)	28	15.4	90	3.0	1.0	0	8.0	3.5	2.4	0.2
13461	Light, made with pork and chicken	1	slice(s)	28	—	60	3.0	2.0	0	4.0	1.0	2.0	0.4
13458	Made with chicken and pork	1	slice(s)	28	15.0	90	3.0	1.0	0	8.0	3.0	2.6	0.7
3260	Turkey	1	slice(s)	57	36.6	119	6.5	2.7	0.3	9.1	2.5	3.9	2.2
	Chicken												
56941	Deli-sliced, oven roasted	1	slice(s)	9	6.3	13	1.2	0.3	0	0.8	0.3	0.2	0.1
	Ham												
7127	Deli-sliced, honey	1	slice(s)	10	—	10	1.5	0.5	0	0.3	0	—	—
7126	Deli-sliced, smoked	1	slice(s)	9	—	10	1.5	0.2	0	0.2	0.1	—	—
8614	**Mortadella, beef & pork, sliced**	2	slice(s)	46	24.1	143	7.5	1.4	0	11.7	4.4	5.2	1.4
1323	**Pork olive loaf**	2	slice(s)	57	33.1	133	6.7	5.2	0	9.4	3.3	4.5	1.1
1324	**Pork pickle & pimento loaf**	2	slice(s)	57	34.2	128	6.4	4.8	0.9	9.1	3.0	4.0	1.6
	Sausages & frankfurters												
37296	Beerwurst beef, beer salami (bierwurst)	1	slice(s)	29	16.6	74	4.1	1.2	0	5.7	2.5	2.7	0.2
37257	Beerwurst pork beer salami	1	slice(s)	21	12.9	50	3.0	0.4	0	4.0	1.3	1.9	0.5
35338	Berliner, pork & beef	1	ounce(s)	28	17.3	65	4.3	0.7	0	4.9	1.7	2.3	0.4
37298	Bratwurst pork, cooked	1	piece(s)	74	42.3	181	10.4	1.9	0	14.3	5.1	6.7	1.5
37299	Braunschweiger pork liver sausage	1	slice(s)	15	7.7	50	2.2	0.5	0	4.3	1.4	1.9	0.5
1329	Cheesefurter or cheese smokie, beef & pork	1	item(s)	43	22.6	141	6.1	0.6	0	12.5	4.5	5.9	1.3
1330	Chorizo, beef & pork	2	ounce(s)	57	18.1	258	13.7	1.1	0	21.7	8.2	10.4	2.0
8600	Frankfurter, beef	1	item(s)	45	24.3	141	5.0	1.7	0	12.5	4.9	5.4	0.3
202	Frankfurter, beef & pork	1	item(s)	45	25.2	137	5.2	0.8	0	12.4	4.8	6.2	1.2
1293	Frankfurter, chicken	1	item(s)	45	28.1	100	7.0	1.2	0.2	7.3	1.7	2.7	1.7
42303	Frankfurter, low sodium	1	item(s)	57	32.3	178	6.8	1.0	0	16.3	6.9	7.8	0.8

PAGE KEY: A-6 5 Breads/Baked Goods A-12 = Cereal/Rice/Pasta A-16 = Fruit A-22 = Vegetables/Legumes A-32 = Nuts/Seeds A-34 = Vegetarian A-36 = Dairy A-44 = Eggs A-44 = Seafood A-46 = Meats A-50 = Poultry A-52 = Processed Meats A-54 = Beverages A-58 = Fats/Oils A-60 = Sweets A-62 = Spices/Condiments/Sauces A-66 = Mixed Foods/Soups/Sandwiches A-72 = Fast Food A-90 = Convenience A-92 = Baby Foods

Chol (mg)	Calc (mg)	Iron (mg)	Magn (mg)	Pota (mg)	Sodi (mg)	Zinc (mg)	Vit A (µg)	Thia (mg)	Vit E (mg α)	Ribo (mg)	Niac (mg)	Vit B$_6$ (mg)	Fola (µg)	Vit C (mg)	Vit B$_{12}$ (µg)	Sele (µg)
64	11	0.92	19.6	200.7	43.4	0.66	6.8	0.05	0.23	0.08	8.90	0.46	2.6	0	0.3	21.9
64	10	1.03	17.9	194.7	63.8	1.29	10.2	0.05	—	0.13	6.70	0.35	4.3	0	0.2	20.9
315	14	2.71	2.6	152.2	47.6	3.76	0	0.02	0.17	0.18	2.65	0.06	4.3	0	0.9	35.0
479	9	9.89	21.3	223.7	64.6	3.38	3385.4	0.25	0.70	1.69	9.39	0.64	491.5	23.7	14.3	70.1
71	12	0.99	17.9	153.1	59.5	1.69	12.8	0.04	0.23	0.14	5.20	0.22	5.1	0	0.2	17.8
71	9	2.30	13.6	173.5	50.2	1.58	53.6	0.15	0.60	0.23	4.10	0.15	5.1	0	0.3	17.0
76	10	2.30	17.0	214.3	55.3	2.21	19.6	0.22	0.60	0.40	4.34	0.21	8.5	0	0.3	19.0
77	11	2.41	18.7	279.8	59.5	2.23	17.9	0.07	1.48	0.27	3.54	0.31	1.7	0	0.3	18.5
82	12	2.44	21.3	330.0	64.6	2.70	10.2	0.08	—	0.33	3.47	0.40	10.2	0	0.4	21.7
78	36	2.86	6.8	71.8	362.4	0.48	520.5	0.05	—	0.16	1.31	0.03	31.2	0	4.9	22.9
79	24	1.29	25.5	250.0	66.3	2.64	20.4	0.07	0.09	0.18	7.42	0.54	6.0	0	1.1	26.4
71	13	2.07	14.1	258.5	533.0	1.35	9.4	0.09	0.87	0.18	2.16	0.19	57.3	0	0.2	20.8
109	14	1.22	23.0	193.0	88.4	2.98	4.3	0.05	0.06	0.32	5.69	0.37	7.7	0	1.4	26.7
71	10	1.30	24.7	248.3	44.2	1.48	0	0.04	0.08	0.11	6.37	0.48	5.1	0	0.3	27.3
68	8	0.60	27.2	211.7	84.2	1.46	2.6	0.03	0.05	0.17	9.99	0.69	8.5	0	0.3	25.7
31	18	0.77	10.2	153.1	270.5	1.13	0	0.05	0.19	0.16	2.72	0.15	2.8	0	0.1	16.6
28	5	0.20	11.3	281.8	526.2	0.48	0	0.01	0.07	0.03	4.23	0.11	2.3	0	0.3	10.8
27	6	1.16	6.2	57.3	540.4	2.32	0	0	—	0.06	1.00	0.07	4.5	0	0.7	9.8
20	0	0.36	4.0	47.6	310.0	0.58	0	0.01	—	0.03	0.69	0.05	3.7	0	0.4	—
20	40	0.36	—	45.6	300.0	—	0	—	—	—	—	—	—	0	—	—
30	20	0.36	6.0	43.1	300.0	0.40	—	—	—	—	—	—	—	0	—	—
43	70	1.70	9.1	76.5	607.3	0.74	5.1	0.03	0.26	0.05	1.48	0.14	5.1	7.5	0.1	8.7
5	0	0.06	2.2	27.2	108.3	0.10	0.8	—	—	—	—	—	—	0	—	—
5	0	0.06	—	—	125.0	—	0	—	—	—	—	—	—	0	—	—
5	0	0.06	—	—	111.6	—	0	—	—	—	—	—	—	0	—	—
26	8	0.64	5.1	75.0	573.2	0.97	0	0.05	0.10	0.07	1.23	0.06	1.4	0	0.7	10.4
22	62	0.31	10.8	168.7	547.6	0.78	34.1	0.17	0.14	0.15	1.04	0.13	1.1	0	0.7	9.3
33	62	0.76	19.3	210.7	590.7	0.95	44.3	0.22	0.23	0.07	1.41	0.24	21.0	4.4	0.3	4.5
18	3	0.44	3.5	66.5	264.9	0.71	0	0.02	0.06	0.04	0.99	0.05	0.9	0	0.6	4.7
12	2	0.16	2.7	53.3	261.0	0.36	0	0.12	0.04	0.04	0.68	0.07	0.6	0	0.2	4.4
13	3	0.33	4.3	80.2	367.7	0.70	0	0.11	—	0.06	0.88	0.06	1.4	0	0.8	4.0
44	33	0.95	11.1	156.9	412.2	1.70	0	0.37	0.01	0.14	2.37	0.16	1.5	0.7	0.7	15.7
27	1	1.70	1.7	30.2	176.2	0.43	641.0	0.04	0.05	0.23	1.27	0.05	6.7	0	3.1	8.8
29	25	0.46	5.6	88.6	465.3	0.97	2.6	0.11	0.10	0.07	1.25	0.06	1.3	0	0.7	6.8
50	5	0.90	10.2	225.6	700.1	1.93	0	0.36	0.12	0.17	2.91	0.30	1.1	0	1.1	12.0
25	6	0.56	4.9	130.5	466.6	0.93	0	0.01	0.09	0.02	0.94	0.08	4.5	0	0.6	5.0
23	5	0.52	4.5	75.2	368.5	0.83	8.1	0.09	0.11	0.05	1.18	0.06	1.8	0	0.6	6.2
43	33	0.53	9.0	90.9	340.2	0.50	0	0.03	0.10	0.12	2.11	0.15	4.9	0	0.2	10.4
35	11	0.82	1.7	94.6	177.3	1.24	0	0.03	0.10	0.06	1.38	0.07	2.3	0	0.9	6.8

TABLE A-2 Table of Food Composition *(continued)*   (Computer code is for Cengage Diet Analysis program)   (For purposes of calculations, use "0" for t, <1, <0.1, <0.01)

DA+ Code	Food Description	Quantity	Measure	Wt (g)	H₂O (g)	Ener (kcal)	Prot (g)	Carb (g)	Fiber (g)	Fat (g)	Fat Breakdown (g) Sat	Mono	Poly
Processed Meats—*continued*													
3261	Frankfurter, turkey	1	item(s)	45	28.3	100	5.5	1.7	0	7.8	1.8	2.6	1.8
37275	Italian sausage, pork, cooked	1	item(s)	68	32.0	235	13.0	2.9	0.1	18.6	6.6	8.7	2.4
37307	Kielbasa, kolbassa, pork & beef	1	slice(s)	30	16.6	94	3.7	0.9	0	8.3	2.8	3.6	1.2
1333	Knockwurst or knackwurst, beef & pork	2	ounce(s)	57	31.3	174	6.3	1.8	0	15.7	5.8	7.3	1.7
37285	Pepperoni, beef & pork	1	slice(s)	11	3.4	54	2.5	0	0	4.8	1.6	1.9	0.4
37313	Polish sausage, pork	1	slice(s)	21	11.1	68	2.9	0.3	0	6.0	2.2	2.8	0.6
206	Salami, beef, cooked, sliced	2	slice(s)	52	31.2	136	6.6	1.0	0	11.5	5.1	5.5	0.5
54045	Salami, pork & beef, dry, sliced, 50% less sodium	1	slice(s)	6	2.3	20	1.2	0.4	0	1.5	0.5	0.7	0.1
37272	Salami, pork, dry or hard	1	slice(s)	13	4.6	52	2.9	0.2	0	4.3	1.5	2.0	0.5
40987	Sausage, turkey, cooked	2	ounce(s)	57	36.9	111	13.5	0.0	0	5.9	1.3	1.7	1.5
8620	Smoked sausage, beef & pork	2	ounce(s)	57	30.6	181	6.8	1.4	0	16.3	5.5	6.9	2.2
8619	Smoked sausage, pork	2	ounce(s)	57	32.0	175	6.8	0.5	0	16.0	5.3	6.4	2.1
37273	Smoked sausage, pork link	1	piece(s)	76	42.8	233	9.1	0.1	0	21.4	7.1	8.5	2.7
1336	Summer sausage, thuringer, or cervelat, beef & pork	2	ounce(s)	57	25.6	205	9.9	1.9	0	17.3	6.5	7.4	0.7
37294	Vienna sausage, cocktail, beef & pork, canned	1	piece(s)	16	10.4	37	1.7	0.4	0	3.1	1.1	1.5	0.2
Spreads													
1318	Ham salad spread	¼	cup(s)	60	37.6	130	5.2	6.4	0	9.3	3.0	4.3	1.6
32419	Pork and beef sandwich spread	4	tablespoon(s)	60	36.2	141	4.6	7.2	0.1	10.4	3.6	4.6	1.5
Turkey													
71632	Breast, honey roasted & smoked, presliced	1	slice(s)	28	—	30	5.0	2.0	0	0.5	0	—	—
71612	Breast, oven roasted deli slices, lower sodium	1	slice(s)	28	—	25	5.0	0.5	0	0.5		—	—
71631	Breast, oven roasted, presliced	1	slice(s)	28	—	30	5.0	1.0	0	0.5	0	—	—
7124	Breast, oven-roasted	1	slice(s)	9	—	8	1.5	0.3	0	0.1	0	—	—
71633	Breast, smoked, presliced	1	slice(s)	28	—	30	5.0	1.0	0	0.5	0	—	—
71629	Ham	1	slice(s)	28	—	40	5.0	0.5	0	2.0	0.5	—	—
37270	Pastrami	1	slice(s)	28	20.3	38	4.6	0.5	0	1.8	0.5	0.6	0.5
3262	Salami	2	slice(s)	57	39.1	98	10.9	0.9	0.1	5.2	1.6	1.8	1.4
37318	Salami, cooked	1	slice(s)	28	19.5	49	5.5	0.4	0	2.6	0.8	0.9	0.7
Beverages													
Beer													
866	Ale, mild	12	fluid ounce(s)	360	331.1	155	1.7	12.8	0	0	0	0.0	0
686	Beer	12	fluid ounce(s)	356	327.7	153	1.6	12.7	0	0	0	0	0
16886	Beer, non alcoholic	12	fluid ounce(s)	360	328.1	133	0.8	29.0	0	0.4	0.1	0.1	0.2
31609	Bud Light beer	12	fluid ounce(s)	355	337.3	110	0.9	6.6	0	0	0	0	0
31608	Budweiser beer	12	fluid ounce(s)	355	329.3	145	1.3	10.6	0	0	0	0	0
869	Light beer	12	fluid ounce(s)	354	335.9	103	0.8	5.8	0	0	0	0.0	0
31613	Michelob Beer	12	fluid ounce(s)	355	326.5	164	1.7	15.0	0	0	0	0	0
31614	Michelob Light beer	12	fluid ounce(s)	355	336.8	123	1.4	8.8	0	0	0	0	0
Gin, rum, vodka, whiskey													
687	Distilled alcohol, 80 proof	1	fluid ounce(s)	28	18.5	64	0	0	0	0	0	0	0
688	Distilled alcohol, 86 proof	1	fluid ounce(s)	28	17.8	70	0	0	0	0	0	0	0
689	Distilled alcohol, 90 proof	1	fluid ounce(s)	28	17.3	73	0	0	0	0	0	0	0
856	Distilled alcohol, 94 proof	1	fluid ounce(s)	28	16.8	76	0	0	0	0	0	0.0	0
857	Distilled alcohol, 100 proof	1	fluid ounce(s)	28	16.0	82	0	0	0	0	0	0.0	0
Liqueurs													
33187	Coffee liqueur, 53 proof	1	fluid ounce(s)	35	10.8	113	0	16.3	0	0.1	0	0	0
3142	Coffee liqueur, 63 proof	1	fluid ounce(s)	35	14.4	107	0	11.2	0	0.1	0	0	0
736	Cordials, 54 proof	1	fluid ounce(s)	30	8.9	104	0	13.3	0	0.1	0	0	0
Wine													
861	California red wine	5	fluid ounce(s)	150	133.4	125	0.3	3.7	0	0	0	0	0
858	Domestic champagne	5	fluid ounce(s)	150	—	105	0.3	3.8	0	0	0	0	0
690	Sweet dessert wine	5	fluid ounce(s)	147	103.7	235	0.3	20.1	0	0	0	0	0
1481	White wine	5	fluid ounce(s)	148	128.1	121	0.1	3.8	0	0	0.0	0	0
1811	Wine cooler	10	fluid ounce(s)	300	266.8	165	0.2	19.6	0	0.1	0	0	0

Chol (mg)	Calc (mg)	Iron (mg)	Magn (mg)	Pota (mg)	Sodi (mg)	Zinc (mg)	Vit A (µg)	Thia (mg)	Vit E (mg α)	Ribo (mg)	Niac (mg)	Vit B$_6$ (mg)	Fola (µg)	Vit C (mg)	Vit B$_{12}$ (µg)	Sele (µg)
35	67	0.66	6.3	176.4	410.0	0.83	0	0.02	0.28	0.08	1.66	0.06	4.5	0	0.4	6.8
39	14	0.97	12.2	206.7	820.8	1.63	6.8	0.42	0.17	0.16	2.83	0.22	3.4	0.1	0.9	15.0
20	5	0.25	4.0	91.4	275.4	0.48	0	0.06	0.07	0.06	1.00	0.06	0.3	0	0.2	5.9
34	6	0.37	6.2	112.8	527.2	0.94	0	0.19	0.32	0.08	1.55	0.10	1.1	0	0.7	7.7
12	2	0.18	2.3	30.7	181.8	0.28	0	0.04	0	0.03	0.51	0.04	0.6	0.1	0.2	3.8
15	2	0.30	2.9	49.4	182.5	0.40	0	0.10	0.05	0.03	0.72	0.04	0.4	0.2	0.2	3.7
37	3	1.14	6.8	97.8	592.8	0.92	0	0.05	0.10	0.10	1.68	0.09	1.0	0	1.6	7.6
5	0	0.08	1.0	21.2	52.4	0.18	0	0.03	0.02	0.02	0.27	0.03	0.1	0	0.1	1.5
10	2	0.17	2.8	48.4	289.3	0.54	0	0.12	0.03	0.04	0.72	0.07	0.3	0	0.4	3.3
52	12	0.84	11.9	169.0	377.1	2.20	7.4	0.05	0.10	0.14	3.24	0.18	3.4	0.4	0.7	0
33	7	0.43	7.4	101.5	516.6	0.71	7.4	0.11	0.07	0.06	1.67	0.09	1.1	0	0.3	0
35	6	0.33	6.2	273.8	468.8	0.74	0	0.12	0.14	0.10	1.59	0.10	0.6	0	0.4	10.4
46	8	0.45	8.3	366.0	626.6	0.99	0	0.16	0.19	0.14	2.13	0.14	0.8	0	0.5	13.9
42	5	1.16	7.9	147.4	737.0	1.45	0	0.09	0.12	0.19	2.44	0.15	1.1	9.4	3.1	11.5
14	2	0.14	1.1	16.2	155.0	0.26	0	0.01	0.04	0.02	0.26	0.02	0.6	0	0.2	2.7
22	5	0.35	6.0	90.0	645.0	0.66	0	0.26	1.04	0.07	1.26	0.09	0.6	0	0.5	10.7
23	7	0.47	4.8	66.0	607.8	0.61	15.6	0.10	1.04	0.08	1.04	0.07	1.2	0	0.7	5.8
10	0	0	—	—	240.0	—	0	—	—	—	—	—	—	0	—	—
15	0	0.18	—	—	175.0	—	0	—	—	—	—	—	—	0	—	—
10	0	0	—	—	240.0	—	0	—	—	—	—	—	—	0	—	—
3	0	0.06	—	—	103.3	—	0	—	—	—	—	—	—	0	—	—
10	0	0	—	—	240.0	—	0	—	—	—	—	—	—	0	—	—
18	0	0.72	—	—	315.0	—	0	—	—	—	—	—	—	0	—	—
19	3	1.19	4.0	97.8	278.1	0.61	1.1	0.02	0.06	0.07	1.00	0.08	1.4	2.3	0.1	4.6
43	23	0.71	12.5	122.5	627.7	1.32	1.1	0.24	0.14	0.17	2.26	0.24	5.7	0	0.6	15.0
22	11	0.35	6.2	61.2	284.6	0.66	0.6	0.12	0.07	0.09	1.13	0.12	2.8	0	0.3	7.5
0	14	0.07	21.6	97.2	14.4	0.04	0	0.02	0	0.09	1.85	0.17	21.6	0	0.1	2.2
0	14	0.07	21.4	96.2	14.3	0.04	0	0.02	0	0.09	1.83	0.16	21.4	0	0.1	2.1
0	25	0.22	25.2	28.8	46.8	0.07	0	0.06	0	0.17	4.01	0.10	50.4	1.8	0.1	4.3
0	14	0.11	24.9	92.3	10.6	0	0	0.02	0	0.05	1.39	0.12	21.3	0	0.1	1.4
0	14	0	24.9	117.2	10.6	0	0	0.02	0	0.09	1.82	0.16	21.3	0	0.1	2.1
0	14	0.11	17.7	74.3	14.2	0.04	0	0.02	0	0.05	1.38	0.12	21.2	0	0.1	1.4
0	14	0.07	21.3	95.8	9.0	0.04	0	0.02	0	0.09	1.82	0.16	21.3	0	0.1	2.1
0	14	0.11	17.8	74.6	9.0	0.04	0	0.02	0	0.05	1.39	0.12	21.3	0	0.1	1.4
0	0	0.01	0	0.6	0.3	0.01	0	0	0	0	0	0	0	0	0	0
0	0	0.01	0	0.6	0.3	0.01	0	0	0	0	0	0	0	0	0	0
0	0	0.01	0	0.6	0.3	0.01	0	0	0	0	0	0	0	0	0	0
0	0	0.01	0	0.6	0.3	0.01	0	0	—	0	0	0	0	0	0	0
0	0	0.01	0	0.6	0.3	0.01	0	0	—	0	0	0	0	0	0	0
0	0	0.02	1.0	10.4	2.8	0.01	0	0	0	0	0.05	0	0	0	0	0.1
0	0	0.02	1.0	10.4	2.8	0.01	0	0	—	0	0.05	0	0	0	0	0.1
0	0	0.02	0.6	4.5	1.8	0.01	0	0	0	0	0.02	0	0	0	0	0.1
0	12	1.43	16.2	170.6	15.0	0.15	0	0.02	0	0.04	0.12	0.05	—	0	0	—
0	—	—	—	—	—	—	—	—	—	—	—	—	—	—	0	—
0	12	0.35	13.2	135.4	13.2	0.10	0	0.03	0	0.03	0.31	0	0	0	0	0.7
0	13	0.40	14.8	104.7	7.4	0.18	0	0.01	0	0.02	0.16	0.07	1.5	0	0	0.1
0	18	0.78	18.0	147.0	21.0	0.24	0	0.02	0.03	0.03	0.25	0.08	3.0	5.4	0	0.3

TABLE A-2 Table of Food Composition (*continued*)   (Computer code is for Cengage Diet Analysis program)   (For purposes of calculations, use "0" for t, <1, <0.1, <0.01)

DA+ Code	Food Description	Quantity	Measure	Wt (g)	H₂O (g)	Ener (kcal)	Prot (g)	Carb (g)	Fiber (g)	Fat (g)	Fat Breakdown (g) Sat	Mono	Poly
Beverages—*continued*													
	Carbonated												
31898	7 Up	12	fluid ounce(s)	360	320.4	150	0	39.0	0	0	0	0	0
692	Club soda	12	fluid ounce(s)	355	354.8	0	0	0	0	0	0	0	0
12010	Coca-Cola Classic cola soda	12	fluid ounce(s)	360	325.1	210	0	58.5	0	0	0	0	0
693	Cola	12	fluid ounce(s)	368	332.7	136	0.3	35.2	0	0.1	0	0	0
2391	Cola or pepper-type soda, low calorie with saccharin	12	fluid ounce(s)	355	354.5	0	0	0.4	0	0	0	0	0
9522	Cola soda, decaffeinated	12	fluid ounce(s)	372	333.4	153	0.0	39.4	0	0	0	0	0
9524	Cola, decaffeinated, low calorie with aspartame	12	fluid ounce(s)	355	354.3	4	0.4	0.5	0	0	0	0	0
1415	Cola, low calorie with aspartame	12	fluid ounce(s)	355	353.6	7	0.4	1.0	0	0.1	0	0	0
1412	Cream soda	12	fluid ounce(s)	371	321.5	189	0	49.3	0	0	0	0	0
31899	Diet 7 Up	12	fluid ounce(s)	360	—	0	0	0	0	0	0	0	0
12031	Diet Coke cola soda	12	fluid ounce(s)	360	358.3	2	0	0.2	0	0	0	0	0
29392	Diet Mountain Dew soda	12	fluid ounce(s)	354	—	0	0	0	0	0	0	0	0
29389	Diet Pepsi cola soda	12	fluid ounce(s)	354	352.8	0	0	0	0	0	0	0	0
12034	Diet Sprite soda	12	fluid ounce(s)	360	—	4	0	0	0	0	0	0	0
695	Ginger ale	12	fluid ounce(s)	366	333.9	124	0	32.1	0	0	0	0	0
694	Grape soda	12	fluid ounce(s)	372	330.3	160	0	41.7	0	0	0	0	0
1876	Lemon lime soda	12	fluid ounce(s)	368	330.7	147	0.2	37.4	0	0.1	0	0	0
29391	Mountain Dew soda	12	fluid ounce(s)	354	—	170	0	46.0	0	0	0	0	0
3145	Orange soda	12	fluid ounce(s)	372	325.9	179	0	45.8	0	0	0	0	0
1414	Pepper-type soda	12	fluid ounce(s)	368	329.3	151	0	38.3	0	0.4	0.3	0	0
29388	Pepsi regular cola soda	12	fluid ounce(s)	354	313.3	150	0	41.0	0	0	0	0	0
696	Root beer	12	fluid ounce(s)	370	330.1	152	0	39.2	0	0	0	0	0
12044	Sprite soda	12	fluid ounce(s)	360	323.2	144	0	39.0	0	0	0	0	0
	Coffee												
731	Brewed	8	fluid ounce(s)	237	235.6	2	0.3	0	0	0	0	0	0
9520	Brewed, decaffeinated	8	fluid ounce(s)	237	234.3	5	0.3	1.0	0	0	0	0	0
16882	Cappuccino	8	fluid ounce(s)	240	224.5	77	4.0	6.2	0.2	4.0	2.3	1.0	0.2
16883	Cappuccino, decaffeinated	8	fluid ounce(s)	240	224.4	74	4.0	6.2	0.2	4.0	2.3	1.0	0.2
16880	Espresso	8	fluid ounce(s)	237	231.8	5	0.3	0	0	0.4	0.2	0	0.2
16881	Espresso, decaffeinated	8	fluid ounce(s)	237	231.8	0	0.2	0	0	0.4	0.2	0	0.2
732	Instant, prepared	8	fluid ounce(s)	239	236.5	5	0.2	0.8	0	0	0	0	0
67526	Starbucks Doubleshot Energy, coffee, canned	15	fluid ounce(s)	443	—	210	12.0	36.0	0	2.0	2.5	—	—
67525	Starbucks Doubleshot, canned	6.5	fluid ounce(s)	192	—	138	4.1	17.9	—	5.7	3.7	—	—
32561	Starbucks Frappuccino, bottled, coffee	9.5	fluid ounce(s)	281	—	200	6.0	37.0	0	3.0	2.0	—	—
32562	Starbucks Frappuccino, bottled, mocha	9.5	fluid ounce(s)	281	—	180	7.0	33.0	0	3.0	2.0	—	—
	Fruit drinks												
29357	Crystal Light sugar-free lemonade drink	8	fluid ounce(s)	237	—	592	0	0	0	0	0	0	0
6012	Fruit punch drink with added vitamin C, canned	8	fluid ounce(s)	248	218.2	119	0	29.7	0	0	0	0	0
31143	Gatorade Thirst Quencher, all flavors	8	fluid ounce(s)	240	—	50	0	14.0	0	0	0	0	0
260	Grape drink, canned	8	fluid ounce(s)	250	210.5	153	0	39.4	0	0	0	0	0
17372	Kool-Aid (lemonade/punch/fruit drink)	8	fluid ounce(s)	248	220.0	108	0.1	27.8	0.2	0	0	0	0
17225	Kool-Aid sugar-free, low-calorie tropical punch drink mix, prepared	8	fluid ounce(s)	240	—	5	0	0	0	0	0	0	0
266	Lemonade, prepared from frozen concentrate	8	fluid ounce(s)	248	221.6	99	0.2	25.8	0	0.1	0	0	0
268	Limeade, prepared from frozen concentrate	8	fluid ounce(s)	247	212.6	128	0	34.1	0	0	0	0	0
57054	Odwalla Pomegranate Limeade	8	fluid ounce(s)	240	—	122	0	29.7	0	0	0	0	0
14266	Odwalla Strawberry C Monster smoothie blend	8	fluid ounce(s)	240	—	240	0	56.0	1.0	0	0	0	0
10099	Snapple fruit punch fruit drink	8	fluid ounce(s)	240	—	110	0	27.0	0	0	0	0	0

Chol (mg)	Calc (mg)	Iron (mg)	Magn (mg)	Pota (mg)	Sodi (mg)	Zinc (mg)	Vit A (µg)	Thia (mg)	Vit E (mg α)	Ribo (mg)	Niac (mg)	Vit B$_6$ (mg)	Fola (µg)	Vit C (mg)	Vit B$_{12}$ (µg)	Sele (µg)
0	7	0.07	3.6	3.6	37.5	0.04	0	0	0	0	0.05	0	0	0	0	0
0	18	0.04	3.6	7.1	74.6	0.36	0	0	0	0	0	0	0	0	0	0
0	7	0.00	0	0	67.5	0.07	0	0	0	0	0	0	0	0	0	0.4
0	7	0.41	0	7.4	14.7	0.07	0	0	0	0	0	0	0	0	0	0.4
0	14	0.07	3.6	14.2	56.8	0.11	0	0	0	0	0	0	0	0	0	0.4
0	7	0.07	0	11.2	14.9	0.04	0	0	0	0	0	0	0	0	0	0.4
0	11	0.07	0	24.9	14.2	0.04	0	0.02	0	0.08	0	0	0	0	0	0.4
0	11	0.39	3.6	28.4	28.4	0.04	0	0.02	0	0.08	0	0	0	0	0	0
0	19	0.19	3.7	3.7	44.5	0.26	0	0	0	0	0	0	0	0	0	0
0	—	—	—	—	45.0	—	—	—	—	—	—	—	—	—	—	—
0	11	0.40	3.6	18.0	42.0	0.04	0	0.02	0	0.08	0	0	0	0	0	0
0	0	0	—	80.0	50.0	—	0	—	—	—	—	—	—	0	—	—
0	0	0	3.6	30.0	35.0	0.04	0	0.02	0	0.08	0	0	0	0	0	0
0	0	0.00	—	109.5	36.0	—	0	—	—	—	—	—	—	0	—	—
0	11	0.66	3.7	3.7	25.6	0.18	0	0	0	0	0	0	0	0	0	0.4
0	11	0.30	3.7	3.7	55.8	0.26	0	0	—	0	0	0	0	0	0	0
0	7	0.41	3.7	3.7	33.2	0.15	0	0	0	0	0.06	0	0	0	0	0
0	0	0	—	5.0	65.0	—	0	—	—	—	—	—	—	0	—	—
0	19	0.22	3.7	7.4	44.6	0.37	0	0	—	0	0	0	0	0	0	0
0	11	0.15	0	3.7	36.8	0.15	0	0	—	0	0	0	0	0	0	0.4
0	0	0	0.0	10.0	30.0	0.07	0	0	0	0	0	0	0	0	0	0.4
0	18	0.18	3.7	3.7	48.0	0.26	0	0	0	0	0	0	0	0	0	0.4
0	7	0.40	3.6	0	70.5	0.14	0	0	0	0	0.05	0	0	0	0	0
0	5	0.02	7.1	116.1	4.7	0.05	0	0.03	0.02	0.18	0.45	0	4.7	0	0	0
0	9	0.09	9.5	85.2	9.5	0.02	0	0	0	0.03	0.67	0	0	0	0	0.5
12	144	0.10	16.8	220.8	55.2	0.48	55.2	0.07	0.10	0.29	0.34	0.04	7.2	0	0.4	4.6
12	144	0.14	19.2	225.6	55.2	0.48	55.2	0.05	0.10	0.21	0.38	0.04	4.8	0	0.4	4.6
0	5	0.31	189.6	272.5	33.2	0.12	0	0	0.02	0.42	12.34	0	2.4	0.5	0	0
0	5	0.31	189.6	272.5	33.2	0.12	0	0	0	0.42	12.34	0	2.4	0.5	0	0
0	10	0.10	9.5	71.6	9.5	0.02	0	0	0	0	0.56	0	0	0	0	0.2
15	4	0	—	—	170.0	—	0	—	—	1.70	20.00	2.00	—	0.3	3.0	—
20	162	0	—	20.3	69.1	—	0	—	—	—	—	—	—	0	—	—
15	3	0	—	—	100.0	—	0	—	—	—	—	—	—	0	—	—
15	2	0	—	—	95.0	—	0	—	—	—	—	—	—	0	—	—
0	0	0	—	—	4140.5	—	0	—	—	—	—	—	—	0	—	—
0	20	0.22	7.4	62.0	24.8	0.03	1.7	0.05	0.05	0.06	0.05	0.03	9.9	89.3	0	0.5
0	2	0	—	30.0	110.0	—	0	—	—	—	—	—	—	0	—	—
0	130	0.17	2.5	30.0	40.0	0.30	0	0	0	0.01	0.03	0	0	78.5	0	0.3
0	14	0.46	5.0	49.6	31.0	0.20	—	0.04	—	0.05	0.05	0.01	—	41.6	0	1.0
0	0	0	—	10.1	10.1	—	0	—	—	—	—	—	—	6.0	—	—
0	10	0.40	5.0	37.2	9.9	0.05	0	0.01	0.02	0.05	0.04	0.01	2.5	9.7	0	0.2
0	5	0	4.9	24.7	7.4	0.02	0	0	0	0.01	0.02	0.01	2.5	7.7	0	0.2
0	0	0	—	—	10.1	—	0	—	—	—	—	—	—	0	—	—
0	40	1.08	—	600.0	30.0	—	0	—	—	—	—	—	—	900.0	—	—
0	0	0	—	20.0	5.0	—	0	—	—	—	—	—	—	0	—	—

TABLE A-2 **Table of Food Composition** (continued)   (Computer code is for Cengage Diet Analysis program)   (For purposes of calculations, use "0" for t, <1, <0.1, <0.01)

DA+ Code	Food Description	Quantity	Measure	Wt (g)	H₂O (g)	Ener (kcal)	Prot (g)	Carb (g)	Fiber (g)	Fat (g)	Sat	Mono	Poly
Beverages—*continued*													
10096	Snapple kiwi strawberry fruit drink	8	fluid ounce(s)	240	211.2	110	0	27.0	0	0	0	0	0
14818	SunnyD Tangy Original	6 ¾	fluid ounce(s)	203	—	76	0	18.6	0	0	0	0	0
	Slim Fast ready-to-drink shake												
16054	French Vanilla	10	fluid ounce(s)	325	—	220	10.0	40.0	5.0	2.5	0.5	1.5	0.5
10095	Rich Chocolate Royale	10	fluid ounce(s)	325	—	220	10.0	40.0	5.0	3.0	1.0	1.5	0.5
16055	Strawberries 'n' Cream	10	fluid ounce(s)	325	—	220	10.0	40.0	5.0	2.5	0.5	1.5	0.5
	Tea												
33179	Decaffeinated, prepared	8	fluid ounce(s)	237	236.3	2	0	0.7	0	0	0	0	0
1877	Herbal, prepared	8	fluid ounce(s)	237	236.1	2	0	0.5	0	0	0	0	0
735	Instant tea mix, lemon flavored with sugar, prepared	8	fluid ounce(s)	259	236.2	91	0	22.3	0.3	0.2	0	0	0
734	Instant tea mix, unsweetened, prepared	8	fluid ounce(s)	238	237.1	2	0.1	0.4	0	0	0	0	0
16097	Nestea with lemon, canned	12	fluid ounce(s)	360	328.2	125	0	34.5	0	0	0	0	0
733	Prepared	8	fluid ounce(s)	237	236.3	2	0	0.7	0	0	0	0	0
	Water												
1413	Mineral water, carbonated	8	fluid ounce(s)	237	236.8	0	0	0	0	0	0	0	0
33183	Poland spring water, bottled	8	fluid ounce(s)	237	237.0	0	0	0	0	0	0	0	0
1821	Tap water	8	fluid ounce(s)	237	236.8	0	0	0	0	0	0	0	0
1879	Tonic water	8	fluid ounce(s)	244	222.3	83	0	21.5	0	0	0	0	0
Fats and Oils													
	Butter												
104	Butter	1	tablespoon(s)	14	2.3	102	0.1	0	0	11.5	7.3	3.0	0.4
2522	Butter Buds, dry butter substitute	1	teaspoon(s)	2	0.1	7	0	1.6	0	0.1	0.1	—	—
921	Unsalted	1	tablespoon(s)	14	2.5	102	0.1	0	0	11.5	7.3	3.0	0.4
107	Whipped	1	tablespoon(s)	9	1.5	67	0.1	0	0	7.6	4.7	2.2	0.3
944	Whipped, unsalted	1	tablespoon(s)	9	1.7	67	0.1	0	0	7.6	4.8	2.0	0.3
	Fats, cooking												
2671	Beef tallow, semisolid	1	tablespoon(s)	13	0	115	0	0	0	12.8	6.4	5.4	0.5
922	Chicken fat	1	tablespoon(s)	13	0	115	0	0	0	12.8	3.8	5.7	2.7
5454	Household shortening with vegetable oil	1	tablespoon(s)	13	0	115	0	0	0	13.0	3.4	5.5	3.5
111	Lard	1	tablespoon(s)	13	0	115	0	0	0	12.8	5.0	5.8	1.4
	Margarine												
114	Margarine	1	tablespoon(s)	14	2.3	101	0	0.1	0	11.4	2.1	5.5	3.4
5439	Soft	1	tablespoon(s)	14	2.3	103	0.1	0.1	0	11.6	1.7	4.4	2.1
928	Unsalted	1	tablespoon(s)	14	2.6	101	0.1	0.1	0	11.3	2.1	5.2	3.5
119	Whipped	1	tablespoon(s)	9	1.5	67	0	0.1	0	7.5	1.3	3.3	2.4
	Spreads												
54657	I Can't Believe It's Not Butter!, tub, soya oil (non-hydrogenated)	1	tablespoon(s)	14	2.3	102	0.1	0.1	0	11.4	2.8	2.0	5.1
2708	Mayonnaise with soybean and safflower oils	1	tablespoon(s)	14	2.1	99	0.2	0.4	0	11.0	1.2	1.8	7.6
57582	Promise buttery spread	1	tablespoon(s)	14	—	80	0	0	0	8.0	1.5	2.5	4.0
	Oils												
2681	Canola	1	tablespoon(s)	14	0	120	0	0	0	13.6	1.0	8.6	3.8
120	Corn	1	tablespoon(s)	14	0	122	0	0	0	13.6	1.8	3.8	7.4
122	Olive	1	tablespoon(s)	14	0	119	0	0	0	13.5	1.9	9.8	1.4
124	Peanut	1	tablespoon(s)	14	0	119	0	0	0	13.5	2.3	6.2	4.3
2693	Safflower	1	tablespoon(s)	14	0	120	0	0	0	13.6	1.0	10.2	1.7
923	Sesame	1	tablespoon(s)	14	0	120	0	0	0	13.6	1.9	5.4	5.7
128	Soybean, hydrogenated	1	tablespoon(s)	14	0	120	0	0	0	13.6	2.0	5.8	5.1
130	Soybean, with soybean and cottonseed oil	1	tablespoon(s)	14	0	120	0	0	0	13.6	2.4	4.0	6.5
2700	Sunflower	1	tablespoon(s)	14	0	120	0	0	0	13.6	1.8	6.3	5.0
357	**Pam original no stick cooking spray**	1	serving(s)	0	—	0	0	0	0	0	0	0	0
	Salad dressing												
132	Blue cheese	2	tablespoon(s)	30	11.9	143	0.4	1.4	0.1	15.3	2.5	4.0	8.3
133	Blue cheese, low-calorie	2	tablespoon(s)	31	25.4	32	1.6	0.9	0	2.3	0.8	0.6	0.8

Chol (mg)	Calc (mg)	Iron (mg)	Magn (mg)	Pota (mg)	Sodi (mg)	Zinc (mg)	Vit A (µg)	Thia (mg)	Vit E (mg α)	Ribo (mg)	Niac (mg)	Vit B$_6$ (mg)	Fola (µg)	Vit C (mg)	Vit B$_{12}$ (µg)	Sele (µg)
0	0	0	—	40.0	10.0	—	0	—	—	—	—	—	—	0	—	—
0	0	0	—	—	143.4	—	0	0.19	—	—	—	—	—	50.6	—	—
5	400	2.70	140.0	600.0	220.0	2.25	525.1	0.52	—	0.60	7.00	0.70	—	60.0	2.1	17.5
5	400	2.70	140.0	600.0	220.0	2.25	525.1	0.53	—	0.60	7.00	0.70	—	60.0	2.1	17.5
5	400	2.70	140.0	600.0	220.0	2.25	525.1	0.52	—	0.60	7.00	0.70	—	60.0	2.1	17.5
0	0	0.05	7.1	87.7	7.1	0.05	0	0	0	0.03	0	0	11.9	0	0	0
0	5	0.19	2.4	21.3	2.4	0.09	0	0.02	0	0.01	0	0	2.4	0	0	0
0	5	0.05	2.6	38.8	5.2	0.03	0	0	0	0	0.03	0	0	0	0	0.3
0	7	0.02	4.8	42.8	9.5	0.02	0	0	0	0.01	0.08	0	0	0	0	0
0	11	0	3.6	68.4	46.5	0.22	0	—	—	—	—	—	—	—	—	—
0	0	0.05	7.1	87.7	7.1	0.05	0	0	0	0.03	0	0	11.9	0	0	0
0	33	0	0	0.0	2.4	0	0	0	—	0	0	0	0	0	0	0
0	2	0.02	2.4	0	2.4	0	0	0	—	0	0	0	0	0	0	0
0	7	0	2.4	2.4	7.1	0	0	0	0	0	0	0	0	0	0	0
0	2	0.02	0	0	29.3	0.24	0	0	0	0	0	0	0	0	0	0
31	3	0.00	0.3	3.4	101.4	0.01	97.1	0	0.33	0	0.01	0	0.4	0	0	0.1
0	8	0	0	—	80.2	0	0	0	0	0	0	0	—	0	0	0
31	3	0	0.3	3.4	1.6	0.01	97.1	0	0.33	0	0.01	0	0.4	0	0	0.1
21	2	0.02	0.2	2.4	77.7	0	64.3	0	0.22	0	0	0	0.3	0	0	0.1
20	2	0	0.2	2.3	1.0	0.01	64.3	0	0.22	0	0	0	0.3	0	0	0.1
14	0	0	0	0	0	0	0	0	0.35	0	0	0	0	0	0	0
11	0	0	0	0	0	0	0	0	0.35	0	0	0	0	0	0	0
0	0	0	0	0	0	0	0	0	0	0	0	0	0	0	0	0
12	0	0	0	0	0	0.01	0	0	0.08	0	0	0	0	0	0	0
0	4	0.01	0.4	5.9	133.0	0	115.5	0	1.27	0.01	0	0	0.1	0	0	0
0	4	0	0.3	5.5	155.4	0	142.7	0	1.01	0	0	0	0.1	0	0	0
0	2	0	0.3	3.5	0.3	0	115.5	0	1.80	0	0	0	0.1	0	0	0
0	0	0	0.1	1.5	59.1	0	73.7	0	1.39	0	0	0	0.1	0	0	0
0	4	0	0.3	5.4	153.1	0	140.6	0	0.71	0	0	0	0.1	0	0	0
8	2	0.07	0.1	4.7	78.4	0.02	11.6	0	3.04	0	0	0.08	1.1	0	0	0.2
0	0	0	—	—	85.0	—	—	—	2.01	—	—	0.70	—	0	1.2	—
0	0	0	0	0	0	0	0	0	2.37	0	0	0	0	0	0	0
0	0	0	0	0	0	0	0	0	1.94	0	0	0	0	0	0	0
0	0	0.08	0	0.1	0.3	0	0	0	1.94	0	0	0	0	0	0	0
0	0	0	0	0	0	0	0	0	2.12	0	0	0	0	0	0	0
0	0	0	0	0	0	0	0	0	4.64	0	0	0	0	0	0	0
0	0	0	0	0	0	0	0	0	0.19	0	0	0	0	0	0	0
0	0	0	0	0	0	0	0	0	1.10	0	0	0	0	0	0	0
0	0	0	0	0	0	0	0	0	1.65	0	0	0	0	0	0	0
0	0	0	0	0	0	0	0	0	5.59	0	0	0	0	0	0	0
0	0	0	—	—	0	—	—	—	—	—	—	—	—	0	—	—
9	11	0.03	2.4	26.4	312.3	0.06	5.7	0	1.28	0.03	0.03	0.01	2.4	0.2	0	0.3
0	28	0.16	2.2	1.6	300.5	0.08	0	0.01	0.08	0.03	0.02	0.01	1.0	0.1	0.1	0.5

TABLE A-2 Table of Food Composition (*continued*)   (Computer code is for Cengage Diet Analysis program)   (For purposes of calculations, use "0" for t, <1, <0.1, <0.01)

DA+ Code	Food Description	Quantity	Measure	Wt (g)	H₂O (g)	Ener (kcal)	Prot (g)	Carb (g)	Fiber (g)	Fat (g)	Fat Breakdown (g) Sat	Mono	Poly
Fats and Oils—*continued*													
1764	Caesar	2	tablespoon(s)	30	10.3	163	0.7	1.0	0.2	17.4	2.6	4.1	9.9
29654	Creamy, reduced-calorie, fat-free, cholesterol free, sour cream and/or buttermilk and oil	2	tablespoon(s)	33	24.7	35	0.5	6.6	0	0.9	0.2	0.2	0.5
29617	Creamy, reduced calorie, sour cream and/or buttermilk and oil	2	tablespoon(s)	30	22.2	48	0.4	2.1	0	4.2	0.6	1.0	2.4
134	French	2	tablespoon(s)	32	11.7	146	0.2	5.0	0	14.3	1.8	2.7	6.7
135	French, low-fat	2	tablespoon(s)	32	17.4	71	0.2	10.0	0.5	3.7	0.3	1.4	1.2
136	Italian	2	tablespoon(s)	29	18.6	71	0.1	3.6	0	6.2	0.9	1.7	3.2
137	Italian, diet	2	tablespoon(s)	30	24.0	31	0.1	3.0	0	2.0	0.2	0.5	1.0
139	Mayonnaise-type	2	tablespoon(s)	29	11.7	115	0.3	7.0	0	9.8	1.4	2.6	5.3
942	Oil and vinegar	2	tablespoon(s)	32	15.2	144	0	0.8	0	16.0	2.9	4.7	7.7
1765	Ranch	2	tablespoon(s)	30	11.5	145	0.3	2.0	0.2	15.4	2.4	3.4	8.5
3666	Ranch, reduced calorie	2	tablespoon(s)	30	20.5	63	0.1	2.0	0	6.1	1.6	3.6	0.6
940	Russian	2	tablespoon(s)	30	11.6	107	0.2	9.6	0.2	7.9	0.7	1.8	4.4
939	Russion, low-calorie	2	tablespoon(s)	32	20.8	45	0.2	8.8	0.1	1.3	0.2	0.3	0.7
941	Sesame seed	2	tablespoon(s)	30	11.8	133	0.9	2.6	0.3	13.6	1.9	3.6	7.5
142	Thousand Island	2	tablespoon(s)	32	14.9	118	0.3	4.7	0.3	11.2	1.6	2.5	5.8
143	Thousand Island, low-calorie	2	tablespoon(s)	30	18.2	59	0.2	7.2	0.4	3.4	0.2	1.9	0.8
	Sandwich spreads												
140	Mayonnaise, low-calorie	1	tablespoon(s)	16	8.9	52	0.1	1.3	0	5.3	0.8	1.3	2.9
138	Mayonnaise with soybean oil	1	tablespoon(s)	14	3.0	94	0.1	0.1	0	10.3	1.6	2.3	6.2
141	Tartar sauce	2	tablespoon(s)	29	18.8	59	0.3	3.7	0.1	4.7	0.9	1.0	2.5
Sweets													
4799	**Butterscotch or caramel topping**	2	tablespoon(s)	41	13.1	103	0.6	27.0	0.4	0	0	0	0
	Candy												
1786	Almond Joy candy bar	1	item(s)	45	3.7	220	2.0	26.0	2.0	13.0	8.0	2.4	0.5
1785	Bit-O-Honey candy	6	item(s)	40	—	150	1.0	32.0	0	3.0	2.0	—	—
33375	Butterscotch candy	2	piece(s)	12	0.6	47	0	10.8	0	0.4	0.2	0.1	0
1701	Chewing gum, stick	1	item(s)	3	0.1	11	0	2.9	0.1	0	0	0	0
33378	Chocolate fudge with nuts, prepared	2	piece(s)	38	2.9	175	1.7	25.8	0.9	7.2	2.5	1.5	2.9
1787	Jelly beans	15	item(s)	43	2.7	159	0	39.8	0.1	0	0	0	0
1784	Kit Kat wafer bar	1	item(s)	42	0.7	210	3.0	27.0	1.0	11.0	7.0	2.5	0.4
4674	Krackel candy bar	1	item(s)	41	0.6	210	2.0	28.0	0.5	10.0	6.0	3.9	0.4
4934	Licorice	4	piece(s)	44	7.3	154	1.1	35.1	0	1.0	0	0.1	0
1780	Life Savers candy	1	item(s)	2	—	6	0	1.4	—	0	0	0	0
1790	Lollipop	1	item(s)	28	—	108	0	28.0	0	0	0	0	0
4679	M & Ms peanut chocolate candy, small bag	1	item(s)	49	1.2	250	5.0	30.0	2.0	13.0	5.0	4.0	1.7
1781	M & Ms plain chocolate candy, small bag	1	item(s)	48	0.8	240	2.0	34.0	1.0	10.0	6.0	2.5	0.4
4673	Milk chocolate bar, Symphony	1	item(s)	91	0.9	483	7.7	52.8	1.5	27.8	16.7	7.2	0.6
1783	Milky Way bar	1	item(s)	58	3.7	260	2.0	41.0	1.0	10.0	7.0	1.3	0.2
1788	Peanut brittle	1 ½	ounce(s)	43	0.3	207	3.2	30.3	1.1	8.1	1.8	3.4	1.9
1789	Reese's peanut butter cups	2	piece(s)	42	0.6	210	5.0	24.0	1.0	13.0	4.5	5.5	2.3
4689	Reese's pieces candy, small bag	1	item(s)	43	0.4	200	5.0	25.0	2.0	9.0	8.0	1.9	0.8
33399	Semisweet chocolate candy, made with butter	½	ounce(s)	14	0.1	68	0.6	9.0	0.8	4.2	2.5	1.4	0.1
1782	Snickers bar	1	item(s)	59	3.3	280	4.0	35.0	1.0	14.0	5.0	4.6	1.8
4694	Special Dark chocolate bar	1	item(s)	41	—	190	2.0	25.0	3.0	12.0	8.0	—	—
4695	Starburst fruit chews, original fruits	1	package(s)	40	3.5	160	0	33.0	0	3.5	3.0	0	0
4698	Taffy	3	piece(s)	45	2.2	179	0	41.2	0	1.5	0.9	0.4	0.1
4699	Three Musketeers bar	1	item(s)	60	3.5	260	2.0	46.0	1.0	8.0	5.0	1.4	0.2
11764	Turtles	1	piece(s)	17	—	86	1.0	10.1	0.5	5.0	2.0	—	—
4702	Twix caramel cookie bars	2	item(s)	51	2.4	250	2.0	33.0	1.0	12.0	9.0	1.7	0.4
4705	York Peppermint Pattie	1	item(s)	39	3.5	140	1.0	31.0	1.0	2.5	1.5	0.2	0
	Frosting, icing												
4760	Chocolate frosting, ready to eat	2	tablespoon(s)	31	5.2	122	0.3	19.4	0.3	5.4	1.7	2.8	0.7

Chol (mg)	Calc (mg)	Iron (mg)	Magn (mg)	Pota (mg)	Sodi (mg)	Zinc (mg)	Vit A (µg)	Thia (mg)	Vit E (mg α)	Ribo (mg)	Niac (mg)	Vit B6 (mg)	Fola (µg)	Vit C (mg)	Vit B12 (µg)	Sele (µg)
12	14	0.32	0.6	8.7	362.7	0.03	2.7	0	1.42	0	0.01	0.01	0.6	0.1	0	0.5
0	12	0.08	1.6	43.9	296.0	0.06	0.3	0	0.22	0.02	0.01	0.01	2.0	0	0	0.5
0	2	0.04	0.6	10.8	336.0	0.01	0	0	0.72	0	0.01	0.01	0	0.1	0	0.5
0	8	0.26	1.6	21.4	267.5	0.09	7.4	0.01	1.60	0.02	0.06	0	0	1.2	0	0
0	4	0.23	2.6	34.2	268.2	0.06	8.6	0.01	0.32	0.02	0.15	0.02	0.6	1.5	0	0.5
0	4	0.08	1.5	24.7	291.9	0.02	0.6	0.01	0.64	0	0.04	0.02	0	0.1	0	0.6
0	5	0.08	1.2	27.0	300.9	0.02	0.3	0	1.28	0	0.03	0.02	0.9	0	0	0.5
8	4	0.06	0.6	2.6	209.0	0.05	6.2	0	0.61	0.01	0	0	1.8	0	0.1	0.5
0	0	0	0	2.6	0.3	0	0	0	1.48	0	0	0	0	0	0	0.5
10	9	0.19	1.5	18.6	328.2	0.12	3.0	0.03	1.27	0.02	0	0.01	1.2	1.0	0.1	0.6
0	5	0.01	0.9	8.1	414.0	0.02	0.6	0	0.73	0.01	0	0	0.3	0.1	0	0.1
0	4	0.18	3.0	51.9	339.9	0.07	8.7	0.01	1.00	0.01	0.18	0.03	1.5	1.8	0	0.5
2	6	0.19	0	50.2	277.8	0.03	0.6	0	0.13	0	0	0	1.0	1.9	0	0.5
0	6	0.18	0	47.1	300.0	0.03	0.6	0	1.50	0	0	0	0	0	0	0.5
8	5	0.38	2.6	34.2	276.2	0.08	4.5	0.46	1.28	0.02	0.13	0	0	0	0	0.5
3	8	0.27	2.1	60.6	286.5	0.06	4.8	0.01	0.30	0.01	0.13	0	0	0.4	0	0
6	1	0.05	0.3	6.4	107.7	0.03	3.4	0	0.49	0	0	0	0.6	0	0	0.4
6	1	0.03	0.1	2.8	87.6	0.02	2.2	0	0.45	0	0	0	0.7	0	0	0.3
2	7	0.07	1.7	19.0	186.8	0.03	3.1	0	0.47	0.01	0.03	0.01	1.4	0.6	0	0.3
0	22	0.08	2.9	34.4	143.1	0.08	11.1	0	—	0.04	0.02	0.01	0.8	0.1	0	0
0	18	0.33	—	114.3	50.0	—	0	—	—	—	—	—	—	0	—	—
0	20	0	—	—	120.0	—	0	—	—	—	—	—	—	0	—	—
1	0	0	0	0.4	46.9	0.01	3.4	0	0.01	0	0	0	0	0	0	0.1
0	0	0	0	0.1	0	0	0	0	0	0	0	0	0	0	0	0
5	22	0.75	20.9	69.5	14.8	0.54	14.4	0.03	0.10	0.04	0.12	0.03	6.1	0.1	0	1.1
0	1	0.06	0.9	15.7	21.3	0.02	0	0	0	0	0	0	0	0	0	0.5
5	60	0.36	15.5	97.0	30.0	0.04	0	0.05	0.14	0.09	0.21	0.01	7.6	0	0.2	2.1
3	40	0.37	—	168.8	50.0	—	0	—	—	—	—	—	—	0	—	—
0	0	0.22	2.6	28.2	126.3	0.07	0	0.01	0.08	0.02	0.04	0	0	0		
0	0	0	—	—	0	—	0	—	—	—	—	—	—	0	—	—
0	0	0	—	—	10.8	0	0	—	—	0	0	—	—	0	—	1.0
5	40	0.36	34.0	171.1	25.0	0.87	—	0.03	1.40	0.07	1.60	0.04	27.1	0.6	0.2	2.0
5	40	0.36	21.1	125.0	30.0	0.77	13.3	0.04	0.17	0.07	0.13	0.01	3.8	0.6	0.3	1.6
22	228	0.83	61.0	398.6	91.9	1.00	—	0.06	—	0.25	0.15	0.10	—	2.0	0.4	—
5	60	0.18	11.6	72.1	95.0	0.40	14.0	0.03	0.52	0.07	0.09	0.01	2.3	0.6	0.1	1.2
5	11	0.52	17.9	71.4	189.2	0.37	16.6	0.06	1.09	0.02	1.13	0.03	19.6	0	0	1.1
5	20	0.72	26.0	144.1	150.0	0.54	0	0.07	0.06	0.05	1.89	0.04	21.0	0	0.1	0.6
0	0	0.72	37.8	154.4	55.0	0.50	0	0.08	0.43	0.09	2.61	0.05	23.6	0	0	0.3
3	5	0.44	16.3	51.7	1.6	0.23	0.4	0.01	—	0.01	0.06	0.01	0.4	0	0	0.5
5	40	0.36	42.3	189.6	140.0	1.47		0.03	0.88	0.08	2.11	0.05	18.2	0	0.1	4.6
5	0	1.80	—	—	15.0	—	0	—	—	—	—	—	—	0	—	—
0	0	0	0.6	1.2	0	0	0	0	0.19	0	0	0	0.6	23.5	0	0.5
4	4	0	0	1.4	23.4	0.09	12.1	0.01	0.04	0.01	0	0	0	0	0	0.3
5	20	0.36	17.5	80.3	110.0	0.33	14.9	0.02	0.59	0.03	0.14	0.01	2.4	0.6	0.1	1.1
0	20	0.36	—	—	15.1	—	0	—	—	—	—	—	—	0	—	—
5	39	0.35	15.2	104.5	100.0	0.60	—	0.08	0.42	0.11	0.57	0.01	19.9	0.6	0.2	2.4
0	0	0.33	—	43.3	10.0	—	0	—	—	—	—	—	—	0	—	—
0	2	0.43	6.4	60.0	56.1	0.09	0	0	0.48	0.01	0.04	0	0.3	0	0	0.2

TABLE A-2 **Table of Food Composition** (*continued*)   (Computer code is for Cengage Diet Analysis program)   (For purposes of calculations, use "0" for t, <1, <0.1, <0.01)

DA+ Code	Food Description	Quantity	Measure	Wt (g)	H₂O (g)	Ener (kcal)	Prot (g)	Carb (g)	Fiber (g)	Fat (g)	Fat Breakdown (g)		
											Sat	Mono	Poly
Sweets—*continued*													
4771	Creamy vanilla frosting, ready to eat	2	tablespoon(s)	35	5.3	146	0	23.8	0	5.7	1.0	1.7	2.8
536	White icing	2	tablespoon(s)	40	6.0	167	0	27.2	0	6.5	1.2	1.9	3.2
	Gelatin												
13697	Gelatin snack, all flavors	1	item(s)	96	—	70	1.0	17.0	0	0	0	0	0
2616	Sugar-free, low-calorie mixed fruit gelatin mix, prepared	½	cup(s)	121	—	10	1.0	0	0	0	0	0	0
548	**Honey**	1	tablespoon(s)	21	3.6	64	0.1	17.3	0	0	0	0	0
	Jams, jellies												
550	Jam or preserves	1	tablespoon(s)	20	6.1	56	0.1	13.8	0.2	0	0	0	0
42199	Jams, preserves, dietetic, all flavors, w/sodium saccarin	1	tablespoon(s)	14	6.4	18	0	7.5	0.3	0	0	0	0
552	Jelly	1	tablespoon(s)	21	6.3	56	0	14.7	0.2	0	0	0	0
545	**Marshmallows**	4	item(s)	29	4.7	92	0.5	23.4	0	0.1	0	0	0
4800	**Marshmallow cream topping**	2	tablespoon(s)	40	7.9	129	0.3	31.6	0	0.1	0	0	0
555	**Molasses**	1	tablespoon(s)	20	4.4	58	0	14.9	0	0	0	0	0
4780	**Popsicle or ice pop**	1	item(s)	59	47.5	47	0.0	11.3	0	0.1	0	0	0
	Sugar												
559	Brown sugar, packed	1	teaspoon(s)	5	0.1	17	0	4.5	0	0	0	0	0
563	Powdered sugar, sifted	⅓	cup(s)	33	0.1	130	0	33.2	0	0	0	0	0
561	White granulated sugar	1	teaspoon(s)	4	0	16	0	4.2	0	0	0	0	0
	Sugar substitute												
1760	Equal sweetener, packet size	1	item(s)	1	—	0	0	0.5	0	0	0	0	0
13029	Splenda granular no-calorie sweetener	1	teaspoon(s)	1	—	0	0	0.5	0	0	0	0	0
1759	Sweet N Low sugar substitute, packet	1	item(s)	1	0.1	4	0	0.5	0	0	0	0	0
	Syrup												
3148	Chocolate syrup	2	tablespoon(s)	39	12.1	109	0.8	25.4	1.0	0.4	0.2	0.1	0
29676	Maple syrup	¼	cup(s)	79	25.5	205	0	52.8	0	0	0	0	0
4795	Pancake syrup	¼	cup(s)	80	30.4	187	0	49.2	0	0	0	0	0
Spices, Condiments, Sauces													
	Spices												
807	Allspice, ground	1	teaspoon(s)	2	0.2	5	0.1	1.4	0.4	0.2	0	0	0
1171	Anise seeds	1	teaspoon(s)	2	0.2	7	0.4	1.1	0.3	0.3	0	0.2	0.1
729	Bakers' yeast, active	1	teaspoon(s)	4	0.2	13	1.6	1.6	1.1	0.3	0	0.2	0
683	Baking powder, double acting with phosphate	1	teaspoon(s)	5	0.2	2	0	1.1	0	0	0	0	0
1611	Baking soda	1	teaspoon(s)	5	0	0	0	0	0	0	0	0	0
8552	Basil	1	teaspoon(s)	1	0.8	0	0	0	0	0	0	0	0
34959	Basil, fresh	1	piece(s)	1	0.5	0	0	0	0	0	0	0	0
808	Basil, ground	1	teaspoon(s)	1	0.1	3	0.3	0.7	0.5	0.1	0	0	0
809	Bay leaf	1	teaspoon(s)	1	0	2	0	0.4	0.2	0.1	0	0	0
11720	Betel leaves	1	ounce(s)	28	—	17	1.8	2.4	0	0	—	—	—
11710	Capers	1	teaspoon(s)	5	—	0	0	0	0	0	0	0	0
1172	Caraway seeds	1	teaspoon(s)	2	0.2	7	0.4	1.0	0.8	0.3	0	0.1	0.1
1173	Celery seeds	1	teaspoon(s)	2	0.1	8	0.4	0.8	0.2	0.5	0	0.3	0.1
1174	Chervil, dried	1	teaspoon(s)	1	0	1	0.1	0.3	0.1	0	0	0	0
810	Chili powder	1	teaspoon(s)	3	0.3	7	0.3	1.3	0.9	0.4	0.1	0.1	0.2
8553	Chives, chopped	1	teaspoon(s)	1	0.9	0	0	0	0	0	0	0	0
51420	Cilantro (coriander)	1	teaspoon(s)	0	0.3	0	0	0	0	0	0	0	0
811	Cinnamon, ground	1	teaspoon(s)	2	0.2	6	0.1	1.9	1.2	0	0	0	0
812	Cloves, ground	1	teaspoon(s)	2	0.2	6	0.1	1.4	0.7	0.3	0.1	0	0.2
1175	Coriander leaf, dried	1	teaspoon(s)	1	0	2	0.1	0.3	0.1	0	0	0	0
1176	Coriander seeds	1	teaspoon(s)	2	0.2	5	0.2	1.0	0.8	0.3	0	0.2	0
1706	Cornstarch	1	tablespoon(s)	8	0.7	30	0	7.3	0.1	0	0	0	0
1177	Cumin seeds	1	teaspoon(s)	2	0.2	8	0.4	0.9	0.2	0.5	0	0.3	0.1
11729	Cumin, ground	1	teaspoon(s)	5	—	11	0.4	0.8	0.8	0.4	—	—	—
1178	Curry powder	1	teaspoon(s)	2	0.2	7	0.3	1.2	0.7	0.3	0	0.1	0.1
1179	Dill seeds	1	teaspoon(s)	2	0.2	6	0.3	1.2	0.4	0.3	0	0.2	0
1180	Dill weed, dried	1	teaspoon(s)	1	0.1	3	0.2	0.6	0.1	0	0	0	0

PAGE KEY: A-6 5 Breads/Baked Goods A-12 = Cereal/Rice/Pasta A-16 = Fruit A-22 = Vegetables/Legumes A-32 = Nuts/Seeds A-34 = Vegetarian A-36 = Dairy A-44 = Eggs A-44 = Seafood A-46 = Meats A-50 = Poultry
A-52 = Processed Meats A-54 = Beverages A-58 = Fats/Oils A-60 = Sweets A-62 = Spices/Condiments/Sauces A-66 = Mixed Foods/Soups/Sandwiches A-72 = Fast Food A-90 = Convenience A-92 = Baby Foods

Chol (mg)	Calc (mg)	Iron (mg)	Magn (mg)	Pota (mg)	Sodi (mg)	Zinc (mg)	Vit A (µg)	Thia (mg)	Vit E (mg α)	Ribo (mg)	Niac (mg)	Vit B$_6$ (mg)	Fola (µg)	Vit C (mg)	Vit B$_{12}$ (µg)	Sele (µg)
0	1	0.06	0.3	11.9	64.4	0.02	0	0	0.54	0.11	0.08	0	2.8	0	0	0
0	1	0.06	0.4	13.6	73.6	0.03	0	0	0.61	0.12	0.09	0	3.2	0	0	0
0	0	0	—	0	40.0	—	0	—	—	—	—	—	—	0	—	—
0	0	0	0	0	45.0	0	0	0	0	0	0	0	0	0	0	—
0	1	0.09	0.4	10.9	0.8	0.05	0	0	0	0.01	0.03	0.01	0.4	0.1	0	0.2
0	4	0.10	0.8	15.4	6.4	0.01	0	0	0.02	0.02	0.01	0	2.2	1.8	0	0.4
0	1	0.06	0.7	9.7	0	0.01	0	0	0.01	0	0	0	1.3	0	0	0.2
0	1	0.04	1.3	11.3	6.3	0.01	0	0	0	0	0.01	0	0.4	0.2	0	0.1
0	1	0.07	0.6	1.4	23.0	0.01	0	0	0	0	0.02	0	0.3	0	0	0.5
0	1	0.09	0.8	2.0	32.0	0.02	0	0	0	0	0.03	0	0.4	0	0	0.8
0	41	0.94	48.4	292.8	7.4	0.06	0	0.01	0	0	0.19	0.13	0	0	0	3.6
0	0	0.32	0.6	8.9	4.1	0.09	0	0	0	0	0	0	0	0.4	0	0.1
0	4	0.03	0.4	6.1	1.3	0	0	0	0	0	0.01	0	0	0	0	0.1
0	0	0.02	0.0	0.7	0.7	0	0	0	0	0	0.01	0	0	0	0	0.2
0	0	0.0	0.0	0.1	0	0	0	0	0	0	0	0	0	0	0	0
0	0	0	—	0	0	—	0	—	—	—	—	—	—	0	—	—
0	0	0	—	—	0	—	0	—	—	—	—	—	—	0	—	—
0	0	0	—	—	0	—	—	—	—	—	—	—	—	0	—	—
0	5	0.82	25.4	87.4	28.1	0.28	0	0	0.01	0.02	0.13	0	0.8	0.1	0	0.5
0	80	0.09	16.5	166.9	9.4	1.16	0	0.05	0	1.00	0.06	0	0	0	0	0.5
0	2	0.02	1.6	12.0	65.6	0.06	0	0.02	0	0.01	0	0	0	0	0	0
0	13	0.13	2.6	19.8	1.5	0.02	0.5	0	—	0	0.05	0	0.7	0.7	0	0.1
0	14	0.78	3.6	30.3	0.3	0.11	0.3	0.01	—	0.01	0.06	0.01	0.2	0.4	0	0.1
0	1	0.09	2.2	38.2	2.0	0.32	0	0.44	0	0.16	1.61	0.06	93.6	0	0	0.3
0	339	0.52	1.8	0.2	363.1	0	0	0	0	0	0	0	0	0	0	0
0	0	0	0	0	1258.6	0	0	0	0	0	0	0	0	0	0	0
0	2	0.03	0.6	2.6	0	0.01	2.3	0	0.01	0	0.01	0	0.6	0.2	0	0
0	1	0.02	0.3	1.5	0	0	1.3	0	—	0	0	0	0.3	0.1	0	0
0	31	1.26	10.0	36.8	1.1	0.10	0.5	0	0.15	0.02	0.07	0.02	4.3	0	0	0
0	5	0.26	0.7	3.2	0.1	0.02	1.9	0	—	0	0.01	0.01	1.1	0.3	0	0
0	110	2.29	—	155.9	2.0	—	—	0.04	—	0.07	0.20	—	—	0.9	0	—
0	—	—	—	105.0	—	—	—	—	—	—	—	—	—	—	0	—
0	14	0.34	5.4	28.4	0.4	0.12	0.4	0.01	0.05	0.01	0.08	0.01	0.2	0.4	0	0.3
0	35	0.90	8.8	28.0	3.2	0.14	0.1	0.01	0.02	0.01	0.06	0.02	0.2	0.3	0	0.2
0	8	0.19	0.8	28.4	0.5	0.05	1.8	0	—	0	0.03	0.01	1.6	0.3	0	0.2
0	9	0.45	3.9	50.7	42.6	0.11	38.6	0.01	0.99	0.02	0.30	0.05	0.7	0	0	0.5
0	1	0.02	0.4	3.0	0	0.01	2.2	0	0	0	0.01	0	1.0	0.6	0	0
0	0	0.01	0.1	1.7	0.2	0	1.1	0	0.01	0	0	0	0.2	0.1	0	0
0	23	0.19	1.4	9.9	0.3	0.02	0.4	0	0.05	0	0.03	0	0.1	0.1	0	0.1
0	13	0.25	5.4	21.4	5.8	0.05	0.2	0	0.19	0	0.03	0.01	0.5	0.3	0	0.3
0	7	0.25	4.2	26.8	1.3	0.03	1.8	0.01	0.01	0.01	0.06	0	1.6	3.4	0	0.2
0	13	0.29	5.9	22.8	0.6	0.08	0	0	—	0.01	0.04	—	0	0.4	0	0.5
0	0	0.04	0.2	0.2	0.7	0	0	0	0	0	0	0	0	0	0	0.2
0	20	1.39	7.7	37.5	3.5	0.10	1.3	0.01	0.07	0.01	0.10	0.01	0.2	0.2	0	0.1
0	20	—	—	43.6	4.8	—	—	—	—	—	—	—	—	—	—	—
0	10	0.59	5.1	30.9	1.0	0.08	1.0	0.01	0.44	0.01	0.07	0.02	3.1	0.2	0	0.3
0	32	0.34	5.4	24.9	0.4	0.11	0.1	0.01	—	0.01	0.06	0.01	0.2	0.4	0	0.3
0	18	0.49	4.5	33.1	2.1	0.03	2.9	0	—	0	0.03	0.02	—	0.5	0	—

TABLE A-2 Table of Food Composition (continued)   (Computer code is for Cengage Diet Analysis program)   (For purposes of calculations, use "0" for t, <1, <0.1, <0.01)

DA+ Code	Food Description	Quantity	Measure	Wt (g)	H₂O (g)	Ener (kcal)	Prot (g)	Carb (g)	Fiber (g)	Fat (g)	Sat	Mono	Poly
											Fat Breakdown (g)		
Spices, Condiments, Sauces—*continued*													
34949	Dill weed, fresh	5	piece(s)	1	0.9	0	0	0.1	0	0	0	0	0
1181	Fennel seeds	1	teaspoon(s)	2	0.2	7	0.3	1.0	0.8	0.3	0	0.2	0
1182	Fenugreek seeds	1	teaspoon(s)	4	0.3	12	0.9	2.2	0.9	0.2	0.1	—	—
11733	Garam masala, powder	1	ounce(s)	28	—	107	4.4	12.8	0	4.3	—	—	—
1067	Garlic clove	1	item(s)	3	1.8	4	0.2	1.0	0.1	0	0	0	0
813	Garlic powder	1	teaspoon(s)	3	0.2	9	0.5	2.0	0.3	0	0	0	0
1068	Ginger root	2	teaspoon(s)	4	3.2	3	0.1	0.7	0.1	0	0	0	0
1183	Ginger, ground	1	teaspoon(s)	2	0.2	6	0.2	1.3	0.3	0.1	0	0	0
35497	Leeks, bulb and lower-leaf, freeze-dried	¼	cup(s)	1	0	3	0.1	0.6	0.1	0	0	0	0
1184	Mace, ground	1	teaspoon(s)	2	0.1	8	0.1	0.9	0.3	0.6	0.2	0.2	0.1
1185	Marjoram, dried	1	teaspoon(s)	1	0	2	0.1	0.4	0.2	0.0	0	0	0
1186	Mustard seeds, yellow	1	teaspoon(s)	3	0.2	17	0.9	0.9	0.4	1.2	0.1	0.7	0.3
814	Nutmeg, ground	1	teaspoon(s)	2	0.1	12	0.1	1.1	0.5	0.8	0.6	0.1	0
2747	Onion flakes, dehydrated	1	teaspoon(s)	2	0.1	6	0.1	1.4	0.2	0	0	0	0
1187	Onion powder	1	teaspoon(s)	2	0.1	7	0.2	1.7	0.3	0	0	0	0
815	Oregano, ground	1	teaspoon(s)	2	0.2	5	0.2	1.2	0.8	0.1	0	0	0
816	Paprika	1	teaspoon(s)	2	0.2	6	0.3	1.1	0.7	0.3	0	0	0.2
817	Parsley, dried	1	teaspoon(s)	0	0	1	0.1	0.2	0.1	0	0	0	0
818	Pepper, black	1	teaspoon(s)	2	0.3	5	0.2	1.3	0.5	0.1	0	0	0
819	Pepper, cayenne	1	teaspoon(s)	2	0.1	6	0.2	1.0	0.5	0.3	0.1	0	0.2
1188	Pepper, white	1	teaspoon(s)	2	0.3	7	0.2	1.6	0.6	0.1	0	0	0
1189	Poppy seeds	1	teaspoon(s)	3	0.2	15	0.5	0.8	0.5	1.2	0.1	0.2	0.8
1190	Poultry seasoning	1	teaspoon(s)	2	0.1	5	0.1	1.0	0.2	0.1	0	0	0
1191	Pumpkin pie spice, powder	1	teaspoon(s)	2	0.1	6	0.1	1.2	0.3	0.2	0.1	0	0
1192	Rosemary, dried	1	teaspoon(s)	1	0.1	4	0.1	0.8	0.5	0.2	0.1	0	0
11723	Rosemary, fresh	1	teaspoon(s)	1	0.5	1	0	0.1	0.1	0	0	0	0
2722	Saffron powder	1	teaspoon(s)	1	0.1	2	0.1	0.5	0	0	0	0	0
11724	Sage	1	teaspoon(s)	1	—	1	0	0.1	0	0	—	—	—
1193	Sage, ground	1	teaspoon(s)	1	0.1	2	0.1	0.4	0.3	0.1	0	0	0
30189	Salt substitute	¼	teaspoon(s)	2	—	0	0	0	0	0	0	0	0
30195	Salt, kosher	¼	teaspoon(s)	2	—	0	0	0	0	0	0	0	0
822	Salt, table	¼	teaspoon(s)	2	0	0	0	0	0	0	0	0	0
1194	Savory, ground	1	teaspoon(s)	1	0.1	4	0.1	1.0	0.6	0.1	0	—	—
820	Sesame seed kernels, toasted	1	teaspoon(s)	3	0.1	15	0.5	0.7	0.5	1.3	0.2	0.5	0.6
11725	Sorrel	1	teaspoon(s)	3	—	1	0.1	0.1	0	0	0	—	—
11721	Spearmint	1	teaspoon(s)	2	1.6	1	0.1	0.2	0.1	0	0	0	0
35498	Sweet green peppers, freeze-dried	¼	cup(s)	2	0	5	0.3	1.1	0.3	0	0	0	0
11726	Tamarind leaves	1	ounce(s)	28	—	33	1.6	5.2	0	0.6	—	—	—
11727	Tarragon	1	ounce(s)	28	—	14	1.0	1.8	0	0.3	—	—	—
1195	Tarragon, ground	1	teaspoon(s)	2	0.1	5	0.4	0.8	0.1	0.1	0	0	0.1
11728	Thyme, fresh	1	teaspoon(s)	1	0.5	1	0	0.2	0.1	0	0	0	0
821	Thyme, ground	1	teaspoon(s)	1	0.1	4	0.1	0.9	0.5	0.1	0	0	0
1196	Turmeric, ground	1	teaspoon(s)	2	0.2	8	0.2	1.4	0.5	0.2	0.1	—	—
11995	Wasabi	1	tablespoon(s)	14	10.7	10	0.7	2.3	0.2	0	—	—	—
	Condiments												
674	Catsup or ketchup	1	tablespoon(s)	15	10.4	17	0.2	3.9	0	0	0	0	0
5812	Catsup or ketchup, low-sodium	1	tablespoon(s)	15	10.4	15	0.3	3.8	0.3	0	0	0	0
703	Dill pickle	1	ounce(s)	28	26.7	3	0.2	0.7	0.3	0	0	0	0
32128	Guacamole	2	tablespoon(s)	32	25.1	42	0.7	2.1	1.1	3.8	0.6	2.4	0.4
1814	Hummus	½	cup(s)	123	79.8	218	6.0	24.7	4.9	10.6	1.4	6.0	2.6
138	Mayonnaise with soybean oil	1	tablespoon(s)	14	3.0	94	0.1	0.1	0	10.3	1.6	2.3	6.2
140	Mayonnaise, low-calorie	1	tablespoon(s)	16	8.9	52	0.1	1.3	0	5.3	0.8	1.3	2.9
1682	Mustard, brown	1	teaspoon(s)	5	4.1	5	0.3	0.3	0	0.3	—	—	—
700	Mustard, yellow	1	teaspoon(s)	5	4.1	3	0.2	0.3	0.2	0.2	0	0.1	0
706	Sweet pickle relish	1	tablespoon(s)	15	9.3	20	0.1	5.3	0.2	0.1	0	0	0
141	Tartar sauce	2	tablespoon(s)	29	18.8	59	0.3	3.7	0.1	4.7	0.9	1.0	2.5
	Sauces												
685	Barbecue sauce	2	tablespoon(s)	31	17.1	54	0.3	12.7	0.3	0.2	0	0	0
40849	Barbecue sauce, low-sodium	2	tablespoon(s)	31	17.1	54	0.3	12.7	0.3	0.2	0	0	0
834	Cheese sauce	¼	cup(s)	63	44.4	110	4.2	4.3	0.3	8.4	3.8	2.4	1.6

PAGE KEY: A-6 5 Breads/Baked Goods A-12 = Cereal/Rice/Pasta A-16 = Fruit A-22 = Vegetables/Legumes A-32 = Nuts/Seeds A-34 = Vegetarian A-36 = Dairy A-44 = Eggs A-44 = Seafood A-46 = Meats A-50 = Poultry A-52 = Processed Meats A-54 = Beverages A-58 = Fats/Oils A-60 = Sweets A-62 = Spices/Condiments/Sauces A-66 = Mixed Foods/Soups/Sandwiches A-72 = Fast Food A-90 = Convenience A-92 = Baby Foods

Chol (mg)	Calc (mg)	Iron (mg)	Magn (mg)	Pota (mg)	Sodi (mg)	Zinc (mg)	Vit A (μg)	Thia (mg)	Vit E (mg α)	Ribo (mg)	Niac (mg)	Vit B_6 (mg)	Fola (μg)	Vit C (mg)	Vit B_{12} (μg)	Sele (μg)
0	2	0.07	0.6	7.4	0.6	0.01	3.9	0	0.02	0	0.02	0	1.5	0.9	0	—
0	24	0.37	7.7	33.9	1.8	0.07	0.1	0.01	—	0.01	0.12	0.01	—	0.4	0	—
0	7	1.24	7.1	28.5	2.5	0.09	0.1	0.01	—	0.01	0.06	0.02	2.1	0.1	0	0.2
0	215	9.24	93.6	411.1	27.5	1.07	—	0.10	—	0.09	0.71	—	—	0	0	—
0	5	0.05	0.8	12.0	0.5	0.03	0	0.01	0	0	0.02	0.04	0.1	0.9	0	0.4
0	2	0.16	2.2	33.4	1.7	0.08	0	0.01	0.02	0	0.02	0.05	1.3	0	0	0.7
0	1	0.02	1.7	16.6	0.5	0.01	0	0	0.01	0	0.03	0.01	0.4	0.2	0	0
0	2	0.36	3.9	23.8	0.5	0.07	0	0	0	0	0.17	0.01	0.2	0	0	1.0
0	3	0.06	1.3	19.2	0.3	0.01	0.1	0.01	—	0	0.03	0.01	2.9	0.9	0	—
0	4	0.24	2.8	7.9	1.4	0.04	0.7	0.01	—	0.01	0.02	0	1.3	0.4	0	0
0	12	0.50	2.1	9.1	0.5	0.02	2.4	0	0.01	0	0.02	0.01	1.6	0.3	0	0
0	9	0.30	12.2	24.4	0.4	0.20	0.1	0.03	0.17	0.01	0.16	0.01	5.3	0.2	0	6.9
0	4	0.07	4.0	7.7	0.4	0.05	0.1	0.01	0	0	0.03	0	1.7	0.1	0	0.1
0	4	0.03	1.5	27.1	0.4	0.03	0	0.01	0	0	0.02	0.03	2.8	1.3	0	0.1
0	8	0.08	2.4	20.7	1.5	0.09	0	0.01	0.01	0	0.01	0.02	1.3	0.5	0	0.3
0	29	0.66	4.9	22.7	0.5	0.05	1.5	0	0.33	0.01	0.08	0.02	4.3	0	0	0.1
0	5	0.44	3.7	47.9	1.4	0.09	51.7	0.01	0.61	0.03	0.21	0.04	1.0	0	0	0.1
0	3	0.07	1.2	8.0	1.4	0.02	0.3	0	0.03	0.01	0.03	0	0.5	0.4	0	0
0	9	0.20	3.6	27.9	0.4	0.02	0.6	0	0.02	0	0.02	0.01	0.4	0	0	0.1
0	3	0.14	2.7	36.3	0.5	0.04	37.5	0.01	0.54	0.02	0.16	0.04	1.9	1.4	0	0.2
0	6	0.34	2.2	1.8	0.1	0.03	0	0	—	0	0.01	0	0.2	0.5	0	0.1
0	40	0.27	9.7	20.1	0.7	0.22	0	0.02	0.05	0	0.03	0.01	2.3	0	0	0.4
0	15	0.53	3.4	10.3	0.4	0.05	2.0	0	0.02	0	0.04	0.02	2.1	0.2	0	0.1
0	12	0.34	2.3	11.3	0.9	0.04	0.2	0	0.03	0	0.04	0.01	0.4	0.4	0	0.2
0	15	0.35	2.6	11.5	0.6	0.04	1.9	0.01	—	0.01	0.01	0.02	3.7	0.7	0	0.1
0	2	0.05	0.6	4.7	0.2	0.01	1.0	0	0	0	0.01	0	0.8	0.2	0	—
0	1	0.08	1.8	12.1	1.0	0.01	0.2	0	0	0	0.01	0.01	0.7	0.6	0	0
0	4	—	1.1	2.7	0	0.01	—	0	—	—	—	—	—	—	—	—
0	12	0.20	3.0	7.5	0.1	0.03	2.1	0.01	0.05	0	0.04	0.02	1.9	0.2	0	0
0	8	0	0	754.5	0.1	—	0	—	—	—	—	—	—	0	—	—
0	0	0	—	—	600.0	—	0	—	—	—	—	—	—	0	—	—
0	0	0	0	0.1	581.4	0	0	0	0	0	0	0	0	0	0	0
0	30	0.53	5.3	14.7	0.3	0.06	3.6	0.01	—	—	0.06	0.03	—	0.7	0	0.1
0	3	0.21	9.2	10.8	1.0	0.27	0.1	0.03	0.01	0.01	0.15	0	2.6	0	0	0.9
0	—	—	—	0.1	—	—	—	—	—	—	—	—	—	—	0	—
0	4	0.23	1.2	8.7	0.6	0.02	3.9	0	—	0	0.02	0	2.0	0.3	0	—
0	2	0.17	3.0	50.7	3.1	0.04	4.5	0.02	0.06	0.02	0.12	0.04	3.7	30.4	0	0.1
0	85	1.48	20.2	—	—	—	—	0.07	—	0.03	1.16	—	—	0.9	0	—
0	48	—	14.5	128.1	2.6	0.17	—	0.04	—	—	—	—	—	0.6	0	—
0	18	0.52	5.6	48.3	1.0	0.06	3.4	0	—	0.02	0.14	0.04	4.4	0.8	0	0.1
0	3	0.14	1.3	4.9	0.1	0.01	1.9	0	—	0	0.01	0	0.4	1.3	0	—
0	26	1.73	3.1	11.4	0.8	0.09	2.7	0.01	0.10	0.01	0.07	0.01	3.8	0.7	0	0.1
0	4	0.91	4.2	55.6	0.8	0.10	0	0	0.07	0.01	0.11	0.04	0.9	0.6	0	0.1
0	13	0.11	—	—	—	—	—	0.02	—	0.01	0.07	—	—	11.2	0	—
0	2	0.06	2.3	47.3	136.1	0.04	3.9	0	0.22	0.03	0.22	0.02	1.4	0.6	0	0
0	3	0.08	2.8	57.3	3.0	0.04	7.0	0	0.22	0.02	0.21	0.02	1.5	2.3	0	0
0	12	0.10	2.0	26.1	248.1	0.03	2.6	0.01	0.03	0.01	0.03	0.01	0.3	0.2	0	0
1	12	0.27	10.2	152.1	79.1	0.13	—	0.03	0.28	0.04	0.43	0.07	—	2.5	0	0
0	60	1.92	35.7	212.8	297.7	1.34	0	0.11	0.92	0.06	0.49	0.49	72.6	9.7	0	3.0
6	1	0.03	0.1	2.8	87.6	0.02	2.2	0	0.45	0	0	0	0.7	0	0	0.3
6	1	0.05	0.3	6.4	107.7	0.03	3.4	0	0.49	0	0	0	0.6	0	0	0.4
0	6	0.09	0.9	6.8	68.1	0.02	0	0	0.09	0	0.01	0	—	0.1	0	—
0	3	0.08	2.5	6.9	56.8	0.03	0.2	0.02	0.02	0	0.03	0	0.3	0.1	0	1.6
0	0	0.13	0.8	3.8	121.7	0.02	9.1	0	0.09	0	0.03	0	0.2	0.2	0	0
2	7	0.07	1.7	19.0	186.8	0.03	3.1	0	0.47	0.01	0.03	0.01	1.4	0.6	0	0.3
0	10	0.20	4.1	72.5	320.9	0.05	3.4	0.01	0.25	0.02	0.19	0.02	0.6	0.2	0	0.4
0	10	0.20	4.1	72.5	41.6	0.05	3.4	0.01	0.25	0.02	0.19	0.02	2.5	0.2	0	0.4
18	116	0.13	5.7	18.9	521.6	0.62	50.4	0	—	0.07	0.02	0.01	2.5	0.3	0.1	2.0

TABLE A-2 Table of Food Composition *(continued)* (Computer code is for Cengage Diet Analysis program) (For purposes of calculations, use "0" for t, <1, <0.1, <0.01)

DA+ Code	Food Description	Quantity	Measure	Wt (g)	H₂O (g)	Ener (kcal)	Prot (g)	Carb (g)	Fiber (g)	Fat (g)	Fat Breakdown (g) Sat	Mono	Poly

(column headers: Fat Breakdown (g) spans Sat, Mono, Poly)

Spices, Condiments, Sauces—*continued*

32123	Chili enchilada sauce, green	2	tablespoon(s)	57	53.0	15	0.6	3.1	0.7	0.3	0	0	0.1
32122	Chili enchilada sauce, red	2	tablespoon(s)	32	24.5	27	1.1	5.0	2.1	0.8	0.1	0	0.4
29688	Hoisin sauce	1	tablespoon(s)	16	7.1	35	0.5	7.1	0.4	0.5	0.1	0.2	0.3
1641	Horseradish sauce, prepared	1	teaspoon(s)	5	3.5	9	0.1	0.1	0	0.9	0.5	0.2	0
16670	Mole poblano sauce	½	cup(s)	133	102.8	156	5.4	10.9	2.7	11.6	2.7	5.2	3.0
29689	Oyster sauce	1	tablespoon(s)	16	12.8	8	0.2	1.7	0	0	0	0	0
1655	Pepper sauce or Tabasco	1	teaspoon(s)	5	4.5	1	0.1	0	0	0	0	0	0
347	Salsa	2	tablespoon(s)	32	28.5	9	0.5	2.2	0.6	0.1	0	0	0
2835	Soy sauce, low-sodium	1	tablespoon(s)	18	12.8	10	0.9	1.5	0.1	0	0	0	0
52206	Soy sauce, tamari	1	tablespoon(s)	18	11.8	11	1.9	1.0	0.1	0	0	0	0
25292	Sweet and sour sauce	2	tablespoon(s)	35	29.0	22	0.5	5.0	0.1	0.1	0	0	0
1613	Teriyaki sauce	1	tablespoon(s)	18	12.2	16	1.1	2.8	0	0	0	0	0
25294	Tomato sauce	½	cup(s)	150	133.4	61	2.4	11.2	2.7	1.6	0.2	0.4	0.8
42233	Tomato sauce, no salt added	½	cup(s)	122	111.2	35	1.6	8.2	1.8	0.2	0	0	0.1
5187	White sauce, medium-thick	¼	cup(s)	59	44.3	87	2.3	5.4	0.1	6.3	1.7	2.6	1.7
1654	Worcestershire sauce	1	teaspoon(s)	6	4.5	4	0	1.1	0	0	0	0	0
	Vinegar												
30853	Balsamic	1	tablespoon(s)	15	—	10	0	2.0	0	0	0	0	0
727	Cider	1	tablespoon(s)	15	14.0	3	0	0.1	0	0	0	0	0
5176	Distilled	1	tablespoon(s)	15	14.0	3	0	0	0	0	0	0	0
12948	Tarragon	1	tablespoon(s)	15	14.3	3	0	0.1	0	0	0	0	0

Mixed Foods, Sandwiches, and Soups

Mixed dishes

16652	Almond chicken	1	cup(s)	242	187.5	283	20.4	15.9	3.4	15.6	2.1	7.1	5.2
25224	Barbecued chicken	1	serving(s)	177	100.1	325	27.2	15.1	0.1	17.1	4.8	6.8	3.8
25227	Bean burrito	1	item(s)	147	81.7	318	16.2	30.9	5.7	14.9	8.3	4.7	1.0
9516	Beef and vegetable fajita	1	item(s)	223	145.3	377	23.3	34.9	2.7	15.7	5.1	6.9	2.5
16796	Beef or pork egg roll	2	item(s)	128	59.6	355	12.0	35.6	2.6	18.3	4.2	8.6	4.1
73314	Beef stew w/potatoes & vegetables	1	cup(s)	252	214.4	161	18.0	12.9	1.7	4.0	1.6	1.9	0.3
30233	Beef stroganoff with noodles	1	cup(s)	256	192.9	330	19.7	22.1	1.5	18.0	6.6	5.5	3.2
16651	Cashew chicken	1	cup(s)	242	187.5	283	20.4	15.9	3.4	15.6	2.1	7.1	5.2
30274	Cheese pizza with vegetables, thin crust	2	slice(s)	224	101.7	603	25.4	63.0	5.4	27.8	12.2	7.2	6.0
30330	Cheese quesadilla	1	item(s)	142	51.9	484	20.0	37.3	1.8	28.2	13.8	9.7	3.5
25240	Chicken and noodles	1	cup(s)	227	163.7	176	18.3	15.2	0.8	4.2	1.0	1.7	1.0
30239	Chicken and vegetables with broccoli, onion, bamboo shoots in soy based sauce	1	cup(s)	217	164.8	289	22.9	10.6	2.8	17.2	3.0	6.6	6.4
25093	Chicken cacciatore	1	cup(s)	244	176.2	283	29.8	5.4	1.3	15.3	4.3	6.2	3.3
28020	Chicken fried turkey steak	3	ounce(s)	85	62.7	115	12.7	11.3	0.7	1.8	0.5	0.3	0.7
218	Chicken pot pie	1	cup(s)	252	147.9	539	15.3	58.0	3.0	27.3	9.1	9.3	3.5
30240	Chicken teriyaki	1	cup(s)	244	153.2	451	66.5	4.7	0	16.6	4.6	5.9	3.8
25119	Chicken waldorf salad	½	cup(s)	100	67.5	179	14.0	6.5	1.0	10.9	1.8	3.2	5.0
25099	Chili con carne	¾	cup(s)	215	174.7	196	13.7	20.9	6.6	6.9	2.6	3.0	0.5
1062	Coleslaw	¾	cup(s)	90	73.4	70	1.2	11.2	1.3	2.3	0.3	0.6	1.2
1574	Crab cakes, from blue crab	1	item(s)	60	42.6	93	12.1	0.3	0	4.5	0.9	1.7	1.4
32144	Enchiladas with green chili sauce (enchiladas verdes)	1	item(s)	144	103.8	207	9.3	17.6	2.6	11.7	6.4	3.6	1.0
2793	Falafel patty	3	item(s)	51	17.7	170	6.8	16.2	—	9.1	1.2	5.2	2.1
28546	Fettuccine Alfredo	1	cup(s)	240	87.2	267	12.3	45.8	1.8	3.5	1.8	0.8	0.4
32146	Flautas	3	item(s)	162	78.0	438	24.9	36.3	4.1	21.6	8.2	8.8	2.3
29629	Fried rice with meat or poultry	1	cup(s)	198	122.0	323	17.1	52.2	1.8	4.9	1.1	1.4	1.8
16649	General Tso chicken	1	cup(s)	146	65.9	431	18.8	35.0	1.3	23.9	4.0	5.7	11.0
1826	Green salad	¾	cup(s)	104	98.9	17	1.3	3.3	2.2	0.1	0	0	0
16650	Kung Pao chicken	1	cup(s)	162	87.1	436	28.9	11.4	2.3	30.7	4.5	13.0	11.8
16622	Lamb curry	1	cup(s)	236	157.6	474	25.6	11.1	2.6	37.1	6.7	14.9	13.3
25253	Lasagna with ground beef	1	cup(s)	238	157.2	288	17.6	22.2	2.5	14.6	7.6	4.8	0.8
442	Macaroni and cheese, prepared	1	cup(s)	243	144.7	484	18.5	54.2	2.7	21.0	8.4	7.2	3.7
29637	Meat filled ravioli with tomato or meat sauce, canned	1	cup(s)	251	196.5	248	8.6	34.5	4.0	8.6	3.6	4.0	0.6
25105	Meat loaf	1	slice(s)	115	84.6	244	17.0	6.6	0.4	15.9	6.1	6.9	0.8

PAGE KEY: A-6 5 Breads/Baked Goods A-12 = Cereal/Rice/Pasta A-16 = Fruit A-22 = Vegetables/Legumes A-32 = Nuts/Seeds A-34 = Vegetarian A-36 = Dairy A-44 = Eggs A-44 = Seafood A-46 = Meats A-50 = Poultry
A-52 = Processed Meats A-54 = Beverages A-58 = Fats/Oils A-60 = Sweets A-62 = Spices/Condiments/Sauces A-66 = Mixed Foods/Soups/Sandwiches A-72 = Fast Food A-90 = Convenience A-92 = Baby Foods

Chol (mg)	Calc (mg)	Iron (mg)	Magn (mg)	Pota (mg)	Sodi (mg)	Zinc (mg)	Vit A (µg)	Thia (mg)	Vit E (mg α)	Ribo (mg)	Niac (mg)	Vit B$_6$ (mg)	Fola (µg)	Vit C (mg)	Vit B$_{12}$ (µg)	Sele (µg)
0	5	0.36	9.5	125.7	61.9	0.11	—	0.03	0	0.02	0.63	0.06	—	43.9	0	0
0	7	1.05	11.1	231.3	113.8	0.14	—	0.02	0	0.22	0.61	0.34	—	0.3	0	0.3
0	5	0.16	3.8	19.0	258.4	0.05	0	0	0.04	0.03	0.19	0.01	3.7	0.1	0	0.3
2	5	0.01	0.5	6.6	15.8	0.02	8.0	0	0.02	0.01	0	0	0.3	0.1	0	0.1
1	36	1.56	58.3	278.3	294.1	1.06	13.3	0.07	1.76	0.09	1.95	0.09	14.6	3.6	0.1	2.1
0	5	0.03	0.6	8.6	437.3	0.01	0	0	0	0.02	0.24	0	2.4	0	0.1	0.7
0	1	0.05	0.6	6.0	29.8	0.01	3.9	0	0	0	0.01	0.01	0.1	0.2	0	0
0	10	0.13	4.8	91.2	225.6	0.06	7.7	0.01	0.39	0.01	0.36	0.06	1.3	0.6	0	0.3
0	3	0.36	6.1	32.4	599.9	0.07	0	0.01	0	0.02	0.60	0.03	2.9	0	0	0.1
0	4	0.43	7.2	37.9	999.3	0.08	0	0.01	0	0.03	0.71	0.04	3.2	0	0	0.1
0	5	0.20	3.1	51.2	183.6	0.05	0	0.01	0.09	0.01	0.33	0.02	2.3	1.4	0	1.4
0	5	0.31	11.0	40.5	689.9	0.02	0	0.01	0	0.01	0.23	0.02	1.4	0	0	0.2
0	28	1.36	26.2	573.3	265.2	0.40	0	0.06	2.11	0.07	1.58	0.16	20.4	19.6	0	1.9
0	16	1.24	19.5	403.8	13.4	0.24	26.8	0.03	1.73	0.08	1.19	0.12	13.4	8.5	0	0.2
4	70	0.20	8.3	92.3	209.4	0.24	61.5	0.04	0.17	0.11	0.24	0.02	6.0	0.5	0.2	2.4
0	6	0.30	0.7	45.4	55.6	0.01	0.3	0	0	0.01	0.04	0	0.5	0.7	0	0
—	0	0	—	—	0	—	—	—	—	—	—	—	—	0	—	—
0	1	0.03	0.7	10.9	0.7	0.01	0	0	0	0	0	0	0	0	0	0
0	1	0	0.1	0.3	0.3	0	0	0	0	0	0	0	0	0.0	0	0.1
0	0	0.08		2.4	0.8	—	—	0.08		0.08	0.08	—	—	0.3	0	
44	63	1.55	55.7	617.1	532.4	1.33	33.9	0.07	3.97	0.24	9.03	0.53	29.0	5.8	0.2	23.2
120	26	1.56	30.0	372.8	476.7	2.68	0	0.07	1.12	0.26	6.89	0.39	25.8	5.0	0.3	19.3
38	331	2.91	47.3	451.1	548.1	1.85	0	0.27	1.42	0.27	1.80	0.20	132.3	4.4	0.3	15.3
58	98	3.46	35.7	468.3	876.4	3.66	17.8	0.35	1.07	0.17	7.01	0.44	133.8	23.0	0.8	33.9
17	41	1.87	24.3	256.0	633.6	1.09	471.0	0.29	0.41	0.13	2.72	0.21	124.2	35.3	0.2	27.5
38	30	2.20	32.8	484.2	589.5	4.31	178.4	0.13	0.24	0.23	5.02	0.24	25.1	8.7	1.5	15.6
74	77	2.82	35.8	378.9	829.4	3.58	66.6	0.24	1.36	0.25	6.39	0.28	87.0	1.0	0.7	33.5
44	63	1.55	55.7	617.1	532.4	1.33	33.9	0.07	3.97	0.24	9.03	0.53	29.0	5.8	0.2	23.2
54	569	3.65	49.3	436.8	1480.6	3.18	143.4	0.41	2.64	0.33	5.32	0.17	266.6	12.5	1.1	39.6
60	487	2.77	31.2	215.8	1036.6	2.17	154.8	0.28	0.89	0.30	2.42	0.08	102.2	6.2	0.3	24.9
49	45	1.34	25.3	275.7	399.5	0.96	58.2	0.18	0.41	0.18	8.21	0.31	71.4	0.7	0.4	25.4
61	54	1.59	34.7	429.7	557.7	1.87	342.9	0.10	2.52	0.21	5.54	0.41	54.3	26.9	0.2	16.9
109	49	2.35	39.4	471.4	488.9	2.14	0	0.11	1.39	0.22	9.75	0.59	25.3	8.6	0.3	22.2
25	64	1.21	17.7	205.8	129.7	1.03	4.0	0.14	0.06	0.17	3.28	0.20	29.1	0.4	0.3	14.8
60	73	2.77	35.3	312.5	957.6	1.41	138.6	0.58	0.40	0.28	5.62	0.30	126.0	0.8	0.8	17.9
200	41	3.22	75.6	612.4	1361.5	4.73	36.6	0.16	0.61	0.42	20.90	1.03	14.6	0	0.7	49.5
42	20	0.78	23.7	196.1	245.7	1.13	0	0.04	0.58	0.10	4.05	0.25	13.1	1.7	0.2	10.6
27	44	3.17	50.0	645.1	788.7	3.44	0	0.13	1.38	0.24	3.02	0.24	31.0	10.2	0.6	6.6
7	41	0.53	9.0	162.9	20.7	0.18	47.7	0.06	—	0.06	0.24	0.11	24.3	29.4	0	0.6
90	63	0.65	19.8	194.4	198.0	2.45	34.2	0.05	—	0.05	1.74	0.10	36.6	1.7	3.6	24.4
27	266	1.08	38.5	251.4	276.3	1.27	—	0.07	0.03	0.16	1.28	0.18	—	59.3	0.2	6.0
0	28	1.74	41.8	298.4	149.9	0.76	0.5	0.07	—	0.08	0.53	0.06	53.0	0.8	0	0.5
10	181	1.55	36.3	167.2	412.1	1.36	0	0.34	0.09	0.34	2.69	0.10	221.3	0.8	0.5	38.4
73	146	2.66	61.3	222.9	885.7	3.44	0	0.10	0.10	0.17	3.00	0.27	—	0	1.2	36.7
63	28	1.52	25.7	223.7	689.0	1.58	17.8	0.05	0.34	0.08	5.14	0.23	11.9	0	0.1	22.2
77	18	1.69	26.3	293.5	635.1	1.90	16.1	0.04	1.77	0.17	4.16	0.29	21.9	2.3	0.3	21.0
0	13	0.65	11.4	178.0	26.9	0.22	59.0	0.03	—	0.05	0.57	0.08	38.3	24.0	0	0.4
65	50	1.94	63.2	432.5	895.9	1.52	38.9	0.15	3.73	0.15	13.05	0.58	42.1	7.5	0.3	23.0
78	45	3.68	54.3	835.4	1064.4	6.04	30.7	0.10	5.90	0.31	7.52	0.28	30.7	14.6	2.5	28.1
66	226	2.22	39.6	438.3	495.6	2.87	0	0.20	1.14	0.29	3.07	0.20	91.1	9.6	1.1	26.1
39	671	2.55	48.6	301.3	928.3	1.99	226.0	0.40	1.36	0.52	2.73	0.12	126.4	0	0.6	44.2
13	33	2.63	32.6	424.2	888.5	1.13	37.7	0.14	1.38	0.15	3.23	0.16	70.3	0	0.4	24.1
85	63	1.95	21.8	295.6	422.2	3.42	0	0.08	0.09	0.29	3.77	0.14	29.0	0.4	1.6	17.2

TABLE A-2 **Table of Food Composition** (*continued*)   (Computer code is for Cengage Diet Analysis program)   (For purposes of calculations, use "0" for t, <1, <0.1, <0.01)

DA+ Code	Food Description	Quantity	Measure	Wt (g)	H₂O (g)	Ener (kcal)	Prot (g)	Carb (g)	Fiber (g)	Fat (g)	Sat	Mono	Poly
Mixed Foods, Sandwiches, and Soups—*continued*													
16646	Moo shi pork	1	cup(s)	151	77.6	504	18.9	5.2	0.6	45.4	6.8	18.2	18.6
16788	Nachos with beef, beans, cheese, tomatoes and onions	1	serving(s)	195	102.8	505	23.0	35.4	4.9	30.8	12.2	10.2	5.6
6116	Pepperoni pizza	2	slice(s)	142	66.1	362	20.2	39.7	2.9	13.9	4.5	6.3	2.3
29601	Pizza with meat and vegetables, thin crust	2	slice(s)	232	97.7	698	30.0	60.5	4.9	37.2	15.5	11.3	6.7
655	Potato salad	½	cup(s)	125	95.0	179	3.3	14.0	1.6	10.3	1.8	3.1	4.7
25109	Salisbury steaks with mushroom sauce	1	serving(s)	135	101.8	250	17.0	9.5	0.5	15.4	6.0	6.7	0.8
16637	Shrimp creole with rice	1	cup(s)	243	178.2	296	24.7	27.6	1.7	8.9	1.6	3.6	3.0
41866	Spaghetti and meatballs, canned	1	cup(s)	248	196.7	241	11.1	27.0	—	9.9	3.6	4.0	1.2
28585	Spicy thai noodles (pad thai)	8	ounce(s)	227	72.7	218	8.8	35.1	3.0	6.4	0.8	3.4	1.7
33073	Stir fried pork and vegetables with rice	1	cup(s)	236	173.9	351	15.4	33.7	1.8	16.3	5.6	7.0	2.6
28588	Stuffed shells	2 ½	item(s)	249	157.6	242	15.1	27.7	2.7	8.2	3.1	3.0	1.3
16821	Sushi with egg in seaweed	6	piece(s)	156	116.7	192	8.9	20.0	0.3	7.8	2.1	3.2	1.9
16819	Sushi with vegetables and fish	6	piece(s)	156	97.6	236	6.9	48.1	0.6	0.8	0.2	0.2	0.2
16820	Sushi with vegetables in seaweed	6	piece(s)	156	109.4	187	3.5	41.0	0.8	0.4	0.1	0.1	0.1
25266	Sweet and sour pork	¾	cup(s)	249	206.0	265	29.3	16.9	1.0	8.1	2.7	3.6	1.4
16824	Tabouli, tabbouleh or tabuli	1	cup(s)	160	124.1	198	2.6	15.5	3.7	15.0	2.1	10.7	1.7
25276	Three bean salad	½	cup(s)	99	82.3	96	1.9	9.6	2.6	6.0	0.8	1.6	3.2
160	Tuna salad	½	cup(s)	103	64.7	192	16.4	9.6	0	9.5	1.6	3.0	4.2
25241	Turkey and noodles	1	cup(s)	227	162.4	193	17.1	15.2	0.8	6.6	1.7	2.5	1.6
16794	Vegetable egg roll	2	item(s)	128	63.3	323	8.0	38.6	3.3	15.3	3.2	7.3	3.8
16818	Vegetable sushi, no fish	6	piece(s)	156	92.1	256	4.2	56.7	0.9	0.4	0.1	0.1	0.1
	Sandwiches												
1744	Bacon, lettuce and tomato with mayonnaise	1	item(s)	164	95.8	346	11.7	35.7	2.5	17.4	3.7	5.4	6.6
30287	Bologna and cheese with margarine	1	item(s)	111	45.7	339	13.6	29.9	1.4	18.0	7.0	5.7	3.3
30286	Bologna with margarine	1	item(s)	83	33.4	251	8.8	27.2	1.4	11.6	3.3	3.9	2.9
16546	Cheese	1	item(s)	83	31.2	254	9.4	27.9	1.4	11.5	4.5	2.9	3.1
8789	Cheeseburger, large, plain	1	item(s)	166	70.8	506	28.7	34.5	2.3	28.3	11.2	9.2	0.9
8624	Cheeseburger, large, with bacon, vegetables and condiments	1	item(s)	195	91.4	550	30.8	36.8	2.5	30.9	11.9	10.6	1.3
1745	Club with bacon, chicken, tomato, lettuce and mayonnaise	1	item(s)	246	137.8	546	40.4	40.1	2.7	24.0	5.6	7.6	8.5
1908	Cold cut submarine with cheese and vegetables	1	item(s)	228	131.8	456	21.8	51.0	2.0	18.6	6.8	8.2	2.3
30247	Corned beef	1	item(s)	130	74.1	268	18.8	25.6	1.7	9.4	3.6	3.4	1.2
25283	Egg salad	1	item(s)	126	72.0	278	10.4	28.5	1.5	13.4	3.0	4.0	4.8
16686	Fried egg	1	item(s)	96	49.2	225	10.7	26.2	1.4	8.1	2.2	3.0	2.3
16547	Grilled cheese	1	item(s)	83	27.8	282	9.4	28.0	1.4	14.6	5.2	5.2	3.2
16659	Gyro with onion and tomato	1	item(s)	390	255.6	593	44.2	73.7	3.9	12.2	4.4	4.3	1.6
1906	Ham and cheese	1	item(s)	146	74.2	352	20.7	33.3	2.0	15.5	6.4	6.7	1.4
31890	Ham with mayonnaise	1	item(s)	112	55.8	272	13.7	28.0	2.1	11.4	2.7	3.9	4.0
756	Hamburger, double patty, large, with condiments and vegetables	1	item(s)	226	121.5	540	34.3	40.3	—	26.6	10.5	10.3	2.8
8793	Hamburger, large, plain	1	item(s)	137	57.7	426	22.6	31.7	1.5	22.9	8.4	9.9	2.1
8795	Hamburger, large, with vegetables and condiments	1	item(s)	218	121.4	512	25.8	40.0	3.1	27.4	10.4	11.4	2.2
25134	Hot chicken salad	1	item(s)	98	48.8	239	15.6	23.4	1.1	8.8	2.8	2.6	2.8
25133	Hot turkey salad	1	item(s)	98	50.4	221	16.0	23.4	1.1	6.6	2.2	1.8	2.3
1411	Hotdog with bun, plain	1	item(s)	98	52.9	242	10.4	18.0	1.6	14.5	5.1	6.9	1.7
30249	Pastrami	1	item(s)	134	82.6	221	16.5	26.6	1.7	4.8	1.8	1.4	0.9
16701	Peanut butter	1	item(s)	93	24.2	337	13.0	37.4	3.4	16.1	3.4	7.1	5.0
30306	Peanut butter and jelly	1	item(s)	93	24.7	323	11.0	41.6	3.1	13.7	2.9	6.1	4.2
1909	Roast beef submarine with mayonnaise and vegetables	1	item(s)	216	127.4	410	28.6	44.3	—	13.0	7.1	1.8	2.6
1910	Roast beef, plain	1	item(s)	139	67.6	346	21.5	33.4	1.2	13.8	3.6	6.8	1.7
1907	Steak with mayonnaise and vegetables	1	item(s)	204	104.2	459	30.3	52.0	2.3	14.1	3.8	5.3	3.3
25288	Tuna salad	1	item(s)	179	102.2	415	24.1	28.9	1.6	22.2	3.6	5.5	11.4

PAGE KEY: A-6 5 Breads/Baked Goods A-12 = Cereal/Rice/Pasta A-16 = Fruit A-22 = Vegetables/Legumes A-32 = Nuts/Seeds A-34 = Vegetarian A-36 = Dairy A-44 = Eggs A-44 = Seafood A-46 = Meats A-50 = Poultry
A-52 = Processed Meats A-54 = Beverages A-58 = Fats/Oils A-60 = Sweets A-62 = Spices/Condiments/Sauces A-66 = Mixed Foods/Soups/Sandwiches A-72 = Fast Food A-90 = Convenience A-92 = Baby Foods

Chol (mg)	Calc (mg)	Iron (mg)	Magn (mg)	Pota (mg)	Sodi (mg)	Zinc (mg)	Vit A (µg)	Thia (mg)	Vit E (mg α)	Ribo (mg)	Niac (mg)	Vit B$_6$ (mg)	Fola (µg)	Vit C (mg)	Vit B$_{12}$ (µg)	Sele (µg)
157	32	1.40	27.2	350.3	1051.0	1.78	54.4	0.51	5.54	0.41	4.04	0.44	18.1	7.9	0.5	31.0
74	310	2.89	93.6	481.6	520.7	4.60	115.1	0.09	2.42	0.26	2.92	0.37	50.7	5.7	1.6	17.5
28	129	1.87	17.0	305.3	533.9	1.04	105.1	0.27	—	0.47	6.09	0.11	92.7	3.3	0.4	26.1
79	554	3.83	51.0	471.0	1719.1	3.85	136.9	0.47	2.55	0.38	6.20	0.20	257.5	9.0	1.4	45.0
85	24	0.81	18.8	317.5	661.3	0.39	40.0	0.10	—	0.08	1.11	0.18	8.8	12.5	0	5.1
60	77	2.00	23.7	308.4	369.1	3.47	0	0.11	0.03	0.30	4.00	0.14	33.3	0.3	1.7	16.9
262	192	4.59	51.0	291.6	984.2	2.48	75.3	0.24	2.45	0.09	3.19	0.24	136.1	14.8	0.8	58.3
17	89	3.03	34.7	498.5	781.2	1.36	47.1	0.24	1.17	0.21	5.54	0.18	—	5.5	0.6	23.6
37	32	1.55	49.2	183.9	587.1	1.06	0	0.17	1.29	0.13	1.85	0.17	55.7	16.0	0.1	3.2
46	40	2.66	32.8	400.0	569.4	2.08	0	0.51	0.60	0.20	5.00	0.30	163.1	18.3	0.4	22.5
30	194	2.50	54.3	382.8	466.6	1.48	0	0.24	1.87	0.30	3.77	0.28	161.0	9.8	0.2	29.9
187	45	1.79	18.7	137.3	455.5	1.06	115.4	0.12	0.89	0.28	1.31	0.15	82.7	1.9	0.5	20.0
12	23	2.12	18.7	115.4	424.3	0.65	7.8	0.23	0.23	0.04	2.37	0.11	135.7	0.9	0.3	14.8
0	17	1.54	17.2	85.8	154.4	0.69	10.9	0.20	0.08	0.04	1.89	0.13	120.1	2.2	0	10.1
74	41	1.72	34.0	612.1	623.9	2.52	0	0.80	0.73	0.37	6.69	0.65	14.6	9.8	0.7	49.6
0	32	1.20	35.2	246.4	798.4	0.48	54.4	0.07	2.43	0.04	1.12	0.11	32.0	25.3	0	0.5
0	27	0.96	15.5	145.0	207.4	0.53	0	0.04	0.94	0.06	0.26	0.06	25.0	9.2	0	2.5
13	17	1.02	19.5	182.4	412.0	0.57	24.6	0.03	—	0.07	6.87	0.08	8.2	2.3	1.2	42.2
53	50	1.74	23.3	283.1	396.6	1.85	84.2	0.17	0.30	0.22	4.60	0.22	78.0	0.8	0.8	27.1
0	55	2.36	32.0	302.1	677.1	0.67	199.7	0.30	0.73	0.18	2.40	0.17	130.6	16.5	0.1	15.6
0	20	2.43	17.2	90.5	425.9	0.70	0	0.27	0.06	0.04	2.47	0.10	156.0	0.2	0	9.7
21	82	2.43	29.5	344.4	944.6	1.08	42.6	0.34	1.16	0.26	4.42	0.21	108.2	10.2	0.2	27.9
39	518	2.47	26.6	213.1	894.7	1.64	73.3	0.35	0.57	0.29	3.25	0.18	96.6	0.2	0.9	22.8
17	159	2.21	17.4	143.6	534.5	1.05	10.0	0.34	0.34	0.18	3.17	0.15	91.3	0.2	0.5	18.1
22	486	2.11	21.6	126.2	627.5	1.00	66.4	0.29	0.58	0.23	2.53	0.10	93.8	0	0.4	15.9
93	277	4.02	39.8	360.2	884.8	5.16	—	0.32	—	0.69	7.42	0.44	129.5	0.0	2.5	34.9
98	267	4.04	44.8	464.1	1314.3	5.21	—	0.34	—	0.68	8.25	0.47	122.8	1.4	2.4	6.6
96	221	4.08	54.1	511.7	949.6	2.24	36.9	0.57	1.35	0.35	17.36	0.74	147.6	4.7	0.6	51.7
36	189	2.51	68.4	394.4	1650.7	2.58	70.7	1.00	—	0.80	5.49	0.14	109.4	12.3	1.1	30.8
44	139	3.02	20.8	135.2	1099.8	2.28	2.6	0.28	0.21	0.20	3.69	0.11	92.3	0.3	0.8	33.4
217	106	2.58	18.6	145.0	494.1	0.94	0	0.27	1.10	0.44	2.27	0.16	112.1	0.7	0.6	24.5
174	164	2.71	19.2	126.7	348.5	1.05	95.0	0.30	0.68	0.34	2.56	0.13	112.3	0	0.4	25.9
21	491	2.13	21.6	128.6	669.0	1.00	131.1	0.22	1.09	0.22	2.30	0.06	62.3	0	0.2	15.9
98	179	5.66	78.0	799.5	873.6	7.99	35.1	0.85	1.09	0.69	14.11	0.62	234.0	12.5	2.5	70.2
58	130	3.24	16.1	290.5	770.9	1.37	96.4	0.31	0.29	0.48	2.69	0.20	78.8	2.8	0.5	23.1
32	150	2.44	24.6	213.9	986.7	1.16	5.6	0.61	0.49	0.22	4.05	0.26	94.1	2.1	0.2	22.6
122	102	5.85	49.7	569.5	791.0	5.67	—	0.36	—	0.38	7.57	0.54	110.7	1.1	4.1	25.5
71	74	3.58	27.4	267.1	474.0	4.11	0	0.29	—	0.29	6.25	0.23	80.8	0	2.1	27.1
87	96	4.93	43.6	479.6	824.0	4.88	—	0.41	—	0.37	7.28	0.33	115.5	2.6	2.4	33.6
39	114	1.93	20.4	150.3	469.7	1.22	0	0.20	0.31	0.23	4.94	0.20	79.5	0.2	0.3	16.9
37	113	2.04	21.8	166.9	459.2	1.09	0	0.19	0.25	0.21	4.36	0.23	79.6	0.2	0.3	20.3
44	24	2.31	12.7	143.1	670.3	1.98	0	0.24	—	0.27	3.65	0.05	60.8	0.1	0.5	26.0
36	142	3.19	22.8	178.2	1069.3	3.10	4.0	0.31	0.20	0.22	4.78	0.17	93.8	0.4	1.0	21.0
0	181	2.86	59.5	255.8	447.3	1.36	0	0.37	2.65	0.19	6.85	0.21	132.1	0	0	15.9
0	154	2.45	51.2	225.1	384.1	1.16	0	0.31	2.25	0.16	5.82	0.18	112.5	0.1	0	13.6
73	41	2.81	67.0	330.5	844.6	4.38	30.2	0.41	—	0.41	5.96	0.32	88.6	5.6	1.8	25.7
51	54	4.23	30.6	315.5	792.3	3.39	11.1	0.38	—	0.31	5.87	0.26	68.1	2.1	1.2	29.2
73	92	5.16	49.0	524.3	797.6	4.53	—	0.41	—	0.37	7.30	0.37	128.5	5.5	1.6	42.0
53	97	3.23	35.6	296.5	794.9	1.09	0	0.27	1.76	0.27	12.29	0.48	99.6	1.1	2.4	71.5

TABLE A-2 **Table of Food Composition** (continued)   (Computer code is for Cengage Diet Analysis program)   (For purposes of calculations, use "0" for t, <1, <0.1, <0.01)

DA+ Code	Food Description	Quantity	Measure	Wt (g)	H₂O (g)	Ener (kcal)	Prot (g)	Carb (g)	Fiber (g)	Fat (g)	Sat	Mono	Poly
											\multicolumn{3}{Fat Breakdown (g)}		

DA+ Code	Food Description	Quantity	Measure	Wt (g)	H₂O (g)	Ener (kcal)	Prot (g)	Carb (g)	Fiber (g)	Fat (g)	Sat	Mono	Poly
Mixed Foods, Sandwiches, and Soups—*continued*													
30283	Turkey submarine with cheese, lettuce, tomato and mayonnaise	1	item(s)	277	167.2	529	29.3	50.9	3.0	22.9	6.5	5.8	8.3
31891	Turkey with mayonnaise	1	item(s)	143	73.9	330	29.1	26.7	1.4	11.1	2.4	2.5	4.9
	Soups												
25296	Bean	1	cup(s)	243	204.8	153	10.8	23.2	8.2	1.9	0.5	0.7	0.6
711	Bean with pork, condensed, prepared with water	1	cup(s)	266	227.0	168	7.7	22.1	7.7	5.7	1.5	2.1	1.8
713	Beef noodle, condensed, prepared with water	1	cup(s)	244	224.9	83	4.7	8.7	0.7	3.0	1.1	1.2	0.5
825	Cheese, condensed, prepared with milk	1	cup(s)	251	206.9	231	9.5	16.2	1.0	14.6	9.1	4.1	0.5
826	Chicken broth, condensed, prepared with water	1	cup(s)	244	234.1	39	4.9	0.9	0	1.4	0.4	0.6	0.3
25297	Chicken noodle soup	1	cup(s)	241	218.2	99	9.1	9.2	0.8	2.5	0.7	0.9	0.6
827	Chicken noodle, condensed, prepared with water	1	cup(s)	248	232.7	62	3.1	7.3	0.5	2.4	0.6	1.0	0.7
724	Chicken noodle, dehydrated, prepared with water	1	cup(s)	245	230.7	56	2.1	9.0	0.2	1.3	0.3	0.5	0.4
1769	Chicken noodle, low-sodium, condensed, prepared with water	1	cup(s)	248	232.7	62	3.1	7.3	0.5	2.4	0.6	1.0	0.7
823	Cream of asparagus, condensed, prepared with milk	1	cup(s)	248	213.3	161	6.3	16.4	0.7	8.2	3.3	2.1	2.2
824	Cream of celery, condensed, prepared with milk	1	cup(s)	248	214.4	164	5.7	14.5	0.7	9.7	3.9	2.5	2.7
708	Cream of chicken, condensed, prepared with milk	1	cup(s)	248	210.4	191	7.5	15.0	0.2	11.5	4.6	4.5	1.6
715	Cream of chicken, condensed, prepared with water	1	cup(s)	244	221.1	117	3.4	9.3	0.2	7.4	2.1	3.3	1.5
709	Cream of mushroom, condensed, prepared with milk	1	cup(s)	252	219.3	161	5.9	14.5	0.8	9.0	2.8	2.2	3.6
716	Cream of mushroom, condensed, prepared with water	1	cup(s)	248	229.3	97	1.6	8.3	0.7	6.4	1.2	1.5	3.5
9558	Cream of mushroom, low-sodium, canned, ready to serve	1	cup(s)	244	218.1	139	2.5	15.6	0	7.4	2.0	1.6	3.3
25298	Cream of vegetable	1	cup(s)	260	229.2	151	6.4	13.8	1.7	7.9	1.4	4.2	1.8
16689	Egg drop	1	cup(s)	244	226.6	66	2.8	10.5	1.0	1.5	0.4	0.5	0.3
25138	Golden squash	1	cup(s)	258	224.0	144	7.5	20.6	1.5	3.9	0.7	2.1	0.9
16663	Hot and sour	1	cup(s)	244	221.2	95	6.3	10.6	1.2	3.0	0.6	0.7	0.8
28054	Lentil chowder	1	cup(s)	248	204.1	168	10.8	30.9	13.2	0.6	0.1	0.1	0.3
28560	Macaroni and bean	1	cup(s)	246	138.8	147	6.6	23.3	5.0	3.5	0.5	2.2	0.5
714	Manhattan clam chowder, condensed, prepared with water	1	cup(s)	249	229.7	75	2.1	11.9	1.5	2.1	0.4	0.4	1.3
28561	Minestrone	1	cup(s)	240	184.6	105	5.2	17.3	4.8	2.2	0.3	1.4	0.3
717	Minestrone, condensed, prepared with water	1	cup(s)	241	220.1	82	4.3	11.2	1.0	2.5	0.6	0.7	1.1
53690	Minestrone, reduced sodium, canned, ready to serve	1	cup(s)	241	210.4	120	4.8	21.7	5.8	1.9	0.3	0.7	0.6
28038	Mushroom & wild rice	1	cup(s)	241	196.6	88	4.7	13.3	1.6	0.3	0.1	0	0.1
828	New England clam chowder, condensed, prepared with milk	1	cup(s)	252	215.4	154	8.2	18.8	0.8	5.1	2.8	0.7	1.3
75714	New England clam chowder, reduced sodium, canned, ready to serve	1	cup(s)	256	221.5	179	6.0	14.5	2.0	10.8	1.8	2.3	5.1
28036	New England style clam chowder	1	cup(s)	254	235.0	67	3.0	11.5	1.2	0.1	0	0	0
28566	Old country pasta	1	cup(s)	245	175.9	151	6.5	21.0	3.4	3.4	1.6	2.1	0.7
725	Onion, dehydrated, prepared with water	1	cup(s)	230	220.3	28	0.7	6.4	0.7	0	0	0	0
16667	Shrimp gumbo	1	cup(s)	244	207.2	163	8.9	18.3	2.9	6.8	3.9	1.6	0.6
28037	Southwestern corn chowder	1	cup(s)	240	211.2	109	4.8	19.7	2.2	0.5	0.1	0.1	0.2
30282	Soybean (miso)	1	cup(s)	240	218.8	84	6.0	7.8	1.9	3.4	0.6	1.2	1.3
25140	Split pea	1	cup(s)	165	116.6	83	4.5	18.5	1.5	0.4	0.1	0	0.2
718	Split pea with ham, condensed, prepared with water	1	cup(s)	253	206.9	190	10.3	28.0	2.3	4.4	1.8	1.8	0.6
32411	Split pea with ham, reduced sodium & fat, ready to serve	1	cup(s)	243	196.8	185	12.6	27.5	—	2.7	0.7	1.0	0.5

PAGE KEY: A-6 5 Breads/Baked Goods A-12 = Cereal/Rice/Pasta A-16 = Fruit A-22 = Vegetables/Legumes A-32 = Nuts/Seeds A-34 = Vegetarian A-36 = Dairy A-44 = Eggs A-44 = Seafood A-46 = Meats A-50 = Poultry
A-52 = Processed Meats A-54 = Beverages A-58 = Fats/Oils A-60 = Sweets A-62 = Spices/Condiments/Sauces A-66 = Mixed Foods/Soups/Sandwiches A-72 = Fast Food A-90 = Convenience A-92 = Baby Foods

Chol (mg)	Calc (mg)	Iron (mg)	Magn (mg)	Pota (mg)	Sodi (mg)	Zinc (mg)	Vit A (µg)	Thia (mg)	Vit E (mg α)	Ribo (mg)	Niac (mg)	Vit B$_6$ (mg)	Fola (µg)	Vit C (mg)	Vit B$_{12}$ (µg)	Sele (µg)
66	521	4.68	52.6	567.8	1795.0	2.63	105.3	0.70	1.36	0.60	4.38	0.33	166.2	11.6	0.7	44.9
64	162	3.42	34.3	307.5	471.9	3.00	5.7	0.34	0.74	0.28	7.05	0.46	98.7	0	0.3	42.2
4	63	2.35	45.2	491.2	539.4	1.12	28.0	0.24	0.23	0.13	3.00	0.16	116.2	2.1	0.2	4.3
3	82	2.00	45.2	391.0	928.3	1.01	45.2	0.09	1.14	0.03	0.55	0.04	31.9	1.6	0	8.2
5	20	1.07	7.3	97.6	793.0	1.51	12.2	0.07	1.22	0.06	1.04	0.04	29.3	0.5	0	7.3
48	289	0.80	20.1	341.4	1019.1	0.68	358.9	0.06	—	0.33	0.50	0.08	10.0	1.3	0.4	7.0
0	10	0.51	2.4	209.8	746.6	0.24	0	0.01	0.05	0.07	3.35	0.02	4.9	0	0.2	0
19	22	1.03	13.6	283.4	631.4	0.68	54.2	0.13	0.18	0.13	4.74	0.12	46.8	1.1	0.3	10.3
12	15	1.64	9.9	54.6	865.5	0.40	27.3	0.14	0.07	0.11	1.34	0.05	29.8	0	0	11.9
10	5	0.49	7.3	31.9	561.0	0.20	2.5	0.20	0.12	0.07	1.06	0.02	27.0	0	0	9.3
12	15	1.64	9.9	54.6	429.0	0.40	27.3	0.14	0.07	0.11	1.34	0.05	29.8	0	0	11.9
22	174	0.87	19.8	359.6	1041.6	0.92	62.0	0.10	—	0.28	0.88	0.06	29.8	4.0	0.5	8.0
32	186	0.69	22.3	310.0	674.6	0.20	114.1	0.07	—	0.25	0.44	0.06	7.4	1.5	0.5	4.7
27	181	0.67	17.4	272.8	897.8	0.67	178.6	0.07	—	0.26	0.92	0.07	7.4	1.2	0.5	8.0
10	34	0.61	2.4	87.8	846.7	0.63	163.5	0.03	—	0.06	0.82	0.02	2.4	0.2	0.1	7.0
10	171	0.25	17.6	259.6	899.6	0.78	75.6	0.07	0.65	0.26	0.54	0.07	7.6	0.3	0.7	6.8
0	17	0.22	5.0	76.9	843.2	0.15	2.5	0.01	0.60	0.02	0.42	0.02	2.5	0	0	3.5
8	33	0	—	155.6	61.4	—	0	—	—	—	—	—	—	0	—	—
1	71	1.10	16.3	311.2	694.3	0.55	202.3	0.10	1.35	0.19	2.99	0.10	49.2	9.2	0.3	4.5
56	17	0.63	4.9	53.7	902.8	0.22	48.8	0.05	0.32	0.05	0.38	0.05	17.1	15.9	0.1	1.0
4	261	0.76	42.4	522.3	496.7	0.92	0	0.18	1.39	0.38	1.15	0.16	42.9	10.5	0.9	7.9
51	46	1.56	22.0	134.2	917.4	0.54	22.0	0.06	0.95	0.08	1.24	0.16	19.5	0	0.2	1.0
0	54	3.86	64.9	660.5	28.3	2.00	0	0.38	0.98	0.11	1.82	0.33	195.9	13.1	0	3.7
0	70	1.92	35.6	270.1	519.7	0.89	0	0.14	1.33	0.14	1.42	0.13	92.3	4.9	0	9.3
2	27	1.59	10.0	184.3	562.7	0.90	49.8	0.03	1.25	0.04	0.79	0.10	10.0	4.0	3.9	9.2
0	71	1.80	31.8	264.9	434.9	0.74	0	0.10	1.12	0.10	0.69	0.10	61.8	10.9	0	4.0
2	34	0.92	7.2	313.3	612.1	0.75	118.1	0.05	—	0.04	0.94	0.10	50.6	1.2	0	8.0
0	48	1.73	31.3	448.2	518.1	0.77	79.5	0.14	1.69	0.10	1.54	0.14	37.8	13.7	0	5.1
0	29	1.11	27.3	347.4	281.1	0.93	0	0.06	0.16	0.22	3.03	0.15	26.9	3.8	0.1	4.9
18	176	3.05	30.2	451.1	688.0	1.08	93.2	0.20	0.55	0.44	2.00	0.18	22.7	5.3	12.2	11.1
8	36	1.43	33.3	862.7	496.6	0.69	20.5	0.04	1.02	0.04	1.08	0.33	15.4	8.4	2.4	11.0
4	74	1.06	29.6	465.3	349.9	0.45	0	0.07	0.41	0.11	0.93	0.17	16.1	10.0	6.1	6.2
7	55	2.44	50.7	472.7	346.8	0.76	0	0.20	0.94	0.16	2.55	0.26	102.3	18.8	0.1	9.2
0	21	0.12	9.2	71.3	795.8	0.12	0	0.03	0.02	0.03	0.14	0.06	0	0.2	0	0.5
90	132	2.90	46.4	429.4	646.6	1.12	65.9	0.17	1.63	0.13	2.21	0.24	104.9	18.5	0.2	17.6
1	83	0.94	26.1	417.2	208.9	0.58	0	0.09	0.28	0.15	1.75	0.24	32.9	35.9	0.3	2.1
0	62	1.82	38.4	367.2	976.8	0.77	230.4	0.06	0.96	0.16	2.62	0.16	55.2	4.6	0.2	1.4
0	30	1.25	32.7	352.3	607.9	0.57	0	0.12	0.14	0.09	1.67	0.21	72.0	8.8	0	0.4
8	23	2.28	48.1	399.7	1006.9	1.32	22.8	0.15	—	0.08	1.47	0.07	2.5	1.5	0.3	8.0
15	—	2.24	—	—	833.5	—	318.3	—	—	—	—	—	—	10.2	—	—

TABLE A-2 Table of Food Composition *(continued)*   (Computer code is for Cengage Diet Analysis program)   (For purposes of calculations, use "0" for t, <1, <0.1, <0.01)

DA+ Code	Food Description	Quantity	Measure	Wt (g)	H₂O (g)	Ener (kcal)	Prot (g)	Carb (g)	Fiber (g)	Fat (g)	Fat Breakdown (g) Sat	Mono	Poly
Mixed Foods, Sandwiches, and Soups—*continued*													
726	Tomato vegetable, dehydrated, prepared with water	1	cup(s)	245	230.9	54	1.9	9.9	0.7	0.8	0.4	0.3	0.1
710	Tomato, condensed, prepared with milk	1	cup(s)	252	216.7	139	6.3	22.6	1.5	3.3	1.8	0.8	0.3
719	Tomato, condensed, prepared with water	1	cup(s)	248	226.6	74	2.0	16.3	1.5	0.7	0.2	0.2	0.2
40840	Tomato, low-sodium, prepared wtih water	1	cup(s)	244	223.0	73	1.9	16.0	1.5	0.7	0.2	0.2	0.2
28595	Turkey noodle	1	cup(s)	244	217.0	113	8.1	14.9	1.9	2.4	0.3	1.2	0.7
28051	Turkey vegetable	1	cup(s)	241	215.4	106	12.1	9.0	1.9	1.1	0.3	0.2	0.3
25141	Vegetable	1	cup(s)	252	225.3	92	4.5	19.6	4.3	0.4	0.1	0	0.2
720	Vegetable beef, condensed, prepared with water	1	cup(s)	244	224.0	76	5.4	9.9	2.0	1.9	0.8	0.8	0.1
28598	Vegetable gumbo	1	cup(s)	244	179.4	162	4.2	27.5	3.4	4.6	0.7	3.1	0.6
40841	Vegetable, low-sodium, prepared with water	1	cup(s)	253	231.1	83	2.8	15.3	2.8	1.1	0.2	0.3	0.5
721	Vegetarian vegetable, condensed, prepared with water	1	cup(s)	241	222.7	67	2.1	11.8	0.7	1.9	0.3	0.8	0.7
Fast Food													
	Arby's												
751	Beef 'n cheddar sandwich	1	item(s)	195	—	440	23.0	47.0	2.0	18.0	5.0	—	
36131	Chocolate shake, regular	1	serving(s)	468	—	570	14.0	99.0	1.0	15.0	10.0	—	—
80611	Cravin' chicken sandwich, crispy	1	item(s)	221	—	510	26.0	51.0	4.0	22.0	4.0	—	—
36045	Curly fries, large size	1	serving(s)	210	—	658	7.3	77.3	8.4	36.6	5.2	—	—
36044	Curly fries, medium size	1	serving(s)	170	—	540	6.0	62.0	7.0	29.0	4.0	—	—
57171	French dip & Swiss sandwich w/ au jus sauce	1	item(s)	286	—	430	26.0	52.0	2.0	14.0	6.0	—	—
34778	Jalapeno bites, 5-piece	1	serving(s)	110	—	280	5.0	31.0	2.0	16.0	6.0	—	—
9296	Jamocha shake, regular	1	serving(s)	468	—	560	14.0	98.0	1.0	15.0	10.0	—	—
9249	Junior roast beef sandwich	1	item(s)	87	—	210	12.0	25.0	1.0	6.0	2.0	—	—
9251	Large roast beef sandwich	1	item(s)	281	—	580	45.0	49.0	3.0	22.0	9.0	—	—
56537	Market Fresh crispy chicken farmhouse chopped salad	1	serving(s)	337	—	430	29.0	26.0	4.0	24.0	9.0	—	—
34769	Market Fresh roast turkey & Swiss sandwich	1	serving(s)	326	—	700	39.0	77.0	5.0	27.0	7.0	—	—
80607	Market Fresh roast turkey & Swiss wrap	1	item(s)	272	—	490	34.0	39.0	7.0	25.0	6.0	—	—
80608	Market Fresh roast turkey farmhouse chopped salad	1	serving(s)	300	—	240	22.0	10.0	3.0	13.0	7.0	—	—
9267	Market Fresh roast turkey ranch & bacon sandwich	1	serving(s)	344	—	800	45.0	78.0	5.0	36.0	9.0	—	—
34780	Mozzarella sticks, 4-piece	1	serving(s)	137	—	420	21.0	35.0	2.0	21.0	9.0	—	—
9275	Potato cakes	1	serving(s)	100	—	230	2.0	25.0	3.0	14.0	2.0	—	—
750	Roast beef sandwich, regular	1	item(s)	154	—	350	23.0	39.0	2.0	12.0	4.0	—	—
2009	Super roast beef sandwich	1	item(s)	229	—	430	23.0	45.0	3.0	17.0	5.0	—	—
36130	Vanilla shake, regular	1	serving(s)	425	—	470	14.0	75.0	0	15.0	10.0	—	—
	Auntie Anne's												
35351	Almond soft pretzel	1	item(s)	127	—	350	8.0	74.0	2.0	2.0	1.0	—	—
35371	Cheese dipping sauce	1	serving(s)	31	—	78	2.3	1.6	0	6.2	2.3	—	—
35353	Cinnamon sugar soft pretzel	1	item(s)	136	—	380	8.0	84.0	2.0	1.0	0	—	—
35354	Cinnamon sugar soft pretzel with butter	1	item(s)	147	—	470	8.0	84.0	2.0	12.0	7.0	—	—
56651	Garlic soft pretzel	1	item(s)	119	—	310	8.0	65.0	2.0	1.0	0	—	—
35372	Marinara dipping sauce	1	serving(s)	37	—	45	2.0	6.0	1.0	2.0	0	—	—
35357	Original soft pretzel	1	serving(s)	119	—	310	8.0	65.0	2.0	1.0	0	—	—
35358	Original soft pretzel with butter	1	item(s)	123	—	340	8.0	65.0	2.0	5.0	3.0	—	—
56653	Original soft preztel without salt	1	item(s)	117	—	310	8.0	65.0	2.0	1.0	0	—	—
35361	Sesame soft pretzel	1	item(s)	128	—	360	10.0	67.0	3.0	6.0	1.0	—	—
35362	Sesame soft pretzel with butter	1	item(s)	132	—	400	10.0	67.0	3.0	10.0	3.5	—	—
35364	Sour cream & onion soft pretzel	1	item(s)	123	—	330	9.0	68.0	2.0	1.5	0	—	—
35366	Sour cream & onion soft pretzel with butter	1	item(s)	127	—	360	9.0	68.0	2.0	5.0	3.0	—	—
35373	Sweet mustard dipping sauce	1	serving(s)	35	—	60	2.0	10.0	0	2.0	1.0	—	—

PAGE KEY: A-6 5 Breads/Baked Goods A-12 = Cereal/Rice/Pasta A-16 = Fruit A-22 = Vegetables/Legumes A-32 = Nuts/Seeds A-34 = Vegetarian A-36 = Dairy A-44 = Eggs A-44 = Seafood A-46 = Meats A-50 = Poultry
A-52 = Processed Meats A-54 = Beverages A-58 = Fats/Oils A-60 = Sweets A-62 = Spices/Condiments/Sauces A-66 = Mixed Foods/Soups/Sandwiches A-72 = Fast Food A-90 = Convenience A-92 = Baby Foods

Chol (mg)	Calc (mg)	Iron (mg)	Magn (mg)	Pota (mg)	Sodi (mg)	Zinc (mg)	Vit A (µg)	Thia (mg)	Vit E (mg α)	Ribo (mg)	Niac (mg)	Vit B_6 (mg)	Fola (µg)	Vit C (mg)	Vit B_{12} (µg)	Sele (µg)
0	20	0.59	9.8	164.1	323.4	0.20	9.8	0.06	0.42	0.09	1.22	0.06	12.3	2.9	0	2.0
10	174	1.39	30.2	461.2	529.2	0.93	95.8	0.10	0.45	0.32	1.37	0.15	5.0	15.9	0.7	9.3
0	20	1.34	17.4	277.8	471.2	0.30	24.8	0.05	0.42	0.08	1.25	0.10	0	15.6	0	6.2
0	20	1.32	17.1	273.3	80.5	0.29	24.4	0.05	0.41	0.08	1.23	0.10	0	15.4	0	6.1
25	31	1.44	23.7	217.1	398.4	0.76	0	0.22	0.63	0.11	2.91	0.16	65.1	5.9	0.1	16.1
21	38	1.37	23.5	405.4	347.8	0.96	0	0.09	0.21	0.09	3.55	0.30	26.1	10.5	0.2	10.0
0	41	2.44	39.4	684.8	720.6	0.67	0	0.12	1.82	0.13	2.37	0.27	38.0	23.5	0.1	1.8
5	20	1.10	7.3	168.4	851.6	1.51	190.3	0.04	0.59	0.05	1.01	0.07	9.8	2.4	0.3	2.7
0	56	2.05	37.3	334.5	501.9	0.60	0	0.18	1.13	0.08	1.72	0.16	104.1	18.8	0	3.9
0	30	0.83	32.9	549.0	490.8	0.51	108.8	0.14	1.82	0.12	1.95	0.21	15.2	1.0	0	5.1
0	24	1.06	7.2	207.3	814.6	0.46	171.1	0.05	1.40	0.05	0.90	0.06	9.6	1.4	0	4.3
45	150	4.50	—	—	1290.0	—	—	—	—	—	—	—	—	1.2	—	—
50	500	1.08	—	—	450.0	—	—	—	—	—	—	—	—	4.8	—	—
50	100	2.70	—	—	1110.0	—	—	—	—	—	—	—	—	9.0	—	—
0	42	2.82	—	—	1483.6	—	0	—	—	—	—	—	—	0	—	—
0	20	1.80	—	—	1200.0	—	0	—	—	—	—	—	—	0	—	—
55	150	4.50	—	—	2120.0	—	—	—	—	—	—	—	—	4.8	—	—
25	40	0.72	—	—	600.0	—	—	—	—	—	—	—	—	0	—	—
50	500	0.72	—	—	440.0	—	—	—	—	—	—	—	—	4.8	—	—
25	40	2.70	—	—	520.0	—	0	—	—	—	—	—	—	0	—	—
110	80	8.10	—	—	1870.0	—	0	—	—	—	—	—	—	0	—	—
65	250	1.44	—	—	1000.0	—	—	—	—	—	—	—	—	12.0	—	—
80	450	5.40	—	—	1770.0	—	—	—	—	—	—	—	—	6.0	—	—
80	350	3.60	—	—	1550.0	—	—	—	—	—	—	—	—	6.0	—	—
60	250	1.44	—	—	760.0	—	—	—	—	—	—	—	—	12.0	—	—
105	450	5.40	—	—	2200.0	—	—	—	—	—	—	—	—	6.0	—	—
50	600	0.72	—	—	1690.0	—	—	—	—	—	—	—	—	0	—	—
0	20	0.36	—	—	460.0	—	0	—	—	—	—	—	—	0	—	—
45	60	4.50	—	—	950.0	—	0	—	—	—	—	—	—	0	—	—
45	80	4.50	—	—	1060.0	—	—	—	—	—	—	—	—	6.0	—	—
50	500	0.36	—	—	390.0	—	—	—	—	—	—	—	—	4.8	—	—
0	20	0.72	—	—	400.0	—	0	—	—	—	—	—	—	0	—	—
12	78	0	—	—	364.3	—	23.3	—	—	—	—	—	—	0	—	—
0	20	0.72	—	—	400.0	—	0	—	—	—	—	—	—	0	—	—
25	20	0.72	—	—	400.0	—	—	—	—	—	—	—	—	0	—	—
0	20	0.72	—	—	990.0	—	0	—	—	—	—	—	—	0	—	—
0	0	1.08	—	—	140.0	—	20.0	—	—	—	—	—	—	36.0	—	—
0	20	0.72	—	—	990.0	—	0	—	—	—	—	—	—	0	—	—
10	20	0.72	—	—	990.0	—	—	—	—	—	—	—	—	0	—	—
0	20	0.72	—	—	400.0	—	0	—	—	—	—	—	—	0	—	—
0	100	1.80	—	—	990.0	—	0	—	—	—	—	—	—	0	—	—
10	100	1.80	—	—	990.0	—	0	—	—	—	—	—	—	0	—	—
0	60	0.72	—	—	1180.0	—	0	—	—	—	—	—	—	0	—	—
10	60	0.72	—	—	1180.0	—	—	—	—	—	—	—	—	0	—	—
35	0	0	—	—	0	—	0	—	—	—	—	—	—	0	—	—

TABLE A-2 Table of Food Composition *(continued)*   (Computer code is for Cengage Diet Analysis program)   (For purposes of calculations, use "0" for t, <1, <0.1, <0.01)

DA+ Code	Food Description	Quantity	Measure	Wt (g)	H₂O (g)	Ener (kcal)	Prot (g)	Carb (g)	Fiber (g)	Fat (g)	Fat Breakdown (g)		
											Sat	Mono	Poly
Fast Food—*continued*													
	Boston Market												
51194	Apple pie	1	slice(s)	163	—	580	43.0	74.0	3.0	30.0	13.0	—	—
35058	Brownie, chocolate	1	item(s)	85	—	320	5.0	49.0	3.0	13.0	3.0	—	—
35013	Chicken Carver sandwich with cheese and sauce	1	item(s)	321	—	750	57.0	64.0	3.0	29.0	8.0	—	—
34979	Chicken gravy	4	ounce(s)	113	—	50	0	7.0	0	2.0	0.5	—	—
35053	Chicken noodle soup	¾	cup(s)	171	—	103	9.1	9.5	0.8	3.3	1.0	—	—
34973	Chicken pot pie	1	item(s)	425	—	800	32.0	59.0	4.0	48.0	18.0	—	—
35054	Chicken tortilla soup with toppings	¾	cup(s)	171	—	193	8.0	14.1	0.9	12.2	3.3	—	—
35064	Chocolate cake	1	slice(s)	145	—	580	5.0	67.0	3.0	34.0	11.0	—	—
35057	Cornbread	1	item(s)	57	—	180	2.0	31.0	0	5.0	1.5	—	—
35008	Cranberry walnut relish	¾	cup(s)	210	—	350	3.0	75.0	3.0	4.5	0	—	—
34980	Creamed spinach	¾	cup(s)	191	—	280	9.0	12.0	4.0	23.0	15.0	—	—
34998	Fresh vegetable stuffing	1	cup(s)	136	—	190	3.0	25.0	2.0	8.0	1.0	—	—
34991	Garlic dill new potatoes	¾	cup(s)	156	—	140	3.0	24.0	3.0	3.0	1.0	—	—
34982	Green beans	¾	cup(s)	91	—	60	2.0	7.0	3.0	3.5	1.5	—	—
34984	Homestyle mashed potatoes	¾	cup(s)	221	—	270	5.0	36.0	4.0	11.0	5.0	—	—
34985	Homestyle mashed potatoes and gravy		cup(s)	227	—	153	3.4	22.4	2.0	6.4	4.1	—	—
34988	Hot cinnamon apples	¾	cup(s)	145	—	210	0	47.0	3.0	3.0	0	—	—
34989	Macaroni and cheese	¾	cup(s)	221	—	300	11.0	35.0	2.0	11.0	7.0	—	—
34970	Meatloaf	1	serving(s)	218	—	520	29.0	21.0	0	36.0	16.0	—	—
39383	Nestle Toll House chocolate chip cookie	1	item(s)	78	—	370	4.0	49.0	2.0	19.0	9.0	—	—
34963	Quarter chicken, white meat, no skin or wing	1	item(s)	173	—	250	41.0	4.0	0	8.0	2.5	—	—
34964	Quarter chicken, white meat, with skin and wing	1	item(s)	110	—	330	50.0	3.0	0	12.0	4.0	—	—
34968	Roasted turkey breast	5	ounce(s)	141	—	188	38.8	0	0	3.1	1.3	—	—
35011	Seasonal fresh fruit salad	1	serving(s)	142	—	60	1.0	15.0	1.0	0	0	0	0
51192	Spinach with garlic butter sauce	1	serving(s)	170	—	130	5.0	9.0	5.0	9.0	6.0	—	—
34999	Squash casserole	¾	cup(s)	187	—	330	7.0	20.0	3.0	24.0	13.0	—	—
35003	Steamed vegetables	1	cup(s)	136	—	60	2.0	8.0	3.0	2.0	0	—	—
35005	Sweet corn	¾	cup(s)	176	—	170	6.0	37.0	2.0	4.0	1.0	—	—
35004	Sweet potato casserole	¾	cup(s)	198	—	460	4.0	77.0	3.0	16.0	4.5	—	—
	Burger King												
29731	Biscuit with sausage, egg & cheese	1	item(s)	191	—	550	20.0	34.0	1.0	37.0	19.0	—	—
14249	Cheeseburger	1	item(s)	121	—	310	16.0	28.0	1.0	15.0	7.0	—	—
14251	Chicken sandwich	1	item(s)	218	—	630	24.0	46.0	3.0	39.0	7.0	—	—
14259	Chocolate shake, 12 ounces	1	item(s)	340	—	340	7.0	60.0	1.0	9.0	7.0	—	—
29732	Croissanwich with sausage & cheese	1	item(s)	106	37.2	380	14.0	26.0	0	24.0	10.0	12.7	3.3
14261	Croissanwich with sausage, egg & cheese	1	item(s)	159	71.4	460	19.0	27.0	0	31.0	11.0	15.8	6.1
3809	Double cheeseburger	1	item(s)	171	—	460	27.0	28.0	1.0	27.0	13.0	—	—
14244	Double Whopper sandwich	1	item(s)	373	—	920	48.0	51.0	3.0	58.0	19.0	—	—
14245	Double Whopper with cheese sandwich	1	item(s)	398	—	1010	53.0	53.0	3.0	65.0	24.0	—	—
14250	Fish sandwich	1	item(s)	248	—	640	23.0	67.0	3.0	31.0	5.0	—	—
14255	French fries, medium, salted	1	serving(s)	148	—	440	5.0	56.0	5.0	22.0	4.5	—	—
14262	French toast sticks (5)	1	serving(s)	109	37.6	380	5.0	49.0	2.0	18.0	3.0	10.6	2.9
14248	Hamburger	1	item(s)	110	—	260	14.0	27.0	1.0	11.0	4.0	—	—
14263	Hash brown rounds, small	1	serving(s)	78	27.1	240	2.0	23.0	3.0	15.0	3.5	—	—
14256	Onion rings, medium	1	serving(s)	117	—	400	6.0	47.0	4.0	21.0	3.5	—	—
39000	Tendercrisp chicken sandwich	1	item(s)	284	—	800	32.0	68.0	3.0	46.0	8.0	—	—
37514	TenderGrill chicken sandwich	1	item(s)	259	—	410	38.0	49.0	2.0	7.0	1.5	—	—
14258	Vanilla shake, 12 ounces	1	item(s)	340	—	290	7.0	46.0	0	9.0	7.0	—	—
1736	Whopper sandwich	1	item(s)	290	—	670	29.0	51.0	3.0	40.0	11.0	—	—
14243	Whopper with cheese sandwich	1	item(s)	315	—	770	33.0	52.0	3.0	48.0	16.0	—	—
	Carl's Jr.												
33962	Carl's bacon Swiss crispy chicken sandwich	1	item(s)	330	—	800	39.0	67.0	5.0	41.0	10.0	—	—

Chol (mg)	Calc (mg)	Iron (mg)	Magn (mg)	Pota (mg)	Sodi (mg)	Zinc (mg)	Vit A (µg)	Thia (mg)	Vit E (mg α)	Ribo (mg)	Niac (mg)	Vit B$_6$ (mg)	Fola (µg)	Vit C (mg)	Vit B$_{12}$ (µg)	Sele (µg)
0	—	—	—	—	690.0	—	—	—	—	—	—	—	—	—	—	—
50	—	—	—	—	220.1	—	—	—	—	—	—	—	—	—	—	—
160	211	2.85	—	—	1960.0	—	—	—	—	—	—	—	—	15.8	—	—
0	0	0	—	—	690.0	—	—	—	—	—	—	—	—	0	—	—
39	—	—	—	—	584.8	—	—	—	—	—	—	—	—	—	—	—
140	40	4.50	—	—	1090.0	—	—	—	—	—	—	—	—	1.2	—	—
33	—	—	—	—	986.4	—	—	—	—	—	—	—	—	—	—	—
45	36	1.64	—	—	360.0	—	—	—	—	—	—	—	—	0	—	—
10	0	0.71	—	—	320.0	—	—	—	—	—	—	—	—	0	—	—
0	0	5.40	—	—	0	—	0	—	—	—	—	—	—	0	—	—
70	264	2.85	—	—	580.0	—	—	—	—	—	—	—	—	9.5	—	—
0	—	—	—	—	580.0	—	—	—	—	—	—	—	—	—	—	—
0	0	0.86	—	—	120.0	—	—	—	—	—	—	—	—	14.3	—	—
0	43	0.38	—	—	180.0	—	—	—	—	—	—	—	—	5.1	—	—
25	51	0.46	—	—	820.0	—	—	—	—	—	—	—	—	19.2	—	—
17	68	0.41	—	—	834.1	—	—	—	—	—	—	—	—	16.9	—	—
0	16	0.29	—	—	15.0	—	—	—	—	—	—	—	—	0	—	—
30	345	1.66	—	—	1100.0	—	—	—	—	—	—	—	—	0	—	—
145	140	3.78	—	—	1030.0	—	—	—	—	—	—	—	—	1.8	—	—
20	0	1.32	—	—	340.0	—	—	—	—	—	—	—	—	0	—	—
125	0	0.89	—	—	480.0	—	0	—	—	—	—	—	—	0	—	—
165	0	0.78	—	—	960.0	—	0	—	—	—	—	—	—	0	—	—
69	25	2.25	—	—	625.0	—	—	—	—	—	—	—	—	0	—	—
0	16	0.29	—	—	20.0	—	—	—	—	—	—	—	—	29.5	—	—
20	—	0	—	—	200.0	—	—	—	—	—	—	—	—	—	—	—
70	200	0.72	—	—	1110.0	—	—	—	—	—	—	—	—	4.8	—	—
0	53	0.47	—	—	40.0	—	—	—	—	—	—	—	—	24.0	—	—
0	0	0.43	—	—	95.0	—	—	—	—	—	—	—	—	5.8	—	—
5	44	1.18	—	—	270.0	—	—	—	—	—	—	—	—	9.8	—	—
210	250	2.70	—	—	1520.0	—	—	—	—	—	—	—	—	0	—	—
40	150	2.70	—	—	740.0	—	—	0.25	—	0.32	4.18	—	—	1.2	—	—
65	64	2.90	—	—	1390.0	—	—	0.50	—	0.32	10.29	—	—	0	—	—
30	333	0.80	—	—	270.0	—	—	0.12	—	0.62	0.26	—	—	2.7	0	—
50	99	1.78	20.1	—	780.0	1.52	—	0.35	1.04	0.34	4.34	—	—	0	0.6	22.2
215	146	2.63	28.6	—	1000.0	2.08	—	0.39	1.67	0.52	4.72	0.29	—	0	1.1	38.0
80	250	4.50	—	—	990.0	—	—	0.26	—	0.45	6.37	—	—	1.2	—	—
140	150	8.08	—	—	1090.0	—	—	0.40	—	0.60	11.05	—	—	9.0	—	—
160	299	8.08	—	—	1530.0	—	—	0.40	—	0.67	11.04	—	—	9.0	—	—
45	101	3.63	—	—	1560.0	—	—	—	—	—	—	—	—	3.6	—	—
0	20	0.71	—	—	670.0	—	0	0.16	—	0.48	2.30	—	—	8.9	—	—
0	60	1.80	21.3	—	430.0	0.57	0	0.32	0.99	0.20	2.88	0.06	—	0	0	13.7
30	80	2.70	—	—	520.0	—	—	0.25	—	0.28	4.26	—	—	1.2	—	—
0	0	0.36	—	—	380.0	—	0	0.12	0.83	0.06	1.36	0.17	—	1.2	—	—
0	100	0	—	—	630.0	—	0	0.14	—	0.09	2.33	—	—	0	—	—
70	79	4.44	—	—	1640.0	—	—	—	—	—	—	—	—	8.9	—	—
75	57	6.83	—	—	1310.0	—	—	—	—	—	—	—	—	5.7	—	—
30	348	0	—	—	230.0	—	—	0.11	—	0.63	0.21	—	—	2.4	0	—
75	100	5.38	—	—	1020.0	—	—	0.39	—	0.44	7.30	—	—	9.0	—	—
100	249	5.38	—	—	1450.0	—	—	0.39	—	0.51	7.29	—	—	9.0	—	—
75	200	4.50	—	—	2130.0	—	—	—	—	—	—	—	—	4.8	—	—

TABLE A-2 Table of Food Composition *(continued)*   (Computer code is for Cengage Diet Analysis program)   (For purposes of calculations, use "0" for t, <1, <0.1, <0.01)

DA+ Code	Food Description	Quantity	Measure	Wt (g)	H₂O (g)	Ener (kcal)	Prot (g)	Carb (g)	Fiber (g)	Fat (g)	Fat Breakdown (g)		
											Sat	Mono	Poly
Fast Food—*continued*													
10801	Carl's Catch Fish sandwich	1	item(s)	298	—	730	20.0	77.0	5.0	37.0	6.0	—	—
10862	Carl's Famous Star hamburger	1	item(s)	269	—	620	25.0	56.0	3.0	34.0	10.0	—	—
10785	Charbroiled chicken club sandwich	1	item(s)	269	—	570	42.0	45.0	3.0	26.0	7.0	—	—
10866	Charbroiled chicken salad	1	item(s)	417	—	260	32.0	15.0	5.0	8.0	3.0	—	—
10855	Charbroiled Santa Fe Chicken sandwich	1	item(s)	273	—	640	39.0	45.0	3.0	33.0	8.0	—	—
10790	Chicken stars (6 pieces)	6	item(s)	84	—	320	12.0	14.0	2.0	24.0	6.0	—	—
34864	Chocolate shake, small	1	serving(s)	397	260.7	710	14.0	86.0	1.0	33.0	23.0	4.3	0.6
10797	Crisscut fries	1	serving(s)	139	—	450	5.0	42.0	4.0	29.0	5.0	—	—
10799	Double Western Bacon cheeseburger	1	item(s)	326	—	980	52.0	73.0	3.0	53.0	23.0	—	—
14238	French fries, small	1	serving(s)	119	—	320	4.0	42.0	4.0	15.0	3.0	—	—
10798	French toast dips without syrup, 5 pieces	1	serving(s)	110	—	430	8.0	51.0	2.0	22.0	4.0	—	—
10802	Onion rings	1	serving(s)	128	—	530	8.0	61.0	3.0	28.0	4.5	—	—
34858	Spicy chicken sandwich	1	item(s)	206	—	550	17.0	61.0	4.0	28.0	5.0	—	—
34867	Strawberry shake, small	1	serving(s)	397	—	700	14.0	85.0	0	33.0	23.0	—	—
10865	Super Star hamburger	1	item(s)	358	—	820	41.0	58.0	3.0	49.0	17.0	—	—
38925	The Six Dollar burger	1	item(s)	406	—	910	46.0	63.0	3.0	54.0	20.0	—	—
10818	Vanilla shake, small	1	item(s)	397	260.9	710	14.0	86.0	0	33.0	23.0	7.1	1.3
10770	Western Bacon cheeseburger	1	item(s)	225	—	667	30.6	67.6	2.8	30.6	12.0	—	—
10770	Western Bacon cheeseburger	1	item(s)	243	—	720	33.0	73.0	3.0	33.0	13.0	—	—
	Chick-Fil-A												
38746	Biscuit with bacon, egg & cheese	1	item(s)	159	—	500	21.0	43.0	2.0	27.0	12.0	—	—
38747	Biscuit with egg	1	item(s)	127	—	420	14.0	42.0	2.0	21.0	8.5	—	—
38748	Biscuit with egg & cheese	1	item(s)	154	—	470	17.0	43.0	2.0	25.0	11.0	—	—
38752	Biscuit with sausage, egg & cheese	1	item(s)	204	—	760	28.0	43.0	2.0	52.0	20.0	—	—
72643	Chargrilled chicken and fruit salad	1	item(s)	347	—	230	22.0	23.0	4.0	6.0	3.5	—	—
38760	Chargrilled chicken club sandwich	1	item(s)	258	—	410	37.0	39.0	3.0	12.0	5.0	—	—
38761	Chargrilled chicken Cool Wrap	1	item(s)	291	—	410	33.0	50.0	9.0	12.0	4.0	—	—
38758	Chargrilled chicken sandwich	1	item(s)	228	—	300	29.0	38.0	3.0	3.5	1.0	—	—
38763	Chick-n-Strips	4	item(s)	218	—	500	47.0	24.0	1.0	24.0	4.5	—	—
38742	Chicken biscuit	1	item(s)	143	—	440	17.0	47.0	3.0	20.0	8.0	—	—
38743	Chicken biscuit with cheese	1	item(s)	157	—	490	20.0	48.0	3.0	24.0	10.5	—	—
38764	Chicken salad sandwich on wheat bun	1	item(s)	233	—	500	29.0	52.0	4.0	20.0	3.5	—	—
38756	Chicken sandwich	1	item(s)	179	—	430	31.0	39.0	3.0	17.0	3.5	—	—
38757	Chicken sandwich, deluxe	1	item(s)	257	—	490	35.0	43.0	3.0	21.0	6.0	—	—
38770	Cole slaw	1	item(s)	298	—	580	3.0	31.0	5.0	50.0	8.0	—	—
38776	Diet lemonade, small	1	cup(s)	226	—	11	0	4.2	0	0.0	0	0	0
50867	Fruit cup, large	1	item(s)	194	—	100	1.0	27.0	3.0	0.0	0	0	0
38755	Hashbrowns	1	serving(s)	77	—	280	3.0	25.0	2.0	19.0	4.0	—	—
38765	Hearty breast of chicken soup	1	cup(s)	226	—	114	5.7	15.4	1.6	3.3	0.8	—	—
38741	Hot buttered biscuit	1	item(s)	86	—	310	5.0	41.0	2.0	13.0	6.0	—	—
38778	IceDream, small cone	1	item(s)	135	—	170	5.0	31.0	0	4.0	2.0	—	—
38774	IceDream, small cup	1	serving(s)	227	—	290	8.0	50.0	0	7.0	4.5	—	—
38775	Lemonade, small	1	cup(s)	226	—	120	0	32.5	0	0.0	0	0	0
38777	Nuggets	8	item(s)	113	—	270	28.0	12.0	1.0	12.0	2.5	—	—
38769	Side salad	1	item(s)	113	—	70	5.0	5.0	2.0	4.5	3.0	—	—
72642	Spicy chicken sandwich	1	item(s)	196	—	490	31.0	46.0	4.0	20.0	4.0	—	—
72626	Spicy chicken sandwich, deluxe	1	item(s)	281	—	580	36.0	48.0	4.0	27.0	8.0	—	—
38772	Waffle potato fries, small, salted	1	serving(s)	85	—	290	3.0	34.0	3.0	16.0	3.0	—	—
72633	Yogurt parfait w/ granola	1	item(s)	227	—	290	7.0	54.0	2.0	5.0	2.0	—	—
	Cinnabon												
39571	Cinnabon Bites	1	serving(s)	149	—	510	8.0	77.0	2.0	19.0	5.0	—	—
39570	Cinnabon Stix	5	item(s)	85	—	379	6.0	41.0	1.0	21.0	6.0	—	—
39567	Classic roll	1	item(s)	221	—	813	15.0	117.0	4.0	32.0	8.0	—	—

PAGE KEY: A-6 5 Breads/Baked Goods A-12 = Cereal/Rice/Pasta A-16 = Fruit A-22 = Vegetables/Legumes A-32 = Nuts/Seeds A-34 = Vegetarian A-36 = Dairy A-44 = Eggs A-44 = Seafood A-46 = Meats A-50 = Poultry
A-52 = Processed Meats A-54 = Beverages A-58 = Fats/Oils A-60 = Sweets A-62 = Spices/Condiments/Sauces A-66 = Mixed Foods/Soups/Sandwiches A-72 = Fast Food A-90 = Convenience A-92 = Baby Foods

Chol (mg)	Calc (mg)	Iron (mg)	Magn (mg)	Pota (mg)	Sodi (mg)	Zinc (mg)	Vit A (µg)	Thia (mg)	Vit E (mg α)	Ribo (mg)	Niac (mg)	Vit B$_6$ (mg)	Fola (µg)	Vit C (mg)	Vit B$_{12}$ (µg)	Sele (µg)
40	100	3.60	—	—	1320.0	—	—	—	—	—	—	—	—	4.8	—	—
65	100	4.50	—	—	1060.0	—	—	—	—	—	—	—	—	6.0	—	—
90	150	3.60	—	—	1310.0	—	—	—	—	—	—	—	—	6.0	—	—
70	200	2.70	—	—	620.0	—	—	—	—	—	—	—	—	27.0	—	—
95	200	3.60	—	—	1440.0	—	—	—	—	—	—	—	—	6.0	—	—
35	19	0.72	—	—	460.0	—	0	—	—	—	—	—	—	0	—	—
100	500	0.72	67.5	794.0	300.0	1.63	419.4	0.23	0.44	0.97	0.64	0.20	19.9	0	1.4	6.7
0	20	1.08	—	—	900.0	—	—	—	—	—	—	—	—	0	—	—
140	250	5.40	—	—	1790.0	—	—	—	—	—	—	—	—	0	—	—
0	20	1.08	—	—	830.0	—	0	—	—	—	—	—	—	1.2	—	—
0	80	1.44	—	—	480.0	—	0	—	—	—	—	—	—	0	—	—
0	20	1.08	—	—	590.0	—	—	—	—	—	—	—	—	1.2	—	—
25	100	3.60	—	—	1220.0	—	—	—	—	—	—	—	—	1.2	—	—
100	500	0	—	—	250.0	—	—	—	—	—	—	—	—	0	—	—
115	100	5.40	—	—	1120.0	—	—	—	—	—	—	—	—	9.0	—	—
130	250	5.40	—	—	2080.0	—	—	—	—	—	—	—	—	9.0	—	—
100	500	0.00	51.6	659.2	240.1	2.26	449.1	0.10	0.99	2.62	0.85	0.24	0	0	0.9	12.7
69	185	4.17	—	—	1342.6	—	—	—	—	—	—	—	—	0	—	—
75	200	4.50	—	—	1450.0	—	—	—	—	—	—	—	—	0	—	—
230	150	3.60	—	—	1370.0	—	—	—	—	—	—	—	—	0	—	—
260	—	—	—	—	830.0	—	—	—	—	—	—	—	—	—	—	—
275	—	—	—	—	1070.0	—	—	—	—	—	—	—	—	—	—	—
325	—	—	—	—	1620.0	—	—	—	—	—	—	—	—	—	—	—
55	150	1.80	—	—	650.0	—	—	—	—	—	—	—	—	96.0	—	—
80	250	3.60	—	—	1460.0	—	—	—	—	—	—	—	—	12.0	—	—
55	200	4.50	—	—	1300.0	—	—	—	—	—	—	—	—	24.0	—	—
55	100	3.60	—	—	1120.0	—	—	—	—	—	—	—	—	12.0	—	—
95	60	3.60	—	—	1630.0	—	—	—	—	—	—	—	—	0	—	—
25	80	1.80	—	—	1240.0	—	—	—	—	—	—	—	—	0	—	—
40	—	—	—	—	1480.0	—	—	—	—	—	—	—	—	—	—	—
80	200	4.50	—	—	1240.0	—	—	—	—	—	—	—	—	4.8	—	—
65	150	2.70	—	—	1370.0	—	0	—	—	—	—	—	—	0	—	—
75	250	2.70	—	—	1620.0	—	—	—	—	—	—	—	—	9.0	—	—
35	80	1.08	—	—	450.0	—	—	—	—	—	—	—	—	72.0	—	—
0	—	—	—	—	7.1	—	—	—	—	—	—	—	—	—	—	—
0	20	0.36	—	—	0	—	0	—	—	—	—	—	—	186.0	—	—
0	20	0.72	—	—	410.0	—	0	—	—	—	—	—	—	6.0	—	—
20	—	—	—	—	902.4	—	—	—	—	—	—	—	—	—	—	—
0	60	1.08	—	—	700.0	—	—	—	—	—	—	—	—	0	—	—
15	150	0.36	—	—	115.0	—	—	—	—	—	—	—	—	1.2	—	—
25	—	—	—	—	200.0	—	—	—	—	—	—	—	—	—	—	—
0	—	—	—	—	3.5	—	—	—	—	—	—	—	—	—	—	—
70	—	—	—	—	990.0	—	—	—	—	—	—	—	—	—	—	—
15	150	0.72	—	—	110.0	—	—	—	—	—	—	—	—	24.0	—	—
60	150	4.50	—	—	1730.0	—	—	—	—	—	—	—	—	0	—	—
80	300	4.50	—	—	1880.0	—	—	—	—	—	—	—	—	9.0	—	—
0	—	—	—	—	140.1	—	—	—	—	—	—	—	—	—	—	—
10	200	0.72	—	—	70.0	—	—	—	—	—	—	—	—	30.0	—	—
35	—	—	—	—	530.0	—	—	—	—	—	—	—	—	—	—	—
16	—	—	—	—	413.2	—	—	—	—	—	—	—	—	—	—	—
67	—	—	—	—	801.0	—	—	—	—	—	—	—	—	—	—	—

TABLE A-2 Table of Food Composition (continued)   (Computer code is for Cengage Diet Analysis program)   (For purposes of calculations, use "0" for t, <1, <0.1, <0.01)

DA+ Code	Food Description	Quantity	Measure	Wt (g)	H₂O (g)	Ener (kcal)	Prot (g)	Carb (g)	Fiber (g)	Fat (g)	Fat Breakdown (g)		
											Sat	Mono	Poly
Fast Food—*continued*													
39568	Minibon	1	item(s)	92	—	339	6.0	49.0	2.0	13.0	3.0	—	—
39573	Mochalatta Chill with whipped cream	16	fluid ounce(s)	473	—	425	10.0	63.0	2.0	17.0	11.0	—	—
39569	Pecanbon	1	item(s)	272	—	1100	16.0	141.0	8.0	56.0	10.0	—	—
	Dairy Queen												
1466	Banana split	1	item(s)	374	—	520	9.0	94.0	3.0	13.0	10.0	—	—
38561	Chocolate chip cookie dough Blizzard, small	1	item(s)	319	—	710	13.0	103.0	1.0	27.0	14.0	—	—
1464	Chocolate malt, small	1	item(s)	427	—	650	15.0	110.0	0	16.0	10.0	—	—
38541	Chocolate shake, small	1	item(s)	406	—	570	13.0	92.0	0	15.0	10.0	—	—
1463	Chocolate sundae, small	1	item(s)	163	—	280	5.0	48.0	0	7.0	4.5	—	—
1462	Dipped cone, small	1	item(s)	156	—	330	6.0	36.0	0	15.0	6.0	—	—
58376	Mint Oreo Blizzard, small	1	item(s)	297	—	580	12.0	89.0	1.0	20.0	10.0	—	—
38552	Oreo Brownie Earthquake	1	serving(s)	304	—	760	11.0	117.0	2.0	27.0	16.0	—	—
38555	Oreo cookies Blizzard, small	1	item(s)	283	—	550	12.0	81.0	1.0	20.0	10.0	—	—
38547	Royal Treats Peanut Buster Parfait	1	item(s)	304	—	700	16.0	94.0	2.0	30.0	16.0	—	—
17256	Vanilla soft serve	½	cup(s)	94	—	145	4.0	21.5	0	4.5	3.0	—	—
	Domino's												
31604	Breadsticks	1	item(s)	30	—	110	2.0	11.0	0	6.0	1.5	—	—
31605	Cheesy bread	1	item(s)	36	—	120	4.0	11.0	0	6.0	2.0	—	—
37548	CinnaStix	1	item(s)	33	—	120	2.0	14.0	1.0	6.0	1.0	—	—
31606	Wings w/ barbecue sauce	1	item(s)	30	—	63	4.3	3.5	0.3	3.3	0.9	—	—
31607	Wings w/ hot sauce	1	item(s)	30	—	50	4.3	1.3	0.3	3.3	0.9	—	—
	Domino's Artisan pizza												
81942	Chicken & Bacon Carbonara	1	slice(s)	76	—	150	8.0	18.0	1.0	6.0	2.5	—	—
81939	Italian Sausage & Pepper Trio	1	slice(s)	74	—	160	7.0	18.0	1.0	7.0	2.5	—	—
81940	Spinach & Feta	1	slice(s)	62	—	150	6.0	17.0	1.0	7.0	3.0	—	—
81941	Tuscan Salami & Roasted Veggie	1	slice(s)	64	—	150	5.0	17.0	1.0	6.0	2.0	—	—
	Domino's hand-tossed pizza												
31573	America's favorite feast, 12"	1	slice(s)	109	—	250	10.0	27.0	2.0	12.0	5.0	—	—
31574	America's favorite feast, 14"	1	slice(s)	151	—	350	14.0	36.0	2.0	17.0	7.0	—	—
37543	Bacon Cheeseburger Feast, 12"	1	slice(s)	106	—	270	12.0	26.0	2.0	13.0	5.5	—	—
37545	Bacon Cheeseburger Feast, 14"	1	slice(s)	146	—	380	17.0	36.0	2.0	19.0	9.0	—	—
81919	Cali Chicken Bacon Ranch, 12"	1	slice(s)	114	—	320	14.0	25.0	1.0	18.0	6.5	—	—
81920	Cali Chicken Bacon Ranch, 14"	1	slice(s)	154	—	430	19.0	33.0	1.0	25.0	9.0	—	—
31569	Cheese, 12"	1	slice(s)	93	—	210	8.0	25.0	1.0	8.0	3.5	—	—
31570	Cheese, 14"	1	slice(s)	128	57.4	290	12.0	35.0	2.0	11.0	5.5	2.8	2.3
31685	Deluxe Feast, 12"	1	slice(s)	106	—	226	9.0	26.0	2.0	9.5	3.5	—	—
31694	Deluxe Feast, 14"	1	slice(s)	145	—	320	13.0	36.0	2.0	14.0	6.0	—	—
31686	ExtravaganZZa Feast, 12"	1	slice(s)	132	—	290	13.0	28.0	2.0	14.0	6.5	—	—
31695	ExtravaganZZa Feast, 14"	1	slice(s)	176	89.4	390	17.0	37.0	2.0	19.0	8.0	6.4	2.5
81931	Fiery Hawaiian, 12"	1	slice(s)	118	—	250	12.0	27.0	2.0	11.0	5.0	—	—
81932	Fiery Hawaiian, 14"	1	slice(s)	160	—	350	15.0	36.0	2.0	16.0	6.5	—	—
39033	Ham and pineapple, 12"	1	slice(s)	100	—	200	8.0	26.0	1.0	6.5	2.5	—	—
39034	Ham and pineapple, 14"	1	slice(s)	128	—	290	12.0	35.0	2.0	11.0	5.5	—	—
31687	MeatZZa Feast, 12"	1	slice(s)	117	—	280	12.0	27.0	2.0	14.0	5.5	—	—
31696	MeatZZa Feast, 14"	1	slice(s)	160	—	380	18.0	36.0	2.0	19.0	8.0	—	—
81923	Memphis BBQ Chicken, 12"	1	slice(s)	103	—	260	13.0	28.0	1.0	12.0	5.5	—	—
81924	Memphis BBQ Chicken, 14"	1	slice(s)	140	—	360	16.0	37.0	1.0	15.0	7.5	—	—
31571	Pepperoni Feast, 12"	1	slice(s)	99	—	260	11.0	25.0	1.0	13.0	5.5	—	—
31572	Pepperoni Feast, 14"	1	slice(s)	136	—	360	15.0	34.0	2.0	18.0	8.0	—	—
81927	Philly Cheese Steak, 12"	1	slice(s)	101	—	260	11.0	24.0	1.0	12.0	6.0	—	—
81928	Philly Cheese Steak, 14"	1	slice(s)	135	—	330	15.0	32.0	1.0	16.0	8.0	—	—
81935	Wisconsin 6 Cheese, 12"	1	slice(s)	101	—	250	12.0	25.0	1.0	12.0	6.0	—	—
81936	Wisconsin 6 Cheese, 14"	1	slice(s)	137	—	340	15.0	34.0	2.0	16.0	7.5	—	—
	Domino's thin crust pizza												
31583	America's Favorite Feast, 12"	1	slice(s)	81	—	210	8.0	15.0	1.0	13.0	5.0	—	—
31584	America's Favorite Feast, 14"	1	slice(s)	112	—	280	11.0	21.0	2.0	17.5	6.5	—	—
31579	Cheese, 12"	1	slice(s)	64	—	165	7.0	15.0	1.5	9.0	3.5	—	—
31580	Cheese, 14"	1	slice(s)	88	36.6	230	9.0	20.0	1.0	11.5	5.0	3.3	3.3
31688	Deluxe Feast, 12"	1	slice(s)	79	—	190	7.0	15.5	1.0	11.0	4.0	—	—

PAGE KEY: A-6 5 Breads/Baked Goods A-12 = Cereal/Rice/Pasta A-16 = Fruit A-22 = Vegetables/Legumes A-32 = Nuts/Seeds A-34 = Vegetarian A-36 = Dairy A-44 = Eggs A-44 = Seafood A-46 = Meats A-50 = Poultry
A-52 = Processed Meats A-54 = Beverages A-58 = Fats/Oils A-60 = Sweets A-62 = Spices/Condiments/Sauces A-66 = Mixed Foods/Soups/Sandwiches A-72 = Fast Food A-90 = Convenience A-92 = Baby Foods

Chol (mg)	Calc (mg)	Iron (mg)	Magn (mg)	Pota (mg)	Sodi (mg)	Zinc (mg)	Vit A (µg)	Thia (mg)	Vit E (mg α)	Ribo (mg)	Niac (mg)	Vit B$_6$ (mg)	Fola (µg)	Vit C (mg)	Vit B$_{12}$ (µg)	Sele (µg)
27	—	—	—	—	337.0	—	—	—	—	—	—	—	—	—	—	—
63	—	—	—	—	287.0	—	—	—	—	—	—	—	—	—	—	—
63	—	—	—	—	600.0	—	—	—	—	—	—	—	—	—	—	—
30	250	2.70	—	—	160.0	—	—	—	—	—	—	—	—	18.0	—	—
55	350	2.70	—	—	350.0	—	—	—	—	—	—	—	—	0	—	—
55	500	3.60	—	—	310.0	—	—	—	—	—	—	—	—	0	—	—
50	500	1.80	—	—	250.0	—	—	—	—	—	—	—	—	0	—	—
25	200	1.80	—	—	115.0	—	—	—	—	—	—	—	—	0	—	—
25	200	1.44	—	—	105.0	—	—	—	—	—	—	—	—	0	—	—
40	350	3.60	—	—	410.0	—	—	—	—	—	—	—	—	0	—	—
60	250	3.60	—	—	400.0	—	—	—	—	—	—	—	—	0	—	—
40	350	2.70	—	—	410.0	—	—	—	—	—	—	—	—	0	—	—
35	400	3.60	—	—	360.0	—	—	—	—	—	—	—	—	0	—	—
15	125	0.90	—	—	65.0	—	112.6	—	—	—	—	—	—	0	—	—
0	0	0.72	—	—	100.0	—	0	—	—	—	—	—	—	1.2	—	—
5	40	0.72	—	—	140.0	—	—	—	—	—	—	—	—	1.2	—	—
0	0	0.72	—	—	85.0	—	0	—	—	—	—	—	—	1.2	—	—
21	5	0.36	—	—	162.5	—	—	—	—	—	—	—	—	0.6	—	—
21	5	0.27	—	—	340.0	—	—	—	—	—	—	—	—	0.9	—	—
20	60	1.44	—	—	360.0	—	—	—	—	—	—	—	—	3.6	—	—
15	60	1.44	—	—	330.0	—	—	—	—	—	—	—	—	9.0	—	—
10	80	1.08	—	—	250.0	—	—	—	—	—	—	—	—	2.4	—	—
10	60	1.08	—	—	280.0	—	—	—	—	—	—	—	—	6.0	—	—
25	100	2.16	—	—	630.0	—	—	—	—	—	—	—	—	3.6	—	—
35	150	2.52	—	—	870.0	—	—	—	—	—	—	—	—	6.0	—	—
35	150	1.80	—	—	590.0	—	—	—	—	—	—	—	—	6.0	—	—
45	203	2.56	—	—	830.0	—	—	—	—	—	—	—	—	8.5	—	—
40	190	1.80	—	—	660.0	—	—	—	—	—	—	—	—	4.8	—	—
55	260	2.52	—	—	900.0	—	—	—	—	—	—	—	—	7.2	—	—
20	150	1.44	—	—	460.0	—	—	—	—	—	—	—	—	3.6	—	—
25	220	1.80	30.7	206.1	640.0	1.59	78.1	0.41	1.27	0.22	4.29	0.10	—	6.0	0.6	29.4
15	80	1.80	—	—	505.0	—	—	—	—	—	—	—	—	6.0	—	—
30	150	2.52	—	—	730.0	—	—	—	—	—	—	—	—	11.4	—	—
35	150	2.52	—	—	770.0	—	—	—	—	—	—	—	—	7.2	—	—
45	200	2.88	38.7	306.2	1020.0	2.23	89.8	0.24	1.41	0.39	5.72	—	—	11.4	1.0	42.2
25	170	1.80	—	—	760.0	—	—	—	—	—	—	—	—	10.2	—	—
35	240	2.52	—	—	1030.0	—	—	—	—	—	—	—	—	14.4	—	—
20	100	1.47	—	—	490.0	—	—	—	—	—	—	—	—	4.9	—	—
25	220	1.80	—	—	640.0	—	—	—	—	—	—	—	—	6.0	—	—
35	150	2.16	—	—	760.0	—	—	—	—	—	—	—	—	3.6	—	—
50	200	2.52	—	—	1030.0	—	—	—	—	—	—	—	—	6.0	—	—
30	210	1.80	—	—	500.0	—	—	—	—	—	—	—	—	2.4	—	—
40	260	2.16	—	—	680.0	—	—	—	—	—	—	—	—	4.8	—	—
30	150	1.80	—	—	650.0	—	—	—	—	—	—	—	—	3.6	—	—
40	200	2.52	—	—	880.0	—	—	—	—	—	—	—	—	6.0	—	—
30	190	1.80	—	—	540.0	—	—	—	—	—	—	—	—	4.8	—	—
40	260	2.16	—	—	690.0	—	—	—	—	—	—	—	—	6.0	—	—
25	220	1.80	—	—	500.0	—	—	—	—	—	—	—	—	3.6	—	—
35	290	2.16	—	—	690.0	—	—	—	—	—	—	—	—	6.0	—	—
25	120	0.72	—	—	500.0	—	—	—	—	—	—	—	—	3.0	—	—
35	170	1.08	—	—	690.0	—	—	—	—	—	—	—	—	3.6	—	—
20	170	0.54	—	—	330.0	—	—	—	—	—	—	—	—	2.4	—	—
25	240	0.72	21.1	177.8	460.0	1.36	—	0.05	1.31	0.07	0.89	0.06	—	3.6	0.6	17.4
20	120	0.72	—	—	410.0	—	—	—	—	—	—	—	—	6.0	—	—

TABLE A-2 Table of Food Composition (continued)   (Computer code is for Cengage Diet Analysis program).   (For purposes of calculations, use "0" for t, <1, <0.1, <0.01)

DA+ Code	Food Description	Quantity	Measure	Wt (g)	H₂O (g)	Ener (kcal)	Prot (g)	Carb (g)	Fiber (g)	Fat (g)	Fat Breakdown (g) Sat	Mono	Poly
Fast Food—*continued*													
31697	Deluxe Feast, 14"	1	slice(s)	106	—	250	10.0	21.0	2.0	14.5	5.5	—	—
31689	ExtravaganZZa Feast, 12"	1	slice(s)	103	—	240	10.5	16.0	1.5	15.0	6.0	—	—
31698	ExtravaganZZa Feast, 14"	1	slice(s)	137	—	320	14.0	22.0	2.0	19.5	7.5	—	—
39037	Ham and pineapple, 12"	1	slice(s)	71	—	155	6.5	16.0	1.0	7.5	2.8	—	—
39038	Ham and pineapple, 14"	1	slice(s)	97	—	220	8.0	21.0	1.0	10.0	3.5	—	—
31690	MeatZZa Feast, 12"	1	slice(s)	89	—	235	10.5	15.5	1.0	14.5	6.0	—	—
31699	MeatZZa Feast, 14"	1	slice(s)	121	—	310	15.0	21.0	2.0	19.5	7.5	—	—
31581	Pepperoni Feast, 12"	1	slice(s)	71	—	215	9.0	14.0	1.0	13.5	5.5	—	—
31582	Pepperoni Feast, 14"	1	slice(s)	97	—	290	12.0	19.0	2.0	18.5	7.5	—	—
In-n-Out Burger													
34391	Cheesburger with mustard & ketchup	1	serving(s)	268	—	400	22.0	41.0	3.0	18.0	9.0		
34374	Cheeseburger	1	serving(s)	268	—	480	22.0	39.0	3.0	27.0	10.0	—	—
34390	Cheeseburger, lettuce leaves instead of buns	1	serving(s)	300	—	330	18.0	11.0	3.0	25.0	9.0	—	—
34377	Chocolate shake	1	serving(s)	425	—	690	9.0	83.0	0	36.0	24.0	—	—
34375	Double-Double cheeseburger	1	serving(s)	330	—	670	37.0	39.0	3.0	41.0	18.0	—	—
34393	Double-Double cheeseburger with mustard & ketchup	1	serving(s)	330	—	590	37.0	41.0	3.0	32.0	17.0	—	—
34392	Double-Double cheeseburger, lettuce leaves instead of buns	1	serving(s)	362	—	520	33.0	11.0	3.0	39.0	17.0	—	—
34376	French fries	1	serving(s)	125	—	400	7.0	54.0	2.0	18.0	5.0	—	—
34373	Hamburger	1	item(s)	243	—	390	16.0	39.0	3.0	19.0	5.0	—	—
34389	Hamburger with mustard & ketchup	1	serving(s)	243	—	310	16.0	41.0	3.0	10.0	4.0	—	—
34388	Hamburger, lettuce leaves instead of buns	1	serving(s)	275	—	240	13.0	11.0	3.0	17.0	4.0	—	—
34379	Strawberry shake	1	serving(s)	425	—	690	9.0	91.0	0	33.0	22.0	—	—
34378	Vanilla shake	1	serving(s)	425	—	680	9.0	78.0	0	37.0	25.0	—	—
Jack in the Box													
30392	Bacon ultimate cheeseburger	1	item(s)	315	—	980	43.0	52.0	2.0	67.0	27.0	—	—
1740	Breakfast Jack	1	item(s)	113	—	300	16.0	29.0	1.0	14.0	5.0	—	—
14074	Cheeseburger	1	item(s)	118	—	320	16.0	30.0	1.0	15.0	7.0	—	—
14106	Chicken breast strips, 4 piece	4	piece(s)	201	—	500	35.0	36.0	3.0	25.0	6.0	—	—
37241	Chicken club salad, plain, without salad dressing	1	serving(s)	415	—	480	33.0	28.0	6.0	27.0	10.0	—	—
14064	Chicken sandwich	1	item(s)	145	—	400	15.0	38.0	2.0	21.0	4.5	—	—
14111	Chocolate ice cream shake, small	1	serving(s)	351	—	750	12.0	95.0	1.0	36.0	24.0	—	—
14073	Hamburger	1	item(s)	106	—	280	14.0	29.0	1.0	12.0	4.5	—	—
14090	Hash browns	1	serving(s)	73	—	230	2.0	20.0	2.0	16.0	4.0	—	—
14072	Jack's Spicy Chicken sandwich	1	item(s)	251	—	550	24.0	59.0	4.0	24.0	5.0	—	—
1468	Jumbo Jack hamburger	1	item(s)	249	—	580	20.0	51.0	2.0	33.0	11.0	—	—
1469	Jumbo Jack hamburger with cheese	1	item(s)	274	—	670	24.0	53.0	2.0	40.0	15.0	—	—
14099	Natural cut french fries, large	1	serving(s)	229	—	620	9.0	75.0	8.0	32.0	7.0	—	—
14098	Natural cut french fries, medium	1	serving(s)	169	—	460	6.0	55.0	6.0	24.0	6.0	—	—
1470	Onion rings	1	serving(s)	119	—	500	6.0	51.0	3.0	30.0	6.0	—	—
33141	Sausage, egg & cheese biscuit	1	item(s)	184	—	590	20.0	38.0	2.0	40.0	16.0	—	—
14095	Seasoned curly fries, medium	1	serving(s)	130	—	420	6.0	46.0	5.0	24.0	5.0	—	—
14077	Sourdough Jack	1	item(s)	228	—	680	26.0	41.0	2.0	46.0	17.0	—	—
37249	Southwest grilled chicken salad, plain, w/o salad dressing	1	serving(s)	442	—	310	31.0	28.0	7.0	12.0	5.0	—	—
14112	Strawberry ice cream shake, small	1	serving(s)	349	—	730	11.0	90.0	0	35.0	24.0	—	—
14078	Ultimate cheeseburger	1	item(s)	304	—	920	38.0	52.0	2.0	63.0	26.0	—	—
14110	Vanilla ice cream shake, small	1	serving(s)	314	—	650	11.0	70.0	0	35.0	24.0	—	—
Jamba Juice													
55682	Acai Super-Antioxidant smoothie	24	fluid ounce(s)	680	—	415	5.5	85.1	5.5	6.5	2.2	—	—
31645	Aloha Pineapple smoothie	24	fluid ounce(s)	680	—	447	6.5	105.8	4.4	1.6	0.5	—	—
31646	Banana Berry smoothie	24	fluid ounce(s)	680	—	436	4.4	102.5	4.4	1.6	0.5	—	—
31647	Carribean Passion smoothie	24	fluid ounce(s)	680	—	393	3.3	89.5	3.3	1.6	0.5	—	—
38422	Carrot juice	16	fluid ounce(s)	473	—	130	4.0	30.0	0	0.5	0	—	—

PAGE KEY: A-6 5 Breads/Baked Goods A-12 = Cereal/Rice/Pasta A-16 = Fruit A-22 = Vegetables/Legumes A-32 = Nuts/Seeds A-34 = Vegetarian A-36 = Dairy A-44 = Eggs A-44 = Seafood A-46 = Meats A-50 = Poultry
A-52 = Processed Meats A-54 = Beverages A-58 = Fats/Oils A-60 = Sweets A-62 = Spices/Condiments/Sauces A-66 = Mixed Foods/Soups/Sandwiches A-72 = Fast Food A-90 = Convenience A-92 = Baby Foods

Chol (mg)	Calc (mg)	Iron (mg)	Magn (mg)	Pota (mg)	Sodi (mg)	Zinc (mg)	Vit A (µg)	Thia (mg)	Vit E (mg α)	Ribo (mg)	Niac (mg)	Vit B$_6$ (mg)	Fola (µg)	Vit C (mg)	Vit B$_{12}$ (µg)	Sele (µg)
30	170	1.08	—	—	550.0	—	—	—	—	—	—	—	—	9.0	—	—
35	170	1.08	—	—	640.0	—	—	—	—	—	—	—	—	6.0	—	—
45	220	1.44	—	—	840.0	—	—	—	—	—	—	—	—	9.0	—	—
15	120	0.36	—	—	350.0	—	—	—	—	—	—	—	—	3.0	—	—
25	190	0.72	—	—	485.0	—	—	—	—	—	—	—	—	4.8	—	—
35	170	0.90	—	—	630.0	—	—	—	—	—	—	—	—	3.0	—	—
50	220	1.08	—	—	850.0	—	—	—	—	—	—	—	—	3.6	—	—
30	145	0.72	—	—	510.0	—	—	—	—	—	—	—	—	3.0	—	—
40	220	1.08	—	—	700.0	—	—	—	—	—	—	—	—	3.6	—	—
60	200	3.60	—	—	1080.0									12.0		
60	200	3.60	—	—	1000.0	—	—	—	—	—	—	—	—	9.0	—	—
60	200	2.70	—	—	720.0	—	—	—	—	—	—	—	—	12.0	—	—
95	300	0.72	—	—	350.0	—	—	—	—	—	—	—	—	0	—	—
120	350	5.40	—	—	1440.0	—	—	—	—	—	—	—	—	9.0	—	—
115	350	5.40	—	—	1520.0	—	—	—	—	—	—	—	—	12.0	—	—
120	350	4.50	—	—	1160.0	—	—	—	—	—	—	—	—	12.0	—	—
0	20	1.80	—	—	245.0	—	0	—	—	—	—	—	—	0	—	—
40	40	3.60	—	—	650.0	—	—	—	—	—	—	—	—	9.0	—	—
35	40	3.60	—	—	730.0	—	—	—	—	—	—	—	—	12.0	—	—
40	40	2.70	—	—	370.0	—	—	—	—	—	—	—	—	12.0	—	—
85	300	0	—	—	280.0	—	—	—	—	—	—	—	—	0	—	—
90	300	0	—	—	390.0	—	—	—	—	—	—	—	—	0	—	—
135	308	7.39	—	490.0	1880.0	—	—	—	—	—	—	—	—	0.6	—	—
215	145	3.49	—	180.0	730.0	—	—	—	—	—	—	—	—	3.5	—	—
45	151	3.61	—	230.0	730.0	—	—	—	—	—	—	—	—	0	—	—
80	18	1.60	—	530.0	1260.0	—	—	—	—	—	—	—	—	1.1	—	—
75	280	3.36	—	790.0	1050.0	—	—	—	—	—	—	—	—	50.4	—	—
35	100	2.70	—	240.0	740.0	—	—	—	—	—	—	—	—	4.8	—	—
115	460	0.47	—	740.0	280.0	—	—	—	—	—	—	—	—	0	—	—
30	100	3.60	—	210.0	540.0	—	0	—	—	—	—	—	—	0	—	—
0	10	0.18	—	160.0	330.0	—	0	—	—	—	—	—	—	0	—	—
50	150	1.80	—	420.0	1050.0	—	—	—	—	—	—	—	—	9.0	—	—
50	164	4.92	—	350.0	920.0	—	—	—	—	—	—	—	—	9.8	—	—
75	234	4.21	—	380.0	1290.0	—	—	—	—	—	—	—	—	8.4	—	—
0	20	1.42	—	1580.0	1150.0	—	0	—	—	—	—	—	—	8.9	—	—
0	19	1.01	—	1160.0	850.0	—	0	—	—	—	—	—	—	5.6	—	—
0	40	2.70	—	140.0	420.0	—	9.8	—	—	—	—	—	—	18.0	—	—
245	88	2.37	—	260.0	1140.0	—	—	—	—	—	—	—	—	0	—	—
0	40	1.80	—	610.0	920.0	—	—	—	—	—	—	—	—	0	—	—
75	200	4.50	—	390.0	1200.0	—	—	—	—	—	—	—	—	9.0	—	—
90	274	4.11	—	930.0	820.0	—	—	—	—	—	—	—	—	43.8	—	—
115	466	0	—	630.0	240.0	—	—	—	—	—	—	—	—	0	—	—
120	308	7.39	—	440.0	1530.0	—	—	—	—	—	—	—	—	0.6	—	—
115	532	0	—	630.0	230.0	—	—	—	—	—	—	—	—	0	—	—
5	109	1.96	—	—	60.0	—	—	—	—	—	—	—	—	—	—	—
5	164	1.96	—	—	60.0	—	—	—	—	—	—	—	—	98.2	—	—
5	164	1.18	—	—	98.2	—	—	—	—	—	—	—	—	16.2	—	—
5	106	1.57	—	—	54.5	—	—	—	—	—	—	—	—	72.0	—	—
0	100	2.72	—	—	230.0	—	2325.0	—	—	—	—	—	—	18.1	—	—

TABLE A-2 **Table of Food Composition** *(continued)* (Computer code is for Cengage Diet Analysis program) (For purposes of calculations, use "0" for t, <1, <0.1, <0.01)

DA+ Code	Food Description	Quantity	Measure	Wt (g)	H₂O (g)	Ener (kcal)	Prot (g)	Carb (g)	Fiber (g)	Fat (g)	Fat Breakdown (g) Sat	Mono	Poly
Fast Food—*continued*													
31648	Chocolate Moo'd smoothie	24	fluid ounce(s)	680	—	622	16.4	126.5	3.3	5.5	2.7	—	—
31657	Mango-a-go-go smoothie	24	fluid ounce(s)	680	—	436	3.3	102.5	3.3	1.6	0.5	—	—
55684	Matcha Green Tea Blast smoothie	24	fluid ounce(s)	680	—	458	10.9	99.3	2.2	0	0	0	0
55673	Mega Mango smoothie	24	fluid ounce(s)	680	—	371	4.4	92.7	5.5	0.5	0	—	—
36945	Orange Dream Machine smoothie	24	fluid ounce(s)	680	—	513	10.9	112.4	1.1	1.6	1.1	—	—
38424	Orange juice, freshly squeezed	16	fluid ounce(s)	473	—	200	3.0	52.0	1.0	1.0	0	—	—
31660	Orange-a-peel smoothie	24	fluid ounce(s)	680	—	404	7.6	92.7	3.3	0	0	—	—
55675	Peach Perfection smoothie	24	fluid ounce(s)	680	—	327	2.2	81.8	5.5	0.5	0	—	—
31662	Peach Pleasure smoothie	24	fluid ounce(s)	680	—	404	3.3	96.0	4.4	1.6	1.1	—	—
55676	Pomegranate Paradise smoothie	24	fluid ounce(s)	680	—	371	2.2	92.7	5.5	0.5	0	—	—
55665	Protein Berry Workout smoothie w/ soy protein	24	fluid ounce(s)	680	—	412	18.2	84.3	4.8	1.4	0	—	—
31668	Razzmatazz smoothie	24	fluid ounce(s)	680	—	425	3.3	99.3	4.4	1.6	1.1	—	—
31669	Strawberries Wild smoothie	24	fluid ounce(s)	680	—	404	5.5	94.9	3.3	0	0	—	—
38421	Strawberry Surf Rider smoothie	24	fluid ounce(s)	680	—	469	3.3	112.4	4.4	1.6	0.5	—	—
55674	Strawberry Whirl smoothie	24	fluid ounce(s)	680	—	327	2.2	81.8	6.5	0.5	0	—	—
38428	Wheatgrass juice, freshly squeezed	1	ounce(s)	28	—	5	1.0	1.0	0	0	0	0	0
	Kentucky Fried Chicken (KFC)												
31850	BBQ baked beans	1	serving(s)	130	—	200	8.0	39.0	9.0	1.5	0	—	—
31853	Biscuit	1	item(s)	57	—	220	4.0	24.0	1.0	11.0	2.5	—	—
31851	Cole slaw	1	serving(s)	130	—	180	1.0	22.0	3.0	10.0	1.5	—	—
31849	Corn on the cob	1	item(s)	146	—	140	5.0	33.0	4.0	1.0	0	—	—
31842	Crispy strips	3	item(s)	151	—	370	28.0	17.0	1.0	20.0	4.0	—	—
74456	Doublicious chicken sandwich, Original Recipe	1	item(s)	188	—	520	32.0	40.0	2.0	25.0	7.0	—	—
3761	Extra Crispy chicken, breast	1	item(s)	176	—	510	39.0	16.0	0	33.0	7.0	—	—
3762	Extra Crispy chicken, drumstick	1	item(s)	60	—	150	12.0	4.0	0	10.0	2.5	—	—
3763	Extra Crispy chicken, thigh	1	item(s)	114	—	290	17.0	16.0	1.0	18.0	4.0	—	—
3764	Extra Crispy chicken, whole wing	1	item(s)	52	—	150	11.0	11.0	1.0	7.0	1.5	—	—
51218	Famous Bowls mashed potatoes with gravy	1	serving(s)	525	—	680	26.0	74.0	6.0	31.0	8.0	—	—
39387	Green beans	1	serving(s)	86	—	20	1.0	3.0	1.0	0	0	—	—
31841	Honey BBQ chicken sandwich	1	item(s)	162	—	310	23.0	42.0	1.0	4.0	1.0	—	—
10859	Hot wings	6	piece(s)	132	—	420	24.0	24.0	0	24.0	3.0	—	—
51223	Hot wings, fiery buffalo	6	item(s)	204	—	480	30.0	36.0	6.0	21.0	3.0	—	—
39386	Hot wings, honey BBQ	6	item(s)	198	—	480	30.0	42.0	6.0	21.0	3.0	—	—
31848	Macaroni & cheese	1	serving(s)	135	—	160	5.0	19.0	1.0	7.0	2.5	—	—
31847	Mashed potatoes with gravy	1	serving(s)	145	—	120	2.0	19.0	1.0	4.0	1.0	—	—
74460	Original Recipe chicken filet	1	item(s)	100	—	200	22.0	8.0	1.0	9.0	1.5	—	—
10825	Original Recipe chicken, breast	1	item(s)	161	—	340	38.0	9.0	2.0	17.0	4.0	—	—
10826	Original Recipe chicken, drumstick	1	item(s)	59	—	140	13.0	3.0	0	8.0	2.0	—	—
10827	Original Recipe chicken, thigh	1	item(s)	126	—	350	19.0	7.0	1.0	27.0	7.0	—	—
10828	Original Recipe chicken, whole wing	1	item(s)	47	—	140	10.0	4.0	0	9.0	2.0	—	—
31844	Popcorn chicken, small or individual	1	item(s)	114	—	370	19.0	21.0	2.0	24.0	4.5	—	—
31852	Potato salad	1	serving(s)	128	—	200	2.0	24.0	3.0	10.0	2.0	—	—
10845	Potato wedges, small	1	serving(s)	102	—	250	4.0	32.0	3.0	12.0	2.0	—	—
	Long John Silver's												
3777	Batter dipped fish sandwich	1	item(s)	176	—	470	18.0	49.0	3.0	23.0	5.0	—	—
37568	Battered fish	1	item(s)	92	—	260	12.0	17.0	0	16.0	4.0	—	—
37569	Breaded clams	1	serving(s)	85	—	320	9.0	29.0	2.0	19.0	4.5	—	—
39398	Cocktail sauce	1	ounce(s)	28	—	25	0	6.0	0	0	0	0	0
3770	Coleslaw	1	serving(s)	113	—	200	1.0	15.0	3.0	15.0	2.5	—	—
39401	Crab cake, lobster stuffed	1	item(s)	62	—	170	6.0	16.0	1.0	9.0	2.0	—	—
78975	Fish taco	1	item(s)	117	—	360	9.0	30.0	3.0	23.0	4.5	—	—
39400	French fries, large	1	item(s)	113	—	310	3.0	45.0	4.0	14.0	3.5	—	—
3774	Fries, regular	1	serving(s)	85	—	230	3.0	34.0	3.0	10.0	2.5	—	—

PAGE KEY: A-6 5 Breads/Baked Goods A-12 = Cereal/Rice/Pasta A-16 = Fruit A-22 = Vegetables/Legumes A-32 = Nuts/Seeds A-34 = Vegetarian A-36 = Dairy A-44 = Eggs A-44 = Seafood A-46 = Meats A-50 = Poultry A-52 = Processed Meats A-54 = Beverages A-58 = Fats/Oils A-60 = Sweets A-62 = Spices/Condiments/Sauces A-66 = Mixed Foods/Soups/Sandwiches A-72 = Fast Food A-90 = Convenience A-92 = Baby Foods

Chol (mg)	Calc (mg)	Iron (mg)	Magn (mg)	Pota (mg)	Sodi (mg)	Zinc (mg)	Vit A (µg)	Thia (mg)	Vit E (mg α)	Ribo (mg)	Niac (mg)	Vit B$_6$ (mg)	Fola (µg)	Vit C (mg)	Vit B$_{12}$ (µg)	Sele (µg)
16	545	—	—	—	414.5	—	—	—	—	—	—	—	—	1.3	—	—
5	112	0.79	—	—	49.1	—	—	—	—	—	—	—	—	72.0	—	—
0	164	1.57	—	—	229.1	—	—	—	—	—	—	—	—	9.8	—	—
0	44	1.96	—	—	10.9	—	354.5	—	—	—	—	—	—	183.3	—	—
11	218	0.79	—	—	218.2	—	—	—	—	—	—	—	—	52.4	—	—
0	57	1.03	—	—	0	—	49.8	—	—	—	—	—	—	246.0	—	—
0	218	1.57	—	—	136.4	—	—	—	—	—	—	—	—	150.5	—	—
0	65	1.18	—	—	32.7	—	245.5	—	—	—	—	—	—	65.5	—	—
5	87	0.77	—	—	54.5	—	—	—	—	—	—	—	—	16.4	—	—
0	109	1.96	—	—	38.2	—	245.5	—	—	—	—	—	—	85.1	—	—
0	1054	3.45	76.7	690.0	220.4	0.86	—	0.11	0.39	0.16	1.15	0.67	76.7	51.7	0	5.4
5	109	1.57	—	—	60.0	—	—	—	—	—	—	—	—	58.9	—	—
5	218	1.92	—	—	152.7	—	—	—	—	—	—	—	—	52.4	—	—
5	87	1.13	—	—	10.9	—	—	—	—	—	—	—	—	85.1	—	—
0	87	1.96	—	—	27.3	—	5.5	—	—	—	—	—	—	78.5	—	—
0	—	1.73	—	—	0	—	—	—	—	—	—	—	—	3.7	—	—
0	—	—	—	—	680.0	—	—	—	—	—	—	—	—	—	—	—
0	40	1.80	—	—	640.0	—	—	—	—	—	—	—	—	0	—	—
5	40	0.72	—	—	270.0	—	—	—	—	—	—	—	—	12.0	—	—
0	—	—	—	—	5.0	—	—	—	—	—	—	—	—	—	—	—
65	40	1.44	—	—	1220.0	—	0	—	—	—	—	—	—	1.2	—	—
85	—	—	—	—	1300.0	—	—	—	—	—	—	—	—	—	—	—
110	—	—	—	—	1010.0	—	—	—	—	—	—	—	—	—	—	—
55	0	1.44	—	—	300.0	—	0	—	—	—	—	—	—	0	—	—
95	20	2.70	—	—	700.0	—	—	—	—	—	—	—	—	—	—	—
45	20	1.08	—	—	340.0	—	—	—	—	—	—	—	—	0	—	—
45	—	—	—	—	2130.0	—	—	—	—	—	—	—	—	—	—	—
0	—	—	—	—	290.0	—	—	—	—	—	—	—	—	—	—	—
70	—	—	—	—	810.0	—	—	—	—	—	—	—	—	—	—	—
120	—	—	—	—	840.0	—	—	—	—	—	—	—	—	—	—	—
60	—	—	—	—	2340.0	—	—	—	—	—	—	—	—	—	—	—
60	—	—	—	—	2040.0	—	—	—	—	—	—	—	—	—	—	—
5	—	—	—	—	720.0	—	—	—	—	—	—	—	—	—	—	—
0	—	—	—	—	530.0	—	—	—	—	—	—	—	—	—	—	—
55	—	—	—	—	670.0	—	—	—	—	—	—	—	—	—	—	—
135	20	2.70	—	—	960.0	—	—	—	—	—	—	—	—	6.0	—	—
70	20	1.08	—	—	340.0	—	—	—	—	—	—	—	—	0	—	—
110	20	2.70	—	—	870.0	—	—	—	—	—	—	—	—	1.2	—	—
50	20	1.44	—	—	350.0	—	0	—	—	—	—	—	—	1.2	—	—
25	40	1.80	—	—	1110.0	—	0	—	—	—	—	—	—	0	—	—
5	—	—	—	—	540.0	—	—	—	—	—	—	—	—	—	—	—
0	20	1.08	—	—	700.0	—	0	—	—	—	—	—	—	0	—	—
40	60	1.80	—	—	1180.0	—	—	—	—	—	—	—	—	1.2	—	—
35	0	0	—	—	790.0	—	0	—	—	—	—	—	—	0	—	—
35	20	1.44	—	—	1190.7	—	0	—	—	—	—	—	—	0	—	—
0	0	0	—	—	250.0	—	0	—	—	—	—	—	—	0	—	—
20	40	0.36	—	—	340.0	—	—	—	—	—	—	—	—	18.0	—	—
30	60	0.72	—	—	390.0	—	0	—	—	—	—	—	—	—	—	—
25	60	1.44	—	—	810.0	—	0	—	—	—	—	—	—	0	—	—
0	0	0	—	—	460.0	—	—	—	—	—	—	—	—	18.0	—	—
0	0	0	—	370.2	350.2	—	0	—	—	—	—	—	—	15.0	—	—

TABLE A-2 Table of Food Composition *(continued)*   (Computer code is for Cengage Diet Analysis program)   (For purposes of calculations, use "0" for t, <1, <0.1, <0.01)

DA+ Code	Food Description	Quantity	Measure	Wt (g)	H₂O (g)	Ener (kcal)	Prot (g)	Carb (g)	Fiber (g)	Fat (g)	Fat Breakdown (g) Sat	Mono	Poly
Fast Food—*continued*													
3779	Hushpuppy	1	piece(s)	23	—	60	1.0	9.0	1.0	2.5	0.5	—	—
56963	Shrimp scampi	1	serving(s)	130	—	200	17.0	3.0	0	13.0	2.5	—	—
3781	Shrimp, batter-dipped, 1 piece	1	piece(s)	14	—	43	1.7	2.7	0	3.0	0.8	—	—
39399	Tartar sauce	1	ounce(s)	28	—	100	0	4.0	0	9.0	1.5	—	—
39395	Ultimate Fish sandwich	1	item(s)	206	—	530	21.0	50.0	3.0	27.0	8.0	—	—
	McDonald's												
2262	Baked apple pie	1	item(s)	77	28.5	250	2.0	32.0	4.0	13.0	7.0	7.1	0.8
2247	Barbecue sauce	1	item(s)	28	16.1	50	0	12.0	0	0	0	0	0
737	Big Mac hamburger	1	item(s)	215	112.3	550	25.0	46.0	3.0	29.0	10.0	7.5	0.7
738	Cheeseburger	1	item(s)	114	45.0	300	15.0	33.0	2.0	12.0	6.0	4.1	0.4
1873	Chicken McNuggets 6 piece	6	item(s)	97	44.8	280	13.0	18.0	1.0	18.0	3.0	7.7	5.3
3792	Chicken McNuggets, 4 piece	4	item(s)	65	30.2	190	9.0	12.0	1.0	12.0	2.0	5.2	3.6
2264	Chocolate shake, large	1	item(s)	356	223.2	580	13.0	102.0	1.0	14.0	8.0	4.0	0.8
29774	Crispy chicken sandwich	1	item(s)	213	110.7	510	24.0	55.0	3.0	22.0	3.5	6.8	7.9
743	Egg McMuffin	1	item(s)	138	72.6	300	18.0	30.0	2.0	12.0	5.0	3.8	2.4
742	Filet-O-Fish sandwich	1	item(s)	142	65.0	390	15.0	39.0	2.0	19.0	4.0	5.7	8.5
2257	French fries, large	1	serving(s)	154	58.0	500	6.0	63.0	6.0	25.0	3.5	12.0	7.2
1872	French fries, small	1	serving(s)	71	27.1	230	3.0	29.0	3.0	11.0	1.5	5.5	3.3
33822	Fruit 'n Yogurt Parfait	1	item(s)	149	110.9	150	4.0	30.0	1.0	2.0	1.0	0.2	0.1
739	Hamburger	1	item(s)	100	44.5	250	12.0	31.0	2.0	9.0	3.5	3.8	1.4
2003	Hash browns	1	item(s)	56	29.5	150	1.0	15.0	2.0	9.0	1.5	4.8	2.8
2260	Hot fudge sundae	1	item(s)	179	105.3	330	8.0	53.0	1.0	9.0	7.0	1.9	0.4
1874	Plain Hotcakes with syrup and margarine	3	item(s)	221	89.7	570	8.0	105.0	3.0	13.0	3.5	1.9	4.6
38388	Premium Bacon Ranch salad with grilled chicken, no dressing	1	serving(s)	306	249.1	230	30.0	10.0	4.0	9.0	4.0	3.1	1.3
38391	Premium Caesar salad with grilled chicken, no dressing	1	serving(s)	296	245.5	190	27.0	10.0	4.0	5.0	3.0	1.5	0.6
38393	Premium Caesar salad, no dressing	1	serving(s)	213	191.1	90	7.0	9.0	3.0	4.0	2.5	1.0	0.3
29775	Premium Grilled Chicken Classic sandwich	1	item(s)	200	114.6	350	28.0	42.0	3.0	9.0	2.0	2.3	4.1
57683	Premium Southwest salad w/grilled chicken	1	item(s)	335	—	290	27.0	28.0	7.0	8.0	2.5	—	—
740	Quarter Pounder hamburger	1	item(s)	173	87.1	420	25.0	38.0	2.0	19.0	7.0	7.3	0.5
741	Quarter Pounder hamburger with cheese	1	item(s)	202	98.8	520	30.0	41.0	3.0	26.0	12.0	9.3	0.9
2005	Sausage McMuffin with egg	1	item(s)	164	81.9	450	21.0	30.0	2.0	27.0	10.0	10.8	4.5
50831	Side salad	1	item(s)	87	81.7	20	1.0	4.0	1.0	0.0	0	0	0
	Pizza Hut												
39009	Hot chicken wings	2	item(s)	44	—	100	10.0	1.0	0	6.0	2.0	—	—
14025	Meat Lovers hand-tossed pizza	1	slice(s)	105	—	300	14.0	26.0	1.0	16.0	7.0	—	—
14026	Meat Lovers pan pizza	1	slice(s)	113	—	330	14.0	27.0	1.0	18.0	7.0	—	—
31009	Meat Lovers stuffed crust pizza	1	slice(s)	165	—	480	22.0	39.0	2.0	26.0	11.0	—	—
14024	Meat Lovers thin 'n crispy pizza	1	slice(s)	85	—	280	13.0	22.0	1.0	16.0	6.0	—	—
14031	Pepperoni Lovers hand-tossed pizza	1	slice(s)	95	—	270	13.0	26.0	1.0	13.0	6.0	—	—
14032	Pepperoni Lovers pan pizza	1	slice(s)	101	—	290	13.0	27.0	1.0	14.0	6.0	—	—
31011	Pepperoni Lovers stuffed crust pizza	1	slice(s)	149	—	430	20.0	40.0	2.0	21.0	10.0	—	—
14030	Pepperoni Lovers thin 'n crispy pizza	1	slice(s)	75	—	250	12.0	22.0	1.0	13.0	6.0	—	—
10834	Personal Pan pepperoni pizza	1	slice(s)	50	—	153	6.5	16.8	0.8	6.5	2.5	—	—
10842	Personal Pan supreme pizza	1	slice(s)	64	—	180	7.5	17.3	1.0	9.0	3.5	—	—
39013	Personal Pan Veggie Lovers pizza	1	slice(s)	58	—	138	5.5	17.5	1.0	5.0	2.0	—	—
14028	Veggie Lovers hand-tossed pizza	1	slice(s)	102	—	200	9.0	27.0	2.0	6.0	3.0	—	—
14029	Veggie Lovers pan pizza	1	slice(s)	107	—	230	9.0	28.0	2.0	9.0	3.5	—	—
31010	Veggie Lovers stuffed crust pizza	1	slice(s)	155	—	330	15.0	41.0	2.0	12.0	6.0	—	—
14027	Veggie Lovers thin 'n crispy pizza	1	slice(s)	86	—	180	8.0	23.0	1.0	6.0	3.0	—	—
39012	Wing blue cheese dipping sauce	1	item(s)	43	—	230	1.0	2.0	0	24.0	4.5	—	—
39011	Wing ranch dipping sauce	1	item(s)	43	—	220	0	2.0	0	23.0	3.5	—	—

Chol (mg)	Calc (mg)	Iron (mg)	Magn (mg)	Pota (mg)	Sodi (mg)	Zinc (mg)	Vit A (µg)	Thia (mg)	Vit E (mg α)	Ribo (mg)	Niac (mg)	Vit B_6 (mg)	Fola (µg)	Vit C (mg)	Vit B_{12} (µg)	Sele (µg)
0	20	0.36	—	—	200.0	—	0	—	—	—	—	—	—	0	—	—
135	60	0.72	—	—	650.0	—	—	—	—	—	—	—	—	0	—	—
15	0	0	—	—	160.0	—	0	—	—	—	—	—	—	0	—	—
15	0	0	—	—	250.0	—	0	—	—	—	—	—	—	0	—	—
55	100	1.80	—	—	1500.0	—	—	—	—	—	—	—	—	1.2	—	—
0	20	1.08	5.4	48.5	170.0	0.18	—	0.23	1.49	0.16	2.03	0.04	—	15.0	—	—
0	0	0	3.6	55.2	260.0	0.05	3.4	0.01	0.30	0.01	0.19	0.02	—	0	—	—
75	250	4.50	43.0	396.0	970.0	4.11	—	0.38	—	0.45	7.28	—	—	1.2	1.9	—
40	202	2.72	22.8	200.0	680.0	2.18	—	0.25	—	0.30	4.59	—	—	1.2	1.0	—
40	20	0.72	23.0	239.0	540.0	0.56	0	0.15	—	0.10	7.03	0.38	—	1.2	0.3	—
25	0	0.36	15.0	161.0	360.0	0.38	0	0.10	—	0.07	4.74	0.25	—	1.2	0.2	—
50	450	1.80	57.0	804.6	250.0	1.78	324.0	0.14	0	0.76	0.47	0.18	—	0	1.9	—
45	150	3.60	57.5	483.5	990.0	1.41	38.3	0.42	—	0.36	11.80	—	—	3.6	—	—
260	300	2.70	27.6	238.7	780.0	1.78	—	0.36	0.81	0.51	4.28	0.20	—	0	—	—
40	150	1.80	38.3	312.4	590.0	0.82	—	0.30	1.66	0.19	3.15	—	—	0	1.5	36.2
0	20	1.44	49.3	862.4	350.0	0.68	0	0.50	—	0.05	4.25	0.80	—	12.0	—	—
0	20	0.72	22.7	397.6	160.0	0.31	0	0.23	—	0.03	1.96	0.37	—	4.8	—	—
5	100	0.67	20.9	248.8	70.0	0.54	—	0.07	—	0.17	0.35	—	—	9.0	0.3	—
25	100	2.70	21.0	192.0	480.0	1.95	—	0.25	—	0.24	4.54	—	—	1.2	0.8	26.2
0	0	0.36	11.8	219.0	310.0	0.19	0	0.06	—	0.01	1.26	0.14	—	1.2	—	—
25	249	1.44	34.0	440.3	170.0	1.00	145.0	0.08	0.34	0.41	0.27	0.09	—	0	1.0	—
20	150	2.70	28.7	276.3	660.0	0.64	—	0.45	—	0.40	3.23	0.12	—	0	0	—
85	150	1.80	—	—	700.0	—	—	0.17	—	0.25	11.33	—	—	21.0	—	—
70	200	1.78	—	754.8	580.0	—	—	0.17	—	0.20	11.31	—	—	21.0	—	—
10	200	1.44	19.2	460.1	180.0	—	—	0.09	—	0.08	0.45	—	—	18.0	0	0.4
65	150	3.60	56.0	456.0	820.0	1.38	—	0.39	1.06	0.38	13.04	0.61	—	4.8	0.3	—
70	150	2.70	—	—	650.0	—	—	—	—	—	—	—	—	21.0	—	—
65	150	4.50	38.1	392.7	700.0	4.65	—	0.32	—	0.60	7.70	—	—	1.2	2.2	—
95	300	4.50	44.4	442.4	1100.0	5.31	—	0.33	—	0.71	7.78	—	—	1.2	2.5	—
285	300	3.60	29.5	280.4	890.0	2.00	—	0.43	0.82	0.56	4.80	0.24	—	1.2	1.1	—
0	20	0.72	—	191.4	10.0	—	—	0.04	—	0.03	0.18	—	—	15.0	0	—
55	—	—	—	—	430.0	—	—	—	—	—	—	—	—	—	—	—
40	—	—	—	—	860.0	—	—	—	—	—	—	—	—	—	—	—
40	—	—	—	—	830.0	—	—	—	—	—	—	—	—	—	—	—
70	—	—	—	—	1380.0	—	—	—	—	—	—	—	—	—	—	—
40	—	—	—	—	860.5	—	—	—	—	—	—	—	—	—	—	—
35	—	—	—	—	770.0	—	—	—	—	—	—	—	—	—	—	—
35	—	—	—	—	730.0	—	—	—	—	—	—	—	—	—	—	—
60	—	—	—	—	1230.0	—	—	—	—	—	—	—	—	—	—	—
35	—	—	—	—	760.0	—	—	—	—	—	—	—	—	—	—	—
14	—	—	—	—	352.5	—	—	—	—	—	—	—	—	—	—	—
20	—	—	—	—	420.0	—	—	—	—	—	—	—	—	—	—	—
9	—	—	—	—	297.5	—	—	—	—	—	—	—	—	—	—	—
15	—	—	—	—	530.0	—	—	—	—	—	—	—	—	—	—	—
15	—	—	—	—	500.0	—	—	—	—	—	—	—	—	—	—	—
35	—	—	—	—	880.0	—	—	—	—	—	—	—	—	—	—	—
15	—	—	—	—	530.0	—	—	—	—	—	—	—	—	—	—	—
20	—	—	—	—	420.0	—	—	—	—	—	—	—	—	—	—	—
10	—	—	—	—	420.0	—	—	—	—	—	—	—	—	—	—	—

TABLE A-2 Table of Food Composition *(continued)*   (Computer code is for Cengage Diet Analysis program)   (For purposes of calculations, use "0" for t, <1, <0.1, <0.01)

DA+ Code	Food Description	Quantity	Measure	Wt (g)	H₂O (g)	Ener (kcal)	Prot (g)	Carb (g)	Fiber (g)	Fat (g)	Fat Breakdown (g) Sat	Mono	Poly
Fast Food—*continued*													
	Starbucks												
33107	Caffè mocha, tall nonfat, w/o whipped cream	12	fluid ounce(s)	354	—	170	10.0	32.0	0.5	2.0	1.0	—	—
33108	Caffè mocha, tall whole milk, w/whipped cream	12	fluid ounce(s)	354	—	290	10.0	34.0	0.5	16.0	9.0	—	—
38052	Cappuccino, tall	12	fluid ounce(s)	354	—	110	6.0	9.0	0	6.0	3.0	—	—
38053	Cappuccino, tall nonfat	12	fluid ounce(s)	354	—	60	6.0	9.0	0	0	0	0	0
38054	Cappuccino, tall soymilk	12	fluid ounce(s)	354	—	100	5.0	12.0	0.5	3.0	0	—	—
68043	Caramel Apple Spice, tall, w/o whipped cream	12	fluid ounce(s)	354	—	210	0	53.0	0	0	0	0	0
68256	Espresso, single shot	1	fluid ounce(s)	30	—	5	0	0.5	0	0	0	0	0
38088	Flavored syrup, 1 pump	1	serving(s)	10	—	20	0	5.0	0	0	0	0	0
38067	Frappuccino, tall caramel w/o whipped cream	12	fluid ounce(s)	354	—	200	3.0	42.0	0	2.5	1.5	—	—
39891	Frappuccino, tall caramel, light	12	fluid ounce(s)	354	—	130	4.0	25.0	2.0	1.0	0	—	—
67330	Frappuccino, tall Cinnamon Dolce, light	12	fluid ounce(s)	354	—	105	3.7	21.7	2.2	0.4	0.0	—	—
67329	Frappuccino, tall Cinnamon Dolce, w/whipped cream	12	fluid ounce(s)	354	—	270	3.0	42.0	0	11.0	6.0	—	—
38070	Frappuccino, tall coffee	12	fluid ounce(s)	354	—	180	3.0	36.0	0	2.5	1.5	—	—
39894	Frappuccino, tall coffee, light	12	fluid ounce(s)	354	—	90	3.0	18.0	0	0	0	—	—
67339	Frappuccino, tall Double Chocolaty Chip, w/whipped cream	12	fluid ounce(s)	354	—	300	5.0	42.0	0.5	14.0	9.0	—	—
38071	Frappuccino, tall espresso	12	fluid ounce(s)	354	—	150	2.0	34.0	0	1.0	0	—	—
39883	Frappuccino, tall Java Chip, w/o whipped cream	12	fluid ounce(s)	354	—	240	4.0	47.0	0.5	5.0	3.5	—	—
38073	Frappuccino, tall mocha w/o whipped cream	12	fluid ounce(s)	354	—	200	3.0	42.0	0.5	3.0	2.0	—	—
39897	Frappuccino, tall mocha, light	12	fluid ounce(s)	354	—	110	3.0	23.0	0.5	0.5	0	—	—
39887	Frappuccino, tall Strawberries & Creme, w/o whipped cream	12	fluid ounce(s)	354	—	190	3.0	38.0	0	3.0	1.5	—	—
38063	Frappuccino, tall Tazo chai creme w/o whipped cream	12	fluid ounce(s)	354	—	160	3.0	32.0	0	2.0	1.0	—	—
38080	Frappuccino, tall vanilla w/o whipped cream	12	fluid ounce(s)	354	—	200	3.0	39.0	0	3.5	2.0	—	—
39898	Frappuccino, tall white chocolate mocha, light blend	12	fluid ounce(s)	354	—	210	4.0	37.0	0	5.0	3.0	—	—
38074	Frappuccino, tall white chocolate w/o whipped cream	12	fluid ounce(s)	354	—	240	4.0	48.0	0	4.0	2.5	—	—
68822	Hot chocolate, tall soy, w/o whipped cream	12	fluid ounce(s)	354	—	230	9.0	40.0	2.0	6.0	1.5	—	—
67421	Iced mocha, tall white chocolate, nonfat, w/whipped cream	12	fluid ounce(s)	354	—	230	8.0	42.0	0	4.5	3.5	—	—
33111	Latte, tall w/nonfat milk	12	fluid ounce(s)	354	—	100	10.0	15.0	0	0	0	0	0
33112	Latte, tall w/whole milk	12	fluid ounce(s)	354	—	180	10.0	14.0	0	9.0	5.0	—	—
33109	Macchiato, tall caramel w/nonfat milk	12	fluid ounce(s)	354	—	140	7.0	25.0	0	1.0	1.0	—	—
33110	Macchiato, tall caramel w/whole milk	12	fluid ounce(s)	354	—	200	8.0	25.0	0	8.0	5.0	—	—
38089	Mocha syrup	1	serving(s)	17	—	25	1.0	6.0	0	0.5	0	—	—
67546	Tazo black shaken iced tea lemonade, tall	12	fluid ounce(s)	354	—	100	0	25.0	0	0	0	0	0
38076	Tazo black shaken iced tea, tall	12	fluid ounce(s)	354	—	60	0	15.0	0	0	0	—	—
67551	Tazo iced chai tea latte, tall w/nonfat milk	12	fluid ounce(s)	354	—	150	6.0	33.0	0	0	0	—	—
67417	Tazo iced green tea latte, tall w/nonfat milk	12	fluid ounce(s)	354	—	180	7.0	37.0	0.5	0	0	0	0
38090	Whipped cream	1	serving(s)	30	—	90	1.0	3.0	0	9.0	5.0	—	—
38062	White chocolate mocha, tall nonfat w/o whipped cream	12	fluid ounce(s)	354	—	270	12.0	47.0	0	4.5	3.5	—	—
38061	White chocolate mocha, tall w/ whipped cream	12	fluid ounce(s)	354	—	390	11.0	48.0	0	18.0	11.0	—	—
38048	White hot chocolate, tall nonfat w/o whipped cream	12	fluid ounce(s)	354	—	270	12.0	47.0	0	4.5	3.5	—	—

Chol (mg)	Calc (mg)	Iron (mg)	Magn (mg)	Pota (mg)	Sodi (mg)	Zinc (mg)	Vit A (µg)	Thia (mg)	Vit E (mg α)	Ribo (mg)	Niac (mg)	Vit B$_6$ (mg)	Fola (µg)	Vit C (mg)	Vit B$_{12}$ (µg)	Sele (µg)
2	300	2.70	—	—	0	—	—	—	—	—	—	—	—	0	—	—
45	300	2.70	—	—	0	—	—	—	—	—	—	—	—	0	—	—
15	200	0	—	—	0	—	—	—	—	—	—	—	—	0	—	—
2	200	0	—	—	0	—	—	—	—	—	—	—	—	0	—	—
0	200	1.08	—	—	0	—	—	—	—	—	—	—	—	0	—	—
0	0	0	—	—	0	—	0	—	—	—	—	—	—	0	—	—
0	0	0	—	—	0	—	0	—	—	—	—	—	—	0	—	—
0	0	0	—	—	0	—	0	—	—	—	—	—	—	0	0	—
10	100	0	—	—	0	—	—	—	—	—	—	—	—	0	—	—
2	100	0	—	—	180.0	—	0	—	—	—	—	—	—	0	—	—
0	112	0	—	—	0	—	0	—	—	—	—	—	—	0	—	—
35	100	0	—	—	0	—	—	—	—	—	—	—	—	0	—	—
10	100	0	—	—	0	—	—	—	—	—	—	—	—	0	—	—
0	100	0	—	—	0	—	—	—	—	—	—	—	—	0	—	—
40	150	2.70	—	—	0	—	—	—	—	—	—	—	—	0	—	—
2	60	0	—	—	0	—	—	—	—	—	—	—	—	0	—	—
10	100	2.70	—	—	0	—	—	—	—	—	—	—	—	0	—	—
10	100	0.72	—	—	0	—	—	—	—	—	—	—	—	0	—	—
0	100	0.72	—	—	0	—	—	—	—	—	—	—	—	0	—	—
10	100	0.36	—	—	0	—	—	—	—	—	—	—	—	3.6	—	—
10	100	0	—	—	0	—	—	—	—	—	—	—	—	0	—	—
10	100	0	—	—	0	—	—	—	—	—	—	—	—	0	—	—
10	150	0	—	—	0	—	—	—	—	—	—	—	—	0	—	—
10	2	0	—	—	0	—	—	—	—	—	—	—	—	0	—	—
0	300	3.60	—	—	0	—	—	—	—	—	—	—	—	0	—	—
2	300	0	—	—	0	—	—	—	—	—	—	—	—	1.2	—	—
2	350	0	—	—	0	—	—	—	—	—	—	—	—	0	—	—
30	300	0	—	—	0	—	—	—	—	—	—	—	—	0	—	—
2	250	0	—	—	0	—	—	—	—	—	—	—	—	0	—	—
25	250	0	—	—	0	—	—	—	—	—	—	—	—	0	—	—
0	0	0.72	—	—	0	—	0	—	—	—	—	—	—	0	—	—
0	0	0	—	—	10.0	—	0	—	—	—	—	—	—	6.0	—	—
0	0	0	—	—	0	—	0	—	—	—	—	—	—	0	—	—
2	200	0.36	—	—	0	—	—	—	—	—	—	—	—	0	—	—
2	250	0.36	—	—	0	—	—	—	—	—	—	—	—	6.0	—	—
30	20	0.36	—	—	10.0	—	90.1	—	—	—	—	—	—	0	—	—
2	400	0	—	—	0	—	—	—	—	—	—	—	—	1.2	0	—
50	400	0	—	—	0	—	—	—	—	—	—	—	—	1.2	—	—
2	450	0	—	—	0	—	—	—	—	—	—	—	—	1.2	—	—

TABLE A-2 **Table of Food Composition** (continued)   (Computer code is for Cengage Diet Analysis program)   (For purposes of calculations, use "0" for t, <1, <0.1, <0.01)

DA+ Code	Food Description	Quantity	Measure	Wt (g)	H₂O (g)	Ener (kcal)	Prot (g)	Carb (g)	Fiber (g)	Fat (g)	Fat Breakdown (g) Sat	Mono	Poly
Fast Food—*continued*													
38050	White hot chocolate, tall soymilk w/whipped cream	12	fluid ounce(s)	354	—	380	11.0	52.0	0.5	14.0	8.0	—	—
38047	White hot chocolate, tall w/whipped cream	12	fluid ounce(s)	354	—	410	12.0	48.0	0	19.0	12.0	—	—
	Subway												
80576	Breakfast BMT Melt	1	item(s)	142	—	240	16.0	25.0	6.0	10.0	4.0	—	—
80594	Buffalo chicken sandwich, 6", wheat bread	1	item(s)	268	—	420	25.0	46.0	5.0	15.0	3.0	—	—
15842	Cheese steak sandwich, 6", wheat bread	1	item(s)	297	—	500	38.0	51.0	6.0	17.0	9.0	—	—
40478	Chicken & bacon ranch sandwich, 6", white or wheat bread	1	serving(s)	292	—	570	35.0	47.0	5.0	28.0	10.0	—	—
32045	Chocolate chip cookie	1	item(s)	45	—	220	2.0	30.0	1.0	10.0	5.0	—	—
32048	Chocolate chip M&M cookie	1	item(s)	45	—	210	2.0	32.0	0.5	10.0	5.0	—	—
32049	Chocolate chunk cookie	1	item(s)	45	—	220	2.0	30.0	0.5	10.0	5.0	—	—
4024	Classic Italian B.M.T. sandwich, 6", white bread	1	item(s)	221	—	400	19.0	44.0	2.0	16.0	6.0	—	—
15838	Classic tuna sandwich, 6", wheat bread	1	item(s)	233	—	470	20.0	44.0	5.0	24.0	4.0	—	—
15837	Classic tuna sandwich, 6", white bread	1	item(s)	228	—	460	19.0	42.0	2.0	24.0	4.0	—	—
32043	Club sandwich, 6", wheat bread	1	item(s)	347	—	420	39.0	50.0	4.0	8.0	3.5	—	—
4030	Cold cut combo sandwich, 6", white bread	1	item(s)	228	—	360	17.0	44.0	2.0	13.0	4.0	—	—
385	Ham sandwich, 6", wheat bread	1	item(s)	219	—	290	18.0	46.0	5.0	4.5	1.0	—	—
3888	Meatball marinara sandwich, 6", wheat bread	1	item(s)	301	—	480	21.0	59.0	8.0	18.0	7.0	—	—
4651	Meatball sandwich, 6", white bread	1	item(s)	296	—	470	20.0	57.0	5.0	18.0	7.0	—	—
80596	Melt sandwich, 6", wheat bread	1	item(s)	240	—	370	23.0	47.0	5.0	11.0	5.0	—	—
32046	Oatmeal raisin cookie	1	item(s)	45	—	200	3.0	30.0	1.0	8.0	4.0	—	—
16379	Oven-roasted chicken breast sandwich, 6", wheat bread	1	item(s)	233	—	320	23.0	47.0	5.0	5.0	1.5	—	—
32047	Peanut butter cookie	1	item(s)	45	—	220	4.0	26.0	1.0	12.0	5.0	—	—
4655	Roast beef sandwich, 6", wheat bread	1	item(s)	233	—	320	24.0	45.0	5.0	5.0	1.5	—	—
3957	Roast beef sandwich, 6", white bread	1	item(s)	228	—	310	23.0	43.0	2.0	5.0	1.5	—	—
16378	Roasted chicken breast sandwich, 6", white bread	1	item(s)	228	—	310	22.0	45.0	2.0	5.0	1.5	—	—
4032	Spicy Italian sandwich, 6", white bread	1	item(s)	216	—	470	19.0	44.0	2.0	24.0	9.0	—	—
4031	Steak & cheese sandwich, 6", white bread	1	item(s)	239	—	370	25.0	46.0	2.0	10.0	4.5	—	—
32050	Sugar cookie	1	item(s)	45	—	220	2.0	28.0	0.5	12.0	6.0	—	—
80579	Sunrise Melt with egg	1	item(s)	149	—	230	18.0	26.0	6.0	8.0	3.0	—	—
40477	Sweet onion chicken teriyaki sandwich, 6", white or wheat bread	1	serving(s)	276	—	380	26.0	59.0	5.0	4.5	1.0	—	—
15834	Turkey breast & ham sandwich, 6", white bread	1	item(s)	214	—	270	17.0	44.0	2.0	4.0	1.0	—	—
16376	Turkey breast sandwich, 6", white bread	1	item(s)	214	—	270	17.0	44.0	2.0	3.5	1.0	—	—
15843	Veggie Delite salad	1	item(s)	271	—	50	3.0	9.0	4.0	1.0	0	—	—
15841	Veggie Delite sandwich, 6", wheat bread	1	item(s)	162	—	230	8.0	44.0	5.0	2.5	0.5	—	—
16375	Veggie Delite sandwich, 6", white bread	1	item(s)	157	—	220	7.0	42.0	2.0	2.5	0	—	—
32051	White chip macadamia nut cookie	1	item(s)	45	—	220	2.0	29.0	0.5	11.0	5.0	—	—
	Taco Bell												
29906	7-Layer burrito	1	item(s)	283	—	510	18.0	68.0	12.0	18.0	6.0	—	—
744	Bean burrito	1	item(s)	198	105.3	370	13.0	56.0	10.0	10.0	3.5	2.1	3.7
749	Beef burrito supreme	1	item(s)	248	—	420	17.0	52.0	9.0	15.0	7.0	—	—
33417	Beef Chalupa Supreme	1	item(s)	153	—	370	14.0	31.0	3.0	21.0	6.0	—	—
29910	Beef Gordita Supreme	1	item(s)	153	—	300	13.0	31.0	4.0	13.0	5.0	—	—

Chol (mg)	Calc (mg)	Iron (mg)	Magn (mg)	Pota (mg)	Sodi (mg)	Zinc (mg)	Vit A (µg)	Thia (mg)	Vit E (mg α)	Ribo (mg)	Niac (mg)	Vit B$_6$ (mg)	Fola (µg)	Vit C (mg)	Vit B$_{12}$ (µg)	Sele (µg)
25	400	1.44	—	—	0	—	—	—	—	—	—	—	—	1.2	—	—
50	400	0	—	—	0	—	—	—	—	—	—	—	—	1.2	—	—
130	200	1.44	—	—	830.0	—	—	—	—	—	—	—	—	1.2	—	—
55	300	3.60	—	—	1190.0	—	—	—	—	—	—	—	—	15.0	—	—
85	500	4.50	—	—	1310.0	—	—	—	—	—	—	—	—	12.0	—	—
95	500	3.60	—	—	1080.0	—	—	—	—	—	—	—	—	15.0	—	—
15	0	1.08	—	—	130.0	—	—	—	—	—	—	—	—	0	—	—
15	20	1.00	—	—	100.0	—	0	—	—	—	—	—	—	0	—	—
10	0	1.00	—	—	100.0	—	0	—	—	—	—	—	—	0	—	—
45	300	3.60	—	—	1280.0	—	—	—	—	—	—	—	—	12.0	—	—
35	300	3.60	—	—	620.0	—	—	—	—	—	—	—	—	12.0	—	—
35	300	3.60	—	—	600.0	—	—	—	—	—	—	—	—	12.0	—	—
70	80	7.20	—	—	2100.0	—	—	—	—	—	—	—	—	18.0	—	—
50	350	4.50	—	—	1120.0	—	—	—	—	—	—	—	—	12.0	—	—
25	300	2.70	—	—	830.0	—	—	—	—	—	—	—	—	12.0	—	—
30	350	4.50	—	—	950.0	—	—	—	—	—	—	—	—	21.0	—	—
30	350	4.50	—	—	930.0	—	—	—	—	—	—	—	—	21.0	—	—
45	400	2.70	—	—	1210.0	—	—	—	—	—	—	—	—	12.0	—	—
15	20	1.08	—	—	130.0	—	0	—	—	—	—	—	—	0	—	—
45	300	2.70	—	—	640.0	—	—	—	—	—	—	—	—	18.0	—	—
10	20	1.08	—	—	130.0	—	—	—	—	—	—	—	—	0	—	—
45	300	4.50	—	—	700.0	—	—	—	—	—	—	—	—	12.0	—	—
45	300	4.50	—	—	680.0	—	—	—	—	—	—	—	—	12.0	—	—
45	300	2.70	—	—	620.0	—	—	—	—	—	—	—	—	18.0	—	—
50	300	3.60	—	—	1500.0	—	—	—	—	—	—	—	—	12.0	—	—
50	400	4.50	—	—	1040.0	—	—	—	—	—	—	—	—	12.0	—	—
15	0	0.72	—	—	130.0	—	0	—	—	—	—	—	—	0	—	—
130	200	1.44	—	—	810.0	—	—	—	—	—	—	—	—	1.2	—	—
50	350	3.60	—	—	900.0	—	—	—	—	—	—	—	—	18.0	—	—
20	300	3.60	—	—	800.0	—	—	—	—	—	—	—	—	12.0	—	—
20	300	3.60	—	—	790.0	—	—	—	—	—	—	—	—	12.0	—	—
0	40	1.08	—	—	65.0	—	—	—	—	—	—	—	—	27.0	—	—
0	300	2.70	—	—	310.0	—	—	—	—	—	—	—	—	12.0	—	—
0	300	2.70	—	—	290.0	—	—	—	—	—	—	—	—	12.0	—	—
15	20	0.72	—	—	130.0	—	—	—	—	—	—	—	—	0	—	—
20	—	—	—	—	1410.0	—	—	—	—	—	—	—	—	—	—	—
5	246	4.69	67.3	516.8	980.0	1.70	5.9	0.38	0.99	0.20	4.00	0.20	134.6	0.8	0.3	20.6
35	—	—	—	—	1380.0	—	—	—	—	—	—	—	—	—	—	—
35	—	—	—	—	610.0	—	—	—	—	—	—	—	—	—	—	—
35	—	—	—	—	590.0	—	—	—	—	—	—	—	—	—	—	—

TABLE A-2 Table of Food Composition (continued)   (Computer code is for Cengage Diet Analysis program)   (For purposes of calculations, use "0" for t, <1, <0.1, <0.01)

DA+ Code	Food Description	Quantity	Measure	Wt (g)	H₂O (g)	Ener (kcal)	Prot (g)	Carb (g)	Fiber (g)	Fat (g)	Fat Breakdown (g) Sat	Mono	Poly
Fast Food—continued													
2014	Beef soft taco	1	item(s)	99	—	210	10.0	21.0	3.0	9.0	4.0	—	—
10860	Beef soft taco supreme	1	item(s)	135	—	240	11.0	24.0	3.0	11.0	5.0	—	—
66167	Cheesy Fiesta potatoes	1	serving(s)	135	—	270	4.0	28.0	3.0	16.0	2.5	—	—
34472	Chicken burrito supreme	1	item(s)	248	—	390	21.0	51.0	7.0	12.0	5.0	—	—
33418	Chicken Chalupa Supreme	1	item(s)	153	—	350	17.0	30.0	2.0	18.0	4.0	—	—
29909	Chicken quesadilla	1	item(s)	184	—	520	28.0	41.0	4.0	28.0	12.0	—	—
50171	Chicken soft taco	1	item(s)	99	57.8	187	13.2	19.5	1.2	6.3	2.5	1.6	1.6
29907	Chili cheese burrito	1	item(s)	156	—	370	16.0	40.0	4.0	16.0	8.0	—	—
10794	Cinnamon twists	1	serving(s)	35	—	170	1.0	26.0	1.0	7.0	0.0	—	—
66033	Fresco bean burrito	1	item(s)	213	—	340	12.0	56.0	11.0	8.0	2.5	—	—
66025	Fresco chicken burrito supreme	1	item(s)	241	—	340	18.0	50.0	8.0	8.0	2.5	—	—
66020	Fresco crunchy taco	1	item(s)	92	—	150	7.0	13.0	3.0	7.0	2.5	—	—
66026	Fresco steak burrito supreme	1	item(s)	241	—	330	16.0	49.0	8.0	8.0	3.0	—	—
29911	Grilled chicken Gordita Supreme	1	item(s)	153	—	270	17.0	29.0	2.0	10.0	3.5	—	—
29912	Grilled Steak Gordita Supreme	1	item(s)	153	—	270	14.0	29.0	2.0	11.0	4.0	—	—
29904	Grilled steak soft taco	1	item(s)	128	—	250	11.0	20.0	2.0	14.0	4.0	—	—
2021	Mexican pizza	1	serving(s)	213	—	540	21.0	47.0	8.0	30.0	8.0	—	—
10772	Meximelt	1	serving(s)	128	—	280	15.0	23.0	4.0	14.0	7.0	—	—
2011	Nachos	1	serving(s)	99	33.9	330	4.0	31.0	2.0	20.0	2.0	12.6	2.6
2012	Nachos BellGrande	1	serving(s)	305	—	770	20.0	78.0	15.0	42.0	7.0	—	—
2023	Pintos 'n cheese	1	serving(s)	128	—	180	10.0	19.0	9.0	7.0	3.0	—	—
34473	Steak burrito supreme	1	item(s)	248	—	380	18.0	51.0	7.0	12.0	5.0	—	—
33419	Steak Chalupa Supreme	1	item(s)	153	—	340	15.0	29.0	2.0	18.0	4.0	—	—
747	Taco	1	item(s)	78	—	170	8.0	12.0	3.0	10.0	3.5	—	—
2015	Taco salad with salsa, with shell	1	serving(s)	463	—	770	27.0	75.0	12.0	41.0	10.0	—	—
748	Tostada	1	item(s)	170	—	250	11.0	29.0	10.0	10.0	3.5	—	—
Convenience Meals													
Banquet													
14788	Boneless white fried chicken meal	1	item(s)	286	—	350	12.0	35.0	5.0	17.0	4.0	—	—
14773	Chicken pasta marinara meal	1	item(s)	184	—	290	12.0	29.0	3.0	14.0	3.0	—	—
29960	Fish sticks meal	1	item(s)	207	—	310	11.0	44.0	4.0	10.0	2.5	—	—
29957	Lasagna with meat sauce meal	1	item(s)	227	—	250	12.0	34.0	4.0	7.0	2.5	—	—
14777	Macaroni and cheese meal	1	item(s)	227	—	260	10.0	39.0	3.0	6.0	3.0	—	—
1741	Meatloaf meal	1	item(s)	269	—	280	12.0	28.0	4.0	13.0	5.0	—	—
39418	Pepperoni pizza meal	1	item(s)	163	—	340	11.0	47.0	4.0	12.0	3.5	—	—
1743	Salisbury steak meal	1	item(s)	269	—	290	11.0	25.0	4.0	16.0	7.0	—	—
14772	Turkey meal	1	item(s)	262	—	250	13.0	32.0	5.0	7.0	2.0	—	—
Healthy Choice													
9337	Beef pot roast complete meal	1	item(s)	312	—	290	17.0	45.0	6.0	4.5	1.5	2.0	1.0
57075	Café Steamers Cajun style chicken & shrimp	1	item(s)	295	—	250	17.0	33.0	5.0	5.0	1.0	—	—
57078	Café Steamers chicken linguini with red pepper Alfredo	1	item(s)	292	—	280	22.0	35.0	5.0	6.0	2.5	—	—
57074	Café Steamers sweet sesame chicken	1	item(s)	292	—	330	17.0	50.0	6.0	6.0	1.0	2.5	2.0
9316	Lemon pepper fish meal	1	item(s)	303	—	310	14.0	50.0	5.0	5.0	1.0	—	—
9322	Traditional salisbury steak meal	1	item(s)	354	—	310	18.0	46.0	9.0	6.0	2.5	2.0	1.0
9359	Traditional turkey breast meal	1	item(s)	298	—	290	18.0	44.0	8.0	4.5	1.0	2.0	1.5
Lean Cuisine													
11043	Culinary Collection baked chicken	1	item(s)	245	—	240	15.0	34.0	3.0	4.5	1.0	1.0	2.0
360	Simple Favorites chicken chow mein	1	item(s)	255	—	260	14.0	41.0	3.0	4.0	1.0	1.5	1.5
11054	Simple Favorites chicken enchilada suiza	1	serving(s)	255	190.9	270	12.0	47.0	3.0	4.0	1.5	1.0	1.0
9467	Simple Favorites fettuccini Alfredo	1	item(s)	262	—	280	14.0	42.0	1.0	6.0	3.0	1.5	1.0
9479	Simple Favorites French bread deluxe pizza	1	item(s)	174	—	340	16.0	46.0	4.0	10.0	3.5	2.5	1.5
11055	Simple Favorites lasagna with meat sauce	1	item(s)	298	—	320	20.0	43.0	4.0	7.0	3.5	2.0	1.0
58267	Spa Collection ginger garlic stir fry with chicken	1	item(s)	280	—	290	17.0	46.0	4.0	4.0	1.0	1.0	1.5

PAGE KEY: A-6 5 Breads/Baked Goods A-12 = Cereal/Rice/Pasta A-16 = Fruit A-22 = Vegetables/Legumes A-32 = Nuts/Seeds A-34 = Vegetarian A-36 = Dairy A-44 = Eggs A-44 = Seafood A-46 = Meats A-50 = Poultry
A-52 = Processed Meats A-54 = Beverages A-58 = Fats/Oils A-60 = Sweets A-62 = Spices/Condiments/Sauces A-66 = Mixed Foods/Soups/Sandwiches A-72 = Fast Food A-90 = Convenience A-92 = Baby Foods

Chol (mg)	Calc (mg)	Iron (mg)	Magn (mg)	Pota (mg)	Sodi (mg)	Zinc (mg)	Vit A (µg)	Thia (mg)	Vit E (mg α)	Ribo (mg)	Niac (mg)	Vit B$_6$ (mg)	Fola (µg)	Vit C (mg)	Vit B$_{12}$ (µg)	Sele (µg)
30	—	—	—	—	620.0	—	—	—	—	—	—	—	—	—	—	—
35	—	—	—	—	650.0	—	—	—	—	—	—	—	—	—	—	—
5	—	—	—	—	840.0	—	—	—	—	—	—	—	—	—	—	—
40	—	—	—	—	1420.0	—	—	—	—	—	—	—	—	—	—	—
40	—	—	—	—	650.0	—	—	—	—	—	—	—	—	—	—	—
75	—	—	—	—	1420.0	—	—	—	—	—	—	—	—	—	—	—
29	121	1.57	23.8	214.8	606.9	0.75	1.0	0.16	0.35	0.11	5.12	0.11	68.3	0.2	0.1	12.6
40	—	—	—	—	1080.0	—	—	—	—	—	—	—	—	—	—	—
0	—	—	—	—	200.0	—	—	—	—	—	—	—	—	—	—	—
0	—	—	—	—	1290.0	—	—	—	—	—	—	—	—	—	—	—
25	—	—	—	—	1410.0	—	—	—	—	—	—	—	—	—	—	—
20	—	—	—	—	350.0	—	—	—	—	—	—	—	—	—	—	—
15	—	—	—	—	1340.0	—	—	—	—	—	—	—	—	—	—	—
35	—	—	—	—	620.0	—	—	—	—	—	—	—	—	—	—	—
30	—	—	—	—	550.0	—	—	—	—	—	—	—	—	—	—	—
30	—	—	—	—	710.0	—	—	—	—	—	—	—	—	—	—	—
45	—	—	—	—	1020.0	—	—	—	—	—	—	—	—	—	—	—
45	—	—	—	—	870.0	—	—	—	—	—	—	—	—	—	—	—
5	88	1.11	51.5	180.2	370.0	1.14	1.0	0.12	1.04	0.13	0.90	0.18	12.9	—	—	3.4
30	—	—	—	—	1300.0	—	—	—	—	—	—	—	—	—	—	—
15	—	—	—	—	720.0	—	—	—	—	—	—	—	—	—	—	—
30	—	—	—	—	1340.0	—	—	—	—	—	—	—	—	—	—	—
30	—	—	—	—	580.0	—	—	—	—	—	—	—	—	—	—	—
30	—	—	—	—	330.0	—	—	—	—	—	—	—	—	—	—	—
60	—	—	—	—	1650.0	—	—	—	—	—	—	—	—	—	—	—
15	—	—	—	—	730.0	—	—	—	—	—	—	—	—	—	—	—
35	100	1.08	40.0	450.0	930.0	1.50	0	0.09	—	0.14	1.20	0.12	—	4.8	0.5	—
15	60	1.80	40.0	380.0	550.0	0.90	—	—	—	0.10	1.60	0.08	—	2.4	1.8	—
25	100	1.80	40.0	290.0	540.0	0.60	—	0.12	—	0.17	0.80	—	—	0	3.0	—
10	60	2.70	40.0	420.0	510.0	1.20	—	0.30	—	0.25	3.00	—	—	1.2	2.7	—
15	100	1.44	32.0	220.0	760.0	0.90	—	0.30	—	0.51	0.80	—	—	0	0.4	—
40	20	1.08	32.0	420.0	1000.0	1.50	0	—	—	—	—	0.16	—	0	0.6	—
10	150	1.80	40.0	310.0	730.0	1.50	—	0.12	—	0.34	0.80	0.12	—	—	—	—
30	20	1.44	32.0	380.0	1100.0	1.50	0	0.06	—	0.14	1.60		—	0	0.9	—
25	40	1.80	32.0	360.0	1060.0	1.20	—	0.15	—	0.17	3.00	0.12	—	6.0	0.9	—
40	40	1.80	40.0	720.0	500.0	3.00	—	0.03	—	0.17	3.00	0.20	—	30.0	1.5	21.0
45	40	1.08	40.0	480.0	590.0	1.20	—	0.22	—	0.25	6.00	0.20	—	6.0	0.5	0
35	100	1.80	40.0	440.0	570.0	1.50	—	0.22	—	0.34	5.00	0.20	—	30.0	0.6	63.0
30	40	0.72	40.0	440.0	400.0	0.90	—	0.09	—	0.14	4.00	0.30	—	1.2	0.6	0
25	60	1.08	40.0	480.0	450.0	0.60	—	0.22	—	0.07	2.00	0.40	—	24.0	1.2	14.0
35	100	2.70	60.0	880.0	590.0	3.00	—	0.15	—	0.17	3.00	0.16	—	24.0	1.2	21.0
25	60	1.80	40.0	680.0	450.0	1.20	—	0.22	—	0.25	5.00	0.20	—	4.8	0.5	31.5
25	40	1.17	—	500.0	650.0	—	—	—	—	—	—	—	—	3.6	—	—
25	60	1.08	—	380.0	550.0	—	—	—	—	—	—	—	—	3.6	—	—
20	150	1.08	—	380.0	550.0	—	—	0.20	—	0.15	1.68	—	—	1.2	—	—
15	200	0.72	—	270.0	690.0	—	0	—	—	—	—	—	—	0	—	—
20	150	2.70	—	330.0	760.0	—	—	—	—	—	—	—	—	12.0	—	—
30	200	2.70	—	710.0	590.0	—	—	—	—	—	—	—	—	3.6	—	—
30	60	1.44	—	550.0	640.0	—	—	—	—	—	—	—	—	15.0	—	—

TABLE A-2 **Table of Food Composition** (continued)   (Computer code is for Cengage Diet Analysis program)   (For purposes of calculations, use "0" for t, <1, <0.1, <0.01)

DA+ Code	Food Description	Quantity	Measure	Wt (g)	H₂O (g)	Ener (kcal)	Prot (g)	Carb (g)	Fiber (g)	Fat (g)	Fat Breakdown (g) Sat	Mono	Poly
Convenience Meals—continued														
	Michelina's												
55332	Cheese manicotti with marinara sauce entrée	1	item(s)	227	—	270	11.0	34.0	3.0	11.0	5.0	—	—
1915	Fettuccini Alfredo with chicken & broccoli entrée	1	item(s)	241	—	310	15.0	38.0	2.0	10.0	6.0	—	—
55320	Lean Gourmet five cheese lasagna entrée	1	item(s)	227	—	290	13.0	50.0	8.0	5.0	2.0	—	—
55329	Lean Gourmet Meatloaf entrée	1	item(s)	227	—	180	11.0	21.0	2.0	6.0	3.0	—	—
55325	Lean Gourmet Santa Fe style rice & beans entrée	1	item(s)	255	—	320	10.0	52.0	3.0	8.0	3.5	—	—
	Stouffer's												
36564	Beef pot roast entrée	1	item(s)	255	—	210	14.0	30.0	2.0	4.0	1.5	—	—
2313	Cheese French bread pizza	1	serving(s)	294	—	370	14.0	44.0	4.0	15.0	6.0	—	—
2366	Chicken pot pie entrée	1	item(s)	454	—	590	19.0	54.0	1.0	34.0	13.0	—	—
11116	Homestyle baked chicken breast with mashed potatoes and gravy entrée	1	item(s)	252	—	250	20.0	20.0	1.0	10.0	3.0	—	—
11152	Homestyle roast turkey breast with stuffing and mashed potatoes entrée	1	item(s)	273	—	290	16.0	30.0	2.0	12.0	3.5	—	—
41781	Lasagna with meat & sauce entrée	1	item(s)	595	441.9	690	47.8	74.8	6.5	22.4	11.3	7.6	1.4
	Weight Watchers												
11164	Smart Ones chicken enchiladas suiza entrée	1	item(s)	255	—	290	11.0	49.0	3.0	5.0	2.0	1.5	1.0
39763	Smart Ones chicken oriental entrée	1	item(s)	255	—	230	14.0	41.0	2.0	1.5	0	0	0
11187	Smart Ones pepperoni pizza	1	item(s)	173	—	410	19.0	63.0	4.0	9.0	3.0	2.5	1.5
58556	Smart Ones spaghetti with meat sauce entrée	1	item(s)	326	—	290	14.0	44.0	5.0	6.0	1.5	2.0	1.0
31512	Smart Ones spicy szechuan style vegetables & chicken	1	item(s)	255	—	240	11.0	38.0	4.0	5.0	1.0	2.0	2.5
Baby Foods														
787	Apple juice	4	fluid ounce(s)	127	111.6	60	0	14.8	0.1	0.1	0	0	0
778	Applesauce, strained	4	tablespoon(s)	64	56.7	26	0.1	6.9	1.1	0.1	0	0	0
779	Bananas with tapioca, strained	4	tablespoon(s)	60	50.4	34	0.2	9.2	1.0	0.1	0	0	0
604	Carrots, strained	4	tablespoon(s)	56	51.7	15	0.4	3.4	1.0	0.1	0	0	0
770	Chicken noodle dinner, strained	4	tablespoon(s)	64	54.8	42	1.7	5.8	1.3	1.3	0.4	0.5	0.3
801	Green beans, strained	4	tablespoon(s)	60	55.1	16	0.7	3.8	1.3	0.1	0	0	0.1
910	Human milk, mature	2	fluid ounce(s)	62	53.9	43	0.6	4.2	0	2.7	1.2	1.0	0.3
760	Mixed cereal, prepared with whole milk	4	ounce(s)	113	89.8	109	4.7	13.9	0.9	3.8	2.0	1.0	0.4
772	Mixed vegetable dinner, strained	2	ounce(s)	57	50.3	23	0.7	5.4	0.9	0.1	—	—	0.1
762	Rice cereal, prepared with whole milk	4	ounce(s)	113	92.9	96	3.9	11.7	0	3.8	2.0	1.0	0.4
758	Teething biscuits	1	item(s)	11	0.7	43	1.2	8.4	0.2	0.5	0.1	0.2	0.1

PAGE KEY: A-6 5 Breads/Baked Goods A-12 = Cereal/Rice/Pasta A-16 = Fruit A-22 = Vegetables/Legumes A-32 = Nuts/Seeds A-34 = Vegetarian A-36 = Dairy A-44 = Eggs A-44 = Seafood A-46 = Meats A-50 = Poultry
A-52 = Processed Meats A-54 = Beverages A-58 = Fats/Oils A-60 = Sweets A-62 = Spices/Condiments/Sauces A-66 = Mixed Foods/Soups/Sandwiches A-72 = Fast Food A-90 = Convenience A-92 = Baby Foods

Chol (mg)	Calc (mg)	Iron (mg)	Magn (mg)	Pota (mg)	Sodi (mg)	Zinc (mg)	Vit A (µg)	Thia (mg)	Vit E (mg α)	Ribo (mg)	Niac (mg)	Vit B$_6$ (mg)	Fola (µg)	Vit C (mg)	Vit B$_{12}$ (µg)	Sele (µg)
30	200	1.08	—	—	980.0	—	—	—	—	—	—	—	—	12.0	—	—
45	150	1.80	—	—	700.0	—	—	—	—	—	—	—	—	9.0	—	—
10	150	3.60	—	—	560.0	—	—	—	—	—	—	—	—	12.0	—	—
35	40	1.44	—	—	860.0	—	—	—	—	—	—	—	—	6.0	—	—
20	150	1.44	—	—	670.0	—	—	—	—	—	—	—	—	6.0	—	—
25	20	1.80	—	—	710.0	—	—	—	—	—	—	—	—	4.8	—	—
20	250	1.80	—	—	600.0	—	—	—	—	—	—	—	—	2.4	—	—
50	100	3.60	—	—	930.0	—	—	—	—	—	—	—	—	1.2	—	—
60	40	0.36	—	—	730.0	—	0	—	—	—	—	—	—	0	—	—
45	40	1.08	—	490.0	970.0	—	—	—	—	—	—	—	—	3.6	—	—
77	411	3.63	—	940.1	1856.4	—	—	0.36	—	0.30	3.81	—	—	3.6	—	—
25	100	0.72	—	—	640.0	—	—	—	—	—	—	—	—	6.0	—	—
25	20	0.36	—	—	700.0	—	—	—	—	—	—	—	—	2.4	—	—
30	100	1.44	—	—	730.0	—	—	—	—	—	—	—	—	0	—	—
10	100	2.70	—	—	520.0	—	—	—	—	—	—	—	—	12.0	—	—
10	60	2.70	—	—	710.0	—	—	—	—	—	—	—	—	0	—	—
0	5	0.72	3.8	115.4	10.1	0.04	1.3	0.01	0.76	0.02	0.11	0.04	0	73.4	0	0.1
0	3	0.14	1.9	45.4	0	0.01	0.6	0.01	0.38	0.02	0.04	0.02	1.3	24.5	0	0.2
0	3	0.12	6.0	52.8	0	0.04	1.2	0.01	0.36	0.02	0.11	0.07	3.6	10.0	0	0.4
0	12	0.21	5.0	109.8	38.6	0.08	320.9	0.01	0.29	0.02	0.26	0.04	8.4	3.2	0	0.1
10	17	0.41	9.0	89.0	24.3	0.35	70.4	0.03	0.13	0.04	0.46	0.04	8.3	0.1	0	2.4
0	23	0.40	12.0	87.6	4.2	0.13	10.8	0.02	0.04	0.05	0.22	0.02	14.4	0.2	0	0.1
9	20	0.02	1.8	31.4	10.5	0.10	37.6	0.01	0.05	0.02	0.11	0.01	3.1	3.1	0	1.1
10	249	11.83	22.7	188.2	47.6	0.67	46.5	0.35	0.53	0.51	4.40	0.06	10.2	0.3	0.5	6.9
—	12	0.19	6.2	68.6	21.5	0.09	77.1	0.01	—	0.02	0.28	0.04	4.5	1.6	0	0.4
11	191	4.12	28.4	171.2	47.6	0.56	47.6	0.28	0.50	0.37	2.78	0.08	6.8	0.2	0.5	4.9
1	29	0.39	3.8	35.5	25.0	0.10	3.1	0.03	0.12	0.06	0.48	0.01	7.6	1.0	0	2.6

Appendix B

WHO: Nutrition Recommendations; Canada: Guidelines and Meal Planning

This appendix presents nutrition recommendations from the World Health Organization (WHO) and details for Canadians on the *Eating Well with Canada s Food Guide* and the *Beyond the Basics* meal-planning system.

Nutrition Recommendations from WHO

The World Health Organization (WHO) has assessed the relationships between diet and the development of chronic diseases. Its recommendations include:

▯ Energy: sufficient to support growth, physical activity, and a healthy body weight (BMI between 18.5 and 24.9) and to avoid weight gain greater than 11 pounds (5 kilograms) during adult life

▯ Total fat: 15 to 30 percent of total energy

▯ Saturated fatty acids: <10 percent of total energy

▯ Polyunsaturated fatty acids: 6 to 10 percent of total energy

▯ Omega-6 polyunsaturated fatty acids: 5 to 8 percent of total energy

▯ Omega-3 polyunsaturated fatty acids: 1 to 2 percent of total energy

▯ *Trans*-fatty acids: <1 percent of total energy

▯ Total carbohydrate: 55 to 75 percent of total energy

▯ Sugars: <10 percent of total energy, preferably <5 percent of total energy

▯ Protein: 10 to 15 percent of total energy

▯ Cholesterol: <300 mg per day

▯ Salt (sodium): <5 g salt per day (<2 g sodium per day), appropriately iodized

▯ Potassium: ≥3510 mg per day

▯ Fruits and vegetables: ≥400 g per day (about 1 pound)

▯ Total dietary fiber: >25 g per day from foods

▯ Physical activity: one hour of moderate-intensity activity, such as walking, on most days of the week

Eating Well with Canada's Food Guide

Figure B-1 presents the 2007 *Eating Well with Canada s Food Guide*. Additional publications, which are available from Health Canada through its website, provide many more details.

Search for "Canada's food guide" at Health Canada: *www.hc-sc.gc.ca*

FIGURE B-1 **Eating Well with Canada's Food Guide**

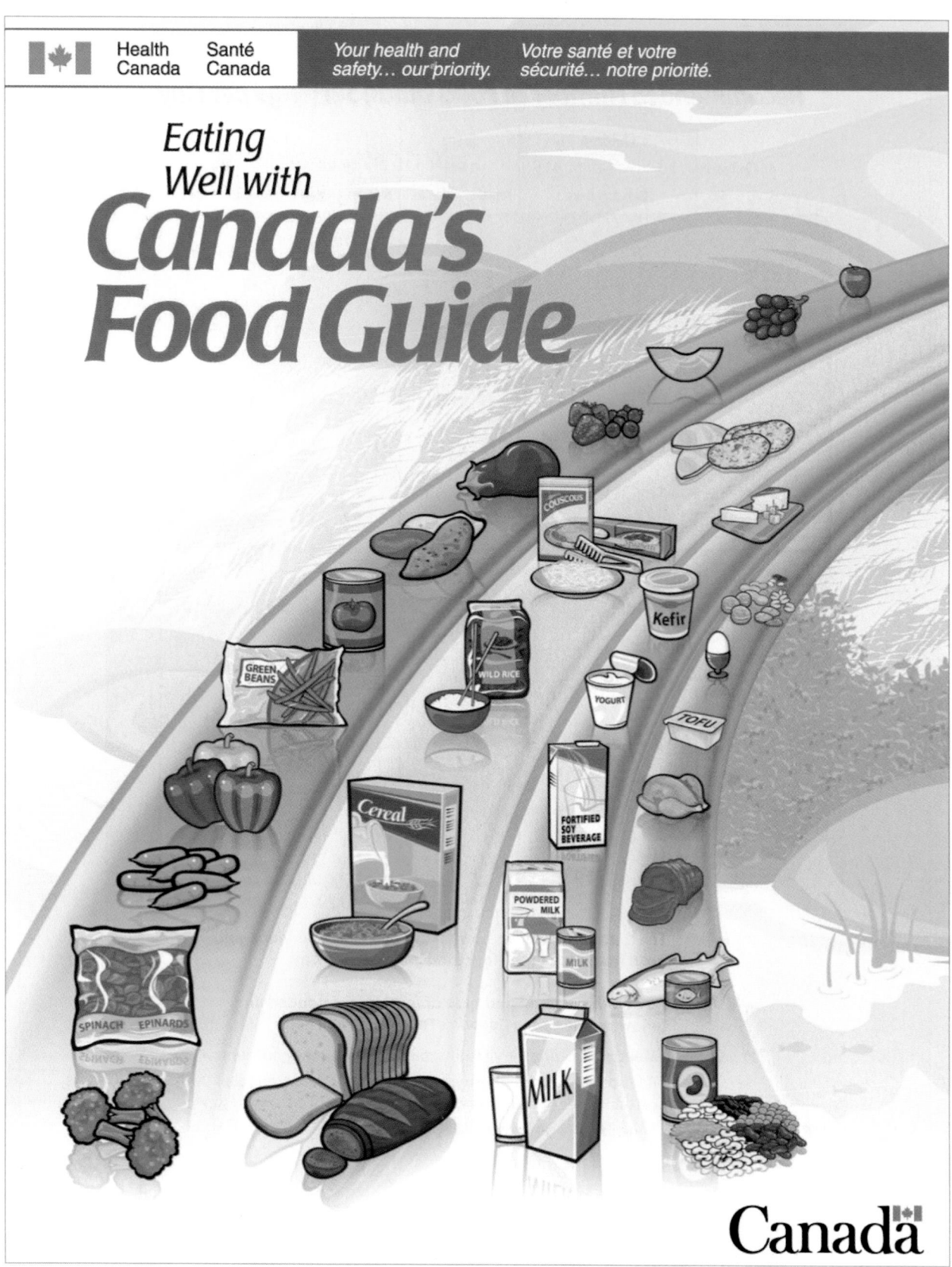

FIGURE B-1 **Eating Well with Canada's Food Guide** (continued)

Recommended Number of *Food Guide Servings* per Day

	Children			Teens		Adults			
Age in Years	2-3	4-8	9-13	14-18		19-50		51+	
Sex	Girls and Boys			Females	Males	Females	Males	Females	Males
Vegetables and Fruit	4	5	6	7	8	7-8	8-10	7	7
Grain Products	3	4	6	6	7	6-7	8	6	7
Milk and Alternatives	2	2	3-4	3-4	3-4	2	2	3	3
Meat and Alternatives	1	1	1-2	2	3	2	3	2	3

The chart above shows how many Food Guide Servings you need from each of the four food groups every day.

Having the amount and type of food recommended and following the tips in *Canada's Food Guide* will help:

• Meet your needs for vitamins, minerals and other nutrients.

• Reduce your risk of obesity, type 2 diabetes, heart disease, certain types of cancer and osteoporosis.

• Contribute to your overall health and vitality.

FIGURE B-1 **Eating Well with Canada's Food Guide** (*continued*)

What is One Food Guide Serving?
Look at the examples below.

Fresh, frozen or canned vegetables
125 mL (½ cup)

Leafy vegetables
Cooked: 125 mL (½ cup)
Raw: 250 mL (1 cup)

Fresh, frozen or canned fruits
1 fruit or 125 mL (½ cup)

100% Juice
125 mL (½ cup)

Bread
1 slice (35 g)

Bagel
½ bagel (45 g)

Flat breads
½ pita or ½ tortilla (35 g)

Cooked rice, bulgur or quinoa
125 mL (½ cup)

Cereal
Cold: 30 g
Hot: 175 mL (¾ cup)

Cooked pasta or couscous
125 mL (½ cup)

Milk or powdered milk (reconstituted)
250 mL (1 cup)

Canned milk (evaporated)
125 mL (½ cup)

Fortified soy beverage
250 mL (1 cup)

Yogurt
175 g
(¾ cup)

Kefir
175 g
(¾ cup)

Cheese
50 g (1 ½ oz.)

Cooked fish, shellfish, poultry, lean meat
75 g (2 ½ oz.)/125 mL (½ cup)

Cooked legumes
175 mL (¾ cup)

Tofu
150 g or
175 mL (¾ cup)

Eggs
2 eggs

Peanut or nut butters
30 mL (2 Tbsp)

Shelled nuts and seeds
60 mL (¼ cup)

Oils and Fats
- Include a small amount – 30 to 45 mL (2 to 3 Tbsp) – of unsaturated fat each day. This includes oil used for cooking, salad dressings, margarine and mayonnaise.
- Use vegetable oils such as canola, olive and soybean.
- Choose soft margarines that are low in saturated and trans fats.
- Limit butter, hard margarine, lard and shortening.

FIGURE B-1 **Eating Well with Canada's Food Guide** *(continued)*

Make each Food Guide Serving count...
wherever you are – at home, at school, at work or when eating out!

▶ **Eat at least one dark green and one orange vegetable each day.**
- · Go for dark green vegetables such as broccoli, romaine lettuce and spinach.
- · Go for orange vegetables such as carrots, sweet potatoes and winter squash.

▶ **Choose vegetables and fruit prepared with little or no added fat, sugar or salt.**
- · Enjoy vegetables steamed, baked or stir-fried instead of deep-fried.

▶ **Have vegetables and fruit more often than juice.**

▶ **Make at least half of your grain products whole grain each day.**
- · Eat a variety of whole grains such as barley, brown rice, oats, quinoa and wild rice.
- · Enjoy whole grain breads, oatmeal or whole wheat pasta.

▶ **Choose grain products that are lower in fat, sugar or salt.**
- · Compare the Nutrition Facts table on labels to make wise choices.
- · Enjoy the true taste of grain products. When adding sauces or spreads, use small amounts.

▶ **Drink skim, 1%, or 2% milk each day.**
- · Have 500 mL (2 cups) of milk every day for adequate vitamin D.
- · Drink fortified soy beverages if you do not drink milk.

▶ **Select lower fat milk alternatives.**
- · Compare the Nutrition Facts table on yogurts or cheeses to make wise choices.

▶ **Have meat alternatives such as beans, lentils and tofu often.**

▶ **Eat at least two Food Guide Servings of fish each week.***
- · Choose fish such as char, herring, mackerel, salmon, sardines and trout.

▶ **Select lean meat and alternatives prepared with little or no added fat or salt.**
- · Trim the visible fat from meats. Remove the skin on poultry.
- · Use cooking methods such as roasting, baking or poaching that require little or no added fat.
- · If you eat luncheon meats, sausages or prepackaged meats, choose those lower in salt (sodium) and fat.

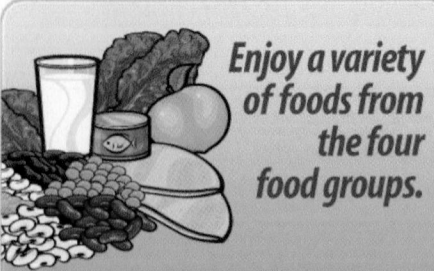

Enjoy a variety of foods from the four food groups.

Satisfy your thirst with water!

Drink water regularly. It's a calorie-free way to quench your thirst. Drink more water in hot weather or when you are very active.

* Health Canada provides advice for limiting exposure to mercury from certain types of fish. Refer to www.hc-sc.gc.ca for the latest information.

FIGURE B-1 **Eating Well with Canada's Food Guide** (*continued*)

Advice for different ages and stages...

Children

Following *Canada's Food Guide* helps children grow and thrive.

Young children have small appetites and need calories for growth and development.

- Serve small nutritious meals and snacks each day.
- Do not restrict nutritious foods because of their fat content. Offer a variety of foods from the four food groups.
- Most of all... be a good role model.

Women of childbearing age

All women who could become pregnant and those who are pregnant or breastfeeding need a multivitamin containing **folic acid** every day. Pregnant women need to ensure that their multivitamin also contains **iron**. A health care professional can help you find the multivitamin that's right for you.

Pregnant and breastfeeding women need more calories. Include an extra 2 to 3 Food Guide Servings each day.

Here are two examples:
- Have fruit and yogurt for a snack, or
- Have an extra slice of toast at breakfast and an extra glass of milk at supper.

Men and women over 50

The need for **vitamin D** increases after the age of 50.

In addition to following *Canada's Food Guide*, everyone over the age of 50 should take a daily vitamin D supplement of 10 µg (400 IU).

How do I count Food Guide Servings in a meal?

Here is an example:

Vegetable and beef stir-fry with rice, a glass of milk and an apple for dessert		
250 mL (1 cup) mixed broccoli, carrot and sweet red pepper	=	2 **Vegetables and Fruit** Food Guide Servings
75 g (2 ½ oz.) lean beef	=	1 **Meat and Alternatives** Food Guide Serving
250 mL (1 cup) brown rice	=	2 **Grain Products** Food Guide Servings
5 mL (1 tsp) canola oil	=	part of your **Oils and Fats** intake for the day
250 mL (1 cup) 1% milk	=	1 **Milk and Alternatives** Food Guide Serving
1 apple	=	1 **Vegetables and Fruit** Food Guide Serving

FIGURE B-1 **Eating Well with Canada's Food Guide** (*continued*)

Eat well and be active today and every day!

The benefits of eating well and being active include:

- Better overall health.
- Feeling and looking better.
- Lower risk of disease.
- More energy.
- A healthy body weight.
- Stronger muscles and bones.

Be active

To be active every day is a step towards better health and a healthy body weight.

Canada's Physical Activity Guide recommends building 30 to 60 minutes of moderate physical activity into daily life for adults and at least 90 minutes a day for children and youth. You don't have to do it all at once. Add it up in periods of at least 10 minutes at a time for adults and five minutes at a time for children and youth.

Start slowly and build up.

Eat well

Another important step towards better health and a healthy body weight is to follow *Canada's Food Guide* by:

- Eating the recommended amount and type of food each day.
- Limiting foods and beverages high in calories, fat, sugar or salt (sodium) such as cakes and pastries, chocolate and candies, cookies and granola bars, doughnuts and muffins, ice cream and frozen desserts, french fries, potato chips, nachos and other salty snacks, alcohol, fruit flavoured drinks, soft drinks, sports and energy drinks, and sweetened hot or cold drinks.

Read the label

- Compare the Nutrition Facts table on food labels to choose products that contain less fat, saturated fat, trans fat, sugar and sodium.
- Keep in mind that the calories and nutrients listed are for the amount of food found at the top of the Nutrition Facts table.

Limit trans fat

When a Nutrition Facts table is not available, ask for nutrition information to choose foods lower in trans and saturated fats.

Nutrition Facts
Per 0 mL (0 g)

Amount	% Daily Value
Calories 0	
Fat 0 g	0 %
Saturates 0 g	0 %
+ Trans 0 g	
Cholesterol 0 mg	
Sodium 0 mg	0 %
Carbohydrate 0 g	0 %
Fibre 0 g	0 %
Sugars 0 g	
Protein 0 g	

Vitamin A	0 %	Vitamin C	0 %
Calcium	0 %	Iron	0 %

Take a step today...

✓ Have breakfast every day. It may help control your hunger later in the day.

✓ Walk wherever you can – get off the bus early, use the stairs.

✓ Benefit from eating vegetables and fruit at all meals and as snacks.

✓ Spend less time being inactive such as watching TV or playing computer games.

✓ Request nutrition information about menu items when eating out to help you make healthier choices.

✓ Enjoy eating with family and friends!

✓ Take time to eat and savour every bite!

For more information, interactive tools, or additional copies visit Canada's Food Guide on-line at:
www.hc-sc.gc.ca

or contact:

Publications
Health Canada
Ottawa, Ontario K1A 0K9
E-Mail: publications@hc-sc.gc.ca
Tel.: 1-866-225-0709
Fax: (613) 941-5366
TTY: 1-800-267-1245

Également disponible en français sous le titre : Bien manger avec le Guide alimentaire canadien

This publication can be made available on request on diskette, large print, audio-cassette and braille.

Beyond the Basics: Meal Planning for Healthy Eating, Diabetes Prevention and Management

Beyond the Basics: Meal Planning for Healthy Eating, Diabetes Prevention and Management is Canada's system of meal planning.[1] Similar to the U.S. *Choose Your Foods: Food Lists for Diabetes, Beyond the Basics* sorts foods into groups and defines portion sizes to help people manage their blood glucose and maintain a healthy weight. Because foods that contain carbohydrate raise blood glucose, the food groups are organized into two sections—those that contain carbohydrate (presented in Table B-1) and those that contain little or no carbohydrate (shown in Table B-2). One portion from any of the food groups listed in Table B-1 provides about 15 grams of available carbohydrate (total carbohydrate minus fiber) and counts as one carbohydrate choice. Within each group, foods are identified as those to "choose more often" (generally higher in vitamins, minerals, and fiber) and those to "choose less often" (generally higher in sugar, saturated fat, or *trans* fat).

[1]The tables for the Canadian meal planning system are adapted from *Beyond the Basics: Meal Planning for Healthy Eating, Diabetes Prevention and Management,* copyright 2005, with permission of the Canadian Diabetes Association. Additional information is available from *www.diabetes.ca*.

TABLE B-1 Food Groups That Contain Carbohydrate

Key:
● Choose more often
▲ Choose less often

1 serving = 15 g carbohydrate or 1 carbohydrate choice	
Food	**Measure**
Grains and starches: 15 g carbohydrate, 3 g protein, 0 g fat, 286 kJ (68 kcal)	
▲ Bagel, large (11 cm, 4.5")	¼
▲ Bagel, small (8 cm, 3")	½
▲ Bannock, fried	1.5" × 2.5"
● Bannock, whole grain baked	1.5" × 2.5"
● Barley, pearled, cooked	125 mL (½ c)
▲ Bread, white	1 slice (30 g)
● Bread, whole grain	1 slice (30 g)
● Bulghur, cooked	125 mL (½ c)
▲ Bun, hamburger or hotdog	½
▲ Cereal, flaked unsweetened	125 mL (½ c)
● Cream of Wheat, cooked	175 mL (¾ c)
● Red River, cooked	125 mL (½ c)
● Chapati (15 cm, 6")	1 (44 g)
● Corn	125 mL (½ c)
● Couscous, cooked	125 mL (½ c)
▲ Crackers, soda type	7
▲ Croutons	175 mL (¾ c)
● English muffin, whole grain	½ (28 g)
▲ French fries	10 (50 g)
● Millet, cooked	⅓ c (75 mL)

TABLE B-1 Food Groups That Contain Carbohydrate (*continued*)

Food	Measure
Grains and starches: 15 g carbohydrate, 3 g protein, 0 g fat, 286 kJ (68 kcal)	
▲ Naan bread (15 cm, 6″)	¼
▲ Pancake (10 cm, 4″)	1
● Pasta, cooked	125 mL (½ c)
▲ Pita bread, white (15 cm, 6″)	½
● Pita bread, whole-wheat (15 cm, 6″)	½
▲ Pizza crust (30 cm, 12″)	1/12 (90 g)
● Plantain, cooked, mashed	⅓ c (75 mL)
● Potatoes, boiled or baked	½ medium (84 g)
● Rice, white or brown, cooked	⅓ c (75 mL)
● Roti (15 cm, 6″)	1 (44 g)
● Soup, thick, chunky type	250 mL (1 c)
● Sweet potato, mashed	⅓ c (75 mL)
▲ Taco shells (13 cm, 5″)	2 (17 g)
● Tortilla, wheat flour (25 cm, 10″)	½
▲ Waffle (medium)	1 (39 g)
Fruits: 15 g carbohydrate, 1–2 g protein, 0 g fat, 269 kJ (64 kcal)	
● Apple	1 medium (138 g)
● Applesauce, unsweetened	125 mL (½ c)
● Banana	1 small or ½ large
● Blackberries	500 mL (2 c)
● Cherries	15 (102 g)
● Fruit, canned in juice	125 mL (½ c)
▲ Fruit, dried	60 mL (¼ c)
● Grapefruit	1 small
● Grapes	15 or ½ c (80 g)
● Kiwi	2 medium (150 g)
▲ Juice	125 mL (½ c)
● Mango	½ medium
● Melon	250 mL (1 c)
● Orange	1 medium
● Other berries	250 mL (1 c)
● Pear	1 medium
● Pineapple	175 mL (¾ c)
● Plum	2 medium
● Raspberries	500 mL (2 c)
● Strawberries	500 mL (2 c)

(*continued*)

TABLE B-1 **Food Groups That Contain Carbohydrate** (*continued*)

Food	Measure
Milk and alternatives: 15 g carbohydrate, 7 g protein, variable fat, 386–651 kJ (92–155 kcal)	
● Evaporated milk, canned	125 mL (½ c)
● Milk, fluid	250 mL (1 c)
● Milk powder, skim	60 mL (4 tbs)
● Soy beverage, flavoured	125 mL (½ c)
● Soy beverage, plain	250 mL (1 c)
● Soy yogourt, flavoured	75 mL (⅓ c)
● Yogourt, nonfat, plain	175 mL (¾ c)
● Yogourt, skim, artificially sweetened	250 mL (1 c)
Other choices (sweet foods and snacks): 15 g carbohydrate, variable protein and fat	
▲ Brownies, unfrosted	5 cm × 5 cm (2″ × 2″)
▲ Cake, unfrosted	5 cm × 5 cm (2″ × 2″)
▲ Cookies, arrowroot or gingersnap	3–4
▲ Jam, jelly, marmalade	15 mL (1 tbs)
● Milk pudding, skim, no sugar added	125 mL (½ c)
▲ Muffin, plain	1 small (45 g)
▲ Oatmeal granola bar	1 (28 g)
● Popcorn, low-fat, air-popped	750 mL (3 c)
▲ Pretzels, low-fat, large	7
▲ Pretzels, low-fat, sticks	30
▲ Sugar, white	15 mL (1 tbs, 3 tsp, or 3 packets)
▲ Syrup, honey, molasses	1 tbs (15 mL)

Key:
● Choose more often
▲ Choose less often

TABLE B-2 **Food Groups That Contain Little or No Carbohydrate**

Food	Measure
Vegetables: To encourage consumption, most vegetables are considered "free"	
▲ Artichokes, Jerusalem[a]	
● Asparagus	
● Beans, yellow or green	
● Bean sprouts	

Key:
● Choose more often
▲ Choose less often

[a]These vegetables contain enough carbohydrate to be counted as one carbohydrate choice (15 g of available carbohydrate) when the portion size eaten is 1 cup (250 mL) or more.

TABLE B-2 Food Groups That Contain Little or No Carbohydrate
(*continued*)

Food	Measure
Vegetables: To encourage consumption, most vegetables are considered "free"	
● Beets	
● Broccoli	
● Cabbage	
● Carrots	
● Cauliflower	
● Celery	
● Cucumber	
● Eggplant	
● Kale	
● Leeks	
● Mushrooms	
● Okra	
● Onions	
▲ Parsnips[a]	
▲ Peas[a]	
● Peppers	
● Rutabagas	
● Salad vegetables	
▲ Squash, Hubbard, pumpkin, spaghetti	
▲ Squash, acorn[a], butternut[a]	
● Tomatoes, fresh	
● Tomatoes, canned, regular	
▲ Tomatoes, canned, stewed[a]	
● Turnips	
Meat and alternatives: 0 g carbohydrate, 7 g protein, 3–5 g fat, 307 kJ (73 kcal)	
● Cheese, skim (<7% milk fat)	2.5 cm × 2.5 cm × 2.5 cm (1″ × 1″ × 1″)
● Cheese, light (<20% milk fat)	2.5 cm × 2.5 cm × 2.5 cm (1″ × 1″ × 1″)
▲ Cheese, regular (≥21% milk fat)	2.5 cm × 2.5 cm × 2.5 cm (1″ × 1″ × 1″)
● Cottage cheese (1–2% milk fat)	60 mL (¼ c)
● Egg	1 medium-large
● Fish, canned in oil or water	60 mL (¼ c)
● Fish, fresh or frozen, cooked	30 g (1 oz)
● Hummus	90 g (⅓ c)
● Legumes, cooked	125 mL (½ c)
● Meat, game, cooked	30 g (1 slice)
● Meat, ground, lean or extra lean, cooked	30 g (2 tbs)

(*continued*)

TABLE B-2   Food Groups That Contain Little or No Carbohydrate
(*continued*)

Food	Measure
Meat and alternatives: 0 g carbohydrate, 7 g protein, 3–5 g fat, 307 kJ (73 kcal)	
● Meat, lean, cooked	30 g (1 slice)
● Meat, organ or tripe, cooked	30 g (1 slice)
● Meat, prepared, low-fat	30 g (1–3 slices)
▲ Meat, prepared, regular fat	30 g (1–3 slices)
▲ Meat, regular, cooked	30 g (1–3 slices)
● Peameal/back bacon, cooked	30 g (1–2 slices)
● Poultry, ground, lean, cooked	30 g (2 tbs)
● Poultry, skinless, cooked	30 g (1 slice)
▲ Poultry/wings, skin on, cooked	45 g (2)
● Shellfish, cooked	30 g (3 medium)
● Tofu (soybean)	½ block (100 g)
● Vegetarian meat alternatives	30 g (1 oz)
Fats: 0 g carbohydrate, 0 g protein, 5 g fat, 189 kJ (45 kcal)	
▲ Avocado	34 g (⅙)
▲ Bacon	30 g (1 slice)
▲ Butter	5 mL (1 tsp)
▲ Cheese, spreadable	15 mL (1 tbs)
▲ Margarine, non-hydrogenated, regular	5 mL (1 tsp)
▲ Mayonnaise, light	15 mL (1 tbs)
▲ Nuts	15 mL (1 tbs)
▲ Oil, canola or olive	5 mL (1 tsp)
▲ Salad dressing, regular	5 mL (1 tsp)
▲ Seeds	15 g (1 tbs)
▲ Tahini	8 mL (½ tbs)
Extras: <5 g carbohydrate, 84 kJ (20 kcal)	
Broth	
Coffee	
Herbs and spices	
Ketchup	
Mustard	
Relish	
Sugar-free gelatin	
Sugar-free soft drinks	
Tea	

Key:
● Choose more often
▲ Choose less often

Appendix C

Choose Your Foods: Food Lists for Diabetes

Chapter 21 describes how a meal-planning system based on food lists can be used to control carbohydrate intakes, and this appendix provides details from the 2014 publication *Choose Your Foods: Food Lists for Diabetes*. Appendix B presents Canada's meal-planning system.

These food lists can help people with diabetes to manage their blood glucose levels by controlling the amount and kinds of carbohydrates they consume. These lists can also help in planning diets for weight management by controlling kcalorie and fat intake.

The Food Lists

The food lists sort foods into groups by their proportions of carbohydrate, fat, and protein (Table C-1 on p. C-2). These major groups may be organized into several lists of foods (Tables C-2 through C-12 on pp. C-3–C-17). For example, the carbohydrate group includes these food lists:

- Starch
- Fruits
- Milk and Milk Substitutes (fat-free/low-fat, reduced-fat, and whole)
- Nonstarchy Vegetables
- Sweets, Desserts, and Other Carbohydrates

Then any food on a list can be substituted for any other on that same list. Note that some foods on the lists may count as choices from more than one group; in this case, the choices per specified serving will also be stated. For example, chocolate nonfat milk counts as 1 fat-free milk plus 1 carbohydrate choice, and ½ cup black beans counts as 1 starch plus 1 lean protein choice. Another group for alcohol has been included as a reminder that these beverages often deliver substantial carbohydrate and kcalories and therefore warrant their own list.

Serving Sizes

The serving sizes have been carefully adjusted and defined so that a serving of any food on a given list provides roughly the same amount of carbohydrate, fat, and protein, and, therefore, total energy. Any food on a list can thus be traded for any other food on the same list without significantly affecting the diet's energy–nutrient balance or total kcalories. For example, a person may select 17 small grapes or ½ large grapefruit as one fruit choice and either would provide roughly 15 grams of carbohydrate and 60 kcalories. A whole grapefruit, however, would count as 2 fruit choices.

To apply the system successfully, users must become familiar with the specified serving sizes. A convenient way to remember the serving sizes and energy values is to keep in mind a typical item from each list (review Table C-1).

The Foods on the Lists

Foods do not always appear on the food list where you might first expect to find them. They are grouped according to their energy–nutrient contents rather than by their source (such as milks), their outward appearance, or their vitamin and mineral contents. For example, cheeses are grouped with proteins (not milk) because, like medium- and high-fat meats, cheeses contribute energy from protein and fat but provide negligible carbohydrate.

For similar reasons, starchy vegetables such as corn, green peas, and potatoes are found on the Starch list with breads and cereals, not with the nonstarchy vegetables. Likewise, bacon is grouped with both saturated fats and high-fat meats.

Diet planners learn to view mixtures of foods, such as casseroles and soups, as combinations of foods from different food lists. They also learn to interpret food labels with the food lists in mind.

Controlling Energy, Fat, and Sodium

The food lists help people control their energy intakes by paying close attention to serving sizes. People wanting to lose weight can limit foods from the Sweets, Desserts, and Other Carbohydrates and Fats lists, and they might choose to avoid the Alcohol list altogether. The Free Foods list provides low-kcalorie choices.

By assigning items like bacon to the High-Fat Protein and Saturated Fats lists, the food lists alert consumers to foods that are high in fat. Even the Starch list specifies which grain products contain added fat (such as biscuits, cornbread, and waffles) by marking them with a symbol to indicate added fat (the symbols are explained in the table keys). In addition, the food lists encourage users to think of fat-free milk as milk and of whole milk as milk with added fat, and to think of lean meats as meats and of medium-fat and high-fat meats as meats with added fat. To that end, foods on the milk and meat lists are separated into categories based on their fat contents (review Table C-1). The Milk and Milk Substitutes list is subdivided for fat-free/low-fat, reduced-fat, and whole; the Proteins list is subdivided for lean, medium-fat, and high-fat. The Proteins

TABLE C-1 The Food Lists

Lists	Typical Item/Portion Size	Carbohydrate (g)	Protein (g)	Fat (g)	Energy[a] (kcal)
Carbohydrates					
Starch[b]	1 slice bread	15	3	1	80
Fruits	1 small apple	15	—	—	60
Milk and Milk Substitutes					
Fat-free, low-fat (1%)	1 c fat-free milk	12	8	0–3	100
Reduced-fat (2%)	1 c reduced-fat milk	12	8	5	120
Whole	1 c whole milk	12	8	8	160
Nonstarchy vegetables	½ c cooked carrots	5	2	—	25
Sweets, desserts, and other carbohydrates[c]	5 vanilla wafers	15	varies	varies	varies
Proteins					
Lean	1 oz chicken (no skin)	—	7	2	45
Medium-fat	1 oz ground beef	—	7	5	75
High-fat	1 oz pork sausage	—	7	8	100
Plant-based	½ c tofu	varies	7	varies	varies
Fats	1 tsp olive oil	—	—	5	45
Alcohol	12 fl oz beer	varies	—	—	100

[a]The energy value for each food list represents an approximate average for the group and does not reflect the precise number of grams of carbohydrate, protein, and fat. For example, a slice of bread contains 15 grams of carbohydrate (60 kcalories), 3 grams protein (12 kcalories), and a little fat—rounded to 80 kcalories for ease in calculating. A ½ cup of vegetables (not including starchy vegetables) contains 5 grams carbohydrate (20 kcalories) and 2 grams protein (8 more), which has been rounded down to 25 kcalories.
[b]The Starch list includes cereals, grains, breads, crackers, snacks, starchy vegetables (such as corn, peas, and potatoes), and legumes (dried beans, peas, and lentils).
[c]The Sweets, Desserts, and Other Carbohydrates list includes foods that contain added sugars and fats such as sodas, candy, cakes, cookies, doughnuts, ice cream, pudding, syrup, and frozen yogurt.

list also includes plant-based proteins, which tend to be rich in fiber. Notice that many of these foods (p. C-7) bear the symbol for "good source of fiber."

People wanting to control the sodium in their diets can begin by eliminating any foods bearing the "high in sodium" symbol. In most cases, the symbol identifies foods that, in one serving, provide 480 milligrams or more of sodium. Foods on the Combination Foods or Fast Foods lists that bear the symbol provide more than 600 milligrams of sodium. Other foods may also contribute substantially to sodium (consult Chapter 9 for details).

Planning a Healthy Diet

To obtain a daily variety of foods that provide healthful amounts of carbohydrate, protein, and fat, as well as vitamins, minerals, and fiber, the meal plan for adults and teenagers should include at least:

- Two to three servings of nonstarchy vegetables
- Two servings of fruits
- Six servings of grains (at least three of whole grains), beans, and starchy vegetables
- Two servings of low-fat or fat-free milk
- About 6 ounces of protein foods
- *Small* amounts of fat and sugar

The actual amounts are determined by age, gender, activity levels, and other factors that influence energy needs.

TABLE C-2 **Starch**

The Starch list includes breads, cereals, grains and pasta, starchy vegetables, crackers and snacks, and legumes (beans, peas, and lentils). 1 starch choice = 15 grams carbohydrate, 3 grams protein, 1 gram fat, and 80 kcalories.

NOTE: In general, one starch choice is ½ cup cooked cereal, grain, or starchy vegetable; ⅓ cup cooked rice or pasta; 1 ounce of bread products; ¾ ounce to 1 ounce of most snack foods.

Food	Serving Size	Food	Serving Size
Bread		**Bread** *(continued)*	
Bagel	¼ large bagel (1 oz)	tortilla, flour (white or whole-wheat)	1 small (6 in. across) or ⅓ large (10 in. across)
! Biscuit	1 (2½ in. across)	Cornbread	1¾-in. cube (1½ oz)
Breads, loaf-type		English muffin	½ muffin
white, whole-grain, French, Italian, pumpernickel, rye, sourdough, unfrosted raisin or cinnamon	1 slice (1 oz)	Hot dog bun or hamburger bun	½ bun (¾ oz)
		Pancake	1 (4 in. across, ¼ in. thick)
✓ reduced-calorie, light	2 slices (1½ oz)	Roll, plain	1 small (1 oz)
Breads, flat-type		! Stuffing, bread	⅓ cup
chapatti	1 oz	Waffle	1 (4-in. square or 4 in. across)
ciabatta	1 oz	**Cereals**	
naan	3¼-in. square (1 oz)	✓ Bran cereal (twigs, buds, or flakes)	½ cup
pita (6 in across)	½ pita	Cooked cereals (oats, oatmeal)	½ cup
roti	1 oz	Granola cereal	¼ cup
✓ sandwich flat buns, whole-wheat	1 bun (1½ oz)	Grits, cooked	½ cup
! taco shell	2 (each 5 in. across)	Muesli	¼ cup
tortilla, corn	1 small (6 in. across)	Puffed cereal	1½ cups

(continued)

TABLE C-2 Starch (*continued*)

Food	Serving Size	Food	Serving Size
Cereals (*continued*)		**Starchy Vegetables**[b] (*continued*)	
Shredded wheat, plain	½ cup	✓ Squash, winter (acorn, butternut)	1 cup
Sugar-coated cereal	½ cup	✓ Succotash	½ cup
Unsweetened, ready-to-eat cereal	¾ cup	Yam or sweet potato, plain	½ cup (3½ oz)
Grains[a]		**Crackers and Snacks**	
Barley	⅓ cup	Crackers	
Bran, dry		animal	8
✓ oat	¼ cup	✓ crispbread	2–5 pieces (¾ oz)
✓ wheat	½ cup	graham, 2 ½-in. square	3
✓ Bulgur	½ cup	nut and rice	10
Couscous	⅓ cup	oyster	20
Kasha	½ cup	! round, butter-type	6
Millet	⅓ cup	saltine-type	6
Pasta, white or whole-wheat	⅓ cup	! sandwich-style, cheese or peanut butter filling	3
Polenta	⅓ cup	whole-wheat, baked	5 regular 1½-in. squares or 10 thins (¾ oz)
Quinoa, all colors	⅓ cup		
Rice, all colors and types	⅓ cup	Granola or snack bar	1 (¾ oz)
Tabbouleh (tabouli), prepared	½ cup	Matzoh, all shapes and sizes	¾ oz
Wheat germ, dry	3 Tbsp	Melba toast	4 (2 by 4 in.)
Wild rice	½ cup	Popcorn	
Starchy Vegetables[b]		✓ no fat added	3 cups
Breadfruit	¼ cup	!! with butter added	3 cups
Cassava or dasheen	⅓ cup	Pretzels	¾ oz
Corn	½ cup	Rice cakes	2 (4 in. across)
on cob	4- to 4 ½-in. piece (½ large)	Snack chips	
✓ Hominy	¾ cup	baked (potato, pita)	~8 (¾ oz)
✓ Mixed vegetables with corn or peas	1 cup	!! regular (tortilla, potato)	~13 (1 oz)
Marinara, pasta, or spaghetti sauce	½ cup	**Beans, Peas, and Lentils**[d]	
✓ Parsnips	½ cup	The choices on this list count as 1 starch + 1 lean protein.	
✓ Peas, green	½ cup	✓ Baked beans, canned	⅓ cup
Plantain	⅓ cup	✓ Beans (black, garbanzo, kidney, lima, navy, pinto, white), cooked or canned, drained and rinsed	½ cup
Potato			
baked with skin	¼ large (3 oz)		
boiled, all kinds	½ cup or ½ medium (3 oz)	✓ Lentils (any color), cooked	½ cup
! mashed, with milk and fat	½ cup	✓ Peas (black-eyed and split), cooked or canned, drained and rinsed	½ cup
french-fried (oven-baked)[c]	1 cup (2 oz)		
✓ Pumpkin puree, canned, no sugar added	¾ cup	🧂 ✓ Refried beans, canned	½ cup

[a]Cooked unless otherwise noted. [b]Serving sizes are for cooked vegetables. [c]Restaurant-style french fries are on the Fast Foods list. [d]Also found on the Proteins list.

Key:

✓ = Good source of fiber: >3 g/serving

! = Extra fat

!! = Added fat: 2 extra fat choices or prepared with added fat

🧂 = High in sodium: ≥480 mg/serving

TABLE C-3 **Fruits**

Fruit[a]

The Fruits list includes fresh, frozen, canned, and dried fruits and fruit juices. 1 fruit choice = 15 grams carbohydrate, 0 grams protein, 0 grams fat, and 60 kcalories.

NOTE: In general, one fruit choice is ½ cup canned or fresh fruit or unsweetened fruit juice; 1 small fresh fruit (4 ounces); 2 tablespoons dried fruit.

Food	Serving Size	Food	Serving Size
Apple, unpeeled	1 small (4 oz)	Mango	½ small (5½ oz) or ½ cup
Apples, dried	4 rings	Nectarine	1 medium (5½ oz)
Applesauce, unsweetened	½ cup	✓ Orange	1 medium (6½ oz)
Apricots		Papaya	½ (8 oz) or 1 cup cubed
canned	½ cup	Peaches	
dried	8 halves	canned	½ cup
fresh	4 (5½ oz total)	fresh	1 medium (6 oz)
Banana	1 extra-small, ~4 in. long (4 oz)	Pears	
✓ Blackberries	1 cup	canned	½ cup
Blueberries	¾ cup	✓ fresh	½ large (4 oz)
Cantaloupe	1 cup diced	Pineapple	
Cherries		canned	½ cup
sweet, canned	½ cup	fresh	¾ cup
sweet, fresh	12 (3½ oz)	Plantain, extra-ripe (black), raw	¼ (2¼ oz)
Dates	3 small (deglet noor) or 1 large (medjool)	Plums	
Dried fruits (blueberries, cherries, cranberries, mixed fruit, raisins)	2 Tbsp	canned	½ cup
		dried (prunes)	3
		fresh	2 small (5 oz)
Figs		Pomegranate seeds (arils)	½ cup
dried	3 small	✓ Raspberries	1 cup
✓ fresh	1½ large or 2 medium (3½ oz)	✓ Strawberries	1¼ cup whole
		Tangerine	1 large (6 oz)
Fruit cocktail	½ cup	Watermelon	1¼ cups diced
Grapefruit		**Fruit Juice**	
fresh	½ large (5½ oz)	Apple juice/cider	½ cup
sections, canned	¾ cup	Fruit juice blends, 100% juice	⅓ cup
Grapes	17 small (3 oz)	Grape juice	⅓ cup
✓ Guava	2 small (2½ oz)	Grapefruit juice	½ cup
Honeydew melon	1 cup diced	Orange juice	½ cup
Kiwi	½ cup sliced	Pineapple juice	½ cup
Loquat	¾ cup cubed	Pomegranate juice	½ cup
Mandarin oranges, canned	¾ cup	Prune juice	⅓ cup

[a]The weights listed include skin, core, seeds, and rind.

Key:

✓ = Good source of fiber: >3 g/serving

TABLE C-4 Milk and Milk Substitutes

The Milk and Milk Substitutes list groups milks and yogurts based on the amount of fat they have (fat-free/low fat, reduced fat, and whole). Cheeses are found on the Proteins list and cream and other dairy fats are found on the Fats list.

1 fat-free or low-fat milk choice = 12 g carbohydrate, 8 g protein, 0–3 g fat, and 100 kcal.

1 reduced-fat milk choice = 12 g carbohydrate, 8 g protein, 5 g fat, and 120 kcal.

1 whole milk choice has 12 g carbohydrate, 8 g protein, 8 g fat, and 160 kcal.

NOTE: In general, one milk choice is 1 cup (8 fluid ounces or ½ pint) milk or yogurt.

Food	Serving Size	Choices per Serving
Milk and Yogurts		
Fat-free (skim) or low-fat (1%)		
milk, buttermilk, acidophilus milk, lactose-free milk	1 cup	1 fat-free milk
evaporated milk	½ cup	1 fat-free milk
yogurt, plain or Greek; may be sweetened with artificial sweetener	⅔ cup (6 oz)	1 fat-free milk
chocolate milk	1 cup	1 fat-free milk + 1 carbohydrate
Reduced-fat (2%)		
milk, acidophilus milk, kefir, lactose-free milk	1 cup	1 reduced-fat milk
yogurt, plain	⅔ cup (6 oz)	1 reduced-fat milk
Whole		
milk, buttermilk, goat's milk	1 cup	1 whole milk
evaporated milk	½ cup	1 whole milk
yogurt, plain	1 cup (8 oz)	1 whole milk
chocolate milk	1 cup	1 whole milk + 1 carbohydrate
Other Milk Foods and Milk Substitutes[a]		
Eggnog		
fat-free	⅓ cup	1 carbohydrate
low-fat	⅓ cup	1 carbohydrate + ½ fat
whole milk	⅓ cup	1 carbohydrate + 1 fat
Rice drink		
plain, fat-free	1 cup	1 carbohydrate
flavored, low-fat	1 cup	2 carbohydrates
Soy milk		
light or low-fat, plain	1 cup	½ carbohydrate + ½ fat
regular, plain	1 cup	½ carbohydrate + 1 fat
Yogurt with fruit, low-fat	⅔ cup (6 oz)	1 fat-free milk + 1 carbohydrate

[a]Unsweetened nut milks (such as almond and coconut milks) are on the Fats list.

TABLE C-5 **Nonstarchy Vegetables**

The Nonstarchy Vegetables list includes vegetables that have few grams of carbohydrates or kcalories; starchy vegetables are found on the Starch list. Salad greens (like arugula, chicory, endive, escarole, lettuce, radicchio, romaine, and watercress) are on the Free Foods list.

1 nonstarchy vegetable choice = 5 grams carbohydrate, 2 grams protein, 0 grams fat, and 25 kcalories.

NOTE: In general, one nonstarchy vegetable choice is ½ cup cooked vegetables or vegetable juice or 1 cup raw vegetables. Count 3 cups of raw vegetables or 1½ cups of cooked vegetables as one carbohydrate choice.

Amaranth leaves (Chinese spinach)	Hearts of palm
Artichoke	✓ Jicama
Artichoke hearts (no oil)	Kale
Asparagus	Kohlrabi
Baby corn	Leeks
Bamboo shoots	Mixed vegetables (without starchy vegetables, legumes, or pasta)
Bean sprouts (alfalfa, mung, soybean)	
Beans (green, wax, Italian, yard-long)	Mushrooms, all kinds, fresh
Beets	Okra
Broccoli	Onions
Broccoli slaw, packaged, no dressing	Pea pods
✓ Brussels sprouts	Peppers (all varieties)
Cabbage (green, red, bok choy, Chinese)	Radishes
✓ Carrots	Rutabaga
Cauliflower	▩ Sauerkraut, drained and rinsed
Celery	Spinach
Chayote	Squash, summer varieties (yellow, pattypan, crookneck, zucchini)
Coleslaw, packaged, no dressing	Sugar snap peas
Cucumber	Swiss chard
Daikon	Tomato
Eggplant	Tomatoes, canned
Fennel	▩ Tomato sauce (unsweetened)
Gourds (bitter, bottle, luffa, bitter melon)	Tomato/vegetable juice
Green onions or scallions	Turnips
Greens (collard, dandelion, mustard, purslane, turnip)	Water chestnuts

Key:

✓ = Good source of fiber: >3 g/serving

▩ = High in sodium: ≥ 480 mg/serving

TABLE C-6 Sweets, Desserts, and Other Carbohydrates

1 other carbohydrate choice = 15 grams carbohydrate, variable grams protein, variable grams fat, and variable kcalories.

NOTE: In general, one choice from this list can substitute for foods on the Starch, Fruits, or Milk and Milk Substitutes lists.

Food	Serving Size	Choices per Serving
Beverages, Soda, and Sports Drinks		
Cranberry juice cocktail	½ cup	1 carbohydrate
Food drink or lemonade	1 cup (8 oz)	2 carbohydrates
Hot chocolate, regular	1 envelope (2 Tbsp or ¾ oz) added to 8 oz water	1 carbohydrate
Soft drink (soda), regular	1 can (12 oz)	2½ carbohydrates
Sports drink (fluid replacement type)	1 cup (8 oz)	1 carbohydrate
Brownies, Cake, Cookies, Gelatin, Pie, and Pudding		
Biscotti	1 oz	1 carbohydrate + 1 fat
Brownie, small, unfrosted	1¼-in. square, ⅞-in. high (~1 oz)	1 carbohydrate + 1 fat
Cake		
angel food, unfrosted	$\frac{1}{12}$ of cake (~2 oz)	2 carbohydrates
frosted	2-in. square (~2 oz)	2 carbohydrates + 1 fat
unfrosted	2-in. square (~1 oz)	1 carbohydrate + 1 fat
Cookies		
100-kcalorie pack	1 oz	1 carbohydrate + ½ fat
chocolate chip cookies	2, 2¼ in. across	1 carbohydrate + 2 fats
gingersnaps	3 small, 1½ in. across	1 carbohydrate
large cookie	1, 6 in. across (~3 oz)	4 carbohydrates + 3 fats
sandwich cookies with crème filling	2 small (~⅔ oz)	1 carbohydrate + 1 fat
sugar-free cookies	1 large or 3 small (¾ to 1 oz)	1 carbohydrate + 1–2 fats
vanilla wafer	5	1 carbohydrate + 1 fat
Cupcake, frosted	1 small (~1¾ oz)	2 carbohydrates + 1–1½ fats
Flan	½ cup	2½ carbohydrates + 1 fat
Fruit cobbler	½ cup (3½ oz)	3 carbohydrates + 1 fat
Gelatin, regular	½ cup	1 carbohydrate
Pie		
commercially prepared fruit, 2 crusts	⅙ of 8-in. pie	3 carbohydrates + 2 fats
pumpkin or custard	⅛ of 8-in. pie	1½ carbohydrates + 1½ fats
Pudding		
regular (made with reduced-fat milk)	½ cup	2 carbohydrates
sugar-free or sugar- and fat-free (made with fat-free milk)	½ cup	1 carbohydrate
Candy, Spreads, Sweets, Sweeteners, Syrups, and Toppings		
Blended sweeteners (mixtures of artificial sweeteners and sugar)	1½ Tbsp	1 carbohydrate
Candy		
chocolate, dark or milk type	1 oz	1 carbohydrate + 2 fats
chocolate "kisses"	5 pieces	1 carbohydrate + 1 fat
hard	3 pieces	1 carbohydrate

TABLE C-6 **Sweets, Desserts, and Other Carbohydrates** (*continued*)

Food	Serving Size	Choices per Serving
Candy, Spreads, Sweets, Sweeteners, Syrups, and Toppings (*continued*)		
Coffee creamer, nondairy type		
powdered, flavored	4 tsp	½ carbohydrate + ½ fat
liquid, flavored	2 Tbsp	1 carbohydrate
Fruit snacks, chewy (pureed fruit concentrate)	1 roll (¾ oz)	1 carbohydrate
Fruit spreads, 100% fruit	1½ Tbsp	1 carbohydrate
Honey	1 Tbsp	1 carbohydrate
Jam or jelly, regular	1 Tbsp	1 carbohydrate
Sugar	1 Tbsp	1 carbohydrate
Syrup		
chocolate	2 Tbsp	2 carbohydrates
light (pancake-type)	2 Tbsp	1 carbohydrate
regular (pancake-type)	1 Tbsp	1 carbohydrate
Condiments and Sauces		
Barbecue sauce	3 Tbsp	1 carbohydrate
Cranberry sauce, jellied	¼ cup	1½ carbohydrates
🗉 Curry sauce	1 oz	1 carbohydrate + 1 fat
🗉 Gravy, canned or bottled	½ cup	½ carbohydrate + ½ fat
Hoisin sauce	1 Tbsp	½ carbohydrate
Marinade	1 Tbsp	½ carbohydrate
Plum sauce	1 Tbsp	½ carbohydrate
Salad dressing, fat-free, cream-based	3 Tbsp	1 carbohydrate
Sweet-and-sour sauce	3 Tbsp	1 carbohydrate
Doughnuts, Muffins, Pastries, and Sweet Breads		
Banana nut bread	1-in. slice (2 oz)	2 carbohydrates + 1 fat
Doughnut		
cake, plain	1 medium (1½ oz)	1½ carbohydrates + 2 fats
hole	2 (1 oz)	1 carbohydrate + 1 fat
yeast-type, glazed	1, 3¾ in. across (2 oz)	2 carbohydrates + 2 fats
Muffin		
regular	1 (4 oz)	4 carbohydrates + 2½ fats
lower-fat	1 (4 oz)	4 carbohydrates + ½ fat
Scone	1 (4 oz)	4 carbohydrates + 3 fats
Sweet roll or Danish	1 (2½ oz)	2½ carbohydrates + 2 fats
Frozen Bars, Frozen Desserts, Frozen Yogurt, and Ice Cream		
Frozen pops	1	½ carbohydrate
Fruit juice bars, frozen, 100% juice	1 (3 oz)	1 carbohydrate
Ice cream		
fat-free	½ cup	1½ carbohydrates
light	½ cup	1 carbohydrate + 1 fat

(*continued*)

TABLE C-6 **Sweets, Desserts, and Other Carbohydrates** (continued)

Food	Serving Size	Choices per Serving
Frozen Bars, Frozen Desserts, Frozen Yogurt, and Ice Cream (continued)		
no-sugar-added	½ cup	1 carbohydrate + 1 fat
regular	½ cup	1 carbohydrate + 2 fats
Sherbet, sorbet	½ cup	2 carbohydrates
Yogurt, frozen		
fat-free	⅓ cup	1 carbohydrate
regular	½ cup	1 carbohydrate + 0–1 fat
Greek, lower-fat or fat-free	½ cup	1½ carbohydrates

Key:

🧂 = High in sodium: ≥ 480 mg/serving

TABLE C-7 **Proteins**

The Proteins list groups foods based on the amount of fat they have (lean meat, medium-fat meat, high-fat meat, and plant-based proteins).

Food	Serving Size	Food	Serving Size
Lean Protein		**Lean Protein** (continued)	
1 lean protein choice = 0 g carbohydrate, 7 g protein, 2 g fat, and 45 kcal.		Pork, lean	
Beef: ground (90% or higher lean/10% or lower fat); select or choice grades trimmed of fat: roast (chuck, round, rump, sirloin), steak (cubed, flank, porterhouse, T-bone), tenderloin	1 oz	🧂 Canadian bacon	1 oz
		🧂 ham	1 oz
		rib or loin chop/roast, tenderloin	1 oz
🧂 Beef jerky	½ oz	Poultry, without skin: chicken; Cornish hen; domestic duck or goose (well-drained of fat); turkey; lean ground turkey or chicken	1 oz
Cheeses with ≤3 g fat/oz	1 oz		
Curd-style cheeses: cottage-type (all kinds); ricotta (fat-free or light)	¼ cup (2 oz)	🧂 Processed sandwich meats with ≤3 g fat/oz: chipped beef, thin-sliced deli meats, turkey ham, turkey pastrami	1 oz
Egg substitutes, plain	¼ cup		
Egg whites	2	🧂 Sausage with ≤3 g fat/oz	1 oz
Fish		Shellfish: clams, crab, imitation shellfish, lobster, scallops, shrimp	1 oz
fresh or frozen, such as catfish, cod, flounder, haddock, halibut, orange roughy, tilapia, trout	1 oz		
		Veal: cutlet (no breading), loin chop, roast	1 oz
salmon, fresh or canned	1 oz	**Medium-Fat Protein**	
sardines, canned	2 small	1 medium-fat protein choice = 0 g carbohydrate, 7 g protein, 5 g fat, and 75 kcal.	
tuna, fresh or canned in water or oil and drained	1 oz		
🧂 smoked: herring or salmon (lox)	1 oz	Beef trimmed of visible fat: ground beef (85% or lower lean/15% or higher fat), corned beef, meatloaf, prime cuts of beef (rib roast), short ribs, tongue	1 oz
Game: buffalo, ostrich, rabbit, venison	1 oz		
🧂 Hot dog[a] with ≤3 g fat/oz	1 (1¾ oz)	Cheeses with 4–7 g fat/oz: feta, mozzarella, pasteurized processed cheese spread, reduced-fat cheeses	1 oz
Lamb: chop, leg, or roast	1 oz		
Organ meats: heart, kidney, liver[b]	1 oz	Cheese, ricotta (regular or part-skim)	¼ cup (2 oz)
Oysters, fresh or frozen	6 medium	Egg	1
		Fish: any fried	1 oz
		Lamb: ground, rib roast	1 oz
		Pork: cutlet, ground, shoulder roast	1 oz

TABLE C-7 Proteins (*continued*)

Food	Serving Size	Food	Serving Size
Medium-Fat Protein (*continued*)		**High-Fat Protein** (*continued*)	
Poultry with skin: chicken, dove, pheasant, turkey, wild duck, or goose; fried chicken	1 oz	Cheese, regular: American, blue-veined, brie, cheddar, hard goat, Monterey jack, Parmesan, queso, and Swiss	1 oz
🅢 Sausage with 4–7 g fat/oz	1 oz	! Hot dog: beef, pork, or combination	1 (10 per 1 lb-sized package)
High-Fat Protein		Hot dog: turkey or chicken	1 (10 per 1 lb-sized package)
1 high-fat protein choice = 0 g carbohydrate, 7 g protein, 8 g fat, and 100 kcal. These foods are high in saturated fat, cholesterol, and kcalories and may raise blood cholesterol levels if eaten on a regular basis. Try to eat 3 or fewer choices from this group per week.		Pork: sausage, spareribs	1 oz
Bacon, pork	2 slices (1 oz each before cooking)	🅢 Processed sandwich meats with ≥ 8 g fat/oz: bologna, hard salami, pastrami	1 oz
🅢 Bacon, turkey	3 slices (½ oz each before cooking)	🅢 Sausage with ≥ 8 g fat/oz: bratwurst, chorizo, Italian, knockwurst, Polish, smoked, summer	1 oz

ᵃMay contain carbohydrate.
ᵇMay be high in cholesterol.

Key:

! = Extra fat

🅢 = High in sodium: ≥ 480 mg/serving (based on the sodium content of a typical 3-oz serving of meat, unless 1 oz or 2 oz is the normal serving size)

Plant-Based Protein

1 plant-based protein choice = variable grams carbohydrate, 7 grams protein, variable grams fat, and variable kcalories. Because carbohydrate content varies among plant-based proteins, you should read the food label.

Food	Serving Size	Choices per Serving
"Bacon" strips, soy-based	2 (½ oz)	1 lean protein
✓ Baked beans, canned	⅓ cup	1 starch + 1 lean protein
✓ Beans (black, garbanzo, kidney, lima, navy, pinto, white), cooked or canned, drained and rinsed	½ cup	1 starch + 1 lean protein
"Beef" or "sausage" crumbles, meatless	1 oz	1 lean protein
"Chicken" nuggets, soy-based	2 (1½ oz)	½ carbohydrate + 1 medium-fat protein
✓ Edamame, shelled	½ cup	½ carbohydrate + 1 lean protein
Falafel (spiced chickpea and wheat patties)	3 patties (~2 in. across)	1 carbohydrate + 1 high-fat protein
Hot dog, meatless, soy-based	1 hot dog (1½ oz)	1 lean protein
✓ Hummus	⅓ cup	1 carbohydrate + 1 medium-fat protein
✓ Lentils, any color, cooked or canned, drained and rinsed	½ cup	1 starch + 1 lean protein
Meatless burger, soy-based	3 oz	½ carbohydrate + 2 lean proteins
✓ Meatless burger, vegetable- and starch-based	1 patty (~2½ oz)	½ carbohydrate + 1 lean protein
Meatless deli slices	1 oz	1 lean protein
Mycoprotein ("chicken" tenders or crumbles), meatless	2 oz	½ carbohydrate + 1 lean protein
Nut spreads: almond butter, cashew butter, peanut butter, soy nut butter	1 tbs	1 high-fat protein
✓ Peas (black-eyed and split peas), cooked or canned, drained and rinsed	½ cup	1 starch + 1 lean protein

(continued)

TABLE C-7 **Proteins** (*continued*)

Food	Serving Size	Choices per Serving
Plant-Based Protein (continued)		
✓ 🅢 Refried beans, canned	½ cup	1 starch + 1 lean protein
"Sausage" breakfast-type patties, meatless	1 (1½ oz)	1 medium-fat protein
Soy nuts, unsalted	¾ oz	½ carbohydrate + 1 medium-fat protein
Tempeh, plain, unflavored	¼ cup (1½ oz)	1 medium-fat protein
Tofu	½ cup (4 oz)	1 medium-fat protein
Tofu, light	½ cup (4 oz)	1 lean protein

Key:

✓ = Good source of fiber: >3 g/serving   🅢 = High in sodium: ≥480 mg/serving

TABLE C-8 **Fats**

Fats and oils have mixtures of unsaturated (polyunsaturated and monounsaturated) and saturated fats. Foods on the Fats list are grouped together based on the major type of fat they contain. 1 fat choice = 0 grams carbohydrate, 0 grams protein, 5 grams fat, and 45 kcalories.

Note: In general, one fat choice is 1 teaspoon of regular margarine, vegetable oil, or butter; 1 tablespoon of regular salad dressing.

When used in large amounts, bacon and peanut butter are counted as high-fat meat choices (see Proteins list). Fat-free salad dressings are found on the Sweets, Desserts, and Other Carbohydrates list. Fat-free products such as margarines, salad dressings, mayonnaise, sour cream, and cream cheese are found on the Free Foods list.

Food	Serving Size	Food	Serving Size
Unsaturated Fats—Monounsaturated Fats		**Unsaturated Fats—Polyunsaturated Fats**	
Almond milk (unsweetened)	1 cup	Margarine	
Avocado, medium	2 Tbsp (1 oz)	lower-fat spread (30–50% vegetable oil, *trans* fat-free)	1 Tbsp
Nut butters (*trans* fat-free): almond butter, cashew butter, peanut butter (smooth or crunchy)	1½ tsp	stick, tub, or squeeze (trans fat-free)	1 tsp
Nuts		Mayonnaise	
almonds	6 nuts	reduced-fat	1 Tbsp
Brazil	2 nuts	regular	1 tsp
cashews	6 nuts	Mayonnaise-style salad dressing	
filberts (hazelnuts)	5 nuts	reduced-fat	1 Tbsp
macadamia	3 nuts	regular	2 tsp
mixed (50% peanuts)	6 nuts	Nuts	
peanuts	10 nuts	pignolia (pine nuts)	1 Tbsp
pecans	4 halves	walnuts, English	4 halves
pistachios	16 nuts	Oil: corn, cottonseed, flaxseed, grapeseed, safflower, soybean, sunflower	1 tsp
Oil: canola, olive, peanut	1 tsp	Salad dressing	
Olives		reduced-fat[a]	2 Tbsp
black (ripe)	8	regular	1 Tbsp
green, stuffed	10 large	Seeds	
Spread, plant stanol ester-type		flaxseed, ground	1½ Tbsp
light	1 Tbsp	pumpkin, sesame, sunflower	1 Tbsp
regular	2 tsp	Tahini or sesame paste	2 tsp

TABLE C-8 **Fats** (*continued*)

Food	Serving Size	Food	Serving Size
Saturated Fats		**Saturated Fats** (*continued*)	
Bacon, cooked, regular or turkey	1 slice	Cream	
Butter		half-and-half	2 Tbsp
reduced-fat	1 Tbsp	heavy	1 Tbsp
stick	1 tsp	light	1½ Tbsp
whipped	2 tsp	whipped	2 Tbsp
Butter blends made with oil		Cream cheese	
reduced-fat or light	1 Tbsp	reduced-fat	1½ Tbsp (¾ oz)
regular	1½ tsp	regular	1 Tbsp (½ oz)
Chitterlings, boiled	2 Tbsp (½ oz)	Lard	1 tsp
Coconut, sweetened, shredded	2 Tbsp	Oil: coconut, palm, palm kernel	1 tsp
Coconut milk, canned, thick		Salt pork	¼ oz
light	⅓ cup	Shortening, solid	1 tsp
regular	1½ Tbsp	Sour cream	
Coconut milk beverage (thin), unsweetened	1 cup	reduced-fat or light	3 Tbsp
		regular	2 Tbsp

ᵃMay contain carbohydrate.

TABLE C-9 **Free Foods**

A "free" food is any food or drink choice that has less than 20 kcalories and 5 grams or less of carbohydrate per serving.

▪ Most foods on this list should be limited to 3 servings (as listed here) per day. Spread out the servings throughout the day. If you eat all 3 servings at once, it could raise your blood glucose level.

▪ Food and drink choices listed here without a serving size can be eaten whenever you like.

Food	Serving Size	Food	Serving Size
Low-Carbohydrate Foods		**Low-Carbohydrate Foods** (*continued*)	
Candy, hard (regular or sugar-free)	1 piece	Vegetables: any **cooked** nonstarchy vegetables (such as carrots, cauliflower, green beans)	¼ cup
Fruits: cranberries or rhubarb, sweetened with sugar substitute	½ cup		
Gelatin dessert, sugar-free, any flavor		**Reduced-Fat or Fat-Free Foods**	
Gum, sugar-free		Cream cheese, fat-free	1 Tbsp (½ oz)
Jam or jelly, light or no-sugar-added	2 tsp	Coffee creamers, nondairy	
Salad greens (such as arugula, chicory, endive, escarole, leaf or iceberg lettuce, purslane, romaine, radicchio, spinach, watercress)		liquid, flavored	1½ tsp
		liquid, sugar-free, flavored	4 tsp
		powdered, flavored	1 tsp
		powdered, sugar-free, flavored	2 tsp
Sugar substitutes (artificial sweeteners)		Margarine spread	
Syrup, sugar-free	2 Tbsp	fat-free	1 Tbsp
Vegetables: any **raw** nonstarchy vegetables (such as broccoli, cabbage, carrots, cucumber, tomato)	½ cup	reduced-fat	1 tsp
		Mayonnaise	
		fat-free	1 Tbsp

(continued)

TABLE C-9 **Free Foods**

Food	Serving Size	Food	Serving Size
Reduced-Fat or Fat-Free Foods (*continued*)		**Condiments** (*continued*)	
reduced-fat	1 tsp	Pimento	
Mayonnaise-style salad dressing		Salsa	¼ cup
fat-free	1 Tbsp	🧂 Soy sauce, light or regular	1 Tbsp
reduced-fat	2 tsp	Sweet-and-sour sauce	2 tsp
Salad dressing		Taco sauce	1 Tbsp
fat-free	1 Tbsp	Vinegar	
fat-free, Italian	2 Tbsp	Worcestershire sauce	
Sour cream, fat-free or reduced fat	1 Tbsp	Yogurt, any type	2 Tbsp
Whipped topping		**Drinks/Mixes**	
light or fat-free	2 Tbsp	🧂 Bouillon, broth, consommé	
regular	1 Tbsp	Bouillon or broth, low-sodium	
Condiments		Carbonated or mineral water	
Barbecue sauce	2 tsp	Club soda	
Catsup (ketchup)	1 Tbsp	Cocoa powder, unsweetened (1 Tbsp)	
Chili sauce, sweet, tomato-type	2 tsp	Coffee, unsweetened or with sugar substitute	
Horseradish		Diet soft drinks, sugar-free	
Hot pepper sauce		Drink mixes (powder or liquid drops), sugar-free	
Lemon juice		Tea, unsweetened or with sugar substitute	
Miso	1½ tsp	Tonic water, sugar-free	
Mustard		Water	
honey	1 Tbsp	Water, flavored, sugar-free	
brown, Dijon, horseradish-flavored, wasabi-flavored, or yellow		**Seasonings**	
Parmesan cheese, grated	1 Tbsp	Flavoring extracts (for example, vanilla, almond, or peppermint)	
Pickle relish (dill or sweet)	1 Tbsp	Garlic, fresh or powder	
Pickles		Herbs, fresh or dried	
🧂 dill	1½ medium	Kelp	
sweet, bread and butter	2 slices	Nonstick cooking spray	
sweet, gherkin	¾ oz	Spices	
		Wine, used in cooking	

Key:

🧂 = High in sodium: ≥480 mg/serving

TABLE C-10 Combination Foods

Many foods are eaten in various combinations, such as casseroles. Because "combination" foods do not fit into any one choice list, this list of choices provides some typical combination foods.

Food	Serving Size	Choices per Serving
Entrees		
▤ Casserole-type entrees (tuna noodle, lasagna, spaghetti with meatballs, chili with beans, macaroni and cheese)	1 cup (8 oz)	2 carbohydrates + 2 medium-fat proteins
▤ Stews (beef/other meats and vegetables)	1 cup (8 oz)	1 carbohydrate + 1 medium-fat protein + 0–3 fats
Frozen Meals/Entrees		
▤ ✓ Burrito (beef and bean)	1 (5 oz)	3 carbohydrates + 1 lean protein + 2 fats
Dinner-type healthy meal (includes dessert and is usually <400 kcal)	~9–12 oz	2–3 carbohydrates + 1–2 lean proteins + 1 fat
"Healthy"-type entree (usually <300 kcal)	~7–10 oz	2 carbohydrates + 2 lean proteins
Pizza		
▤ cheese/vegetarian, thin crust	¼ of a 12-in. pizza (4½–5 oz)	2 carbohydrates + 2 medium-fat proteins
▤ meat topping, thin crust	¼ of a 12-in. pizza (5 oz)	2 carbohydrates + 2 medium-fat proteins + 1½ fats
▤ cheese/vegetarian or meat topping, rising crust	⅙ of a 12-in. pizza (4 oz)	2½ carbohydrates + 2 medium-fat proteins
▤ Pocket sandwich	1 sandwich (4½ oz)	3 carbohydrates + 1 lean protein + 1–2 fats
▤ Pot pie	1 (7 oz)	3 carbohydrates + 1 medium-fat protein + 3 fats
Salads (Deli-Style)		
Coleslaw	½ cup	1 carbohydrate + 1½ fats
Macaroni/pasta salad	½ cup	2 carbohydrates + 3 fats
▤ Potato salad	½ cup	1½–2 carbohydrates + 1–2 fats
Tuna salad or chicken salad	½ cup (3½ oz)	½ carbohydrate + 2 lean proteins + 1 fat
Soups		
▤ ✓ Bean, lentil, or split pea soup	1 cup (8 oz)	1½ carbohydrates + 1 lean protein
▤ Chowder (made with milk)	1 cup (8 oz)	1 carbohydrate + 1 lean protein + 1½ fats
▤ Cream soup (made with water)	1 cup (8 oz)	1 carbohydrate + 1 fat
▤ Miso soup	1 cup (8 oz)	½ carbohydrate + 1 lean protein
▤ Ramen noodle soup	1 cup (8 oz)	2 carbohydrates + 2 fats
Rice soup/porridge (congee)	1 cup (8 oz)	1 carbohydrate
▤ Tomato soup (made with water), borscht	1 cup (8 oz)	1 carbohydrate
▤ Vegetable beef, chicken, noodle, or other broth-type soup (including "healthy"-type soups, such as those lower in sodium and/or fat)	1 cup (8 oz)	1 carbohydrate + 1 lean protein

Key:

✓ = Good source of fiber: >3 g/serving

▤ = High in sodium: ≥600 mg/serving for main dishes or ≥480 mg/serving for side dishes

TABLE C-11 **Fast Foods**

The choices in the Fast Foods list are not specific fast-food meals or items, but are estimates based on popular foods. Ask the restaurant or check its website for nutrition information about your favorite fast foods.

Food	Serving Size	Choices per Serving
Main Dishes/Entrees		
Chicken		
▣ breast, breaded and fried[a]	1 (~7 oz)	1 carbohydrate + 6 medium-fat proteins
breast, meat only[b]	1	4 lean proteins
drumstick, breaded and fried[a]	1 (~2½ oz)	½ carbohydrate + 2 medium-fat proteins
drumstick, meat only[b]	1	1 lean protein + ½ fat
▣ nuggets or tenders	6 (~3½ oz)	1 carbohydrate + 2 medium-fat proteins + 1 fat
▣ thigh, breaded and fried[a]	1 (~5 oz)	1 carbohydrate + 3 medium-fat proteins + 2 fats
thigh, meat only[b]	1	2 lean proteins + ½ fat
wing, breaded and fried[a]	1 wing (~2 oz)	½ carbohydrate + 2 medium-fat proteins
wing, meat only[b]	1 wing	1 lean protein
▣ ✓ Main dish salad (grilled chicken-type, no dressing or croutons)	1 salad (~11½ oz)	1 carbohydrate + 4 lean proteins
Pizza		
▣ cheese, pepperoni, or sausage, regular or thick crust	⅛ of a 14-in. pizza (~4 oz)	2½ carbohydrates + 1 high-fat protein + 1 fat
▣ cheese, pepperoni, or sausage, thin crust	⅛ of a 14-in. pizza (~2¾ oz)	1½ carbohydrates + 1 high-fat protein + 1 fats
▣ cheese, meat, and vegetable, regular crust	⅛ of a 14-in. pizza (~5 oz)	2½ carbohydrates + 2 high-fat proteins
Asian		
▣ Beef/chicken/shrimp with vegetables in sauce	1 cup (~6 oz)	1 carbohydrate + 2 lean proteins + 1 fat
Egg roll, meat	1 egg roll (~3 oz)	1½ carbohydrates + 1 lean protein + 1½ fats
Fried rice, meatless	1 cup	2½ carbohydrates + 2 fats
Fortune cookie	1	½ carbohydrate
▣ Hot-and-sour soup	1 cup	½ carbohydrate + ½ fat
▣ Meat with sweet sauce	1 cup (~6 oz)	3½ carbohydrates + 3 medium-fat proteins + 3 fats
▣ Noodles and vegetables in sauce (chow mein, lo mein)	1 cup	2 carbohydrates + 2 fats
Mexican		
▣ ✓ Burrito with beans and cheese	1 small (~6 oz)	3½ carbohydrates + 1 medium-fat protein + 1 fat
▣ Nachos with cheese	1 small order (~8)	2½ carbohydrates + 1 high-fat protein + 2 fats
▣ Quesadilla, cheese only	1 small order (~5 oz)	2½ carbohydrates + 3 high-fat proteins
Taco, crisp, with meat and cheese	1 small (~3 oz)	1 carbohydrate + 1 medium-fat protein + ½ fat
▣ ✓ Taco salad with chicken and tortilla bowl	1 salad (1 lb including bowl)	3½ carbohydrates + 4 medium-fat proteins + 3 fats
▣ Tostada with beans and cheese	1 small (~5 oz)	2 carbohydrates + 1 high-fat protein
Sandwiches		
Breakfast sandwiches		
▣ breakfast burrito with sausage, egg, cheese	1 (~4 oz)	1½ carbohydrates + 2 high-fat proteins
▣ egg, cheese, meat on an English muffin	1	2 carbohydrates + 3 medium-fat proteins + ½ fat

TABLE C-11 **Fast Foods** (*continued*)

Food	Serving Size	Choices per Serving
Sandwiches (*continued*)		
🗚 egg, cheese, meat on a biscuit	1	2 carbohydrates + 3 medium-fat proteins + 2 fats
🗚 sausage biscuit sandwich	1	2 carbohydrates + 1 high-fat protein + 4 fats
Chicken sandwiches		
🗚 grilled with bun, lettuce, tomatoes, spread	1 (~7½ oz)	3 carbohydrates + 4 lean proteins
🗚 crispy, with bun, lettuce, tomatoes, spread	1 (~6 oz)	3 carbohydrates + 2 lean proteins + 3½ fats
Fish sandwich with tartar sauce and cheese	1 (5 oz)	2½ carbohydrates + 2 medium-fat proteins + 1½ fats
Hamburger		
regular with bun and condiments (catsup, mustard, onion, pickle)	1 (~3½ oz)	2 carbohydrates + 1 medium-fat protein + 1 fat
🗚 4 oz meat with cheese, bun, and condiments (catsup, mustard, onion, pickle)	1 (~8½ oz)	3 carbohydrates + 4 medium-fat proteins + 2½ fats
Hot dog with bun, plain	1 (~3½ oz)	1½ carbohydrates + 1 high-fat protein + 2 fats
Submarine sandwich (no cheese or sauce)		
🗚 <6 g fat	1 6-in. sub	3 carbohydrates + 2 lean proteins
🗚 regular	1 6-in. sub	3 carbohydrates + 2 lean proteins + 1 fat
🗚 Wrap, grilled chicken, vegetables, cheese, and spread	1 small (~4–5 oz)	2 carbohydrates + 2 lean proteins + 1½ fats
Sides/Appetizers		
🗚 ! French fries	1 small order (~3½ oz)	2½ carbohydrates + 2 fats
	1 medium order (~5 oz)	3½ carbohydrates + 3 fats
	1 large order (~6 oz)	4½ carbohydrates + 4 fats
🗚 Hash browns	1 cup/medium order (~5 oz)	3 carbohydrates + 6 fats
🗚 Onion rings	1 serving (8–9 rings, ~4 oz)	3½ carbohydrates + 4 fats
Salad, side (no dressing, croutons, or cheese)	1 small	1 nonstarchy vegetable
Beverages and Desserts		
Coffee, latte (fat-free milk)	1 small (~12 oz)	1 fat-free milk
Coffee, mocha (fat-free milk, no whipped cream)	1 small (~12 oz)	1 fat-free milk + 1 carbohydrate
Milkshake, any flavor	1 small (~12 oz)	5½ carbohydrates + 3 fats
	1 medium (~16 oz)	7 carbohydrates + 4 fats
	1 large (~22 oz)	10 carbohydrates + 5 fats
Soft-serve ice cream cone	1 small	2 carbohydrates + ½ fat

[a]Definition and weight refer to food **with** bone, skin, and breading.
[b]Definition refers to above food **without** bone, skin, and breading.

Key:

✓ = Good source of fiber: >3 g/serving

! = Extra fat

🗚 = High in sodium: ≥600 mg/serving for main dishes or ≥480 mg/serving for side dishes

TABLE C-12 Alcohol

1 alcohol equivalent = variable grams carbohydrate, 0 grams protein, 0 grams fat, and 100 kcalories.

Note: In general, one alcohol choice (½ ounce absolute alcohol) has about 100 kcalories. For those who choose to drink alcohol, guidelines suggest limiting alcohol intake to 1 drink or less per day for women, and 2 drinks or less per day for men. To reduce your risk of low blood glucose (hypoglycemia), especially if you take insulin or a diabetes pill that increases insulin, always drink alcohol with food. While alcohol, by itself, does not directly affect blood glucose, be aware of the carbohydrate (for example, in mixed drinks, beer, and wine) that may raise your blood glucose.

Alcoholic Beverage[a]	Serving Size	Choices per Serving
Beer		
light (<4.5% abv)	12 fl oz	1 alcohol equivalent + ½ carbohydrate
regular (~5% abv)	12 fl oz	1 alcohol equivalent + 1 carbohydrate
dark (>5.7% abv)	12 fl oz	1 alcohol equivalent + 1–1½ carbohydrates
Distilled spirits (80 or 86 proof): vodka, rum, gin, whiskey, tequila	1½ fl oz	1 alcohol equivalent
Liqueur, coffee (53 proof)	1 fl oz	½ alcohol equivalent + 1 carbohydrate
Sake	1 fl oz	½ alcohol equivalent
Wine		
champagne/sparkling	5 fl oz	1 alcohol equivalent
dessert (sherry)	3½ fl oz	1 alcohol equivalent + 1 carbohydrate
dry, red or white (10% abv)	5 fl oz	1 alcohol equivalent

[a] "%abv" refers to the percentage of alcohol by volume.

The Food Lists are the basis of a meal planning system designed by a committee of the American Diabetes Association and the Academy of Nutrition and Dietetics. While designed primary for people with diabetes and others who must follow special diets, the Food Lists are based on principles of good nutrition that apply to everyone. (c) 2014 by the American Diabetes Association and the Academy of Nutrition and Dietetics.

Appendix D

Physical Activity and Energy Requirements

Chapter 6 described how to calculate your estimated energy requirements by using an equation that accounts for your gender, age, weight, height, and physical activity level. This appendix presents tables that provide a shortcut to estimating total energy requirements, as developed by the *Dietary Guidelines for Americans 2010*, and based on the equations of the Committee on Dietary Reference Intakes.

Table D-1 describes activity levels for three groups of people: sedentary, moderately active, or active. Once you have found an activity level that approximates your own, find your daily kcalorie need in Table D-2.

TABLE D-1 Sedentary, Moderately Active, and Active People

Sedentary	A lifestyle that includes only the light physical activity associated with typical day-to-day life.
Moderately active	A lifestyle that includes physical activity equivalent to walking about 1.5 to 3 miles per day at 3 to 4 miles per hour in addition to the light physical activity associated with typical day-to-day life.
Active	A lifestyle that includes physical activity equivalent to walking more than 3 miles per day at 3 to 4 miles per hour in addition to the light physical activity associated with typical day-to-day life.

© Cengage Learning 2014

TABLE D-2 Estimated kCalorie Needs per Day by Age, Gender, and Physical Activity Level (Detailed)

Estimated amounts of kcalories needed to maintain kcalorie balance for various gender and age groups at three different levels of physical activity. The estimates are rounded to the nearest 200 kcalories. An individual's kcalorie needs may be higher or lower than these average estimates.[a]

Age (years)	Gender/Activity Level					
	Male/Sedentary	Male/Moderately Active	Male/Active	Female[b]/Sedentary	Female[b]/Moderately Active	Female[b]/Active
2	1000	1000	1000	1000	1000	1000
3	1200	1400	1400	1000	1200	1400
4	1200	1400	1600	1200	1400	1400
5	1200	1400	1600	1200	1400	1600
6	1400	1600	1800	1200	1400	1600
7	1400	1600	1800	1200	1600	1800
8	1400	1600	2000	1400	1600	1800
9	1600	1800	2000	1400	1600	1800
10	1600	1800	2200	1400	1800	2000
11	1800	2000	2200	1600	1800	2000
12	1800	2200	2400	1600	2000	2200
13	2000	2200	2600	1600	2000	2200
14	2000	2400	2800	1800	2000	2400

© Cengage Learning

(continued)

TABLE D-2 **Estimated kCalorie Needs per Day by Age, Gender, and Physical Activity Level (Detailed)** *(continued)*

Age (years)	Male/Sedentary	Male/ Moderately Active	Male/Active	Female[b]/ Sedentary	Female[b]/ Moderately Active	Female[b]/ Active
			Gender/Activity Level			
15	2200	2600	3000	1800	2000	2400
16–18	2400	2800	3200	1800	2000	2400
19–20	2600	2800	3000	2000	2200	2400
21–25	2400	2800	3000	2000	2200	2400
26–30	2400	2600	3000	1800	2000	2400
31–35	2400	2600	3000	1800	2000	2200
36–40	2400	2600	2800	1800	2000	2200
41–45	2200	2600	2800	1800	2000	2200
46–50	2200	2400	2800	1800	2000	2200
51–55	2200	2400	2800	1600	1800	2200
56–60	2200	2400	2600	1600	1800	2200
61–65	2000	2400	2600	1600	1800	2000
66–75	2000	2200	2600	1600	1800	2000
76+	2000	2200	2400	1600	1800	2000

[a]Based on Estimated Energy Requirements (EER) equations, using reference heights (average) and reference weights (healthy) for each age-gender group. For children and adolescents, reference height and weight vary. For adults the reference man is 5 feet 10 inches tall and weighs 154 pounds. The reference woman is 5 feet 4 inches tall and weighs 126 pounds. EER equations are from the Institute of Medicine. *Dietary Reference Intakes for Energy, Carbohydrate, Fiber, Fat, Fatty Acids, Cholesterol, Protein, and Amino Acids*. Washington, D.C.: The National Academies Press; 2002.

[b]Estimates for females do not include women who are pregnant or breastfeeding.

Source: U.S. Department of Agriculture and U.S. Department of Health and Human Services, *Dietary Guidelines for Americans 2010*, www.dietaryguidelines.gov.

Appendix E

Nutrition Assessment: Supplemental Information

Chapter 14 describes data from nutrition assessments that allow health professionals to evaluate their patients' nutrition status and nutritional needs. This appendix provides additional information that may be useful for complete assessments.

Weight Gain during Pregnancy

Chapter 11 describes desirable weight-gain patterns during pregnancy. Figure E-1 shows prenatal weight-gain grids, which are used to plot the rate of weight gain during pregnancy.

BOX E-1

The *body mass index (BMI)* is a measure of body size, determined by dividing a person's weight by the square of their height:

$$BMI = \frac{Weight\ (kg)}{Height\ (m)^2}$$

Growth Charts

Health professionals evaluate physical development by monitoring growth rates of children and comparing these rates with those on standard growth charts. Standard charts compare length or height to age, weight to age, weight to length, head circumference to age, and body mass index (BMI) to age (see Box E-1). Although individual growth patterns vary, a child's growth curve will generally stay at about the same percentile throughout childhood. In children whose growth has been impaired, nutrition rehabilitation will ideally allow height and weight to increase to higher percentiles. In overweight children, the goal is for weight to remain stable as height increases, until weight becomes appropriate for height.

FIGURE E-1 Recommended Prenatal Weight Gain Based on Prepregnancy Weight

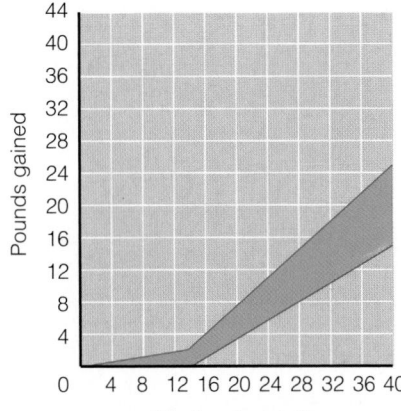

Normal-weight women should gain about 3½ pounds in the first trimester and just under 1 pound/week thereafter, achieving a total gain of 25 to 35 pounds by term.

Underweight women should gain about 5 pounds in the first trimester and just over 1 pound/week thereafter, achieving a total gain of 28 to 40 pounds by term.

Overweight women should gain about 2 pounds in the first trimester and ⅔ pound/week thereafter, achieving a total gain of 15 to 25 pounds.

To evaluate growth in infants, the assessor uses a chart such as those in Figures E-2 through E-5 (pp. E-3 to E-6). For example, the assessor follows the steps in Box E-2 to determine the weight percentile. For other measures, the assessor follows a similar procedure using the appropriate chart. (When length is measured, use the chart for birth to 36 months; when height is measured, use the chart for 2 to 20 years.) Once all of the values are plotted on growth charts, a skilled clinician can begin to interpret the data. Ideally, the height, weight, and head circumference should be in roughly the same percentile.

Head circumference is generally measured in children under 2 years of age. Since the brain grows rapidly before birth and during early infancy, extreme and chronic malnutrition during these periods can impair brain development, curtailing the number of brain cells and reducing head circumference. Nonnutritional factors, such as certain disorders and genetic variation, can also influence head circumference.

Measures of Body Fat and Lean Tissue

Significant weight changes in both children and adults can reflect overnutrition or undernutrition with respect to energy and protein. To estimate the degree to which fat stores or lean tissues are affected by malnutrition, several anthropometric measurements are useful.

Skinfold Measures Skinfold measures provide a good estimate of total body fat and a fair assessment of the fat's location (see Box E-3). Most body fat lies directly beneath the skin, and the thickness of this subcutaneous fat correlates with total body fat. In some parts of the body, such as the back of the arm over the triceps muscle, this fat is loosely attached. As illustrated in Figure E-6 (p. E-7), an assessor can measure the thickness of the fat with calipers that apply a fixed amount of pressure. If a person gains body fat, the skinfold increases proportionately; if the person loses fat, it decreases. Measurements taken from central-body sites reflect changes in fatness better than those taken from upper sites (arm and back). Because subcutaneous fat may be thicker in one area than in another, skinfold measurements are often taken at three or four different places on the body (including upper-, central-, and lower-body sites); the sum of these measures is then compared to standard values. In some situations, the triceps skinfold measurement alone may be used because it is easily accessible. Triceps skinfold measures greater than 15 millimeters in men or 25 millimeters in women suggest excessive body fat.

Waist Circumference Chapter 6 explains how fat distribution correlates with health risks and mentions that the waist circumference is a valuable indicator of abdominal fat. To measure waist circumference, the assessor places a nonstretchable tape around the person's body, crossing just above the upper hip bones and making sure that the tape remains on a level horizontal plane on all sides (see Figure E-7, p. E-7). The tape is tightened slightly, but without compressing the skin.

Waist-to-Hip Ratio The waist-to-hip ratio assesses abdominal obesity but offers no advantage over the waist circumference alone. To calculate the waist-to-hip ratio, divide the waist measurement by the hip measurement (in a woman with a 28-inch waist and 38-inch hips, the waist-to-hip ratio would be $28 \div 38 = 0.74$). In general, women and men with waist-to-hip ratios above 0.8 and 0.9, respectively, are at increased risk of developing diabetes and cardiovascular diseases.

BOX E-2

How To Determine a Child's Weight Percentile

▌ Select the appropriate chart based on age and gender.

▌ Locate the child's age along the horizontal axis on the bottom of the chart.

▌ Locate the child's weight in pounds or kilograms along the vertical axis.

▌ Mark the chart where the age and weight lines intersect, and read off the percentile.

BOX E-3

Common sites for skinfold measures:

▌ Triceps

▌ Biceps

▌ Subscapular (below shoulder blade)

▌ Suprailiac (above hip bone)

▌ Abdomen

▌ Upper thigh

FIGURE E-2 Length-for-Age and Weight-for-Age Percentiles

Length-for-Age and Weight-for-Age Percentiles: NAME ——— RECORD # ———
Boys, Birth to 36 Months

Published May 30, 2000 (modified 4/20/01).
SOURCE: Developed by the National Center for Health Statistics in collaboration with
the National Center for Chronic Disease Prevention and Health Promotion (2000).
www.cdc.gov/growthcharts.

Length-for-Age and Weight-for-Age Percentiles: NAME ——— RECORD # ———
Girls, Birth to 36 Months

Published May 30, 2000 (modified 4/20/01).
SOURCE: Developed by the National Center for Health Statistics in collaboration with
the National Center for Chronic Disease Prevention and Health Promotion (2000).
www.cdc.gov/growthcharts.

FIGURE E-3 Head Circumference-for-Age and Weight-for-Length Percentiles

Head Circumference-for-Age and
Weight-for-Length Percentiles: Boys, Birth to 36 Months

Head Circumference-for-Age and
Weight-for-Length Percentiles: Girls, Birth to 36 Months

Published May 30, 2000 (modified 10/16/00).
SOURCE: Developed by the National Center for Health Statistics in collaboration with
the National Center for Chronic Disease Prevention and Health Promotion (2000).
www.cdc.gov/growthcharts.

FIGURE E-4 Stature-for-Age and Weight-for-Age Percentiles

Stature-for-Age and Weight-for-Age
Percentiles: Boys, 2 to 20 Years

Stature-for-Age and Weight-for-Age
Percentiles: Girls, 2 to 20 Years

FIGURE E-5 Body Mass Index-for-Age Percentiles

**Body Mass Index-for-Age Percentiles:
Boys, 2 to 20 Years**

NAME _____ RECORD # _____

**Body Mass Index-for-Age Percentiles:
Girls, 2 to 20 Years**

NAME _____ RECORD # _____

Published May 30, 2000 (modified 10/16/00).
SOURCE: Developed by the National Center for Health Statistics in collaboration with
the National Center for Chronic Disease Prevention and Health Promotion (2000).
www.cdc.gov/growthcharts.

Published May 30, 2000 (modified 10/16/00).
SOURCE: Developed by the National Center for Health Statistics in collaboration with
the National Center for Chronic Disease Prevention and Health Promotion (2000).
www.cdc.gov/growthcharts.

FIGURE E-6 How to Measure the Triceps Skinfold

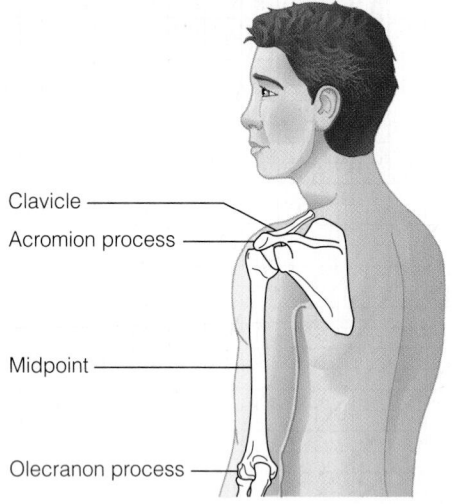

Clavicle
Acromion process

Midpoint

Olecranon process

A. Find the midpoint of the arm:
  1. Ask the subject to bend his or her arm at the elbow and lay the hand across the stomach. (If he or she is right-handed, measure the left arm, and vice versa.)
  2. Feel the shoulder to locate the acromion process. It helps to slide your fingers along the clavicle to find the acromion process. The olecranon process is the tip of the elbow.
  3. Place a measuring tape from the acromion process to the tip of the elbow.

Divide this measurement by 2 and mark the midpoint of the arm with a pen.
B. Measure the skinfold:
  1. Ask the subject to let his or her arm hang loosely to the side.
  2. Grasp a fold of skin and subcutaneous fat between the thumb and forefinger slightly above the midpoint mark. Gently pull the skin away from the underlying muscle. (This step takes a lot of practice. If you want to be sure you don't have muscle as well as fat, ask the subject to

contract and relax the muscle. You should be able to feel if you are pinching muscle.)
  3. Place the calipers over the skinfold at the midpoint mark, and read the measurement to the nearest 1.0 millimeter in two to three seconds. (If using plastic calipers, align pressure lines, and read the measurement to the nearest 1.0 millimeter in two to three seconds.)
  4. Repeat steps 2 and 3 twice more. Add the three readings, and then divide by 3 to find the average.

FIGURE E-7 How to Measure Waist Circumference
Place the measuring tape around the waist just above the bony crest of the hip. The tape runs parallel to the floor and is snug (but does not compress the skin). The measurement is taken at the end of normal expiration.

Source: National Institutes of Health Obesity Education Initiative, *Clinical Guidelines on the Identification, Evaluation, and Treatment of Overweight and Obesity in Adults* (Washington, D.C.: U.S. Department of Health and Human Services, 1998), p. 59.

TABLE E-1 Selected Methods for Estimating Body Fat Content

Air-displacement plethysmography (Bod Pod®): Estimates body density by measuring the body's volume (density = mass/volume); the density value allows derivation of the body's fat and lean tissue contents

Bioelectrical impedance assay: Measures the magnitude of an electrical current passed through the body; electrical conductivity is higher in lean tissues than in fat tissue

Dual energy X-ray absorptiometry: Analyzes the change in X-rays after they contact body tissues; fat and lean tissue have different effects on X-rays, allowing quantification of these tissues

Hydrodensitometry: Estimates body density by comparing the body's weight on land and in water or by measuring the body's volume (density = mass/volume); the density value allows derivation of the body's fat and lean tissue contents

Isotope dilution—deuterated water: Measures total body water content by analyzing the dilution of heavy water (water with a heavy form of hydrogen) in body tissues; allows an estimate of lean tissue (and by difference, the body fat content)

Skinfold: Estimates subcutaneous fat in several regions of the body by using calipers to measure skinfold thicknesses

Ultrasound: Estimates subcutaneous fat in several regions of the body by using ultrasound to measure skinfold thicknesses

Waist-to-Height Ratio The waist-to-height ratio helps to assess the health risks associated with excessive abdominal fat. To calculate the waist-to-height ratio, divide the waist measurement by the height measurement (in a woman with a 28-inch waist who is 63 inches tall, the waist-to-height ratio would be $28 \div 63 = 0.44$). Women and men with waist-to-height ratios above 0.5 may be at increased risk of developing diabetes and cardiovascular diseases.

Hydrodensitometry To estimate body density using hydrodensitometry, the person is weighed twice—first on land and then again when submerged in water. Underwater weighing usually generates a good estimate of body fat and is useful in research, although the technique has drawbacks: it requires bulky, expensive, and nonportable equipment. Furthermore, submerging some people in water (especially those who are very young, very old, ill, or fearful) is difficult and not well tolerated.

Bioelectrical Impedance To measure body fat using the bioelectrical impedance method, a very low-intensity electrical current is briefly sent through the body by way of electrodes placed on the wrist and ankle. Fat impedes the flow of electricity; thus, the magnitude of the current is influenced by the body-fat content. Recent food intake and hydration status can influence results. As with other anthropometric methods, bioelectrical impedance requires standardized procedures and calibrated instruments.

A number of other methods are sometimes used to estimate the body's content of body fat. Table E-1 describes common techniques often used in the clinical or research setting.

Nutritional Anemias

Anemia, which can result from a wide variety of medical problems, is characterized by a significant reduction in the blood's oxygen-carrying capacity. Iron, folate, and vitamin B_{12} deficiencies—caused by inadequate intake, poor absorption, or abnormal metabolism of these nutrients—are the most common causes of the nutrition-related anemias. Some nonnutritional causes of anemia include massive blood loss, infection, hereditary blood disorders such as sickle-cell anemia, and chronic liver or kidney

TABLE E-2 Laboratory Tests for Anemia

Test or Test Result	What It Reflects
For Anemia (general)	
Hemoglobin (Hb)	Total amount of hemoglobin in the red blood cells (RBCs)
Hematocrit (Hct)	Percentage of RBCs in the total blood volume
Red blood cell (RBC) count	Number of RBCs
Mean corpuscular volume (MCV)	RBC size; helps to determine if anemia is microcytic (iron deficiency) or macrocytic (folate or vitamin B_{12} deficiency)
Mean corpuscular hemoglobin concentration (MCHC)	Hemoglobin concentration within the average RBC; helps to determine if anemia is hypochromic (iron deficiency) or normochromic (folate or vitamin B_{12} deficiency)
Bone marrow aspiration	The manufacture of blood cells in different developmental states
For Iron-Deficiency Anemia	
↓ Serum ferritin	Early deficiency state with depleted iron stores
↓ Transferrin saturation	Progressing deficiency state with diminished transport iron
↑ Erythrocyte protoporphyrin	Later deficiency state with limited hemoglobin production
For Folate-Deficiency Anemia	
↓ Serum folate	Progressing deficiency state
↓ RBC folate	Later deficiency state
For Vitamin B_{12}–Deficiency Anemia	
↓ Serum vitamin B_{12}	Progressing deficiency state
↑ Serum methylmalonic acid	Vitamin B_{12} deficiency
Schilling test	Adequacy of vitamin B_{12} absorption

disease. Table E-2 lists laboratory tests that are useful for diagnosing or evaluating anemia.

Assessment of Iron Status

Chapter 9 describes the progression of iron deficiency in detail, as well as the roles of some of the proteins involved in iron metabolism. This section describes the various tests that assess iron status, and Table E-3 (p. E-10) provides acceptable values. Although other tests are more specific for detecting the early stages of iron deficiency, hemoglobin levels and hematocrit values are most often used to detect iron-deficiency anemia because they are inexpensive and easily measured.

Serum Ferritin In the initial stage of iron deficiency, iron stores diminish (see Box E-4). Iron is stored in the protein ferritin, which is located in the liver, spleen, and bone marrow. Serum ferritin values provide a noninvasive estimate of iron stores because the ferritin levels in blood reflect the amounts present in tissues. Serum ferritin is not a reliable indicator of iron deficiency, however, because its concentrations are increased by infection, inflammation, alcohol consumption, and liver disease.

Serum Iron and Total Iron-Binding Capacity (TIBC) Early stages of iron deficiency are characterized by reduced levels of serum iron, which represent the amount of iron bound to transferrin, the iron transport protein. Total iron-binding

BOX E-4

Iron deficiency progresses as follows:

1 Iron stores diminish

2 Transport iron decreases

3 Hemoglobin production falls

TABLE E-3 **Criteria for Assessing Iron Status**

Laboratory Test	Acceptable Values	Effect of Iron Deficiency
Serum ferritin	Male: 20–250 ng/mL Female: 10–120 ng/mL	Lower than normal
Serum iron	Male: 60–175 μg/dL Female: 50–170 μg/dL	Lower than normal
Total iron-binding capacity	250–450 μg/dL	Higher than normal
Transferrin saturation	Male: 20–50% Female: 15–50%	Lower than normal
Erythrocyte protoporphyrin	<70 μg/dL red blood cells	Higher than normal
Hemoglobin (Hb), whole blood	Male: 13.5–17.5 g/dL Female: 12.0–16.0 g/dL	Lower than normal
Hematocrit (Hct)	Male: 39–49% Female: 35–45%	Lower than normal
Mean corpuscular volume (MCV)	80–100 fL	Lower than normal

Note: ng = nanogram, μg = microgram, dL = deciliter, nmol = nanomole, fL = femtoliter
Source: L. Goldman and A. I. Schafer, eds., *Goldman's Cecil Medicine* (Philadelphia: Saunders, 2012), pp. 2558–2569.

capacity (TIBC) is a measure of the total amount of iron that the blood can carry; thus, it is an indirect measure of the transferrin content of blood. During iron deficiency, the liver produces more transferrin in an effort to increase iron transport capacity, and therefore iron depletion is characterized by an increase in TIBC. TIBC reflects liver function as well as changes in iron metabolism.

Transferrin Saturation The percentage of transferrin that is saturated with iron is an indirect measure derived from the serum iron and total iron-binding capacity measures, as follows:

$$\% \text{ Transferrin saturation} = \frac{\text{serum iron}}{\text{total iron-binding capacity}} \times 100$$

During iron deficiency, transferrin saturation decreases. The transferrin saturation value is a useful indicator of iron status because it includes information about both the iron and transferrin content of the blood.

Erythrocyte Protoporphyrin The iron-containing molecule in hemoglobin is heme, which is formed from iron and protoporphyrin. Protoporphyrin accumulates in the blood when iron supplies are inadequate for the formation of heme. However, levels of protoporphyrin may increase when hemoglobin synthesis is impaired for other reasons, such as lead poisoning or inflammation.

Hemoglobin When iron stores are depleted, hemoglobin production is impaired, and symptoms of anemia may eventually develop. Hemoglobin's usefulness in evaluating iron status is limited, however, because hemoglobin concentrations drop fairly late in the development of iron deficiency, and other nutrient deficiencies and medical conditions can also alter hemoglobin concentrations.

Hematocrit The hematocrit value reflects the percentage of the total blood volume occupied by red blood cells. To measure the hematocrit, a clinician spins the blood samples in a centrifuge to separate the red blood cells from the plasma. Low values indicate a reduced number or size of red blood cells. Although this test is not specific for iron status, it can help to detect the presence of iron-deficiency anemia.

Mean Corpuscular Volume (MCV) The hematocrit value divided by the red blood cell count provides a measure of the average size of a red blood cell, referred to as the mean corpuscular volume (MCV). This measure helps to classify the type of anemia that is present. In iron deficiency, the red blood cells are smaller than average (microcytic cells).

Assessment of Folate and Vitamin B_{12} Status

Folate deficiency and vitamin B_{12} deficiency present a similar clinical picture—an anemia characterized by abnormally large, misshapen, and immature red blood cells (megaloblastic cells). Distinguishing between folate and vitamin B_{12} deficiency is essential, however, because their treatments differ. Giving folate to a person with vitamin B_{12} deficiency can improve many of the test results indicative of vitamin B_{12} deficiency, but this would be a dangerous treatment because vitamin B_{12} deficiency causes nerve damage that folate cannot correct. Thus, inappropriate folate administration can mask vitamin B_{12}–deficiency anemia, and nerve damage could worsen. For this reason, it is critical to determine whether an anemia characterized by macrocytic cells results from a folate deficiency or from a vitamin B_{12} deficiency. Several of the following assessment measures can help to make this distinction.

Mean Corpuscular Volume (MCV) As previously mentioned, MCV is a measure of red blood cell size. In folate and vitamin B_{12} deficiencies, the red blood cells are larger than average, or macrocytic. Macrocytic cells are not necessarily indicative of nutrient deficiency, however, as they may also result from a high alcohol intake, liver disease, or various medications.

Serum Folate and Vitamin B_{12} Levels Analyses of serum folate and vitamin B_{12} levels are usually among the first tests conducted to determine the cause of macrocytic red blood cells. The presence of low serum levels of either nutrient is consistent with a deficiency of that nutrient, whereas adequate levels can help to rule out deficiency. Folate levels are not a specific measure of folate status, however, as they may increase after folate consumption, and decrease due to alcohol consumption, pregnancy, or use of anticonvulsants. The folate level in red blood cells—called erythrocyte folate—correlates well with folate stores and can help in the diagnosis of folate deficiency, but this test is not available at all institutions. Table E-4 (p. E-12) shows acceptable ranges for the tests used in assessing folate and vitamin B_{12} status.

Homocysteine and Methylmalonic Acid Levels To determine whether a nutrient deficiency is present, clinicians can measure the levels of substances that accumulate when the functions of that nutrient are impaired. For example, blood levels of the amino acid homocysteine are usually increased by both folate and vitamin B_{12} deficiency because both nutrients are needed for its metabolism. Methylmalonic acid, a breakdown product of several amino acids, requires vitamin B_{12} for its metabolism; hence, serum levels increase as a result of vitamin B_{12} deficiency. Because methylmalonic acid levels are not influenced by folate status, this measure is useful in distinguishing between folate and vitamin B_{12} deficiency.

Schilling Test As Chapter 8 explains, vitamin B_{12} deficiency most often results from malabsorption, not poor intake. The Schilling test can help to diagnose malabsorption

TABLE E-4 Criteria for Assessing Folate and Vitamin B$_{12}$ Status

Laboratory Test	Acceptable Range	Effect of Folate or Vitamin B$_{12}$ Deficiency
Serum folate	3–16 ng/mL	Reduced in folate deficiency
Erythrocyte folate	140–628 ng/mL packed cells	Reduced in folate deficiency
Serum vitamin B$_{12}$	200–835 pg/mL	Reduced in vitamin B$_{12}$ deficiency
Serum methylmalonic acid	150–370 nmol/L	Increased in vitamin B$_{12}$ deficiency
Serum homocysteine	Male: 4–16 μmol/L Female: 3–14 μmol/L	Increased in folate or vitamin B$_{12}$ deficiency

Note: ng = nanogram, pg = picogram, nmol = nanomole, μmol = micromole

Sources: L. Goldman and A. I. Schafer, eds., *Goldman's Cecil Medicine* (Philadelphia: Saunders, 2012), pp. 2558–2569; R. S. Porter and J. L. Kaplan, eds., *Merck Manual of Diagnosis and Therapy* (Whitehouse Station, NJ: Merck Sharp and Dohme, 2011), pp. 3491–3502.

of vitamin B$_{12}$: after the patient takes an oral dose of radioactive vitamin B$_{12}$, a urine test determines whether the vitamin B$_{12}$ was absorbed. The Schilling test is rarely performed at present because it involves the administration of a radioactive reagent.

Antibodies to Intrinsic Factor The presence of serum antibodies to intrinsic factor can help to confirm a diagnosis of pernicious anemia, an autoimmune disease characterized by destruction of the cells that produce intrinsic factor (a protein required for vitamin B$_{12}$ absorption; see Chapter 8). Serum antibodies to the parietal cells that produce and release intrinsic factor may also indicate pernicious anemia, but these antibodies may be present in various other conditions as well.

Cautions about Nutrition Assessment

The tests outlined in this appendix yield information that becomes meaningful only when they are conducted and interpreted by a skilled clinician. Potential sources of error may be introduced at any step, from the collection of samples to the analysis and reporting of data. Equipment must be regularly calibrated to ensure accuracy of measurements. In addition, the assessor must keep in mind that few tests may be specific to the nutrient of interest alone, and lab results may reflect physiological processes other than the ones being tested. Furthermore, because many tests are not sensitive enough to detect the early stages of deficiency, follow-up testing is often necessary to identify a nutrition problem.

Appendix F

Aids to Calculation

Many mathematical problems have been worked out in the "How To" boxes within the text. These pages provide additional help and examples.

Conversion Factors

A *conversion factor* is a numerical factor—expressed as a ratio—that can convert a quantity expressed in one unit to another unit; for example, the factor may be used to convert pounds to kilograms or feet to inches. To create a conversion factor, an equality (such as *1 kilogram = 2.2 pounds*) is expressed as a fraction:

$$\frac{1\ kg}{2.2\ lb} \quad and \quad \frac{2.2\ lb}{1\ kg}.$$

Because a conversion factor has a value of *1* (the value in the numerator is equal to the value in the denominator), it can be used as a multiplier to change the *unit* of measure without changing the *value* of the measurement. To convert the units of a measurement, the fraction must have the desired unit in the numerator, as the unit in the denominator will cancel out the original unit.

Example 1 Convert the weight of 130 pounds to kilograms.

▌ Multiply 130 pounds by a conversion factor (fraction) that includes both pounds and kilograms and is arranged so that the desired unit (kilograms) is in the numerator:

$$130\ lb \times \frac{1\ kg}{2.2\ lb} = \frac{130\ kg}{2.2} = 59\ kg.$$

As this example shows, the unit for *pounds* cancels out and the unit for *kilograms* remains in the solution.

Example 2 The food label on a bottle of apple juice shows the contents in both fluid ounces and liters. How many liters are contained in a bottle that holds 64 fluid ounces?

▌ Multiply 64 ounces by a conversion factor that includes both fluid ounces and liters, with the desired unit (liters) in the numerator:

$$64\ fl\ oz \times \frac{1\ L}{33.8\ fl\ oz} = \frac{64\ L}{33.8} = 1.89\ L.$$

Percentages

A percentage expresses a fraction that has 100 in the denominator; for example, the term *50 percent* is equivalent to the fraction 50/100. Similar to other fractions, percentages are used to express a *proportion* of the *whole;* therefore, the units in the numerator and denominator must be similar. Any fraction can be expressed in hundredths and converted to a percentage by dividing the numerator by the denominator and multiplying by 100:

$$¼ = 0.25.$$
$$0.25 \times 100 = 25\%.$$

Example 3 Suppose your energy intake for the day is 2000 kcalories (kcal) and your recommended energy intake is 2400 kcalories. What percent of the recommended energy intake did you consume?

▊ Divide your intake by the recommended intake:

$$2000 \text{ kcal (your intake)} \div 2400 \text{ kcal (recommended intake)} = 0.83.$$

▊ Multiply by 100 to express the decimal as a percentage:

$$0.83 \times 100 = 83\%.$$

Example 4 A percentage can also be greater than 100. Suppose your intake of vitamin C is 120 milligrams and your RDA (male) is 90 milligrams. What percent of the RDA for vitamin C did you consume?

$$120 \text{ mg (your intake)} \div 90 \text{ mg (RDA)} = 1.33.$$
$$1.33 \times 100 = 133\%.$$

Weights and Measures

Length
1 meter (m) = 39 in
1 centimeter (cm) = 0.4 in
1 inch (in) = 2.5 cm
1 foot (ft) = 30 cm

Temperature

	Celsius*			Fahrenheit
Boiling point	100°C		212°F	Boiling point
Body temperature	37°C		98.6°F	Body temperature
Freezing	0°C		32°F	Freezing

▊ To find degrees Fahrenheit (°F) when you know degrees Celsius (°C), multiply by 9/5 and then add 32.

▊ To find degrees Celsius (°C) when you know degrees Fahrenheit (°F), subtract 32 and then multiply by 5/9.

Volume
1 liter (L) = 1000 mL, 0.26 gal, 1.06 qt, 2.1 pt, or 33.8 fl oz
1 milliliter (mL) = 1/1000 L or 0.03 fl oz
1 gallon (gal) = 128 oz, 16 c, or 3.8 L
1 quart (qt) = 32 fl oz, 4 c, or 0.95 L
1 pint (pt) = 16 fl oz, 2 c, or 0.47 L
1 cup (c) = 8 fl oz, 16 tbs, about 250 mL, or 0.25 L

*Also known as centigrade.

1 fluid ounce (fl oz) = 30 mL
1 tablespoon (tbs) = 3 tsp or 15 mL
1 teaspoon (tsp) = 5 mL

Weight
1 kilogram (kg) = 1000 g or 2.2 lb
1 gram (g) = 1/1000 kg, 1000 mg, or 0.035 oz
1 milligram (mg) = 1/1000 g or 1000 μg
1 microgram (μg) = 1/1000 mg
1 pound (lb) = 16 oz, 454 g, or 0.45 kg
1 ounce (oz) = about 28 g

Energy
1 megajoule (MJ) = 240 kcal
1 kilojoule (kJ) = 0.24 kcal
1 kcalorie (kcal) = 4.2 kJ
1 g carbohydrate = 4 kcal = 17 kJ
1 g fat = 9 kcal = 37 kJ
1 g protein = 4 kcal = 17 kJ
1 g alcohol = 7 kcal = 29 kJ

Appendix G

Enteral Formulas

The large number of enteral formulas available allows patients to meet a wide variety of medical needs. The first step in narrowing the choice of formulas is to determine the patient's ability to digest and absorb nutrients. Table G–1 (pp. G-2 to G-3) lists examples of standard formulas for patients who can adequately digest and absorb nutrients, and Table G–2 (p. G-4) provides examples of elemental formulas for patients with a limited ability to digest or absorb nutrients. Each formula is listed only once, although a formula may have more than one use. A high-protein formula, for example, may also be a fiber-containing formula. Tables G–3 and G–4 (p. G-4) list modules that can be used to prepare modular formulas or enhance enteral formulas.

The information shown in this appendix reflects the literature provided by manufacturers and does not suggest endorsement by the authors. Manufacturers frequently add new formulas, discontinue old ones, and change formula composition. Consult the manufacturers' literature and websites for updates and additional examples of enteral formulas.[a] The following products are listed in this appendix:

▌ *Abbott Nutrition:* Glucerna 1.0 Cal, Jevity 1 Cal, Jevity 1.5 Cal, Nepro with Carb Steady, Osmolite 1 Cal, Oxepa, Pivot 1.5 Cal, Polycose, Promote, Promote with Fiber, Pulmocare, Suplena with Carb Steady, Vital 1.0 Cal

▌ *Nestlé Nutrition:* Beneprotein, Compleat, Compleat Pediatric, Diabetisource AC, Fibersource HN, Impact, Impact Peptide 1.5, Impact Glutamine, Isosource HN, MCT Oil, Microlipid, Novasource Renal, Nutren 1.0, Nutren 1.0 Fiber, Nutren 1.5, Nutren 2.0, Nutren Glytrol, Nutren Junior, Nutren Pulmonary, Nutren Replete, Nutren Replete Fiber, NutriHep, Peptamen, Peptamen Junior, Vivonex Pediatric, Vivonex T.E.N.

---

[a]Sources for the information in this appendix: Abbott Nutrition, www.abbottnutrition.com; Nestlé Nutrition, www.nestle-nutrition.com.

TABLE G-1 Standard Formulas

Product[a]	Volume to Meet 100% RDI[b] (mL)	Energy (kcal/mL)	Protein or Amino Acids (g/L)	Carbohydrate (g/L)	Fat (g/L)	Notes
General-Use Adult Formulas						
Compleat	1400	1.06	48	132	40	Blenderized formula, 6 g fiber/L
Nutren 1.0	1500	1.00	40	128	38	25% fat from MCT
Osmolite 1 Cal	1321	1.06	44	144	35	20% fat from MCT
Fiber-Enhanced Formulas						
Jevity 1 Cal	1321	1.06	44	155	35	14 g fiber/L
Nutren 1.0 Fiber	1500	1.00	40	128	38	14 g fiber/L
Promote with Fiber	1000	1.00	63	138	28	14 g fiber/L
High-kCalorie Formulas						
Jevity 1.5 Cal	1000	1.50	64	216	50	22 g fiber/L
Nutren 1.5	1000	1.50	60	168	68	50% fat from MCT
Nutren 2.0	750	2.00	80	196	104	75% fat from MCT
High-Protein Formulas						
Fibersource HN	1250	1.20	54	160	39	20% fat from MCT, 10 g fiber/L
Isosource HN	1165	1.20	54	160	39	20% fat from MCT, low fiber
Promote	1000	1.00	63	130	26	19% fat from MCT, low fiber
Specialized Formulas: Pediatric (1 to 10 years)						
Compleat Pediatric	1–8 yr: 1000 mL; 9–13 yr: 1500 mL	1.00	38	132	39	Blenderized formula, 7 g fiber/L
Nutren Junior	1–8 yr: 1000 mL; 9–13 yr: 1500 mL	1.00	30	110	50	20% fat from MCT
Specialized Formulas: Glucose Intolerance						
Diabetisource AC	1250	1.20	60	100	59	36% kcal from carbohydrate, 15 g fiber/L
Glucerna 1.0 Cal	1420	1.00	42	96	54	34% kcal from carbohydrate, 14 g fiber/L
Nutren Glytrol	1500	1.00	45	100	48	40% kcal from carbohydrate, 15 g fiber/L
Specialized Formulas: Immune System Support						
Impact	1500	1.00	56	132	28	Enriched with arginine, nucleotides, and omega-3 fatty acids
Impact Peptide 1.5	1000	1.50	94	140	64	Same as above
Impact Glutamine	1000	1.30	78	148	43	Same as above, and enriched with glutamine

TABLE G-1 Standard Formulas (*continued*)

Product[a]	Volume to Meet 100% RDI[b] (mL)	Energy (kcal/mL)	Protein or Amino Acids (g/L)	Carbohydrate (g/L)	Fat (g/L)	Notes
Specialized Formulas: Chronic Kidney Disease (CKD)						
Nepro with Carb Steady	944	1.80	81	161	96	Low in potassium and phosphorus; to be used after dialysis has been instituted
Novasource Renal	1000	2.00	91	183	100	Low in electrolytes; to be used after dialysis has been instituted
Suplena with Carb Steady	1000	1.80	45	196	96	Low in protein, potassium, phosphorus, and calcium; for stage 3 and 4 CKD
Specialized Formulas: Respiratory Insufficiency						
Nutren Pulmonary	1000	1.50	68	100	95	56% kcal from fat, 40% fat from MCT
Oxepa	946	1.50	63	105	94	Enriched with omega-3 fatty acids and antioxidants; for mechanically ventilated patients
Pulmocare	947	1.50	63	106	93	55% kcal from fat, 20% fat from MCT, enriched with antioxidant nutrients
Specialized Formulas: Wound Healing						
Nutren Replete	1000	1.00	62	112	34	Enhanced with vitamins and minerals; for patients recovering from surgery, burns, or pressure ulcers
Nutren Replete Fiber	1000	1.00	62	112	34	Same as above; 14 g fiber/L

Note: MCT = Medium-chain triglycerides

[a]All formulas listed are both gluten free and suitable for patients with lactose intolerance.
[b]RDI = Reference Daily Intakes, which are labeling standards for vitamins, minerals, and protein. Consuming 100% of the RDI will meet the nutrient needs of most people using the product.

TABLE G-2 Elemental Formulas

Product[a]	Volume to Meet 100% RDI[b] (mL)	Energy (kcal/mL)	Protein or Amino Acids (g/L)	Carbohydrate (g/L)	Fat (g/L)	Notes
Specialized Elemental Formula: Hepatic Insufficiency						
NutriHep	1000	1.50	40	290	21	High in branched-chain amino acids and low in aromatic amino acids; 70% fat from MCT
Specialized Elemental Formula: Immune System Support						
Pivot 1.5 Cal	1000	1.50	94	172	51	Enriched with arginine, glutamine, omega-3 fatty acids, and antioxidant nutrients
Specialized Elemental Formulas: Malabsorption						
Peptamen	1500	1.00	40	128	39	70% fat from MCT
Vital 1.0 Cal	1422	1.00	40	130	38	Enhanced with prebiotics and antioxidants
Vivonex T.E.N.	2000	1.00	38	204	3	Powder form, 100% free amino acids, very low fat
Specialized Elemental Formulas: Pediatric (1 to 10 years)						
Peptamen Junior	1–8 yr: 1000 mL; 9–13 yr: 1500 mL	1.00	30	136	38	60% fat from MCT
Vivonex Pediatric	1–8 yr: 1000 mL; 9–13 yr: 1500 mL	0.80	24	126	23	Powder form, 100% free amino acids

Note: MCT = Medium-chain triglycerides

[a]All formulas listed are both gluten free and suitable for patients with lactose intolerance.
[b]RDI = Reference Daily Intakes, which are labeling standards for vitamins, minerals, and protein. Consuming 100% of the RDI will meet the nutrient needs of most people using the product.

TABLE G-3 Protein and Carbohydrate Modules

Product	Major Ingredient	Energy (kcal/g)	Nutrient Content (g/100 g)
Beneprotein	Whey protein powder	3.6	86 g protein
Polycose	Hydrolyzed cornstarch (powder)	3.8	94 g carbohydrate

TABLE G-4 Fat Modules

Product	Major Ingredient	Energy (kcal/mL)	Fat Content (g/100 mL)
MCT Oil	Coconut and/or palm kernel oil	7.7	93
Microlipid	Safflower oil	4.5	50

Appendix H

Answers to Self-Check Questions

Chapter 1
1. d, 2. d, 3. c, 4. d, 5. c, 6. b,
7. c, 8. b, 9. c, 10. c

Chapter 2
1. b, 2. b, 3. c, 4. a, 5. a, 6. a,
7. b, 8. a, 9. d, 10. c

Chapter 3
1. b, 2. c, 3. a, 4. d, 5. a, 6. a,
7. d, 8. d, 9. b, 10. a

Chapter 4
1. c, 2. b, 3. d, 4. d, 5. a, 6. d,
7. c, 8. b, 9. c, 10. d

Chapter 5
1. b, 2. a, 3. d, 4. a, 5. c, 6. a,
7. d, 8. c, 9. d, 10. d

Chapter 6
1. d, 2. b, 3. c, 4. d, 5. d, 6. a,
7. a, 8. b, 9. c, 10. c

Chapter 7
1. b, 2. a, 3. a, 4. c, 5. b, 6. c,
7. d, 8. b, 9. c, 10. b

Chapter 8
1. d, 2. d, 3. c, 4. a, 5. d, 6. d,
7. b, 8. c, 9. c, 10. a

Chapter 9
1. d, 2. b, 3. a, 4. d, 5. c, 6. d,
7. a, 8. d, 9. d, 10. b

Chapter 10
1. b, 2. a, 3. b, 4. c, 5. d, 6. c,
7. d, 8. b, 9. a, 10. d

Chapter 11
1. a, 2. d, 3. c, 4. c, 5. b, 6. d,
7. b, 8. c, 9. b, 10. c

Chapter 12
1. c, 2. b, 3. a, 4. b, 5. d, 6. c,
7. d, 8. c, 9. b, 10. c

Chapter 13
1. d, 2. c, 3. d, 4. d, 5. d, 6. d,
7. b, 8. b, 9. a, 10. b

Chapter 14
1. b, 2. c, 3. d, 4. a, 5. b, 6. d,
7. c, 8. a, 9. c, 10. b

Chapter 15
1. d, 2. a, 3. a, 4. b, 5. d, 6. c,
7. b, 8. b, 9. d, 10. c

Chapter 16
1. d, 2. b, 3. c, 4. a, 5. b, 6. d,
7. a, 8. b, 9. a, 10. c

Chapter 17
1. a, 2. c, 3. b, 4. d, 5. a, 6. c,
7. d, 8. b, 9. b, 10. c

Chapter 18
1. b, 2. c, 3. d, 4. c, 5. d, 6. a,
7. b, 8. b, 9. a, 10. c

Chapter 19
1. d, 2. c, 3. b, 4. b, 5. a, 6. c,
7. a, 8. c, 9. a, 10. d

Chapter 20
1. d, 2. a, 3. b, 4. a, 5. b, 6. c,
7. d, 8. a, 9. b, 10. c

Chapter 21
1. b, 2. d, 3. d, 4. c, 5. a, 6. c,
7. d, 8. c, 9. a, 10. b

Chapter 22
1. a, 2. d, 3. c, 4. c, 5. b, 6. d,
7. b, 8. d, 9. b, 10. c

Chapter 23
1. a, 2. c, 3. b, 4. d, 5. a, 6. a,
7. b, 8. b, 9. c, 10. d

Chapter 24
1. d, 2. a, 3. b, 4. c, 5. d, 6. b,
7. c, 8. c, 9. d, 10. a

Chapter 25
1. d, 2. c, 3. c, 4. b, 5. d, 6. b,
7. b, 8. a, 9. a, 10. d

Glossary

2-in-1 solution: a parenteral solution that contains dextrose and amino acids, but excludes lipids.

24-hour dietary recall: a record of foods consumed during the previous day or in the past 24 hours; sometimes modified to include foods consumed in a typical day.

abscesses (AB-sess-es): accumulations of pus.

Acceptable Daily Intake (ADI): the amount of a nonnutritive sweetener that individuals can safely consume each day over the course of a lifetime without adverse effect. It includes a 100-fold safety factor.

Acceptable Macronutrient Distribution Ranges (AMDR): ranges of intakes for the energy-yielding nutrients that provide adequate energy and nutrients and reduce the risk of chronic disease.

acetaldehyde (ah-set-AL-deh-hide): an intermediate in alcohol metabolism that, in excess, can damage the body's tissues and interfere with cellular functions.

acetate (AH-seh-tate): the product of alcohol metabolism that is used as a source of energy by many tissues in the body.

acetone breath: a distinctive fruity odor on the breath of a person with ketosis.

acetyl CoA (ASS-eh-teel, or ah-SEET-il, coh-AY): a 2-carbon compound (acetate, or acetic acid) with a molecule of CoA attached to it.

achalasia (ack-ah-LAY-zhah): an esophageal disorder characterized by weakened peristalsis and impaired relaxation of the lower esophageal sphincter.

achlorhydria (AY-clor-HIGH-dree-ah): absence of gastric acid secretions.

acid–base balance: the balance maintained between acid and base concentrations in the blood and body fluids.

acidosis: acid accumulation in body tissues; depresses the central nervous system and may lead to disorientation and, eventually, coma.

acids: compounds that release hydrogen ions in a solution.

acquired immune deficiency syndrome (AIDS): the late stage of illness caused by infection with the human immunodeficiency virus (HIV); characterized by severe damage to immune function.

acute kidney injury: the rapid decline of kidney function over a period of hours or days; potentially a cause of acute renal failure.

acute respiratory distress syndrome (ARDS): respiratory failure triggered by severe lung injury; a medical emergency that causes dyspnea and pulmonary edema and usually requires mechanical ventilation.

acute-phase response: changes in body chemistry resulting from infection, inflammation, or injury; characterized by alterations in plasma proteins.

added sugars: sugars, syrups, and other kcaloric sweeteners that are added to foods during processing or preparation or at the table; excludes the naturally occurring sugars found in fruits and milk products.

adequacy: the characteristic of a diet that provides all the essential nutrients, fiber, and energy necessary to maintain health and body weight.

Adequate Intakes (AI): a set of values that are used as guides for nutrient intakes when scientific evidence is insufficient to determine an RDA.

adipokines (AD-ih-poh-kynz): protein hormones made and released by adipose tissue (fat) cells.

adiponectin (AH-dih-poe-NECK-tin): a hormone produced by adipose cells that improves insulin sensitivity.

adipose tissue: the body's fat, which consists of masses of fat-storing cells called adipose cells.

adolescence: the period of growth from the beginning of puberty until full maturity. Timing of adolescence varies from person to person.

advance health care directive: written or oral instructions regarding one's preferences for medical treatment to be used in the event of becoming incapacitated; also called an *advance medical directive* or a *living will*.

advanced glycation end products (AGEs): reactive compounds formed after glucose combines with protein; AGEs can damage tissues and lead to diabetic complications.

adverse reactions: unusual responses to food (including intolerances and allergies).

aerobic physical activity: activity in which the body's large muscles move in a rhythmic manner for a sustained period of time (e.g., brisk walking, running, swimming, bicycling), which improves cardiorespiratory fitness; also called *endurance activity*.

AIDS-defining illnesses: diseases and complications associated with the later stages of an HIV infection, including wasting, recurrent bacterial pneumonia, opportunistic infections, and certain cancers.

albuminuria: the presence of albumin (a blood protein) in the urine, a sign of diabetic nephropathy.

alcohol abuse: the continued use of alcohol despite the development of social, legal, or health problems. Individuals who abuse alcohol are called *alcoholics*.

alcohol-related birth defects (ARBD): a condition caused by prenatal alcohol exposure that is diagnosed when there is a history of substantial, regular maternal alcohol intake or heavy episodic drinking and birth defects known to be associated with alcohol exposure.

alcohol-related neurodevelopmental disorder (ARND): a condition caused by prenatal alcohol exposure that is diagnosed when there is a confirmed history of substantial, regular maternal alcohol intake or heavy episodic drinking and behavioral, cognitive, or central nervous system abnormalities known to be associated with alcohol exposure.

alcoholic liver disease: liver disease that is related to excessive alcohol consumption. Disorders that may develop include fatty liver, hepatitis, and cirrhosis, which may lead to liver failure.

aldosterone: a steroid hormone secreted by the adrenal cortex that promotes sodium (and therefore water) retention and potassium excretion.

alkalosis: excessive base in the blood and body fluids.

alpha-lactalbumin (lact-AL-byoo-min): a major protein in human breast milk.

alveoli (al-VEE-oh-lie): air sacs in the lungs. One air sac is an *alveolus*.

Alzheimer's disease: a progressive, degenerative disease that attacks the brain and impairs thinking, behavior, and memory.

amenorrhea (ay-MEN-oh-RE-ah): the absence of or cessation of menstruation. Primary amenorrhea is menarche delayed beyond 16 years of age. Secondary amenorrhea is the absence of three to six consecutive menstrual cycles.

amino (a-MEEN-oh) **acids:** building blocks of protein; each contains an amino group, an acid group, a hydrogen atom, and a distinctive side group, all attached to a central carbon atom.

amniotic (am-nee-OTT-ic) **sac:** the "bag of waters" in the uterus in which the fetus floats.

amylase (AM-uh-lace): an enzyme (carbohydrase) that splits amylose (a form of starch).

anabolic steroids: drugs related to the male sex hormone, testosterone, that stimulate the development of lean body mass.

anabolism (an-AB-o-lism): reactions that require energy in which small molecules are put together to build larger ones.

anaerobic (AN-air-ROH-bic): not requiring oxygen.

analgesic: a drug that relieves pain.

anaphylactic (AN-ah-feh-LAC-tic) **shock:** a life-threatening whole-body allergic reaction to an offending substance.

anemia of chronic disease: anemia that develops in persons with chronic illness; may resemble iron-deficiency anemia even though iron stores are often adequate. Also called *anemia of chronic inflammation*.

anencephaly (AN-en-SEF-a-lee): an uncommon and always fatal type of neural tube defect; characterized by the absence of a brain.

aneurysm (AN-you-rih-zum): an abnormal enlargement or bulging of a blood vessel (usually an artery) caused by weakness in the blood vessel wall.

angina (an-JYE-nah or AN-ji-nah) **pectoris:** a condition caused by ischemia in the heart muscle that results in discomfort or dull pain in the chest region. The pain often radiates to the left shoulder and arm or to the back, neck, and lower jaw.

anorexia nervosa: an eating disorder characterized by a refusal to maintain a minimally normal body weight, self-starvation to the extreme, and a disturbed perception of body weight and shape; seen (usually) in adolescent girls and young women.

anorexia: lack of appetite.

anthropometric (AN-throw-poe-MEH-trik): related to physical measurements of the human body, such as height, weight, body circumferences, and percentage of body fat.

antibodies: large proteins of the blood and body fluids, produced in response to invasion of the body by unfamiliar molecules (mostly proteins) called *antigens*; they inactivate the invaders and so protect the body.

anticonvulsants: drugs that treat epileptic seizures.

antiemetics: drugs that prevent vomiting.

antigens: substances that elicit the formation of antibodies or an inflammation reaction from the immune system (e.g., bacteria, viruses, toxins, and proteins in food that cause an allergy).

antineoplastic drugs: drugs that control or kill cancer cells.

antioxidant (anti-OX-ih-dant): (1) a compound that protects other compounds from oxygen by itself reacting with oxygen. (2) A food additive (preservative) that delays or prevents rancidity of foods and other damage to food caused by oxygen.

antiretroviral drugs: drugs that treat retrovirus infections, such as infection with human immunodeficiency virus (HIV).

anuria (ah-NOO-ree-ah): the absence of urine; clinically identified as urine output less than 50 mL/day.

anus (AY-nus): the terminal outlet of the GI tract.

aplastic anemia: anemia characterized by the inability of bone marrow to produce adequate numbers of blood cells; causes include drug toxicity, viruses, and genetic defects.

appendix: a narrow blind sac extending from the beginning of the colon that stores lymph cells.

appetite: the psychological desire to eat; a learned motivation that is experienced as a pleasant sensation that accompanies the sight, smell, or thought of appealing foods.

aromatic amino acids: the amino acids phenylalanine, tyrosine, and tryptophan, which have carbon rings in their side groups.

artery: a vessel that carries blood away from the heart.

arthritis: inflammation of a joint, usually accompanied by pain, swelling, and structural changes.

artificial fats: zero-energy fat replacers that are chemically synthesized to mimic the sensory and cooking qualities of naturally occurring fats but are totally or partially resistant to digestion.

ascites (ah-SIGH-teez): an abnormal accumulation of fluid in the abdominal cavity.

ascorbic acid: one of the two active forms of vitamin C.

aspiration: drawing in by suction or inhalation; a common complication of enteral feedings in which substances from the GI tract are drawn into the lungs.

atherogenic: able to initiate or promote atherosclerosis.

atherosclerosis (ATH-er-oh-scler-OH-sis): an arterial disease characterized by a buildup of lipids and fibrous scar tissue on the inner walls of arteries.

ATP or adenosine (ah-DEN-oh-seen) **triphosphate** (tri-FOS-fate): a common high-energy compound that contains three phosphate groups; the bonds between the phosphate groups are

often described as "high-energy" because of their readiness to release energy.

atrophic gastritis (a-TROH-fik gas-TRY-tis): a chronic inflammation of the stomach accompanied by a diminished size and functioning of the stomach's mucous membrane and glands; eventually the gastric epithelium may be replaced with another type of tissue.

atrophy (AT-tro-fee): a decrease in size (for example, of a muscle) because of disuse.

autoimmune: refers to an immune response directed against the body's own tissues.

azotemia: the accumulation of nitrogenous wastes in the blood.

bacterial cholangitis (KOH-lan-JYE-tis): bacterial infection involving the bile ducts.

bacterial overgrowth: excessive bacterial colonization of the stomach and small intestine; may be due to low gastric acidity, altered GI motility, mucosal damage, contamination, or changes in intestinal anatomy due to surgical reconstruction.

bacterial translocation: movement of bacteria across the intestinal mucosa, allowing access to body tissues.

balance: the dietary characteristic of providing foods in proportion to one another and in proportion to the body's needs.

bariatric (BAH-ree-AH-trik) **surgery:** surgery that treats severe obesity.

Barrett's esophagus: a condition in which esophageal cells damaged by chronic exposure to stomach acid are replaced by cells that resemble those in the stomach or small intestine, sometimes becoming cancerous.

basal metabolic rate (BMR): the rate of energy use for metabolism under specified conditions: after a 12-hour fast and restful sleep, without any physical activity or emotional excitement, and in a comfortable setting; usually expressed as kcalories per kilogram of body weight per hour.

basal metabolism: the energy needed to maintain life when a person is at complete digestive, physical, and emotional rest; normally the largest part of a person's daily energy expenditure.

bases: compounds that accept hydrogen ions in a solution.

behavior modification: the changing of behavior by the manipulation of *antecedents* (cues or environmental factors that trigger behavior), the behavior itself, and *consequences* (the penalties or rewards attached to behavior).

beneficence (be-NEF-eh-sense): the act of performing beneficial services rather than harmful ones.

beriberi: the thiamin-deficiency disease; characterized by loss of sensation in the hands and feet, muscular weakness, advancing paralysis, and abnormal heart action.

beta-alanine: a nonessential amino acid that is the rate-limiting precursor for the synthesis of the dipeptide carnosine.

beta-carotene: a vitamin A precursor made by plants and stored in human fat tissue; an orange pigment.

beta-hydroxymethylbutyrate (HMB): a metabolite of the amino acid leucine promoted to increase muscle mass and strength.

BHA, BHT: preservatives commonly used to slow the development of "off" flavors, odors, and color changes caused by oxidation.

bicarbonate: an alkaline secretion of the pancreas (part of the pancreatic juice); also occurs widely in all cell fluids.

bile: an emulsifier that prepares fats and oils for digestion; made by the liver, stored in the

gallbladder, and released into the small intestine when needed.

biliary system: the gallbladder and ducts that deliver bile from the liver and gallbladder to the small intestine.

binge eating disorder: an eating disorder characterized by recurring episodes of eating a significant amount of food in a short period of time with marked feelings of lack of control.

bioactive food components: compounds in foods (either nutrients or phytochemicals) that alter physiological processes in the body.

bioavailability: the rate and extent to which a nutrient is absorbed and used.

biopsy: removal of a tissue sample to determine the cause of an illness.

blastocyst (BLASS-toe-sist): the developmental stage of the zygote when it is about 5 days old and ready for implantation.

blenderized formulas: enteral formulas that are prepared by using a food blender to mix and puree whole foods.

body composition: the proportions of muscle, bone, fat, and other tissues that make up a person's total body weight.

body mass index (BMI): an index of a person's weight in relation to height; determined by dividing the weight (in kilograms) by the square of the height (in meters).

bolus (BOH-lus): the portion of food swallowed at one time.

bolus (BOH-lus) **feeding:** delivery of about 250 to 500 milliliters of formula over a 5- to 15-minute period.

Bowman's (BOE-minz) **capsule:** a cuplike component of the nephron that surrounds the glomerulus and collects the filtrate that is passed to the tubules.

branched-chain amino acids: the essential amino acids leucine, isoleucine, and valine, which have side groups with a branched structure.

bronchi (BRON-key), **bronchioles** (BRON-key-oles): the main airways of the lungs. The singular form of bronchi is *bronchus*.

buffalo hump: the accumulation of fatty tissue at the base of the neck.

buffers: compounds that can reversibly combine with hydrogen ions to help keep a solution's acidity or alkalinity constant.

built environment: the buildings, roads, utilities, homes, fixtures, parks, and all other manufactured entities that form the physical characteristics of a community.

bulimia (byoo-LEE-mee-uh) **nervosa:** recurring episodes of binge eating combined with a morbid fear of becoming fat, usually followed by self-induced vomiting or purging.

C-reactive protein: an acute-phase protein produced in substantial amounts during acute inflammation and considered the best clinical indicator of the acute-phase response (although it is elevated during many chronic illnesses). It binds dead or dying cells to activate certain immune responses.

caffeine: a natural stimulant found in many common foods and beverages, including coffee, tea, and chocolate; may enhance endurance by stimulating fatty acid release. High doses cause headaches, trembling, rapid heart rate, and other undesirable side effects.

calciferol (kal-SIF-er-ol): vitamin D.

calories: a measure of *heat* energy. Food energy is measured in **kilocalories** (1000 calories equal 1 kilocalorie), abbreviated **kcalories** or kcal.

cancer cachexia (ka-KEK-see-ah): a wasting syndrome associated with cancer that is characterized by anorexia, weight loss, muscle wasting, and fatigue.

cancers: diseases characterized by the uncontrolled growth of a group of abnormal cells, which can destroy adjacent tissues and spread to other areas of the body via the lymph or blood.

candidiasis: a fungal infection on the mucous membranes of the oral cavity and elsewhere; usually caused by *Candida albicans*.

capillaries: small vessels that branch from an artery, connecting arteries to veins; oxygen, nutrients, and waste materials are exchanged across capillary walls.

carbohydrate loading: a regimen of moderate exercise, followed by eating a high-carbohydrate diet, which enables muscles to temporarily store glycogen beyond their normal capacity; also called *glycogen loading* or *glycogen supercompensation*.

carbohydrate-to-insulin ratio: the amount of carbohydrate that can be handled per unit of insulin; on average, every 15 grams of carbohydrate requires about 1 unit of rapid- or short-acting insulin.

carbohydrates: energy nutrients composed of monosaccharides.

carcinogenesis (CAR-sin-oh-JEN-eh-sis): the process of cancer development.

carcinogens (CAR-sin-oh-jenz or car-SIN-oh-jenz): substances that can cause cancer (the adjective is *carcinogenic*).

cardiac cachexia: severe malnutrition that develops in heart failure patients; characterized by weight loss and tissue wasting.

cardiac output: the volume of blood discharged by the heart each minute.

cardiopulmonary resuscitation (CPR): life-sustaining treatment that supplies oxygen and restores a person's ability to breathe and pump blood.

cardiorespiratory conditioning: improvements in heart and lung function and increased blood volume, brought about by aerobic training.

cardiorespiratory endurance: the ability to perform large-muscle dynamic exercise of moderate-to-high intensity for prolonged periods.

cardiovascular disease (CVD): a general term for all diseases of the heart and blood vessels.

cariogenic (KAH-ree-oh-JEN-ic): conducive to development of dental caries.

carnitine: a nonessential nonprotein amino acid made in the body from lysine that helps transport fatty acids across the mitochondrial membrane.

catabolism (ca-TAB-o-lism): energy-releasing reactions in which large molecules are broken down to smaller ones.

cataracts: clouding of the eye lenses that impairs vision and can lead to blindness.

cathartic: a strong laxative.

catheter: a thin tube placed within a narrow lumen (such as a blood vessel) or body cavity; can be used to infuse or withdraw fluids or keep a passage open.

celiac (SEE-lee-ack) **disease:** an immune disorder characterized by an abnormal immune response to wheat gluten and related proteins; also called *gluten-sensitive enteropathy* or *celiac sprue*.

central obesity: excess fat around the trunk of the body; also called *abdominal fat* or *upper-body fat*.

central veins: the large-diameter veins located close to the heart.

cerebral cortex: the outer surface of the cerebrum, which is the largest part of the brain.

Certified Diabetes Educator (CDE): a health care professional who specializes in diabetes management education; certification is obtained from the National Certification Board for Diabetes Educators.

cesarean (see-ZAIR-ee-un) **section:** surgical childbirth, in which the infant is taken through an incision in the woman's abdomen.

chemotherapy: the use of drugs to arrest or destroy cancer cells; these drugs are called *antineoplastic agents*.

cholecystectomy (KOH-leh-sis-TEK-toe-mee): surgical removal of the gallbladder.

cholecystitis (KOH-leh-sih-STY-tis): inflammation of the gallbladder, usually caused by obstruction of the cystic duct by gallstones.

cholelithiasis (KOH-leh-lih-THIGH-ah-sis): formation of gallstones.

choline: a nutrient that can be made in the body from an amino acid.

chromium picolinate (CROW-mee-um pick-oh-LYN-ate): a trace mineral supplement; falsely promoted as building muscle, enhancing energy, and burning fat.

chronic bronchitis (bron-KYE-tis): a lung disorder characterized by persistent inflammation and excessive secretions of mucus in the main airways of the lungs.

chronic diseases: diseases characterized by slow progression, long duration, and degeneration of body organs due in part to such personal lifestyle elements as poor food choices, smoking, alcohol use, and lack of physical activity.

chronic hypertension: in pregnant women, hypertension that is present and documented before pregnancy; in women whose prepregnancy blood pressure is unknown, the presence of sustained hypertension before 20 weeks of gestation.

chronic kidney disease: kidney disease characterized by gradual, irreversible deterioration of the kidneys; also called *chronic renal failure*.

chronic malnutrition: malnutrition caused by long-term food deprivation; characterized in children by short height for age (stunting).

chronic obstructive pulmonary disease (COPD): a group of lung diseases characterized by persistent obstructed airflow through the lungs and airways; includes chronic bronchitis and emphysema.

chronological age: a person's age in years from his or her date of birth.

chylomicrons (kye-lo-MY-crons): the lipoproteins that transport lipids from the intestinal cells into the body; body cells remove the lipids they need, leaving chylomicron remnants to be picked up by the liver cells.

chyme (KIME): the semiliquid mass of partly digested food expelled by the stomach into the duodenum (the top portion of the small intestine).

cirrhosis (sih-ROE-sis): an advanced stage of liver disease in which extensive scarring replaces healthy liver tissue, causing impaired liver function and liver failure.

claudication (CLAW-dih-KAY-shun): pain in the legs while walking; usually due to an inadequate supply of blood to muscles.

clear liquid diet: a diet that consists of foods that are liquid at room temperature, require minimal digestion, and leave little residue (undigested material) in the colon.

clinical pathways: coordinated programs of treatment that merge the care plans of different health practitioners; also called *care pathways*, *care maps*, or *critical pathways*.

clinically severe obesity: a BMI of 40 or greater, or a BMI of 35 or greater with one or more serious conditions such as hypertension; also called *morbid obesity*.

closed feeding system: a formula delivery system in which the sterile formula comes prepackaged in a container that can be attached directly to the feeding tube for administration.

CoA (coh-AY): coenzyme A; the coenzyme derived from the B vitamin pantothenic acid and central to energy metabolism.

coenzymes (co-EN-zimes): small molecules that work with enzymes to facilitate the enzymes' activity; most have B vitamins as part of their structures.

cognitive skills: as taught in behavior therapy, changes to conscious thoughts with the goal of improving adherence to lifestyle modifications; examples are problem-solving skills or the correction of false negative thoughts, termed *cognitive restructuring*.

cognitive therapy: psychological therapy aimed at changing undesirable behaviors by changing underlying thought processes contributing to these behaviors.

colectomy: removal of a portion or all of the colon.

collagen: the characteristic protein of connective tissue.

collateral vessels: blood vessels that enlarge or newly form to allow an alternative pathway for diverted blood.

colostomy (co-LAH-stoe-me): a surgical passage through the abdominal wall into the colon.

colostrum (co-LAHS-trum): a milklike secretion from the breasts, present during the first few days after delivery before milk appears; rich in protective factors.

complement: a group of plasma proteins that assist the activities of antibodies.

complementary and alternative medicine (CAM): health care practices that have not been proved to be effective and consequently are not included as part of conventional treatment (see Nutrition in Practice 15).

complementary proteins: two or more proteins whose amino acid assortments complement each other in such a way that the essential amino acids limited in one are supplied by the other.

conditionally essential amino acid: an amino acid that is normally nonessential but must be supplied by the diet in special circumstances when the need for it becomes greater than the body's ability to produce it.

conjugated linoleic acid: a collective term for several fatty acids that have the same chemical formulas as linoleic acid but with different configurations.

continuous ambulatory peritoneal dialysis (CAPD): the most common method of peritoneal dialysis; involves frequent exchanges of dialysate, which remains in the peritoneal cavity throughout the day.

continuous feedings: slow delivery of formula at a constant rate over an 8- to 24-hour period.

continuous glucose monitoring: continuous monitoring of tissue glucose levels using a small sensor placed under the skin.

continuous parenteral nutrition: continuous administration of parenteral solutions over a 24-hour period.

continuous renal replacement therapy (CRRT): a slow, continuous method of removing solutes and/or fluids from the blood by gently pumping the blood across a filtration membrane over a prolonged time period.

convenient dietary supplements: liquid meal replacers, energy drinks, energy bars, and energy gels that athletes and active people use to replenish energy and nutrients when time is limited.

cornea (KOR-nee-uh): the hard, transparent membrane covering the outside of the eye.

coronary heart disease (CHD): a chronic, progressive disease characterized by obstructed blood flow in the coronary arteries; also called *coronary artery disease*.

creatine (KREE-ah-teen): a nitrogen-containing compound that combines with phosphate to form the high-energy compound creatine phosphate (or phosphocreatine) in muscles.

creatinine: the waste product of creatine, a nitrogen-containing compound in muscle cells that supplies energy for muscle contraction.

critical period: a finite period during development in which certain events occur that will have irreversible effects on later developmental stages; usually a period of rapid cell division.

Crohn's disease: an inflammatory bowel disease that usually occurs in the lower portion of the small intestine and the colon; the inflammation may pervade the entire intestinal wall.

cross-contamination: the contamination of food by bacteria that occurs when the food comes into contact with surfaces previously touched by raw meat, poultry, or seafood.

cryptosporidiosis (KRIP-toe-spor-ih-dee-OH-sis): a foodborne illness caused by the parasite *Cryptosporidium parvum*.

cultural competence: an awareness and acceptance of one's own and others' cultures combined with the skills needed to interact effectively with people of diverse cultures.

cyanosis (sigh-ah-NOH-sis): a bluish cast in the skin due to the color of deoxygenated hemoglobin. It is most evident in individuals with lighter, thinner skin; it is mostly seen on lips, cheeks, and ears and under the nails.

cyclic feedings: continuous tube feedings conducted for 8 to 16 hours daily, allowing patient mobility and bowel rest during the remaining hours of the day.

cyclic parenteral nutrition: administration of parenteral solutions over a 10- to 14-hour period each day.

cystic fibrosis: an inherited disorder that affects the transport of chloride across epithelial cell membranes and is characterized by abnormal chloride and sodium levels in exocrine secretions; primarily affects the gastrointestinal and respiratory systems.

cystinuria (SIS-tin-NOO-ree-ah): a genetic disorder characterized by the elevated urinary excretion of several amino acids, including cystine.

cytokines (SIGH-toe-kines): signaling proteins produced by the body's cells; many cytokines are produced by immune cells and regulate immune responses.

Daily Values: reference values developed by the FDA specifically for use on food labels.

dawn phenomenon: morning hyperglycemia that is caused by the early-morning release of growth hormone, which reduces insulin sensitivity.

deamination: removal of the amino group (NH_2) from a compound such as an amino acid.

debridement: the surgical removal of dead, damaged, or contaminated tissue resulting from burns or wounds; helps to prevent infection and hasten healing.

decision-making capacity: the ability to understand pertinent information and make appropriate decisions; known as *decision-making competency* within the legal system.

deep vein thrombosis: formation of a stationary blood clot (thrombus) in a deep vein, usually in the leg, which causes inflammation, pain, and swelling, and is potentially fatal.

defibrillation: life-sustaining treatment in which an electronic device is used to shock the heart and reestablish a pattern of normal contractions; used when the heart has arrhythmias or has experienced cardiac arrest.

deficient: in regard to nutrient intake, describes the amount below which almost all healthy people can be expected, over time, to experience deficiency symptoms.

denaturation (dee-nay-cher-AY-shun): the change in a protein's shape brought about by heat, acid, or other agents.

dental calculus: mineralized dental plaque, often associated with inflammation and bleeding.

dental caries (KAH-reez): infectious disease of the teeth that causes the gradual decay and disintegration of tooth structures.

dental plaque (PLACK): a film of bacteria and bacterial by-products that accumulates on the tooth surface.

dermatitis herpetiformis: a gluten-sensitive disorder characterized by a severe skin rash.

DHA: docosahexaenoic (DOE-cosa-HEX-ee-NO-ick) acid, an omega-3 fatty acid made from linolenic acid.

DHEA (dehydroepiandrosterone) and **androstenedione:** hormones made in the adrenal glands that serve as precursors to the male sex hormone, testosterone; falsely promoted as burning fat, building muscle, and slowing aging.

diabetes (DYE-ah-BEE-teez) **mellitus:** a group of metabolic disorders characterized by hyperglycemia and disordered insulin metabolism.

diabetic coma: a coma that occurs in uncontrolled diabetes; may be due to diabetic ketoacidosis, the hyperosmolar hyperglycemic syndrome, or severe hypoglycemia.

diabetic nephropathy (neh-FRAH-pah-thee): damage to the kidneys that results from long-term diabetes.

diabetic neuropathy (nur-RAH-pah-thee): nerve damage that results from long-term diabetes.

diabetic retinopathy (REH-tih-NAH-pah-thee): retinal damage that results from long-term diabetes.

dialysate (dye-AL-ih-sate): the solution used in dialysis to draw wastes and fluids from the blood.

dialysis (dye-AH-lih-sis): life-sustaining treatment in which a patient's blood is filtered using selective diffusion through a semipermeable membrane; substitutes for kidney function.

dialyzer (DYE-ah-LYE-zer): a machine used in hemodialysis to filter the blood; also called an *artificial kidney*.

diet manual: a resource that specifies the foods or preparation methods to include in or exclude from modified diets and provides sample menus.

diet orders: specific instructions regarding dietary management; also called *nutrition prescriptions*.

diet progression: a change in diet as a patient's tolerances permit.

dietary antioxidants: compounds typically found in plant foods that significantly decrease the adverse effects of oxidation on living tissues (e.g., vitamin E, vitamin C, and beta-carotene).

dietary fibers: a general term denoting in plant foods the polysaccharides cellulose, hemicellulose, pectins, gums, and mucilages, as well as the nonpolysaccharide lignins, which are not digested by human digestive enzymes, although some are digested by GI tract bacteria.

dietary folate equivalents (DFE): the amount of folate available to the body from naturally occurring sources, fortified foods, and supplements, accounting for differences in bioavailability from each source.

Dietary Reference Intakes (DRI): a set of values for the dietary nutrient intakes of healthy people in the United States and Canada; used for planning and assessing diets.

dietary supplements: products that are added to the diet and contain any of the following ingredients: a vitamin, a mineral, an herb or other botanical, an amino acid, a metabolite, a constituent, or an extract.

differentiation: the development of specific functions different from those of the original.

diffusion: movement of solutes from an area of high concentration to one of low concentration.

digestion: the process by which complex food particles are broken down to smaller, absorbable particles.

digestive system: all the organs and glands associated with the ingestion and digestion of food.

dipeptide: two amino acids bonded together.

disaccharides (dye-SACK-uh-rides): pairs of sugar units bonded together.

disclosure: the act of revealing pertinent information.

discretionary kcalories: the kcalories remaining in a person's energy allowance after consuming enough nutrient-dense foods to meet all nutrient needs for a day.

disordered eating: eating behaviors that are neither normal nor healthy, including restrained eating, fasting, binge eating, and purging.

distributive justice: the equitable distribution of resources.

diuresis (DYE-uh-REE-sis): increased urine production.

diuretics: drugs that promote urine production.

diverticulitis (dye-ver-tic-you-LYE-tis): an inflammation or infection involving diverticula.

diverticulosis (dye-ver-tic-you-LOH-sis): an intestinal condition characterized by the presence of small herniations (called diverticula) in the intestinal wall.

do-not-resuscitate (DNR) order: a request by a patient or surrogate to withhold cardiopulmonary resuscitation.

drink: volume of an alcoholic beverage containing about ½ ounce of pure ethanol; equivalent to 12 ounces of beer, 5 ounces of wine, or 1½ ounces of 80-proof distilled spirits such as gin, rum, vodka, and whiskey.

dumping syndrome: a cluster of symptoms that result from the rapid emptying of an osmotic load from the stomach into the small intestine.

duodenum (doo-oh-DEEN-um, doo-ODD-num): the top portion of the small intestine (about "12 fingers' breadth long" in ancient terminology).

durable power of attorney: a legal document (sometimes called a *health care proxy*) that gives legal authority to another (a *health care agent*) to make medical decisions in the event of incapacitation.

dyspepsia: symptoms of pain or discomfort in the upper abdominal area, often called "indigestion"; a symptom of illness rather than a disease itself.

dysphagia (dis-FAY-jah): difficulty swallowing.

dyspnea (DISP-nee-ah): shortness of breath.

eating disorder: a disturbance in eating behavior that jeopardizes a person's physical and psychological health.

eating pattern: customary intake of foods and beverages over time.

eclampsia (eh-KLAMP-see-ah)**:** a severe complication during pregnancy in which seizures occur.

edema (eh-DEEM-uh)**:** the swelling of body tissue caused by leakage of fluid from the blood vessels and accumulation of the fluid in the interstitial spaces.

eicosanoids (eye-KO-sa-noids)**:** 20-carbon molecules derived from dietary fatty acids that help to regulate blood pressure, blood clotting, and other body functions.

electron transport chain: the final pathway in energy metabolism that transports electrons from hydrogen to oxygen and captures the energy released in the bonds of a high-energy compound, ATP.

elemental formulas: enteral formulas that contain proteins and carbohydrates that are partially or fully hydrolyzed; also called *hydrolyzed, chemically defined*, or *monomeric formulas.*

embolism (EM-boh-lizm)**:** the obstruction of a blood vessel by an embolus, causing sudden tissue death.

embolus (EM-boh-lus)**:** an abnormal particle, such as a blood clot or air bubble, that travels in the blood.

embryo (EM-bree-oh)**:** the developing infant from two to eight weeks after conception.

emergency kitchens: programs that provide meals to be eaten on-site; often called *soup kitchens.*

emetic (em-ET-ic)**:** an agent that causes vomiting.

emphysema (EM-fih-ZEE-mah)**:** a progressive lung disease characterized by the breakdown of the lungs' elastic structure and destruction of the walls of the bronchioles and alveoli, reducing the surface area involved in respiration.

empty-kcalorie foods: a popular term used to denote foods that contribute energy but lack protein, vitamins, and minerals.

emulsifier: a substance that mixes with both fat and water and that disperses the fat in the water, forming an emulsion.

end-stage renal disease: an advanced stage of chronic kidney disease in which dialysis or a kidney transplant is necessary to sustain life.

endocrine: pertains to hormonal secretions into the blood.

endoscope: a flexible fiber optic tube used for viewing internal cavities of the body.

endothelial cells: cells that line the inner surfaces of blood vessels, lymphatic vessels, and body cavities.

energy density: a measure of the energy a food provides relative to the amount of food (kcalories per gram).

energy metabolism: all the reactions by which the body obtains and expends the energy from food.

energy-yielding nutrients: the nutrients that break down to yield energy the body can use. The three energy-yielding nutrients are carbohydrate, protein, and fat.

engorgement: overfilling of the breasts with milk.

enhanced water: water that is fortified with ingredients such as vitamins, minerals, protein, oxygen, or herbs.

enrichment: the addition to a food of nutrients to meet a specified standard; e.g., in the case of refined bread or cereal, the addition of thiamin, riboflavin, niacin, and folate in amounts approximately equivalent to, or higher than, those

originally present and iron in amounts to alleviate the prevalence of iron-deficiency anemia.

enteral (EN-ter-al) **nutrition:** the provision of nutrients using the GI tract; usually refers to the use of tube feedings.

enteric coated: refers to medications or enzyme preparations that are coated to withstand gastric acidity and dissolve only at the higher pH of the small intestine.

enterostomy (EN-ter-AH-stoe-mee)**:** an opening into the GI tract through the abdominal wall.

environmental tobacco smoke (ETS): the combination of exhaled smoke (mainstream smoke) and smoke from lighted cigarettes, pipes, or cigars (sidestream smoke) that enters the air and may be inhaled by other people.

enzymes: protein catalysts (compounds that facilitate chemical reactions without being changed in the process).

EPA: eicosapentaenoic (EYE-cosa-PENTA-ee-NO-ick) acid, an omega-3 fatty acid made from linolenic acid.

epiglottis (epp-ih-GLOTT-iss)**:** cartilage in the throat that guards the entrance to the trachea and prevents fluid or food from entering it when a person swallows.

epinephrine (EP-ih-NEFF-rin)**:** the major hormone that elicits the stress response; prescribed therapeutically to relax the bronchioles during allergy or asthma attacks.

epithelial (ep-i-THEE-lee-ul) **cells:** cells on the surface of the skin and mucous membranes.

epithelial tissue: tissue composing the layers of the body that serve as selective barriers between the body's interior and the environment (examples are the cornea, the skin, the respiratory lining, and the lining of the digestive tract).

ergogenic (ER-go-JEN-ick) **aids:** substances or techniques used in an attempt to enhance physical performance.

erythrocyte (er-REETH-ro-cite) **hemolysis** (he-MOLL-uh-sis)**:** rupture of the red blood cells, caused by vitamin E deficiency.

erythropoiesis (eh-RIH-throh-poy-EE-sis)**:** production of red blood cells within the bone marrow.

erythropoietin (eh-RIH-throh-POY-eh-tin)**:** a hormone produced by kidney cells that stimulates red blood cell production.

esophageal dysphagia: an inability to move food through the esophagus; usually caused by an obstruction or a motility disorder.

esophageal (ee-SOF-a-GEE-al) **sphincter:** a sphincter muscle at the upper or lower end of the esophagus; also called the **cardiac sphincter**.

esophagus (ee-SOFF-ah-gus)**:** the food pipe; the conduit from the mouth to the stomach.

essential amino acids: amino acids that the body cannot synthesize in amounts sufficient to meet physiological need; for human adults, these are: histidine (HISS-tuh-deen), isoleucine (eye-so-LOO-seen), leucine (LOO-seen), lysine (LYE-seen), methionine (meh-THIGH-oh-neen), phenylalanine (fen-il-AL-uh-neen), threonine (THREE-oh-neen), tryptophan (TRIP-toe-fane, TRIP-toe-fan), and valine (VAY-leen).

essential fatty acids: fatty acids that the body requires but cannot make and so must be obtained through the diet.

essential nutrients: nutrients a person must obtain from food because the body cannot make them for itself in sufficient quantities to meet physiological needs.

Estimated Average Requirements (EAR): the average daily nutrient intake levels estimated to meet the requirements of half of the healthy individuals in a given age and gender group;

used in nutrition research and policymaking and as the basis on which RDA values are set.

Estimated Energy Requirement (EER): the dietary energy intake level that is predicted to maintain energy balance in a healthy adult of a defined age, gender, weight, and physical activity level consistent with good health.

ethical: in accordance with accepted principles of right and wrong.

ethnic diets: foodways and cuisines typical of national origins, races, cultural heritages, or geographic locations.

exclusive breastfeeding: an infant's consumption of human milk with no supplementation of any type (no water, no juice, no nonhuman milk, and no foods) except for vitamins, minerals, and medications.

exercise: planned, structured, and repetitive bodily movement that promotes or maintains physical fitness.

exocrine: pertains to external secretions, such as those of the mucous membranes or the skin.

fasting hyperglycemia: hyperglycemia that typically develops in the early morning after an overnight fast of at least eight hours.

fat replacers: ingredients that replace some or all of the functions of fat in foods and may or may not provide energy.

fats: lipids that are solid at room temperature (70°F or 21°C).

fatty acids: organic compounds composed of a chain of carbon atoms with hydrogen atoms attached and an acid group at one end.

fatty liver: an accumulation of fat in liver tissue; also called *hepatic steatosis* (STEE-ah-TOE-sis).

fatty streaks: initial lesions of atherosclerosis that form on the artery wall, characterized by accumulations of foam cells, lipid material, and connective tissue.

fermentation: the anaerobic (without oxygen) breakdown of carbohydrates by microorganisms that releases small organic compounds along with carbon dioxide and energy.

fertility: the capacity of a woman to produce a normal ovum periodically and of a man to produce normal sperm; the ability to reproduce.

fetal alcohol spectrum disorders (FASD): a spectrum of physical, behavioral, and cognitive disabilities caused by prenatal alcohol exposure.

fetal alcohol syndrome (FAS): the cluster of symptoms seen in an infant or child whose mother consumed excessive alcohol during her pregnancy. FAS includes, but is not limited to, brain damage, growth retardation, mental retardation, and facial abnormalities.

fetus (FEET-us)**:** the developing infant from eight weeks after conception until its birth.

fibrinogen (fye-BRIN-oh-jen)**:** a liver protein that promotes blood clot formation.

filtrate: the substances that pass through the glomerulus and travel through the nephron's tubules, eventually forming urine.

fistulas (FIST-you-luz)**:** abnormal passages between organs or tissues (or between an internal organ and the body's surface) that permit the passage of fluids or secretions.

fitness: the characteristics that enable the body to perform physical activity; more broadly, the ability to meet routine physical demands with enough reserve energy to rise to a physical challenge; the body's ability to withstand stress of all kinds.

flatulence: the condition of having excessive intestinal gas, which causes abdominal discomfort.

flexibility: the capacity of the joints to move through a full range of motion; the ability to bend and recover without injury.

flora: the bacteria that normally reside in a person's body.

fluid and electrolyte balance: maintenance of the necessary amounts and types of fluid and minerals in each compartment of the body fluids.

foam cells: swollen cells in the artery wall that accumulate lipids.

follicle (FOLL-i-cul): a group of cells in the skin from which a hair grows.

food allergy: an adverse reaction to food that involves an immune response; also called *food-hypersensitivity reactions*.

food aversions: strong desires to avoid particular foods.

food banks: facilities that collect and distribute food donations to authorized organizations feeding the hungry.

food cravings: deep longings for particular foods.

food deserts: urban and rural low-income areas with limited access to affordable and nutritious foods.

food frequency questionnaire: a survey of foods routinely consumed. Some questionnaires ask about the types of food eaten and yield only qualitative information; others include questions about portions consumed and yield semiquantitative data as well.

food group plan: a diet-planning tool that sorts foods into groups based on nutrient content and then specifies that people should eat certain amounts of food from each group.

food insecurity: limited or uncertain access to foods of sufficient quality or quantity to sustain a healthy and active life (categorized as *low* or *very low food security*).

food intolerances: adverse reactions to foods or food additives that do not involve the immune system.

food pantries: community food collection programs that provide groceries to be prepared and eaten at home.

food poverty: hunger occurring when enough food exists in an area but some of the people cannot obtain it because they lack money, are being deprived for political reasons, live in a country at war, or suffer from other problems such as lack of transportation.

food record: a detailed log of food eaten during a specified time period, usually several days; also called a *food diary*. A food record may also include information regarding medications, disease symptoms, and physical activity.

food recovery: the collection of wholesome food for distribution to low-income people who are hungry.

food security: access to enough food to sustain a healthy and active life (categorized as *high* or *marginal food security*).

foodborne illness: illness transmitted to human beings through food and water, caused by either an infectious agent (foodborne infection) or a poisonous substance (foodborne intoxication); commonly known as food poisoning.

foodways: the eating habits and culinary practices of a people, region, or historical period.

fortification: the addition to a food of nutrients that were either not originally present or present in insignificant amounts.

free radicals: highly reactive chemical forms that can cause destructive changes in nearby compounds, sometimes setting up a chain reaction.

French units: units of measure for a feeding tube's outer diameter; 1 French equals 1/3 millimeter.

fructose: a monosaccharide; sometimes known as *fruit sugar*.

full liquid diet: a liquid diet that includes clear liquids, milk, yogurt, ice cream, and liquid nutritional supplements (such as Ensure).

functional foods: foods that have a potentially beneficial effect on health when consumed as part of a varied diet on a regular basis at effective levels.

futile: describes medical care that will not improve the medical circumstances of a patient.

galactose: a monosaccharide; part of the disaccharide lactose.

galactosemia (ga-LAK-toe-SEE-me-ah): an inherited disorder that impairs galactose metabolism; may cause damage to the brain, liver, kidneys, and lens in untreated patients.

gallbladder: the organ that stores and concentrates bile; when it receives the signal that fat is present in the duodenum, the gallbladder contracts and squirts bile through the bile duct into the duodenum.

gallstones: stones that form in the gallbladder from crystalline deposits of cholesterol or bilirubin; also called *choleliths*.

gangrene: death of tissue due to a deficient blood supply and/or infection.

gastrectomy (gah-STREK-ta-mie): the surgical removal of part of the stomach (partial gastrectomy) or the entire stomach (total gastrectomy).

gastric banding: a surgical means of producing weight loss by restricting stomach size with a constricting band.

gastric bypass: surgery that restricts stomach size and reroutes food from the stomach to the lower part of the small intestine; creates a chronic, lifelong state of malabsorption by preventing normal digestion and absorption of nutrients.

gastric decompression: the removal of stomach contents (such as GI secretions, air, or blood) in patients with motility problems or obstructions that prevent stomach emptying.

gastric glands: exocrine glands in the stomach wall that secrete gastric juice into the stomach.

gastric juice: the digestive secretion of the gastric glands containing a mixture of water, hydrochloric acid, and enzymes (principally pepsin, which acts on proteins, and lipase, which acts on emulsified fats).

gastric outlet obstruction: an obstruction that prevents the normal emptying of stomach contents into the duodenum.

gastric residual volume: the volume of formula and GI secretions remaining in the stomach after a previous feeding.

gastritis: inflammation of stomach tissue.

gastroesophageal reflux disease (GERD): condition characterized by frequent reflux (backward flow) of the stomach's acidic contents into the esophagus.

gastrointestinal (GI) tract: the digestive tract; the principal organs are the stomach and intestines.

gastrointestinal motility: spontaneous motion in the digestive tract accomplished by involuntary muscular contractions.

gastroparesis (GAS-tro-pah-REE-sis): delayed stomach emptying caused by nerve damage in stomach tissue.

gastrostomy (gah-STRAH-stoe-mee): an opening into the stomach through which a feeding tube can be passed.

gatekeeper: with respect to nutrition, a key person who controls other people's access to foods and thereby exerts a profound impact on their nutrition.

gene therapy: treatment for inherited disorders in which DNA sequences are introduced into the chromosomes of affected cells, prompting the cells to express the protein needed to correct the disease.

generic drug: a drug that lacks patent protection.

genetic counseling: support for families at risk of genetic disorders; involves diagnosis of disease, identification of inheritance patterns within the family, and review of reproductive options.

gestation: the period of about 40 weeks (three trimesters) from conception to birth; the term of a pregnancy.

gestational diabetes: glucose intolerance with first onset or first recognition during pregnancy.

gestational hypertension: high blood pressure that develops in the second half of pregnancy and usually resolves after childbirth.

ghrelin (GRELL-in): a hormone produced primarily by the stomach cells; it signals the hypothalamus of the brain to stimulate appetite and food intake.

gingiva (jin-JYE-va, JIN-jeh-va): the gums.

gingivitis (jin-jeh-VYE-tus): inflammation of the gums, characterized by redness, swelling, and bleeding.

glands: cells or groups of cells that secrete materials for special uses in the body.

glomerular filtration rate (GFR): the rate at which filtrate is formed within the kidneys, normally about 125 mL/min in healthy young adults.

glomerulus (gloh-MEHR-yoo-lus): a tuft of capillaries within the nephron that filters water and solutes from the blood as urine production begins (plural: *glomeruli*).

glucagon (GLOO-ka-gon): a hormone that is secreted by special cells in the pancreas in response to low blood glucose concentration and that elicits release of glucose from storage.

gluconeogenesis (gloo-co-nee-oh-GEN-ih-sis): the making of glucose from a noncarbohydrate source.

glucose: a monosaccharide; the sugar common to all disaccharides and polysaccharides; also called *blood sugar* in the body or *dextrose* in foods.

glucose polymers: compounds that supply glucose, not as single molecules, but linked in chains somewhat like starch. The objective is to attract less water from the body into the digestive tract.

glycated hemoglobin (HbA$_{1c}$): hemoglobin that has nonenzymatically attached to glucose; the level of HbA$_{1c}$ in the blood helps to diagnose diabetes and evaluate long-term glycemic control. Also called *glycosylated hemoglobin*.

glycemic (gly-SEE-mic): pertaining to blood glucose.

glycemic index (GI): a method of classifying foods according to their potential for raising blood glucose; low-GI foods are those with a lesser glycemic effect whereas high-GI foods have a greater glycemic effect.

glycemic response: the extent to which a food raises the blood glucose concentration and elicits an insulin response.

glycerol (GLISS-er-ol): an organic compound, three carbons long, that can form the backbone of triglycerides and phospholipids.

glycogen (GLY-co-gen): a polysaccharide composed of glucose, made and stored by liver and muscle tissues of human beings and animals as a storage form of glucose; not a significant food source of carbohydrate.

glycolysis (gligh-COLL-ih-sis): the metabolic breakdown of glucose to pyruvate.

glycosuria (GLY-co-SOOR-ee-ah): the presence of glucose in the urine.

gout (GOWT): a metabolic disorder characterized by elevated uric acid levels in the blood and urine and the deposition of uric acid in and around the joints, causing acute joint inflammation.

graft rejection: destruction of donor tissue by the recipient's immune system, which recognizes the donor cells as foreign.

graft-versus-host disease: a condition in which the immune cells in transplanted tissue (the graft) attack recipient (host) cells, leading to widespread tissue damage.

half-life: in blood tests, refers to the time it takes for the concentration of a substance to be reduced by half.

Hazard Analysis Critical Control Points (HACCP): a systematic plan to identify and correct potential microbial hazards in the manufacturing, distribution, and commercial use of food products; commonly referred to as "HASS-ip."

health: a range of states with physical, mental, emotional, spiritual, and social components. At a minimum, health means freedom from physical disease, mental disturbances, emotional distress, spiritual discontent, social maladjustment, and other negative states. At a maximum, health means *wellness*.

health care agent: a person given legal authority to make medical decisions for another in the event of incapacitation.

health care communities: living environments for people with chronic conditions, functional limitations, or need for supervision or assistance; they include assisted living facilities, group homes, short-term rehabilitation facilities, skilled nursing facilities, and hospice facilities.

health claims: statements that characterize the relationship between a nutrient or other substance in food and a disease or health-related condition.

Healthy People: a national public health initiative under the jurisdiction of the U.S. Department of Health and Human Services (DHHS) that identifies the most significant preventable threats to health and focuses efforts toward eliminating them.

heart failure: a condition characterized by the heart's inability to pump adequate blood to the body's cells, resulting in fluid accumulation in the tissues; also called *congestive heart failure*.

heat stroke: an acute and life-threatening reaction to heat buildup in the body.

Helicobacter pylori (H. pylori): a species of bacterium that colonizes the GI mucosa; a primary cause of gastritis and peptic ulcer disease.

helper T cells: lymphocytes that have a specific protein called CD4 on their surfaces and therefore are also known as *CD4+ T cells*; these are the cells most affected in HIV infection.

hematopoietic stem cell transplantation: transplantation of the stem cells that produce red blood cells and white blood cells; the stem cells are obtained from bone marrow (*bone marrow transplantation*) or circulating blood.

hematuria (HE-mah-TOO-ree-ah): blood in the urine.

hemodialysis (HE-moe-dye-AL-ih-sis): a treatment that removes fluids and wastes from the blood by passing the blood through a dialyzer.

hemofiltration: removal of fluid and solutes from the blood by pumping the blood across a membrane; no osmotic gradients are created during the process.

hemolytic (HE-moh-LIT-ick) **anemia:** the condition of having too few red blood cells as a result of erythrocyte hemolysis.

hemophilia (HE-moh-FEEL-ee-ah): an inherited bleeding disorder characterized by deficiency or malfunction of a plasma protein needed for clotting blood.

hemorrhagic (hem-oh-RAJ-ik) **disease:** the vitamin K–deficiency disease in which blood fails to clot.

hemorrhagic strokes: strokes caused by bleeding within the brain, which destroys or compresses brain tissue.

hepatic coma: loss of consciousness resulting from severe liver disease.

hepatic encephalopathy (en-sef-ah-LOP-ah-thie): a neurological complication of advanced liver disease that is characterized by changes in personality, mood, behavior, mental ability, and motor functions.

hepatic portal vein: the vein that collects blood from the GI tract and conducts it to capillaries in the liver.

hepatic vein: the vein that collects blood from the liver capillaries and returns it to the heart.

hepatitis (hep-ah-TYE-tis): inflammation of the liver.

hepatomegaly (HEP-ah-toe-MEG-ah-lee): enlargement of the liver.

hepcidin: an acute-phase protein involved in the regulation of iron metabolism.

herpes simplex virus: a common virus that can cause blisterlike lesions on the lips and in the mouth.

hGH (human growth hormone): a hormone produced by the brain's pituitary gland that regulates normal growth and development; also called *somatotropin*.

hiatal hernia: a condition in which the upper portion of the stomach protrudes above the diaphragm; most cases are asymptomatic.

high-density lipoproteins (HDL): the type of lipoproteins that transport cholesterol back to the liver from peripheral cells; composed primarily of protein.

high energy density: a high number of kcalories per unit weight of food; foods of high energy density are generally high in fat and low in water content.

high food security: food security with no indications of food-access problems or limitations.

high-fructose corn syrup: a widely used commercial kcaloric sweetener made by adding enzymes to cornstarch to convert a portion of its glucose molecules into sweet-tasting fructose.

high-quality proteins: dietary proteins containing all the essential amino acids in relatively the same amounts that human beings require.

high-risk pregnancy: a pregnancy characterized by risk factors that make it likely the birth will be surrounded by problems such as premature delivery, difficult birth, retarded growth, birth defects, and early infant death.

histamine-2 receptor blockers: a class of drugs that suppress acid secretion by inhibiting receptors on acid-producing cells; commonly called *H2 blockers*. Examples include cimetidine (Tagamet), ranitidine (Zantac), and famotidine (Pepcid).

homeostasis (HOME-ee-oh-STAY-sis): the maintenance of constant internal conditions (such as chemistry, temperature, and blood pressure) by the body's control system.

homocysteine: an amino acid produced during the conversion of methionine to cysteine; blood homocysteine levels are influenced by intakes of folate, vitamin B$_{12}$, and vitamin B$_6$.

hormones: chemical messengers that are secreted by a variety of glands in the body in response to altered conditions; each travels to one or more target tissues or organs and elicits specific responses to restore normal conditions.

hourly sweat rate: the amount of weight lost plus fluid consumed during exercise per hour.

human genome (GEE-nome): the complete set of genetic material (DNA) in a human being.

human immunodeficiency virus (HIV): the virus that causes acquired immune deficiency syndrome (AIDS); it destroys immune cells and progressively impedes the body's ability to fight infections and certain cancers.

hunger: the physiological need to eat, experienced as a drive to obtain food; an unpleasant sensation that demands relief.

hydrochloric acid (HCl): an acid composed of hydrogen and chloride atoms; normally produced by the gastric glands.

hydrogenation (high-dro-gen-AY-shun): a chemical process by which hydrogen atoms are added to monounsaturated or polyunsaturated fats to reduce the number of double bonds, making the fats more saturated (solid) and more resistant to oxidation (protecting against rancidity); produces *trans*-fatty acids.

hyperactivity: inattentive and impulsive behavior that is more frequent and severe than is typical of others of a similar age; professionally called *attention deficit/hyperactivity disorder (ADHD)*.

hypercalcemia (HIGH-per-kal-SEE-me-ah): elevated serum calcium levels.

hypercalciuria (HIGH-per-kal-see-YOO-ree-ah): elevated urinary calcium levels.

hypercapnia (high-per-CAP-nee-ah): excessive carbon dioxide in the blood.

hyperglycemia: elevated blood glucose concentrations. Normal fasting plasma glucose levels are less than 100 mg/dL. Fasting plasma glucose levels between 100 and 125 mg/dL suggest prediabetes; values of 126 mg/dL and above suggest diabetes.

hyperinsulinemia: abnormally high levels of insulin in the blood.

hyperkalemia (HIGH-per-ka-LEE-me-ah): elevated serum potassium levels.

hypermetabolism: a higher-than-normal metabolic rate.

hyperosmolar: having an abnormally high osmolarity.

hyperosmolar hyperglycemic syndrome: a condition of extreme hyperglycemia associated with dehydration, hyperosmolar blood, and altered mental status; sometimes called the *hyperosmolar hyperglycemic nonketotic state*.

hyperoxaluria (HIGH-per-ox-ah-LOO-ree-ah): elevated urinary oxalate levels.

hyperphosphatemia (HIGH-per-fos-fa-TEE-me-ah): elevated serum phosphate levels.

hyperthermia: an above-normal body temperature.

hypertonic formula: a formula with an osmolality greater than that of blood serum.

hypertriglyceridemia: elevated blood triglyceride levels.

hypertrophy (high-PURR-tro-fee): an increase in size (for example, of a muscle) in response to use.

hypoalbuminemia: low plasma albumin concentrations. Plasma proteins such as albumin help to maintain fluid balance within the blood; thus, low levels contribute to edema.

hypocaloric feedings: reduced-kcalorie feedings that usually include sufficient protein and micronutrients to maintain nitrogen balance and prevent malnutrition.

hypochlorhydria (HIGH-poe-clor-HIGH-dree-ah): abnormally low gastric acid secretions.

hypoglycemia: abnormally low blood glucose concentrations. In diabetes, hypoglycemia is treated when plasma glucose falls below 70 mg/dL.

hypokalemia (HIGH-po-ka-LEE-me-ah): low serum potassium levels.

hyponatremia (HIGH-poh-na-TREE-mee-ah): an abnormally low concentration of sodium in the blood.

hypothalamus (high-po-THAL-ah-mus): a brain center that controls activities such as maintenance of water balance, regulation of body temperature, and control of appetite.

hypothermia: a below-normal body temperature.

hypoxemia (high-pock-SEE-me-ah): a low level of oxygen in the blood.

hypoxia (high-POCK-see-ah): a low amount of oxygen in body tissues.

ileocecal (ill-ee-oh-SEEK-ul) **valve:** the sphincter separating the small and large intestines.

ileostomy (ill-ee-AH-stoe-me): a surgical passage through the abdominal wall into the ileum.

ileum (ILL-ee-um): the last segment of the small intestine.

immunity: the body's ability to defend itself against diseases.

implantation: the stage of development in which the blastocyst embeds itself in the wall of the uterus and begins to develop; occurs during the first 2 weeks after conception.

inborn error of metabolism: an inherited trait (one that is present at birth) that causes the absence, deficiency, or malfunction of a protein that has a critical metabolic role.

indirect calorimetry: a method of estimating resting energy expenditure by measuring a person's oxygen consumption and carbon dioxide production.

inflammation: an immunological response to cellular injury characterized by an increase in white blood cells.

inflammatory response: a group of nonspecific immune responses to infection or injury.

informed consent: a patient's or caregiver's agreement to undergo a treatment that has been adequately disclosed.

inorganic: not containing carbon or pertaining to living organisms.

insoluble fibers: the tough, fibrous structures of fruits, vegetables, and grains; indigestible food components that do not dissolve in water.

insulin: a pancreatic hormone that regulates glucose metabolism; it promotes glucose uptake and storage; its actions are countered mainly by the hormone *glucagon*.

insulin resistance: subnormal response to insulin in muscle, adipose, and liver cells.

intermittent feedings: delivery of about 250 to 400 milliliters of formula over 30 to 45 minutes.

intestinal adaptation: physiological changes in the small intestine that increase its absorptive capacity after resection.

intestinal flora: the bacterial inhabitants of the GI tract.

intestinal juice: the secretion of the intestinal glands; contains enzymes for the digestion of carbohydrate and protein and a minor enzyme for fat digestion.

intractable: not easily managed or controlled.

intractable vomiting: vomiting that is not easily managed or controlled.

intradialytic parenteral nutrition: the infusion of nutrients during hemodialysis, often providing amino acids, dextrose, lipids, and some trace minerals.

intrinsic factor: a substance secreted by the stomach cells that binds with vitamin B_{12} in the small intestine to aid in the absorption of vitamin B_{12}.

irritable bowel syndrome: an intestinal disorder of unknown cause that disturbs the functioning of the large intestine; symptoms include abdominal pain, flatulence, diarrhea, and constipation.

ischemia (iss-KEE-mee-a): inadequate blood supply within a tissue due to obstructed blood flow.

ischemic strokes: strokes caused by the obstruction of blood flow to brain tissue.

isotonic formula: a formula with an osmolality similar to that of blood serum (about 300 milliosmoles per kilogram).

jaundice (JAWN-dis): yellow discoloration of the skin and eyes due to an accumulation of bilirubin, a breakdown product of hemoglobin that normally exits the body via bile secretions.

jejunostomy (JEH-ju-NAH-stoe-mee): an opening into the jejunum through which a feeding tube can be passed.

jejunum (je-JOON-um): the first two-fifths of the small intestine beyond the duodenum.

Joint Commission: a nonprofit organization that sets standards for health care performance and safety and confers accreditation to health care organizations and programs that meet those standards.

Kaposi's (kah-POH-seez) **sarcoma:** a common cancer in HIV-infected persons that is characterized by lesions in the skin, lungs, and GI tract.

kcalorie (energy) control: management of food energy intake.

kcalorie counts: estimates of food energy (and often, protein) consumed by patients for one or more days.

keratin (KERR-uh-tin): a water-insoluble protein; the normal protein of hair and nails.

keratomalacia (KARE-ah-toe-ma-LAY-shuh): softening of the cornea that leads to irreversible blindness; a sign of severe vitamin A deficiency

ketoacidosis (KEY-to-ass-ih-DOE-sis): an acidosis (lowering of blood pH) that results from the excessive production of ketone bodies.

ketone bodies: acidic, water-soluble products of fat metabolism within the liver; accumulate in the blood when abnormally high amounts of fatty acids are released from adipose tissue; also known as *ketones*.

ketonuria (KEY-to-NOOR-ee-ah): the presence of ketone bodies in the urine.

ketosis (key-TOE-sis): the combination of a high blood concentration of ketone bodies (*ketonemia*) and ketone bodies in the urine (*ketonuria*).

kidney stones: crystalline masses that form in the urinary tract; also called *renal calculi* or *nephrolithiasis*.

kwashiorkor (kwash-ee-OR-core or kwash-ee-or-CORE): severe malnutrition characterized by failure to grow and develop, edema, changes in the pigmentation of the hair and skin, fatty liver, anemia, and apathy.

lactate: a compound produced during the breakdown of glucose in anaerobic metabolism.

lactation: production and secretion of breast milk for the purpose of nourishing an infant.

lacto-ovo vegetarian diet: an eating pattern that includes milk, milk products, eggs, vegetables, grains, legumes, fruits, and nuts; excludes meat, poultry, and seafood.

lacto-vegetarian diet: an eating pattern that includes milk, milk products, vegetables, grains, legumes, fruits, and nuts; excludes meat, poultry, seafood, and eggs.

lactose: a disaccharide composed of glucose and galactose; commonly known as *milk sugar*.

lactose intolerance: intolerance to lactose-containing foods due to the loss or reduction of intestinal lactase; symptoms may include flatulence, bloating, and diarrhea.

laparoscopic: pertaining to procedures that use a laparoscope (a narrow surgical telescope, usually with a video camera attached) inserted through a small incision for internal examination or surgery.

laparoscopic weight-loss surgery: a weight-loss surgery procedure in which surgeons gain access to the abdomen via several small incisions. A tiny video camera is inserted through one of the incisions and surgical instruments through the others. The surgeons watch their work on a large-screen monitor.

lapses: periods of returning to old habits.

large intestine or **colon** (COAL-un): the lower portion of intestine that completes the digestive process; its segments are the ascending colon, the transverse colon, the descending colon, and the sigmoid colon.

lecithins: one type of phospholipid.

legumes (lay-GYOOMS, LEG-yooms): plants of the bean and pea family with seeds that are rich in protein compared with other plant-derived foods.

length: the distance from the top of the head to the soles of the feet while a person is recumbent (lying down).

leptin: a hormone produced by fat cells under the direction of the (*ob*) gene; it decreases appetite and increases energy expenditure.

letdown reflex: the reflex that forces milk to the front of the breast when the infant begins to nurse.

life expectancy: the average number of years lived by people in a given society.

life span: the maximum number of years of life attainable by a member of a species.

limiting amino acid: an essential amino acid that is present in dietary protein in the shortest supply relative to the amount needed for protein synthesis in the body.

linoleic acid: a polyunsaturated omega-6 fatty acid that is essential for human beings.

linolenic acid: a polyunsaturated omega-3 fatty acid that is essential for human beings.

lipids: a family of compounds that includes triglycerides (fats and oils), phospholipids, and sterols. Lipids are characterized by their insolubility in water.

lipodystrophy (LIP-oh-DIS-tro-fee): abnormalities in body fat and fat metabolism that may result from drug treatments for HIV infection. The accumulation of abdominal fat is sometimes called *protease paunch*.

lipomas (lih-POE-muz): benign tumors composed of fatty tissue.

lipoprotein lipase (LPL): an enzyme mounted on the surface of fat cells (and other cells) that hydrolyzes triglycerides in the blood into fatty acids and glycerol for absorption into the cells.

lipoproteins: clusters of lipids associated with proteins that serve as transport vehicles for lipids in the lymph and blood.

listeriosis: a serious foodborne infection that can cause severe brain infection or death in a fetus or newborn; caused by the bacterium *Listeria monocytogenes*, which is found in soil and water.

liver: a body organ with multiple metabolic functions; it processes and stores nutrients, produces bile, synthesizes plasma proteins and hormones, and detoxifies drugs and alcohol.

longevity: long duration of life.

low birthweight (LBW): a birthweight less than 5½ pounds (2500 grams); indicates probable poor health in the newborn and poor nutrition status of the mother during pregnancy.

low-density lipoproteins (LDL): the type of lipoproteins derived from VLDL as cells remove triglycerides from them; they carry cholesterol and triglycerides from the liver to the cells of the body and are composed primarily of cholesterol.

low food security: food insecurity characterized by reduced dietary quality, variety, or desirability but with little or no indication of reduced food intake.

low-microbial diet: a diet that contains foods that are unlikely to be contaminated with bacteria or other microbes.

low-risk pregnancy: a pregnancy characterized by factors that make it likely the birth will be normal and the infant healthy.

lymph (LIMF)**:** the body fluid found in lymphatic vessels; consists of all the constituents of blood except red blood cells.

lymphatic system: a loosely organized system of vessels and ducts that conveys the products of digestion toward the heart.

macrobiotic diet: an eating pattern composed mostly of whole grains, beans, and certain vegetables; taken to extremes, macrobiotic diets can compromise nutrient status.

macrocytic anemia: large-cell anemia; also known as *megaloblastic anemia.*

macrophages: immune cells that engulf pathogens and cellular debris; they are derived from white blood cells called *monocytes.*

macrosomia (MAK-roh-SOH-mee-ah)**:** the condition of having an abnormally large body; in infants, refers to birth weights of 4000 grams (8 pounds 13 ounces) and above.

macrovascular complications: disorders that affect large blood vessels, including the coronary arteries and arteries of the limbs.

macula: a small, oval, yellowish region in the center of the retina that provides the sharp, straight-ahead vision so critical to reading and driving.

macular (MACK-you-lar) **degeneration:** deterioration of the macular area of the eye that can lead to loss of central vision and eventual blindness.

maleficence (mah-LEF-eh-sense)**:** the act of doing evil or harm.

malignant (ma-LIG-nent)**:** describes a cancerous cell or tumor, which can injure healthy tissue and spread cancer to other regions of the body.

malnutrition: any condition caused by deficient or excess energy or nutrient intake or by an imbalance of nutrients.

maltose: a disaccharide composed of two glucose units; sometimes known as *malt sugar.*

marasmus (ma-RAZZ-mus)**:** severe malnutrition characterized by poor growth, dramatic weight loss, loss of body fat and muscle, and apathy.

marginal food security: food security with one or two indications of food-access problems but with little or no change in food intake.

mast cells: cells within connective tissue that produce and release histamine.

mastitis: infection of a breast.

mechanical ventilation: life-sustaining treatment in which a mechanical ventilator is used to substitute for a patient's failing lungs.

mechanically altered diets: diets that contain foods that have been mechanically altered to modify texture or consistency; foods may be liquid, pureed, ground, chopped, minced, or tenderized.

medical nutrition therapy: nutrition care provided by a registered dietitian nutritionist; includes assessing nutrition status, diagnosing nutrition problems, and providing nutrition care.

medium-chain triglycerides (MCT): triglycerides with fatty acids that are 8 to 10 carbons in length. MCT do not require digestion and can be absorbed in the absence of lipase or bile.

megaloblastic anemia: anemia characterized by large (macrocytic), immature red blood cells, as occurs in folate or vitamin B_{12} deficiency; also called *macrocytic anemia.*

metabolic stress: a disruption in the body's chemical environment due to the effects of disease or injury; characterized by changes in metabolic rate, heart rate, blood pressure, hormonal status, and nutrient metabolism.

metabolic syndrome: a cluster of interrelated disorders, including abdominal obesity, insulin resistance, high blood pressure, and abnormal blood lipids, which together increase risk of diabetes and cardiovascular disease; also known as *insulin resistance syndrome* or *syndrome X.*

metabolism: the sum total of all the chemical reactions that go on in living cells.

metabolites: products of metabolism; compounds produced by a biochemical pathway.

metastasize (meh-TAS-tah-size)**:** to spread from one part of the body to another; refers to cancer cells.

methotrexate: an anticancer drug that inhibits cell division; it closely resembles the B vitamin folate, which is needed for DNA synthesis, and works by blocking activity of the enzyme that converts folate to its active form.

microcytic anemia: anemia characterized by small, hypochromic (pale) red blood cells, as occurs in iron deficiency.

microvascular complications: disorders that affect small blood vessels, including those in the retina and kidneys.

microvilli (MY-cro-VILL-ee or MY-cro-VILL-eye)**:** tiny, hairlike projections on each cell of every villus that can trap nutrient particles and transport them into the cells (singular form is microvillus).

moderate-intensity physical activity: physical activity that requires some increase in breathing and/or heart rate and expends 3.5 to 7 kcalories per minute (e.g., walking at a speed of 3 to 4.5 miles per hour).

moderation: the provision of enough, but not too much, of a substance.

modified diet: a diet that contains foods altered in texture, consistency, or nutrient content or that includes or omits specific foods; may also be called a *therapeutic diet.*

modular formulas: enteral formulas prepared in the hospital from *modules* that contain single macronutrients; used for people with unique nutrient needs.

monosaccharides (mon-oh-SACK-uh-rides)**:** single sugar units.

monounsaturated fatty acid (MUFA): a fatty acid that has one point of unsaturation; for example, the oleic acid found in olive oil.

mouth: the oral cavity containing the tongue and teeth.

mucous membrane: membrane composed of mucus-secreting cells that lines the surfaces of body tissues.

mucus (MYOO-cuss)**:** a mucopolysaccharide (a relative of carbohydrate) secreted by cells of the stomach wall that protects the cells from exposure to digestive juices (and other destructive agents). (The noun is *mucus*; the adjective is *mucous*.)

muscle endurance: the ability of a muscle to contract repeatedly within a given time without becoming exhausted.

muscle power: the product of force generation (strength) and movement velocity (speed); the speed at which a given amount of exertion is completed.

muscle strength: the ability of muscles to work against resistance.

mutation: an heritable change in the DNA sequence of a gene.

myocardial (MY-oh-CAR-dee-al) **infarction** (in-FARK-shun)**, or MI:** death of heart muscle caused by a sudden reduction in coronary blood flow; also called a *heart attack* or *cardiac arrest.*

nasoduodenal (ND) feeding tube: a feeding tube placed into the duodenum via the nose.

nasoenteric feeding tube: a feeding tube placed into the GI tract via the nose; most often refers to *nasoduodenal* and *nasojejunal* feeding routes (also known as *nasointestinal* feeding routes).

nasogastric (NG) feeding tube: a feeding tube placed into the stomach via the nose.

nasojejunal (NJ) feeding tube: a feeding tube placed into the jejunum via the nose.

naturally occurring sugars: sugars that are not added to a food but are present as its original constituents, such as the sugars of fruit or milk.

nephron (NEF-ron)**:** the functional unit of the kidneys, consisting of a glomerulus and tubules.

nephrotic (neh-FROT-ik) **syndrome:** a syndrome caused by significant urinary protein losses (more than 3 to 3½ grams daily), as a result of severe glomerular damage.

nephrotoxic: toxic to the kidneys.

neural tube: the embryonic tissue that later forms the brain and spinal cord.

neural tube defects (NTD): malformations of the brain, spinal cord, or both that occur during embryonic development; the two main types are *spina bifida* and *anencephaly.*

neurofibrillary tangles: snarls of the thread-like strands that extend from the nerve cells, commonly found in the brains of people with Alzheimer's dementia.

neurons: nerve cells; the structural and functional units of the nervous system. Neurons initiate and conduct nerve transmissions.

neutropenia: a low white blood cell (neutrophil) count, which increases susceptibility to infection.

niacin equivalents (NE): the amount of niacin present in food, including the niacin that can theoretically be made from tryptophan, its precursor, present in the food.

night blindness: the slow recovery of vision after exposure to flashes of bright light at night; an early symptom of vitamin A deficiency.

nitrogen balance: the amount of nitrogen consumed (N in) as compared with the amount of nitrogen excreted (N out) in a given period of time.

nonessential amino acids: amino acids that the body can synthesize.

nonnutritive sweeteners: synthetic or natural food additives that offer sweet flavor but with negligible or no kcalories per serving; also called *artificial sweeteners, intense sweeteners, noncaloric sweeteners,* and *very-low-calorie sweeteners.*

nonpathogenic: not capable of causing disease.

nursing bottle tooth decay: extensive tooth decay due to prolonged tooth contact with formula, milk, fruit juice, or other carbohydrate-rich liquid offered to an infant in a bottle.

nutrient claims: statements that characterize the quantity of a nutrient in a food.

nutrient density: a measure of the nutrients a food provides relative to the energy it provides. The more nutrients and the fewer kcalories, the higher the nutrient density.

nutrient profiling: ranking foods based on their nutrient composition.

nutrients: substances obtained from food and used in the body to provide energy and structural materials and to serve as regulating agents to promote growth, maintenance, and repair; may also reduce the risks of some diseases.

nutrition: the science of foods and the nutrients and other substances they contain, and of their ingestion, digestion, absorption, transport, metabolism, interaction, storage, and excretion. A broader definition includes the study of the environment and of human behavior as it relates to these processes.

nutrition care plans: strategies for meeting an individual's nutritional needs.

nutrition care process: a systematic approach used by dietetics professionals to evaluate and treat nutrition-related problems.

nutrition screening: a brief assessment of health-related variables to identify patients who are malnourished or at risk for malnutrition.

nutrition support: the delivery of nutrients using a feeding tube or intravenous infusions.

nutrition support teams: health care professionals responsible for the provision of nutrients by tube feeding or intravenous infusion.

nutritive sweeteners: sweeteners that yield energy, including both the sugars and the sugar alcohols.

obese: having too much body fat with adverse health effects; BMI 30 or more.

obesogenic (oh-BEES-oh-JEN-ick) **environment:** all the factors surrounding a person that promote weight gain, such as an increased food intake—especially of unhealthy choices—and decreased physical activity.

oils: lipids that are liquid at room temperature (70°F or 21°C).

olestra: a synthetic fat made from sucrose and fatty acids that provides zero kcalories per gram; also known as *sucrose polyester*.

oliguria (OL-lih-GOO-ree-ah): an abnormally low amount of urine, often less than 400 mL/day.

omega-3 fatty acids: polyunsaturated fatty acids in which the endmost double bond is three carbons back from the end of the carbon chain (e.g., linolenic acid).

omega-6 fatty acid: a polyunsaturated fatty acid with its endmost double bond six carbons back from the end of its carbon chain (e.g., linoleic acid).

oncotic pressure: the pressure exerted by fluid on one side of a membrane as a result of osmosis.

open feeding system: a formula delivery system that requires the transfer of the formula from its original packaging to a feeding container.

opportunistic infections: infections caused by microorganisms that normally do not cause disease in healthy people but are damaging to persons with compromised immune function.

opsin (OP-sin): the protein portion of the visual pigment molecule.

oral glucose tolerance test: a test that evaluates a person's ability to tolerate an oral glucose load.

oral mucositis: inflammation of the oral mucosa; signs may include swelling, redness, mouth sores, bleeding, or ulcerations in mucosal tissue.

organic: in chemistry, substances or molecules containing carbon-carbon bonds or carbon-hydrogen bonds. The four organic nutrients are carbohydrate, fat, protein, and vitamins.

orogastric feeding tube: a feeding tube inserted into the stomach through the mouth. This method is often used to feed infants because a nasogastric tube may hinder the infant's breathing.

oropharyngeal dysphagia (OR-oh-fah-ren-JEE-al diss-FAY-jah): an inability to transfer food from the mouth and pharynx to the esophagus; . usually caused by a neurological or muscular disorder.

osmolality (OZ-moe-LAL-ih-tee): the concentration of osmotically active solutes in a solution, expressed as milliosmoles (mOsm) per kilogram of solvent. Osmotically active solutes affect *osmosis*, the movement of water across semipermeable membranes.

osmolarity: the concentration of osmotically active solutes in a solution, expressed as milliosmoles per liter of solution (mOsm/L). *Osmolality* (mOsm/kg) is an alternative measure used to describe a solution's osmotic properties.

osmosis: movement of water across a membrane toward the side where solutes are more concentrated.

osteoarthritis: a painful, chronic disease of the joints that occurs when the cushioning cartilage in a joint breaks down; joint structure is usually altered, with loss of function; also called *degenerative arthritis*.

osteomalacia (os-tee-oh-mal-AY-shuh): a bone disease characterized by softening of the bones that occurs most often in adults with renal failure or malabsorption disorders; symptoms include bending of the spine and bowing of the legs.

osteoporosis: (os-tee-oh-pore-OH-sis): literally, porous bones; reduced density of the bones, also known as *adult bone loss*.

outbreaks: two or more cases of a similar illness resulting from the ingestion of a common food.

overload: an extra physical demand placed on the body; an increase in the frequency, duration, or intensity of an activity.

overnutrition: overconsumption of food energy or nutrients sufficient to cause disease or increased susceptibility to disease; a form of malnutrition.

overweight: body weight greater than the weight range that is considered healthy; BMI 25.0 to 29.9.

ovo-vegetarian diet: an eating pattern that includes eggs, vegetables, grains, legumes, fruits, and nuts; excludes meat, poultry, seafood, and milk and milk products.

ovum (OH-vum): the female reproductive cell, capable of developing into a new organism upon fertilization; commonly referred to as an egg.

oxidation (ok-si-DEY-shun): the process of a substance combining with oxygen.

pancreas: a gland that (1) secretes digestive enzymes and juices into the duodenum and (2) secretes hormones into the blood that help to maintain glucose homeostasis.

pancreatic (pank-ree-AT-ic) **juice:** the exocrine secretion of the pancreas, containing enzymes for the digestion of carbohydrate, fat, and protein; it enters the small intestine through the pancreatic duct.

paracentesis (pah-rah-sen-TEE-sis): a surgical puncture of a body cavity with an aspirator to draw out excess fluid.

parathyroid hormone: a protein hormone secreted by the parathyroid glands that helps to regulate serum concentrations of calcium and phosphate.

parenteral (par-EN-ter-al) **nutrition:** the intravenous provision of nutrients that bypasses the GI tract.

partial vegetarian diet: a term sometimes used to describe an eating pattern that includes seafood, poultry, eggs, milk and milk products, vegetables, grains, legumes, fruits, and nuts; excludes or strictly limits certain meats, such as red meat. Also called *semi-vegetarian*.

pasteurization: heat processing of food that inactivates some, but not all, microorganisms in the food; not a sterilization process.

pathogenic: capable of causing disease.

pathogens (PATH-oh-jens): microorganisms capable of producing disease.

patient autonomy: a principle of self-determination, such that patients (or surrogate decision makers) are free to choose the medical interventions that are acceptable to them, even if they choose to refuse interventions that may extend their lives.

pellagra (pell-AY-gra): the niacin-deficiency disease. Symptoms include the "4 Ds": diarrhea, dermatitis, dementia, and, ultimately, death.

pepsin: a protein-digesting enzyme (gastric protease) in the stomach; its precursor, pepsinogen, is converted to pepsin by the action of stomach acid.

peptic ulcer: an open sore in the gastrointestinal mucosa; may develop in the esophagus, stomach, or duodenum.

periodontal disease: disease that involves the connective tissue that supports the teeth.

periodontitis: inflammation or degeneration of the tissues that support the teeth.

periodontium: the tissues that support the teeth, including the gums, cementum (bonelike material covering the dentin layer of the tooth), periodontal ligament, and underlying bone.

peripheral artery disease: impaired blood flow in the arteries of the legs; may cause pain or discomfort in the legs and feet.

peripheral blood smear: a blood sample spread on a glass slide and stained for analysis under a microscope; circulating blood is used.

peripheral parenteral nutrition (PPN): the infusion of nutrient solutions into peripheral veins, usually a vein in the arm or back of the hand.

peripheral vascular disease: a condition characterized by impaired blood circulation in the limbs.

peripheral veins: the small-diameter veins that carry blood from the limbs.

peristalsis (peri-STALL-sis): successive waves of involuntary muscular contractions passing along the walls of the GI tract that push the contents along.

peritoneal (PEH-rih-toe-NEE-al) **dialysis:** a treatment that removes fluids and wastes from the blood by using the body's peritoneal membrane as a filter.

peritonitis: inflammation of the peritoneal membrane, which lines the abdominal cavity.

pernicious (per-NISH-us) **anemia:** a blood disorder that reflects a vitamin B$_{12}$ deficiency caused by lack of intrinsic factor and characterized by large, immature red blood cells and damage to the nervous system.

persistent vegetative state: a vegetative mental state (loss of awareness and thinking ability) resulting from brain injury that persists for at least one month.

PES statement: a statement that describes a nutrition problem in a format that includes the problem (P), the etiology or cause (E), and the signs and symptoms (S).

pH: the concentration of hydrogen ions; the lower the pH, the stronger the acid.

phagocytes (FAG-oh-sites): immune cells (neutrophils and macrophages) that have the ability to engulf and destroy antigens.

pharynx (FAIR-inks): the passageway leading from the nose and mouth to the larynx and esophagus, respectively.

phenylketonuria (FEN-il-KEY-toe-NU-ree-ah) or **PKU:** an inherited disorder characterized by a defect in the enzyme phenylalanine hydroxylase, which normally converts the essential amino acid phenylalanine to the amino acid tyrosine.

phlebitis (fleh-BYE-tiss)**:** inflammation of a vein.

phospholipids: one of the three main classes of lipids; compounds that are similar to triglycerides but have *choline* (or another compound) and a phosphorus-containing acid in place of one of the fatty acids.

physical activity: bodily movement produced by muscle contractions that substantially increase energy expenditure.

physiological age: a person's age as estimated from her or his body's health and probable life expectancy.

phytochemicals (FIGH-toe-CHEM-ih-cals)**:** compounds in plants that confer color, taste, and other characteristics; some are bioactive food components in functional foods.

pigment: a molecule capable of absorbing certain wavelengths of light so that it reflects only those that we perceive as a certain color.

placenta (pla-SEN-tuh)**:** an organ that develops inside the uterus early in pregnancy, in which maternal and fetal blood circulate in close proximity and exchange materials. The fetus receives nutrients and oxygen across the placenta; the mother's blood picks up carbon dioxide and other waste materials to be excreted via her lungs and kidneys.

plant sterols: steroid compounds produced in plants; those added to commercial food products are extracted from soybeans and pine tree oils and can be hydrogenated to produce *plant stanols*.

plaque (PLACK)**:** an accumulation of fatty deposits, fibrous connective tissue, and smooth muscle cells in blood vessels. See also: *dental plaque*.

plasminogen activator inhibitor-1: a protein that promotes blood clotting by inhibiting blood clot degradation within blood vessels.

polydipsia (POL-ee-DIP-see-ah)**:** excessive thirst.

polypeptide: 10 or more amino acids bonded together.

polyphagia (POL-ee-FAY-jee-ah)**:** excessive appetite or hunger.

polysaccharides: long chains of monosaccharide units arranged as starch, glycogen, or fiber.

polyunsaturated fatty acids (PUFA): fatty acids with two or more points of unsaturation (e.g., linoleic acid has two such points, and linolenic acid has three).

polyuria (POL-ee-YOOR-ee-ah)**:** excessive urine production.

portal hypertension: elevated blood pressure in the hepatic portal vein due to obstructed blood flow through the liver and a greater inflow of portal blood.

portion size: the quantity of food served or eaten at one meal or snack; *not* a standard amount.

prebiotics: indigestible substances in foods that stimulate the growth of nonpathogenic bacteria within the large intestine.

precursors: compounds that can be converted into other compounds; with regard to vitamins, compounds that can be converted into active vitamins; also known as *provitamins*.

prediabetes: the state of having plasma glucose levels that are higher than normal but not high enough to be diagnosed as diabetes (100–125 mg/dL when fasting or 140–199 mg/dL when measured two hours after ingesting 75 grams of glucose); occurs in individuals who have metabolic defects that often lead to type 2 diabetes.

preeclampsia (PRE-ee-KLAMP-see-ah)**:** a condition characterized by hypertension and protein in the urine during pregnancy.

preformed vitamin A: vitamin A in its active form.

pregame meal: a meal eaten three to four hours before athletic competition.

prenatal supplements: nutrient supplements specifically designed to provide the nutrients needed during pregnancy, particularly folate, iron, and calcium, without excesses or unneeded constituents.

pressure gradient: the change in pressure over a given distance. In dialysis, a pressure gradient is created between the blood and the dialysate.

pressure sores: regions of skin and tissue that are damaged due to prolonged pressure on the affected area by an external object, such as a bed, wheelchair, or cast; vulnerable areas of the body include buttocks, hips, and heels. Also called *decubitus* (deh-KYU-bih-tus) *ulcers*.

probiotics: live microorganisms provided in foods and dietary supplements for the purpose of preventing or treating disease.

protein digestibility: a measure of the amount of amino acids absorbed from a given protein intake.

protein-energy malnutrition (PEM): a state of malnutrition characterized by depletion of tissue proteins and energy stores, usually accompanied by micronutrient deficiencies.

protein isolates: proteins that have been isolated from foods.

protein turnover: the continuous breakdown and synthesis of body proteins involving the recycling of amino acids.

proteins: compounds made from strands of amino acids composed of carbon, hydrogen, oxygen, and nitrogen atoms. Some amino acids also contain sulfur atoms.

proteinuria (PRO-teen-NOO-ree-ah)**:** the presence of protein in the urine.

proton-pump inhibitors: a class of drugs that inhibit the enzyme that pumps hydrogen ions (protons) into the stomach. Examples include omeprazole (Prilosec) and lansoprazole (Prevacid).

pruritis: itchy skin.

puberty: the period in life in which a person becomes physically capable of reproduction.

purines (PYOO-reens)**:** products of nucleotide metabolism that degrade to uric acid.

pyloric (pie-LORE-ic) **sphincter:** the circular muscle that separates the stomach from the small intestine and regulates the flow of partially digested food into the small intestine; also called **pylorus** or **pyloric valve**.

pyruvate (PIE-roo-vate)**:** a 3-carbon compound that plays a key role in energy metabolism.

quality of life: a person's perceived physical and mental well-being.

radiation enteritis: inflammation of intestinal tissue caused by radiation therapy.

radiation therapy: the use of X-rays, gamma rays, or atomic particles to destroy cancer cells.

rancid: the term used to describe fats when they have deteriorated, usually by oxidation.

rebound hyperglycemia: hyperglycemia that results from the release of counterregulatory hormones following nighttime hypoglycemia; also called the **Somogyi effect**.

Recommended Dietary Allowances (RDA): a set of values reflecting the average daily amounts of nutrients considered adequate to meet the known nutrient needs of practically all healthy people in a particular life stage and gender group; a goal for dietary intake by individuals.

rectum: the muscular terminal part of the intestine, extending from the sigmoid colon to the anus.

RED-S (relative energy deficiency in sport): a syndrome of impaired physiological function including, but not limited to, metabolic rate, menstrual function, bone health, immunity, protein synthesis, and cardiovascular health caused by relative energy deficiency.

refeeding syndrome: a group of metabolic abnormalities that may result from aggressive refeeding in severely malnourished persons; characterized by shifts in fluid and electrolyte levels that can lead to organ failure and other complications.

refined grain: a product from which the bran, germ, and husk have been removed, leaving only the endosperm.

reflux esophagitis: inflammation in the esophagus resulting from the reflux of acidic stomach contents.

registered dietitian nutritionist: a food and nutrition expert who has completed the education and training specified by the Academy of Nutrition and Dietetics (or Dietitians of Canada), including a bachelor's degree in nutrition or dietetics, a supervised internship, and a national registration examination; also called *registered dietitian*.

regular diet: a diet that includes all foods and meets the nutrient needs of healthy people; may also be called a *standard diet* or *house diet*.

renal (REE-nal)**:** pertaining to the kidneys.

renal colic: the intense pain that occurs when a kidney stone passes through the ureter; the pain typically begins in the back and intensifies as the stone travels toward the bladder.

renal osteodystrophy: a bone disorder that develops in patients with chronic kidney disease as a result of increased secretion of parathyroid hormone, reduced serum calcium, acidosis, and impaired vitamin D activation in the kidneys.

renal threshold: the blood concentration of a substance that exceeds the kidneys' capacity for reabsorption, causing the substance to be passed into the urine.

requirement: the lowest continuing intake of a nutrient that will maintain a specified criterion of adequacy.

resection: the surgical removal of part of an organ or body structure.

residue: material left in the intestine after digestion; includes mostly dietary fiber and undigested starches and proteins.

resistance training: physical activity that develops muscle strength, power, endurance, and mass using resistance provided by body weight, free weights, weight machines, elastic bands, or other objects; also called *weight training*.

resistant starches: starches that escape digestion and absorption in the small intestine of healthy people.

resistin (re-ZIST-in)**:** a hormone produced by adipose cells that promotes insulin resistance.

respiratory failure: a potentially life-threatening condition in which inadequate respiratory function impairs gas exchange between the air and circulating blood, resulting in abnormal levels of tissue gases.

respiratory stress: a condition characterized by abnormal oxygen and carbon dioxide levels in body tissues due to abnormal gas exchange between the air and blood.

resting metabolic rate (RMR): a measure of the energy use of a person at rest in a comfortable setting—similar to the BMR but with less stringent criteria for recent food intake and physical activity.

reticulocytes: immature red blood cells released into blood by bone marrow.

retina (RET-in-uh)**:** the layer of light-sensitive nerve cells lining the back of the inside of the eye; consists of rods and cones.

retinol activity equivalents (RAE): a measure of vitamin A activity; the amount of retinol that the body will derive from a food containing preformed retinol or its precursor beta-carotene.

retinol-binding protein (RBP): the specific protein responsible for transporting retinol. Measurement of the blood concentration of RBP is a sensitive test of vitamin A status.

rheumatoid arthritis: a disease of the immune system involving painful inflammation of the joints and related structures.

rhodopsin (ro-DOP-sin)**:** a light-sensitive pigment of the retina; contains the retinal form of vitamin A and the protein opsin.

ribose: a naturally occurring 5-carbon sugar needed for the synthesis of ATP.

rickets: the vitamin D–deficiency disease in children.

rooting reflex: a reflex that causes an infant to turn toward whichever cheek is touched, in search of a nipple.

saliva: the secretion of the salivary glands; contains salivary amylase.

salivary glands: exocrine glands that secrete saliva into the mouth.

sarcopenia (SAR-koh-PEE-nee-ah)**:** age-related loss of skeletal muscle mass, muscle strength, and muscle function.

satiation (say-she-AY-shun)**:** the feeling of satisfaction and fullness that occurs during a meal and halts eating.

satiety: the feeling of fullness and satisfaction that occurs after a meal and inhibits eating until the next meal.

saturated fatty acid: a fatty acid carrying the maximum possible number of hydrogen atoms (having no points of unsaturation).

screen time: sedentary time spent using an electronic device, such as a television, computer, or video game player.

scurvy: the vitamin C–deficiency disease.

sedentary: physically inactive (literally "sitting down a lot").

segmentation: a periodic squeezing or partitioning of the intestine by its circular muscles that both mixes and slowly pushes the contents along.

self-efficacy: a person's belief in his or her ability to succeed in an undertaking.

self-monitoring of blood glucose: home monitoring of blood glucose levels using a glucose meter.

semipermeable membrane: a membrane that allows some, but not all, particles to pass through.

senile dementia: the loss of brain function beyond the normal loss of physical adeptness and memory that occurs with aging.

senile plaques: clumps of the protein fragment beta-amyloid on the nerve cells, commonly found in the brains of people with Alzheimer's dementia.

sepsis: a whole-body inflammatory response caused by infection; characterized by signs and symptoms similar to those of systemic inflammatory response syndrome.

set-point theory: the theory that the body tends to maintain a certain weight by means of its own internal controls.

severe acute malnutrition (SAM): malnutrition caused by recent severe food restriction; characterized in children by underweight for height (wasting).

shear stress: a stress that occurs sideways against a surface rather than perpendicular to a surface.

shock-wave lithotripsy: a nonsurgical procedure that uses high-amplitude sound waves to fragment gallstones or kidney stones.

shock: a severe reduction in blood flow that deprives the body's tissues of oxygen and nutrients; characterized by reduced blood pressure, raised heart and respiratory rates, and muscle weakness.

short bowel syndrome: the malabsorption syndrome that follows resection of the small intestine; characterized by inadequate absorptive capacity in the remaining intestine.

sinusoids: the small capillary-like passages that carry blood through liver tissue.

Sjögren's (SHOW-grenz) **syndrome:** an autoimmune disease characterized by the destruction of secretory glands, resulting in dry mouth and dry eyes.

skinfold measure: a clinical estimate of total body fatness in which the thickness of a fold of skin on the back of the arm (over the triceps muscle), below the shoulder blade (subscapular), or in other places is measured with a caliper.

sludge: literally, a semisolid mass. Biliary sludge is made up of mucus, cholesterol crystals, and bilirubin granules.

small intestine: a 10-foot length of small-diameter intestine that is the major site of digestion of food and absorption of nutrients; its segments are the duodenum, jejunum, and ileum.

soaps: chemical compounds formed from fatty acids and positively charged minerals.

sodium bicarbonate (baking soda): a white crystalline powder that is used to buffer acid that accumulates in the muscles and blood during high-intensity exercise.

solid fats: fats that are not usually liquid at room temperature; commonly found in most foods derived from animals and vegetable oils that have been hydrogenated; typically contain more saturated and *trans* fats than most oils.

soluble fibers: indigestible food components that readily dissolve in water and often impart gummy or gel-like characteristics to foods. An example is pectin from fruit, which is used to thicken jellies.

Special Supplemental Nutrition Program for Women, Infants, and Children (WIC): a high-quality, cost-effective health care and nutrition services program administered by the U.S. Department of Agriculture for low-income women, infants, and children who are nutritionally at risk. WIC provides supplemental foods, nutrition education, and referrals to health care and other social services.

specialized formulas: enteral formulas for patients with specific illnesses; also called *disease-specific formulas* or *specialty formulas*.

sphincter (SFINK-ter)**:** a circular muscle surrounding, and able to close, a body opening.

spina (SPY-nah) **bifida** (BIFF-ih-dah)**:** one of the most common types of neural tube defects; characterized by the incomplete closure of the spinal cord and its bony encasement.

standard formulas: enteral formulas that contain mostly intact proteins and polysaccharides; also called *polymeric formulas*.

starch: a plant polysaccharide composed of glucose and digestible by human beings.

steatohepatitis (STEE-ah-to-HEP-ah-TYE-tis)**:** liver inflammation that is associated with fatty liver.

steatorrhea (stee-AH-tor-REE-ah)**:** excessive fat in the stool due to fat malabsorption; characterized by stools that are loose, frothy, and foul smelling due to a high fat content.

sterile: free of microorganisms such as bacteria.

sterols: one of the main classes of lipids; includes cholesterol, vitamin D, and the sex hormones (such as testosterone).

stoma (STOE-ma)**:** a surgically created opening in a body tissue or organ.

stomach: a muscular, elastic, saclike portion of the digestive tract that grinds and churns swallowed food, mixing it with acid and enzymes to form chyme.

stress fractures: bone damage or breaks caused by stress on bone surfaces during exercise.

stress response: the chemical and physical changes that occur within the body during stress.

stricture: abnormal narrowing of a passageway; often due to inflammation, scarring, or a congenital abnormality.

stroke: a sudden injury to brain tissue resulting from impaired blood flow through an artery that supplies blood to the brain; also called a *cerebrovascular accident*.

structure-function claims: statements that describe how a product may affect a structure or function of the body; for example, "calcium builds strong bones."

struvite (STROO-vite)**:** crystals of magnesium ammonium phosphate.

subcutaneous (sub-cue-TAY-nee-us)**:** beneath the skin.

subcutaneous fat: fat stored directly under the skin.

sucrose: a disaccharide composed of glucose and fructose; commonly known as *table sugar, beet sugar,* or *cane sugar.*

sugar alcohols: sugarlike compounds in the chemical family *alcohol* derived from fruits or manufactured from carbohydrates (e.g., maltitol, mannitol, sorbitol, isomalt, lactitol, xylitol); they are absorbed more slowly than other sugars, are metabolized differently, and do not elevate the risk of dental caries.

surrogate: a substitute; a person who takes the place of another.

sushi: vinegar-flavored rice and raw or cooked seafood, typically wrapped in seaweed and stuffed with colorful vegetables.

syringe: a device used for injecting medications; consists of a hypodermic needle attached to a hollow tube with a plunger inside.

systemic (sih-STEM-ic)**:** relating to the entire body.

systemic inflammatory response syndrome (SIRS): a whole-body inflammatory response caused by severe illness or trauma; characterized by raised heart and respiratory rates, abnormal white blood cell counts, and fever.

TCA cycle or tricarboxylic (try-car-box-ILL-ick) **acid cycle:** a series of metabolic reactions that break down molecules of acetyl CoA to carbon dioxide and hydrogen atoms; also called the *Krebs cycle.*

teratogenic (ter-AT-oh-jen-ik)**:** causing abnormal fetal development and birth defects.

thermic effect of food: an estimation of the energy required to process food (digest, absorb, transport, metabolize, and store ingested nutrients).

thrombosis (throm-BOH-sis)**:** the formation or presence of a blood clot in blood vessels. A *coronary thrombosis* occurs in a coronary artery, and a *cerebral thrombosis* occurs in an artery that supplies blood to the brain.

thrombus: a blood clot formed within a blood vessel that remains attached to its place of origin.

tocopherol (tuh-KOFF-er-ol)**:** a general term for several chemically related compounds, one of which has vitamin E activity.

Tolerable Upper Intake Levels (UL): a set of values reflecting the highest average daily nutrient intake levels that are likely to pose no risk of toxicity to almost all healthy individuals in a particular life stage and gender group.

tolerance level: the maximum amount of residue permitted in a food when a pesticide is used according to the label directions.

total nutrient admixture (TNA): a parenteral solution that contains dextrose, amino acids, and lipids; also called a **3-in-1 solution** or an **all-in-one solution.**

total parenteral nutrition (TPN): the infusion of nutrient solutions into a central vein.

training: regular practice of an activity, which leads to physical adaptations of the body with improvement in flexibility, strength, or endurance.

***trans*-fatty acids:** fatty acids in which the hydrogen atoms next to the double bond are on opposite sides of the carbon chain.

transient ischemic attacks (TIAs): brief ischemic strokes that cause short-term neurological symptoms.

transjugular intrahepatic portosystemic shunt: a passage within the liver that connects a portion of the portal vein to the hepatic vein using a stent; access to the liver is gained via the jugular vein in the neck.

transnasal feeding tube: a feeding tube that is inserted through the nose.

traveler's diarrhea: nausea, vomiting, and diarrhea caused by consuming food or water contaminated by any of several organisms, most commonly, *E. coli, Shigella, Campylobacter jejuni,* and *Salmonella.*

triglycerides (try-GLISS-er-rides)**:** one of the main classes of lipids; the chief form of fat in foods and the major storage form of fat in the body; composed of glycerol with three fatty acids attached.

trimester: a period representing one-third of the term of gestation (about 13–14 weeks).

tripeptide: three amino acids bonded together.

tube feedings: liquid formulas delivered through a tube placed in the stomach or intestine.

tubules: tubelike structures of the nephron that process filtrate during urine production; they are surrounded by capillaries that reabsorb substances retained by tubule cells.

tumor: an abnormal tissue mass that has no physiological function; also called a *neoplasm* (NEE-oh-plazm). Tumors may be malignant (cancerous) or benign (noncancerous).

type 1 diabetes: diabetes that is characterized by absolute insulin deficiency, usually resulting from the autoimmune destruction of pancreatic beta cells.

type 2 diabetes: diabetes that is characterized by insulin resistance coupled with insufficient insulin secretion.

ulcerative colitis (ko-LYE-tis)**:** an inflammatory bowel disease that involves the rectum and colon; the inflammation affects the mucosa and submucosa of the intestinal wall.

ultrafiltration: removal of fluids and solutes from the blood by using pressure to transfer the blood across a semipermeable membrane.

umbilical (um-BIL-ih-cul) **cord:** the ropelike structure through which the fetus's veins and arteries reach the placenta; the route of nourishment and oxygen into the fetus and the route of waste disposal from the fetus.

undernutrition: underconsumption of food energy or nutrients severe enough to cause disease or increased susceptibility to disease; a form of malnutrition.

underweight: body weight lower than the weight range that is considered healthy; BMI below 18.5.

unsaturated fatty acid: a fatty acid with one or more points of unsaturation where hydrogen atoms are missing (includes monounsaturated and polyunsaturated fatty acids).

urea (yoo-REE-uh)**:** the principal nitrogen-excretion product of protein metabolism.

urea kinetic modeling: a method of determining the adequacy of dialysis treatment by calculating the urea clearance from blood.

uremia (you-REE-me-ah)**:** the accumulation of nitrogenous and various other waste products in the blood; may also be used to indicate the toxic state that results when wastes are retained in the blood.

uremic syndrome: the cluster of disorders caused by inadequate kidney function; complications include fluid, electrolyte, and hormonal imbalances; altered heart function; neuromuscular disturbances; and other metabolic derangements.

USDA Food Patterns: the USDA's food group plan for ensuring dietary adequacy that assigns foods to five major food groups.

uterus (YOO-ter-us)**:** the womb, the muscular organ within which the infant develops before birth.

varices (VAH-rih-seez)**:** abnormally dilated blood vessels (singular: *varix*).

variety (dietary): consumption of a wide selection of foods within and among the major food groups (the opposite of monotony).

vegan diet: an eating pattern that includes only plant-based foods: vegetables, grains, legumes, fruits, seeds, and nuts; also called *strict vegetarian.*

vegetarian diet: a general term used to describe an eating pattern that includes plant-based foods and eliminates some or all animal-derived foods.

vein: a vessel that carries blood back to the heart.

very-low-density lipoproteins (VLDL): lipoproteins, composed primarily of triglycerides, that transport triglycerides from the liver to other tissues; in clinical practice, VLDL are commonly referred to as *blood triglycerides.*

very low food security: food insecurity with multiple indications of disrupted eating patterns and reduced food intake.

vigorous-intensity physical activity: physical activity that requires a large increase in breathing and/or heart rate and expends more than 7 kcalories per minute (e.g., walking at a very brisk pace [>4.5 miles per hour] or running at a pace of at least 5 miles per hour).

villi (VILL-ee or VILL-eye)**:** fingerlike projections from the folds of the small intestine (singular form is *villus*).

visceral fat: fat stored within the abdominal cavity in association with the internal abdominal organs, as opposed to fat stored directly under the skin (subcutaneous fat); also called *intra-abdominal fat.*

viscous: having a gel-like consistency.

vitamin A: a fat-soluble vitamin with three chemical forms: *retinol* (the alcohol form), *retinal* (the aldehyde form), and *retinoic acid* (the acid form).

vitamin D$_2$: vitamin D derived from plants in the diet; also called *ergocalciferol* (ER-go-kal-SIF-er-ol).

vitamin D$_3$: vitamin D derived from animals in the diet or made in the skin from 7-dehydrocholesterol, a precursor of cholesterol, with the help of sunlight; also called *cholecalciferol* (KO-lee-kal-SIF-er-ol).

vitamins: essential, nonkaloric, organic nutrients needed in tiny amounts in the diet.

VO$_2$ max: the maximum rate of oxygen consumption by an individual (measured at sea level).

voluntary activities: the component of a person's daily energy expenditure that involves conscious and deliberate muscular work: walking, lifting, climbing, and other physical activities.

waist circumference: a measurement used to assess a person's abdominal fat.

wasting: the gradual atrophy (loss) of body tissues; associated with protein-energy malnutrition or chronic illness.

wean: to gradually replace breast milk with infant formula or other foods appropriate to an infant's diet.

weight cycling: repeated rounds of weight loss and subsequent regain, with reduced ability to lose weight with each attempt; also called *yo-yo dieting.*

wellness: maximum well-being; the top range of health states; the goal of the person who strives toward realizing his or her full potential physically, mentally, emotionally, spiritually, and socially.

Wernicke-Korsakoff syndrome: severe thiamin deficiency in alcohol abusers; symptoms include disorientation, loss of short-term memory, jerky eye movements, and staggering gait.

wheat gluten (GLU-ten)**:** a family of water-insoluble proteins in wheat; includes the gliadin (GLY-ah-din) fractions that are toxic to persons with celiac disease.

whole grains: grains or foods made from them that contain all the essential parts and naturally occurring nutrients of the entire grain seed (except the inedible husk).

xerophthalmia (zer-off-THAL-mee-uh)**:** progressive blindness caused by inadequate mucus production due to severe vitamin A deficiency.

xerosis (zee-ROW-sis)**:** abnormal drying of the skin and mucous membranes; a sign of vitamin A deficiency

xerostomia (ZEE-roh-STOE-me-ah)**:** dry mouth caused by reduced salivary flow.

zygote (ZY-goat)**:** the product of the union of ovum and sperm; a fertilized ovum.

Index

Daily Values (DV) for Food Labels

The Daily Values (DV) are standards developed by the Food and Drug Administration (FDA) for use on food labels. The values are based on 2000 kcalories a day for adults and children 4 years and older.

Nutrient	Current DV	Proposed DV
Vitamins		
Biotin	300 μg	30 μg
Choline	550 mg	550 mg
Folate	400 μg	400 μg DFE
Niacin	20 mg NE	16 mg NE
Pantothenic acid	10 mg	5 mg
Riboflavin	1.7 mg	1.3 mg
Thiamin	1.5 mg	1.2 mg
Vitamin A	1500 μg (5000 IU)	900 μg RAE
Vitamin B$_6$	2 mg	1.7 mg
Vitamin B$_{12}$	6 μg	2.4 μg
Vitamin C	60 mg	90 mg
Vitamin D	10 μg (400 IU)	20 μg
Vitamin E (α-tocopherol)	20 mg (30 IU)	15 mg
Vitamin K	80 μg	120 μg
Minerals		
Calcium	1000 mg	1300 mg
Chloride	3400 mg	2300 mg
Chromium	120 μg	35 μg
Copper	2 mg	0.9 mg
Iodine	150 μg	150 μg
Iron	18 mg	18 mg
Magnesium	400 mg	420 mg
Manganese	2 mg	2.3 mg
Molybdenum	75 μg	45 μg
Phosphorus	1000 mg	1250 mg
Potassium	3500 mg	4700 mg
Selenium	70 μg	55 μg
Sodium	2400 mg	2300 mg
Zinc	15 mg	11 mg

Food Component	Amount	Calculation Factors
Fat	65 g	30% of kcalories
Saturated fat	20 g	10% of kcalories
Cholesterol	300 mg	Same regardless of kcalories
Carbohydrate (total)	300 g	60% of kcalories
Fiber[a]	25 g	11.5 g per 1000 kcalories
Protein	50 g	10% of kcalories

[a]For fiber, the proposed value is 28 g (14 g per 1000 kcalories).

Glossary of Nutrient Measures

kcal: kcalories; a unit by which energy is measured (Chapter 1 provides more details).

g: grams; a unit of weight equivalent to about 0.03 ounces.

mg: milligrams; one-thousandth of a gram.

µg: micrograms; one-millionth of a gram.

IU: international units; an old measure of vitamin activity determined by biological methods (as opposed to new measures that are determined by direct chemical analyses). For those still using IU, the following factors can be used for conversions.
- For vitamin A, 1 IU = 0.3 µg retinol, 3.6 µg β-carotene, or 7.2 µg other vitamin A carotenoids.
- For vitamin D, 1 IU = 0.025 µg cholecalciferol.
- For vitamin E, 1 IU = 0.67 mg α-tocopherol.

mg NE: milligrams niacin equivalents; a measure of niacin activity (Chapter 8 provides more details).
- 1 NE = 1 mg niacin.
    = 60 mg tryptophan (an amino acid).

µg DFE: micrograms dietary folate equivalents; a measure of folate activity (Chapter 8 provides more details).
- 1 µg DFE = 1 µg food folate.
    = 0.6 µg fortified food or supplement folate.
    = 0.5 µg supplement folate taken on an empty stomach.

µg RAE: micrograms retinol activity equivalents; a measure of vitamin A activity (Chapter 8 provides more details).
- 1 µg RE = 1 µg retinol.
    = 12 µg β-carotene.
    = 24 µg other vitamin A carotenoids.

mmol: millimoles; one-thousanth of a mole, the molecular weight of a substance. To convert mmol to mg, multiply by the atomic weight of the substance.
- For sodium, mmol = 23 = mg Na.
- For chloride, mmol = 35.5 = mg Cl.
- For sodium chloride, mmol = 58.5 = mg NaCl.

Body Mass Index (BMI)

Height	18	19	20	21	22	23	24	25	26	27	28	29	30	31	32	33	34	35	36	37	38	39	40
								Body Weight (pounds)															
4'10"	86	91	96	100	105	110	115	119	124	129	134	138	143	148	153	158	162	167	172	177	181	186	191
4'11"	89	94	99	104	109	114	119	124	128	133	138	143	148	153	158	163	168	173	178	183	188	193	198
5'0"	92	97	102	107	112	118	123	128	133	138	143	148	153	158	163	168	174	179	184	189	194	199	204
5'1"	95	100	106	111	116	122	127	132	137	143	148	153	158	164	169	174	180	185	190	195	201	206	211
5'2"	98	104	109	115	120	126	131	136	142	147	153	158	164	169	175	180	186	191	196	202	207	213	218
5'3"	102	107	113	118	124	130	135	141	146	152	158	163	169	175	180	186	191	197	203	208	214	220	225
5'4"	105	110	116	122	128	134	140	145	151	157	163	169	174	180	186	192	197	204	209	215	221	227	232
5'5"	108	114	120	126	132	138	144	150	156	162	168	174	180	186	192	198	204	210	216	222	228	234	240
5'6"	112	118	124	130	136	142	148	155	161	167	173	179	186	192	198	204	210	216	223	229	235	241	247
5'7"	115	121	127	134	140	146	153	159	166	172	178	185	191	198	204	211	217	223	230	236	242	249	255
5'8"	118	125	131	138	144	151	158	164	171	177	184	190	197	203	210	216	223	230	236	243	249	256	262
5'9"	122	128	135	142	149	155	162	169	176	182	189	196	203	209	216	223	230	236	243	250	257	263	270
5'10"	126	132	139	146	153	160	167	174	181	188	195	202	209	216	222	229	236	243	250	257	264	271	278
5'11"	129	136	143	150	157	165	172	179	186	193	200	208	215	222	229	236	243	250	257	265	272	279	286
6'0"	132	140	147	154	162	169	177	184	191	199	206	213	221	228	235	242	250	258	265	272	279	287	294
6'1"	136	144	151	159	166	174	182	189	197	204	212	219	227	235	242	250	257	265	272	280	288	295	302
6'2"	141	148	155	163	171	179	186	194	202	210	218	225	233	241	249	256	264	272	280	287	295	303	311
6'3"	144	152	160	168	176	184	192	200	208	216	224	232	240	248	256	264	272	279	287	295	303	311	319
6'4"	148	156	164	172	180	189	197	205	213	221	230	238	246	254	263	271	279	287	295	304	312	320	328
6'5"	151	160	168	176	185	193	202	210	218	227	235	244	252	261	269	277	286	294	303	311	319	328	336
6'6"	155	164	172	181	190	198	207	216	224	233	241	250	259	267	276	284	293	302	310	319	328	336	345

Underweight	Healthy Weight	Overweight	Obese
(<18.5)	(18.5–24.9)	(25–29.9)	(≥30)

Find your height along the left-hand column and look across the row until you find the number that is closest to your weight. The number at the top of that column identifies your BMI. Chapter 6 describes how BMI correlates with disease risks and defines obesity. The area shaded in blue represents healthy weight ranges.

Recommended Dietary Allowances (RDA) and Adequate Intakes (AI) for Vitamins

Age (yr)	Thiamin RDA (mg/day)	Riboflavin RDA (mg/day)	Niacin RDA (mg/day)[a]	Biotin AI (µg/day)	Pantothenic acid AI (mg/day)	Vitamin B_6 RDA (mg/day)	Folate RDA (µg/day)[b]	Vitamin B_{12} RDA (µg/day)	Choline AI (mg/day)	Vitamin C RDA (mg/day)	Vitamin A RDA (µg/day)[c]	Vitamin D RDA (µg/day)[d]	Vitamin E RDA (mg/day)[e]	Vitamin K AI (µg/day)
Infants														
0–0.5	0.2	0.3	2	5	1.7	0.1	65	0.4	125	40	400	10	4	2.0
0.5–1	0.3	0.4	4	6	1.8	0.3	80	0.5	150	50	500	10	5	2.5
Children														
1–3	0.5	0.5	6	8	2	0.5	150	0.9	200	15	300	15	6	30
4–8	0.6	0.6	8	12	3	0.6	200	1.2	250	25	400	15	7	55
Males														
9–13	0.9	0.9	12	20	4	1.0	300	1.8	375	45	600	15	11	60
14–18	1.2	1.3	16	25	5	1.3	400	2.4	550	75	900	15	15	75
19–30	1.2	1.3	16	30	5	1.3	400	2.4	550	90	900	15	15	120
31–50	1.2	1.3	16	30	5	1.3	400	2.4	550	90	900	15	15	120
51–70	1.2	1.3	16	30	5	1.7	400	2.4	550	90	900	15	15	120
>70	1.2	1.3	16	30	5	1.7	400	2.4	550	90	900	20	15	120
Females														
9–13	0.9	0.9	12	20	4	1.0	300	1.8	375	45	600	15	11	60
14–18	1.0	1.0	14	25	5	1.2	400	2.4	400	65	700	15	15	75
19–30	1.1	1.1	14	30	5	1.3	400	2.4	425	75	700	15	15	90
31–50	1.1	1.1	14	30	5	1.3	400	2.4	425	75	700	15	15	90
51–70	1.1	1.1	14	30	5	1.5	400	2.4	425	75	700	15	15	90
>70	1.1	1.1	14	30	5	1.5	400	2.4	425	75	700	20	15	90
Pregnancy														
≤18	1.4	1.4	18	30	6	1.9	600	2.6	450	80	750	15	15	75
19–30	1.4	1.4	18	30	6	1.9	600	2.6	450	85	770	15	15	90
31–50	1.4	1.4	18	30	6	1.9	600	2.6	450	85	770	15	15	90
Lactation														
≤18	1.4	1.6	17	35	7	2.0	500	2.8	550	115	1200	15	19	75
19–30	1.4	1.6	17	35	7	2.0	500	2.8	550	120	1300	15	19	90
31–50	1.4	1.6	17	35	7	2.0	500	2.8	550	120	1300	15	19	90

Note: For all nutrients, values for infants are AI. The glossary on the inside back cover defines units of nutrient measure.
[a] Niacin recommendations are expressed as niacin equivalents (NE), except for recommendations for infants younger than 6 months, which are expressed as preformed niacin.
[b] Folate recommendations are expressed as dietary folate equivalents (DFE).
[c] Vitamin A recommendations are expressed as retinol activity equivalents (RAE).
[d] Vitamin D recommendations are expressed as cholecalciferol and assume an absence of adequate exposure to sunlight.
[e] Vitamin E recommendations are expressed as α-tocopherol.

Recommended Dietary Allowances (RDA) and Adequate Intakes (AI) for Minerals

Age (yr)	Sodium AI (mg/day)	Chloride AI (mg/day)	Potassium AI (mg/day)	Calcium RDA (mg/day)	Phosphorus RDA (mg/day)	Magnesium RDA (mg/day)	Iron RDA (mg/day)	Zinc RDA (mg/day)	Iodine RDA (µg/day)	Selenium RDA (µg/day)	Copper RDA (µg/day)	Manganese AI (mg/day)	Fluoride AI (mg/day)	Chromium AI (µg/day)	Molybdenum RDA (µg/day)
Infants															
0–0.5	120	180	400	200	100	30	0.27	2	110	15	200	0.003	0.01	0.2	2
0.5–1	370	570	700	260	275	75	11	3	130	20	220	0.6	0.5	5.5	3
Children															
1–3	1000	1500	3000	700	460	80	7	3	90	20	340	1.2	0.7	11	17
4–8	1200	1900	3800	1000	500	130	10	5	90	30	440	1.5	1.0	15	22
Males															
9–13	1500	2300	4500	1300	1250	240	8	8	120	40	700	1.9	2	25	34
14–18	1500	2300	4700	1300	1250	410	11	11	150	55	890	2.2	3	35	43
19–30	1500	2300	4700	1000	700	400	8	11	150	55	900	2.3	4	35	45
31–50	1500	2300	4700	1000	700	420	8	11	150	55	900	2.3	4	35	45
51–70	1300	2000	4700	1000	700	420	8	11	150	55	900	2.3	4	30	45
>70	1200	1800	4700	1200	700	420	8	11	150	55	900	2.3	4	30	45
Females															
9–13	1500	2300	4500	1300	1250	240	8	8	120	40	700	1.6	2	21	34
14–18	1500	2300	4700	1300	1250	360	15	9	150	55	890	1.6	3	24	43
19–30	1500	2300	4700	1000	700	310	18	8	150	55	900	1.8	3	25	45
31–50	1500	2300	4700	1000	700	320	18	8	150	55	900	1.8	3	25	45
51–70	1300	2000	4700	1200	700	320	8	8	150	55	900	1.8	3	20	45
>70	1200	1800	4700	1200	700	320	8	8	150	55	900	1.8	3	20	45
Pregnancy															
≤18	1500	2300	4700	1300	1250	400	27	12	220	60	1000	2.0	3	29	50
19–30	1500	2300	4700	1000	700	350	27	11	220	60	1000	2.0	3	30	50
31–50	1500	2300	4700	1000	700	360	27	11	220	60	1000	2.0	3	30	50
Lactation															
≤18	1500	2300	5100	1300	1250	360	10	13	290	70	1300	2.6	3	44	50
19–30	1500	2300	5100	1000	700	310	9	12	290	70	1300	2.6	3	45	50
31–50	1500	2300	5100	1000	700	320	9	12	290	70	1300	2.6	3	45	50

NOTE: For all nutrients, values for infants are AI. The glossary on the inside back cover defines units of nutrient measure.

Tolerable Upper Intake Levels (UL) for Vitamins

Age (yr)	Niacin (mg/day)[a]	Vitamin B_6 (mg/day)	Folate (µg/day)[a]	Choline (mg/day)	Vitamin C (mg/day)	Vitamin A (µg/day)[b]	Vitamin D (µg/day)	Vitamin E (mg/day)[c]
Infants								
0–0.5	—	—	—	—	—	600	25	—
0.5–1	—	—	—	—	—	600	38	—
Children								
1–3	10	30	300	1000	400	600	63	200
4–8	15	40	400	1000	650	900	75	300
9–13	20	60	600	2000	1200	1700	100	600
Adolescents								
14–18	30	80	800	3000	1800	2800	100	800
Adults								
19–70	35	100	1000	3500	2000	3000	100	1000
>70	35	100	1000	3500	2000	3000	100	1000
Pregnancy								
≤18	30	80	800	3000	1800	2800	100	800
19–50	35	100	1000	3500	2000	3000	100	1000
Lactation								
≤18	30	80	800	3000	1800	2800	100	800
19–50	35	100	1000	3500	2000	3000	100	1000

[a]The UL for niacin and folate apply to synthetic forms obtained from supplements, fortified foods, or a combination of the two.
[b]The UL for vitamin A applies to the preformed vitamin only.
[c]The UL for vitamin E applies to any form of supplemental α-tocopherol, fortified foods, or a combination of the two.

Tolerable Upper Intake Levels (UL) for Minerals

Age (yr)	Sodium (mg/day)	Chloride (mg/day)	Calcium (mg/day)	Phosphorus (mg/day)	Magnesium (mg/day)[d]	Iron (mg/day)	Zinc (mg/day)	Iodine (µg/day)	Selenium (µg/day)	Copper (µg/day)	Manganese (mg/day)	Fluoride (mg/day)	Molybdenum (µg/day)	Boron (mg/day)	Nickel (mg/day)	Vanadium (mg/day)
Infants																
0–0.5	—	—	1000	—	—	40	4	—	45	—	—	0.7	—	—	—	—
0.5–1	—	—	1500	—	—	40	5	—	60	—	—	0.9	—	—	—	—
Children																
1–3	1500	2300	2500	3000	65	40	7	200	90	1000	2	1.3	300	3	0.2	—
4–8	1900	2900	2500	3000	110	40	12	300	150	3000	3	2.2	600	6	0.3	—
9–13	2200	3400	3000	4000	350	40	23	600	280	5000	6	10	1100	11	0.6	—
Adolescents																
14–18	2300	3600	3000	4000	350	45	34	900	400	8000	9	10	1700	17	1.0	—
Adults																
19–50	2300	3600	2500	4000	350	45	40	1100	400	10,000	11	10	2000	20	1.0	1.8
51–70	2300	3600	2000	4000	350	45	40	1100	400	10,000	11	10	2000	20	1.0	1.8
>70	2300	3600	2000	3000	350	45	40	1100	400	10,000	11	10	2000	20	1.0	1.8
Pregnancy																
≤18	2300	3600	3000	3500	350	45	34	900	400	8000	9	10	1700	17	1.0	—
19–50	2300	3600	2500	3500	350	45	40	1100	400	10,000	11	10	2000	20	1.0	—
Lactation																
≤18	2300	3600	3000	4000	350	45	34	900	400	8000	9	10	1700	17	1.0	—
19–50	2300	3600	2500	4000	350	45	40	1100	400	10,000	11	10	2000	20	1.0	—

[d]The UL for magnesium applies to synthetic forms obtained from supplements or drugs only. NOTE: An Upper Limit was not established for vitamins and minerals not listed and for those age groups listed with a dash (—) because of a lack of data, not because these nutrients are safe to consume at any level of intake. All nutrients can have adverse effects when intakes are excessive.

SOURCE: Adapted with permission from the *Dietary Reference Intakes* series, National Academies Press. Copyright 1997, 1998, 2000, 2001, 2002, 2005, 2011 by the National Academies of Sciences.